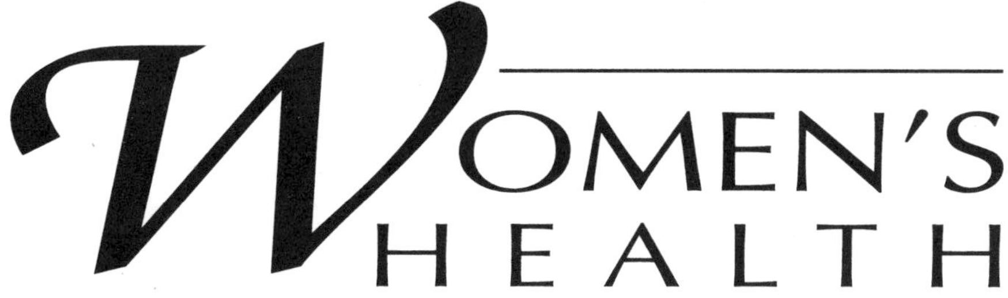


# Women's Health
## A Primary Care Clinical Guide

**Ellis Quinn Youngkin, PhD, RNC, OGNP**
Associate Professor
School of Nursing

Obstetric–Gynecologic Nurse Practitioner
University Student Health Services
Virginia Commonwealth University
Richmond, Virginia

**Marcia Szmania Davis, MS, MSEd, RNC, WHCNP, ANP**
Women's Health Care Nurse Practitioner
Richmond Urban Primary Care Initiative

Faculty
School of Nursing
Virginia Commonwealth University
Richmond, Virginia

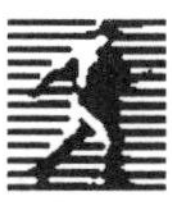

APPLETON & LANGE
Norwalk, Connecticut

Notice: The authors and the publisher of this volume have taken care that the information and recommendations contained herein are accurate and compatible with the standards generally accepted at the time of publication. Nevertheless, it is difficult to ensure that all the information given is entirely accurate for all circumstances. The publisher disclaims any liability, loss, or damage incurred as a consequence, directly or indirectly, of the use and application of any of the contents of this volume.

***Cover: Photomicrography showing estrogen crystal, © Dennis Kunkel, PhD, University of Hawaii. This image of an estrogen (estradiol) crystal viewed under polarized light was part of a display of Dr. Kunkel's photomicrography published in the May 1993 issue of* Smithsonian *magazine.***

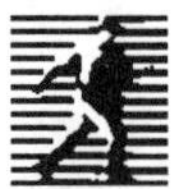



95 96 97 98 / 10 9 8 7 6 5 4 3 2

Prentice Hall International (UK) Limited, *London*
Prentice Hall of Australia Pty. Limited, *Sydney*
Prentice Hall Canada, Inc., *Toronto*
Prentice Hall Hispanoamericana, S.A., *Mexico*
Prentice Hall of India Private Limited, *New Delhi*
Prentice Hall of Japan, Inc., *Tokyo*
Simon & Schuster Asia Pte. Ltd., *Singapore*
Editora Prentice Hall do Brasil Ltda., *Rio de Janeiro*
Prentice Hall, *Englewood Cliffs, New Jersey*

Library of Congress Cataloging-in-Publication Data

Women's health: a primary care clinical guide / [edited by]
Ellis Quinn Youngkin, Marcia Szmania Davis.
p. cm.
Includes index.
ISBN 0-8385-1230-5
1. Women—Health and hygiene—Sociological aspects. 2. Women—Diseases. 3. Women's health services. 4. Gynecology. 5. Obstetrics. I. Younglin, Ellis Quinn. II. Davis, Marcia Szmania.
[DNLM: 1. Women's Health. 2. Primary Health Care. WA 300 W872905 1994]
RA561.85.W6668 1994
613'.04244—dc20
DNLM/DLC
for Library of Congress

94-4953
CIP

Editor-in-Chief: Sally J. Barhydt
Development Editor: Barbara Severs
Production Editor: Karen W. Davis
Designer: Janice Barsevich Bielawa

PRINTED IN THE UNITED STATES OF AMERICA

# CONTRIBUTORS

**Kathleen M. Akridge, MS, RNC, OGNP**
Clinical Faculty
School of Nursing
Virginia Commonwealth University
Richmond, Virginia

OB/GYN Nurse Practitioner
Private OB/GYN Medical Practice
Virginia Beach, Virginia

**Cynthia W. Bailey, MS, RNC, OGNP**
Clinical Faculty
School of Nursing
Virginia Commonwealth University

OB/GYN Nurse Practitioner
Private OB/GYN Medical Practice
Richmond, Virginia

**Sharon Baker, MN, RNC, OGNP**
OB/GYN Nurse Practitioner
Private Family Practice

President and Founder
The Women's Information Network, Inc.
Rome, Georgia

**Emily Coogan Bennett, MS, RNC, OGNP**
Associate Professor
Department of OB/GYN
Virginia Commonwealth University
Richmond, Virginia

**Lynette Galloway Branch, MS, RN, LFNP**
Director
Student Health Service
Virginia State University
Petersburg, Virginia

Clinical Faculty
School of Nursing
Virginia Commonwealth University
Richmond, Virginia

**Kathryn A. Caufield, MS, RN, CFNP**
Adjunct Assistant Professor
Hampton University School of Nursing

Nurse Practitioner Associate
Private Family Medicine Practice
Hampton, Virginia

**Judith B. Collins, MS, RNC, OGNP, FAAN**
Associate Professor
Schools of Nursing and Medicine

Director, Women's Center Stony Point
Virginia Commonwealth University
Richmond, Virginia

**Joan Corder-Mabe, MS, RNC, OGNP**
Perinatal Nurse Consultant
Virginia Department of Health
Division of Women's and Infant's Health
Richmond, Virginia

**Catherine Ingram Fogel, PhD, RNC, OGNP**
Associate Professor
School of Nursing
The University of North Carolina at Chapel Hill
Chapel Hill, North Carolina

**Donna E. Forrest, MS, RNC, OGNP**
OB/GYN Nurse Practitioner
Private OB/GYN Practice
Williamsburg, Virginia

Clinical Faculty
School of Nursing
Virginia Commonwealth University
Richmond, Virginia

**Marion Herndon Fuqua, MS, RNC, OGNP**
OB/GYN Nurse Practitioner
Private OB/GYN and Infertility Practice
Greensboro, North Carolina

**Catherine H. Garner, MSN, MPA, RNC, OGNP**
Affiliated Faculty
University of Missouri at Kansas City
Kansas City, Missouri

President
Mature Strategies, Inc.
Durham, North Carolina

**Linda C. Hancock, MS, RN, CFNP**
Assistant Director
Office of Health Promotion
University Student Health Services

Clinical Faculty
School of Nursing
Virginia Commonwealth University
Richmond, Virginia

**Nancy L. Harris, MS, RNC, OGNP**
Obstetric Gynecologic Nurse Practitioner
Thomas Jefferson Health District
Charlottesville, Virginia

**Martha Edwards Hart, MS, RNC, PNP, NNP**
Pediatric Nurse Practitioner
Infectious Disease Clinic

Clinical Faculty
School of Nursing
Virginia Commonwealth University
Richmond, Virginia

**Mary Beth Bryant McGurin, MS, RNC, CRNP**
Perinatal Services Coordinator
Planned Parenthood of Metropolitan Washington, Inc.
Washington, D.C.

**Maryellen Remich, MSN, RNC, OGNP**
Adjunct Faculty
Old Dominion University
Norfolk, Virginia

OB/GYN Nurse Practitioner
Private OB/GYN Medical Practice
Virginia Beach, Virginia

**Kathleen J. Sawin, DNS, CNS, CPNP**
Family and Pediatric Nurse Practitioner

Associate Professor
School of Nursing
Virginia Commonwealth University
Richmond, Virginia

**Belinda Seimer, MSN, RN, CFNP**
Family Nurse Practitioner
Adolescent Health Services
Children's Hospital
Columbus, Ohio

**Patricia M. Selig, MS, RNC, FNP**
Nurse Practitioner
Division of Primary Care
Department of Internal Medicine

Clinical Faculty
School of Nursing
Virginia Commonwealth University
Richmond, Virginia

**Valerie Johnson South, MS, RNC, OGNP**
Clinical Faculty
School of Nursing
Virginia Commonwealth University

OB/GYN Nurse Practitioner
Private OB/GYN Medical Practice
Richmond, Virginia

**Sue C. Wood, RNC, MS, OGNP**
Clinical Faculty
School of Nursing
Virginia Commonwealth University

In Vitro Fertility Program Coordinator
Private Fertility and Endocrinology Practice
Richmond, Virginia

# CONTENTS

# PREFACE

In this period of rapid change and development in health care, the scope of health care for women becomes a critically important issue. The move into a primary care–based system is the stimulus for the consumer to be better educated and to have high expectations regarding her care. Thus, it is essential that each woman be viewed from a holistic perspective.

Women's health care is, and must be, more than obstetrics and gynecology. Women in this century and the next will ask for the type of health care that offers guidance in a wide variety of issues and needs, far beyond the confines of the reproductive system. The provider, therefore, must be knowledgeable about a wide spectrum of physical and psychosocial factors that can have an impact on the woman's well-being.

Recognizing that the primary care provider may be the only provider a woman will see, it seemed to us that a book providing more than reproductive and gynecologic insights was needed. Thus, this book *Women's Health: A Primary Care Clinical Guide,* was conceived to fill a void; it covers the traditional reproductive content as well as selected common medical and psycho-socio-developmental-political problems and issues.

The book begins with major historical and current changes that relate to women and health care, focusing on important societal and political factors that will affect health needs for the end of this century and for the next. From there, the book moves into women's developmental issues, incidences of diseases, general guidelines for health care screening and interventions, and sexuality facts and issues. In Part II the more traditional health problems and needs of women related to the reproductive system are covered in depth, including fertility management, menstrual concerns, infertility, sexually transmittted diseases and vaginitis, pelvic and abdominal diseases, breast concerns, and the special needs of older women. Part III details uncomplicated and complicated pregnancies, postpartum problems and needs, lactation issues, and fetal surveillance.

Finally, Part IV explores some of the primary care issues associated with more common medical problems, such as headaches, anemia, and respiratory problems, that the provider may encounter in women's health. Selected psychosocial problems, such as violence, depression, and eating disorders, and their impact on women are also discussed, providing insights into related health care needs. The last chapter reviews unique care issues concerning the woman with disabilities.

We particularly want this book to be a handbook, a resource that allows any primary health care provider to retrieve basic information easily. We see it as a reference with enough depth to be useful in a clinical setting, serving as a source of teaching–counseling advice for clients, nursing diagnoses as well as differential medical diagnoses, screening and early intervention measures, and guidelines for referral. The reader will note that some of the chapters more easily fit an outline format for diseases or other conditions, but that many chapters conform to a more traditional text format or a combination format for presentation of issues. In some situations, the information has been supplemented by more in-depth presentations.

We wish to remind the reader that the scope of advanced nursing practice varies from state to state, and the individual practitioner is responsible for knowing her/his legal limits of practice. Also, recognizing the rapidity with which new knowledge becomes available and standards change, the practitioner must stay ever alert to these changes.

Our sincere thanks go to our excellent contributing authors who persevered to meet the numerous demands for this type of book. Without their extraordinary expertise, time, patience, and effort, the book would not exist. Also, we wish to thank all the formal and informal reviewers who helped make this a reality. Last, but not least, our deep appreciation goes to our husbands who supported and encouraged us during the months of preparation and work.

We, with the contributing authors, hope that you, as primary care providers in a rapidly changing world of health care, will find this handbook useful and an effective approach to presenting information for the holistic care of women.

# FOREWORD

*Women's Health.* Until recently, these words have conjured up an image of diseases and disorders that center on women's reproductive organs: breast and ovarian cancers, endometriosis, and uterine leiomyomata. The words have not evoked thoughts of diseases of all the organ systems, nor have they roused visions of health rather than disease. Yet the health of women begins before birth and is affected throughout life by a vast panoply of factors and elements—genetic, lifestyle, and environmental.

*Women's Health.* Until recently many have considered this arena largely the purview of physicians, with some assistance by so-called "allied health professionals." Today, however, the emphasis is on a multidisciplinary approach to health care by a team of health professionals—physicians, nurses, health educators, and others—who join with the woman to realize a compelling objective: her health and well-being.

This change has evolved gradually, but with more persistence and energy in the last two decades. Societal forces have raised awareness and mandated action, action that could not be ignored. Since 1990, the Federal government has legislated action in women's health. The National Institutes of Health (NIH), the preeminent Federal research institution, established the Office of Research on Women's Health and Congress mandated it with the NIH Revitalization Act of 1993.

This office is charged with assuring that diseases, disorders, and conditions that affect women throughout their lives are addressed and that gaps in knowledge are filled. The office is further charged with assuring that women are appropriately included in clinical studies, unless a compelling rationale can be presented as to why such action is not necessary. This latter charge has been strengthened even more vigorously in the NIH Revitalization Act of 1993. That act specifies that clinical trials must now include sufficient numbers of women such that valid analyses can be performed and differences between genders demonstrated where they exist. Working in concert with the twenty institutes and centers of NIH, the office has sought to enhance action on both mandates such that the number and type of studies on women's health has escalated across the biomedical research spectrum from basic to applied and that women are appropriately included in clinical studies of all diseases that affect them.

Furthermore, there has been a surge in activity in areas that were previously neglected. Coronary heart disease, sexually transmitted diseases, urological diseases, autoimmune diseases, and mental health have received special attention to redress the gaps in knowledge. One of the most noted studies recently initiated is the Women's Health Initiative. This study is the largest prevention trial ever conducted and will address the leading causes of death and disability in postmenopausal women: cardiovascular disease, breast and colorectal cancers, and osteoporosis. NIH-wide efforts are being coordinated by the Office of Research on Women's Health, for example, studies on the effects of DES on mothers and offspring and diseases and conditions leading to hysterectomy and their sequelae. Other focal points by NIH institutes and centers include chronic fatigue syndrome, effects of implantation for temporal mandibular joint disorder, and breast cancer.

Action now extends throughout the Department of Health and Human Services (DHHS) with women's health offices having been established to bring resources to bear on understanding health and disease, finding ways to treat disease, and, perhaps most importantly, defining ways to prevent disease and sustain health throughout life. And this action is directed toward all women—not limited by racial and ethnic origin, sexual orientation, or age, wherever they reside. The message is clear and uncompromising: women's health can no longer be denied or ignored.

The National Center for Health Statistics, Centers for Disease Control and Prevention, is enhancing its activities to catalogue and publish information on morbidity and mortality among all racial and ethnic groups of women. The Agency for Health Care Policy and Research is pursuing myriad projects to establish guidelines for clinical intervention as well as efficacy and efficiency of health services delivery. The Health Resources and Services Administration not only addresses enhanced education for health professionals, but monitors health care delivery and works to improve efficiency of all health professionals. The Food and Drug Administration, a regulatory agency, has recently revised its guidelines on the inclusion of women in Phase I and II clinical trials; the action will provide much needed information.

The goal of this unified, yet diverse, effort throughout government and the scientific and clinical communities is to assure that all women receive the best care possible and that their health is protected such that they can live healthy lives. To achieve this goal, it is imperative that valid and tested research findings be placed in the hands of willing, knowledgeable health professionals.

This book provides an excellent vehicle for the transfer of such information. Not only are the myriad factors that affect women's lives presented, but they are presented cogently and thoughtfully such that they can be easily incorporated into clinical practice. That the book has been prepared by a distinguished group of nurses who are clinical experts only underscores the importance and relevance of nurses as experienced diagnosticians and practitioners.

Florence Nightingale is remembered for her extraordinary nursing skills during the Crimean War, but she should be equally noted for her remarkable skills as an epidemiologist. Not only did she clean up the battlefield hospitals, thereby dramatically reducing battlefield mortality, but she brought that same fire and zeal to revitalizing hospitals back in England. This rich tradition is evident in nurses today. Nurses bring a breadth of knowledge and experience to every aspect of health from bench to bedside, from practice to policy, from the bedside nurse to the Director of the National Institute for Nursing Research. This book is another contribution to that tradition and to excellence in health care for all women.

**Judith H. LaRosa, PhD**
*Deputy Director*
*Office of Research on Women's Health*
*National Institutes of Health*

# WOMEN, HEALTH, AND THE HEALTH CARE SYSTEM

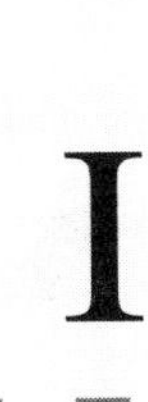

CHAPTER 1

# WOMEN AND THE HEALTH CARE SYSTEM

*Judith B. Collins*

*This spotlight of attention on women's health issues has energized women and organizations across the United States and empowered them to speak out with new force about inequities.*

### *Highlights*

- Historical Perspective
- Barriers to Quality Health Care
- Political Action
- Health Care Policies
- Predictions for the Year 2000

## INTRODUCTION

Many authors have noted that women enter the health care system by their reproductive organs. Often health care for women has focused on the reproductive system to the exclusion of other health needs, leading to the emergence of a narrow definition of women's health care centered on the breasts and the pelvis. A comprehensive approach to women's health care, on the other hand, addresses the physical, social, and emotional needs of women. This holistic approach is sensitive to women's *dis-ease*, not just their *diseases*. Some women may seek care only in a women's health care setting; therefore, health care providers in that setting must think beyond the breasts and the pelvis.

The U.S. Department of Health and Human Services (HHS), at the National Conference on Women's Health in 1986, defined a women's health issue as "any matter that affects the health of women exclusively, that impacts predominately on women's health (at any age), or that affects women's health differently from that of men."[1] This definition of women's health, it is pointed out, is based on a male norm. Thus, "by limiting women's health to a consideration of ways that women are different from men, this definition not only defines women's health incompletely—to the detriment of women—but also ensures that no beneficial effects can accrue to men, because only women's differences from men are legitimate areas of concern."[2] Alternatively, a "woman centered" definition addressing all of women's needs would provide for broader societal changes to benefit everyone.[2]

A comprehensive view of women's health care moves beyond the biomedical approach to the concepts of totality, centrality, and diversity.[2] *Totality* includes women's many roles and contexts. The Rodriquez-Trias totality concept "defines the health problems of women as deeply implanted in the statuses that derive from their multiple social relations."[3] Totality calls for women to be viewed as inextricably connected with their families and communities, not separate from their multiple roles as mothers, sisters, wives, workers, and caretakers.[3]

*Centrality* denotes care that is woman centered. One view of centrality "defines health problems as women themselves experience those problems."[3] This view casts women as "active decision makers in their own lives" and thus rejects and reshapes "the all too common view of women as passive recipients of health care and public health action."[3]

*Diversity* entails meeting the needs of all women. It "requires recognizing not only women's different social roles but also their different races, economic conditions, sexual orientations, and cultures and how these relate to health."[2] Diversity is manifested in "varying rates of diseases among ethnic groups" as well as "in different understandings of what health is and what health needs are, and [these] are shaped by socio-economic status and social roles."[2]

## HISTORICAL PERSPECTIVE

Throughout the ages, an evolution of the health care of women has occurred, often paralleling the changing roles of women in society. Women's consumer health activities began in the United States during the 1830s and 1840s. Suffrage during the mid-19th century was accompanied by the Popular Health Movement, which demanded a total redefinition of health itself and health care. Abrum's[4] historical perspective on women's health care discusses Naphey's 1870 work entitled *The Physical Life of Women: Advice to the Maiden, Wife, and Mother.* Although the book was widely acclaimed as valuable scientific literature, it identified only three phases in a women's life: maidenhood, matrimony, and maternity.[5]

About the turn of the 20th century, it was believed that the ovaries and uterus were the controlling organs and the center of all disease in a woman's body, thus the etiology of most female complaints, including headaches, indigestion, and sore throats.[6] Consequently, the stage was set for decades during which women's health care would be plagued with sexism and ageism. Women felt that they lacked control of their bodies, and many normal physiological processes were viewed by medicine and society as diseases. For example, menstruation was seen as a chronic problem, and pregnancy and menopause as disorders requiring intervention.[6] Sexism in the health care system provided the basis for "oppression of women derived from her 'womanness': her biologic differences and her ability to bear children."[7] These differences have been used to build social structures and a supportive ideology of female submissiveness and to "permit condescension toward women."[7] Further reinforcing this ideology, in 1905, the president of the Oregon State Medical Society stated, "Educated women could not bear children with ease because study arrested the development of the pelvis at the same time it increased the size of the child's brain, and therefore its head."[8]

This ideology was also extended to mature women. In the popular 1970 book *Everything You Always Wanted to Know about Sex*, Dr. David Reuben described the menopausal woman:

> As the estrogen is shut off, a woman comes as close as she can to being a man. Increased facial hair, deepened voice, obesity, and the decline of breasts and female genitalia all contribute to a masculine appearance. Coarsened features, enlargement of the clitoris, and gradual baldness complete the picture. Not really a man but no longer a functional woman, these individuals live in a world of intersex . . . sex no longer interests them. To many women the menopause marks the end of their useful life. They see it as the onset of old age, the beginning of the end. They may be right. Having outlived their ovaries, they may have outlived their usefulness as human beings. The remaining years may be just marking time until they follow their glands into oblivion.[9]

## THE 1960s AND 1970s

Many social changes erupted in the 1960s fueled by societal unrest about the lack of equality for all citizens. Most notable and visible was the civil rights movement. Major changes for women also evolved, catalyzed in 1963 by Betty Friedan's historic book *The Feminine Mystique*, which told of women's disenchantments with their relationships, both personal and institutional.[10] This disenchantment developed into the women's liberation movement, which addressed the cause of equal rights for women. Health care system change was strategic to women's liberation, because the system is an agent of social control equally restrictive as any political or economic system.

The women's health movement grew from the women's liberation movement in the early 1970s as a grassroots organization with a common uniting goal: "a demand for improved health care for all women and an end to sexism in the health system."[7]

"Activities centered around abortion law reform provided the initial cohesion from which the women's health movement could emerge."[7] In January 1973, the landmark Supreme Court decision in *Roe v. Wade* provided a legal right to abortion.

The women's health movement focused on "changing consciousness, providing health related services, and struggling to change established health institutions."[7] The major thrust of concern was that women wanted to own and control their bodies, not just to be cured. In a landmark book published by the Boston Women's Health Collective, *Our Bodies, Ourselves*, women spoke out and asked for something different and better from health care providers.[11]

The women's health movement also raised issues of childbirth education, natural methods of childbirth, and birthing options, including father participation in labor and delivery and home births. Spurred by consumer education in books, magazines, and networking meetings, women's requests from the health care system then grew beyond childbearing issues. Hospitals, awakened to the fact that women were their major customers, began to market women's services by establishing women's health resource centers (either within the hospital or as a freestanding center) to provide specialized care and education in homelike surroundings.

## THE 1980s AND 1990s

More recently, women have demanded participatory health-care decision making, humanistic and holistic preventive care, and a wellness, rather than illness, orientation to care. In the sociopolitical arena women have been advocating for health services and policies that address reproductive freedom, contraceptive options, domestic violence, and research on women's special health problems (e.g., breast disease, menopause, osteoporosis, hormonal replacement therapy, premenstrual syndrome (PMS), heart disease, and human immunodeficiency virus/acquired immunodeficiency syndrome (HIV/AIDS).

Abortion rights remain a major emotional and legal issue for the nation. As *Roe v. Wade* is being debated by the Supreme Court, the implications of reversing the constitutional right to abortion raises questions about state-by-state legislation, reproductive freedom, and access to safe medical care in the future.

Betty Friedan, speaking out on the new feminine mystique,[12] asserts that the women's movement has been halted by the general reversal of social progress in the United States during the 1980s and 1990s. She feels that the rights women have won during the past 20 years are in "grave danger."[12]

Women are the preeminent consumers of health care in the United States, measured by standards such as doctors' visits, medication prescriptions, surgery, hospitalization, and nursing home care.[13] Women are also responsible for spending "two of every three health care dollars."[14] Seventy to 90 percent of all health care decisions are made by women for themselves and their families, and 60 to 70 percent of all hospital beds are filled by women. The National Center for Health Statistics (NCHS) reports that of the 20 most frequently performed surgeries, 11 are performed exclusively on women; none are performed exclusively on men. Women account for 63 to 66 percent of all surgeries.[15] Women, therefore, should have the best health care that the U.S. system can offer.

## SOCIETAL BARRIERS TO QUALITY HEALTH CARE

Not all American women are getting quality health care. Clancy and Massion view American women's health care as "a patchwork quilt with gaps."[16] For many women, access to care still has many barriers,[16] including excessive costs; limited availability of providers and services; insensitive attitudes in the paternalistic, male-dominated medical profession; lack of transportation; and poorly coordinated and disorganized systems for referral.

### DISCOUNTING OF WOMEN'S SYMPTOMS

Women's symptoms, rather than being taken seriously, often are ascribed to hormonal or psychiatric causes. This delays diagnosis and treatment and may have serious consequences. According to Paula Doress, coauthor of *Ourselves, Growing Older*, "If a man comes in with certain symptoms, it's diabetes or heart disease. For women, menopause is the wastebasket diagnosis for everything."[13] The combination of social inequities and a male-dominated medical profession has had a major effect on women's health referred to as "gender bias."[20]

### OVERUSE OF SURGICAL PROCEDURES

The two most common surgical procedures in the United States are cesarean births and hysterectomy. The incidence of cesarean births has increased steadily: from 10 percent in 1975 to 25 percent in 1990.[13] Thus, in the United States, one infant in four is delivered by cesarean.

### RESTRICTED ACCESS TO PRENATAL CARE

Despite technological advances in perinatal health care, many women are still unable to access routine care. In 1989, only 75.5 percent of women received early prenatal care,[18] compared with 76.3 percent in 1980.[19] According to 1989 data, the United States ranked behind 21 other nations in infant mortality, and 30 nations had fewer low birthweight infants.[20,21]

In 1989 the overall U.S. infant mortality rate was 9.8 per 1000 live births.[22] Among African Americans it was 17.7 per 1000, and among whites it was 8.22.[22,23] Historically, the rate of infant mortality among African American infants has been more than double that of white infants.

Multiple social and health problems contribute to these tragic statistics, but to a great extent the dismal record can be attributed to severely inadequate access to prenatal care. The poor health status among rural mothers and infants is indicative of limited availability of obstetric providers and limited access to specialized care for complicated pregnancies and deliveries.[24] In the United States in 1989, 6 percent of births were to women living in counties with no access to prenatal care.[25] As a nation we spent more than $808 billion for health care in 1992,[26] yet we made no commitment to ensuring prenatal care for every pregnant woman in the United States. This is a significant political issue because women and children—who represent more than half of the population—are not our policymakers and often do not vote.

Politics also plays a role in other women's health issues, such as lack of health insurance coverage for in vitro fertilization and bone marrow transplant for breast cancer, lack of research into women's unique diseases, and the ongoing challenge of abortion rights.

## INADEQUATE INSURANCE

Approximately 35 million Americans, about 14 percent of the population, were uninsured in 1992.[26] The uninsured include 8.5 million women of childbearing age and 10 million children.[20] Sixty million Americans are underinsured or have inadequate coverage, which is often comparable to no insurance.[27]

Being underinsured is especially difficult for women. It can include high cost sharing, lengthy waiting periods, restricted coverage for preexisting conditions, and limited services or exclusion from some that are important to women (i.e., Papanicolaou smears, mammograms, infertility services, and family planning services). In addition, lack of long-term care insurance is a special threat to older women, who "live longer than men and suffer more chronic disorders as they age."[28]

## LACK OF RESEARCH

Cancer, cardiovascular disease, and osteoporosis are the three leading causes of death and disability among American women. Each year cardiovascular disease claims the lives of some 500,000 U.S. women. Too little research focuses on women's unique and common health issues, especially studies of chronic diseases and their prevention in older women.[29]

A 1989 study of women's health research revealed three points that were especially disturbing.

- Historically, women have been excluded from large clinical trials, such as the study of aspirin and heart disease. Even when women were included, study results were not routinely analyzed for gender differences.
- No gynecologic unit existed within the entire structure of the National Institutes of Health (NIH) nor was there any central coordinating office for women's health matters.
- Few women have achieved the top echelons of medicine and scientific research.[30]

Thus, even though women make up 52 percent of the U.S. population, research on major diseases and the drugs to treat them has been done mostly on "mice and men." Researchers have excluded women, arguing that pregnancy and women's fluctuating hormone levels could alter study results.[31]

## OTHER INFLUENCES ON WOMEN'S HEALTH

### POVERTY

Poverty and health are significantly interrelated. Low income women are in poorer health and have greater difficulty accessing health care services than affluent women. Poor women face the inability to pay for care, or if they receive Medicaid, the problem of finding a provider who accepts it. Child care, time off from work, and transportation are other issues they face.[28]

Inequities in income between men and women persist. "Women are poorer than men regardless of age, race, ethnicity, education or employment status."[28] Women of all ages continue to earn only 70 percent of what men earn. In 1989, almost three employed women in five worked in low paying sales, services, and clerical jobs.[32] In addition, nearly three-fourths of elderly Americans living in poverty are women.[33]

In addition, after divorce or separation, the average family income of mothers with child custody drops by 23 percent. Families headed by a mother alone are six times as likely to be poor as those with two parents.[34] Women and children are the fastest growing segment of the homeless population.

### MARITAL STATUS

Marital status, standard of living, and health status are also interrelated. Public policy is often developed on the outdated concept of the American family headed by a male wage earner with a spouse at home. Social Security, private pension, and health insurance plans are notable examples.[28] However, only about one U.S. family in four conforms to this model.[35]

### LONGEVITY

American women live an average of 7 years longer than American men; as of 1988, the average life span was 78.3 years for women and 71.4 years for men.[36] By living longer, women may have an increased incidence of chronic diseases that require long-term care. It was estimated that in 1990, more than half of the women who reached age 85 were living in nursing homes.[37]

### CAREGIVING

Women, providing the majority of paid and unpaid family care, have become the safety net for our health care system. Women make up three-fourths of the unpaid caregivers of the elderly.[32] Without these family caregivers, many more elderly would be in health care institutions. "Almost two million women, the 'sandwich generation,' have both elder and child care responsibilities."[28] Women's health can be impacted by the stress of juggling employment, homemaking, and child and elder care. One caregiver in three is age 65 or over, and the impact on one's health may be severe.[38] Because women are nurturers and caregivers, their state of health can also affect their families and society.[24]

## POLITICAL ACTION

### STATUS OF WOMEN'S HEALTH

In 1983, Dr. Edward N. Brandt, Jr., assistant secretary of health, commissioned a Public Health Services (PHS) task force to examine the status of women's health. This action acknowledged that cultural, economic, social, and environmental factors make it necessary to develop different approaches and strategies to provide adequate health care services that meet women's needs. In 1985, the task force findings were published in *Women's Health: Report of the Public Health Service Task Force on Women's Health Issues.*[39] Academics and government policymakers agreed, for the first time, that women were disadvantaged in terms of health care. The task force report made 15 recommendations that focused on six major areas:

- Promoting physical and social environments that are safe and healthful.
- Providing services to prevent and treat disease.
- Conducting research and evaluation.
- Recruiting and training women health care personnel.
- Education and informing the public and disseminating research information.
- Designing guidance for legislative and regulatory measures.

## CONGRESSIONAL CAUCUS ON WOMEN'S ISSUES

Despite the startling conclusions of the PHS task force report, little action was taken, especially in eliminating the inequities in women's health research. In 1989, the Congressional Caucus on Women's Issues (CCWI), a bipartisan group of more than 125 members of Congress, was formed and officially requested an audit of the inclusion of women by the NIH in clinical trials (a policy adopted as a result of the PHS task force recommendations in 1985). The report, issued in June 1990, found that the NIH had failed in several serious ways: policy not well communicated or understood, study results not being analyzed by gender, and policy only applied to extramural, not intramural, research.

When the NIH, Congress, the media, and the public reacted to this report, changes began to occur. Multimedia coverage showed women's omission from research, and reports focused on women's diseases. Meanwhile, the CCWI developed a women's health legislative agenda for research, prevention, and services. It was introduced in Congress as The Women's Health Equity Act in 1990 and continued to 1993.

## OTHER MILESTONES IN WOMEN'S HEALTH

Recent milestones that have contributed to a focus on women's health during the 1990s include the formation of several groups: the Society for the Advancement of Women's Health Research, the Coalition for Women's Health Research, the Office of Research on Women's Health at NIH, and the Office of Women's Health (in the office of the assistant secretary for health, HHS). Furthermore, women have held key positions: Bernadine Healy, M.D., director of NIH; Antonia Novello, M.D., U.S. surgeon general; Jocelyn Elders, M.D., U.S. surgeon general; Vivian Pinn, M.D., director, Office of Research on Women's Health, NIH; Judith H. LaRosa, Ph.D., deputy director, Office of Research on Women's Health, NIH; Agnes Donahue, D.D.S., director, Office on Women's Health, HHS; Donna Shalala, Ph.D., secretary of health and human services.

The NIH Women's Health Initiative is the largest community-based clinical intervention and prevention trial ever conducted. The study has two major parts: first, to evaluate the effectiveness of three preventive approaches (hormonal replacement therapy, vitamin D and calcium supplementation, and low fat diet) on the incidence of breast cancer, cardiovascular disease, and fractures related to osteoporosis; and, second, to evaluate strategies devised to help women achieve healthy lifestyles (improving diet, stopping smoking, achieving and maintaining optimal weight, maintaining physical activity, and having regular cancer screening).[2]

- Recent conferences have addressed the women's health agenda.
  - The Office of Research on Women's Health sponsored Opportunities for Research on Women's Health (1991) and Advancing Women in Bio-Medical Careers (1992).
  - The Center for Research on Women and Gender, of the University of Illinois at Chicago, sponsored Reframing Women's Health: Multidisciplinary Research and Practice (1992).
  - Jacob's Institute for Women's Health sponsored Women's Health Centers: Review, Assessment and Goals (1993).
  - The First Annual Congress on Women's Health was held in Washington, DC (1993).
- Recommendations have been presented for the development of a new multidisciplinary specialty in women's health by Karen Johnson, M.D., and Charlea Massion, M.D.[40]
- Professional journals have focused on women's health.

This spotlight of attention on women's health issues has energized women and organizations across the United States and empowered them to speak out with new force about inequities. For example, the national Breast Cancer Coalition delivered 500,000 letters to Congress in October 1991 to request more money for breast cancer research. One American woman in eight will develop breast cancer. Each year in the United States, 175,000 women are diagnosed with breast cancer and about 45,000 are expected to die.[41]

If this increasing visibility of women's health issues is an indicator, then the 1990s may become the "decade of women's health."[2]

## HEALTH CARE POLICY

### INFLUENCES ON HEALTH POLICY AND WOMEN'S HEALTH CARE

To understand health policy as it relates to women, the subject must be viewed in the context of all health policy, including the major influencing economic, social, and political forces.

#### Health Care Costs

- Health care costs are projected to be $898 billion and 14.3 percent of the gross domestic product (GDP) in 1993.[26]
- If not controlled, health care spending is projected to be $1,679 trillion in the year 2000 and 18 percent of the GDP.[26]

#### Corporate Influence on the Health Industry

- In today's market, a business approach is taken to health care delivery, with a focus on marketing services and the financial bottom line. Women's health care is viewed as a tremendous source of revenue for hospitals. Exploitation of women's services as simply a hospital marketing strategy, without provision of quality services, must be guarded against.
- Economic good competes with social good; emphasis can be on paying for care or on providing care.

#### Competition

- Players in the health care marketplace—patients, providers, payers, purchasers, and policymakers—have competing objectives.
- Prices and costs of services should decrease with competition, but this principle is not reflected in the health care industry.

### Care of the Poor

- The gap between the "haves" and the "have nots" in American society is increasing.
- Women are especially vulnerable to a market oriented system with health insurance linked to employment. Many women work in jobs without health benefits; others do not work outside the home while caring for children.
- Debate is increasing about health care as a right or a privilege for all, including the poor.

### Reproductive Freedom

- A public spotlight is on this women's issue.
- The so-called gag rule on health care providers in federally funded clinics (Title X), which inhibited discussion of abortion as an option for unwanted pregnancies, was rescinded by an executive order of President Bill Clinton in 1993.
- *Roe v. Wade*, which was the basis of the 1973 Supreme Court decision on abortion, is constantly challenged in test cases that seek to limit or reverse it.
- Parental notification and/or consent for abortion is a national issue.
- Funding and availability of abortion services is a major health policy issue.
- Limited contraceptive options for women remain an issue.
  - A 1990 National Academy of Science report stated that contraceptive research in the United States had come to a virtual halt, and that the United States had fallen far behind other countries in developing new techniques.[42]
  - Up to 15 years and $50 million are required for a new contraceptive to move from the laboratory through the U.S. Food and Drug Administration (FDA) approval process.[42]
  - In 1970, nine major firms were conducting contraceptive research; as of 1990, only one firm was doing research.[41]

### Technological Advances

- Advancing technology in areas such as bioengineering, transplantation, and use of fetal tissue raises issues of who shall live, who shall die, and who shall decide.
- With increasing technological ability to save and prolong life, discussions of health care rationing arise, requiring explicit policy decisions of who gets advanced technology care based on age, illness, and so on.

### Aging/Migrant Populations

- The number of elderly and the number of migrants in the United States are growing. Each group has very different needs for health care services.
- The "intergenerational war," or competition for funding of programs and services for the elderly and children, is a major political issue.

### Long-Term Care/Home Care

- 93 percent of the 1.5 million workers in long-term care facilities in the United States are women.[43]
- Women provide the majority of paid and unpaid family care in the United States, including that for elders and children.[28]
- Approximately two-thirds of persons over age 65 who require nursing home care are women.[44]

### HIV/AIDS

- HIV/AIDS is a major public health issue; and public policy and political forces are pushing for funding for research, prevention, education, and treatment.

- HIV/AIDS became the fifth leading cause of death among women of childbearing age (15 to 44 years old) by the end of 1992.[45]
- In the second decade of the AIDS epidemic, the affected population is increasingly heterosexual, young, and female.[46]
- Women and perinatally infected children are the fastest growing subgroups with HIV infection. Approximately 19,000 American women have AIDS, representing 12 percent of U.S. cases.[46]
- Infected women die sooner than infected men. This may be related to delay in diagnosis, lack of access to health care, or possible physiological differences in HIV response to female hormones.[46]

### Substance Abuse

- Substance abuse is a major public health and public safety issue.
- One-third of Americans addicted to alcohol or drugs are women, yet only 12.7 percent of women get treatment.[47]

### Domestic Violence

- Domestic violence may be the largest hidden public health problem facing women.[46]
- It is the single largest cause of injury to women in the United States—more common than automobile accidents, muggings, and rapes combined.[46]
- Four million women are abused each year,[46] and battered women account for 21 percent of the women who use emergency room services.[39]

### Consumerism

- The American public has an increasing knowledge of health issues and is demanding quality health care services.
- Consumer advocates are lobbying at the local, state, and national levels for special interest needs, such as breast cancer, AIDS, infant mortality, and aging.
- Women are becoming more vocal and active, especially regarding reproductive rights and research on women's diseases.

### Liability Insurance

- Increased lawsuits have led to increased defensive medical practices by physicians to protect themselves. Hence a major increase in the cost of liability insurance to providers has occurred.
- High liability insurance premiums have caused some obstetricians to eliminate maternity care or reduce services for high risk women.
- Contrary to public opinion, the American College of Obstetricians and Gynecologists reports that poor women do not sue more often than other patient groups.[48]

## PREDICTIONS FOR THE YEAR 2000

The United States has never enjoyed a comprehensive, internally consistent national health policy.[49] Instead, the nation has been a "clumsy juggler" of diverse policies and objectives trying to achieve equilibrium in access, quality, and cost-effectiveness.[49] A scenario for health policy in the year 2000 has been predicted.

- Cost effectiveness versus access or quality will remain the most urgent and dominant issue influencing health policy decisions. The aims of cost effectiveness include the provision of medically appropriate care in the least costly way.
- A mixture of regulatory and market-based approaches will be evident in emerging health policy. The regulatory approach encompasses governmental regulations, certificate of need, rate review/rate-setting programs, and peer review organizations. The market-based approach encourages competition, alternative delivery systems, and use of management programs.

- Incremental (minor) policy changes will be made rather than fundamental (major) policy changes in response to powerful advocate groups, such as hospitals, professional organizations, consumer organizations, and insurance companies.
- A continuing shift will occur, from treating health care as a social good to treating it as an economic good. Thus, policy emphasis will be on the purchasing and financing of health care versus the provision of accessible, quality care to all individuals.[51]

Health care reform is at the forefront of the Clinton administration agenda, and major changes are being promised. The health care task force, directed by First Lady Hillary Rodham Clinton, has focused discussion to date on access to care for the uninsured, managed competition with Health Alliances (HA) and Accountable Health Plans (AHP) at the state level, and a core of benefits for insurance policies emphasizing preventive care. With a focus on access to care and prevention, women's health care needs should be addressed.

## CONCLUSION

Providers involved in women's health care have a professional responsibility to know the issues and be involved in the political process to exert positive influence over state and national health policy for women, infants, and their families.

The U.S. health care system is in disarray, but the nation is focused on major reform. Women's health care is spotlighted in Congress, the U.S. Public Health Service, the health care marketplace, and the media. "The women's movement in its many forms [has] identified women's health research no longer as a luxury item, but as an entitlement."[6]

Providers of women's health care have an unprecedented opportunity to enter the public policy debate and advocate for new services, new care delivery approaches, and more research in women's health. Vigilance will be important to maintain the momentum of real changes for women and their families. With attention on prevention and personal responsibility, health care providers can also help empower women to become partners in self-care and health care decision making.

## REFERENCES


1. Young, F.E. (1987). Proceedings of the national conference on women's health. *Public Health Reports: Journal of the U.S. Public Health Service, 4*(Suppl. 1).
2. Dan, A.J., & Hemphill, S.T. (1992). Women's health. *Medical and Health Annual.* Chicago: Encyclopedia Britannica.
3. Rodriquez-Trias, H. (1992). Women's health, women's lives, women's rights. *American Journal of Public Health. 82*(5).
4. Abrums, M. (1986). Health care for women. *Journal of Obstetrics, Gynecologic and Neonatal Nursing, 3*, 250–255.
5. Naphey, G. (1870). *The physical life of women: Advice to maiden wife, and mother* (4th ed.). Philadelphia: George Maclean.
6. Ehrenreich, B., & English, D. (1973). *Complaints and disorders: The sexual politics of sickness.* New York: Feminist Press.
7. Marieskind, H. (1975). The women's health movement. *International Journal of Health Services, 5*(2), 217–223.
8. Bullough, V., & Vought, M. (1973). Women, menstruation, and nineteenth century medicine. *Bulletin of Historical Medicine, 47*(1).
9. Reuben, D. (1970). *Everything you always wanted to know about sex.* New York: David McKay.
10. Friedan, B.J. (1963). *The feminine mystique.* New York: W.W. Norton.
11. Boston Women's Health Collective. (1971). *Our bodies, ourselves.* New York: Simon & Schuster.
12. Friedan, B. (1991, November). The dangers of the new feminine mystique. *McCall's*, pp. 78–86.

13. Southwick, K. (1990, August). Women confront second-class care. *Healthweek*, pp. 1, 40–42.
14. Wentz, A.C., & Haseltine, F.P. (1992). Editorial. *Journal of Women's Health, 1*(1).
15. McKinnon, S. (1990, June/July). Women's control of health care dollars. *Richmond Surroundings*, pp. 34–73.
16. Clancy, C.M., & Massion, C.T. (1992). American women's health care: A patchwork quilt with gaps. *Journal of the American Medical Association, 268*(14).
17. Lempert, L.B. (1986). Women's health from a women's point of view: A review of the literature. *Health Care Women International, 7*, 255–275.
18. National Center for Health Statistics. (1991, December). Advance report of final natality statistics, 1989. *Monthly Vital Statistics Report, 40* (8[S]).
19. National Center for Health Statistics. (1978–1988). *Vital statistics of the United States: Vol. I. Natality*. Washington, DC: U.S. Public Health Service, U.S. Government Printing Office.
20. National Commission to Prevent Infant Mortality. (1992). *Troubling trends persist: Shortchanging America's next generation*. Washington, DC: Author.
21. Grant, J.P. (1991). *The state of the world's children 1992, UNICEF*. New York: Oxford University Press.
22. National Center for Health Statistics. (1992, January). Advance report of final mortality statistics, 1989. *Monthly Vital Statistics Report, supplement, 40,* (8[2]).
23. National Center for Health Statistics. (1978–88). *Vital statistics of the United States: Vol. II. Mortality*. Washington, DC: U.S. Public Health Service, U.S. Government Printing Office.
24. Office of Technology Assessment. (1990, September). *Health care in rural America* (OTA Publication No. H435). Washington, DC: U.S. Government Printing Office.
25. Singh, S., Forrest, J., & Torres, A. (1989). *Prenatal care in the U.S.: A state inventory: Vol. 1*. Washington, DC: Alan Guttmacher Institute.
26. Congressional Budget Office (1993, October). *A CBO study: Projections of national health expenditures*, Washington, DC: Author.
27. U.S. Senate Committee on Labor and Human Resources. (1990). *The health care crisis: A report to the American people* (p. 3). Washington, DC: U.S. Government Printing Office.
28. Campaign for Women's Health. (1991). *A challenge for the 1990's: Improving health care for American women*. Washington, DC: Older Women's League.
29. Healy, B.P. (1992). The women's health initiative. *The Female Patient, 17*, 36–38.
30. Bass, M., & Howes, J. (1992). Women's health: The making of a powerful new public issue. *Women's Health Issues, 2*(1), 3.
31. Bhargaua, S.W. (1992, July). Finally, a healthy interest in women. *Business Week*, pp. 88–89.
32. Raymon, R., & Allshouse, K. (undated). *Resiliency amidst inequity: Older women workers in an aging U.S.* (pp. 1–4). Southport, CT: Southport Institute for Policy Analysis, Project for Women and Population Aging.
33. Older Women's League. (1990, May). *Heading for hardship: Retirement income for American women in the next century*. Washington, DC: Author.
34. Waldman, S. (1992, May). Deadbeat dads. *Newsweek*, pp. 46–52.
35. Hartmann, H., & Spalter-Roth, R. (1990, November). *Working parents: Differences, similarities and the implications for a policy agenda*. Paper presented at a meeting on women, work, and the family: Advancing the Policy and Research Agenda, Institute for Research on Women and Center. Columbia University, New York.
36. U.S. Department of Commerce, Bureau of the Census. (1990). *Statistical abstract of the United States: 1990* (110th ed.). (Table 103). Washington, DC: U.S. Government Printing Office.
37. Agency for Health Care Policy and Research. (1990, October). *Research Activities, 134*.
38. Older Women's League. (1989, May). Failing America's caregivers: A status report on women who care. *Mother's Day Report*, p. 3.

39. U.S. Public Health Service. (1985). *Women's health: Report of the public health service task force on women's health issues: Vol. II* (DHHS Publication No. PHS 85-50206). Washington, DC: U.S. Government Printing Office.
40. Johnson, K., & Massion, C. (1991, November/December). Why a women's medical specialty? *Ms. Magazine*, pp. 68–69.
41. Solomon, A. (1991). The politics of breast cancer. *Revolution Premiere Issue, 1*, 51–64.
42. Elmer-DeWitt, P. (1990, February). A better pill to swallow. *Time*, p. 44.
43. Loeb, L. (1990). *Caring for caregivers: Addressing the employment needs of long term care workers*. Washington, DC: Older Women's League.
44. Kemper, P., & Martaugh, C. (1991). Lifetime use of nursing home care. *New England Journal of Medicine, 324*, 595–600.
45. Chu, S.Y., Buehler, J.W., & Berkelman, R.L. (1990). Impact on the human immunodeficiency virus epidemic on mortality in women of reproductive age, United States. *Journal of the American Medical Association, 264*, 225–228.
46. Novello, A.C., & Soto-Torres, L.E. (1992). Women and hidden epidemics: HIV/AIDS and domestic violence. *Female Patient, 17*, 17–31.
47. Tracy, C, Talbert, D., & Steinschneider, J. (1990). *Women, babies, and drugs; Family centered treatment options*. Washington, DC: Center for Policy Alternative, National Conference of State Legislatures.
48. Opinion Research Corporation. (1988, February). Hospital survey on obstetric claim frequency by patient category, prepared for the American College of Obstetricians and Gynecologists, Washington, DC.
49. Longest, B.B. (1988). American health policy in the year 2000. *Hospital and Health Services Administration, 33*(4), 419–434.

## BIBLIOGRAPHY

Ahurdene, P., & Naisbett, J. (1992). *Megatrends for women*. New York: Villard Books.

Horton, J.A. (Ed.). (1992). *The women's health data book: A profile of women's health in the United States*. Washington, DC: Jacob's Institute of Women's Health.

CHAPTER 2

# HEALTH AND DEVELOPMENT THROUGH THE LIFE CYCLE

*Marcia Szmania Davis • Ellis Quinn Youngkin*

*Indeed, women with multiple roles may be the most well adjusted.*

*Highlights*

- Stage Theories
- Historical Psychoanalytic Influence
- Erikson's Stages
- Levinson's Model
- Current Views: Moral and Human Development, A New Psychology
- Major Periods and Tasks: Transitions From Early to Late Adulthood

## INTRODUCTION

In order to define and understand women's development, one must address the societal norms that prevail over time (see Chapter 1). One important change during the late 1960s and early 1970s was women's realization that many important individual concerns they had previously been hesitant to discuss were actually widespread and political in nature. "The personal is political" slogan reflected an energy borne out in consciousness-raising groups where women talked about their lived experiences, learning that their innermost feelings were shared by women in general. A period of self-discovery began as women began to break out of socially constrictive stereotypes.

Earlier, in the 1950s, remarkable changes in women's lives were associated with fewer births, extended longevity, greater acceptance of lifestyle options in marriage and family formation, and attachment to the labor force.[1] Affirmative action movements eventually developed into academic programs in women's studies beginning in the 1960s, often with reluctant acceptance by universities.[2] These courses reflected limitations set on women by patriarchal societies, and women contemplated the reasons. Recent history books celebrated women's influences that had largely been ignored or downplayed.

Is the contemporary view of society toward women indeed different from the past? The answer must be an equivocal yes, in part because traditional sex-role stereotypes continue to pervade the thinking of many men and women. Women who do not marry and reproduce may be viewed as having failed to develop their fullest potential. Moreover, femininity has long been, and to a great extent continues to be, equated with passivity, dependency, and pleasing men.[3]

## GROWTH AND DEVELOPMENT

Growth and development are often viewed according to a person's stage in the life cycle. Whereas *growth* refers to quantitative physical and physiological changes, *development* encompasses more qualitative changes, including functional, psychosocial, and cognitive behaviors.[4] Both areas need to be assessed so that the health care provider can offer anticipatory guidance to women as they adapt to personal and environmental changes. The developmental theories most closely linked to sequential ages and life stages have frequently been used for clinical evaluation. Controversy exists, however, about the applicability of such theories to women, particularly because cultural biases may be a problem. For example, Erikson studied primarily white, middle class males. Also, developmental norms may not apply to all cultural backgrounds; and stage theories may promote ageism if one does not fulfill expectations, such as marriage, by a given point in life.[4]

## STAGE THEORIES OF DEVELOPMENT

Investigation of developmental change across the life span has gained prominence over the past 50 years, largely as a result of psychoanalytic influence. The resulting developmental theories emerged from the body of knowledge in child psychology. Although the life-span developmental framework focused primarily on men, the resulting theories were generalized to apply to all adults. Women's development, which was seldom alluded to, was viewed narrowly and judged aberrant if gender development did not conform to the accepted male pattern.[5]

Characteristics commonly attributed to women, such as being less aggressive, more emotional, and less independent, were seen to be less healthy. Although the majority of psychoanalytic clients were women, little was known about their experiences as women. Virtually no attention was directed towards the effects of the societal environment on women. Feminists thus came to view traditional psychotherapy as an agent of social control, reinforcing the traditional sex roles and traditional values that led to a devaluation of women.

## HISTORICAL PSYCHOANALYTIC INFLUENCE

Freudian psychosexual theory and practice—the largest influence on psychotherapeutic knowledge—gave therapists a largely antifeminine orientation.[6–8] Freud espoused that biological drives influence a person's psychological and personality development. In his view, superiority of men was largely derived from the possession of a penis. Penis envy purportedly led to feminine aggression. According to Freud, limitations of women inherent in their biology ("anatomy is destiny") included women's innate dependency, passivity, and masochism, which were required for their primary fulfilling role, successful motherhood. Women were viewed as more narcissistic, more prone to jealousy, and having a weaker sense of justice.[9] Women were labeled "frigid" if they were incapable of mature (phallocentric) vaginal orgasm, versus clitoral orgasm. The studies of Masters and Johnson proved this concept incorrect.[5]

### Feminist Views on Psychoanalysis

Critics condemned Freud for deriding women who displayed qualities that would be lauded in men, primarily boldness and independence.[2] Many women also voiced resentment toward the implied foreclosure on women's opportunities.

- Karen Horney (1920s and 1930s) proposed that if penis envy existed, it was because the penis symbolized the social and political power of men.[8]
- Simone de Beauvoir (*The Second Sex*, 1949) caused a great deal of controversy by challenging the ideation of biological and psychological determination of roles for women.
- Betty Friedan (*The Feminine Mystique*, 1963) attempted to broaden society's narrow role of women's place being in the home.
- Kate Millet (*Sexual Politics*, 1969) continued to scorn Freud for upholding the male body as the norm and questioned the validity of Freud's concept of female fear of castration while ignoring issues such as rape.

## ADULT DEVELOPMENTAL THEORIES

Although developmental changes during childhood and adolescence have been studied, relatively little attention has been paid to the adult years,[10] and the study of women's development is still in its infancy and is controversial. The climate exists for an interdisciplinary approach to the study of human development, and social scientists have shown us that societal issues must be closely addressed.

### ERIKSON'S STAGES OF PSYCHOSOCIAL DEVELOPMENT (1950S TO 1960S)

One of the earliest contributors to the study of adult development, Erikson suggested the normalcy and necessity of growth and change during adult years and not just in childhood.[11,12] His theories, grounded in conceptions of the life cycle and the life course, addressed stages in ego development. According to Erikson,

- Each stage is primary at a particular age level, or segment of the life cycle, from infancy to old age.
- If a task that is appropriate to a given phase of life is not resolved, then development in subsequent phases of life may be impaired.
- A patterned sequence of stages occurs, each with appropriate physical, emotional, and cognitive tasks.
- A person who successfully passes through each stage eventually attains ego integrity, which is associated with high self-esteem and a positive outlook on life.
- A major difference for a woman is that her identity is enmeshed in a married state, which is viewed as necessary for her mature integration of personality[13] (see Chapter 1, Other Influences on Women's Health, Marital Status.)

Erikson's eight stages of development, composed of bipolar tasks at various stages of life, include *Trust versus Mistrust*, infancy; *Autonomy versus Shame and Doubt*, early childhood; *Initiative versus Guilt*, preschool age; *Industry versus Inferiority*, school age; *Identity versus Identity Diffusion*, adolescence; *Intimacy versus Isolation or Self-Absorption*, young adulthood; *Generativity versus Stagnation*, middle adulthood; and *Integrity versus Despair and Disdain*, late adulthood.

### LEVINSON'S MODEL OF ADULT DEVELOPMENT (1970S TO PRESENT)

This well-known model of adult development, which is grounded in psychoanalytic theory, is applied in research and psychotherapy. Levinson believes that women go through the same developmental periods that men do; however, he included only male subjects up to age 45 in his early, extensive study. More recent work including women is cited in publications, but the full study is not yet released.[10,14] Levinson expanded on Erikson's notion of development and characterized each segment of adulthood in terms of intrinsic tasks.[10,14] This theory proposes an underlying set of developmental periods and tasks along with transition crises that involve reassessment of one's life. Adult development is an evolving process of mutual interaction between self and the world, of which family and work are central components. Career choice and work are paramount in terms of goals, social roles, ethical standards and values, and development of self-concept. The assumption is that we desire self-actualization, which requires psychological and realistic change in controllable measures. To this extent, men and women are similar. (Women's adult development is addressed in Major Periods and Tasks: The Women's Perspective).

***Early Adult Transition (Ages 17 to 22).*** The shaky start toward maturity involves taking new steps in individuation. Choices are made concerning career, lifestyle, and modification of existing family and social relationships. This is the adult era of greatest energy and abundance—and of greatest contradiction and stress.

***Entering the Adult World (Ages 22 to 28).*** Through the establishment of an independent living situation, exploration, and commitment to adult roles, the 20s reflect structure building.

***Age 30 Transition (Ages 28 to 33).*** During the transition period, the sense of being young, especially in terms of options, is given up. Current lifestyles, values, family situations, and career choices are evaluated. Biologically, the 20s and 30s are the peak years of life.

***Settling Down (Ages 33 to 40).*** Affirming personal integrity, realizing oneself as a full-fledged adult, and goal achievement are characteristic of this period.

***Midlife Transition (Ages 40 to 45).*** Lifestyle is critically examined, and the need arises to recognize time limitations for goal achievement. Polarities, including young–old and destruction–creation, are integrated. Levinson believes that the character of living always changes appreciably between early and middle childhood.

***Entering Middle Adulthood (Ages 45 to 50).*** Undergoing restabilization after midlife transition, individuals in middle adulthood have biological capacities below earlier years but normally are still sufficiently fit for energetic, personally satisfying, and socially valuable lives.

***Age 50 Transition (Ages 50 to 53).*** Once more lifestyle and major goals are reevaluated.

***Middle Adulthood Culmination (Ages 53 to 60).*** Work continues toward achieving life goals and contributing to society.

***Late Adulthood (Ages 60 to 80) and the Late Adult Transition (60 to 65).*** Although the character of one's life is fundamentally altered as a result of biological, psychological, and social changes, the individual recognizes that this period can be distinctive and fulfilling.

***Late, Late Adulthood (Age 80 and Older).*** At this time, the process of aging may be more obvious than the process of growth. The individual must make peace with dying; development occurs as one gives new meaning to life and death. These oldest adults may be an example for others by demonstrating wisdom and personal nobility.[14]

# CURRENT VIEWS ON WOMEN'S DEVELOPMENT

## WOMEN'S CONTRIBUTIONS

Women's influence has been largely absent in many areas, including art, literature, social sciences, and psychological research.[6,15] Even though women have devoted their lives to supporting the lifelong development of others, their own development experiences are still essentially untold.[15] Women's life experiences and viewpoints may indeed be different from men's as a result of complex factors such as social status, power and reproductive biology.[6,16]

### Gilligan's Theory of Moral Development

Gilligan, a clinical psychologist, traced women's voices as she studied the development of morality.[6] She found that existing psychological accounts failed to describe the progression of relationships toward a maturity of interdependence, or to trace the evolution of the capacity for responsible care. Gilligan challenged Freud, Piaget, and Kohlberg, who studied boys and men and then assumed that women's ability to make moral judgments was inferior.[17] Gilligan's work asserts that

- Women have learned, from their early socialization, to place priority on responsibility toward others in important relationships (the ethics of care) rather than on individual welfare and concerns.
- When faced with a dilemma, women are interested in understanding individual circumstances.
- The standard of moral judgment that women use for self-assessment also has to do with relationships: the ability to nurture, to care for others, and to bear responsibility.
- Women's differing modes of moral reasoning lead to different forms of self-definition and different views of relationships.[6] Gilligan's work has been criticized as perpetuating gender stereotypes during the socially conservative 1980s.[18]

### Bardwick's Model of Human Development

Bardwick's model addresses women's adult development while incorporating much of Levinson's model of adult maturation. Bardwick maintains that psychological growth and change are intertwined and never cease.[19] Moreover, the goals and values of one's life reflect changing societal and cultural values.[10] The transition from one developmental stage to the next includes a process of self-evaluation. For women, transitions to new values and lifestyles are likely to be more extreme and more emotionally volatile than in previous generations, as options provided to women become more numerous.[19]

Bardwick defines the self in terms of dependent, interdependent, and egocentric mental stances. A woman may maintain a *dependent* sense of self, which is basically relational, or move toward a more *interdependent* stance, in which a sense of self exists simultaneously with a keen awareness of being a contributing and receiving member of an affectional relationship. Bardwick, however, contends that for a woman to develop a permanent *egocentric* stance is rare, because socialization of women in our society and the definition of femininity tend much more toward an interdependent or dependent sense of self.

## A NEW PSYCHOLOGY OF WOMEN

### Equality

Caring for others is valued less in our society than are individuation and individual achievement; thus women's concern with relationships is often viewed as a weakness.[16] The need for social equality is reflected in problems that arise when affiliation and relationships are molded by domination and subordination.[16] A new language in psychology should describe the structuring of women's sense of self, that is, the need to make and then maintain relationships. Caring and connection must be separated from the resulting inequality and oppression. Women judge themselves in terms of their ability to care, so much so that professional and academic endeavors may be seen as jeopardizing their own sense of themselves.[6] Personal conflict may arise when women have to choose between achievement and caring, if being successful is at the expense of another's failure.

### Valuing Self

The psychology of women is distinct in relationships of temporary and permanent inequality.[16] A woman may be temporarily dominant in relationships of nurturance, yet subservient in relationships of permanently unequal social status and power. Women are subordinate in social position to men, yet at the same time entwined with them in the intimate and intense relationships of adult sexuality and family life. Feminist therapy involves the individual's recognition of the restrictive social binds that influence many women, including an overdependence on men for self-esteem and financial, psychological, and social needs.[5] Women traditionally have taken care of men, but men have tended to assume or devalue that care.[6] Women need to learn to nurture and value themselves and other women, rather than nurturing only men and children. Women's psychology reflects both sides of relationships of interdependence.

### Empowerment

Women need power to advance their own development and maintain an identity characterized by self-determination and a diminished need for continuous approval.[16] Too often women find their lives being dominated by prevalent societal values.[16] Often, women and men experience enormous differences in access to power and control of resources,[20] and for women, a stance of less power may result in an emphasis on relatedness to others and compassion.[18] Powerlessness, or learned helplessness, in femininity may be exhibited in relationships of battering and more subtly as depression.[5]

Many women have learned to demystify aspects of their lives, finding strength in the shared experiences of other women. Their strength is reflected in greater self-sufficiency, assertiveness, and self-knowledge. Consider the example of violence against women. Issues such as rape, battering of women, child sexual abuse, and incest were largely ignored, or their existence disbelieved, before the collected efforts of enraged women.[16] Women have effected changes in medical/gynecologic care and will no longer accept care that is limited to their reproductive organs to the exclusion of concerns such as cardiac disease or to the discounting of entities such as premenstrual syndrome (PMS).

### A Different Starting Point in Defining Women's Development

Women develop in a context of their attachment to others. Women's sense of self, as well as their perceived strength, is based on the ability to form affiliations and relationships.[6,16] Many women perceive the threat of a disrupted affiliation as a total loss of self.

Perhaps there is a more ideal midpoint where affiliation is valued along with self-sufficiency. Possibilities exist for a more advanced approach to living and functioning in which affiliation is valued as highly, or more highly, than self-enhancement.[16]

## THE WAYS THAT WOMEN KNOW

The intellectual development of women has become another topic of study.[15,21] The inability for women to "gain a voice" reflects their image of being powerless, subjugated, and inadequate. Indeed, more women than men pose questions, listen to others, and refrain from speaking out, but women's pattern of discourse may be suitable for a maternal, caring, relationship-oriented role. For example, a mother may refrain from sharing ideas too quickly with her child in order to foster the child's own ability to form ideas. Thus, women may value drawing out the voices of others as a means of enhancing others' development. This mode of discourse, similar to Socratic thinking, could serve as a model for promoting human development.[21]

## SOCIETAL ISSUES

Ambiguity in the language of adult development stems from the lack of a cultural definition of *adulthood* and how people's lives evolve within it.[10] Controversies in the study of adult development include whether the use of separate, gender-specific, and age-status criteria is still relevant.[22] In fact, age norms today are more fluid than in the past; for example, many people divorce, or never marry, and many adults choose to have no children or to have children later in life.

Furthermore, in our society women as well as men are economically productive and not isolated in the home. The 1980s witnessed a remarkable increase in the number of employed women, especially married working mothers. Both men and women may aspire for social power, social privileges, and dominant social status. Meanwhile, many of the baby boomer generation, born during the 1950s and 1960s, men and women alike, are taking another look at the importance of work and family life.[23] A substantial portion claim that family life will become more important to them, a trend sometimes referred to as "downshifting," including earlier retirement for both men and women and more leisure activities for greater family contact.

An alternative approach to the study of adult development is to focus on changing social contexts surrounding human development and the normative life crises marking individual and family lifestyle.[22] The individual's inner developmental changes and outer contextual life changes can be viewed as dynamically interdependent; consequently, age diminishes as the focus of our attention in a complex social structure.

## WOMEN'S ISSUES AND CONFLICTING VALUES

### Value Changes

The value changes that occurred most dramatically during the 1970s redefined and expanded choices for women in their roles related to work and family.[13,19] Many women must now address both modern and traditional patterns of lifestyle in their decision making. Facing conflicting life choices and societal norms, women grapple with cultural ambiguity and personal uncertainty. Traditional norms regarding femininity prevail, even for women in less traditional roles. For example, despite reduced gender separation of work and family roles in the 1990s, couples still tend to make decisions concerning geographical locations and timing of major family events according to the husband's career needs. On the other hand, women are choosing to have fewer children. This fact, combined with increasing longevity, means that a substantially shorter percentage of women's lives are spent childrearing.

### Cultural Ambiguity and Personal Uncertainty

Although women's choices can create ambiguity and uncertainty, the freedom of choice is perhaps less frustrating than the restrictions of the recent past.[19] Often, however, change may be an illusion for women; the reality of the social foundation of power still leans strongly toward enhanced status for traditional feminine values.[18] Modern women also face significant challenges to "have it all," as the social changes necessary to allow for ample choices have not been resolved.[13] Barriers still exist to equitable pay, adequate child care, and breaking through "old boy" networks. Women may have adequate drive to achieve; however, they may feel limited to a level of achievement that society deems appropriate for their gender difference or, some would argue, their social status.[13,19] Conflict may arise between the need for affiliation or the desire for approval from other people, and the pursuit of achievement for its own sake. Competition may be viewed as contrary to the feminine ideal and may lead to social rejection. Although women and men tend to be compared favorably in neutral situations, women tend to have less internal hope for success in more competitive situations. A particular dilemma for women has been to achieve success in a traditionally "male" occupation.

***Gender Issues.*** Whereas Levinson believes that the timing of developmental periods and tasks are similar for women and men,[10] others hold that gender differences exist in movement through developmental periods.[6,19] Furthermore, women, more than men, tend to avoid evaluating their own lives. Perhaps this is because self-assessment may heighten women's awareness of their lack of self-determination and relative powerlessness, revealed in their tendency to respond to the directives and initiative of others.[19] Women's self-esteem and identity also depend more heavily on validation by others.

***Life Events, Options, and Stress.*** Along with more options, women may also experience discontent, as it is less clear what is expected of them. Stressors occur in traditional homemaker choices, in career options, and in attempts to combine the two. In addition, women may experience developmental periods at later ages and in more irregular sequences, while focusing on different aspects of their life structure.[24] Moreover, developmental tasks may be dealt with very differently at different times, as women themselves may change psychologically over time.

## MAJOR PERIODS AND TASKS: THE WOMEN'S PERSPECTIVE

A well-formed body of knowledge on women's development does not exist; however, issues in women's development are discussed here, using Levinson's framework, where feasible, and other authors' contributions, especially those of Bardwick.[19] The novice phase of early adulthood—individuals as apprentice adults, ages 17 to 33—encompasses several large tasks, including forming a dream, a mentor relationship, an occupation, and an enduring relationship. Women and men may have significant differences in accomplishing these tasks.[25] Timing of major life events is not as important as understanding the importance in forming the life structure. A discussion of key transition periods follows.

## EARLY ADULT TRANSITION (AGES 17 TO 22)

Major tasks for women in this period include value assessment; goal setting for education and work; formation of important peer relationships that focus on sex, love, and commitment; and separation from parents.[10,14] Individuation may be reflected in great differences in values between parents and young adults in areas such as politics and career choices. However, values may more strongly reflect identification with peer groups than true individuation or autonomy. The sense of self is very fluid at this period.

A major conflict exists between making commitments and avoiding them in order to keep options open.[10] Commitments are more easily made if one's peers are doing so. The early adult is often egocentric as she progresses through rapid emotional and physical changes. She may believe that she is invulnerable, unique, and immune, and hence be prone to misconceptions, for example, that sexual activity will not lead to pregnancy.[26]

### Gender Identity

A crucial task is to internalize a sense of gender, which encompasses a sense of one's body in relation to sexuality. To traditional young women, this focus may mean marriage, the prime example of moving into an adult sexual role. Women are essentially dependent at this time, and occasionally interdependent, as the need to form relationships dominates. A great deal of psychological fluidity exists with some sense of egocentrism. Men at this time exhibit comparatively less fluidity and interpersonal dependence and more egocentricity.

Traditional sex-role expectations are still prominent in adolescence and early adulthood.[13] For example, a woman may fear that her own ambitions will cost a relationship. A conflict exists between fulfillment of egocentric and interpersonal/dependent priorities as the early adult tries to define the sense of self.

### Identity and Adult Commitments

Erikson describes the male adolescent as developing an autonomous, initiating, industrious self through the forging of an identity based on the ideal image—ability to support and justify adult commitments.[12] He describes the female adolescent as holding her identity in abeyance while preparing to attract the man she will marry and by whose status she will be defined.[12] Such attitudes predominated well into the 1960s and to a great degree, still exist. Many women, however, have begun to emerge as breadwinners in their own right, often choosing professions once thought of as strictly in the man's domain. These women may have more confusing choices as they struggle with career decisions that will affect their family's life.

### Identity and Intimacy

For men, identity precedes intimacy and generativity in the traditional view of the optimum cycle of human separation and attachment. For women, these tasks are fused, developing together as the woman comes to know herself as she is known, primarily through her relationships with others.[6,13] Most men in their 20s are not ready to form loving, emotionally intimate relationships, or to make an enduring commitment to wives and families.[10] Whereas women resolve the intimacy issue by their 20s,[27] men are still engaged in this task well into their 30s. Traditionally, men view attachment as a developmental impediment. Hence, married women may be "intimacy mentors" to their husbands.

### Factors Influencing Identity

Identity development in women is influenced by communion, connection, relation (to friends and all significant others) embeddedness, spirituality, and affiliation.[28] Men and women differ significantly in the separation–individuation process. Some women may never completely individuate from their mothers. Often they transfer their dependence onto a boyfriend, as their vision of themselves is relational. A process of anchoring in the family of origin, with a partner and children, in a career, or with friends is critical to women's identity formation and provides the anchor for growth, change, or new directions in life. For women, identity and intimacy are developed at the same time.[6]

### Challenges to Women's Independent Goals

Women now in their 20s have grown up in a society different from that of their mothers.[19] A growing number of women today focus on their own careers, as independent goals are articulated more freely. During this period as a woman deals with the demands of egocentric children, it is possible to become engulfed and lose a sense of self, especially if her marital partner is also demanding. Although the majority of women who divorce in their 20s do remarry, they may become more egocentric, unwilling to give anyone else that much power over them again.

### Identity and Parenthood

Women, especially working women or those with difficult infants, experience appreciably more change than do men in the transition to parenthood.[29] Women tend to feel responsible for their children's success and happiness. They also experience the "contagion of stress" as they internalize the distress experienced by those to whom they are closest, particularly family members. During this period, however, if work serves as a visible marker of achievement, it may lessen stress. Indeed, women with multiple roles may be the most well adjusted. The supportive family buffers a woman from endless demands of child care and other family responsibilities.

## ENTRY LIFE STRUCTURE FOR EARLY ADULTHOOD (AGES 22 TO 28)

Life structures for women tend to be less stable than those for men, essentially because of more diverse concerns involving marriage, motherhood, and career.[25]

## AGE THIRTY TRANSITION AND THE SETTLING DOWN PERIOD OF EARLY ADULTHOOD (AGES 28 TO 39)

Both sexes, in settling down, must give up a youthful self-image and the idea that involvements are tentative and options still open. Priorities of the 20s may be reversed; choices and their consequences may be reassessed; and options regarding marriage and especially childbearing may not exist much longer.[10]

- *Men's Success.* Success in work is imperative to men's timetable. A shift in centrality by men—from work to family—may be a reaction to a combination of stress, age, or failure in work. Men sever ties with mentors in order to be seen as knowledgeable and successful in their own right, of "becoming one's own man."[10]
- *Women's Success.* In contrast, few women would define "becoming one's own woman" primarily through success in their work.[19] Those who are successful in their careers may still be anxious about their femininity unless they are also involved in significant relationships and have experienced motherhood. Women may sacrifice success in careers and attain lower financial status as they compromise to maintain relationships. Factors leading to a sense of independence in men, such as career suc-

cess, may instead highlight the dependent needs in women.

- *Prolonged Transition*. Women in their 30s are likely to experience a more prolonged and profound transition period than men are, perhaps most importantly linked to the age limits for childbearing (the "biological clock"). Current technology may permit women to become pregnant well beyond their earlier expectations, however. The age thirty transition can be a time of increased individuation that is self-generated rather then relational. During the period of evaluation and reappraisal (ages 28 to 33), married women may demand that husbands recognize and accommodate their aspirations and interests outside of the home.[25]
- *Career versus Family*. Women reappraise the relative importance of career and family, often adding the missing component rather than reversing priorities (e.g., a mother may begin a career).[19] Women may attempt to lead a life in which they do it all. The mental health stressors of women's multiple roles may be influenced more by marital factors than by work factors. Work often buffers some marital stress, but parenthood exacerbates occupational stress, especially if responsibilities are not shared in the home.[29]
- *Multiple Roles*. Having multiple roles may counterbalance some negative effects of a particular role. Thus, the healthiest women may be those with multiple roles, including having a career, a husband, and often children.[29] "Having it all" may mean "doing it all, " and women may experience strain in attempting to fulfill multiple role obligations. American society does not yet support working women with child care options or pay that is comparable to men's. Often they must choose between family and career. Women's ability to cope with the stresses has been associated with having a high income and job satisfaction, marrying later, and arranging time for family activities.[29]
- *American Values and Women's Sexuality*. The American culture values youth and beauty, and often by age 35, a woman is no longer considered young.[30] Women are labeled old 10 to 15 years earlier than men are, with resulting psychological, sexual, and economic disadvantages.[30]
- *Confusing Choices*. Women in their 30s are facing the growing influence of feminist thinking and more egalitarian life patterns. At the same time they are confronted by others who tell them that their behaviors should be more traditional. Women also struggle with their own psychological tendencies regarding more traditional values, which they internalized early in life.
- *Readjustment in the Thirties*. Demographically, most women now in their 30s are married with school-age children. Those who are employed are not necessarily on a career path. Others who are unemployed have been out of school for about 10 years.[19] As women reach ages 35 to 40, their husband's tremendous involvement in their own careers, and children's decreasing dependence on them, may provide the opportunity for personal change. Women may return to work or school, or look for other relationships in the community. Family members may initially agree to change their lifestyles in order to accommodate the woman's needs; however, when changes impact them directly, they may become resentful or confused.
- *Stress*. Stress is inherent in the reality or the illusion of choice. Some women may sacrifice personal relationships to achieve career success; others may be "doing it all" with very little support from their partners. Partners' expectations of each other in their relationship are not always clear. Many women who divorce in their 30s may become more confident and perhaps more an-

gry. Anger may lead to egocentricism that enables women to formulate obtainable objectives. For married women, responsibilities outside the home—community and career involvement—may help them become less dependent economically, socially, and psychologically. Most women in this age group tend toward interdependence.

## MIDLIFE TRANSITION AND MIDDLE ADULTHOOD (AGES 39 TO 60)

An appreciable change in the character of living occurs between early and middle adulthood. The main tasks of entering middle adulthood are making crucial choices, giving those choices meaning and commitment, and building a life structure around them.[10]

### Midlife Transitions

- Assessment for both men and women may have a sense of urgency; they wish to accomplish their life goals as they confront mortality. Those who do not assess their lives at this point may feel frightened and unable to make changes in their lifestyles or careers. Men assess what they receive and what they give to work, family, friends, and community as they reach the symbolically powerful age of 40.[10,14] Their established autonomy now allows greater compassion, more reflection, less tyranny by inner conflicts and external demands, and more genuine love of self and others. Middle aged men may experience this as their fullest and most creative period.

  By the end of middle adulthood problems may include declining health, aging or death of parents, spousal death, and stagnation at work with no viable options. Although the relationship with one's spouse may only be comfortable, the option of ending it means losing crucial roots. Nonetheless, divorce has increased markedly for both men and women in their 40s. One may see a partner as a reason for discontent, or someone to blame for perceived losses. A new relationship may be viewed as a way to recoup the feelings and pleasure of youth.
- Growth can be seen in women who become more autonomous as they succeed in relationships; both sexes may become more interdependent.[19] Women may grow more comfortable as initiators and become gratified functioning as individuals. Most women now in their 40s grew up in traditional environments in which choices were limited. Consequently, few have been seriously involved in a career. Becoming involved in a career after 40 can be an opportunity for real beginnings, but it also can be frightening. This may be a time for women to generate new values internally, reflecting who they are rather than what they do.
- Losses or adjustments in relationships may cause depression in women beginning the midlife phase; they may experience loneliness as children leave home or they become widowed or divorced.[19] The "empty nest" concept is not totally supported by national data; a dependent woman who faces the loss of her children and her husband at this time may be more vulnerable. Women, but not men, tend to define their age status in terms of the timing of events within their family; even unmarried career women often discuss middle age in terms of the family they might have had. Women with more complex lives may experience sadness and joy in this time of readjustment as they face losses along with new beginnings. Many more men than women remarry at this age.

  A majority of women have made a reality transition, as evidenced by a high employment rate.[19] The expansion of activities, maturing, and increased self-confidence lead many of these women to be more interdependent rather than dependent, as compared with women in their 30s. This is perhaps the most complex of all developmental periods because women are given social permission to work at precisely the time their traditional responsibilities decline.

## Middle Adulthood

Although Levinson's studies ended with men in their 40s, he believed that a major transition phase occurs from ages 50 to 55. A stable period follows from ages 55 to 60, during which rejuvenation in some can result in achieving significant fulfillment and enrichment.[10,14] For men especially whose connection with others depends largely on their jobs, retirement may be associated with a loss of prestige and decreased self-esteem. Women tend to face this loss much earlier if their primary role in life is that of mother, their secondary role that of homemaker, and their tertiary role that of sexual partner.

- The aging process traditionally has been symbolized as retirement for men and menopause for women, although the formerly predominant views regarding women and the menopause have been challenged.[27] Anticipating menopause is often more dreadful than the difficulty experienced with its actual occurrence. Women often feel relief with the loss of menses as well as the loss of tasks associated with rearing young children. The real difficulty may be adjusting to the aging process—a continuum that does not just begin after menses ends. Other changes associated with aging are socially more apparent, such as graying hair and wrinkles. Bifocal glasses and hearing aids may be a threat to self-esteem and a visible admission of aging, which may cause problems in intimate relationships.[27,31]
- "The sandwich generation" refers to the women who are caretakers for their children as well as for their aging parents.

  Aging is a gradual process, and changes of aging are adaptive across the life span. During middle age, women may to some extent lose their roles of mother and sex partner, especially through divorce or death. A partner's retirement may force another adaptation. Distancing from parents in the middle years is replaced by establishing a commitment for parents' care, which allows some women who see themselves primarily as homemakers to reestablish that lifestyle.
- Readjustment in the 50s may be necessary because today's women in that age group were in their 20s when new options for women gained momentum.[19] A few will feel the need to change or reassess values or direction at this stage in their lives; others will reject new values, believing themselves incapable of achieving different goals. Women most at risk for psychological dependence are traditional housewives who lack involvement or outside commitments. Interdependence is more likely to occur among older women who have found fulfillment in their traditional roles and who have assumed varied roles, whether or not through employment. A few older women are egocentric as a result of being widows, divorced, displaced homemakers, or having never married.
- Societal views of aging women include negative stereotypes such as being inactive, unhealthy, asexual, unattractive, and ineffective—despite the diversity of older women who lead interesting, productive lives.[20] Revising expectations about advancing age requires that society move beyond these stereotypes and overcome ageist and sexual biases.[26] Health care providers need to recognize the diversity among women as they age. Older women receive messages that growing older is a

process to be prevented (with face lifts or antiaging facial creams) rather than to be enjoyed.[7] Even professional women view aging as a serious impairment. Discrimination in employment is particularly harmful for women reentering the work force after their children leave home or when the loss of a spouse decreases their income and security. Throughout adulthood, women are increasingly threatened by poverty as a result of greater numbers of female-headed households and the continuing disparity in salaries between men and women. Older women are particularly affected by inadequate spousal retirement plans, especially if they themselves have a history of unemployment. As women live longer, they have more opportunity to develop illness, another stress on their finances.

## LATE ADULT TRANSITION

Ages 60 to 65 mark the end of middle life and entry into the late adult transition.[14] Overall, women feel good about themselves and what they are accomplishing as they use time freed by retirement or other life changes to pursue creative activities, community work, and self-development.[24] When women outlive their husbands, creativity may develop as a response to loss and loneliness, including social and emotional isolation. Women may also return to creative activities they enjoyed in earlier years. During their 60s women are most likely to experience transitions relating to their own illness and the illness and death of significant others.

### Behavioral Shifts with Age

In the last decades, studies have addressed endocrine changes as they affect the physiological and psychological aspects of life, as well as the relationships between women and men, and women and women, and the changes that occur in those relationships over time. The studies are controversial.[27] Some authors propose that a shift to more assertive or controlling behavior among women beginning in midlife is the result of a change in the androgen–estrogen ratio toward more biologically active androgens of greater influence. The reverse pattern is observed in men, with estrogens affecting affiliative and nurturing aspects as androgens drop. Thus, while aging women may become more tolerant of their own aggressive and egocentric impulses, aging men may become more accepting of their nurturant and affiliative impulses.

## LATE ADULTHOOD AND LATE, LATE ADULTHOOD

Women can expect to live well into their 70s and 80s. Ages 76 to 80 may represent a transition toward wisdom as women are challenged to adapt to a number of changes, including loss of health, friends, and family.[24] A surge of creativity may continue as women find pleasurable ways to enrich their lives. Relationships and affiliation with others remain important for women, and their creativity may take the form of altruistic responses to the needs of others. Successful or creative aging may be associated with maintaining meaningful activities, keeping close relationships with persons of all ages, and remaining flexible and adaptable. Nonconformists who are willing to take risks and who sustain a positive outlook on life perhaps experience the greatest success in aging. Psychological development never ends as long as the individual engages in reality; thus the potential for growth and change is always present.[19,24]

## REFERENCES

1. O'Rand, A.M., & Henrette, J.C. (1982). Women at middle age: Development and transitions. *Annals of the American Academy of Political and Social Sciences*. Beverly Hills, CA: Sage.

2. Grosskurth, P. (1991). The new psychology of women. *New York Review of Books, 38*(17).
3. Barnard, J. (1981). Women's educational needs. In A.W. Chickering and Associates (Eds.), *The modern American college: Responding to the new realities of diverse students and a changing society*. San Francisco: Jossey-Bass.
4. Fuller, J., & Schaller-Ayers, J. (1990). *Health assessment: A nursing approach*. Philadelphia: Lippincott.
5. Kaschak, E. (1981). Feminist psychotherapy: The first decade. In S. Cox (Ed.), *Female psychology* (pp. 387–401). New York: St. Martin's Press.
6. Gilligan, C. (1982). *In a different voice: Psychological theory and women's development*. Cambridge, MA: Harvard University Press.
7. Fogel, C.I., & Woods, N.F. (1981). *Health care of women: A nursing perspective*. St. Louis: C.V. Mosby.
8. Hyde, J.S. (1985). *Half the human experience: The psychology of women* (3rd ed.). Lexington, MA: D.C. Heath.
9. Strachey, J. (Ed. and Trans.). (1961). *The standard edition of the complete psychological works of Sigmund Freud*. London: Hogarth Press.
10. Levinson, D.J. (1986). A conception of adult development. *American Psychologist, 41*(1), 3–13.
11. Erikson, E.H. (1950). *Childhood and society*. New York: Norton.
12. Erikson, E.H. (1968). *Identity, youth and crises*. New York: Norton.
13. Evans, N.J. (1985, March). Women's development across the life span. In N.J. Evans (Ed.), *Facilitating the development of women: New directions for student services*, No. 29. San Francisco: Jossey-Bass.
14. Levinson, D.J. (1978). *The seasons of a man's life*. New York: Alfred A. Knopf.
15. Belenky, M.F., et al. (1985). Epistemological development and the politics of talk in family life. *Journal of Education, 167*(3).
16. Miller, J.B. (1986). *Toward a new psychology of women* (2nd ed.). Boston: Beacon Press.
17. Gilligan, C. (1982). New maps of development: New visions of maturity. *American Journal of Orthopsychiatry. 52*(2), 199–212.
18. Mednick, M.T. (1989). On the politics of psychological constructs: Stop the bandwagon, I want to get off. *American Psychologist, 44*(8), 1118–1123.
19. Bardwick, J.M. (1980). The seasons of a woman's life. In D.G. McGuigan (Ed.), *Women's lives: New theory, research, and policy*. Ann Arbor: University of Michigan, Center for Continuing Education of Women.
20. Lott, B. (1987). *Women's lives: Themes and variations in gender learning*. Pacific Grove, CA: Brooks/Cole.
21. Belenky, M.F., et al. (1986). *Women's ways of knowing. The development of self, voice, and mind*. New York: Basic Books.
22. Steitz, J.A. (1982). The female life course: Life situations and perception of control. *International Journal of Aging and Human Development, 14*(3).
23. Hueber, G. (1991, April 7). Baby boomers heading for earlier retirement. *Richmond Times-Dispatch*, p. H-8.
24. Mercer, R.T., Nichols, E.G., & Doyle, G.C. (1989). *Transitions in a woman's life: Major life events in developmental context*. New York: Springer.
25. Roberts, P., & Newton, P.M. (1987). Levinsonian studies of women's adult development. *Psychology & Aging, 2*(2), 154–163.
26. Lichtman, R., & Papera, S. (1990). *Gynecology: Well woman care*. Norwalk, CT: Appleton & Lange.
27. Rossi, A.S. (1980). Life span theories and women's lives. *Signs: Journal of Women in Culture and Society, 6*(1).
28. Josselson, R. (1987). *Finding herself: Pathways to identity development in women*. San Francisco: Jossey-Bass.
29. McBride, A.B. (1990). Mental health effects of women's multiple roles. *American Psychologist, 45*(3), 381–384.
30. Bell, I.P. (1979). The double standard: Age. In Freeman (Ed.), *Women: A feminist perspective* (pp. 145–155). Palo Alto, CA: Mayfield.
31. Eliopoulos, C. (1990). *Health assessment of the older adult* (2nd ed.). Redwood City, CA: Addison-Wesley.

## BIBLIOGRAPHY

Rossi, A.S. (1985). *Gender and the life course.* Hawthorne, NY: Aldine.

Lott, B. (1981). *Becoming a woman: The socialization of gender.* Springfield, IL: Charles C Thomas.

Matlin, M.W. (1987). *The psychology of women.* New York: CBS College Publishing.

McGuigan, D.G. (Ed.). (1980). *Women's lives: New theory, research and policy.* Ann Arbor: University of Michigan, Center for Continuing Education of Women.

CHAPTER 3

# ASSESSING WOMEN'S HEALTH

*Ellis Quinn Youngkin • Marcia Szmania Davis*

*The provider must help the woman become more attuned to her body and its cues, and use the assessment period as an opportunity for teaching and counseling.*

*Highlights*

- Mortality, Morbidity, and Risk Factors
- Screening Methods
  - *Health History*
  - *Special Assessment: Family, Nutrition, Stress, Fitness, Occupation*
  - *Physical Examination*
- Laboratory Tests
  - *Papanicolaou Smear*
  - *Gonorrhea Culture*
  - *Chlamydia Trachomatis Tests*
  - *Wet Mounts*
  - *Urinalysis*
  - *Herpes Culture*

## INTRODUCTION

Women's life span, choice of opportunities and risks, and array of challenges and stresses are ever increasing. As perhaps the only person a woman sees for health care, the women's health care provider must approach assessment holistically. Indeed, all factors impinging on the woman's health and well-being must be considered if significant omissions in detecting problems and offering care are to be avoided. "Wellness isn't a destination but a process."[1] For that reason, the provider must help the woman become more attuned to her body and its cues, and use the assessment period as an opportunity for teaching and counseling.

## MORTALITY, MORBIDITY, AND RISK FACTORS IN AMERICAN WOMEN

### LEADING CAUSES OF MORTALITY IN AMERICAN WOMEN

The causes of death differ significantly for American women depending on age and race. Age groupings in this section are derived from statistical tables for mortality (see Tables 3–1, 3–2, and 3–3).[2,3]

***Adolescence to Young Adulthood (Ages 15 to 24).*** Young women are at greatest risk for death from accidents and violence. However, deaths from human immunodeficiency virus

TABLE 3–1. SELECTED CAUSES OF MORTALITY FOR WOMEN, 1989 (IN 1000S)

| *Age* | *Heart Disease* | *Cancer* | *Accidents* | *Cerebrovascular Disease* | *COPD*[a] | *Pneumonia* | *Suicide* | *Liver Disease* | *DM*[b] | *Homicide and Legal Intervention* |
|---|---|---|---|---|---|---|---|---|---|---|
| <15 | 0.6 | 0.8 | 2.9 | 0.1 | 0.1 | 0.4 | 0.1 | — | — | 0.6 |
| 15–24 | 0.3 | 0.8 | **4.1** | 0.1 | 0.1 | 0.1 | 0.8 | — | 0.1 | **1.1** |
| 25–34 | 1.1 | **2.7** | **3.7** | 0.5 | 0.1 | 0.4 | **1.2** | 0.3 | 0.3 | **1.5** |
| 35–44 | **2.9**[c] | **8.8** | **2.8** | 1.1 | 0.3 | 0.5 | **1.2** | 0.9 | 0.5 | 0.9 |
| 45–54 | **7.9** | **19.4** | 2.0 | 2.2 | 1.1 | 0.6 | 0.9 | 1.3 | 1.2 | 0.4 |
| 55–64 | **25.1** | **42.5** | 2.3 | **4.8** | **4.8** | 1.4 | 0.8 | **2.2** | **3.6** | 0.3 |
| 65–74 | **64.2** | **67.7** | 3.5 | **13.0** | **11.3** | **4.1** | 0.6 | **2.6** | **7.2** | 0.3 |
| 75–84 | **122.0** | **61.3** | **5.0** | **29.9** | **12.7** | **11.9** | 0.4 | 1.6 | **8.7** | 0.2 |
| 85– | **141.5** | 28.8 | **4.8** | **36.5** | **5.7** | **21.4** | 0.1 | 0.4 | **5.4** | 0.1 |
| **Totals for women** | **365.7** | **232.8** | **31.1** | **88.2** | **36.2** | **40.8** | **6.1** | **9.4** | **27.1** | **5.2** |
| **Totals for men** | **368.2** | **263.3** | **63.9** | **57.3** | **48.2** | **35.7** | **24.1** | **17.3** | **19.7** | **17.7** |

[a]Chronic obstructive pulmonary disease.
[b]Diabetes mellitus.
[c]Numerals are boldfaced for emphasis.
*Source: Reference 2.*

**TABLE 3–2. ACCIDENTS AND VIOLENCE MORTALITY FOR WOMEN BY RACE, 1989 (PER 100,000 POPULATION)**

| *Cause of Death* | *Caucasian* | *African American* |
|---|---|---|
| Motor vehicle accidents | 12.1 | 9.3 |
| All other accidents | 12.7 | 15.0 |
| Suicide | 5.2 | 2.4 |
| Homicide | 2.8 | 12.9 |

*Source: Reference 3.*

(HIV) are rising rapidly (see Leading Causes of Mortality in American Women, Cancer).

***Young Adulthood to Mid-Adulthood (Ages 25 to 44).*** Cancer (including HIV deaths), heart diseases, and suicide begin to increase as causes of death. Accidents and violence continue to be important causes, especially among African American women.

***Mid-Adulthood to Older Adulthood (Ages 45 to 64).*** Heart diseases, cancer, cerebrovascular diseases (CVD), chronic obstructive pulmonary disease (COPD), chronic liver diseases/cirrhosis, and diabetes mellitus gain momentum as causes of death. Accidents, violence, and suicide decrease slightly, but remain significant causes. Suicide is highest among Caucasian women in every age group as compared with non-Caucasian women, peaking between ages 45 and 64.

**TABLE 3–3. DEATHS RESULTING FROM ACCIDENTS AND VIOLENCE BY AGE GROUP, 1989 (PER 100,000 POPULATION)**

| *Age (in years)* | *Caucasian* | *African American* |
|---|---|---|
| 15–24 | 32.7 | 33.9 |
| 25–34 | 26.6 | 47.4 |
| 35–44 | 24.7 | 40.8 |
| 45–54 | 25.5 | 30.8 |
| 55–64 | 28.7 | 37.3 |
| 65– | 81.4 | 87.8 |

*Source: Reference 3.*

***Maturity (Ages 65 and Older).*** Heart disease increases dramatically with age, as do cancer, CVD, COPD, pneumonia, and diabetes. Accidents again become a more prevalent cause, but suicides decrease. Each year one-third of all elderly fall; 75 percent of elderly deaths from accidental injury are from falls.[4] Falls occur significantly more often among elderly women than among elderly men.

***Differences in Causes of Death for Women by Race.*** Compared with Caucasian women, African American women have a higher incidence of death from every cause except COPD, motor vehicle accidents, and suicide (see Table 3–4).[5] Deaths from homicides and legal interventions (police interventions, execution), HIV infection, heart diseases, CVD, and cancer (other than breast) are dramatically higher among African American women. Cancer is the leading cause of death for Asian and Pacific Islander women.[6] Although the risk of dying from pregnancy and childbirth-related causes is very low in the United States (i.e., 320 maternal deaths reported in 1989 from 3.8 million live births), nonwhite women are at a greater risk of death (threefold), and African American women are at the greatest risk (i.e., 18.4 per 1000 live births as compared to 5.6 for white women).[6] Pregnancy-induced hypertension, hemorrhage, embolism, and ectopic pregnancy are the major causes of maternal death.

***Cancer.*** Lung cancer peaks at ages 75 to 84; digestive system, breast, genital, blood-related, urologic, and oral cancers rise steadily from age 45 to peak in the 85 and older age group.[7] The death rate from HIV infection

**TABLE 3–4. DIFFERENCES IN DEATH RATES BY SELECTED CAUSE FOR CAUCASIAN AND AFRICAN AMERICAN WOMEN, 1987 OR 1989 (PER 100,000 POPULATION)**

| *Disease/Cause* | *Caucasian* | *African American* |
|---|---|---|
| Heart diseases | 106.6 | 172.9 |
| Cerebrovascular diseases | 24.1 | 44.9 |
| Malignant neoplasms | 110.7 | 130.9 |
| Respiratory cancer (1987) | 23.8[a] | 24.3[a] |
| Breast cancer | 22.8[a] | 26.5[a] |
| Chronic pulmonary obstructive disease | 15.2 | 10.9 |
| Pneumonia/influenza | 10.3 | 13.8 |
| Chronic liver disease and cirrhosis | 5.0 | 8.5 |
| Human immunodeficiency virus | 0.6[a] | 4.7[a] |
| Accidents and adverse effects | 18.5 | 21.6 |
| Motor vehicle accidents | 11.4[a] | 8.7[a] |
| Suicide | 4.8 | 2.4 |
| Homicide and legal intervention | 2.8 | 12.5 |
| Diabetes mellitus | 9.6 | 24.2 |

[a]1987 statistics.
*Source: 1989 statistics from Reference 3. 1987 statistics from Reference 5.*

quadrupled between 1985 and 1988, and HIV related deaths became one of the five leading causes of death among American women 15 to 44 years old, as predicted for 1991.[8] Transmission from injection of drugs caused 46 percent of the deaths from acquired immunodeficiency syndrome (AIDS) in women in 1990.[6] As of December 1991, the highest incidence of AIDS deaths in women was among African Americans, followed next by white women, then Hispanic and other racial/ethnic groups. Lung cancer became the leading cancer killer among white women in 1988, as women's smoking reached an all time high.[6] Smoking contributes to 25 percent of all cancer deaths in women.

***Heart Diseases.*** All major causes of heart disease (ischemic, rheumatic, and hypertensive) rise continuously from middle age through old age, but ischemic heart disease is the dramatic killer.[9] Cardiovascular disease kills 500,000 U.S. women each year; yet until 1991, little research had addressed health issues for women, such as heart disease.[10] Thirty-six percent of all deaths in women are attributed to heart disease.[6] The National Institutes of Health (NIH) are now studying questions such as the relationships between diet, hormonal replacement therapy, exercise, and smoking cessation and the major causes of death and disability in women: cancer, cardiovascular disease, and osteoporosis.

## LEADING CAUSES OF MORBIDITY IN AMERICAN WOMEN

### Acute Conditions

For all of the following acute conditions except injuries, women have a higher incidence than men.[11]

- Infective and parasitic diseases such as diarrhea are more common in late adolescence through mid-adulthood. They become less frequent after age 45.

- Upper respiratory diseases are more common in women younger than 45; lower respiratory diseases are more common in older women.
- Digestive diseases increase with age, except for acute problems in adolescence. Irritable bowel syndrome is frequently seen in women.
- Injuries occur most frequently during adolescence and young adulthood, decrease in middle adulthood, then increase again among older women.

### Chronic Conditions

Heart diseases, hypertension, diabetes mellitus, and arthritis increase steadily in both sexes as they age. Women, however, have higher incidences of all of these conditions. Other chronic conditions more common in women than in men include constipation, abdominal hernia, orthopedic impairments, cataracts, urinary diseases, migraine, itching skin, corns/calluses/ingrown nails, acne and cysts, dermatitis (eczema), hay fever, rhinitis without asthma, sinusitis, chronic bronchitis, asthma, hemorrhoids, and varicose veins.[12] Osteoporosis is considered one of three leading causes of disability in women after age 45;[10] heart disease and cancer are the other two.

## LEADING RISK FACTORS FOR WOMEN

An overall evaluation of risk factors should include assessment of the following behaviors.

### Unsafe Lifestyle Behaviors

Such behaviors are related to personal choices and are amenable to change in most instances.

- Cigarette smoking is associated with lung cancer and other lung disease, heart diseases, lowered estrogen levels, early menopause, cervical cancer, rapid skin aging/wrinkling, and secondhand smoke risk.[13] Assessment should include what the women smokes, the number smoked per day, the number of years she has smoked, ill effects, and others in the household who smoke or are affected. A 1993 U.S. Environmental Protection Agency (EPA) brochure, "What You Can Do about Secondhand Smoke," indicts secondhand smoke in the development of respiratory disease.
- Substance use/abuse involves alcohol, nicotine, caffeine, cocaine, marijuana, and tranquilizers. Alcohol use is associated with cirrhosis, stroke, hypertension, accidents, increased risk of cancer, use of other addicting drugs, and psychosocial behavioral changes and their sequelae. Deaths related to alcohol use in women are primarily from cancer, cardiovascular disease, digestive disorders, and unintentional and intentional injuries.[14] Nicotine, caffeine, cocaine, marijuana, and tranquilizer are each associated with health dangers (see Chapter 18). Damage to psychosocial relationships may be significant with substance use. Assessment includes the type of substance, amount used, years of use, unsafe associated behaviors, and effects.
- Overuse of any medication may occur when clients fail to read warnings or are not cautioned about the excessive use of legal drugs. Some changes that may occur are gastric mucosal irritation with overuse of nonsteroidal anti-inflammatory drugs (NSAID);[15] and neurological abnormalities with excessive vitamin $B_6$ ingestion.[16] Assess the type of drug, amount used, years of use, and effects.
- Sedentary lifestyle and lack of exercise and personal fitness are associated with cardiovascular, respiratory, gastrointestinal, and musculoskeletal problems. Exercise in-

creases endorphins and improves the emotional health. Americans are among the most sedentary people in the world.

- Nutritional excesses and deficits are associated with cancer, cardiovascular disease, diabetes, eating disorders, obesity, malnutrition, and deficiency diseases. Coronary artery disease in women is highly associated with obesity.[17] Binging, purging, and anorexia are significantly more common in women than in men.[18]
- Unsafe automobile driving, inattention to precautions, and lapses in driving safety are associated with a high level of morbidity and mortality for women up to age 64, especially young women. Substance abuse, nonuse of protective devices (seatbelts), and reckless driving need to be assessed.[13]
- Violence encompasses homicide, suicide, sexual assault, physical abuse/battering, and emotional trauma (see Chapter 18). Women are more likely to be the victims of violence than its perpetrators.[6] They are injured most often by domestic violence, which occurs more than rape, muggings, and auto accidents combined. Assessment should include asking about dangerous, conflictual relationships and living conditions (e.g., violent families and neighborhoods). Rape is the second leading violent crime, and it is believed that most rapes are unreported.[19] Women who are young, single, students, African American, and unemployed are at greatest risk.[6] Spousal abuse is anticipated in 66 percent of all marriages.[20] African American women are at a fourfold greater risk of homicide, often from their partners, than Caucasian women are. Elder abuse, now receiving widespread attention, has become a serious problem for older women, with estimates ranging from 1 to 4 percent of the elderly.[6]
- Exposure to HIV, hepatitis, and sexually transmitted diseases may cause life-threatening, incurable, or disabling conditions (see Chapter 8). Assessment should include questions about the frequency of sexual relations, the number of partners currently and in the past, the risk status of partners, forms of sexual expression, and use of barrier and chemical contraception.
- Lack of health directed behaviors, or poor personal care, is associated with a substandard health status and inadequate detection and prevention behaviors, such as immunization status, and use of contraception. Personal assessment should include breast self-exam, regular dental and eye exams, general screening physical exams including pelvic exam, Papanicolaou (Pap) smear and indicated cultures, and vulvar self-exam.
- Inadequate, excessive, or unusual sleep is less a problem for women than for men. A sleep study found that women have better sleep quality than men, equal to a 10-year difference in age. This difference may be associated with women's longer life spans.[21] Sleep apnea occurs more often in men than women (affects 1 woman for every 10 men). The reason may be testosterone effects on the tongue (a muscle), making it heavier and more prone to fall back and block the airway during sleep. Also, progesterone may play a protective role in women, but as yet, this is unproven in research.[21] It is important to note that after menopause, there are fewer sex differences related to sleep between men and women. Women present more often with the complaint of insomnia associated with depression, but this does not indicate if there is a real difference between sexes in relation to this problem since women tend to seek help more readily than men. Evaluation should include breathing difficulties, snoring, smoking, neuroses, alcohol use, medication use, estrogen deficiency, time zone or job shift changes, sleepwalking, stress and depression, heavy exercise near bedtime, and environmental conditions for sleep. Severe sleep apnea has been associated with cardiac arrest.[22]

### Exposure to Environmental Hazards

Unsafe conditions may be found in the home or work environment.

- Unsafe home environment encompasses falls, exposure to chemical/toxic/radon hazards, fire, excessive heat or cold, unsanitary living conditions, unsafe drinking water, lack of running water, rodent or insect infestation, and infections among people living in crowded conditions. Tuberculosis, one example of a serious disease that proliferates in crowded conditions, is on the rise again because of new resistant strains of the causative organism and the deficient immunity of individuals with HIV infection.
- Unsafe occupational situations are associated with life-threatening, damaging, or debilitating conditions, such as asbestosis, lead poisoning, pesticide exposure, and radiation exposure. Assessment should include the individual's type of work, work hazards and conditions, and effects[22] (see Screening Methods, Special Assessment Guides in this chapter and Chapters 12 and 13 on pregnancy).

### Negative Influences on Emotional Health

Such influences vary widely from family crises to unrealistic values of thinness.

- Stress is associated with a wide array of physical and emotional problems. American women are increasingly stressed with multiple roles and pressures. Assessment includes stressors related to work, home, family, and other relationships.
- Family crises mean increased physical and emotional risks for both the individual and the family. Assessment includes family health, values, and health care beliefs, cultural influences, and coping abilities.
- A poor or absent support system is associated with feelings of loneliness, helplessness, hopelessness, and powerlessness. Social networks are known to decrease health risks associated with occupational stress, cancer, and pregnancy.[23] Assessment of supports should include determining recent changes in life (e.g., marriage, divorce, birth, change of residence, change of job); distance from friends, relatives, cultural group, health resources; and access to support systems, such as church.
- Depression is associated with suicide, a leading cause of death among women. In the United States, depression is significantly related to social, psychological, and physical loss. Typical signs and symptoms of depression, such as eating or sleeping difficulties, unusual sadness, and suicidal thoughts are assessed.
- Unrealistic values of youth, beauty, and thinness lead to unhealthy, excessive concerns and behaviors related to appearance. These concerns may also indicate an inability to accept the aging process. Assessment includes appearance, age, weight, height, history of unusual or overuse of plastic/reparative surgery, diet and exercise history, and verbal and nonverbal cues, such as great concern with being overweight when in reality one is underweight (see Chapter 18, Eating Disorders).
- Lack of recreational and relaxation activities can cause stress, overwork, anxiety, and in some instances depression. Assessment includes financial, social, physical, and psychological conditions and barriers.

### Poverty, Insufficient Insurance, and Inadequate Material Resources

These are very much a problem of women and children, often called the "nouveau poor." Most adult welfare recipients are women,[24] and the fastest growing segment of homeless people is women and children. Poor people often delay seeking health care when ill, use fewer measures to prevent or alleviate illness, have less accurate information about health, and have fewer choices for access to health care. As women age, a greater chance for poverty exists. Assessment includes estimated income level, quality of nutrition and living conditions, untreated illnesses or conditions (acute and chronic), dental conditions, disabilities, excessive sleep and sedentary living, depression and stresses associated with lifestyle, and inadequate self-concept and ability to change life. Choices for women are often limited because of family and child care needs.

### Hereditary, Cultural, and Ethnic Influences

Family history and culture impact health.

- Familial diseases may be detected by assessing family history of diseases such as diabetes, cardiovascular disease, and cancer. Significant health problems can be prevented or minimized by careful attention to family history.
- Race is another consideration. Some diseases are more common among people of certain races; for example, osteoporosis is more prevalent in light- or yellow-skinned women; sickle cell disease is found in African Americans; and glucose-6-phosphate dehydrogenase (G-6-PD) deficiency occurs more often in people of Mediterranean descent.
- Ethnic, cultural, and religious influences may be associated with unhealthy practices; for example, eating uncooked meat, refusing to see a health care provider, lacking health directed behaviors, and lacking the understanding or education necessary for good health.

### Current or Past Medical Problems

Of particular concern are the risks of past and present problems, and the potential or real effects of current or past illness on new disease conditions. For example, recent research indicates a past history of smoking, even if the person no longer smokes, increases the risk of multiple myeloma by threefold. Multiple drug interactions may cause increased risks and confusing presentations. Polypharmacy, the use of multiple medications, is seen most in the elderly, and is essential to assess.

# SCREENING METHODS

## HEALTH HISTORY[25–29]

### Interview and Approach Considerations

- Effective interviewing and interpersonal skills are required in order to gather accurate, useful data.
    - Consider any interaction with a client to be a therapeutic intervention by permitting the free expression of issues and concerns. Treat the client with dignity and respect; be nonjudgmental, accepting, supportive, concerned, and an appropriate role model (e.g., do not smoke in a client's presence).
    - Use clear language and terminology matched to the client's level of understanding, culture, and background. Consider the client's age, education, response to the interview, and ethical, cultural, and religious taboos. Avoid medical jargon and clarify by restating confusing information. Use an interpreter if necessary.
    - Appropriate questioning technique includes using open questions early in the interview to facilitate broad information gathering and to assist with mental status and general survey assessment. Open questions draw forth an overview of the client's problems. Ask the client about her concerns. Avoid interrupting, which may cause valuable data to be lost. Use pointed, directive questions to obtain specific data. Avoid leading questions ("You've never had a sexually transmitted disease, have you?"). Phrase sensitive questions in a nonjudgmental man-

ner ("How many partners do I need to notify about the risk of AIDS?").
   - Be aware of nonverbal cues such as facial expressions, body movements, and signs of anxiety. The client may avoid making eye contact or answering questions. She may be reluctant to give information. Such cues may indicate fears or concerns.
- Physical and psychological factors affect interaction.
   - Provide a quiet, private place for the interview. Ideally, the interview should not take place in the examination room. Use measures, such as a sign on the door, to discourage others from walking in during the interview.
   - Maintain the client's comfort. Permit her to remain dressed during the interview, and provide comfortable seating that will allow client and interviewer to be at the same eye level. Never obtain a history with the client in lithotomy position.
   - Maintain a realistic time frame. Keep the interview focused to stay within a reasonable time limit, using more than one session if needed.

## Components of Health History

- Demographic and biographical data, called identifying data (ID), must be accurate. Record the client's full name; street and mailing addresses; telephone numbers for work, home, and contact persons; sex; age; birth date; Social Security number; city, county, state of birth; race, nationality, culture, religion; marital status; dependents and persons living with client; years of formal education; religious preference; occupation; usual sources of medical care; and source and reliability of health information.
- Record the chief complaint (CC) or reason for visit (RFV). Use the client's own words in a brief statement and put into a time frame (e.g., "I've had chest pain for two days," or "I need a Pap test and checkup").
- Probe the history of present illness (HPI) or current health status (CHS). An introductory statement for all women is essential: gravidity (G); parity (P); full-term or premature pregnancies; abortions (A), spontaneous and induced, with reasons and length of gestation; number of living children (LC); dates of last and previous normal menstrual periods based on first day of bleeding (LNMP, PNMP); and methods of contraception used by client and partner, for how long or when stopped. If the woman is older, include date of menopause and use of replacement hormone therapy.

  Write the remainder of the paragraph as a narrative, giving

   - Usual state of health.
   - Clear, chronological development/analysis of complaints: sequencing (starting with onset), causes or associated phenomena, factors worsening/lessening/relieving/aggravating, quality or character of complaint, quantity of problem, effect on activities, location, radiation, severity (on a scale of 1 to 10), timing, past occurrence, others with problem.
   - Relevant family history.
   - Degree of disability.
   - Significant negatives.

  If the visit is related to the menstrual cycle, a complete description of the menstrual cycles is needed, including characteristics before and after the use of hormonal or other contraception that may affect the cycles.

  If the visit is for routine health maintenance, elicit information about the client's usual health, last exams or tests and their results, current medications, habits, and significant problems or negatives, such as diabetes mellitus or cardiac disease.
- Assess and record the past medical history (PMH) or health status (PHS).

  - Childhood Diseases. Measles, mumps, frequent infections, and so on.
  - Immunizations and Screening Tests. Dates of diphtheria, pertussis, tetanus, measles, mumps, rubella, oral polio vaccines; dates of pneumococcus, influenza, hepatitis, tuberculosis, meningococcus, smallpox, typhoid, and other special vaccines for at-risk and older populations; screening tests (HIV, rubella, tuberculosis, sickle cell, G-6-PD).
  - Hospitalizations and Serious Illnesses. Dates, places, health care providers, reasons, courses of recovery, sequelae.
  - Accidents and Injuries. Type of injury, how it occurred, severity, treatment, where, by whom, sequelae.
  - Obstetric History. All pregnancies, regardless of outcome; dates and types of deliveries, sex and weights of infants, lengths of gestations; antepartum, intrapartum, and postpartum complications.
  - Contraceptive History. Types of contraceptives used by client or partner, length of use, complications, side effects, satisfaction with method.
  - Sexual History. See Chapter 4.
  - Allergies. Specific allergens (food, environmental, medication), types of reactions, treatments, and results.
  - Medications. Prescription and over-the-counter, dosages, administration routes, frequencies, reasons for use, side effects.
  - Habits. Recreational of illicit drug use; tobacco, alcohol, caffeine use; type of substances, frequency, duration of use, effects, routes of administration, risk practices such as needle-sharing.
  - Transfusions/Transplants. Dates, reasons, exposure to HIV, hepatitis.
  - Violence History. Incidences of assault, incest, rape, other violence; treatment, counseling, sequelae.

- Family history (FH) includes hereditary, communicable, and environmental family diseases; causes of death of maternal and paternal grandparents, parents, siblings, children, partners, aunts, uncles, and cousins (if indicated). A genogram can be visually helpful (see Special Assessment Guides, Family Assessment). Note if family history is unknown or the client is adopted. Of particular importance is a family history of breast cancer in mother or sister, congenital anomalies or retardation, multiple births, and anemia.
- Psychosocial history taking (PSH) and personal history taking and assessment require sensitivity.
  - Nutrition. (See Special Assessment Guides, Nutritional Assessment.)
  - Family Relationships, Friendships, and Support Systems. Significance and quality of relationships and interactions, areas of concern or conflict, living arrangements, availability of support systems, club and organization memberships, activities enjoyed with friends and relatives (see Special Assessment Guides, Family Assessment).
  - Culture/Ethnicity. Foods, religion, values, and beliefs affecting health.
  - Occupation. Full- or part-time employment, length of employment, type of work, hazards, stressors (see Special Assessment Guides, Occupational Assessment).
  - Education. Highest level obtained (formal and informal); client's feelings of satisfaction and how she learns best.
  - Economic Status. Adequacy of income for basic and recreational needs, monetary concerns, adequacy of insurance.
  - Exercise and Activity. Current levels and types of activity, length of time spent, frequency, tolerance, safety.
  - Developmental Status. Current level of task accomplishment according to developmental stage (see Chapter 2).
  - Self-Concept. Locus of control, positive and negative feelings about self, satisfac-

tion with self, perceived strengths and weaknesses.

- Coping Mechanisms. Stressors and usual methods of coping, perceived effectiveness (see Special Assessment Guides, Stress/Risk Assessment).
- Patterns and Maintenance of Health Care. Types, sources, and frequency of health care visits; home/folk remedies; general experiences and attitudes about health and care.
- Sleep and Wakefulness. Patterns, effects, problems, dreams, medication use to sleep or to stay awake.
- Recreation/Relaxation. Hobbies and activities for fun or relaxation; associated patterns, roles, and relationships.
- Living Environment. Hazards (real or potential), level of comfort; privacy, space.
- Religion. Importance to client, source of strength or stress, level of involvement.
- Daily Profile. Description of a typical day for the client.

■ A review of systems (ROS) includes a thorough past and present history of each system.

- General. General health, fatigue, exercise tolerance, episodes of unusual weight/height loss or gain, malaise, ability to carry out activities of daily living (ADL).
- Skin, Hair, Nails. Diseases; primary or secondary skin lesions, itching, flaking; changes in texture, moisture, color, skin temperature, amount of hair, care practices.
- Head and Neck. Injuries and their treatments, sequelae; headaches (type); range-of-motion limitations, pain, or stiffness; enlarged nodes; swelling.
- Eyes. Use of corrective lenses, reason for prescription, results of last exam and glaucoma test, diseases or infections, pain, itching, discharge, diplopia, cataracts, blurred vision, spots, halos, flashing lights, blind spots.
- Ears. Hearing acuity, test results and dates, use of aids and their effectiveness, diseases, pain, ringing, vertigo, infection, discharge, care habits.
- Mouth, Teeth, and Throat. Diseases; condition of teeth (loose, missing, caries), last exam and results, knowledge of routine care; sore throats, lesions, bleeding, hoarseness, voice changes; chewing, swallowing, or taste problems.
- Nose and Sinuses. Diseases; problems with sense of smell; nosebleeds; allergies/seasonal problems, sneezing, congestion, drainage, pain; trauma; breathing difficulties; infections and their treatments.
- Chest and Lungs. Diseases; dyspnea, cough, hemoptysis, exertion breathing difficulty, wheezing, asthma, pneumonia, bronchitis, tuberculosis (TB), emphysema, orthopnea, night sweats, smoking; time of last chest x-ray, reason, and results; last TB test and results.
- Cardiovascular. Diseases; pain, cyanosis, palpitations, murmurs, bruits, irregular heart rate, mitral valve prolapse, hypertension, edema, varicosities, rheumatic fever; coldness, tingling, color changes, hair loss on extremities; recent cholesterol and lipid screening results.
- Breasts and Axillae. Diseases; pain, masses, changes related to menstrual cycle, discharge, color, characteristics; skin, vascular, temperature changes; breast self-exam (when, how); last provider exam; last mammogram results; breastfeeding history.
- Gastrointestinal. Diseases; abdominal pain, distention, masses, indigestion, food intolerances, belching, nausea, vomiting (character), reflux, jaundice, ascites, diarrhea, constipation, character of stools; hemorrhoids; use of antacids or laxatives; last hemoccult test, results.

- Genitourinary
  *Reproductive.* Onset of puberty, menarche (when, character, regularity of menses), current menstrual pattern (frequency, duration, flow amount); premenstrual syndrome (PMS); dysmenorrhea; tampon or pad use, size, correct use; problems related to menses; use of medications or hormones, reasons, problems; last pelvic exam and Pap smear (if abnormal results, follow-up, sequelae); vaginitis, itching, discharge, lesions, diseases, abnormalities; sexually transmitted disease (STD); diethylstilbestrol (DES) exposure; fertility problems. (Obstetric, sexual, and contraceptive history data may go here, or in HPI or CHS if it relates to the reason for visit; see Chapter 12 for further information about obstetric history.)
  *Urinary.* Character and regularity of urination/urine; diseases, infections (cystitis or pyelonephritis); dysuria, polyuria, oliguria, anuria, incontinence, hematuria, nocturia, urgency, stones.
- Musculoskeletal. Diseases, fractures, or other injuries, cramping, pain, fasciculations, weakness/strength, range-of-motion/activities of daily living limitations, gait problems, joint complaints (swelling, redness, pain, deformity, crepitus); back discomfort, ache, or deformity; loss of height.
- Neurological. Diseases; fainting, loss of consciousness, seizures (and medication for them), sensory problems (numbness, tingling, paresthesia), motor problems (balance, gait, spasm, paralysis), cognitive problems (mood changes, memory loss, disorientation, loss of judgment, hallucinations); sleep disturbances.
- Blood and Immune. Diseases; anemias, bleeding tendencies, easy bruising, transfusions, allergies, treatments; unexplained infections or node enlargement; blood type.
- Endocrine. Diseases; unusual changes in weight, height, glove, or shoe size; increased thirst, urination, appetite; heat/cold intolerance; weakness/fatigue; changes in skin and hair (loss, excessive growth, hirsute, texture).

## SPECIAL ASSESSMENT GUIDES

### Family Assessment

Determine who lives in the family, their relationships, cultural origins, religious preferences, health practices; the role of each member (education, occupation), communication among members, material management (home, money), goals of the family, relaxation and recreational family activities; and strengths, weaknesses, conflicts, problems, past resolution methods.[25,30]

- "Family APGAR" is one quick screening tool for identifying areas of family difficulty.[31] It uses five areas for scoring: *adaptation, partnership, growth, affection,* and *resolve*. Each category receives a score of 0 to 2 points. The provider asks the client to score 2 points for "almost always," 1 point for "some of the time," and 0 points for "hardly ever." The following statements are given to the client for scoring:
  - I am satisfied with the help that I receive from my family* when something is troubling me. (Adaptation)
  - I am satisfied with the way my family* discusses items of common interest and shares problem solving with me. (Partnership)
  - I find that my family* accepts my wishes to take on new activities or make changes in my lifestyle. (Growth)

---

*Substitute spouse, significant other, parents, or children if necessary.

**GOVERNMENTAL DIETARY GUIDELINES FOR DAILY INTAKE[a]**

| Bread/Cereal Rice/Pasta | Meats/Poultry Fish/Dried Beans/Eggs | Milk/Dairy Products | Vegetables | Fruit |
|---|---|---|---|---|
| 6–9 servings. | 2–3 servings, up to total of 6 ounces or less. | 2–3 servings, such as 1 cup milk, 1.5 ounces cheese. | 3–4 servings of dark green leafy, yellow, beans/peas, starchy. | 2–3 servings. |

[a]For nonpregnant, nonlactating women. The lesser amounts for less active or older women.

- I am satisfied with the way my family* expresses affection and responds to my feelings, such as anger, sorrow, and love. (Affection)
- I am satisfied with the amount of time my family* and I spend together. (Resolve)

A score of 0 to 3 is associated with a severely dysfunctional family; 4 to 6 with a moderately dysfunctional family; and 7 to 10 with a highly functional family.

- The *genogram* is a family tree that contains a family's relationships, structure, health, and other important data over three generations.[30] More research is needed on the effectiveness of its use, but this visual picture may be very helpful in identifying tendencies of conditions within families and, thus, risk factors for individual clients.
- The resiliency model of family stress is a theoretical model used to evaluate whether an illness would lead to family crisis. Its practical use in determining a family's adaptability strengths is beyond the scope of this handbook, but the Bibliography at the end of this chapter lists sources for further information.

*Substitute spouse, significant other, parents, or children if necessary.

## Nutritional Assessment

Assess the client's 24-hour diet recall of food/drink intake for balance and adequacy of nutrients. For nonpregnant, nonlactating women, the table of governmental dietary guidelines gives the daily intake (the lesser amounts for less active or older women).[32]

Sugar and salt should be used in moderation; no more than 30 percent of calories should come from fat, and no more than 10 percent of fat should come from saturated fats (i.e., animal fat and tropical oils such as coconut or palm). No more than one alcoholic drink (one ounce of liquor or the equivalent) per day is advised for a woman who drinks. Ideally, no alcohol intake is advised. Six to eight glasses of water are recommended daily for optimal body functioning, and additional calcium is recommended for adolescents and older women.

Determine if the client eats breakfast; skips meals; uses vitamin and mineral supplements; wears dentures; eats snacks (how often and what); drinks caffeinated or carbonated beverages (what and how much); eats more beef than fish and poultry; consumes excessive fat, salt, sugar, or substitutes; eats alone or too quickly; chews adequately; uses alcohol, tobacco, or other substances or medications that could alter nutrient intake; is unable to tolerate some foods, eats charcoal grilled or fried foods; eats what someone else cooks; has wide weight fluctuations; abuses food when stressed; or diets constantly. Be sure that the client knows what is included in a balanced diet.

Correlate diet patterns with other history, physical examination, and diagnostic test findings; for example, high fat intake may be correlated with obesity and abnormal lipid levels. See Chapter 13, for nutritional recommendations during pregnancy.

Appropriate weight is calculated on the basis of the woman's height: 100 pounds for the first 5 feet and an additional 5 pounds for each additional inch.[33] If her body frame is large, add another 5 pounds; if small, subtract 5 pounds.

## Stress/Risk Assessment

Assess the amount of healthy stress in the woman's life, and the amount of distress.[34] Distress is stress overload; therefore, look at factors such as financial problems; changing situations or relationships with family or significant others; and employment, unemployment, or underemployment problems or concerns (such as lack of control or input into the job situation). In addition, assess personal information (age, hereditary factors such as family history of depression, lifestyle, living conditions, habits) and coping strategies. Stress and ineffective coping are associated with hypertension, coronary artery disease, domestic violence, gastrointestinal disease, and substance abuse.[11]

Helpful assessment tools for evaluating stress or anxiety are the Holmes and Rahe Life-Change Index, which measures the degree of change in one's life to predict the chance of illness;[35] and Speilberger's State-Trait Anxiety Inventory,[34] which measures the amount of anxiety a person feels at the time of testing. Signs of excessive stress (mood swings, disposition changes, physical signs and symptoms) must be correlated with other assessment findings (sleep, appearance, nutrition, relaxation, recreation, self-concept, social supports, use of medications/substances, or unusual be-haviors).

## Fitness Assessment

Assess activities at work, home, or play for aerobic quality, stretching/flexibility movement, strength components, and sufficient intensity to meet therapeutic cardiovascular levels without compromising safety. Determine the duration of the exercise session, frequency per week, and the motivation of the client to exercise.[36] To achieve a realistic assessment, evaluate fitness within a framework of life-style, diet, weight, stress, and substance use.

Teach the value of beginning an exercise regimen slowly for short periods of time, then gradually building it, with emphasis on increasing tone, strengthening, reducing stress, enhancing flexibility and coordination, promoting relaxation, preventing injury, and improving self-concept. For a healthy woman who has no contraindications for exercise, advise building up to 20 to 40 minutes of aerobic activity, with a warmup of 5 to 10 minutes before the more vigorous activity. Advise her to stretch after warming up and to cool down slowly for 5 to 10 minutes after exercising, monitoring her heart rate. She should continue a similar program for the rest of her life.

The intensity of exercise is aimed at safely improving cardiovascular function. The formula to determine approximate target heart-rate zones for training, based on age, can be taught; however, referral to an exercise therapist may be necessary for a full assessment and program management. Recommended *target zones* (defined as 60 to 85 percent of the average maximum heart rate) for women, according to age and based on a resting heart rate of 80 are as follows:[36]

| Age | Target Zone (heartbeats per minute) |
|---|---|
| 20 | 120–170 |
| 25 | 117–166 |
| 30 | 114–162 |
| 35 | 111–157 |
| 40 | 108–153 |
| 45 | 105–149 |
| 50 | 102–144 |
| 55 | 99–140 |
| 60 | 96–136 |
| 65 | 93–132 |
| 70 | 90–123 |

Advise the client that for a conditioning response, the objective is to sustain the lower value of the target zone (60 percent) for 20 to 25 minutes. A good rule of thumb is that the client should be able to talk while in the target percentage range, but probably not sing.[36] An individual would have to be in peak fitness to sustain the upper end of the target zone for that extended time; it could cause exhaustion in the average person.[36]

### Occupational Assessment

Assess the type of work, amount, duration, physical labor involved, rest breaks, environmental risks, and stress overload. Problem areas include prolonged standing or sitting, heavy lifting, excessive noise, excessive heat or cold, exposure to toxins, exposure to chemicals or radiation, excessive hours on the job, boredom, low pay, low recognition, and little or no control over work.

Be especially concerned about a pregnant woman (see Chapters 12 and 13): Determine if she has been exposed to chemicals, anesthetic gases, radiation, or infections.[37] Consider the influence of multiple variables, such as secondhand smoke, stress, nutrition, lack of sleep, and exposure to hazardous materials.

## PHYSICAL EXAMINATION[25–29, 38–39]

### Overview

Accurate inspection, palpation, percussion, and auscultation are critical, as is the precise use of appropriate equipment. Understanding the findings is also essential.

- In preparation for the exam, explain all procedures to the client. Ensure privacy, draping, and comfort. Have all necessary equipment available and clean, and use good lighting. Ask the client to void before the exam. *Clean hands and the use of universal precautions are essential.*
- During the exam, give anticipatory advice and information; for example, teach abdominal breathing to help the client relax. Use the exam as an opportunity to teach. Be gentle, systematic, and sensitive. Avoid facial expressions or utterances indicating disgust. Provide tissues for the client after the pelvic exam. When finished, wash hands and allow the client to dress before reviewing findings.
- An abbreviated physical examination of a well woman, as done in some family planning clinics or private offices, includes assessment of blood pressure, height and weight, lymph nodes (head/neck, axillae, groin), thyroid, heart, lungs, breasts, abdomen, extremities, and genitourinary tracts and rectum.

### General Survey

Obtain an overall first impression of the client. Obvious and more subtle clues are obtained primarily by sensory observation and listening with a "sixth sense."

- Note signs of respiratory, cardiac, and emotional distress, along with signs of pain.

- Assess levels of awareness and consciousness through levels of alertness, wakefulness, and appropriate timely response.
- Note the client's facial expression: its mobility, symmetry, and affect in response to questions.
- Observe the symmetry of gait and movements, and how coordinated the woman is when walking, sitting, and moving. Note any involuntary movements and her ability to move purposefully.
- Measure height and weight with clothes on and shoes off; compare findings to standardized charts. Consider racial effects: African Americans tend to be heavier and taller than Caucasians; Asians tend to be slighter and shorter than Caucasians. Consider age and gender effects: Girls tend to reach peak height at puberty; older women tend to lose height after menopause.
- Note body type and posture, whether the woman is obese, slender, average, or stocky; her fat distribution and any deformities. Consider that an older woman may develop a thoracic hump, especially if she is not on hormone replacement therapy. Observe her ability to stand and to sit straight.
- Note the client's speech, the pace at which she speaks, her ability to answer/speak spontaneously, clearly, logically, and with appropriate inflection.
- Observe personal hygiene, grooming, and dress.
- Evaluate the client's affect, manner, and orientation, including the cooperativeness, anxiety, manner toward others and examiner, and nonverbal clues.
- Body and breath odors may indicate problems: alcohol on the breath, urine on clothes, decaying teeth odor, acetone on the breath, halitosis.
- Determine vital signs, including accurate temperature, pulse rate, respiratory rate, and blood pressure. Use appropriate equipment and technique, such as a large cuff for obese clients and, if blood pressure is abnormal, checking both arms with client sitting and lying. Use a rectal thermometer if the client is not alert. Always recheck abnormal findings.
- Assess developmental changes of the breasts and reproductive system (sexual maturity). (See Physical Examination, Developmental Changes of the Breasts and the Reproductive System.)

### Skin

Evaluate color, temperature, vascularity, turgor, moisture, texture, thickness, and primary and secondary lesions. Teach the client to examine moles for changes.

### Hair

Note its color, texture, thickness, and distribution. Observe how the hair is cared for; observe the effects of dyes, permanent waves and other cosmetic changes; and check for nits and lice.

### Nails

Observe for color, texture/consistency, care/cleanliness, clubbing, infection, damage/intactness, and smoothness.

### Scalp, Head, Face

Note lesions, flaking, scaliness, abnormal contours, tenderness, lumps or masses, symmetry, and edema.

### Eyes

Note symmetry, normal appearance, tenderness, lesions, and discharge. Assess intactness and abnormalities of eyes, eyebrows, eyelids, lens, cornea, conjunctiva, sclera, iris, pupil. Test visual acuity, intact extraocular movements, accommodation and convergence, peripheral fields, and corneal light reflex. Do a fundoscopic.

## Ears

Note symmetry, position, tenderness, masses, lesions, discharge, or normal appearance. Assess auditory acuity, internal canal, tympanic membrane, and external structures. If indicated, assess sensorineural/conduction loss.

## Nose/Mucosa

Assess color, edema, discharge, lesions, bleeding, turbinates, and septum deviation.

## Sinuses

Evaluate the frontal and maxillary sinuses for tenderness and swelling. Transillumination is done if indicated.

## Lacrimal Glands and Sacs

Note swelling, tenderness, and punctal regurgitation.

## Mouth, Teeth, Pharynx

Evaluate color, symmetry, texture, lesions, swelling, exudate, bleeding, tenderness, induration, lip moisture, buccal mucosa, gums, palate, ducts, tongue/papillae, pharynx, pillars, tonsils, sublingual area, and uvula. Note the number and condition of teeth.

## Neck, Lymph Nodes, Thyroid, Trachea

Evaluate the range of motion, symmetry, pain, swelling, masses/nodules, lesions, enlarged nodes (mobility, size, shape, consistency, discreteness, tenderness), and tracheal position.

## Thorax and Lungs

Evaluate the respiratory rate, rhythm, and effort; contour, symmetry, and shape of chest; bulges, retractions, deformities; tenderness, masses, lesions, thoracic expansion, tactile fremitus, and diaphragmatic excursion. Percussion and auscultation for adventitious sound are part of the examination.

## Heart, Vessels

Assess chest symmetry, skin and mucous membrane color, pulsations, lifts, heaves, apical impulse, rate, rhythm, intensity, first heart sound ($S_1$), second heart sound ($S_2$), murmurs, and other extra sounds of the heart; amplitude, contour, rate, and rhythm of pulses; symmetry and pressure of jugular veins; color, temperature, hair pattern, and skin/vascular condition of extremities; Homan's sign.

## Breasts, Areolae, Nipples and Axillae

Note sexual maturity, size, symmetry, dimpling, retractions, color, edema, thickening, vascular pattern, lesions/rashes/scaling, discharge, masses/nodules, rash, unusual pigmentation, abnormal lymph nodes. Teach breast self-exam.

## Abdomen

Observe color of skin, lesions, contour, masses, distention, symmetry, vascularity, peristalsis, and pulsations and the umbilicus. Using percussion and/or palpation, assess pulsations, bowel sounds, bruits, ascites, organomegaly, and masses. Note inguinal node enlargement, tenderness/pain, rebound, rigidity. Perform iliopsoas and obturator maneuvers with acute abdomen.

## Musculoskeletal

Evaluate gait (stance, swing, abnormalities), joints and spine (limited range of motion, swelling, tenderness, warmth, redness, crepitation, scoliosis); note symmetry of structures, muscle strength, deformities, abnormal condition of surrounding tissues.

## Neurological

Note mental status (mood, affect, appearance, posture, alertness/consciousness, orientation, facial expression, recent and remote memory, speech, abstract reasoning, judgment, and basic understanding). Test cranial nerves I through XII. Evaluate motor function (gait, posture, muscle tone, balance, muscle mass symmetry, muscle strength), coordination (rapid alternating movements, point-to-point testing), sensory (pain, temperature, light touch, vibration, position, stereognosis, graphesthesia, two point discrimination, extinction, point localization), and deep tendon reflexes (biceps, triceps, brachioradialis, patellar, plantar, Achilles, abdominal, clonus).

### Pelvic

Use gloves on both hands; maintain strict medical aseptic technique to prevent spread of organisms.

- *Inspect and palpate* external genitalia and Bartholin glands, urethra, and Skene's (BUS) glands. This includes, in addition to the Bartholin glands and urethra, the mons pubis, labia minora and majora, clitoris, urethral meatus, and vaginal opening. Assess sexual maturity and check pubic hair for pattern/parasite. Note any swelling, enlargement, inflammation, lesions, discharge, relaxation/celes, and tenderness. Teach self-examination of the vulva.
- *The vagina and cervix* are examined with a warmed speculum; lubricate with water only. Inspect the cervix and os: size, shape, color, lesions, discharge/bleeding, position. Obtain the Pap smear and prepare cultures and wet prep specimens (see Overview of Commonly Indicated Laboratory Tests). Inspect the vagina for color, rugae, lesions, inflammation, discharge.
- *Assess the uterus and adnexa.* Lubricate internal gloved fingers. Note vaginal nodules, masses, or tenderness; note cervical size, consistency, nodules or masses, tenderness, pain with movement of the cervix, and closure of the os. Assess the position, size, shape, consistency, mobility, and tenderness of the uterus, adnexal organs, and any masses.
- *The rectovaginal area* is evaluated after gloves are changed and fingers lubricated again. Inspect the external anal area and palpate the sphincter, rectal walls, septum, posterior surface of the uterus, and palpable adnexal areas. Test any stool on the gloved finger for blood. Retroverted or retroflexed uteri are more accessible by rectal exam.

### Developmental Changes of the Breasts and the Reproductive System

- *Pubertal changes* include functional maturation of the reproductive organs. The breast bud (thelarche) is usually the first sign of puberty, followed soon afterward with the emergence of pubic hair. Axillary hair generally appears about 2 years after pubic hair begins; rarely does it precede pubic hair growth. Menarche (median age 12.8 years, range 9 to 15+ years), occurs after the peak of the growth spurt (median age 11.4 years, range 10–14 years).

  As the external genitalia develop into adult proportions, the clitoris becomes more erectile and the labia minora more vascular. The labia majora and mons pubis become more prominent at the same time as the breasts develop. The internal organs, including the uterus, ovaries, and fallopian tubes, increase in size and weight. The endometrial lining becomes thick in preparation for menarche, and vaginal secretions increase.[27,38]
- *Tanner Staging.* This is widely used to assess adolescent pubertal development.[38,39] The sample used to develop these guidelines comprised white, middle-class English girls; therefore, modifications may be needed when applying the parameters to other groups.

- *Stage I (Prepubertal).* Breasts have elevated papilla only. No pubic hair present.
- *Stage II.* Breast and papilla are elevated and appear as a small mound with enlarged areola diameter (median age 9.8 years, range <8 to 13 years). Sparse, long, pigmented hair develops chiefly along the labia majora (median age 10.5 years, range 8–13 years).
- *Stage III.* Further breast enlargement occurs without separation of breast and areola (median age 11.2 years). Dark, coarse, curled pubic hair is sparsely spread over mons (median age 11.4 years).
- *Stage IV.* Secondary mound of areola and papilla develop above the breast (median age 12.1 years). Adult-type pubic hair is abundant, but limited to the mons pubis (median age 12 years).
- *Stage V (Final Adult Stage).* Recession of areola occurs (median age 14.6 years, range 12–18 years). Pubic hair is of adult type in both quantity and distribution (median age 13.7 years, range 12–18 years).

■ *Although the normal time frame for sexual development varies greatly, deviations do occur.* Variations from normal development are identified by the terms *precocious* and *delayed.* The health care provider must be aware of these aberrations and must ensure that complete family and medical histories are obtained (see Chapter 5).

- *Precocious Puberty.* Development of secondary sexual changes (see preceding discussion of Tanner staging) occurs before age 8, or menarche before age 10.[34,37] This occurs rarely.
- *Delayed Puberty.* Menarche is absent at age 18, or breast budding is completely absent at age 13. This occurs rarely.

■ The reproductive years (Tanner stage V) involve additional changes, for example, cyclic changes in the size, nodularity, and tenderness of the breasts, related to hormonal changes in the menstrual cycle. These changes, along with an increase in total breast volume, occur maximally 3 to 4 days before the onset of menses and minimally in days 4 through 7 of the menstrual cycle.

Structural changes also occur, unrelated to the cycle. Pubic hair may spread onto the inner aspect of the upper thighs. The labia majora increase in prominence; the labia minora and clitoris enlarge. Increased elasticity of vaginal tissue along with attainment of the mature vagina and ovarian size occurs.

■ Older women note profound effects on their breasts and genitalia as ovulation and estrogen production cease.[28] The perimenopause encompasses a 25-year continuum from about age 35 to 60. The average age of menopause is 50, with a normal range of 48 to 55.[38,39] Ovulation usually continues until 1 to 2 years before menopause.[38]

- *Breasts.* Breasts may begin to sag. Glandular tissue atrophies and is replaced by fat.
- *Hair Patterns.* Pubic hair turns gray and decreases in quantity. Axillary hair may also diminish. Hirsutism may develop, with coarse hair on the lip, chin, chest, abdomen, and back.
- *Genitalia and Reproductive Organs.* As estrogen levels decrease, the vulva appears atrophic and the labia flattens. Gradually, the vaginal introitus constricts, the vagina becomes shorter and narrower, and the vaginal epithelium becomes thinner and less vascular, appearing pink, dry, and smooth with fewer rugae. The clitoris, cervix, and uterus become smaller. The uterus may be difficult to palpate or may even prolapse, as the ligaments and connective tissue of the

pelvis sometimes lose their elasticity and tone. The ovaries and fallopian tubes also atrophy. Many changes may be less drastic with hormone replacement therapy.

## GUIDELINES FOR ROUTINE EXAMINATIONS AND SCREENING TESTS

After menarche until death, self-examination of the breasts, vulva, and skin is indicated for all women. Signs and symptoms of cancer should be taught (see Table 3–5).[40–44]

## GUIDELINES FOR GENERAL EDUCATION AND ANTICIPATORY GUIDANCE

Education and guidance in areas such as alcohol use, parenting, fitness, and immunizations are targeted for specific age groups (see Table 3–6).[43,44]

# OVERVIEW OF COMMONLY INDICATED LABORATORY TESTS

## PAPANICOLAOU SMEAR

### Purpose

The Papanicolaou (Pap) smear is a screening test for abnormal/atypical cells suggesting actual or preneoplastic changes. It may help to identify infections of the cervix and vagina, but other definitive testing is needed for diagnosis. Although the Pap smear may be used to evaluate the hormonal status of squamous cells, modern serum hormone levels are more precise.[45] Vaginal pool specimens are no longer considered useful. It is essential to know the reliability of the laboratory that reads the Pap smear; false negative reports may range from 6 to 50 percent.[46]

### Technique

To obtain the best possible specimen, be precise. Be sure that the entire cervix is visible. Use the endocervical cytobrush instead of a cotton-tipped applicator, and the plastic spatula instead of a wooden spatula; the cotton-tipped applicator and wooden spatula may hold the best cells in porous material. If a cotton-tipped applicator must be used, wet in normal saline first so that the cells will be released from the fibers onto the slide. Obtain the brush specimen first, then the spatula specimen. The aim is to get the best possible cells first from the endocervical canal and squamocolumnar junction, because the latter is where cancer begins. The squamocolumnar junction may be out on the ectocervix. If so, use the more rounded end of the spatula to collect cells.

In a study comparing the brush spatula and cotton swab, the cervical brush was significantly better in providing an adequate endocervical specimen.[46] Be sure to rotate each implement a full 360°; roll cells onto a slide with slight pressure. Then obtain a second specimen, rotating the longer pointed end of the spatula to get cells from the ectocervix and endocervix. (*If the woman is pregnant, do not use the longer pointed end of the spatula.*) Paint specimen onto a separate slide or the same one. Spray the slides or drop into fixative within 10 seconds after specimen is applied. Be sure that the specimen is correctly labeled with name, date, and source. If the newer, fan-type implement is used to collect the squamocolumnar junction specimen, rotate it several times in the os to get an adequate number of cells.

### Interpretation of Results and Action

The Bethesda System is the newest test reporting system suggested for nationwide use.[47] Precise terminology tells the provider

**TABLE 3–5. GUIDELINES FOR SELECTED SCREENING EXAMINATIONS AND TESTS FOR WELL NONPREGNANT WOMEN**

| *Exam/Test* | *Ages 18–39* | *Ages 40–59* | *Ages 60–74* | *Ages 75–* |
|---|---|---|---|---|
| Physical (including height/weight) | q3y (Breast examination advised every year) | q1y | q1y | q1y |
| Pelvic and Pap | q1y[a] | q1y | q1–2y | q1–2y |
| Rectal | q1y | q1y | q1y | q1y |
| Mammography | Baseline at age 35–40 | q1–2y | q1y | q1y |
| Hematocrit/hemoglobin | Baseline, q2y | q2y | q5y | q5y |
| Blood glucose | Baseline and [d] | q2y | q2y | q2y |
| Cholesterol, lipids | Baseline and q5y | q3–5y | q3–5y | q3–5y |
| Stool hemoccult | q1y | q1y | q1y | q1y |
| Proctoscopy/ sigmoidoscopy | [d] | q3–5y[b] (Colonoscopy may be indicated) | q3–5y | q3–5y |
| Blood pressure | q2y | q1y | q1y | q1y |
| Urinalysis | [d] | q5y | q5y | q1y |
| Dental | q1y | q1y | q1y | q1y |
| Eye, with tonometry | Baseline, then q3–5y or [d] | q3–5y or [d] | q3–5 y or [d] | q3–5y or [d] |
| Hearing | Baseline at age 40 | repeat at age 50 | q1y[c] | q1y |
| Endometrial sampling | [d] | [d] | [d] | [d] |
| Tuberculosis | [d] | [d] | [d] | [d] |
| Chest x-ray | [d] | [d] | [d] | [d] |
| Thyroid testing | [d] | [d] | q3–5y | q3–5y |

[a] If sexually active begin earlier. Sexually transmitted disease screen advised if history indicates client of any age is at high risk.
[b] After age 50. Should have two consecutive annual negative examinations before having q3–5y.
[c] Audiogram may be needed as the woman ages.
[d] Indicated if risk factors present.
*Source: References 40–44.*

exactly what the findings are, eliminates traditional "class" groupings, includes a category "atypical squamous cells of undetermined significance" to indicate the need for greater concern about atypia, and introduces a new grouping, squamous intraepithelial lesion (SIL). Low grade SIL includes human papilloma virus (HPV) changes and carcinoma in situ (CIS) grade I. High grade SIL includes moderate and severe dysplasia, and cervical intraepithelial neoplasia (CIN). Reporting systems other than the Bethesda System are still being used; therefore, the guidelines in Table 3–7 are presented for interpretation and follow-up of report results.[45,47–49]

Because the Pap smear does not yield a full-thickness specimen, the entire thickness to the basement membrane cannot be examined. Thus, 25 to 77 percent of the women with atypia on Pap smear will have CIN that is not indicated. Consequently, colposcopy is

**TABLE 3–6. ANTICIPATORY GUIDANCE TIME FRAME FOR SELECTED TOPICS BY AGE GROUP**

| *Anticipatory Guidance* | *Ages 15–24* | *Ages 25–39* | *Ages 40–59* | *Ages 60–74* | *Ages 75–* |
|---|---|---|---|---|---|
| Sun exposure | * | * | * | * | * |
| Smoking | * | * | * | * | * |
| Illicit drug use | * | * | | | |
| Alcohol use | * | * | * | * | * |
| Prescription/over-the-counter drug use | * | * | * | * | * |
| Nutrition | * | * | * | * | * |
| Driving accidents | * | * | | | |
| Falls/other accidents | | | | * | * |
| Family/marital/other relationships | * | * | * | * | * |
| Parenting | * | * | * | * | |
| School/work | * | * | * | * | |
| Retirement | | | * | * | * |
| Fitness | * | * | * | * | * |
| Stress | * | * | * | * | * |
| Sleep | * | * | * | * | * |
| Contraception | * | * | * | | |
| Pregnancy | * | * | * | | |
| Breast cancer | * | * | * | * | * |
| Loneliness/grief/loss | | | * | * | * |
| Menopause/climacteric | | * | * | | |
| Bowel/bladder problems | | | * | * | * |
| Self-care problems | | | | * | * |
| Dental care | * | * | * | * | * |
| Sensory deficiency | | | * | * | * |
| Sexuality | * | * | * | * | * |
| Sexually transmitted disease/HIV risks | * | * | * | | |
| Immunizations | * | * | * | * | * |
| Violence/abuse | * | * | * | * | * |

Asterisk indicates that topic should be discussed.
*Source: References 43, 44.*

recommended for all women with atypia.[48] In the controversy over this recommendation, some suggest that a repeat Pap smear in 3 to 6 months would pick up progressive disease. Pregnant women with atypia or dysplasia are referred for colposcopy and biopsy. Generally, treatment is delayed until after pregnancy, unless carcinoma is present.

### Follow-Up of Abnormal Pap Smear

Following treatment for an abnormal Pap smear, repeat Paps should be done every 8 to 12 weeks during the first year, every 6 months in the second year, and annually thereafter as long as the results are normal. It is important to wait at least 8 weeks between Paps to allow for healing and more accurate results.[45]

**TABLE 3–7. PAP SMEAR REPORT FINDINGS, INTERPRETATION, AND ACTION**

| *Report Result* | *Interpretation* | *Action* |
|---|---|---|
| Normal cells, squamous metaplasia or mild inflammation (Class I). | Negative; cells differentiated; infection may be present. | Repeat annually; treat any infection. |
| Significant inflammation and atypia noted; nuclear enlargement, low-grade SIL (Class II). | May indicate infection; no infection or continued atypia or SIL suspicious. | Treat infection and repeat Pap in 8–12 weeks; colposcopy for suspicious atypia or SIL. |
| Mild dysplasia, CIN I, low-grade SIL (Class III). | Suggestive of malignancy, but not conclusive. Less than 10 percent undifferentiated cells. | Colposcopy, biopsy, and treatment if indicated. |
| Moderate dysplasia, CIN II, high-grade SIL (Class III). | Same as 3; 10–20 percent undifferentiated cells. | Colposcopy, biopsy, and treatment if indicated. |
| Severe dysplasia, CIN III, CIS, high-grade SIL (Class IV). | Positive; strongly suggests malignancy. | Colposcopy, biopsy, and treatment if indicated. |
| Malignant cells, squamous carcinoma. | Invasive carcinoma. | Colposcopy, biopsy, and treatment if indicated; and/or conization or hysterectomy. |

If no endocervical cells are found on Pap smear, repeat Pap in 8–12 weeks. Notify woman of results whether negative or positive.

*Note:* CIN = cervical intraepithelial neoplasia; CIS = carcinoma in situ; SIL = squamous intraepithelial lesion.
*Source: References 45, 47–49.*

## GONORRHEA CULTURE

### Purpose

A gonorrhea culture is done to diagnose *Neisseria gonorrhoeae* diplococci.

### Technique

Obtain specimen for culture from each potential site (cervix, urethra, Bartholin glands, Skene's ducts, rectum, pharynx) separately and label. Gently remove excess mucus from the portio of the cervix. Insert sterile cotton-tipped (some recommend synthetic tip over cotton) applicator 0.5 cm into os; rotate half turn; wait 10 seconds. Roll applicator onto Thayer-Martin medium in Z pattern, making slight impression in medium. Medium must be at room temperature. Place in carbon dioxide ($CO_2$) environment within 15 minutes. Keep bottles upright to prevent $CO_2$ from leaking out.[37]

### Results

Positive report indicates need for treatment (see Chapter 8).

## *CHLAMYDIA TRACHOMATIS* TESTS

### Purpose

The tests are carried out to diagnose *Chlamydia trachomatis* intracellular parasite.

### Technique

Definitive diagnosis is done by McCoy cell culture, but this is costly and requires substantial time. Two rapid, nonculture tests using antigen detection are also available as follows:

- *Enzyme immunoassay*: Insert a specially provided swab 0.5 cm into the cervical os; rotate vigorously; place in a tube with transport medium; and send for analysis by spectrophotometer.
- *Monoclonal antibody test*: Insert an endocervical brush 0.5 cm into the cervical os; rotate vigorously; roll onto designated portion of specially provided slide and allow to dry; apply fixative and allow to dry; send for analysis.[25] The slide is read by a medical technologist.

### Results

Positive report indicates need for treatment (see Chapter 8).

## WET MOUNTS. NORMAL SALINE AND POTASSIUM HYDROXIDE

### Purpose

Wet mounts are done to diagnose selected vaginal infections and to assist in determining causes of bleeding.

### Technique

Wear gloves while handling specimens. Dip cotton swab into vaginal/cervical discharge; place in tube with 1 ml saline; mix; drop one drop on clean slide and cover with coverslip. Dip second swab into discharge; place in tube with 1 mL of 10% potassium hydroxide (KOH) and mix; drop one drop on clean slide or same slide at other end; cover. Blue or green food dye may be added to enhance visibility of organisms/cells. Evaluate with low and high power microscope objectives. The value of the specimen is proportional to the effectiveness of the collection techniques and the quality of the provider's interpretation. Vaginal/cervical discharge specimen may also be placed directly on a slide with a drop of solution, rather than placed in a tube, and covered with a coverslip for viewing.

### Results

Clue cells indicate the occurrence of bacterial vaginosis (abundant coccobacilli will be seen in fluid); spores and/or hyphae indicate fungal infection (best seen in KOH suspension); motile trichomonads indicate trichomoniasis vaginitis; leukocytosis (leukocytes in greater number than epithelial cells) indicates infections such as gonorrhea, chlamydia.[25,37] Excessive lactobacilli in epithelial cells indicate overgrowth and acidic vaginitis. Red blood cells indicate obvious or microscopic bleeding. (Because bleeding may be induced by examiner, wet mount specimens may be obtained before Pap and cultures; however, care must be taken not to take cells needed for Pap smear.) A greenish-yellow vaginal/cervical discharge on white background of cotton-tipped swab indicates presence of bacterial infection. "Fishy" odor when discharge and KOH are mixed on slide indicates bacterial vaginosis (positive whiff test). (See Chapter 8 for more details on STD and vaginitis diagnosis.)

## URINALYSIS

### Purpose

A urinalysis provides supportive data in diagnosing urinary complaints; however it should not be used alone if results are negative but other findings indicate that a problem exists.

### Technique

Instruct the client to wash her hands well and collect a midstream urine specimen. A clean-catch specimen is not necessary. Studies indicate that a midstream collection is adequate. Use a tampon or cotton ball in the introitus during collection of urine if heavy vaginal discharge or bleeding is present.[37] Test or culture the specimen within a few minutes, or refrigerate it with a tight cover and test within a few hours.

- If screening for nitrite and normal pH, a dipstick test is done on a first morning urine specimen. Keep dipsticks in cool, dark, tightly closed container. Assess glucose, ketones, blood, leukocytes, protein, and specific gravity.
- Microscopic examination should be done on centrifuged sediment, or a specimen may be sent out for analysis. Look for white blood cells (WBCs, or leukocytes) red blood cells (RBCs, or erythrocytes), crystals, bacteria, epithelial cells, and casts. Use low light to see casts better.
- Culture and sensitivity tests are indicated when the number of WBCs is greater than 5 per high power field or when Microstix indicates infection.

### Results

All findings should be within normal limits (see standard laboratory testing text or manual).

## HERPES CULTURE

### Purpose

Culture is done to diagnose herpes simplex genitalis.

### Technique

*Wear goggles to protect eyes and cover unclothed skin with a mask, gloves, gown, and/or lab coat.* Carefully puncture intact vesicle with sterile tuberculin needle or scrape vesicle with saline-moistened swab to get viral sample. Place specimen in culture medium immediately.[34] Refrigerate and transport within 12 hours. Drainage from new lesions (those that have developed within 24 to 48 hours) can be applied to a glass slide and prepared as for Pap testing or other cytology staining for direct identification of multinucleated giant cells.

### Results

Positive growth of type 1 or type 2 herpes simplex virus (HSV).

## REFERENCES


1. Northrup, C. (Spring, 1988). The road of wellness. *New England Nursing, 1,* 6–9.
2. U.S. Bureau of the Census. (1992). Deaths, by selected cause and selected characteristics: 1989 (No. 115). *Statistical abstracts of the United States, 1992* (112th ed.). Washington, DC: U.S. Government Printing Office.
3. U.S. Bureau of the Census. (1992). Deaths from accidents and violence: 1970–1989 (No. 122). *Statistical abstracts of the United States, 1992* (112th ed.). Washington, DC: U.S. Government Printing Office.
4. Wyman, J. (1991, May 29). *Falls in the elderly.* Paper presented at MCV-VCU Nurse Practitioners meeting, Medical College of Virginia, Virginia Commonwealth University, Richmond.
5. National Center for Health Statistics. (1989). Age-adjusted death rates for selected causes of death, according to sex and race: United States, selected years 1950–1987. *United States, health and prevention profile* (DHHS Publication No. PHS 90-1232). Hyattsville, MD: Author.
6. Horton, J.A. (1992). *The women's health data book: A profile of women's health in the United States.* Washington, DC: Jacob's Institute for Women's Health.
7. U.S. Bureau of the Census. (1992). Death rate from cancer, by sex, age, and selected type: 1970–1989 (No. 121). *Statistical abstracts of the United States, 1992* (112th ed.).

Washington, DC: U.S. Government Printing Office.

8. Chu, S.Y., Buehler, J.W., & Berkelman, R.L. (1990). Impact of the human immunodeficiency virus on mortality in women of reproductive age, United States. *Journal of the American Medical Association, 264*, 225–229.
9. U.S. Bureau of the Census. (1992). Deaths from heart disease, by sex, age, and selected type: 1970–1989 (No. 120). *Statistical abstracts of the United States, 1992* (112th ed.). Washington, DC: U.S. Government Printing Office.
10. Healy, B.P. (1992). The women's health initiative. *Female Patient, 17*, 36–38.
11. U.S. Bureau of the Census. (1992). Acute conditions by type and selected characteristics: 1970–1989 (No. 194). *Statistical abstracts of the United States, 1992* (112th ed.). Washington, DC: U.S. Government Printing Office.
12. U.S. Bureau of the Census. (1992). Prevalence of selected reported chronic conditions, by age and sex: 1980–1989 (No. 195). *Statistical abstracts of the United States, 1992* (112th ed.). Washington, DC: U.S. Government Printing Office.
13. Stewart, F., Guest, F., Stewart, G., & Hatcher, R. (1987). *Understanding your body*. New York: Bantam Books.
14. Alcohol-related mortality estimates by sex, 1987. (1990, March 23). *Mortality and Morbidity Weekly Report, 39*.
15. Bates, N., Bayer, L., Lang, K., & Ravnikar, V. (1986, December 15). Help for the dysmenorrheic adolescent. *Patient Care*, pp. 100–121.
16. Schaumburg, H., Kaplan, J., Windebark, A., Vick, N., Rasmus, S., Pleasure, D., & Brown, M. (1983). Sensory neuropathy from pyridoxine abuse. *New England Journal of Nursing, 309*, 445–448.
17. Manson, J.E., Colditz, G.A., Stampfer, M.J., Willett, W.C., Rosner, B., Monson, R.R., Speizer, F.E., & Nennekens, C.H. (1990). A prospective study of obesity and risk of coronary heart disease in women. *New England Journal of Medicine, 322*, 882–889.
18. Plehn, K.W. (1990). Anorexia nervosa and bulimia: Incidence and diagnosis. *Nurse Practitioner, 15*, 22, 25, 28, 31.
19. Heinrich, L.B. (1987). Care of the female rape victim. *Nurse Practitioner, 12*, 9–10, 12, 16–18, 23, 26–27.
20. Blair, K.A. (1986). The battered woman: Is she a silent victim? *Nurse Practitioner, 11*, 38, 40, 42–44, 47.
21. Ware, J.C., Director, Sleep Disorders Center, Eastern Virginia Medical School and Sentera Norfolk General Hospital, Norfolk, VA. Telephone interview regarding differences in sleep patterns between sexes and relationship to longevity, November 24, 1993.
22. Block, G.J., Nolan, J.W., & Dempsey, M.K. (1981). *Health assessment for professional nursing: A developmental approach*. New York: Appleton-Century-Crofts.
23. Auslander, G.K. (1988). Social networks and the functional health status of the poor: A secondary analysis of data from the national survey of personal health practices and consequences. *Journal of Community Health, 13*, 197–209.
24. McElmurry, B.L. (1986). Health appraisal of low-income women. In D.K. Kjervik and I.M. Martinson (Eds.), *Women in health and illness*. Philadelphia: Saunders.
25. Morton, P.G. (1993). *Health assessment* (2nd ed.). Springhouse, PA: Springhouse.
26. Bates, B. (1991). *A guide to physical examination and history taking* (5th ed.). New York: Lippincott.
27. Seidel, H.M., Ball, J.W., Dains, J.E., & Benedict, G.W. (1991). *Mosby's guide to physical examination* (2nd ed.). St. Louis: Mosby Year Book.
28. Fuller, J., & Schaller-Ayers, J. (1990). *Health assessment: A nursing approach*. New York: Lippincott.
29. Eliopoulos, C. (1990). *Health assessment of the older adult* (2nd ed.). Redwood City, CA: Addison-Wesley Nursing.
30. Berkey, K., & Hanson, S. (1991). *Pocket guide to family assessment and intervention*. St. Louis: Mosby Year Book.
31. Sawin, K., & Harrigan, M. (1994, in press).

Measures of family assessment. *Scholarly Inquiry for Nursing.*

32. U.S. Department of Agriculture. (1992, August). *Food guide pyramid.* Pueblo, CO: Consumer Information Center, Department 159-Y.
33. Star, W.L., Shannon, M.T., Samnors, L.N., Neeson, J.D., & Gutierrez, Y. (1992). *Ambulatory obstetrics: Protocols for nurse practitioners/nurse midwives.* San Francisco: University of California, School of Nursing.
34. Pender, N. (1987). *Health promotion in nursing practice.* Norwalk, CT: Appleton & Lange.
35. Holmes, T., & Rahe, R. (1967). The social readjustment rating scale. *Journal of Psychosomatic Research, 11,* 213.
36. Dunn, M.M. (1987). Guidelines for an effective personal fitness prescription. *Nurse Practitioner, 12,* 9–10, 12, 14–16, 18, 23, 26.
37. Keleher, K.C. (1991). Occupational health: How work environments can affect reproductive capacity and outcome. *Nurse Practitioner, 16,* 23–37.
38. Lichtman, R., & Papera, S. (1990). *Gynecology: Well-woman care.* Norwalk, CT: Appleton & Lange.
39. Speroff, L., Glass, R., & Kase, N. (1989). *Clinical gynecologic endocrinology and infertility* (4th ed.). Baltimore: Williams & Wilkins.
40. Report of task force on routine cancer screening. (1989, April). *ACOG Committee Opinion* (No. 68). Washington, DC: American College of Obstetricians and Gynecologists.
41. Byyny, R.L. (1988). Establishing guidelines for preventive medicine. *Contemporary OB/GYN [Special Issue], 31,* 43–49.
42. Goroll, A.H., May, L.A., & Mulley, A.G. (1987). *Primary care medicine.* Philadelphia: Lippincott.
43. Jones, J.M., Cox, A.R., Levy, E.Y., & Thompson, C.E. (1984). *Women's health management: Guidelines for nurse practitioners.* Reston, VA: Reston.
44. Women's health. (1985). *Report of the Public Health Service task force on women's health issues* (DHHS Publication No. PHS 85-50-206).
45. Beal, M.W. (1987). Understanding cervical cytology. *Nurse Practitioner, 12,* 8–22.
46. Toffler, W.L., Pluedeman, C.K., Sinclair, A.E., Ireland, K.M., & Byrne, S.J. (1993). Comparative cytologic yield and quality of three Pap smear instruments. *Family Medicine, 25*(6), 403–407.
47. Kurman, R.J., Malkasian, G.D., Sedlis, A., & Solomon, D. (1991). From Papanicolaou to Bethesda: The rationale for a new cervical cytologic classification. *Obstetrics & Gynecology, 77,* 779–781.
48. Soper, D. (1992, August 17). Presentation on Pap smears and HPV, Planned Parenthood of Richmond.
49. Baldor, R.A. (1988). The cervical Pap smear: Reducing false-negative results. *Family Practice Recertification, 10,* 20–39.

## BIBLIOGRAPHY

Alpers, D.H., Clouse, R.E., & Stenson, W.F. (1988). *Manual of nutritional therapeutics* (2nd ed.). Boston: Little, Brown.

Aronson, V., Fitzgerald, B., & Hewes, L. (1990). *Guidebook for nutritional counselors* (2nd ed.). Englewood Cliffs, NJ: Prentice-Hall.

Grotevant, H.D., & Carlson, C.I. (1989). *Family assessment: A guide to methods and measures.* New York: Guilford Press.

McCubbin, H.I., & Thompson, A.I. (1991). *Family assessment inventories for research and practice.* Madison, WI: University of Wisconsin-Madison Press.

McCubbin, M.A., & McCubbin, H.I. (1993). Families coping with illness: The resiliency model of family stress, adjustment, and adaptation. In C. Danielson, B. Hamil-Bissell, & P. Winstead-Fry (Eds.), *Families, health and illness,* New York: Mosby.

Ross, V., & Cobb, K. (1990). *Family nursing: A nursing process approach.* Redwood City, CA: Addison-Wesley Nursing.

CHAPTER 4

# WOMEN AND SEXUALITY

*Catherine Ingram Fogel*

*Older women who become celibate due to lack of a partner retain their need for touch and closeness and should be encouraged to seek out opportunities for intimacy with another person.*[1]

### Highlights

- Dimensions of Sexuality
- Age-Related Issues
- Disability
- The Women's Movement
- Sexual Problems and Dysfunction
- Sexual Health Care
- Sexual Assessment and History
- Interventions: PLISSIT Model

## INTRODUCTION

Sexuality is inextricably woven into the fabric of a woman's life and is an important aspect of her health. It is an integrated, unique expression of self that encompasses physiological and psychosocial processes inherent in sexual development, sexual response, sexual desire, view of self as a female, and presentation of self to society as a woman.[2]

Sexuality underlies much of who and what a person is, and it is an inherent, everchanging aspect of life from birth to death. It is expressed in different ways at different times—alone, with one partner, or with different partners.[1] Although experts do not agree on a definition of sexual health or what constitutes normal sexual behavior, the World Health Organization definition provides a starting point: "Sexual health is the integration of somatic, emotional, intellectual, and social aspects of sexual beings in ways that are positively enriching and that enhance personality, communication and love."[3] In short, sexual health may be considered the physical and emotional state of well-being that enables us to enjoy and act on our sexual feelings.[4]

Promoting sexual health is a legitimate role for health professionals and an essential nursing function. The nurse practitioner can have a primary role in promoting and maintaining the sexual health of women.

## DIMENSIONS OF SEXUALITY

*Sexuality* is a broad concept that encompasses the dimensions of sexual desire, sexual response, view of self, and presentation of self.

## SEXUAL DESIRE

*Libido* is the innate urge for sexual activity, produced by the activation of a specific system in the brain and experienced as a specific sensation that motivates a person to seek out or be receptive to sexual experience.[5] The amount of sexual desire experienced can vary across a woman's life span and from woman to woman. Moreover, sexual desire is a response learned through feelings of pleasure, enjoyment, or dissatisfaction during sexual activity. Sexual desire derives from interest in sexual activity, preferred frequency of activity, and gender preference for a sexual partner.[2]

## SEXUAL RESPONSE CYCLE

The sexual response cycle may be divided into *capacity* (i.e., what a woman is able to experience) and activity (i.e., what she actually experiences). The two principal physiological responses to sexual stimulation are vasocongestion and myotonia. Vasocongestion corresponds to sexual excitement, as the tissues and blood vessels become engorged. Myotonia, an increase in muscle tension, peaks with orgasm.

### Four Phase Response Cycle (Masters and Johnson)

The most widely known approach for labeling and identifying the physiological response to sexual stimuli, this cycle has four phases: excitement, plateau, orgasm, and resolution.[6]

- *Excitement* is characterized by vaginal lubrication. This phase may develop from any bodily or psychic stimuli and may be interrupted, prolonged, or ended by distracting stimuli.
- *Plateau* is characterized by vaginal engorgement and clitoral retraction. This phase also may be interrupted by distracting stimuli.
- *Orgasm* is the peak of vasocongestion and myotonia released by involuntary climax.
- *Resolution* is characterized by bodily return to the preexcitement state. With adequate stimulation, a woman may again begin sexual response before complete resolution occurs.

### Diagnostic and Statistical Manual of Mental Disorders, 3rd edition (DSM-III-R)* Response Cycle

This well-known approach that incorporates both biologic and psychological components is useful in categorizing sexual disorders.[7] It comprises four phases: appetitive, excitement, orgasm, and resolution.

- The *appetitive* phase is characterized by sexual fantasy and desire for sexual activity.
- *Excitement* involves pelvic vasocongestion with vaginal lubrication, swelling of external genitalia, narrowing of the lower third of the vagina, and lengthening of the upper two-thirds of the vagina, in addition to breast tumescence. Sensations of pleasure are experienced.
- *Orgasm* is the peaking of sexual pleasure followed by the release of sexual tension and rhythmic contractions of the perineal muscles, uterus, and in some women, the lower third of the vagina.
- *Resolution* is characterized by a sense of general relaxation and well-being.

## VIEW OF SELF AS FEMALE

A woman's view of herself as female incorporates (a) concepts of gender identity (identification of self as female); (b) the sense of

*According to the American Psychiatric Association only a few content changes have been made in the not yet released DSM-IV.

having characteristics customarily defined as female, masculine, or both; and (c) body image (a mental picture of one's body and its relationship to the environment).[2]

### PRESENTATION OF SELF AS A WOMAN

Sex role behaviors encompass all behaviors that women use to present themselves as women, such as dress, hairstyle, speech pattern, and gait. These behaviors reflect a woman's internalization of sociocultural stereotypes and expectations of what a woman's behavior should be.[8]

### SEXUAL LIFESTYLES

Sexual lifestyle provides the pattern and context for a woman's sexuality.[2] Several options exist.

- *Marriage with a Monogamous Partner.* The most frequently acknowledged pattern for women and the one that the majority of society assumes is most desirable.
- *Serial Monogamy.* An established pattern of having one monogamous relationship followed by another.
- *Nonmonogamous Marriage.* A married woman may participate in sexual activity with other individuals or couples—often called "swinging."
- *Heterosexual Coupling without Marriage.*
- *Single State.* Women with this lifestyle may be unmarried, divorced, or widowed. Society often considers this a transition phase.
- *Lesbianism.* Sexual desire for persons of the same sex. A woman may be coupled or single with many sexual partners or one. The most typical pattern is serial monogamy.
- *Bisexuality.* Sexual desire for persons of either sex. A woman may be married, have partners of both sexes serially or simultaneously, or have had lesbian relationships as well as sexual relationships with men.
- *Celibacy.* Consciously chosen abstinence from sexual activity. A woman may view this lifestyle positively, as enabling her to focus all of her time and energy on other activities. Celibacy may also be nonvoluntary when a woman is between relationships.

## FACTORS THAT AFFECT SEXUALITY

### AGE-RELATED ISSUES

#### Adolescence

The period between childhood and adulthood is a time of awareness and change in sexual feelings. The central issue in adolescent sexuality is defining sexuality through activities such as dating. During this time, one selects companions, tests ideas about oneself, and eventually experiences sexual pleasure. Adolescence is a time of developing a capacity for sexual intimacy, and sexual curiosity and experimentation are common.

In the United States, the mean age of first voluntary intercourse is 17.2 years for white women and 16.7 years for African American women.[9] Teenagers often face peer pressure to become sexually active. For girls, a motivation to become sexually active may come from a desire for intimacy, not for the physical act of intercourse. Risks associated with early sexual activity include sexually transmitted diseases (STDs), including acquired immunodeficiency syndrome (AIDS), and pregnancy.

#### Reproductive Years

During the reproductive years, developmental tasks include achieving maturity in a sexual role and in the relationship tasks started in adolescence. Balancing career, children, and relationships is often of concern. For many, sexuality during pregnancy and the postpartum period also is of concern. During that period, women frequently report diminished sexual desire and frequency of intercourse. Fears about the effect of intercourse on the fetus and restrictions associated with high risk pregnancy also may affect sexual activity and satisfaction.

In addition, many lactating women experience a lack of sexual desire, primarily because of low estrogen levels. These women also may experience decreased vaginal secretions and therefore require some form of lubrication to prevent dyspareunia.

Moreover, struggling with infertility or repeated attempts to conceive can adversely affect sexual expression, activity, and desire.

### Midlife

Physiological changes occur in the sexuality of women during midlife as a result of the climacteric or menopause. For some women, sleep disturbances associated with hot flushes and the resulting fatigue may adversely affect sexual desire. Vaginal dryness caused by decreasing estrogen levels may also diminish sexual activity. For some women, however, the lessened fear that they will become pregnant may increase sexual desire.

### Older Adulthood

Patterns of sexual behavior in old age are similar to patterns in midlife (see Chapter 11). A critical issue for women, however, is the availability of a partner. Societal emphasis on youth, beauty, and slimness contributes to the expectation of asexuality in older women—a view that often becomes a self-fulfilling prophecy.

Physiological changes of aging (e.g., decreased estrogen supply, decreased tissue elasticity, thinning of vaginal tissues) can cause irritation or discomfort with penetration and may make the woman more susceptible to vaginitis. Loss of fatty tissue in the labia and mons pubis also may result in tenderness and easily damaged tissueor abrasions.

Orgasms may decrease in intensity, and in some women they may be painful. Breast size also decreases and breasts sag. These changes do not alter a woman's ability to respond sexually, but they may alter her view of her sexual self.

Physiological changes may require that the woman and her partners alter how they engage in sexual activity. A water-soluble lubricant may be used, foreplay increased, different positions used, and intercourse planned for when energy levels are highest.

Although sexual interest and activity may decrease somewhat, most older women do maintain sexual relationships if a partner is available. Older women who become celibate due to lack of a partner retain their need for touch and closeness and should be encouraged to seek out opportunities for intimacy with another person.

## ISSUES OF DISABILITY

The disabled are often perceived as asexual, by health care providers as well as the public. Most disabled persons are not married.[10] How long a woman has had a disability may affect her sexuality: Women with an early onset of physical disability are less likely than those with a later onset to engage in various sexual activities.[11] An important issue is body image. The disabled woman may view her body as a problem and a source of anxiety rather than pleasure (see Chapter 19).

## THE WOMEN'S MOVEMENT

In the 1960s and 1970s, women began to redefine sexuality for themselves. New definitions recognized that sexuality is created by individuals, not anatomically prescribed. Women-centered definitions of sexuality include the ideas of sensuality, closeness, mutuality, and relationships.[2]

## SEXUAL CONCERNS OR PROBLEMS

### ILLNESS

Illness can affect sexuality in a number of ways. Trauma such as spinal cord injury, for example, can negatively affect sexuality. Chronic illness with its associated fatigue, pain, and stress affects sexual desire and arousal more often than it affects orgasm. For example, treatment of gynecologic cancer is associated with less frequent intercourse, sexual excitement, and arousal[12,13]; and studies suggest that diabetic women are likely to have sexual difficulties including orgasmic dysfunction and inadequate lubrication.[14,15] Results of studies on the effect of a hysterectomy on sexuality vary considerably and no longer document negative effects only.[16,17]

In our society where breasts are sexual, a woman with breast cancer may have sexuality concerns; greater sexuality problems may be experienced by women who dislike their breasts, have a negative self-image, have been sexually abused, lack a support system, or are uncomfortable discussing personal or sexual concerns.[18]

In addition, sexually transmitted diseases can have a tremendous impact on a woman's sexuality. Drastic changes may occur in her sexual behavior, including choice of partner, use of condoms, and specific sexual practices.

Medication, such as psychotropic drugs, can impair sexual response in women; the degree of impairment is dose related.[2]

### SEXUAL MYTHS

Sexual myths are common in every culture and society. The list of these myths is long.

- Women should satisfy men; women's needs are secondary.
- Sexual pleasure is the responsibility of the partner. Related to this is the expectation that a partner should somehow sense what a woman's needs are.
- A great deal of stimulation is necessary to sexually arouse a woman; she becomes aroused more slowly than a man.
- Women who are raped asked for it; every woman wants to be raped; when a woman says no she doesn't mean it.
- Little girls should not be told about sex, as that will put ideas in their heads.
- Women are not interested in sex; they are not capable of multiple orgasms.
- Women want sex only for procreative purposes.
- Women are so sexually aggressive they can never be satisfied.
- Sex is intercourse.
- A woman who initiates sex is immoral.
- Older women are neither interested in sexual expression nor capable of it.
- A woman cannot enjoy sex unless she has an orgasm.
- There are absolute norms for sexual expression.
- Masturbation is dirty.
- Women can have an orgasm only with intercourse.

### LOSS OF A PARTNER

Many women define their identity through relationships, and thus the loss of a partner can be a loss of self. Furthermore, the stereotypical view of a widow is of a sad, grieving woman whose sexual life is over. A woman's sexuality after the loss of a partner may be influenced by her past extramarital sexual experiences, age, and sexual satisfaction in her marriage.[19,20] Remarriage is correlated with age; the older a woman, the less likely remarriage.

### FAMILY INFLUENCE

Poor parent–child interactions contribute indirectly to sexual problems; such a child may have lower self-esteem or difficulty coping with intimacy.[21] In addition, less satisfactory relationships with fathers may contribute to orgasmic difficulties.[22] Restrictive family upbringing and the belief that expressions of intimacy or sexuality are shameful or taboo may affect a woman's later ability to express herself sexually. Sexual expression or enjoyment may be inhibited by messages that were taught within a restrictive family—messages such as, "Sex is something to be endured" or "Women who enjoy sex are no good."

Incest contributes to sexual dysfunction particularly if its circumstances were associated with strong negative feelings, such as when threat or force was used, or when the incest victim was an older child and more apt to have feelings of guilt, or when the incest was repeated over time.[21]

### RELATIONSHIP ISSUES

Discord within a relationship may precipitate sexual dysfunction, so much so that many sex therapists believe that sexual dysfunction is a symptom of the underlying relationship problem. One or both partners may experience difficulty after the disclosure of sexual encounters out of their relationship. Communication problems are exacerbated by distrust, feelings of betrayal, and fear of disease. Sexual dysfunction in one's partner may precipitate dysfunction in the other. For example, premature ejaculation is often accompanied by female orgasmic difficulties and lack of desire.

### SOCIOCULTURAL INFLUENCES

Religious and cultural beliefs may contribute to sexual concerns or problems. One such conviction is that using a contraceptive during the fertile period is amoral. In addition, attitudes and expectations exist regarding monogamy for males and females. Quite definitely, cultural practices that physically alter the anatomy of sexual response, such as a clitoridectomy, affect sexuality.

## SEXUAL DYSFUNCTION

### CHARACTERISTICS OF SEXUAL DYSFUNCTION

"Impaired, incomplete, or absent expressions of normally recurring human sexual desires and responses"[23] become dysfunctions only when there is subjective discomfort associated with them. Several factors characterize dysfunction.

- Dysfunction may occur in one or more phases of the sexual response cycle but is less common in the resolution phase.
- Dysfunction may occur during masturbation or, more commonly, during sexual activity with a partner.
- Dysfunction may be lifelong or develop after a period of normal responsiveness; it may occur once or recur.
- Most typically, dysfunction is seen among individuals in their late 20s or early 30s.

### CAUSES OF SEXUAL DYSFUNCTION

Pathophysiological causes of sexual dysfunction are more common than those that are psychogenic[24]; however, traumatic sexual experiences such as incest and rape may precipitate dysfunction. Other associated factors may be depression and life stress. Anxieties, including fear of partner rejection and fear of demand for performance, may also result in dysfunction.[5] An excessive need to please one's partner may cause sexual dysfunction. Poor communication between partners about sexual feelings, needs, and desires is common and can perpetuate an unsatisfying sexual pattern or escalate problems by limiting knowledge of each other or restricting standards of acceptable sexual behavior.

## SEXUAL DYSFUNCTIONS IN WOMEN

Female sexual dysfunctions include inhibited desire, anorgasmia, vaginismus, and dyspareunia. Psychiatrists would add sexual aversion disorder and female sexual arousal disorder.

### Inhibited Sexual Desire

Inhibition occurs when a woman lacks desire for sexual activity, sexual dreams or fantasies, or frustration if sexual activity does not occur. Sexual activity occurs infrequently or only in reluctant compliance with the partner's desire for activity.[25] It is the sexual problem with which women most frequently seek assistance. Although the cause is unknown, the disorder is thought to be associated with high levels of stress.

Treatment is often difficult and frequently incorporates sensate focus and techniques to improve communication between partners.[2] It is essential that health care providers working with these women provide a supportive environment and frequent opportunities for expression of feelings. A client may require referral to a health care professional with advanced training in sexual counseling and therapy.

### Anorgasmia

The inability to experience orgasm is defined as a disorder only if a woman reports receiving sufficient stimulation without orgasm. Anorgasmic women do experience erotic feelings, genital swelling, and vaginal lubrication. Anorgasmia is classified as *primary* (preorgasmia) if a woman has never experienced an orgasm, or *secondary* if a woman has experienced orgasm in the past but is unable to with her current partner or at this time.

Causes include a restrictive home environment, negative cultural conditioning during childhood, unrealistic expectations about performance, current relationship issues, lack of knowledge about female anatomy or the sexual response cycle, and so on. Secondary anorgasmia (anorgasmia that occurs after the woman has established an orgasmic response) may be caused by psychoactive drugs[26]; any physical cause of dyspareunia, such as episiotomy scars or endometriosis; and by oophorectomy.[2]

The most common treatments for this problem are behavioral. For example, the woman is taught to experience orgasm through a series of exercises that increase her awareness of genital sensations and masturbatory techniques.[27] Once she has experienced an orgasm through self-stimulation she is taught to transfer this knowledge to a partner experience. Women with a partner may be given specific couple exercises to practice. Women with an orgasmic dysfunction may also benefit from information about female anatomy and physiology and the differences between male and female response cycles.

### Vaginismus

This disorder involves the involuntary, spasmodic, sometimes painful contractions of the pubococcygeus and other muscles in the lower third of the vagina and the introitus.[28]

Vaginismus can occur during any phase of the sexual response cycle when vaginal entry is attempted. Although the dysfunction is considered rare, sex therapists believe it may be more common than is documented and women do not seek help for it.[2]

Causes of vaginismus are varied and include sexual trauma, strong conservative religious values in the woman's family of origin, dyspareunia, and hostile feelings toward one's sexual partner.[28]

Treatment usually involves a desensitization process including insertion of progressively larger dilators into the vagina by the woman and/or her partner. At the same time she is taught to relax vaginal muscles consciously. Often psychotherapy is needed. Treatment of this sexual dysfunction requires a health professional with advanced training in sexual therapy. Clients should be referred to such an individual.

### Dyspareunia

Pain experienced in the labia, vagina, or pelvis during or after intercourse is called dyspareunia.[29] Its incidence is unknown; some authorities suggest that as many as 60 percent of women experience dyspareunia at some time in their lives.[29]

Physical causes are most common and numerous. They include sexually transmitted disease, bladder disease, diabetes, anatomic defects, and decreased estrogen due to aging. Mechanical causative factors may be excessive douching or the use of irritating soaps or sprays. Dyspareunia can also be caused by psychological factors related to family religious taboos or teachings that the vagina should not be touched; traumatic factors such as rape, incest, or previous painful intercourse; or other factors such as a lack of complete arousal and inadequate vaginal lubrication, personal problems, or negative feelings toward one's partner.[30]

Treatment addresses the specific cause of dyspareunia; for example, suggesting a water-soluble vaginal lubricant for the menopausal woman, treating the sexually transmitted disease, or providing information about techniques for sexual arousal.

### Sexual Aversion Disorder

Extreme repulsion and avoidance of almost all genital sexual contact with a partner is classified as sexual aversion disorder.[7] These women, who experience intense irrational fear of sexual activity and a compelling desire to avoid sexual situations,[31] should be referred to a trained sex therapist for care.

### Female Sexual Arousal Disorder

The disorder is characterized by partial or complete failure to attain or maintain vaginal lubrication and swelling or sexual excitement. Women also report a lack of sexual excitement or pleasure. A woman with this disorder should be referred to a trained sex therapist for care.

## SEXUAL HEALTH CARE ASSESSMENT, AND HISTORY

In order to provide adequate sexual health care, nurse practitioners must be aware of their sexual biases, be comfortable with their sexuality, and have a genuine desire to help the client. The health care provider should know how various health problems, diseases, and their treatment affect sexuality and sexual functioning. When providing sexual health care, it is critical that assumptions not be made about a woman's sexual behavior, feelings, or attitudes.

Sexual assessment includes a physiological, psychological, and sociocultural evaluation. Data are gathered regarding the client's sexual response cycle and any alterations she has noted in its phases. The woman should be asked about attempts to conceive, any previous high-risk pregnancy, postpartum difficulties, and contraceptive choices and any associated problems. In addition, data about past and present illness, surgery, and medications are obtained.

Components of psychological sexual assessment include the client's self-concept and body image; view of self as a sexual being and level of confidence in ability to function sexually; past and current psychiatric problems or illness including anxiety and depression; use of psychotropic medications; satisfaction with current relationship; and history of sexual abuse.

Sociocultural sexual assessment incorporates information about the client's perceptions of sex-appropriate roles for men and women in relationships and her perception of her ability to fulfill those roles competently. Women should be asked about their sources of sexual education, when they received it, and their reactions to the information. The nurse practitioner/primary care provider should assess whether the information that the client received was correct and accurate. The woman's religious affiliation and beliefs and her ethnic and cultural belief system should be noted.

## TECHNIQUES FOR TAKING A SEXUAL HISTORY

The health care provider should take responsibility for introducing the topic of sexual health problems. Choose a private location where the client is comfortable and assure her that the information will be held in strict confidence. It is essential that sufficient time be given to build trust and develop rapport before soliciting information that the client may consider highly personal or intimate. Several meetings may be needed to collect the history, especially if anxiety is high. Continually monitor your own responses to detect negative or embarrassed feelings that may easily be conveyed to the client. Usually you will obtain more information if you begin with open questions that will permit clients to tell their story on their own terms. Closed questions generally facilitate gathering specific information, such as medical history, menstrual history, and drug reactions.

### From Simple to Complex

History taking should always begin with the least threatening material, for example, obstetric history or childhood sexual education, and progress to more sensitive topics, such as current sexual practices. A general guide is to begin with questions about the individual's sexual learning history, proceed to personal attitudes and beliefs about sexuality, and finally assess actual sexual behaviors. Explain to your clients the purpose of your questions. You can set limits on the length of responses if excessive or irrelevant information is offered or provide encouragement if progress is slow. Tell your clients if information becomes tangential.

### Appropriate Terminology

Avoid using excessive medical terminology during an interview; in other words, make sure that both you and the client know the meaning of the terms used. Avoid euphemisms such as "slept with." Pose only one question at a time, and give the client sufficient time to answer it. Questions such as, "How many times a week do you have sexual intercourse?" should not be asked because norms vary widely among individuals.

"Universalizing," or prefacing questions with phrases such as "Many people" or "The Kinsey Report shows" may make a client feel more comfortable when answering sensitive questions.

## SEXUAL HISTORY FORMATS

A sexual history can be incorporated into a total health history (brief sexual history) or it can be more formal and inclusive (sexual problem history).

### Brief Sexual History

When the sexual history is incorporated into the total health history, various formats can be used.

- Two questions that elicit sexual concerns are: "Are you sexually active?" and, "Are you having any sexual difficulties or problems at this time?"[32]
- The three question format is used to gather information about a client's usual sexual roles, views of self as a sexual being, and sexual functioning. These questions are: "Has any [illness, pregnancy, surgery] interfered with your being a [mother, wife, partner]?" "Has any [surgery, medical treatment, illness] changed the way you feel about yourself as a woman?" and, "Has any [surgery, disease, medication] altered your ability to function sexually?"[33]

An additional question that could be added to either of the above formats is "Are you satisfied with your sexual relationship?

Other elements of a *routine* history are also significant for a sexual history. The woman's menstrual history is queried, including her age at menarche and the characteristics of her menstrual cycle (i.e., length, duration of flow, presence or absence of associated premenstrual symptoms, and ovulatory discomfort or dysmenorrhea). Ask your client about the presence of vaginal discharge, discomfort, or itching and about her preferred method of sanitary protection and level of satisfaction with that method. If the woman is beyond her childbearing years, ask when menopause occurred and whether she has experienced any difficulties with sexual functioning, such as vaginal dryness. If problems have occurred, ask her how she dealt with them.

Obstetric history data are significant and include the number of pregnancies, deliveries, and spontaneous and induced abortions. Note any difficulties the client has experienced conceiving and any history of infertility. Questions about her contraceptive history include the methods used, her satisfaction or dissatisfaction and confidence with each, and partner participation. Be sure to record any history of sexually transmitted disease, including pelvic inflammatory disease.

Obtain a brief description of the client's sexual response cycle. It is important to clarify the degree of lubrication that develops during sexual arousal or if pain occurs during sexual intercourse. Ask the client to describe briefly her present relationship and to rate it with respect to communication, affection, sexual needs met, and sexual communication.

### Sexual Problem History

A sexual problem history is used to supplement a brief sexual history and is obtained within the context of sexual counseling and therapy. It is intended to collect information so that the provider can define the character, etiology, onset, severity, duration, and psychosocial effect of presenting sexual dysfunction. Formats may vary; however, certain commonalities should be explored.

- Description of the problem in the client's own words.
- Exploration of the onset and course of the problem.
- Determination of the client's assessment of the cause and persistence of the problem.
- A description of any past treatment and its results.

- The client's expectations of current therapy.[1]

An indepth sexual history generally includes several factors.

- The nature of the presenting distress.
- Information about the client's present relationship, such as duration, other partners.
- Life cycle influences and events in childhood, adolescence, premarital adulthood, and marriage.
- The client's perception of self.
- The client's response to sensory stimuli.[34]

These histories can generate extensive information about experiences, feelings, sexual practices, and perceptions of self-concept. *History taking requires several hours of interviewing and is conducted only by health professionals with* extensive *training in sexual counseling or therapy.*

### PHYSICAL EXAMINATION

A physical examination is done when indicated by history, presenting concern, treatment goals, or need for referral. Components might be determination of vital signs and a general physical examination, especially an abdominal and pelvic exam including external genitalia and internal genitalia (using a speculum and bimanual techniques).

### DIAGNOSTIC TESTS/METHODS

While no tests are specific to determine sexual assessment, laboratory studies may be indicated when infection is evident. For example, cultures may be done for gonorrhea or chlamydia if there is history of purulent discharge. If a woman complains of dyspareunia and a bladder infection is suspected, the nurse practitioner may elect to obtain a clean catch urine specimen for culture and sensitivity.

## SEXUAL HEALTH INTERVENTIONS: PLISSIT MODEL

The PLISSIT model[35] is a schema for ordering levels of intervention for sexual problems, and is the approach to sexual counseling most used by nurses. It incorporates four levels of counseling: permission, limited information, specific suggestions, and intensive therapy. As the complexity of intervention levels increases, more knowledge and skills are needed. All nurses should be able to provide permission and limited information related to many sexual concerns. Many nurses and all advanced nurse practitioners should also be able to intervene at the specific suggestion level. Intensive therapy, however, requires that nurses be specially trained in sexuality and sex therapy or that the client be referred to experts in sex therapy.

### PERMISSION

The provider gives permission to the client to function sexually as she usually does and to accept herself and her desires. Reassurance is offered that such behaviors are normal. The health care professional may also encourage the woman to talk with her partner. It is important never to give permission for activities that are potentially harmful to a woman.

Permission-giving involves answering questions about sexual fantasies, feelings, and dreams. Inquiring about the effect of developmental changes, illness, or lifestyle alterations may give a woman permission to be a sexual being. Permission giving is particularly useful for a client with a nursing diagnosis of anxiety related to sexual adequacy or sexual dysfunction related to guilt over sexual enjoyment. Examples of interventions at this level include providing permission to be sexually aroused by normal feelings; to engage in safe activities that arouse sexual feelings, such as masturbation and fantasizing; and to have sexual intercourse as often as desired.

## LIMITED INFORMATION

Provide the client with specific facts that are directly related to her area of sexual concern, making sure that the information is immediately relevant and limited in scope. Limited information helps to change potentially negative thoughts and attitudes about specific areas of sexuality and to refute sexual myths.

The purpose of providing limited information about sexual matters is to open the topic of sexual health for the client so that she, in turn, can discuss her concerns with the health care provider. This approach is particularly useful when the nursing diagnosis is knowledge deficit related to sexuality or anxiety related to sexual misinformation.

## SPECIFIC SUGGESTIONS

The health care provider using the specific suggestions approach gives direct behavioral suggestions to relieve a sexual problem that is limited in scope or of brief duration. The client and the health care provider agree on specific goals, and the practitioner offers specific behavioral suggestions. These interventions are followed up after a brief period.

Numerous suggestions can be made, but they are always tailored to an individual's needs and particular situation. For example, a woman with a recent mastectomy might be counseled to use a side-lying position for intercourse to avoid putting pressure on her wound. Or the health care provider might suggest that a postmenopausal woman who is experiencing vaginal dryness and dyspareunia use a water-soluble vaginal lubricant prior to penile penetration. Additional examples of specific suggestions include sensate focus exercises (mutual stimulation of erotic areas excluding the genitals); medication specific to the organism causing vaginal infection; and alternative ways of sexual pleasuring (oral–genital contact, mutual masturbation, cuddling, holding, massage).

Specific suggestions are used when the nursing diagnosis is sexual dysfunction related to pain with intercourse secondary to vaginal infection, or pain related to sexual position secondary to pregnancy, surgery, or other interfering factors.

## INTENSIVE THERAPY

Intensive therapy is used when a client's problems are not relieved by interventions included in the first three levels (permission-giving, limited information, and specific suggestions) or when the problems are personal and emotional difficulties that interfere with sexual expression. Intensive therapy is appropriate for women with a nursing diagnosis of sexual dysfunction related to inhibited female orgasm or to vaginismus. This level of intervention is the most complex and should be undertaken only by professionals with advanced training in sexual counseling and therapy. It is essential that nursing professionals recognize the limits of their own knowledge and refer the client appropriately.

## REFERENCES

1. Bernhard, L. (in press). Sexuality in women's lives. In C.I. Fogel & N.F. Woods (Eds.), *Health care of women* (2nd ed.). Springhouse, PA: Springhouse.
2. Fogel, C.I., & Lauver, D. (1990). *Sexual health promotion*. Philadelphia: Saunders.
3. World Health Organization. (1975). Education and treatment in human sexuality: The training of health professionals. Report of WHO meeting. *Technical Report Series, 572.*

4. Boston Women's Health Book Collective. (1985). *The new our bodies, ourselves.* New York: Simon & Schuster.
5. Kaplan, H. (1979). *Disorders of sexual desire and other new concepts and techniques in sex therapy.* New York: Brunner/Mazel.
6. Masters, W., & Johnson, V. (1966). *The human sexual response.* Boston: Little, Brown.
7. American Psychiatric Association. (1987). *Diagnostic and statistical manual of mental disorders, DSM-III-R* (3rd rev. ed.). Washington, DC: American Psychiatric Press.
8. Heilbrun, A.B. (1981). *Human sex role behavior.* New York: Pergamon Press.
9. Wyatt, G.E. (1989). Reexamining factors predicting Afro-American and white American women's age at first coitus. *Archives of Sexual Behavior, 18,* 271–298.
10. Fine, M., & Asch, A. (1981). Disabled women: Sexism without the pedestal. *Journal of Sociology and Social Welfare, 8,* 233–248.
11. DeHaan, C.B., & Wallander, J.L. (1988). Self-concept, sexual knowledge and attitudes and parental support in the sexual adjustment of women with early- and late-onset physical disability. *Archives of Sexual Behavior, 13,* 233–245.
12. Andersen, B.L., Anderson, B., & deProsse, C. (1989). Controlled prospective longitudinal study of women with cancer: I. Sexual functioning outcomes. *Journal of Consulting and Clinical Psychology, 57,* 683–691.
13. Schover, L.R., Fife, M., & Gershenson, D.M. (1989). Sexual dysfunction and treatment for early stage cervical cancer. *Cancer, 63,* 204–212.
14. Schreiner-Engel, P., Schiavi, R.C., Vietorisz, D., & Smith, H. (1987). The differential impact of diabetes type on female sexuality. *Journal of Psychosomatic Research, 31,* 23–33.
15. Bahen-Ayer, N., Wilson, M., & Assalian, P. (1988). Sexual response of type I diabetic women. *Medical Aspects of Human Sexuality, 22,* 94–100.
16. Gath, D., Cooper, P., & Day, A. (1982). Hysterectomy and psychiatric disorder: I. Levels of psychiatric morbidity before and after hysterectomy. *British Journal of Psychiatry, 140,* 335–350.
17. Bernhard, L.A. (1986). *Sexuality expectations and outcomes in women having hysterectomies.* Unpublished dissertation, University of Illinois at Chicago.
18. Schain, W.S. (1985). Breast cancer surgeries and psychosexual sequelae: Implications for remediation. *Seminars in Oncology Nursing, 1,* 200–205.
19. Kansky, J. (1986). Sexuality of widows: A study of the sexual practices of widows during the first fourteen months of bereavement. *Journal of Sex and Marital Therapy, 12,* 307–321.
20. Malatesta, V.J., Chambless, D.L., Pollack, M., & Cantor, A. (1988). Widowhood, sexuality and aging: A life span analysis. *Journal of Sex and Marital Therapy, 14,* 49–62.
21. Sheaham, S.L. (1989). Identifying female sexual dysfunctions. *Nurse Practitioner, 14,* 25–26, 28, 30, 32, 34.
22. Uddenberg, N. (1974). Psychological aspects of sexual inadequacy in women. *Journal of Psychosomatic Research, 18,* 33–47.
23. Renshaw, D.C. (1983). Recognition and treatment of sexual disorders. *Pennsylvania Medicine, 86,* 64–67.
24. Field, M. (1990). In C.I. Fogel & D. Lauver (Eds.), *Sexual health promotion.* Philadelphia: Saunders.
25. Schover, L., & LoPiccolo, J. (1982). Treatment effectiveness for dysfunctions of sexual desire. *Journal of Sex and Marital Therapy, 8,* 179–197.
26. Seagraves, R.T. (1988). Psychiatric drugs and inhibited female orgasm. *Journal of Sex and Marital Therapy, 15,* 202–207.
27. Barbach, L. (1980). *Women discover orgasm.* New York: Free Press.
28. Lieblum, S.R., Pervin, L.A., & Campbell, E.H. (1989). The treatment of vaginismus: Success and failure. In S.R. Leiblum & R.C. Rosen (Eds.), *Principles and practices of sex therapy* (2nd ed.). New York: Guilford Press.
29. Glatt, A.E., Zinner, S.H., & McCormack, W.M. (1990). The prevalence of dyspareunia. *Obstetrics and Gynecology, 75,* 433–436.

30. Lazarus, A.A. (1989). Dyspareunia: A multimodel perspective. In S.R. Leiblum & R.C. Rosen (Eds.), *Principles and practices of sex therapy* (2nd ed.). New York: Guilford Press.
31. Kaplan, H.S., & Klein, D. (1987). *Sexual aversion, sexual phobias, and panic disorder*. New York: Brunner/Mazel.
32. Bachman, G.A., Leiblum, S.R., & Grill, J. (1989). Brief sexual inquiry in gynecologic practice. *Obstetrics and Gynecology, 73*, 425–427.
33. Woods, N.F. (1984). *Human sexuality in health and illness* (3rd ed). St. Louis: Mosby.
34. Masters, W., & Johnson, V. (1970). *Human sexual inadequacy*. Boston: Little, Brown.
35. Annon, J.S. (1974). *Behavioral treatment of sexual problems: Brief therapy*. New York: Harper & Row.

## BIBLIOGRAPHY

Anderson, W.B. (1986). Use of a "permission giving" patient checklist in identification of social and sexual problems. *Henry Ford Hospital Medical Journal, 34*, 267–269.

Bernhard, L.A. (1988). Women's sexuality. In C.J. Leppa & C. Miller (Eds.), *Women's health perspectives: An annual review. Vol 1.* Phoenix, AZ: Oryx Press.

Chapman, J., & Sughrue, J. (1987). A model for sexual assessment and intervention. *Health Care for Women International, 8*, 87–99.

Collier, P. (1986). Education for sexual self-awareness. In V.J. Littlefield (Ed.), *Health education for women*. Norwalk, CT: Appleton-Century-Crofts.

Fogel, C.I. (1990). Sexual health promotion. In C.I. Fogel & D. Lauver (Eds.), *Sexual health promotion.* Philadelphia: Saunders.

Fogel, C.I., Forker, J., & Welch, M.B. (1990). Sexual health care. In C.I. Fogel & D. Lauver (Eds.), *Sexual health promotion.* Philadelphia: Saunders.

Hunt, A.D., Litt, I.F., & Loebner, M. (1988). Obtaining a sexual history from adolescent girls. *Journal of Adolescent Health Care, 9*, 52-54.

MacElveen-Hoehn, P. (1985). Sexual assessment and counseling. *Seminars in Oncology Nursing, 1*, 69–75.

Morrison-Beedy, D., & Robbins, L. (1989). Sexual assessment and the aging female. *Nurse Practitioner, 14*, 35, 38–39, 42, 45.

Muscari, M.E. (1987). Obtaining the adolescent sexual history. *Pediatric Nursing, 13*, 307–310.

# PROMOTION OF GYNECOLOGIC HEALTH CARE

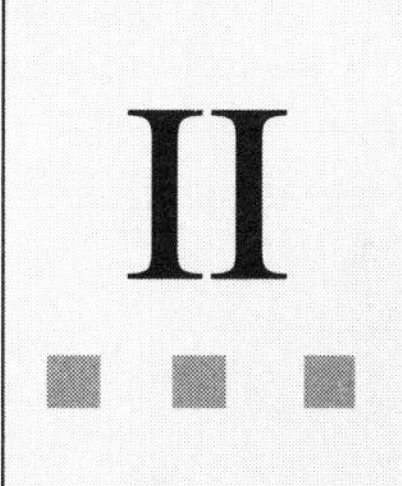

CHAPTER 5

# MENSTRUATION AND RELATED PROBLEMS AND CONCERNS

*Sharon Baker*

*As late as 1985 knowledge of menstrual function remained poor, and attitudes predominantly negative.*

### *Highlights*

- Myths
- Normal Onset and Occurrence
- Amenorrhea
- Dysfunctional Uterine Bleeding
- Dysmenorrhea
- Toxic Shock Syndrome
- Premenstrual Syndrome

## INTRODUCTION

Menstruation is a normal, cyclically recurring event for most women between the approximate ages of 12 and 50. Like childbirth, it usually occurs without major difficulties. Yet our cultural connotation, reflected in lay language describing menstruation as "the curse" or being "on the rag," is predominantly negative. In the past, menstruation was not mentioned openly, but referred to in the code "time of the month." Lack of forthrightness often led to difficulties for young women attempting to access accurate information. The public and professionals alike were uncomfortable discussing the subject, and knowledge about it was generally lacking. But progress has occurred; structured classes about menstruation are being held. Studies, however, continue to demonstrate that knowledge of menstrual function remains poor, and attitudes predominantly negative.[1]

### MYTHS

Historically, menstruation was viewed as a disease rather than a normal condition. Medical treatment during the second half of the 19th century rested on an explicit view of women as fragile and vulnerable, totally dominated by the cyclicity and disability of their reproductive system. Such a view has led many women and men to consider the menstruating woman as weak, suffering, unstable, or physically unable to execute her normal duties competently. Today feminist researchers challenge this view by pointing out many biases in menstrual cycle research. The medical and psychiatric literature on the topic has been charged with sexism and biologic determinism.

### ONSET OF NORMAL MENSES

Events preceding the first menses have a characteristic pattern. *Thelarche*, the development of breast buds, first occurs between ages 9 and 11. It is secondary to the release of pituitary gonadotropins and estrogen. Estrogen lowers vaginal pH to between 4 and 5, and initiates the formation of superficial cells. Then *adrenarche*, the appearance of pubic hair, follows and signals production of androgenic steroids from the adrenal cortex. Axillary hair appears next, followed by the growth spurt. These processes usually take less than 2 years and culminate in *menarche.* American girls usually experience menarche between ages 10 and 14; the average age is 12 years, 9 months.[2,3]

### NORMAL OCCURRENCE OF MENSES

The menstrual cycle will be repeated 300 to 400 times in the life of the human female. Cycles vary in frequency from 21 to 40 days (regularity is normal), bleeding lasts 3 to 8 days; and blood loss averages 30 to 80 mL.[4,5] Small clots are normal; large clots indicate rapid bleeding and inability of fibrinogen to act in the uterus.

*Descriptive Terms for Menstrual Abnormalities*

- Amenorrhea. Absence of menses.
- Oligomenorrhea. Infrequently occurring menses at intervals greater than 35 days.
- Polymenorrhea. Menses at intervals of 21 days or less.
- Hypermenorrhea/Menorrhagia. Regularly occurring bleeding excessive in duration and flow.
- Metrorrhagia. Bleeding occurring irregularly.
- Menometrorrhagia. Excessive, frequent, irregular bleeding.
- Hypomenorrhea. Regular bleeding in less than normal amount.
- Intermenstrual Bleeding. Bleeding at any time between otherwise normal menses.[6]

## ABNORMALITIES RELATED TO THE MENSTRUAL CYCLE

### AMENORRHEA

Amenorrhea is a symptom, not a diagnosis, categorized as primary or secondary. *Primary amenorrhea* is the absence of menses by age 16 whether or not normal growth and secondary sexual characteristics are present, or it is the absence of menses as well as normal growth and signs of secondary sexual characteristics by age 14. *Secondary amenorrhea* is the absence of menses for 3 cycles or 6 months in women who have previously menstruated.[5,7]

#### Epidemiology

***Etiology.*** Etiology includes pregnancy, lactation, and age appropriate menopause, which are by far the most likely causes of amenorrhea and are considered physiological. Among women of reproductive age, amenorrhea that is unrelated to pregnancy may signal stress or a life threatening disease. Causative factors include anatomic deviations, genetic factors, endocrine abnormalities or imbalances, defective enzyme systems, autoimmune diseases, tumors, weight abnormalities, excessive exercise, medications, or past surgery.[7,8]

***Incidence.*** Incidence reports estimate that 5 percent of women of reproductive age have nonphysiological amenorrhea.[8] Irregular menses or the absence of menses is significantly related to severe dieting.[9]

#### Subjective Data

The etiology of amenorrhea is revealed in a woman's history 80 percent of the time. Questions about each of the following areas should be carefully posed.

- Menstrual history includes the following information: age of development of secondary sex characteristics and current status, absence of menarche or age it occurred, date of last menstrual period, symptoms associated with menses, interval between menses, duration and characteristics of flow.
- Past illnesses, hospitalizations, and surgeries should be noted. Chronic diseases such as childhood leukemia, thyroid or adrenal dysfunction, and renal or hepatic disease are recorded, along with a description of radiation therapy, chemotherapy, or surgery, particularly a dilation and curettage (D & C), which can affect the menstrual pattern.
- Obstetric history records the date and course of any pregnancy. Intrauterine or ectopic pregnancy, abortion, and type of delivery are also noted. Postpartum hemorrhage or infection could be a causative factor of amenorrhea.
- Prescription and over-the-counter drugs can affect menstrual function, and a history of oral contraceptives may alter usual patterns. Illicit drug use, smoking, and alcohol intake also can disturb normal cycles.
- Lifestyle evaluation includes eating patterns, weight loss or gain, critical level of body fat, exercise regimens, obesity, anorexia, bulimia, life stressors, and sexual behaviors, including contraception.
- History of present illness (HPI) is an assessment of bodily changes or abnormalities, such as nipple discharge, hirsutism, virilization, absence of menses alternating with heavy bleeding cycles, hot flashes, vaginal dryness, insomnia, headaches, or infertility.[5,8]

## Objective Data

*Physical Examination*

- General Appearance and Skin. Observe carefully and note general body habitus, stage of development of secondary sexual characteristics (see Tanner stages, Chapter 3), amount and distribution of hair and fat, and presence of striae.
- Vital Signs. Gather baseline data, height, weight, and blood pressure and compare with norms.
- Head and Eyes. Perform a complete head-to-toe physical, including a visual field exam.[7]
- Neck. Examine thyroid for nodules or enlargement.
- Breasts. Observe breasts for discharge, then palpate for masses and attempt to express discharge.
- Abdomen. Palpate abdomen for masses or hernias.
- Genitalia/Reproductive. Examine genitalia for obstructive problems, such as imperforate hymen or vaginal septum. Observe the cervix for signs of pregnancy (bluish discoloration or softening). Palpate the uterus and adnexa for signs of pregnancy or tumor.[5,10]
- Endocrine. Assess for signs of androgen excess such as hirsutism, clitoromegaly, or acne. Evaluate hormonal status (estrogen and progesterone) by color of mucous membranes, presence or absence of rugae, amount and consistency of cervical mucus, and presence of ferning. Vaginal cells may be collected for maturation index;[8] however, this test is rarely done today.[5–6] In the normal woman of reproductive age, mucous membranes are pink and moist; rugae are present; and cervical mucus is clear and ferns if estrogen, without progesterone, is present.

*Commonly Recommended Diagnostic Tests and Methods*

- *A pregnancy test should always be done first.* The serum beta human chorionic gonadotropin (β-hCG) test is most accurate, but expensive. Urine testing is usually adequate if the hCG level is not below 25 mIU/mL.

- Thyrotropin (TSH) and thyroxine ($T_4$) are tested to rule out primary hypothyroidism, a relatively rare but easily treatable cause of amenorrhea.[5]
- The prolactin (PRL) test is the primary test for a pituitary tumor.[11] If galactorrhea is present, pituitary or central nervous system lesions are the second most common cause after drugs. Stress can elevate the PRL level; therefore, an elevated result should be confirmed with a second test done in a situation that is as unstressful as possible. If more than 20 ng/dL are detected, repeat the test; if more than 60 ng/dL, order coned down lateral x-ray evaluation of the sella turcica or thin section coronal computed tomography (CT) with intravenous contrast enhancement or magnetic resonance imaging (MRI) head scan to rule out pituitary adenoma.[4,5,8,11]
- If the above three tests—for pregnancy, hypothyroidism, and pituitary tumor—are negative, then administer the progesterone challenge test. Progesterone in oil (100–200 mg I.M.) or medroxyprogesterone acetate (5–10 mg p.o. for 5–10 days) is given to test the presence of estrogen priming and the intactness of the outflow tract (uterus and vagina). If there is no galactorrhea and bleeding occurs in 2–7 days after concluding medication, anovulation is established as the diagnosis.[5]
- If no bleeding occurs with the progesterone challenge, administer estrogen 2.5 mg p.o. for 21 days with the addition of medroxyprogesterone acetate 10 mg p.o. for the last 5 days of estrogen administration. Bleeding after medications rules out defects of the outflow tract.[5]
- If no bleeding occurs after this regimen, repeat medications. Then, if no bleeding occurs, a diagnosis of defective uterus or outflow tract can be made. This is a relatively rare diagnosis with no history of infection or trauma in clients whose pelvic exam findings are normal.[5]
- If the history includes D & C or uterine infection, but no bleeding with an initial administration of estrogen and medroxyprogesterone or repeated regimen, then order a hysterosalpingogram or hysteroscopy to rule out Asherman's syndrome (intrauterine adhesions).
- If withdrawal bleeding occurs with the administration of estrogen and medroxyprogesterone, then the reason for the client's inability to produce adequate levels of estrogen must be determined. Various ovarian and ovarian/adrenal factors are evaluated.

*Ovarian*

- *Follicle-Stimulating Hormone (FSH).* A level greater than 40 mIU/mL indicates ovarian failure.[5,8]
- *Luteinizing Hormone (LH).* A normal LH level with a high FSH level indicates impending ovarian failure.
- *LH–FSH Ratio.* A value of greater than 2.5 mIU/mL suggests polycystic ovaries.[5,8]
- *Autoimmune Dysfunction.* This is associated with premature ovarian failure. Measure thyroid antibodies to rule out thyroiditis; serum calcium and phosphorous to rule out hypoparathyroidism; and random glucose to rule out diabetes. Additional screening may be done to rule out autoimmune dysfunction: sedimentation rate, antinuclear antibodies, complete blood cell (CBC) count with differential, rheumatoid factor, total serum protein, and albumin–globulin ratio.[8]

*Ovarian/Adrenal*

- *Total Testosterone.* Levels greater than 200 ng/dL suggest a tumor; the adrenal or ovarian source should be determined.[5,8]
- *Dehydroepiandrosterone Sulfate (DHEA-S).* A level greater than 700 μg/dL suggests an adrenal disorder or tumor.[5,8]

- *Cortisol Level.* Order this test if Cushing's stigmata are present, in order to screen for adrenal hyperactivity.

- *Karyotype.* Order this test if genetic or chromosomal abnormalities are suspected.[6]
- *CBC, Coagulation Profile, Serum Iron, or Ferritin.* These tests may be ordered to rule out anemia or clotting disorders.

## Differential Medical Diagnoses

*Pregnancy Related*
- Pregnancy, lactation, or pregnancy complications such as ectopic pregnancy, missed abortion, postpartum hemorrhage, or trophoblastic neoplasm.

*Hypothalamic–Pituitary–Ovarian (HPO) Axis Related*
- Anovulation secondary to immature HPO axis, obesity, or polycystic ovaries.
- Premature ovarian failure secondary to genetic conditions, smoking, chemotherapy, radiation, surgery, ovarian insensitivity to gonadotropins (Savage syndrome), or steroidogenic enzyme defect, 17 $\alpha$-hydroxylase deficiency.
- Menopause secondary to age-appropriate follicular depletion.
- Hypoestrogenemia secondary to anorexia nervosa, bulimia, or excessive exercise.
- Hyperprolactinemia secondary to pituitary tumor, stress, or thyroid disorder, or drug induced.
- Inhibited gonadotropin-releasing hormone (GnRH) secondary to discontinuation of oral contraceptives or use of medications such as danazol or hypothalamic defects.

*Obstructive Related*
- Imperforate hymen.
- Transverse vaginal septum.
- Cervical stenosis following instrumentation or trauma.

*Genetic/Chromosome Related*
- Mayer-Rokintansky-Küster-Hauser syndrome (no apparent vagina).
- Testicular feminization (complete or incomplete).
- Gonadal dysgenesis (Turner's syndrome, Swyer's syndrome).

*Autoimmune Disorders*

*Asherman's Syndrome*
- See References 3, 5, 6, 8, 10.

## Plan

***Psychosocial Interventions.*** The health care provider must address the diverse causes of amenorrhea, the relationship to sexual identity, perception of normal menstrual function, possible infertility, tumor, or life-threatening disease. Sensitive listening and interviewing and individualized evaluation are essential. Always consider the possibility of pregnancy and related emergencies, despite the client's history or social situation. If karyotyping is necessary, then order the tests and explain the result with great care to avoid further trauma.

***Medication.*** The medication prescribed varies with the client situation. Combination oral contraceptives are superior to progesterone-only treatment in a sexually active, nonsmoking client who is younger than 35. Cyclic progesterone may be preferred when estrogen is contraindicated.

*Medroxyprogesterone Acetate (MPA)*
- Indications are to prevent endometrial hyperplasia by causing cyclic shedding in anovulatory clients who do not need contraception.[5]
- Administer 10 mg p.o. the first 10 to 14 days of each month or during cycle days 16 to 26.
- Side effects and adverse reactions most commonly reported include spotting, weight gain, fatigue, depression, or acne.

- Contraindications include pregnancy, thromboembolic disorders, liver dysfunction, known or suspected malignancy of breast or reproductive organs, undiagnosed vaginal bleeding, or missed abortion. The use of medroxyprogesterone acetate (MPA) as a diagnostic test for pregnancy is also contraindicated.
- Anticipated outcome on evaluation is that the client begins cyclic withdrawal spotting or bleeding 2 to 7 days after completing medication.
- Client teaching should include information about the possibility of bleeding being heavy when medication is completed. Emphasize the importance of taking the medication to prevent endometrial hyperplasia or cancer, and for long term protection of the breasts and bones. Inform the client of side effects and tell her to report any abnormal bleeding or the absence of withdrawal bleeding. Stress the necessity of consistently using reliable birth control measures.

*Low-Dose Combination Oral Contraceptives*

- Indications are to prevent endometrial hyperplasia *and* to provide contraception for clients with anovulatory cycles (first choice of therapy).
- Administer 21- or 28-day pack cyclic therapy.
- Side effects and adverse reactions most commonly reported include breast tenderness, weight gain, spotting, and scanty menses.
- Contraindications are pregnancy, undiagnosed vaginal bleeding, history of breast or reproductive tract cancer, history of thromboembolism, cerebrovascular or coronary heart disease, liver tumor or malignancy, or smoker older than 35.[12]
- Anticipated outcomes on evaluation are cyclic withdrawal bleeding, contraception, and absence of side effects of MPA.
- Client teaching and counseling should include information about how to take pills and manage missed pills, and the danger signs (see Chapter 6). Instruct the client to chart dates of menses or spotting.

*Hormone Replacement Therapy*

- Indications are premature or physiological menopause to help prevent osteoporosis, vaginal dryness, hot flashes, insomnia, headaches, and mood changes[5,8] (as a first choice of treatment).
- Implications (see Chapter 11).

*Other*

- Other medication regimens should be managed by physician referral or with physician consultation, because of the complex etiology of amenorrhea.

***Surgical Interventions.*** Endometrial biopsy—curette or flushing of endometrial cells for microscopic examination—may be done to evaluate the uterus for atrophy, phase of endometrium, or abnormalities, although the test is not commonly done unless prior tests and treatments yield no answer to the problem. It is an outpatient procedure.

Client teaching and counseling include informing the client about the purpose of the biopsy, how the procedure is to be performed, relaxation techniques, follow-up, and the monetary cost.

***Follow-Up.*** Follow-up is done annually. Prior to refilling medications, evaluate the client's menstrual charts, the client's adherence to the medication schedule, the presence of danger signs or side effects, and the results of the Pap test and breast exam/mammography. Refer all clients with primary amenorrhea for physician evaluation. Reassure young amenorrheic teens and their parents; recommend "watchful waiting" if results of tests are normal. Refer all clients with secondary amenorrhea caused by central lesions, autoimmune diseases, psychiatric problems, or complex endocrine or metabolic diseases to a physician for evaluation and management.

## DYSFUNCTIONAL UTERINE BLEEDING (DUB)

Dysfunctional uterine bleeding (DUB) is uterine bleeding generally associated with a "disruption in normal ovarian function and consequent failure of ovulation."[13] DUB is not related to pregnancy, inflammation, genital tumor, or other anatomic uterine lesion.[13,14] "Anovulatory uterine bleeding" is a more meaningful term than "DUB."

### Epidemiology

***Etiology.*** Etiology is usually a hormonal disturbance, basically, failure of ovarian follicular maturation with resulting lack of progesterone production, limitation of endometrial growth, and synchronous shedding. Chronic anovulation with continuous estrogen production increases endometrial vascularity and thickness without adequate stromal support for maintenance. Irregular spotting and episodes of profuse and usually painless bleeding result. An atrophic endometrium that bleeds irregularly can be formed by lack of estrogen due to menopause or formed pharmacologically through long term use of low-dose birth control pills. Excessive fibrinolytic activity and changes in prostaglandin also appear to be associated with DUB. Excessive use of acetylsalicylic acid (aspirin) can increase bleeding.[14]

***Incidence.*** Incidence of dysfunctional uterine bleeding is attributed to anovulation in 90 percent of cases and occurs most commonly during puberty and the perimenopausal years.[14]

### Subjective Data

A history of irregular menses is typically exhibited as episodes of heavy painless bleeding alternating with periods of amenorrhea. Assess whether excessive blood loss has occurred; dizziness, fainting, and lightheadedness when standing are important clues.[10] Note passing tissue and test specimens if available and suspicious.

### Objective Data

Although no organic problems are associated with DUB, a complete physical examination, including pelvic and rectal exams, is performed to rule out neoplasia.

Diagnostic tests and methods include a CBC and Pap smear to rule out abnormalities. In a woman of reproductive age, particularly if unilateral abdominal pain is present, a serum ß-hCG test and ultrasound should be done to rule out an ectopic pregnancy. If blood dyscrasias are suspected, a coagulation evaluation is done.[7]

*In-Office Endometrial Biopsy*

- This diagnostic evaluation is done to determine the cytologic status of endometrial tissue.[6,14] The biopsy is recommended for all women older than 30 who are chronically anovulatory.
- Test procedure involves helping the client to assume lithotomy position. Then a small curette is passed through the cervix to the endometrium cavity in order to obtain a small amount of tissue for examination.
- Nursing implications and client teaching involve informing the client about the purpose of the test, obtaining her signature on the consent form, and explaining the cost of the procedures. Encourage relaxation breathing and convey the progression of each step to the client to alleviate her discomfort and anxiety.

*Hysteroscopy*

- *Hysteroscopy* is visualization of the endometrium through a scope.[15] The observation and directed tissue sampling is replacing D & C as the diagnostic procedure of choice. (Minor treatments, such as polyp or septal removal, also can be done through the hysteroscope.)
- The procedure is done in the office or operating room. The hysteroscope is inserted

when the cervix is dilated. The uterus is distended with dextran 70, carbon dioxide, or another distention medium to facilitate visualization of the endometrium.

- Nursing implications include teaching the client that some cramps and bleeding are expected following the procedure, and leakage of dextran 70 through the cervix and vagina can be messy. Carbon dioxide distention may cause cramps or shoulder pain. Pain medications should be provided. *Advise the client to report signs of infection, excessive bleeding, or pain—and to report any allergic response that occurs with dextran 70 at once.*

*Hysterosalpingography*

- Hysterosalpingography is done to detect defects of the uterine cavity, tubes, and peritubal area.[14,15]
- The procedure is performed in the operating room with the client in lithotomy position. A radiographic dye is injected through the cervix. The uterine cavity, tubes, and peritubal area are then viewed for defects and the filling and spillage pattern. Usually anesthesia is not required.[15]
- Nursing implications are to explain the procedure, risks, and rationale for the test and to rule out the client's allergy to dye. Obtain the client's written consent. Tell her about possible cramping. Throughout the procedure watch for allergic reactions to dye and encourage relaxation breathing. If cramping or pain occurs, provide pain medications and follow-up instructions—including the need to wear a perineal pad and to report signs of infection and/or excessive bleeding or pain.

*Dilation and Curettage (D & C)*

- Dilation of the cervix and curettage (D & C) may be done for diagnostic evaluation. Endometrial D & C is recommended when medical regimens are ineffective, or if polyps, incomplete abortion, or neoplasia is suspected, or if a more complete biopsy sampling of the endometrium may be desired and hysteroscopy is unavailable.
  - The procedure requires that the client be given local or general anesthesia and that specimens be sent to pathology.
  - Nursing implications are to provide appropriate explanations of the procedure, anesthesia, cost, and risks. Postoperative instructions are given, advising the client to report signs of infection, excessive bleeding, and/or pain. Pain medication is also provided.

## Differential Medical Diagnoses

Any early pregnancy disorder or ectopic pregnancy; fibroids/adenomyosis; endometrial polyps/carcinoma; endometriosis, coagulation defects (diagnosed in 20 percent of adolescents with DUB); ovarian abnormalities (polycystic ovaries, tumors); thyroid dysfunction; massive obesity; stress; drugs (anticoagulants, steroids, phenothiazides, digitalis, diet pills, anticholinergics).[3,5,7,13]

## Plan

***Psychosocial Interventions.*** Educate the client about normal menstrual cycles and possible reasons for her abnormal pattern. Be generous with reassurance. Menstrual calendars are helpful with instruction given about documenting any bleeding or spotting, days and dosages of medications, pad or tampon count, and associated symptoms of dysmenorrhea. By providing information about expected bleeding patterns on discontinuation of medications you will help the client to avoid fears of recurrence or treatment failure. Because some medications are teratogenic, it is important to address birth control.

### *Medication*

- A low dose combination oral contraceptive (OC) is the first choice of therapy for anovulatory bleeding in clients who need contraception.

- A requirement for beginning therapy is to rule out pregnancy prior to prescribing.
- Prescribe one 35 μg pill q.i.d. for from 5 to 7 days. Continue oral contraceptives in usual fashion for 3 to 6 months.[8,13]
- Side effects and adverse reactions most commonly reported include breast tenderness, weight gain, spotting, and scanty menses.
- Contraindications are pregnancy, undiagnosed vaginal bleeding, history of breast or reproductive tract cancer, history of thromboembolism, cerebrovascular or coronary heart disease, liver tumor or malignancy, or smoker older than 35.[12]
- Anticipated outcome on evaluation is that bleeding will abate in 12–14 hours.

  Client Teaching and Counseling. If bleeding does not abate, consult a physician. If an anovulatory pattern returns after discontinuing OCs, then resume the low dose combination pills or progesterone therapy described below.

- Medroxyprogesterone acetate (MPA) is indicated for clients with anovulatory bleeding who do not need contraception.[13] If contraception is needed, barrier methods are advised with this treatment.
  - A requirement for beginning therapy is to rule out pregnancy.
  - Prescribe MPA 10 mg q.d. for 10–14 days for a medical "D & C."

    Endometrial maturation and cyclic shedding can be maintained by prescribing 10 mg of progesterone on days 1 through 10–14 of each month, or cycle days 16–25.[4,13]
  - Side effects and adverse reactions most commonly reported include spotting, weight gain, fatigue, depression, or acne.
  - Contraindications include pregnancy, thromboembolic disorders, liver dysfunction, known or suspected malignancy of breast or reproductive organs, undiagnosed vaginal bleeding, or missed abortion. The use of medroxyprogesterone acetate (MPA) as a diagnostic test for pregnancy is also contraindicated.
  - Anticipated outcome on evaluation is that the first episode of bleeding after progesterone therapy will be heavy.
  - Client teaching should include information about the possibility of bleeding being heavy when medication is completed. Emphasize the importance of taking medication to prevent endometrial hyperplasia or cancer, and for long term protection of the breasts and bones. Inform the client of side effects and tell her to report any abnormal bleeding or the absence of withdrawal bleeding. Stress the necessity of consistently using reliable birth control measures.
- Estrogens may be needed if bleeding is heavy and endometrial support is indicated.[5,13,15,16]
  - Intravenous conjugated estrogen 25 mg q.4h. up to 3 doses until bleeding lessens. If bleeding initially is less, use 1.25 mg q.d. p.o. conjugated estrogen for 7 to 10 days. Follow either of these regimes with progestin treatment.[5]
  - Conjugated estrogens, 0.625–1.25 mg p.o. for days 1–25 of each month with MPA 10 mg p.o. days 12–25 of each month; *or*
  - Conjugated estrogens 1.25/day p.o. for 7–10 days.[13,16]
- Prostaglandin synthetase inhibitors (PGSIs) are a nonhormonal treatment of menorrhagia.
  - A requirement for beginning therapy is that pregnancy be ruled out. Prescribe mefenamic acid (Ponstel) 500 mg p.o. t.i.d. for 3 days *or* naproxen (Naprosyn) 500 mg p.o. stat., then 250 mg p.o. of

same t.i.d. for 5 days beginning the first day of menses. Instruct the client to take the medication with food.[14]

- Side effects and adverse reactions include gastrointestinal upset, rash, and edema.
- Contraindications include pregnancy, peptic ulcers, asthma, sensitivity to aspirin, and inflammatory bowel disease.
- Anticipated outcome on evaluation is a 50 percent reduction in bleeding.
- Client teaching and counseling should include the precaution to take the medication with food. Instruct the client about the dosing regimen and the side effects of the drug.
- GnRH agonist has been used in some women to totally suppress the hypothalamic pituitary axis and stop bleeding. This extreme measure is used if the woman cannot undergo D & C.[17]

#### *Surgical Interventions*

- D & C or hysteroscopy may be used as a treatment intervention as well as a diagnostic procedure.[15]
- Hysterectomy is a radical procedure in which the uterus is removed. The surgery is reserved for perimenopausal women who fail to improve with hormonal therapy or for adolescents with severe blood dyscrasia.
- Endometrial ablation is a technique to end bleeding difficulties by laser destruction of the endometrium through a hysteroscope.[14,16] The uterus is not removed.

Explain all surgical procedures to the client carefully, including their purpose, risks, benefits, and cost. Before and after surgery, give instructions about pain medication, the expected postoperative course, and the follow-up schedule.

***Follow-Up.*** Follow-up and referral may include iron therapy; 300 mg ferrous sulfate may be taken by mouth with orange juice 30 minutes after meals in addition to the therapy described above if the hemoglobin level is below 12 g. Anovulatory patterns tend to recur; therefore, clients should have a regular follow-up schedule and keep a menstrual and medication calendar. If more than a year elapses without a health care visit, notify the client. Cancer prevention should be a priority with this population.

## DYSMENORRHEA

Dysmenorrhea is crampy lower abdominal pain before and/or during menstruation. It is categorized as primary or secondary. Primary dysmenorrhea is usually without pelvic pathology; on the other hand, secondary dysmenorrhea is frequently accompanied by pelvic pathology.[18,19]

### Epidemiology

***Etiology.*** Primary dysmenorrhea occurs once ovulatory cycles are established and results from excessive prostaglandin release. Secondary dysmenorrhea is most frequently caused by endometriosis, intrauterine devices (IUDs), or pelvic infection.[20] Endometriosis is thought to cause nearly half of all cases of secondary dysmenorrhea. Etiology may be obstructive defects, such as cervical stenosis, imperforate hymen, or müllerian defects, if pain begins at menarche rather than after a regular pattern of cycling is established.

***Incidence.*** Incidence of primary dysmenorrhea is approximately 50 percent of menstruating women.[19] Of these women, 10 percent are "incapacitated for from one to three days each month."[19]

### Subjective Data

*Primary dysmenorrhea* typically presents in ovulatory cycles 6–12 months following menarche, and is most commonly diagnosed in adolescents.[20] Pain is suprapubic and described as "crampy;" it starts 12–24 hours before menses and is intermittent, except in severe cases. Pain is most severe during the first day of menses and disappears in 48–72 hours. The lower abdomen is most painful, but frequently pain extends to the back and thighs. Related molimina include fatigue, headaches, abdominal bloating, and occasionally nausea, vomiting, or syncope.[20]

*Secondary dysmenorrhea* typically presents in women with a history of painful menses that are increasingly intense or severe. It occurs most commonly in the third or fourth decades of life. Usually the location or duration of pain changes. Endometriosis presents with suprapubic pain that may begin a few days or weeks prior to menses. Associated symptoms are frequently dyspareunia, painful defecation, rectal pressure, cycle less than 27 days with duration of bleeding more than 7 days, and/or infertility.[15,18,20]

## Objective Data

***Physical Examination.*** A thorough pelvic exam is mandatory to establish a diagnosis. With primary dysmenorrhea pelvic findings will be completely within normal limits.[19] Secondary dysmenorrhea, however, may reveal an assortment of pelvic pathologies, depending on the etiology of the problem:

- Endometriosis may present with a normal pelvic exam[15] or the examination may reveal small bluish endometrial lesions on the labia, cervix, or vaginal walls; a fixed, tender, retroverted uterus; tenderness or nodularity of the uterosacral ligaments, of the cul-de-sac, or above the posterior fornix of the vagina; and/or the ovaries may be enlarged, tender, or fixed.[18,20]
- Adenomyosis will often present as an enlarged globular uterus, particularly in women who are in their 40s or 50s.[19]
- Leiomyoma will present as an irregular or enlarged uterus and may be tender.[15]
- Infection will present with discharge, adnexal tenderness, and/or uterine tenderness. Fever may be present.
- Pelvic inflammation is associated with pelvic tenderness, a history of dyspareunia, and bleeding between cycles.[15]

### *Diagnostic Tests and Methods*

#### Variety of Tests

- Diagnostic evaluation to detect specific infection: Gonorrhea, chlamydia, herpes, tuberculosis, and/or ureaplasma cultures[19]; wet mounts for clue cells and/or white blood cells.
- Test procedure (see Chapters 3 and 8).
- Nursing implications are to explain the purpose of the culture or test, the actual procedure, and the cost of specimen collection.

#### Ultrasound (Vaginal)[19]

- Diagnostic evaluation to diagnose pelvic abnormalities: myomas, ovarian cysts, congenital malformations.
- Nursing implications are to explain the necessity of a full bladder for visualization and to teach the client about ultrasound, its purpose, and its cost.

#### Laparoscopy

- Diagnostic evaluation to stage and grade endometriosis if treatment fails or fertility workup is desired.
- The procedure is done with the client in lithotomy position in the operating room using local or general anesthesia. An intrauterine manipulator is used to promote visibility. A small subumbilical incision is made and the laparoscope inserted to visualize the pelvic organs. Carbon dioxide or nitrous oxide is used to insufflate the pelvic region. Some surgery can be performed through the laparoscope.[15]
- Nursing implications are to explain to the client the types of anesthesia, what the pro-

cedure entails, the risks, recovery, and the activity schedule that will follow surgery. Obtain the client's written consent for the laparoscopy, and prescribe pain medication p.r.n.

***Hysterosalpingogram, Hysteroscopy, or D & C***

See Dysfunctional Uterine Bleeding (DUB), Objective Data.

*Barium Enema*

- Diagnostic evaluation done to rule out bowel pathology.
- Test procedure, generally outpatient, begins with barium enema followed by fluoroscopic and radiographic examination of the large intestine.
- Nursing implications and client teaching include explanations of preparation, procedure, follow-up, and test results.

*Urinalysis*

- Diagnostic evaluation done to rule out bladder pathology.
- Client teaching includes explanations of the procedure and its purpose, the cost, and the results.

## Differential Medical Diagnoses

- Obstructive Defects. Cervical stenosis; imperforate hymen; congenital disorders of the müllerian tract.
- Endometriosis.
- Other Differential Diagnoses. Adenomyosis, pain secondary to an IUD, fibroids, endometrial polyps or carcinoma, pelvic inflammatory disease, urinary tract infection, infected rectal fissures, uterine malformations, ilioinguinal neuralgia, pelvic prolapse, pelvic tumors, pelvic congestion.[3,15]

## Plan

***Psychosocial Interventions.*** Helping the client to understand the normal events surrounding the menstrual cycle and the etiology of the dysmenorrhea is an important part of intervention. In addition, intervention is directed toward pain relief and the coping strategies that will promote a productive lifestyle. Explaining the normal menstrual cycle will provide the client with the vocabulary to communicate more accurately about symptoms, and it will help to dispel myths. Give the client charts to record menses, onset of pain, timing of medication, relief afforded by the medication, and relationship of pain to basal body temperature. Charts are a teaching tool; they provide the client with a realistic picture of her pain and an objective record for modifying future therapy.

Carefully explain the nature and severity of the pathology associated with secondary dysmenorrhea. Discuss in detail the rationales for selecting particular tests, treatments, medications, or surgery; this will enhance client understanding and compliance. Be sure to address the impact that the disease and treatment will have on fertility.

***Medication***

*Prostaglandin Synthetase Inhibitors (PGSIs)*

- First choice of therapy for primary dysmenorrhea in clients not needing contraception. Administer these drugs to relieve pain; they prevent the synthesis of prostaglandins, thereby stopping uterine hypercontractility and ischemia and restoring normal function. Commonly prescribed inhibitors include ibuprofen 200–400 mg p.o. q. 4–6 hours; naproxen sodium 550 mg p.o. stat., then 275 mg p.o. q. 6–12 hours; diflunisal 1000 mg p.o. stat., then 500 mg p.o. b.i.d.; mefenamic acid 500 mg p.o. stat., then 250 mg p.o. q. 6 hours; ketoprofen 25–50 mg p.o. q. 6–8 hours.[4,18] Instruct the client to begin the medication 24 hours prior to menses or at the earliest sign of menses, and to take the medication with food.

- Side effects and adverse reactions include gastrointestinal upset, rash, and edema.
- PGSIs may be teratogenic; therefore, they are contraindicated in pregnancy. Also, peptic ulcers, asthma, aspirin sensitivity, and inflammatory bowel disease are contraindications.
- Anticipated outcome on evaluation is relief of pain. The client should use one drug for a minimum of 2–4 cycles before evaluating effectiveness. If pain is not relieved, choose another PGSI, preferably from a different pharmacological group (e.g., naproxen sodium versus ibuprofen). If no relief occurs after another 2–4 months, initiate oral contraceptive therapy.
- Client teaching and counseling are the same as for DUB. Tell the client to take the medication with food. Give instructions about the dosing regimen and the side effects of the drug.

*Low-Dose Combination Oral Contraceptives*

- Indication as first choice of therapy is for primary dysmenorrhea in clients who need contraception. Among women who have primary dysmenorrhea, 90 percent are relieved by using an oral contraceptive. Its use also can decrease the necessary dose of PGSI.
- Administer low-dose combination oral contraceptives to reduce pain through the suppression of ovulation and endometrial proliferation. This reduces menstrual fluid volume and prostaglandin production to below normal.
- Side effects, adverse reactions, and contraindications are the same as for amenorrhea (see p. 82).
- Anticipated outcome on evaluation is relief of 90 percent of primary dysmenorrhea with oral contraceptives.
- Client teaching and counseling should include information about how to take pills and manage missed pills, and the danger signs (see Chapter 6). Instruct the client to chart dates of menses or spotting.

Combined low-dose oral contraceptives and PGSI treatment may be needed for some women.[4]

***Surgical Interventions.*** One of several surgical procedures may be needed. Laparoscopy is recommended if medical treatment fails after a 6- to 12-month trial period. A D & C to correct cervical stenosis or remove endometrial polyps is sometimes necessary. Uterosacral ligament division or a hysterectomy is considered a last resort therapy to relieve intractable pain.

***Lifestyle Changes.*** Share information about lifestyle factors that can be initiated to restore some sense of control and alleviate the sense of frustration and victimization. For example, exercise increases endorphins, suppresses prostaglandin release, raises the estrone–estradiol ratio that decreases endometrial proliferation, and shunts blood away from the uterus; pelvic congestion and pain are thereby decreased. Menus can be planned to limit salty foods, increase fiber with fresh fruits and vegetables, and increase water to serve as a natural diuretic. Heating pads or warm baths decrease muscle spasms and may increase comfort. Relaxation techniques can supplement medication regimens and enhance the client's ability to deal with pain. Support groups may provide reassurance and alternative methods of pain relief such as massage and effleurage.

***Follow-Up.*** Follow-up of clients with primary dysmenorrhea can be done on a regular gynecologic exam schedule, once a medical regimen has been found that relieves pain adequately and is well tolerated. Follow clients with secondary dysmenorrhea according to the diagnosis, the type of medication prescribed, and the need for investigative or therapeutic surgery. Because treatment of secondary dysmenorrhea is more varied and may involve infertility issues, much client education and reassurance is needed. Explain each procedure carefully, and allow adequate time for questioning.

## TOXIC SHOCK SYNDROME (TSS)

Toxic shock syndrome (TSS) can be a potentially lethal disorder that affects many systems.[21] It is caused in almost all cases by absorption of one or more toxins produced by colonized *Staphylococcus aureus*.[15,22]

### Epidemiology

The etiology of TSS shows that young (particularly ages 15–19), white, menstruating females using tampons are at highest risk.[23] Initial studies found that significantly more women with menstrual TSS had used tampons than women in the control group, and women with TSS used tampons 24 hours per day during menstruation, significantly longer than did controls. Several mechanisms are *implicated* as causative, although no causation has been proved.

- Alterations in the normal vaginal flora.
- Mechanical blockage of menstrual fluids.
- Tampon contamination with *S. aureus*.
- Absorption of bacteriostatic cervical secretions.
- The superabsorbent or synthetic materials of which tampons are made.
- Damaged cervical and vaginal mucosa.
- Enhanced multiplication of the organism in the menstrual efflux.

TSS is usually associated with tampon use, but it also has been reported with prolonged contraceptive sponge or diaphragm use, after laser surgery for condylomata acuminatum, postpartum, and following nongynecologic surgery. It also has been reported in children and adult men.[15,22,24]

Approximately 88 percent of reported cases of TSS among women have occurred during menstruation. Incidence is 1 or 2 per 100,000 per year in women using tampons or barrier contraceptives. The overall fatality rate among persons with TSS has been 4.4 percent. Incidence has decreased steadily as a result of education, altered patterns of tampon use, and removal of extremely high absorbency tampons from the market.[22]

### Subjective Data

An abrupt onset of symptoms occurs, including high fever of about 104° F (40° C), chills, vomiting, watery diarrhea, myalgia, headaches, or abdominal pain in a previously healthy young woman during or shortly after menstruation. Some complaints of watery discharge, aching muscles, bloodshot eyes, or a sore throat may also occur. The most characteristic symptom is a sunburn-like rash that progresses to desquamation. Multisystemic involvement is typical; hemodynamic instability is prominent.

### Objective Data

*Physical Examination*

- Vital signs include a temperature of 102° F or higher; systolic blood pressure of less than 90 mm Hg. An orthostatic drop in pressure of 15 mm Hg or more may occur when moving from a lying to sitting position.
- Skin may show a sunburn-like rash that desquamates 1 or 2 weeks after onset of the illness, especially on the palms and soles. Many clients have conjunctival hyperemia, oropharyngeal erythema, strawberry tongue, vaginal hyperemia.
- Nonspecific abdominal tenderness may be found.
- Neurological findings are general confusion and disorientation without focal neurological findings.

- Multisystemic involvement occurs. At least three organ systems must be involved, with no evidence of another cause.[22]

*Diagnostic Tests and Methods*

- CBC with Differential. A platelet count of 100,000/mm$^3$ or less.
- Serum Electrolyte and Chemistry Determinations. Total bilirubin, serum aspartate aminotransferase, and serum alanine aminotransferase values are twice the upper limit of normal.
- Serology for Syphilis. Negative.
- Cultures. Wound, throat, vagina, cervix, blood, cerebrospinal fluid, and tampons or sponges removed. Ascertain if negative for organisms other than *S. aureus*.

## Differential Medical Diagnoses

Rocky Mountain spotted fever, leptospirosis, meningococcal meningitis, Kawasaki disease, scarlet fever, or septic shock; viral gastroenteritis or pelvic inflammatory disease.[22]

## Plan

***Psychosocial Interventions.*** Stress the importance of seeking care quickly. Most clients require intensive care in the hospital. Reassure the client that most clients suffer no apparent long term effects. Inform her that the menstrual TSS recurrence rate is approximately 30 percent and can be reduced by continuing antibiotics and avoiding tampon use.[22]

### *Medications*

*Antistaphylococcal Antibiotics*

- Indications are to treat *Staphylococcus aureus* toxin.
- Beta-lactamase-resistant antibiotic therapy is used. Included antibiotics are the cephalosporins, clindamycin, vancomycin, and penicillinase-resistant penicillins.[26]
- Administration of nafcillin sodium, cephalosporins, or vancomycin hydrochloride is recommended and given for 7–14 days.
- Side effects and adverse reactions include acute or delayed allergic reaction to therapy, neurotoxicity, hepatotoxicity, or renal damage.
- Contraindications include hypersensitivity to penicillin. Use with caution in clients with significant allergies or asthma.[25]
- Anticipated outcome on evaluation is a decrease in the rate of menstrual TSS recurrence. No drug benefit has been proven for the acute illness.
- Client teaching and counseling should include information about bacteriologic studies that are done to determine causative organisms and susceptibility. With prolonged therapy, periodic assessment of renal, hepatic, and hematopoietic systems should be done. Blood cultures, white blood cell count, and differential cell counts should be obtained prior to therapy and continued at least weekly.

***Intravenous Fluid Replacement.*** Aggressive intravenous fluid replacement is necessary when capillary leakage, fever, vomiting, and diarrhea cause volume depletion.

***Follow-Up.*** Follow-up includes providing the client with information: Inform her that subsequent attacks of TSS usually develop within 2–3 months. Encourage compliance with antibiotics. Discourage tampon use; however, if tampons are used, they should be used intermittently with pads (e.g., tampons during the day and pads at night). Changing tampons more frequently does not decrease the risk of TSS. Advise the client to use caution when using contraceptive sponges or a diaphragm and to adhere to the manufacturer's directions. *Advise her that if fever, vomiting, or diarrhea develops during a menstrual period, she must remove the tampon and seek medical care immediately.*[22]

## PREMENSTRUAL SYNDROME (PMS)

*Premenstrual syndrome* (PMS) is a "cyclic recurrence" of a combination of distressing physical, psychological, and behavioral changes during the luteal phase of the menstrual cycle.[26,27] A range of symptoms is associated with the syndrome, and various techniques are used for diagnosis and treatment. PMS is a cause of personal anguish for many women.

Premenstrual dysphoric disorder (PMDD) is included in the appendix of the *Diagnostic and Statistical Manual of Mental Disorders (DSM-IV).*[28] The appendix is entitled "Criteria Sets and Axes Provided for Further Study." The inclusion does not constitute its designation as an official diagnostic category, according to the American Psychiatric Association, but it does encourage further psychiatric research into PMDD.

Contrary to recent misstatements that have been published and broadcast, PMDD, which is a rare condition, is not comparable to PMS. PMS is not included in *DSM-IV.*[28]

The recommendations for PMDD in *DSM-IV* differ little from those in *DSM-III-R.* In 1986, PMDD was included in *DSM-III-R* as *late luteal phase dysphoric disorder* (LLPDD); PMDD and LLPPD are the same entity.[28]

### Epidemiology

***Etiology.*** The etiology of PMS is nebulous, and many theories abound.[15] Research is inconclusive because many definitions are used. Sampling has been primarily with client populations, rather than a broader sampling of the community, and diagnosis may be by retrospective or prospective reporting and then compared. PMS is "a complex disorder generally agreed to be linked to the cyclic activity of the hypothalamic-pituitary-ovarian axis; interactions between ovarian steroid hormones, endogenous opioid peptides, central neurotransmitters, prostaglandins, and peripheral autonomic and endocrine systems."[29]

The etiologies of PMS that have been proposed and debated include hormone imbalances, particularly an estrogen excess and a progesterone deficiency. More recently, the notion of estrogen deficiency at the time of symptoms, namely midcycle, and during the week prior to menses has been implicated.

Nutritional deficiencies have been proposed; the most popular theories describe a deficiency of B vitamins and/or magnesium.[15,30] Many endocrine imbalances are cited, including hypoglycemia, hyperprolactinemia, and hypothyroidism. Lifestyle factors have been cited as contributory if not causative; these include increased stress, decreased exercise, poor diet, and increased intake of caffeine, nicotine, alcohol, red meat, and salt. Also implicated are overgrowth of *Candida albicans,* amino acid deficiencies, hyperandrogenism, post-tubal ligation interruption in normal blood supply, sleep deprivation, and altered electroencephalogram (EEG) pattern.

Psychiatric hypotheses are that PMS is caused by negative "imprinting" regarding the menstrual cycle, denial of femininity, learned helplessness, attributing bad things in one's life to a physical event, dysfunctional family systems, and poor coping styles.[31] PMS has also been presented as a culture-bound syndrome—a disease of industrialized nations only. Role conflict is implicated, wherein PMS is viewed as a safety valve. With PMS, women can be seen as "victims" who did not "choose" to be sick.[32]

***Incidence.*** One estimate is that PMS occurs in 20 to 80 percent of reproductive-age women.[26,29,33] Statistics depend on how *normal* is defined and whether the physical and behavioral changes that precede or accompany menses are considered normal. In our culture many symptoms, because they are ubiquitous, are "normal" even though they represent a deviation from optimal health. Approximately 5 to 15 percent of women will have symptoms so severe as to disrupt their everyday lives.[33]

## Subjective Data

Typically, clients with PMS have a number of physical symptoms, for example, breast tenderness, fluid retention, abdominal bloating, increased appetite and weight gain, craving for salty or sweet foods—chocolate in particular—acne, fatigue, heart palpitations, dizziness, faintness, and/or headaches premenstrually. These symptoms may be stated as the chief complaint, but are actually incidental when compared with the symptoms that are truly distressing the client. Usually, several of the following symptoms are present: mood swings, irritability, anxiety, hostility, depression, crying spells, thoughts of suicide, relationship conflict and fear of breakup, guilt over yelling at or battering children, feelings of inadequacy, increased or decreased libido, and inability to cope with the ever-recurring symptoms.

Usually clients delay treatment, deny the syndrome, make and cancel several appointments, and finally see a health care professional as a result of a recent crisis or threat from a significant other. The symptoms, usually present in the luteal phase, may present in one of four cyclic patterns.

- They appear at midcycle, disappear, and reappear the week prior to menstruation.
- They begin at midcycle with subtle changes that gradually escalate until menses.
- They appear the week prior to menses and intensify until menstruation ensues.
- They appear in the first or second luteal weeks and do not disappear until the end of menstruation.[31]

## Objective Data

Although no specific physical findings are characteristic, a complete physical examination is required to rule out other causes of the signs and symptoms.[26]

Diagnostic tests and methods to rule out other illnesses may include a CBC, Pap smear, and urinalysis. Hormonal assays may be initiated to rule out menopause, hypothyroidism, hyperprolactinemia, hyperandrogynism, or hypoglycemia.

## Differential Medical Diagnoses

Cyclothymic disorder; dysfunctional marital situation; depression; bipolar depression type I or II; stress, "superwoman syndrome"; perimenopausal status; poor diet; endocrine abnormalities including hypoglycemia, diabetes, hypothyroidism, hyperprolactinemia, and hyperandrogynism; alcoholism; or drug addiction. Brain, breast, adrenal, or ovarian tumors should also be ruled out.

## Plan

### *Psychosocial Interventions*

Assure the client that her symptoms are real, that PMS exists and she is not "crazy." Acceptance and acknowledgment are therapeutic.

Briefly explain PMS. Provide the client with interesting, informative, and accurate articles and books on the topic.

Teach the client the basics of the menstrual cycle, and provide a menstrual symptoms chart for her to record and rate symptoms. This will enhance the client's awareness of her problem and the actual timing of PMS, and it will assist you in planning and evaluating interventions. Symptoms should be prospectively charted for 2–3 months.

Focus on stresses contributing to PMS and ways to adjust lifestyle. Encourage the client to talk with family and friends about her needs and symptoms and to ask for nonthreatening types of support. Suggest assertiveness seminars or books about the subject. Role play new strategies for dealing with troublesome situations that the client presented in her history. Teach her to schedule activities with PMS in mind, namely, not to overschedule when symptoms are worst. Encourage her to get adequate sleep, particularly during times of most severe symptoms.

Lifestyle changes may include beginning a safe exercise program, preferably outdoors, to increase endorphin production, reduce stress, enhance cardiovascular health, and prevent osteoporosis. Encourage the client to exercise three to five times per week. Regular relaxation is effective in reducing symptoms.[40] Assist the client with planning a balanced diet that avoids salts, refined sugars, and includes a nutritious snack. Many symptoms can be relieved simply by eating a morning meal and avoiding self-induced hypoglycemia. Encourage the client to carry small, low calorie snacks in her purse for times when symptoms such as fatigue, difficulty concentrating, or irritability occur. Advise her to decrease caffeine intake gradually to avoid headaches with the goal of total elimination to reduce irritability and enhance sleep. Recommend increasing water intake to achieve natural diuresis.

Give the client permission to set aside time for herself. Teach stress reduction techniques, for example, taking long baths; taking time for pleasurable activity, yoga, Lamaze, biofeedback, meditation, or visual imagery—or refer her to a specialist for instruction. Discuss the "superwoman syndrome" in which women try to excel in all areas of life in a perfectionistic way. Suggest the book *Healing the Shame that Binds You* to help her gain insight into this problem.[34]

Dissuade client from blaming everything on PMS and perpetuating the role of victim. Keep stressing that the client is responsible for herself. She *can* recognize and learn to cope with symptoms as do other chronic disease sufferers.[35] Encourage the client to approach her therapy a little at a time, to seek assistance, and to accept her mistakes. Discourage "all or nothing" thinking patterns.

Review a typical day's communication patterns, sources of conflict, and problematic lifestyle factors. With the client, select one or two realistic goals to begin to pursue right away; accomplishing even small changes enhances self-esteem and the desire to continue making changes. Discourage the client from making too many changes at once.

Stress the importance of *not* smoking because of the overall negative health consequences and toxicity to the ovaries. Encourage limited intake of alcohol or avoiding it, particularly high-sugar beverages such as wine, which may cause rebound hypoglycemia, headaches, palpitations, and fatigue.

Encourage the client to evaluate her coping styles and discard unhealthy habits, such as alcohol consumption, drug abuse, and smoking, for more functional styles. Give the client permission to take care of herself.[35]

Provide information about assertiveness classes, support groups for PMS, Co-Dependency, Al-Anon, Alcoholics Anonymous, counselors, or psychiatrists.

Long-term pharmacological therapy may be needed; therefore, the client should be included in decisions regarding therapy so that concerns about cost and side effects are shared. Women at different ends of the menopausal years may experience quite opposite symptoms and need different therapies.[36]

***Medications.*** Part of the therapeutic effect from any drug used for PMS is due to the placebo effect.[15]

*Vitamin and Mineral Supplements*

- An indication for supplements can be a benign beginning treatment while the client collects data for charts.

- Vitamins and minerals are commonly indicated for PMS therapy; however, because studies have been poorly controlled, use should be carefully monitored.
- No more than 50–100 mg daily of pyridoxine (vitamin $B_6$) is recommended.[37] More than 200 mg daily can cause gastric upset;[26] excessive amounts can cause sensory neuropathy.[29]
- Overdosage of vitamin A must be avoided because research results have not been definitive on its use as a successful treatment. No more than the recommended daily allowance (5,000 units) should be advised.
- Vitamin E, 150–600 units per day, may alleviate breast symptoms.[26]
- Calcium, 1000 mg elemental daily, was found to improve mood and reduce pain and fluid retention.[36] Magnesium, 360 mg daily, also improved those complaints.[37] Magnesium and neurotransmitter actions are related.
- Optivite, a high dose multivitamin-mineral, developed by Abraham, has often been prescribed for PMS. However, there is speculation that the magnesium component is the therapeutic ingredient and that Optivite could potentially be unsafe because of high levels of pyridoxine and vitamin A.[36]
  - Vitamin supplements.
  - Gastrointestinal (GI) upset is a possible side effect.
  - A contraindication is any condition caused by added levels of any vitamins and minerals.
  - Anticipated outcomes on evaluation may be positive effects; however, the placebo effect is proven.[15]
  - Client teaching and counseling should include encouragement to take vitamin and mineral supplements with meals. Phasing in reduces GI upsets and enhances compliance. Caution clients about the possible side effects and the dangers of toxicity and megadoses.

*Prostaglandin Synthetase Inhibitors (PGSIs)*

- Indications for these drugs include premenstrual headaches, tension, irritability, depression, abdominal pain, breast tenderness, abdominal bloating, and ankle edema, depending on the study.[29] Mefenamic acid is the PGSI primarily studied.
- Side effects, and contraindications are the same as for dysmenorrhea. Side effects and adverse reactions include gastrointestinal upset, rash, and edema. PGSIs may be teratogenic; therefore they are contraindicated in pregnancy. Also peptic ulcers, asthma, aspirin sensitivity, and inflammatory bowel disease are contraindications.
- Client teaching and counseling should begin with a discussion of the client's symptom records. It should include information about taking PGSIs with meals to avoid gastric upset or ulcer development. The medication should be initiated on the day of the luteal phase when symptoms and signs are perceived, as recorded on a previous month's symptom record.

*Spironolactone*

- The indication for this potassium-sparing diuretic is severe fluid retention (i.e., weight gain of 5 pounds or more).[36] It has a limited role in PMS therapy.[29] Most fluid retention does not require drug therapy because of favorable response to measures such as a decreased salt diet, use of mineral supplements (calcium and/or magnesium), and increased water intake.
- Administer spironolactone during the luteal phase (q.i.d. p.o. range daily for total does is 25–200 mg). The lowest effective dose is suggested.[36]
- Side effects include gynecomastia, GI upset, drowsiness, headache, rash, mental confusion, irregular menses or amenorrhea, and deepening of the voice.[25]

- Contraindications include anuria, acute renal insufficiency, significant renal impairment, and hyperkalemia.[25]
- Anticipated outcomes on evaluation are decreased bloating, feelings of fullness, and affective/physical symptoms associated with excessive fluid retention.
- Client teaching and counseling should make clear that potassium supplementation in the form of food or medication should not be taken with spironolactone. Furthermore, spironolactone should not be taken with other potassium-sparing diuretics. Follow clients with fluid and electrolyte studies to avoid excessive potassium levels and resulting cardiac arrhythmias.[25] It is better to recommend increasing water intake and reducing sodium rather than to prescribe diuretics.

*Progesterone Oral Micronized Tablets—Oragest (Micronized Progesterone)*

- The indication for progesterone is to relieve a wide variety of PMS symptoms; however, other therapies should be exhausted prior to prescribing progesterone. In clinical trials, it has not performed superiorly to a placebo.[29]
- Oral progesterone is easier to administer and has fewer side effects. The dosage is 100 mg p.o. in A.M. and 200 mg h.s. 10–14 days prior to menses. The nighttime dose enhances sleep. If drowsiness is not desired, Oragest[38] should be taken with food. If significant bleeding occurs, the nighttime dose can be decreased to 100 mg.
- Side effects are drowsiness and spotting.
- A contraindication is undiagnosed vaginal bleeding.[38]
- Client teaching and counseling should include information about how to take the medication and its side effects and symptom charting.

*Estradiol Therapy*

- Indications for estradiol therapy are severe premenstrual headaches.[39] In a double-blind crossover study in Britain, premenstrual migraine frequency was reduced in 60 percent of clients with percutaneous estradiol patch use. The Estraderm patch has not been approved for this therapy in the United States, although some practitioners are having positive individual results using it. As a consequence, *physician consultation is recommended with patch application.*
- Nonpharmacological and/or traditional pharmacological therapies, such as PGSIs, should be tried first, and treatment limited to the days or week when symptoms are unbearable, as documented on the client symptoms charts.
- Administer (apply) a 0.05 mg patch at the time during cycle when symptoms appear; remove it at the onset or completion of menses. In the aforementioned study, the patch was applied 48 hours before headache usually occurred and continued for 7 days.
- Side effects and contraindications. Side effects of estrogen therapy include nausea, headache, breast tenderness and enlargement, fluid retention, cervical ectropion, and an increase in vaginal discharge. More severe adverse effects include thromboembolic development, cerebrovascular accident, pulmonary emboli, liver disease, uterine myoma growth, telangiectasia, hypertension, and myocardial infarction. Estrogen is contraindicated in pregnancy, cancer of the uterus or breast, in the presence of unusual/unexplained vaginal bleeding, endometriosis, or abnormal blood clotting. Women with hypertension, heart or kidney disease, asthma, skin allergies, epilepsy, diabetes, migraine headache, or depression have a relative con-

traindication to estrogen use. Signs/symptoms of concern with estrogen therapy are severe headache, visual disturbance, dizziness, chest pain, shortness of breath, leg cramps, abdominal pain, and irregular bleeding. The Estraderm patch may cause skin irritation, rash, or redness.

- Anticipated outcomes on evaluation are better sleep patterns and mood and fewer headaches.
- Client teaching and counseling should help the client with her essential task of keeping accurate menstrual records and symptom charts. Pap tests and mammography must be current and normal.

*Oral Contraceptives*

- The indication for oral contraception is elimination of cyclic hormonal fluctuations. Prescribe only when all else fails and there are no contraindications. Generally, oral contraceptives are not well tolerated among the PMS population.[36]
- Administration, side effects, and contraindications. Administer oral contraceptives according to manufacturer's guidelines. See Chapter 6 for detailed discussion of administration, side effects, and contraindications. Side effects most commonly include breast tenderness, weight gain, spotting, and scanty menses. Contraindications are pregnancy, undiagnosed vaginal bleeding, history of breast or reproductive tract cancer, history of thromboembolism, cerebrovascular or coronary disease, even tumor or malignancy, or smoker older than 35.[12]
- The anticipated outcome on evaluation is very limited. Little success occurs in reducing symptoms, and oral contraceptives may exacerbate symptoms in some PMS sufferers.[29]
- Client teaching and counseling. Advise regarding appropriate use of oral contraceptives (OC), danger signs, and side effects. Anticipated outcomes relates to OC used for PMS may best be presented as positive, since telling the client they may not help unfairly biases the outcome toward the negative.

*Alprazolam*

- The indication for alprazolam is short term relief of several symptoms.[29] Placebo controlled trials indicate that nervousness, irritability, mood swings, anxiety, depression, fatigue, and cravings for sweets are among the symptoms reduced.
- Administer alprazolam, 0.25 or 0.5 mg p.o., b.i.d. or t.i.d. during the luteal phase. The medication is prescribed in small amounts and refilled with caution. Taper the drug to prevent withdrawal when stopping administration.[29]
- Side effects include addiction potential, drowsiness, and if used with alcohol, a synergistic effect.
- Contraindications include pregnancy, lactation, history of addiction, or acute narrow angle glaucoma. Alprazolam is used cautiously for clients with renal, hepatic, or pulmonary conditions.[25]
- The anticipated outcome on evaluation is that the therapy will allow temporary symptom reduction and enable the client to seek problem resolution through counseling or therapy.
- Client teaching should encourage specialized counseling; therapists may be recommended. Discuss ways to reduce stress and learn coping skills.

*Bromocriptine (Dopamine Agonist)*

- The indication for bromocriptine is breast tenderness, galactorrhea, or hyperprolactinemia.[29]
- Administration of bromocriptine is 2.5 mg p.o., b.i.d. or t.i.d. daily.[29] The initial dose is 2.5 mg q.h.s.; cut in half if the client

shows intolerance. A second dose is added after 1 week.[5]

- Side effects are diarrhea, nausea, fatigue, and headache.[5]
- The anticipated outcome on evaluation is reduced breast symptoms.
- Client teaching and counseling includes discussing the side effects and the gradual addition of a second or third dose. *Physician consultation is recommended.* A serum PRL test and complete breast exam are necessary.[29]

*Danazol (Synthetic Androgen)*

- Indications for danazol include severe breast discomfort, irritability, anxiety, lethargy, weight gain, premenstrual fluid retention, and bloating.[29] Controlled studies report relief of selected symptoms[29]; however, the side effects of danazol can be more distressing than the PMS symptoms.
- Administer 200–400 mg p.o. daily.
- The anticipated outcome on evaluation is reduced symptoms.
- Side effects include masculinizing changes, nausea, changes in libido, tendency toward acne, and edema.
- Danazol is contraindicated in pregnancy and kidney, cardiac, or hepatic disease, and seizure disorder. It can adversely affect serum calcium levels.
- Client teaching and counseling include information about the side effects and contraindications. Advise clients to use effective barrier contraception or an IUD.[29] *Physician consultation is recommended for danazol use.*

*Gonadotropin-Releasing Hormone Agonist (GnRH-a)*

- Indications are extremely severe symptoms. This treatment medically castrates the woman and carries increased risks of heart disease and osteoporosis.[29]
- *Administer with physician consultation only.* Requires daily subcutaneous injections.
- Side effects are menopause induced by complete ovulation cessation (see Chapter 11, Hypoestrogenic Changes, for effects of estrogen deficiency).
- The anticipated outcome on evaluation is effective symptom relief.
- Client teaching and counseling require informed consent and indepth education about the effects of this treatment. Although GnRH-a can reduce symptoms dramatically, other effects may be unacceptable. A trial is suggested.[29]

***Surgical Interventions.*** Oophorectomy is reserved for clients with the most severe cases of PMS and truly should be a last resort. Frequently following surgery, clients who are placed on a hormone replacement regimen develop a chemically induced PMS; therefore, little is gained.

Hysterectomy has *no place* in the treatment of PMS and will not help the syndrome. Clients should be informed of this.

***Follow-Up.*** Follow-up involves rescheduling the client in 1 or 2 months to evaluate her charts and progress and to arrive at a workable diagnosis and plan of care. The first few months involve intense examination of lifestyle, menstrual patterns, and coping strategies. Frequent visits provide time to review and provide more information, reinforce desired changes, give encouragement, assign reading, and discuss referrals. Results of initial lab work can be shared at this time, and continuation of symptom charting is stressed.[35,36] As the client accrues knowledge and coping techniques and begins to see progress, her visits can be less frequent and shorter. The goal is to have yearly visits. An interdisciplinary team approach is useful in the management of PMS.

## NURSING DIAGNOSES

The following nursing diagnoses identified by the author are representative of those used in the health care plan of women with menstrual dysfunction; however, this is by no means an inclusive list:

- Activity limitation secondary to pain
- Anxiety
- Body image disturbance
- Discomfort
- Family coping ineffective
- Family processes altered
- Fatigue
- Fear
- Individual coping ineffective
- Infection, high risk
- Knowledge deficit concerning
  —menstrual cycle and etiology of pain
  —alterations in menstrual cycle
  —safe tampon use
- Nutrition altered: less than body requirements
- Powerlessness
- Role performance altered
- Self-esteem disturbance
- Social interaction impaired
- Tissue perfusion altered, cardiopulmonary and peripherally

## REFERENCES


1. Golub, S. (Ed.). (1985). *Lifting the curse of menstruation: A feminist appraisal of the influences of menstruation on women's lives.* New York: Harrington Park Press.
2. Greydanus, D., & Shearin, R. (1990). *Adolescent sexuality and gynecology.* Philadelphia: Saunders.
3. Wentz, A. (1988). *Gynecologic endocrinology and infertility for the house officer.* Baltimore: Williams & Wilkins.
4. Brown, J.S., & Crombleholme, W.R. (1993). *Handbook of gynecology and obstetrics.* Norwalk: Appleton & Lange.
5. Speroff, L., Glass, R., & Kase, N. (1989). *Clinical gynecologic endocrinology and infertility* (4th ed.). Baltimore: Williams & Wilkins.
6. Connell, A. (1989). Abnormal uterine bleeding. *Nurse Practitioner, 14*(4), 40–57.
7. Murata, J. (1990). Abnormal genital bleeding and secondary amenorrhea. *Journal of Obstetric, Gynecologic, and Neonatal Nursing, 19*(1), 26–36.
8. American College of Obstetrics and Gynecology. (1989). *Technical bulletin: Amenorrhea* (Report No. 128). Washington, DC: Author.
9. Krahn, D., Demitrack, M., Kurta, C., et al. (1992). Dieting and menstrual irregularity. *Journal of Women's Health, 1*, 289–291.
10. Clark-Coller, T. (1991). Dysfunctional uterine bleeding and amenorrhea: Differential diagnosis and management. *Journal of Nurse Midwifery, 36*(1), 49–62.
11. Edge, D.S., & Segatore, M. (1993). Assessment and management of galactorrhea. *Nurse Practitioner, 18*(6), 35–49.
12. Hatcher, R., Guest, F., Stewart, F., Steward, G., Trussell, J., Bowen, S., & Cates, W. (1990). *Contraceptive technology* (15th ed.). Atlanta: Printed Matter.
13. American College of Obstetrics and Gynecology. (1989). Report No. 134. *Technical bulletin: Dysfunctional uterine bleeding.*
14. Field, C. (1988). Dysfunctional uterine bleeding. In R. Avant (Ed.), *Primary care clinics in office practice* (pp. 561–574). Philadelphia: Saunders.
15. Hacker, N.F., & Moore, J. G. (1992). *Essentials of obstetrics and gynecology* (2nd ed.). Philadelphia: Saunders.
16. Johnson, C.A. (1991). Making sense of dysfunctional uterine bleeding. *American Family Physician, 44*(1), 149–157.

17. Freeman, S.B. (1991). Management of perimenopausal symptoms. *NAACOG's Clinical Issues, 2*(4), 429–439.
18. Coupey, S., & Ahlstrom, P. (1989). Common menstrual disorders. In V. Strasburger (Ed.), *Pediatric Clinics of North America, 36*, 551–571.
19. Dawood, M. (1990). Dysmenorrhea. *Clinical Obstetrics and Gynecology, 33*(1), 168–177.
20. Hill, C. (1988). Dysmenorrhea and premenstrual syndrome. In A. Wentz (Ed.), *Gynecologic endocrinology and infertility for the house officer*. Baltimore: Williams & Wilkins.
21. Colbry, S.L. (1992). A review of toxic shock syndrome: The need for education still exists. *Nurse Practitioner, 17*(9).
22. Ciesielski, C., & Broome, C. (1986). Toxic shock syndrome: Still in the differential. *Journal of Critical Illness, 1*(6), 26–40.
23. Broome, C. (1989). Epidemiology of toxic shock syndrome in the United States: Overview. *Reviews of Infectious Diseases, 11*(1), S14–S21.
24. Centers for Disease Control. (1990). *Reduced incidence of menstrual toxic-shock syndrome—United States, 1980–1990* (DHHS Vol. 38, No. 25). Washington, DC: U.S. Government Printing Office.
25. *Physician's desk reference*. (1985). Oradell, NJ: Medical Economics.
26. Lichtman, R., & Papera, S. (1990). *Gynecology: Well-woman care*. Norwalk, CT: Appleton & Lange.
27. Freeman, S.R. (1991). Management of perimenopausal symptoms. *NACCOG's Clinical Issues, 2*(4), 429–439.
28. American Psychiatric Association. (1993, July 10). *Statement from APA Board of Trustees on inclusion of premenstrual dysphoric disorder in appendix of DSM-IV*. News release.
29. Smith, S., & Schiff, I. (1989). The premenstrual syndrome: Diagnosis and management. *Fertility and Sterility, 52*, 527–543.
30. Abraham, G. (1983). Nutritional factors in the etiology of the premenstrual tension syndromes. *Journal of Reproductive Medicine, 28*, 446–464.
31. Reid, R. (1986). Premenstrual syndrome: A time for introspection. *American Journal of Obstetrics and Gynecology, 1*, 921–926.
32. Johnson, T. (1987). Premenstrual syndrome as a Western culture-specific disorder. *Culture, Medicine and Psychiatry, 11*, 337–356.
33. Johnson, S., McChesney, C., & Bean, J. (1988). Epidemiology of premenstrual symptoms in a nonclinical sample. *Journal of Reproductive Medicine, 33*, 340–346.
34. Bradshaw, J. (1988). *Healing the shame that binds you.* Deerfield Beach, FL: Health Communications.
35. Warren, C., & Baker, S. (1992). Coping resources of women with premenstrual syndrome. *Archives of Psychiatric Nursing, 6*(1) 48–53.
36. Johnson, S.R. (1992). Clinician's approach to the diagnosis and management of premenstrual syndrome. *Clinical Obstetrics and Gynecology, 35*, 637–657.
37. Facchinetti, F., Borella, P., Sances, G., Fioroni, L., Nappi, R., Genazzani, A. (1991). Oral magnesium successfully relieves premenstrual mood changes. *Obstetrics and Gynecology, 78*, 177–181.
38. Chakmakjian, A. (1989). Progesterone and progestins: Past, present, and future. *Baylor University Medical Center Proceedings*. Baylor Research Foundation, Dallas.
39. DeLigonieres, B., Vincers, M., & Mauvais-Jarvis, P. (1986). Prevention of menstrual migraine by percutaneous oestradiol. *British Medical Journal, 293*, 1540.
40. Goodale, I., Domar, A., & Benson, H. (1990). Alleviation of premenstrual syndrome symptoms with the relaxation-response. *Obstetrics and Gynecology, 75*, 649–655.

CHAPTER 6

# CONTROLLING FERTILITY

*Kathryn A. Caufield*

*When the goal is to prevent pregnancy, any contraceptive method is better than none.*

### *Highlights*

- Historical and Political Perspectives
- Principles of Fertility Control
- Issues of Control, Safety, and Choice
- "Safer Sex"
- Evaluation of Clients
- Client Education, Informed Consent
- Combined Oral Contraceptives
- Progestin-Only Pills, Implants, Injections, Vaginal Rings
- Postcoital Contraceptive Methods
- Male and Female Condoms
- Spermicides, Foams, Jellies, Creams, Suppositories, Vaginal Film
- Barrier Methods: Diaphragms, Cervical Caps, Sponges
- Intrauterine Devices
- Sterilization
- Cycle Charting and Periodic Abstinence
- Withdrawal
- Induced Abortion
- Outlook for Controlling Fertility: Men and Women

## INTRODUCTION

### HISTORICAL AND POLITICAL PERSPECTIVES ON CONTRACEPTION

The desire of women and men to control their reproductive destinies has been evident since ancient times. Use of primitive barriers, spermicides, condoms, and withdrawal is documented in the writings of many ancient cultures. Until the mid-nineteenth century, however, few reliable methods to prevent or delay pregnancy were available. Herbal and chemical spermicides, condoms, and coitus interruptus (withdrawal) carried high risks of pregnancy; the latter two also depended on the cooperation of men.[1–4]

Margaret Sanger (1883–1966), a nurse and feminist and the most important early leader of the U.S. family planning movement, introduced the diaphragm into the United States and fought for women's rights. She founded the American Birth Control League, which later became the Planned Parenthood Federation of America. A 1965 U.S. Supreme Court decision in the case of *Estelle T. Griswold and C. Lee Buxton v. State of Connecticut* declared birth control to be a basic right under the Bill of Rights.[1–5] In the early 1960s, oral contraceptives and intrauterine devices (IUD) became available, beginning the "contraceptive revolution." The ability to control the timing and circumstances under which they would conceive gave women a higher degree of personal control, more freedom of choice in many dimensions of their lives, and the self-determination to work toward equality.

Not coincidentally, the women's movement gained momentum with the introduction of these more "modern" methods of birth control. In turn, the women's movement provided the stimulus to limit family size through birth control and to move society toward acceptance of different roles for women.[1–4]

Large numbers of women continue to experience unplanned pregnancies, resulting in morbidity, mortality, and social distress. In fact the United States is far behind other countries in varieties of birth control methods available. Numerous factors contribute to this phenomenon. Issues constraining contraceptive availability and research include product liability lawsuits; antifamily-planning activism; pressures from well-intended feminist, consumer, political, and religious groups; cautious and lengthy U.S. Food and Drug Administration (FDA) procedural requirements; too little knowledge about reproductive biology; and too little money.[5–7] Contraceptive technologies, however, are slowly but steadily evolving. Research and development underway in many parts of the world should eventually result in a wider array of contraceptive methods, offering advantages over some currently available contraceptive techniques and wider choices for consumers.

## DEFINITION AND PURPOSE

*Fertility control* may be defined as follows.

1. Purposeful regulation of conception or childbirth.
2. Voluntary avoidance or delay of pregnancy or childbirth.
3. Use of devices, chemicals, abortion, or other techniques to prevent or terminate pregnancy.

Related terms often used interchangeably with fertility control include *birth control, family planning, contraception, pregnancy prevention,* and *planned parenthood.*[2,3,8] The reasons for controlling fertility include personal convenience, economics, social values, and lifestyle.

## SELECTING A METHOD OF CONTRACEPTION

A woman's reproductive life spans almost 40 years, and throughout those years, a variety of contraceptive methods may be used. Table 6–1 summarizes desirable method characteristics according to the stages of a woman's reproductive life.[8,9] Women need assistance in reevaluating contraceptive choices as their needs change over time and in understanding and recognizing the many variables that can influence those choices. Many individual factors may enhance or impair contraceptive behavior and impact the selection of birth control methods.[1,2,8–11]

- Age and maturity.
- Stage of reproductive life (desire for future fertility).
- Marital status.
- Cultural and religious beliefs.
- Health/medical history.
- Presence of physical or mental limitations.
- Motivation of the woman.
- Degree of cooperation of the male partner.
- Wishes and concerns of the partner.
- Degree of comfort with one's body and one's sexuality.
- Individual locus of control.
- Monogamous versus multiple sexual partners (risk of sexually transmitted diseases).

**TABLE 6–1. IMPORTANCE OF CONTRACEPTIVE METHOD CHARACTERISTICS ACCORDING TO STAGES OF REPRODUCTIVE LIFE**

| | Importance of Method Characteristics | | | |
|---|---|---|---|---|
| **Reproductive Life Stage** | ***Pregnancy Prevention*** | ***STD/PID Prevention***[a] | ***Not Coitus Linked*** | ***Reversibility*** |
| I: Menarche to first intercourse | — | — | — | — |
| II: First intercourse to marriage | High | High | High | High |
| III: Marriage to first birth | Moderate | Moderate | Low | High |
| IV: First birth to completion of desired family size | Moderate | Moderate | Low | High |
| V: Completion of desired family size to menopause | High | Low | Moderate | Low |

[a]STD = sexually transmitted disease; PID = pelvic inflammatory disease.

*Source: Adapted with permission from Forrest, J.D. (1988). Contraceptive needs through stages of women's reproductive lives. Contemporary Ob/Gyn [Special Issue: Fertility], Medical Economics Company, 32, 12–22.*

- Lactation status.
- Cost of methods.
- Previous experience with birth control methods (successes, failures, problems, side effects).
- Frequency of intercourse.
- Other patterns of sexual activity.
- Effectiveness of methods.
- Safety of methods.
- Access to health care.
- Noncontraceptive benefits.
- Short term versus long term contraceptive needs.
- Confidence in methods.
- Perceived convenience of methods.

Characteristics that may impact the selection and use of specific contraceptive methods are summarized in Tables 6–2A and 6–2B.

*General Principles of Fertility Control*[2,4,6,8]

- When the goal is to prevent pregnancy, any contraceptive method is better than none.
- *All* sexually active women of every age must have access to effective, confidential, and nonpunitive contraceptive services.
- Women need to know their options, the risks and benefits, and which methods may be contraindicated for them and why.
- Women are entitled to professional assistance when selecting a method that meets their own needs and circumstances.
- Health professionals are obligated to educate clients, without undue bias, about the range of possible methods so that fully informed choices can be made.
- No birth control method is 100 percent effective in preventing pregnancy.
- Information and counseling about acquired immunodeficiency syndrome (AIDS) and human immunodeficiency virus (HIV) infection, sexually transmitted diseases (STDs), use of latex condoms, and "safer sex" must be provided to individuals seeking family planning services.
- Responsibility for preventing pregnancy should ideally be shared by the man and the woman in a relationship.

## ISSUES OF CONTROL, SAFETY, AND CHOICE.[6,8]

A "perfect" contraceptive would be 100 percent effective in preventing pregnancy, highly acceptable, free from health hazards

**TABLE 6–2A. IMPORTANCE OF CHARACTERISTICS IMPACTING CONTRACEPTIVE SELECTION AND USE ACCORDING TO METHOD**

| | Characteristics | | | | | | | |
|---|---|---|---|---|---|---|---|---|
| **Contraceptive Method** | ***Cost*** | ***Ease of Use*** | ***Coitus Linked*** | ***Level of Convenience*** | ***Effectiveness*** | ***Systemic Effects*** | ***Level of Safety*** | ***Availability*** |
| Combined oral contraceptives | Mod | Great | No | High | High | Yes | High for non-smokers | Wide |
| Progestin-only methods | | | | | | | | |
| Progestin-only pills | Mod | Great | No | High | High | Yes | High | Wide |
| Implants | High | Great | No | High | High | Yes | Mod | Limited |
| Vaginal rings | Mod | Great | No | Mod to high | High | High | High | Limited |
| Injections | Mod | Great | No | High | High | Yes | High | Limited |
| Diaphragms | Mod to high | Mod | Yes | Mod | Mod | No | Mod to high | Mod |
| Cervical caps | Mod to high | Mod | Yes | Mod | Mod | No | Mod to high | Low |
| Sponges | Mod | Mod | Yes | Mod | Mod | No | Mod to high | Wide |
| Postcoital methods | High | Difficult | No | Low | High | Yes | Mod | Limited |
| Male condoms | Low to mod | Mod | Yes | Mod to low | Mod | No | High | Wide |
| Female condoms | Mod | Mod | Yes | Low | Mod | No | High | Low |
| Vaginal spermicides | Low to mod | Mod | Yes | Low | Mod | No | High | Wide |
| Intrauterine devices | High | Great | No | High | High | Some | Mod | Limited |
| Fertility awareness methods | Low | Difficult | Yes | Low | Low | No | Mod | Mod |
| Withdrawal | None | Mod | Yes | Mod | Low | No | Mod | Wide |
| Female sterilization | High | Great | No | High | High | No | Mod | Mod |

*Note:* Mod = moderate.
*Source: References 2, 8, 10, 17, 18, 21, 26.*

**TABLE 6–2B. IMPORTANCE OF CHARACTERISTICS IMPACTING CONTRACEPTIVE SELECTION AND USE ACCORDING TO METHOD**

| | Characteristics | | | | | |
|---|---|---|---|---|---|---|
| **Contraceptive Method** | ***Partner Involvement Required*** | ***Protection Against STDs/HIV*** | ***Prescription Required*** | ***Health Care System Contact Required*** | ***Return to Fertility After Discontinued Use*** | ***Can Be Used While Lactating*** |
| Combined oral contraceptives | None | Some | Yes | Yes | Delay—Possibly 2–3 months | No |
| Progestin-only methods | | | | | | |
| Progestin-only pills | None | None | Yes | Yes | Rapid | Yes |
| Implants | None | None | Yes | Yes | Delayed—possibly 2–3 months | Yes |
| Vaginal rings | None | None | Yes | Yes | Slight delay possible | Yes |
| Injections | None | None | Yes | Yes | Delayed, 6–12 months | Yes |
| Diaphragms | None | Mod | Yes | Yes | Immediate | Yes |
| Cervical caps | None | Mod | Yes | Yes | Immediate | Yes |
| Sponges | None | Mod | No | No | Immediate | Yes |
| Postcoital methods | None | None | Yes | Yes | Rapid | Not recom-mended |
| Male condoms | Yes | High | No | No | Immediate | Yes |
| Female condoms | Some | High | No | No | Immediate | Yes |
| Vaginal spermicides | None | Mod | No | No | Immediate | Yes |
| Intrauterine devices | None | None | Yes | Yes | Rapid | Yes |
| Fertility awareness methods | Yes | None | No | Yes for teaching | Immediate | Not reliable |
| Withdrawal | Yes | Limited | No | No | Immediate | Yes |
| Female sterilization | None | None | No | Yes | Not applicable | Yes |

*Note:* STD = sexually transmitted disease; HIV = human immunodeficiency virus; Mod = moderate.
*Source: References 2, 8, 10, 17, 18, 21, 26.*

and side effects, self-administered, and easily reversible. In addition, it would be relatively inexpensive and offer noncontraceptive benefits such as protection against sexually transmitted diseases (STDs). Currently, however, all available methods for controlling fertility carry some risks to users; therefore, disadvantages and risks must be carefully weighed against benefits. In assisting clients with contraceptive choices, it is often helpful to compare method risks with the risks of full term delivery. In most cases, the risks associated with pregnancy and delivery are much greater than those associated with contraceptive use.

In an era when many women wish to delay pregnancy and simultaneously face many hazards to future fertility caused by STDs, choices are indeed difficult. Clients need assistance to select contraceptives that will protect them from both pregnancy and STDs. For young, healthy women, the combination of oral contraceptives and spermicidal condoms is a very sound choice.[8]

## CONTRACEPTION AND "SAFER SEX"

### Responsibility for Prevention and Protection

When seeking birth control, both men and women bear responsibility. Today, the question of whether the method offers any protection against STDs must be added to other selection considerations such as convenience, effectiveness, failure rate, safety, and noncontraceptive benefits. According to a U.S. government report, "Abstinence or sexual intercourse with one mutually faithful, uninfected partner is the only totally effective prevention" strategy against STDs. Individuals with multiple sexual partners must make difficult decisions about responsibility and consequences for actions, sexual expression, communication patterns with partners, and the long term impact of these decisions.[8,12]

### Safer Sex

When the HIV serostatus or STD status of a person is not certain, there is no such entity as "safe sex"; hence the term "safer sex." Condoms are not 100 percent effective in preventing infections. Although two principal problems with condom use are breakage and difficulty integrating use successfully into sexual activity, condoms are the best protection available at this time. Table 6–3 summarizes safer sex options.[8,13]

## EVALUATION OF CLIENTS REQUESTING FERTILITY CONTROL

In many cases, women seeking care or advice about fertility control are in a state of physical wellness; however, they may or may not have been successful in their contraceptive efforts. Several examples of nursing diagnoses applied to clients seeking family planning services or using or attempting to use some method of birth control are listed in the Nursing Diagnoses box at the end of this chapter.[11,14,15]

Health care professionals must be aware that certain clients are at high risk for lack of contraceptive services: teenagers, low income women, and women in underserved areas. These women need services low in cost with convenient hours and accessible locations.[11,16] Other groups with special family planning concerns include women with chronic illnesses, women who are physically or mentally handicapped, and women approaching midlife. All women need individualized plans of care, but these groups deserve special attention in order to meet their contraceptive needs fully (see Chapters 4, 11, and 19).

### Initial Evaluation[8,17–20]

A thorough initial assessment seeks data to identify risk factors and other influences on method selection (as discussed above), and

**TABLE 6–3. SAFER SEX OPTIONS**

| *Safe* | *Possibly Safe* | *Unsafe* |
|---|---|---|
| Massage<br>Body rubbing<br>Masturbation<br>Mutual masturbation<br>Movies<br>Hugging<br>Dry kissing<br>Hand–genital touching<br>Erotic books | Kissing<br>Vaginal/rectal intercourse using a latex condom (use spermicide for extra safety; more effective is use of two spermicidal condoms or two latex condoms with spermicide applied between them<br>Oral sex on a man using a latex condom<br>Oral sex on a woman who does not have her period or a vaginal infection with discharge (use latex barrier such as a dental dam for extra safety) | Any intercourse without a latex condom<br>Oral sex on a man without a latex condom<br>Oral sex on a woman during her period or during a vaginal infection with discharge, without a latex barrier such as a dental dam<br>Semen in the mouth<br>Oral–anal contact<br>Sharing sex toys or douching equipment<br>Blood contact of *any* kind, including menstrual blood, sharing needles, and any sex that causes tissue damage or bleeding |

*Source: Contraceptive Technology 1990–1992, as expanded from Planned Parenthood. New medical standards for HIV testing and counseling. Reproduced by permission of Hatcher, R.A., et al. (1990).* Contraceptive technology, 1990–92 *(15th rev. ed.). New York: Irvington Publishers, Inc.*

contraindications to certain methods. Subsequently, a database is established. During the initial evaluation a complete history is taken, including, but not limited to the following.

- *Medical History.* Smoking, cardiovascular disease (CVD), diabetes mellitus (DM), frequent urinary tract infections (UTIs), and so on.
- *Obstetric and Gynecologic History.* Menstrual, premenstrual syndrome (PMS), contraceptive, STDs and vaginitis, sexual.
- *Family History.* Especially cancer and other significant problems.
- *Review of Systems.*
- *Personal and Social Data.* Comfort with touching one's self, use of tampons and female hygiene products, desire or plans for children.

Objective data are obtained from a complete screening physical examination with special attention to height, weight, blood pressure (BP), and examination of thyroid, breasts, abdomen, and pelvis (noting position of uterus and any anatomic variation), and extremities. Other components of physical examination may also require emphasis, depending on birth control methods being considered.

Diagnostic testing includes the following.

- Cervical cytology (Pap smear) essential.
- Wet mounts (saline and potassium hydroxide [KOH] highly recommended; others as indicated).
- Hematocrit.
- Urinalysis.
- STD (especially gonorrhea and chlamydia).

In addition, consider human papilloma virus (HPV) testing, such as polymerase chain reaction (PCR); and blood chemistries, especially lipid profile and blood glucose.

### Subsequent Evaluations

All women who are sexually active or using a method of contraception that requires a prescription should be evaluated annually to evaluate new risk factors, contraindications, side effects, concerns, or new problems as-sociated with the present birth control method and to identify any other reproductive problems.

Subjective data include a review of the client's history, any significant changes in her health status, and her method of birth control (including satisfaction with the method and any problems). Objective data include the client's weight and blood pressure, screening physical and pelvic exam, and Pap smear. Other lab tests are performed as indicated (see above). Include a mammogram at the recommended intervals after age 35. (See Chapter 10.)

## METHODS OF BIRTH CONTROL

Several birth control methods are currently available.

- Combined oral contraceptives (COCs), also referred to as oral contraceptives (OCs), birth control pills (BCPs).
- Progestin-only methods (pills, implants, injections, vaginal rings).
- Postcoital methods.
- Barriers (male and female condoms, sponges, diaphragms, cervical caps).
- Vaginal spermicides (creams, jellies, suppositories, films).
- Intrauterine devices (IUDs).
- Fertility awareness methods.
- Coitus interruptus (withdrawal).
- Lactation.
- Sterilization.
- Abortion.

### MANAGEMENT CONSIDERATIONS, GUIDELINES FOR CLIENT EDUCATION AND INFORMED CONSENT[2,8,11,17,19]

- The client must participate in choosing the birth control method; she must be an informed user.
- Always obtain informed consent, particularly for a client choosing an intrauterine device (IUD), implant, injection, or sterilization. *Informed consent* implies that client makes a knowledgeable, voluntary choice, receives complete counseling about the procedure and its consequences, and is free to change her mind prior to the procedure.
- When working with a client planning to use any birth control method, carefully screen for contraindications.
- Set aside time for teaching as a routine part of the clinic visit. During the initial visit, use counseling to help the client select a birth control method; then use additional counseling after the visit to learn specific information about the method chosen.
- *For certain methods (diaphragms, cervical caps, IUDs, implants, vaginal rings, sterilization), the health provider must receive formal education, training, and practice in fitting, insertion, and other technical aspects.*
- During the visit, the health professional is responsible for providing client education and the opportunity for practice and validation of skills pertaining to selected methods (as applicable).
- Make all presentations, counseling, and educational materials compatible with the language, culture, and education of the client.
- Be aware of local myths and misperceptions about particular methods. Address misconceptions sensitively but directly. For example, douching, or "washing" semen out of the woman's body, will not

prevent sperm from entering the uterus. Indeed, douching could theoretically enhance the movement of sperm up the cervical canal by washing them deeper into the vagina toward the cervix or by washing away protective mucus.[2]

- To prevent the omission of important information, use a standard teaching checklist outlining key information that the user should know.
- Instruct about female and male anatomy using models and illustrations.
- Provide the client with method-specific teaching and counseling, using models, illustrations, and handouts to describe key information.
  - How the methods work.
  - Effectiveness of methods.
  - Advantages and disadvantages of methods.
  - Noncontraceptive benefits.
  - What to expect during the visit.
  - Recommendations concerning follow-up.
  - Descriptions of short and long-term side effects that can occur, and how to deal with them.
  - Danger signs associated with the method selected.
- Explore factors that could place the client at risk for method failure (e.g., frequent intercourse, age, parity, previous failure of method, sexual or lifestyle patterns that make consistent use difficult). Counsel the client regarding these factors.
- If it is determined that the client is at risk for failure with her chosen method, recommend its use in combination with another method.
- Clients who choose a coitus-associated method need accurate understanding of the timing of ovulation and awareness of days with high risk for conception. An additional method may be employed during high risk times.
- Provide both oral and written instructions. Instruct the client to read specific package literature and follow the instructions carefully.
- Inform the client that regardless of the method chosen, she must always keep a second birth control method available and be familiar with its use.
- Suggest to the client that she keep sufficient quantities of contraceptive products/supplies available at all times in a convenient location. Counsel her about the importance of budgeting for the purchase of products and supplies and for annual exams.
- Teach the proper care and storage of contraceptive devices and supplies.
- For devices requiring insertion, instruct the client to wash her hands before and after insertion to minimize possible introduction of contaminants into the vagina; also to wash applicators with soap and water after each use.
- Ask the client to repeat important information.
- Inform couples about the availability of postcoital protection in the event of method failure.

## EFFECTIVENESS

In this chapter, the effectiveness of birth control methods is reported as estimated failure rates during the first year of use: among couples who used the method perfectly (i.e., correct use at every act of intercourse; lowest expected failure rate); and among typical users, including incorrect and inconsistent use as well as method failures. Table 6–4 shows these failure rates for each method discussed.[8,21]

## COMBINED ORAL CONTRACEPTIVES

Birth control pills (BCPs) or oral contraceptives (OCs), also called "the Pill," have been

**TABLE 6–4. CONTRACEPTIVE METHOD FAILURE RATES DURING THE FIRST YEAR OF USE**

| | Percentage (%) of Women Experiencing Accidental Pregnancy in the First Year of Use | |
|---|---|---|
| ***Method*** | ***Lowest Expected Failure Rate***[a] | ***Typical Use Failure Rate***[b] |
| Chance | 85 | 85 |
| Spermicidal creams or jellies | 3 | 21 |
| Periodic abstinence | | 20 |
| Calendar | 9 | |
| Ovulation method | 3 | |
| Sympto-thermal | 2 | |
| Postovulation | 1 | |
| Withdrawal | 4 | 18 |
| Cervical cap with spermicide | 6 | 18 |
| Sponge | | |
| Parous women | 9 | 28 |
| Nulliparous women | 6 | 18 |
| Diaphragm with spermicide | 6 | 18 |
| Condom without spermicide | 2 | 12 |
| Intrauterine device | | 3 |
| Progestasert | 2.0 | |
| Copper-T-380A | 0.8 | |
| Pills | | 3.0[c] |
| Combined | 0.1 | |
| Progestogen only | 0.5 | |
| Injectable Progestin | | |
| Depo-medroxy progesterone acetate (DMPA) | 0.3 | 0.3 |
| Norethindrone enanthate (NET) | 0.4 | 0.4 |
| Implants | | |
| Norplant (6 capsules) | 0.04 | 0.04 |
| Norplant-2 (2 rods) | 0.03 | 0.03 |
| Female sterilization | 0.2 | 0.4 |
| Male sterilization | 0.1 | 0.15 |

[a]Lowest expected failure rate during the first year of use among couples who use the method perfectly (i.e., consistent and correct use at every act of intercourse).
[b]Failure rate during the first year of use among typical couples; includes incorrect and inconsistent use.
[c]4.7 for women under age 22.
*Source: References 8, 21.*

available in the United States for 30 years. It is estimated that about 60 million women worldwide and 13.8 million American women use OCs.[8] Pill use, its effectiveness, risks, benefits, and side effects have been well researched over the past 30 years. Low dosages of estrogen and progestin in today's pills make them very safe and effective for most women. Many noncontraceptive benefits have been identified.[8,22–25]

Combined OCs contain two primary components, synthetic estrogen and progestin.

The two estrogen compounds currently used in oral contraceptives in the United States are ethinyl estradiol or mestranol. Synthetic progestins are all derived from *19 nortestosterones*. OCs currently available in the United States contain one of several progestins. First generation progestins currently in use include norethindrone, norethindrone acetate, ethynodiol diacetate, norgestrel, levonorgestrel. OCs containing norethynodrel are no longer marketed in this country.[8,17,18,23]

New generation progestins derived from levonorgestrel have been developed. These are gestodene, norgestimate, and desogestrel. Combined OCs containing desogestrel and norgestimate are now available in the United States.[26–29] There appears to be little difference among these new progestins with regard to clinical efficacy. The new progestins are very potent in their ability to inhibit ovulation and to transform estrogen-primed endometrium into secretory endometrium. Of the three new agents, it appears that gestodene is most potent with regard to progestational activity. The new progestins have little estrogenic effect and they are weak antiestrogens. They have far less androgenic activity in animal studies in vivo than currently available progestins.[26–33] Estrogen and progestin are combined in fixed dose combined pills or in variable amounts in relation to one another throughout the pill cycle, as in biphasic or triphasic preparations. Table 6–5 lists the types and dosages of OCs available in the United States and their comparative biologic activities.

### Prescription

OCs are available in 21- or 28-day packs. Active pills are taken for 21 days; 28-day preparations contain 7 inert "spacer" tablets, except for some Parke-Davis products that contain ferrous fumarate in the last 7 brown pills of the 28-day pack.

### Mechanism of Action[8,17,18,23]

Pregnancy is prevented by several effects of estrogen and progestin.

- Gonadotropin-releasing hormone (GnRH) is suppressed, which in turn suppresses follicle-stimulating hormone (FSH) and luteinizing hormone (LH), inhibiting ovulation.
- Ovum/tubal transport is altered.
- Cervical mucus thickens, inhibiting sperm mobility.
- Implantation is inhibited by suppression of the endometrium and alteration of uterine secretions.

### Effectiveness

OCs are considered highly effective in preventing pregnancy (see Table 6–4). Failures are attributed to the following.

- Method failure, improper use, user error.
- Discontinuing the pill without immediate use of another method.
- Drug interactions.

Little difference exists in the failure rates among individual OCs.[8,17,21,33,34]

### Advantages[8,17,18,24,30,34]

- High rate of effectiveness.
- Use not associated with the act of intercourse.
- Use controlled by the woman.
- Easy to use, convenient.
- Rapid reversal of effects after discontinuing its use.
- Very safe for women under age 35 who do not smoke.
- Multiple noncontraceptive benefits.

### Noncontraceptive Benefits[8,17,24,34,35]

- *Improved Menstrual Characteristics.* OCs minimize dysmenorrhea and usually

## TABLE 6–5. ORAL CONTRACEPTIVE TYPES, DOSAGES, AND PHYSIOLOGICAL ACTIVITIES

| Oral Contraceptive | *Progestational Activity* | *Androgenic Activity* | *Endometrial Activity* |
|---|---|---|---|
| *Low Dose Monophasics* | | | |
| Brevicon (Syntex) 21 or 28 day<br>0.5 mg norethindrone<br>0.035 mg ethinyl estradiol | Low | Low | Intermediate |
| Demulen 1/35 (Searle) 21 or 28 day<br>1 mg ethynodiol diacetate<br>0.035 mg ethinyl estradiol | Intermediate/High | Low | Low |
| Desogen (Organon) 28 day<br>0.15 mg desogestrel<br>0.03 mg ethinyl estradiol | Intermediate/High | Low | Low/Intermediate |
| Genora 1/35 (Rugby) 28 day<br>1 mg norethindrone<br>0.035 mg ethinyl estradiol | Intermediate | Low/Intermediate | Intermediate |
| Levlen (Berlex) 21 or 28 day<br>0.15 mg levonorgestrel<br>0.03 mg ethinyl estradiol | Low/Intermediate | Intermediate | Intermediate |
| Loestrin 1/20 (Parke-Davis) 21 day<br>1 mg norethindrone acetate<br>0.02 mg ethinyl estradiol | Intermediate | Intermediate/High | Low |
| Loestrin 1.5/30 (Parke-Davis) 21 day<br>1.5 mg norethindrone acetate<br>0.03 mg ethinyl estradiol | Intermediate/High | Intermediate/High | Low |
| Loestrin Fe 1/20 (Parke-Davis) 28 day<br>1 mg norethindrone acetate<br>0.02 mg ethinyl estradiol<br>7 pills 75 mg ferrous fumarate | Intermediate | Intermediate/High | Low |
| Loestrin Fe 1.5/30 (Parke-Davis) 28 day<br>1.5 mg norethindrone acetate<br>0.03 mg ethinyl estradiol<br>7 pills 75 mg ferrous fumarate | Intermediate/High | Intermediate/High | Low |
| Lo-Ovral (Wyeth) 21 or 28 day<br>0.3 mg norgestrel<br>0.03 mg ethinyl estradiol | Low/Intermediate | Intermediate | Low/Intermediate |
| Modicon (Ortho) 21 or 28 day<br>0.5 mg norethindrone<br>0.035 mg ethinyl estradiol | Low | Low | Intermediate |
| Nelova 1/35E (Warner-Chilcott)<br>1 mg norethindrone<br>0.035 mg ethinyl estradiol | Intermediate | Low/Intermediate | Intermediate |
| Nelova 0.5/35E (Warner-Chilcott)<br>0.5 mg norethindrone<br>0.035 mg ethinyl estradiol | Low | Low | Intermediate |
| Nordette (Wyeth) 21 or 28 day<br>0.15 mg levonorgestrel<br>0.03 mg ethinyl estradiol | Low/Intermediate | Intermediate | Intermediate |
| Norethin 1/35E (Schiapparelli Searle)<br>28 day<br>1 mg norethindrone<br>0.035 mg ethinyl estradiol | Intermediate | Low/Intermediate | Intermediate |

**TABLE 6–5. CONTINUED**

| Oral Contraceptive | *Progestational Activity* | *Androgenic Activity* | *Endometrial Activity* |
|---|---|---|---|
| Norinyl 1+35 (Syntex) 21 or 28 day<br>1 mg norethindrone<br>0.035 mg ethinyl estradiol | Intermediate | Low/Intermediate | Intermediate |
| Ortho-Cept (Ortho) 21 or 28 day<br>0.150 mg desogestrel<br>0.03 mg ethinyl estradiol | Intermediate/High | Low | Intermediate |
| Ortho-Cyclen (Ortho) 21 or 28 day<br>.25 mg norgestimate<br>0.035 mg ethinyl estradiol | Low | Low | Low/Intermediate |
| Ortho-Novum 1/35 (Ortho) 21 or 28 day<br>1 mg norethindrone<br>0.035 mg ethinyl estradiol | Intermediate | Low/Intermediate | Intermediate |
| Ovcon 35 (Mead Johnson) 21 or 28 day<br>0.4 mg norethindrone<br>0.035 mg ethinyl estradiol | Low | Low | Intermediate |
| *Triphasics* | | | |
| Ortho-Novum 7/7/7 (Ortho) 21 or 28 day<br>7 days: 0.5 mg norethindrone<br>0.035 mg ethinyl estradiol<br>7 days: 0.75 mg norethindrone<br>0.035 mg ethinyl estradiol<br>7 days: 1 mg norethindrone<br>0.035 mg ethinyl estradiol | Low/Intermediate | Low/Intermediate | Intermediate |
| Tri-Levlen (Berlex) 21 or 28 day<br>6 days: 0.05 mg levongorgestrel<br>0.03 mg ethinyl estradiol<br>5 days: 0.075 mg levonorgestrel<br>0.04 mg ethinyl estradiol<br>10 days: 0.125 mg levonorgestrel<br>0.03 mg ethinyl estradiol | Low | Low/Intermediate | Intermediate |
| Tri-Cyclen (Ortho) 21 or 28 day<br>7 days: 0.18 mg norgestimate<br>0.035 mg ethinyl estradiol<br>7 days: 0.215 mg norgestimate<br>0.035 mg ethinyl estradiol<br>7 days: 0.25 mg norgestimate<br>0.035 mg ethinyl estradiol | Low | Low | Low/Intermediate |
| Tri-Norinyl (Syntex) 21 or 28 day<br>7 days: 0.5 mg norethindrone<br>0.035 mg ethinyl estradiol<br>9 days: 1 mg norethindrone<br>0.035 mg ethinyl estradiol<br>5 days: 0.5 mg norethindrone<br>0.035 mg ethinyl estradiol | Low/Intermediate | Low/Intermediate | Intermediate |
| Triphasil (Wyeth) 21 or 28 day<br>6 days: .0.05 mg levonorgestrel<br>0.03 mg ethinyl estradiol<br>5 days: 0.075 mg levonorgestrel<br>0.04 mg ethinyl estradiol<br>10 days: 0.125 mg levonorgestrel<br>0.03 mg ethinyl estradiol | Low | Low/Intermediate | Intermediate |

*(continued)*

**TABLE 6–5. CONTINUED**

| Oral Contraceptive | *Progestational Activity* | *Androgenic Activity* | *Endometrial Activity* |
|---|---|---|---|
| *Biphasics* | | | |
| Jenest (Organon) 28 day<br>7 days: 0.5 mg norethindrone<br>0.035 mg ethinyl estradiol<br>14 days: 1 mg norethindrone<br>0.035 mg ethinyl estradiol | Low/Intermediate | Low/Intermediate | Intermediate |
| Ortho-Novum 10/11 (Ortho) 21 or 28 day<br>10 days: 0.5 mg norethindrone<br>0.035 mg ethinyl estradiol<br>11 days: 1 mg norethindrone<br>0.035 mg ethinyl estradiol | Low/Intermediate | Low/Intermediate | Intermediate |
| *Moderate Dose Monophasics* | | | |
| Demulen 1/50 (Searle) 21 or 28 day<br>1 mg ethynodiol diacetate<br>0.050 mg ethinyl estradiol | Intermediate/High | Low | Intermediate |
| Genora 1/50 (Rugby) 28 day<br>1 mg norethindrone<br>0.05 mg mestranol | Intermediate | Low/Intermediate | Intermediate |
| Norethin 1/50M (Schiapparelli Searle) 28 day<br>1 mg norethindrone<br>0.05 mg mestranol | Intermediate | Low/Intermediate | Intermediate |
| Norinyl 1+50 (Syntex) 21 or 28 day<br>1 mg norethindrone<br>0.05 mg mestranol | Intermediate | Low/Intermediate | Intermediate |
| Norlestrin 1/50 (Parke-Davis) 21 day<br>1 mg norethindrone acetate<br>0.05 mg ethinyl estradiol | Intermediate | Intermediate | Intermediate |
| Norlestrin FE 1/50 (Parke-Davis) 28 day<br>1 mg norethindrone acetate<br>0.05 mg ethinyl estradiol<br>7 pills 75 mg ferrous fumerate | Intermediate | Intermediate | Intermediate |
| Norlestrin 2.5/50 (Parke-Davis) 21 day<br>2.5 mg norethindrone acetate<br>0.05 mg ethinyl estradiol | High | High | High |
| Norlestrin Fe 2.5/50 (Parke-Davis) 28 day<br>2.5 mg norethindrone acetate<br>0.05 mg ethinyl estradiol<br>7 pills 75 mg ferrous fumerate | High | High | High |
| Ortho-Novum 1/50 (Ortho) 21 or 28 day<br>1 mg norethindrone<br>0.05 mg mestranol | Intermediate | Low/Intermediate | Intermediate |
| Ovcon 50 (Mead Johnson) 21 or 28 day<br>1 mg norethindrone<br>0.05 mg ethinyl estradiol | Intermediate | Low/Intermediate | Intermediate |

**TABLE 6–5. CONTINUED**

| Oral Contraceptive | *Progestational Activity* | *Androgenic Activity* | *Endometrial Activity* |
|---|---|---|---|
| Ovral (Wyeth) 21 or 28 day<br>0.5 mg norgestrel<br>0.05 mg ethinyl estradiol | High | High | Intermediate/High |
| *Progestin Only* | | | |
| Micronor (Ortho) 28 day<br>0.35 mg norethindrone | Low | Low | Low |
| Nor-QD (Syntex) 42 day<br>0.35 mg norethindrone | Low | Low | Low |
| Ovrette (Wyeth) 28 day<br>0.075 mg norgestrel | Low | Low | Low |

*Source: Adapted from Dickey, R.P.* Managing contraceptive pill patients *(7th ed.). Durant, OK: Essential Medical Information Systems, Inc. 1993.*

*The author wishes to acknowledge the contributions of the following persons in their review of Table 6–5: Carolyn L. Stang, Pharm.D., Assistant Pharmacy Director for Clinical Services, Evanston Hospital, Evanston, Illinois; and Lauwana E. Hollis, Pharm.D., Clinical Instructor, School of Pharmacy, Virginia Commonwealth University, Richmond, Virginia.*

decrease the amount and duration of bleeding, so that periods are regular and predictable. OCs relieve premenstrual syndrome (PMS) in some women, and they lower the incidence of iron deficiency anemia. They can be used to ameliorate amenorrhea and dysfunctional uterine bleeding.

- *Protection against Ovarian and Endometrial Cancer.* Compared with women who never used OCs, users had half the risk of developing these cancers. Protection is noted after a minimum of 12 months of use and persists long after pills are discontinued.
- *Lower Incidence of Ovarian Cysts.* Incidence is reduced by 90 percent, due to the suppression of ovulation.
- *Prevention of Ectopic Pregnancy.* Prevention occurs through the suppression of ovulation.
- *Lower Incidence of Endometriosis.* Incidence is reduced due to the suppression of endometrial growth.
- *Protection against Pelvic Inflammatory Disease (PID).* Incidence of PID is 20 to 50 percent lower among users of OCs than among those who use no contraceptive method. The greatest protection is against PID caused by gonorrhea.
- *Lower Incidence of Benign Breast Cysts and Fibroadenomas.* As a result breast biopsy procedures are decreased.
- *Other Benefits.* OCs may reduce acne in some women; may reduce the incidence of rheumatoid arthritis (refuted in recent studies).[8,16]

## Disadvantages[8,17,24,34]

- Affects all body systems.
- User must remember to take pills daily.
- Some users experience undesirable side effects that cause discontinuance of pills.
- Should not be used while lactating.
- Provides no protection against HIV infection and most other STDs.
- High cost for some women.
- For some women, slight delay in becoming pregnant after discontinuing (2 to 3 months).
- Prescription needed.

- Access to pharmacy needed.
- User must interact with medical system.
- OCs may interact with other drugs (see Table 6–6).
- Many possible side effects.

## Side Effects and Complications

Side effects and complications are caused by systemic effects of OCs, and may be due to estrogenic, progestational, and/or androgenic activities, or their effects on serum lipoproteins. Pills with the lowest feasible biologic activity in each of these three areas should be chosen, because of potential long-term adverse effects on some body systems, particularly the cardiovascular system.[17] Table 6–7 summarizes most common side effects of OCs based on their relation to excess or deficient hormone activity.

## Managing Side Effects[8,17,18,27,35]

- Allow the client time to adjust to the pills (two or three packs).
- Determine that she is taking the pills correctly.
- Determine whether any symptom indicates the possible development of a serious health problem or OC-related complication (especially myocardial infarction, stroke, pulmonary embolism, thrombophlebitis, gallbladder or liver problems). Ask specific questions regarding early pill danger signs, remembering the acronym *ACHES*—severe *A*bdominal pain, severe *C*hest pain, severe *H*eadaches, *E*ye-visual changes, *S*hortness of breath. Other danger signs are severe leg pain, loss of coordination, speech problems, and depression.

**TABLE 6–6. ORAL CONTRACEPTIVE INTERACTIONS WITH OTHER DRUGS**

| Effect | Substances | Comments |
|---|---|---|
| Drugs whose effects may be enhanced in combination with oral contraceptives. | Alcohol, tricyclic antidepressants,[a] some benzodiazepines (alprazolam, chlordiazepoxide, clorazepate, diazepam, flurazepam), ß-blockers, corticosteroids, theophylline, Troleandomycin (Tao).[b] | Monitor blood levels when available and monitor affected body systems. |
| Drugs whose effects may be diminished in combination with oral contraceptives. | Acetaminophen,[b] oral anticoagulants, some benzodiazepines (lorazepam, oxazepam, temazepam), guanethidine,[a] oral hypoglycemic agents (chlorpropamide, glipizide, glyburide, tolazamide, tolbutamide). | Monitor physiological effect of drug, or use alternative drug, or use alternative contraceptive method. |
| Drugs that may diminish the effectiveness of oral contraceptives. | Any antibiotic (especially ampicillin, sulfonamides, tetracyclines), antacids, anticonvulsants (carbamazepine, ethosuximide, phenobarbital, phenytoin, primidone, valproic acid, valproate), barbiturates, griseofulvin, rifampin. | Use additional birth control method during drug use and for one cycle after drug discontinuation, or use alternative contraceptive method. |

*Note:* Vitamin C, 1 g or more daily, may cause increased serum concentrations of estrogen and possibly increased adverse effects of estrogens.
[a] Clinical significance of this interaction is unknown.
[b] Increased risk of hepatotoxicity with simultaneous use.

**TABLE 6–7. HORMONE CONTENT AND RELATED SIDE EFFECTS**

| Estrogen Excess | | | Estrogen Deficiency |
|---|---|---|---|
| *Reproductive System*<br>Hypermenorrhea, menorrhagia, and clotting<br>Cervical extrophy<br>Dysmenorrhea<br>Breast enlargement and tenderness<br>Mucorrhea<br>Uterine fibroid growth<br>Enlargement of uterus<br>Cystic breast changes | *PMS-Type Symptoms*<br>Nausea<br>Edema, leg cramps<br>Nonvascular headaches<br>Irritability<br>Bloating<br>Dizziness, syncope<br>Cyclic weight gain<br>*Miscellaneous Symptoms*<br>Chloasma<br>Hayfever & allergic rhinitis<br>Urinary tract infection<br>Upper respiratory disorders<br>Epigastric distress | *Cardiovascular System*<br>Vascular headaches<br>Hypertension<br>Cerebrovascular accident<br>Deep vein thrombosis<br>Thromboembolic disorders<br>Telangiectasias | Absence of withdrawal bleeding<br>Spotting and bleeding (day 1 to day 9, or continuously)<br>Hypomenorrhea<br>Nervousness<br>Atrophic vaginitis<br>Vasomotor symptoms<br>Pelvic relaxation |
| **Progestin Excess** | | | **Progestin Deficiency** |
| *Progestational*<br>Reproduction Symptoms:<br>Post-pill amenorrhea<br>Libido decrease<br>Light menses<br>Cervicitis<br>Monilial vaginitis<br>Miscellaneous Symptoms:<br>Increased appetite<br>Fatigue/weakness<br>Depression, mood changes<br>Noncyclic weight gain | *Androgenic/Anabolic*<br>Increased libido<br>Acne<br>Hirsutism<br>Oil skin and scalp<br>Cholestatic jaundice<br>Rash<br>Pruritis<br>Edema | *Cardiovascular System*<br>Hypertension<br>Dilation of leg veins<br>Lowered protective forms of high density lipoproteins (HDLs) | Breakthrough bleeding and spotting during late cycle (days 10 to 21)<br>Delayed withdrawal bleeding<br>Dysmenorrhea<br>Menorrhagia and clotting |

*Source: References 2, 8, 17, 18, 27.*

- Determine which hormonal component of the OC is likely to be responsible for the symptom.
- Determine whether the side effect is due to an excess or deficiency of a hormonal component (see Table 6–7). If it is determined that the side effect is due to a deficiency or excess of a particular hormonal component, switch the client to a different OC product that has greater or lesser activity of the offending hormone (Table 6–5).

Table 6–8 lists common side effects, suggested hormone adjustments, and other management considerations. Tables 6–5 and 6–9 include hormonal activities of low and mod-

**TABLE 6–8. MANAGEMENT OF SIDE EFFECTS OF ORAL CONTRACEPTIVES**

| Sign, Symptom, Side Effect | Estrogen Adjustment | Progestin Adjustment | Comments and Other Considerations |
|---|---|---|---|
| Acne | Increase *or* | Decrease—less androgenic | Hygiene, diet, antibiotic therapy |
| Amenorrhea or light menses | Increase | Decrease | Rule out pregnancy; change to pill with higher endometrial activity |
| Anemia | No change | No change or increase | Diet, iron supplements, evaluate anemia |
| Bloating, fluid retention | Decrease | No change | Consider minipill |
| Breakthrough bleeding, spotting | Early cycle (days 1 to 14) increase or give estrogen supplement | No change | Review history for misuse; check for infection, cervical changes, pregnancy |
| | Late cycle (days 15 to 21) No change | Increase or more biologically active | Change to pill with higher endometrial activity |
| Breast tenderness, fullness | Decrease | No change or decrease | Consider minipill; decrease sodium, caffeine intake; Vitamin E 400 IU b.i.d. |
| Breast or uterine cancer | Stop | Stop | Refer |
| Cervical eversion and increased mucus | Decrease | No change or decrease | Examine for infection |
| Chloasma | Decrease or stop | No change or less estrogenic | Consider minipill |
| Contact lens discomfort, refractive changes | Decrease or stop | No change | Consider minipill |
| Cyclic weight gain | Decrease | No change or decrease | |
| Decreased breast milk in nursing mothers | Stop | No change or decrease | Combined OCs not recommended—consider minipill |

| | | | |
|---|---|---|---|
| Decreased libido | Decrease or stop | Decrease or stop, or higher androgenic | Sexual counseling |
| Depression | Decrease or stop | Decrease or stop | Try vitamin $B_6$ 20–25 mg per day; monitor closely |
| Diplopia, any loss of vision, papilledema | Stop | Stop | Evaluate |
| Diabetes, worsening of | Decrease or stop | Decrease or stop | Monitor closely |
| Dizziness | Decrease or stop | No change; or if hypoglycemia present, decrease | If hypoglycemia, eat regularly and avoid simple carbohydrates |
| Dysmenorrhea | Decrease | Increase—higher progestational and androgenic | Rule out infection, other pathology |
| Gallbladder disease | Stop | Stop | Evaluate |
| Increased facial hair, hair changes, thinning scalp hair | Increase | Decrease—less androgenic | Rule out thyroid dysfunction |
| High-density lipoprotein (HDL) cholesterol, decrease | Decrease or stop | Decrease or stop | Triphasic pill or try pill with new generation progestin |
| Headache, migraine | Decrease or stop | Decrease or stop | Evaluate headaches, consult physician |
| Hypermenorrhea | Decrease *and/or* | Increase—higher progestational and androgenic | Rule out pathology first |
| Hypertension | Decrease or stop | Decrease or stop | Consider minipill, stop smoking, increase exercise, lose weight, reduce stress |
| Increased appetite | No change or decrease | Decrease—less androgenic | Dietary counseling |
| Increased growth of benign fibroid tumors | Decrease or stop | No change or decrease | Rule out malignancy |
| Liver disease, jaundice, or benign liver tumor | Stop | Stop | Evaluate |

*(continued)*

**TABLE 6–8. CONTINUED**

| Sign, Symptom, Side Effect | Estrogen Adjustment | Progestin Adjustment | Comments and Other Considerations |
|---|---|---|---|
| Myocardial infarction or stroke | Stop | Stop | Refer |
| Noncyclic weight gain | No change or decrease | Decrease—less androgenic | Avoid norgestrel and levonorgestrel |
| Nausea or vomiting | Decrease or change type | No change | Take after full meal; consider minipill |
| Nervousness | No change | Decrease or stop | Rule out hypoglycemia; try monophasic pill |
| Ovarian cysts | No change | Increase—moderate to high progestational activity | If on minipill, triphasic or very low dose OC, then switch to 35 μg dose monophasic or higher |
| Pelvic inflammatory disease (PID) | No change | No change | Evaluate and treat infection; monitor closely |
| Pulmonary embolism, thromboembolism, thrombophlebitis (or symptoms of) | Stop | Stop | Refer |
| Rheumatoid arthritis | No change | No change | Treat rheumatoid arthritis adequately |
| Thyroid function tests changes | No change | No change | Evaluate for thyroid dysfunction |
| Urinary tract infection | Decrease | No change | Treat infections |
| Vaginal dryness | Increase | Decrease | Use additional lubrication |
| Varicose veins | Decrease | No change | Consider minipill |
| Yeast infections | No change | Decrease | Hygiene measures, treat infection |

*Source: References 2, 8, 17, 18, 24, 26, 27, 34, 35.*

**TABLE 6–9. CONTRACEPTIVE PILL ACTIVITY[a]**

| Drug | Endometrial Activity (%)[b] | Estrogenic Activity μg[c] | Progestational Activity (mg)[d] | Androgenic Activity (mg)[e] |
|---|---|---|---|---|
| *50 μg Estrogen* | | | | |
| Ovral | 4.5[f] | 42 | 1.3 | 0.80 |
| Norlestrin 2.5 | 5.1[f] | 16 | 2.7 | 1.30 |
| Genora/Norethin/Norinyl/ Ortho-Novum 1/50 | 10.6 | 32 | 1.0 | 0.34 |
| Ovcon 50 | 11.9 | 50 | 1.0 | 0.34 |
| Demulen 50 | 13.9[f] | 26 | 1.4 | 0.21 |
| Norlestrin 1/50 | 13.6[f] | 39 | 1.2 | 0.53 |
| *Sub-50 μg Estrogen Monophasic* | | | | |
| Lo-Ovral | 9.6[f] | 25 | 0.8 | 0.46 |
| Desogen/Ortho-Cept | 9.9 | 30 | 1.5 | 0.17 |
| Ovcon 35 | 11.0 | 40 | 0.4 | 0.15 |
| Levlen/Nordette | 14.0[f] | 25 | 0.8 | 0.46 |
| Ortho-Cyclen | 14.3[f] | 35 | 0.3 | 0.18 |
| Brevicon/Modicon/ Nelova 0.5/35 | 14.6 | 42 | 0.5 | 0.17 |
| Genora/Nelova/Norethin/ Norinyl/Ortho-Novum 1/35 | 14.7 | 38 | 1.0 | 0.34 |
| Loestrin 1/5/30 | 25.2[f] | 14 | 1.7 | 0.80 |
| Loestrin 1/20 | 29.7[f] | 13 | 1.2 | 0.53 |
| Demulen 1/35 | 37.4[f] | 19 | 1.4 | 0.21 |
| *Sub-50 μg Estrogen Multiphasic* | | | | |
| Ortho-Novum 7/7/7 | 12.2 | 48 | 0.8 | 0.25 |
| Jenest | 14.1 | 39 | 0.8 | 0.28 |
| Tri-Norinyl | 14.7 | 40 | 0.7 | 0.23 |
| Tri-Levlen/Triphasil | 15.1[f] | 28 | 0.5 | 0.29 |
| Tri-Cyclen | 17.5[f] | 35 | 0.3 | 0.15 |
| Ortho-Novum 10/11 | 19.6 | 40 | 0.8 | 0.25 |
| *Progestin-Only* | | | | |
| Ovrette | 34.9 | 0 | 0.08 | 0.13 |
| Micronor/Nor-QD | 42.3 | 1 | 0.12 | 0.13 |

[a] Listed according to estrogen content and endometrial potency.
[b] Spotting, and bleeding, in third cycle of use. Information submitted to the United States Food and Drug Administration by the manufacturer. These rates are derived from separate studies conducted by different investigators in several population groups, and therefore, a precise comparison cannot be made.
[c] Ethinyl estradiol equivalents per day. Estrogenic activity of entire tablet—mouse uterine assay.
[d] Norethindrone equivalents per day. Induction of glycogen vacuoles in human endometrium.
[e] Methyltestosterone per 28 days. Rat ventral prostate assay.
[f] Includes early withdrawal flow.
*Source: Reprinted with permission of Dickey, R.P.* Managing contraceptive pill patients *(7th ed.). Durant, OK: Essential Medical Information Systems, Inc. 1993.*

erate dose OCs, and may be used when OC dosage and/or potency adjustments are indicated for management of specific side effects.

### Effects of OCs on Blood Lipids

Use of OCs as a factor influencing blood lipoproteins has received a disproportionate amount of attention. No causal link between OC use and cardiovascular morbidity resulting from blood lipid changes has been noted. Interest, however, has focused on lipoprotein changes that occur, because they are known indicators of increased risk for cardiovascular disease (CVD).[18,28,36–37]

It is known that estrogens increase high density lipoproteins (HDLs) and decrease low density lipoproteins (LDLs). Progestins tend to increase total cholesterol and LDLs. Progestins also decrease triglycerides, very-low-density lipoproteins (VLDLs), and HDLs, especially HDL-2, which provides the protective effect against CVD. New generation progestins have shown fewer atherogenic lipid changes over time. These metabolic effects are summarized in Table 6–10.[17,25,26,33–36]

### Effects of OCs on Carbohydrate (CHO) Metabolism

Early studies of OCs demonstrated increases in glucose levels (slight), decreases in glucose tolerance, and increases in plasma levels of insulin; however, low dose OCs currently used show minimal or no changes in CHO metabolism. The progestational component of the OC seems to have greatest effect on CHO metabolism. In a nondiabetic user, the significance of these changes is uncertain, but the issue is important because glucose intolerance may be linked to coronary heart disease and increased levels of insulin may be involved in the atherogenic process. For diabetic women or women with a history of glucose intolerance, it is felt that low dose pills may be given provided that clients are followed closely (refer to Table 6–10).[8,27,28,37–40]

### Effects of OCs on the Risk of Breast Cancer

Whether a relationship exists between OC use and the development of breast cancer remains unclear and controversial. A few studies have suggested a link between the development of breast cancer at a relatively young age and long-term use of OCs; however, other studies refute these findings. Existing data suggest that the overall risk of breast cancer is not increased by the use of OCs. No increased breast cancer risk was noted for women older than 60 years who had used OCs. General conclusions are that the benefits of OCs greatly outweigh the risks for appropriately selected candidates.[38,41–45]

### Contraindications

Table 6–11 lists absolute and relative contraindications to the use of oral contraceptives.

### Management Considerations[8,17,18,46,47]

- All clients taking OCs should be advised to stop smoking. Nonsmoking, healthy women (without contraindications) older than 35 may take low dose OCs.
- Instruct that OCs do not protect against STDs, including HIV infection. If the client is not in a mutually monogamous relationship, advise that condoms with spermicide be used in addition to pills.
- Initial pill selection is based on individual client characteristics. New OC users should generally be started on the lowest dose that is still effective: a 35 μg (or less)

**TABLE 6–10. SELECTED METABOLIC EFFECTS OF ESTROGENS AND PROGESTINS**

| Estrogens | Progestins |
|---|---|
| Increase HDL cholesterol | Increase LDL cholesterol |
| Decrease LDL cholesterol | Decrease HDL cholesterol, especially HDL-2 |
| Increase blood glucose | Increase total cholesterol |
| | Decrease triglycerides |
| | Decrease VLDL |
| | Increase insulin levels |

*Note:* HDL = high density lipoprotein; LDL = low density lipoprotein; VLDL = very-low-density lipoprotein.

The new generation progestins have shown fewer atherogenic lipid changes over time.

The greater the androgenicity and higher the dose of the progestin, the greater the potential to affect lipid and carbohydrate metabolism adversely.

*Source: References 8, 17, 18, 25, 26, 31, 33, 36, 37.*

pill. Since the introduction of triphasic preparations, many practitioners start new users on one of them. The lowest dose monophasic combined OC available, Loestrin 1/20 (Parke-Davis), should be considered for older women. Specific client characteristics that may influence initial OC selection include age, personal and family history, relative contraindications, menstrual patterns, and hormone sensitivity.

New users should be reevaluated after 3 cycles of pill use to determine how they are adjusting. Instruct the client to contact the provider sooner if concerns arise. Early intervention and support when a client experiences bothersome side effects may prevent her from discontinuing the pill for nonmedical reasons.

- Instruct the client about how to take combined OCs. When first initiating pill use, one of the following methods is recommended.
  - Start pack on first Sunday after period begins, regardless of whether bleeding is still present (preferred method). *or*
  - Start pack on first day of menstrual bleeding. *or*
  - Start pack on fifth day after menstrual bleeding begins.

  Pill manufacturers often recommend specific routines for initiating use of their products. Instruct the client to swallow one pill daily, at the same time each day, until the pack is finished.
  - If using 28-day pack, begin new pack immediately. Do not skip any days.
  - If using 21-day pack, stop pills for exactly 7 days, then start new pack.
  - Periods may be very light while on pills. Even slight spotting or bleeding should be considered a period (as long as no pills were missed).
- Instruct the client to use a second birth control method, such as condoms or a diaphragm used with spermicide, until she completes her first pack of OCs. Another method is always kept on hand to use in case of missed pills, when taking another medication that might interfere with pill effectiveness (see Table 6–6), or when vomiting or diarrhea occurs.
- If one or more pills are missed for any reason, the following instructions apply.
  - If one pill is missed, take missed pill as soon as remembered and next pill at usual time. If one missed pill is taken more than 12 hours late, a backup method of contraception must be used for next 2 weeks even if menses occur or a new pill pack is started.
  - If two or more pills are missed, take two pills as soon as remembered and discard remaining missed (forgotten) pills. The next day's pill will be the one normally taken for that day, had no pills been forgotten. Spotting is very likely to occur.

**TABLE 6–11. CONTRAINDICATIONS TO THE USE OF ORAL CONTRACEPTIVES**

*Absolute Contraindications*

- Thrombophlebitis or thromboembolic disorder
- Cerebrovascular disease
- Coronary artery or ischemic heart disease
- Known or suspected breast cancer
- Known or suspected estrogen-dependent neoplasia
- Known or suspected pregnancy
- Benign or malignant liver tumor
- Current impaired liver function
- Previous cholestasis with pregnancy or with previous pill use
- Undiagnosed, abnormal vaginal bleeding

*Relative Contraindications*

- Vascular or migraine headaches, especially if they began or worsened with the use of combined oral contraceptives
- Hypertension
- Acute mononucleosis or recent hepatitis
- Presence of factors predisposing to thromboembolic disorder, such as illness or surgery requiring immobilization, long leg cast, trauma to lower leg
- Cardiac or renal dysfunction (or history of)
- Diabetes or prediabetes
- Obesity (of more than 20 percent of ideal body weight)
- Varicose veins
- Lactation
- Age over 50
- Age over 35 for a smoker (some providers feel that no heavy smoker should take birth control pills)
- Psychic depression
- History of myocardial infarction in an immediate family member before age 50 (especially a mother or a sister)
- Hyperlipidemia
- Active gallbladder disease
- Sickle cell (SS) or sickle C disease
- Completion of a term pregnancy within the past 10 to 14 days
- Ulcerative colitis
- Asthma

*Source: References 8, 17, 18, 23, 37–39.*

Again, use backup method for next 2 weeks.

- If a period is missed and pills were taken correctly, the client should begin a new pack as usual. Pregnancy is unlikely. If two consecutive periods are missed, pills are stopped and a pregnancy test is done.
- If a period is missed and client missed one or more pills, pills are stopped; pregnancy test is done.
- If a decision is made to stop OCs and pregnancy is not desired, begin using another

BC method immediately. If pregnancy is desired, use another method for two or three cycles after stopping pills.

- Birth control pills are considered medication. Always tell any health care provider when OCs are being taken.
- The client who seems to consistently miss pills should consider other methods of contraception.

## PROGESTIN-ONLY PILLS (POPs)

Referred to as "minipills," progestin-only pills (POPs) were introduced 10 years after combined oral contraceptives (COCs). POPs are taken daily with no pill-free interval. Although much less popular than COCs, POPs are well suited to women who want to take contraceptive pills but have contraindications to COCs (e.g., women with a history of thrombophlebitis, or who developed hypertension or severe headaches while taking COCs). Available POPs contain norethindrone or norgestrel[8,17,18]; they contain a fixed dose of progestin in either 28- or 42-day packs (see Table 6–5).

### Mechanisms of Action

There are four mechanisms by which POPs may prevent pregnancy.[8,17,18,23]

- Ovulation is suppressed by inhibition of LH release from the anterior pituitary. Ovulation is inhibited in about 40 percent of cycles.
- Cervical mucus maintains a thick consistency, inhibiting sperm penetration.
- The endometrium becomes thin and atrophic.
- Tubal changes occur, including altered tubal transport, contractility, and histology.

### Effectiveness

POPs are somewhat less effective than combined OCs (see Table 6–4). Efficacy increases significantly in women of older reproductive age and women who are lactating.[21]

### Advantages[8,17,18,39]

- No estrogen-related side effects.
- Overall safer than combined OCs (fewer and less serious complications).
- May be used by lactating women.
- May be used by clients with prior history of thrombophlebitis (no effect on blood clotting) or with history of other estrogen-related contraindications to COC use.
- Minimal effect on carbohydrate metabolism; therefore, may be used (with caution) by diabetic women.
- Rapid reversal of effects after stopping.
- Several noncontraceptive benefits.

### Noncontraceptive Benefits[8,17,18]

Most health benefits are similar to those of combined OCs. Because only a small number of women use POPs, large scale studies are not available. Menstrual cycle benefits include decreased cramping, lighter bleeding, shorter periods, decreased PMS-type symptoms, and lessened breast tenderness.

### Disadvantages[8,17,42]

- Must be taken with meticulous accuracy; no more than 27 hours between pills.
- Less effective than combined OCs.
- May cause irregular bleeding with unpredictable patterns (may include spotting, breakthrough bleeding (BTB), amenorrhea, prolonged bleeding).
- No protection against HIV infection and other STDs.
- Interaction with other drugs can decrease effectiveness (see Table 6–6).
- Higher incidence of functional ovarian cysts.
- Higher incidence of ectopic pregnancy.
- Progestins may adversely affect blood

lipids by decreasing HDLs and increasing LDLs and triglycerides (see Table 6–10).
- Less widely available than combined OCs. Also refer to the section on combined OCs and to Tables 6–7, 6–8, and 6–9 to evaluate and manage side effects.

### Contraindications[8,17,18]

According to the FDA, progestin-only pills are required to carry the same contraindications as combined OCs, even though many of these contraindications are related to estrogen content (see Table 6–11). Several relative contraindications to POPs should be emphasized.

- History of functional ovarian cysts.
- History of ectopic pregnancy.
- Inability to take pills consistently.
- Undiagnosed abnormal vaginal bleeding during the preceding 3 months.
- Hyperlipidemia.

### Management Considerations[8,17,18,34,35]

- All clients taking POPs should be advised to stop smoking. Nonsmoking, healthy women (without contraindications) older than 35 may take low dose OCs.
- Instruct that POPs do not protect against STDs, including HIV infection. If the client is not in a mutually monogamous relationship, advise that condoms with spermicide be used in addition to pills.
- If decision is made to stop POPs and pregnancy is not desired, begin using another BC method immediately. If pregnancy is desired, use another method for two or three cycles after stopping pills.
- Birth control pills are considered medication. Always tell any health care provider when POPs are being taken.
- When taking POPs, it is important to keep track of periods. Tell the client that if more than 45 days pass with no bleeding, a health care professional should be contacted for an examination and pregnancy test.
- Spotting or bleeding between periods is not unusual for a woman on the minipill, especially during the first few months of use. Furthermore, some bleeding is very likely if one or more pills are missed. Heavy bleeding, pain, or fever is reported to the health care professional.
- *Initiating Use.* Pills are started on the first day of the period, or immediately after completing a 21-day pack of combined OC, or after the 21st pill of 28-day pack (placebo pills are discarded). A second birth control method is kept on hand to use for (a) the first 7 days on minipills, (b) times when pills are missed, (c) when on antibiotics, or (d) when experiencing diarrhea or vomiting.
- One pill is swallowed daily until pack is finished; new pack is started the very next day—a day is never skipped. In addition, minipills must be taken at *exactly* the same time every day.
- When minipills are missed or forgotten, instruct the client as follows.
  - If pill is taken more than 3 hours late, use a backup birth control method for the next 48 hours.
  - If one pill is missed, take it as soon as remembered. Take the next pill at the regular time, even if this means taking two pills in 1 day. Use a backup method for the next 48 hours.
  - If two pills or more are missed in a row, there is good chance of pregnancy occurring. Take two pills as soon as remembered and two the next day. Start using a second method of birth control right away. If no period occurs in 4 to 6 weeks, a pregnancy test is needed.

## OTHER PROGESTIN-ONLY CONTRACEPTIVES: IMPLANTS, INJECTIONS, VAGINAL RINGS

The newest methods available (and being tested) for controlling fertility are long acting progestin-only systems. These are ideal for women who desire long term, continuous contraception and who may desire future pregnancies. Among the systems developed or being developed, five are discussed here.

### Norplant

Approved for use in the United States in 1990 and marketed by Wyeth-Ayerst, Norplant is a timed-release implant of levonorgestrel. Once in place, it provides 5 years of continuous, highly effective contraception. The system consists of six Silastic capsules, each measuring 2.4 × 34 mm and containing 36 mg of levonorgestrel. Capsules are implanted in a fanlike pattern through a 3–5 mm incision, usually in the medial aspect of the upper arm. The Norplant System releases 80 μg of le-vonorgestrel per day during the first few weeks after insertion, decreasing over the next 18 months to a constant rate of approximately 30 μg per day over a 5-year period.[8,18,48–50]

### Depo-Provera Injections

Depo-Provera is an intramuscular (I.M.) injection of depo-medroxyprogesterone acetate (DMPA) that provides 3 months of protection. It was approved by the FDA for use as a contraceptive in the United States in November 1992, after many years of controversy. The standard dosage is DMPA 150 mg I.M. every 90 days.[8,18,52]

### Capronor

Still being tested in the United States, Capronor consists of biodegradable capsules that contain levonorgestrel, which provides contraceptive protection for 12 to 18 months. Once placed under the skin, the capsules *cannot* be easily removed. Other biodegradable pellet systems are being developed.[8,18,49,51]

### Norethindrone Enanthate (NET) Injections

Intramuscular injections of NET are given every 2 months. The drug has been tested extensively by the World Health Organization (WHO) but is not currently used in the United States. The dosage is NET 200 mg I.M. every 2 months.[8,18,52]

### Vaginal Ring

Being developed and tested, this Silastic ring containing progesterone or levonorgestrel is placed high in the vagina, much like a diaphragm. The hormone is released gradually and absorbed systemically through the vaginal walls. The ring may be removed at specified intervals only. Protection lasts for 6 months.[8,18,49,53]

### Mechanisms of Action

Progestin-only systems vary in their delivery method, blood levels, and duration of action. The mechanisms of action by which pregnancy is prevented are the same, however.[8,18,49]

- Ovulation is suppressed by inhibition of LH release from the anterior pituitary. Ovulation is inhibited in about 40 percent of cycles.
- Cervical mucus maintains a thick consistency, inhibiting sperm penetration.
- The endometrium becomes thin and atrophic.
- Tubal changes occur, including altered tubal transport, contractility, and histology.

### Effectiveness

Failure of long acting progestins is rare when they are properly administered and used no longer than the specified time limits. Injection systems must be injected within the first 5 days of the menstrual cycle; inserted within the first 7 days for implants and vaginal rings. *It must be determined that the woman is not pregnant.* These methods are considered highly effective (see Table 6–4).[8,21,49]

Note that the body weight of the user may affect the efficacy of implants and vaginal rings. In early studies with Norplant, the pregnancy rate during the second year of use was higher among women who weighed more than 70 kg (154 lb) than it was among women of lower body weight.[8,48]

### Advantages[8,48,50,54]

- Long duration of action.
- Relative low doses of hormone.
- Few systemic complications.
- Low ectopic pregnancy rates.
- Major complications are rare.
- Effects on blood lipids appear to be minimal.
- Some noncontraceptive benefits.

### Disadvantages[8,48,50,54]

- Most women experience some side effects; most are minor and related to menstrual irregularities. If bleeding is heavy, anemia may occur.
- Implants are very expensive.
- Implants may be slightly visible.
- Implants must be inserted and removed by a specially trained clinician.
- Removal of implants may be difficult if scar tissue has formed around implants.
- In rare instances infection can occur at the implant insertion site.
- Partner may feel the vaginal ring. (If so, ring may be removed during intercourse and then replaced.)
- Expulsion of the implant system or vaginal ring can occur.
- Injections may not be effective for up to 2 weeks.
- Return to fertility may be delayed up to 6 or 12 months after injection of Depo-Provera.
- Studies indicate some possible increased risk of breast cancer in young women who use Depo-Provera for 6 years or more.

### Contraindications

Progestin-only methods must carry the same contraindications as COCs, even though many are related to estrogen content (see Table 6–11). Several relative contraindications to long acting progestin-only systems should be emphasized.

- History of undiagnosed abnormal vaginal bleeding during the 3 months prior to use of one of these methods.
- Acute liver disease.
- Jaundice.
- For Depo-Provera injection: when rapid return to fertility is desired.[8,49]

### Management Considerations[8,18,48,53]

- The insertion and removal of implant systems must be done by a professional specifically trained in the proper techniques.
- Teaching and counseling must include information about how long the system is effective; what to expect regarding changes in bleeding patterns; and the importance of continuing annual gynecologic care (see Management Considerations, Guidelines for Client Information, and Informed Consent).
- Danger signs that indicate possible serious problems associated with use of the methods must be taught.
    - Severe abdominal pain.
    - Heavy vaginal bleeding.
    - Frequent urination.

- Depression.
- Severe headache.
- Pus or bleeding at the insertion site.
- Weight gain.
- Expulsion of the implant.

## POSTCOITAL CONTRACEPTIVE METHODS

The terms *postcoital contraception, interception,* and *morning-after contraception* refer to intervention taken to prevent pregnancy after a single act of unprotected intercourse. Indications for use include sexual assault; condom breakage; dislodgement of cervical cap, diaphragm, or sponge; missed OC; or any unexpected event or emotion that leads to unprotected intercourse and the possibility of pregnancy.[8]

### Morning-After Pills

- Combined oral contraceptives in the form of 0.5 mg norgestrel and 0.05 mg ethinyl estradiol (Ovral) tablets. Two tablets are taken within 72 hours (preferably sooner) of unprotected coitus and 2 more tablets are taken in 12 hours. This method carries a high rate of effectiveness. It works by causing luteal phase dysfunction, asynchrony of endometrial development, and disordered tubal transport. Give the client extra pills in case nausea and vomiting occur, and teach pill danger signs (*ACHES*: See page 116). Menses should begin within 2 to 3 weeks; if it does not, a pregnancy test should be performed.
- High dose oral estrogens in the form of diethylstilbestrol (DES) 25 mg twice daily for 5 days *or* ethinyl estradiol (EE) 2.5 mg twice daily for 5 days may also be used for postcoital contraception; however, *DES is no longer approved for this use in the United States.* This method is highly effective. Side effects are nausea and vomiting.[8,17]
  - Conjugated estrogens (Premarin) 10 mg b.i.d. for 5 days is also used, but is slightly less effective.
- High dose progestins are being investigated for postcoital contraceptive use.
- The antiprogesterone drug mifepristone (RU-486) is used in countries other than the United States as a postcoital contraceptive. European studies have shown it highly effective as a morning-after contraceptive when used within 3 days of having unprotected intercourse. Mifepristone induces less nausea or vomiting than other drugs used as a postcoital contraceptive.[55,56]

### Morning-After IUD Insertion

Copper-containing IUDs can be inserted 5 to 7 days after unprotected intercourse to prevent implantation of a fertilized egg. This method has a high success rate for preventing pregnancy when used postcoitally.[8] The same precautions and contraindications apply when an IUD is inserted for this purpose as when used for routine contraception (see Intrauterine Devices, later in this chapter).

### Menstrual Induction

The drug of choice for menstrual induction is 0.5 mg norgestrel and 0.05 mg ethinyl estradiol (Ovral) given within the first 72 hours after unprotected intercourse. Alternatively, the antiprogesterone drug mifepristone (RU-486) is used in other countries as a postcoital contraceptive to induce menses. When administered after ovulation, late in the menstrual cycle, mifepristone acts as a competitive antagonist to progesterone, preventing implantation or causing sloughing of the fertilized zygote. Serious side effects have not been identified, and RU-486 is highly effective. Effectiveness increases when used in combination with prostaglandin ($PGE_2$). That this method may induce early abortion has made it very controversial in the United States.[8,55–57]

## THE MALE CONDOM

The male condom, also referred to as a *rubber, prophylactic,* or *skin*, is a sheath that fits over an erect penis to contain fluid from ejaculation. Made of latex rubber or processed collagenous tissue, condoms are available in many colors, textures, sizes, shapes, and thicknesses. Some condoms feature lubrication, a reservoir tip, and/or a spermicide (nonoxynol-9) on the inside and outside.[8,58]

### Mechanism of Action

A *condom* is a mechanical barrier to prevent sperm from entering the vagina and cervix. Latex condoms prevent transmission of most sexually transmitted infections, including HIV. Spermicidal condoms have the additional action of nonoxynol-9 to immobilize and kill sperm after ejaculation and thus reduce the likelihood of transmitting STDs (see Spermicides, later in this chapter). Infecting organisms can be physically transmitted into the uterus and tubes by sperm.[8,11,58]

### Effectiveness

Condoms are considered *moderately* effective at preventing accidental pregnancy (see Table 6–4). Failure to prevent pregnancy is most frequently attributed to inconsistent use.[21] Condom breakage can occur, but this probably is not a major cause of accidental pregnancy.[8] Effectiveness increases significantly, approaching the effectiveness of oral contraceptives or an IUD, when used concurrently with a vaginal spermicide.[58]

### Advantages[8,58,59]

- Available without a prescription or examination.
- Relatively inexpensive.
- Widely available.
- Physiologically safe.
- No adverse effect on fertility.
- Easily reversible contraception.
- Few side effects.
- Significant protection against most STDs and their consequences, including HIV disease.
- Possible protection against cancer of the cervix.
- Male participation in contraception is encouraged.
- Only reversible contraceptive available for use by men.
- May delay premature ejaculation in men for whom this is a concern.
- May be used during lactation.
- Lubricated condoms may reduce friction, preventing irritation to either partner.
- Postcoital drainage of semen from the vagina, which some women find objectionable, is eliminated.
- Allergic reactions are prevented for women who are sensitive to partner's semen.

### Disadvantages[8,58,59]

- Fairly expensive for frequent use.
- Possible decreased sensation for man.
- Interferes with sexual spontaneity (requires forethought and preparedness).
- Necessity to interrupt foreplay to put condom on.
- "Skin" condoms made from animal membranes may not protect against some STDs, including HIV.
- Some women and men experience irritation with the use of particular lubricants or spermicides on condoms.
- Male partner may be unwilling to cooperate with condom use.

### Contraindications

- Allergy of man or woman to the latex in the condom.

### Management Considerations[8,58,59]

The following instructions will be helpful to partners using condoms.

- Store condoms in a cool, dry place. Heat, even body heat, may weaken the rubber. Always keep the condom in its original package until use. Condoms should keep 5 years when properly stored. Consider using name brands; these may be of more reliable quality.
- The condom is placed on the erect penis (either partner can do this) *before* the penis comes in contact with the woman's genital area.
- Roll the condom all the way down to the base of the penis.
- If the condom does not have a built-in reservoir, leave one-half inch of empty space at the end of it to collect ejaculate. This is accomplished by pinching the tip of the condom as it is rolled on. Leave no air in the tip; this could contribute to tearing.
- Be sure that the vagina and/or condom are well lubricated to prevent condom tearing. If additional lubrication is needed, use only water, saliva, water-based jelly, or contraceptive foam, gel, or cream. Other products, especially petroleum based, will cause rapid deterioration and weakening of the rubber. Other vaginal products that cause condom weakening include miconazole nitrate (Monistat), butoconazole nitrate (Femstat), estradiol (Estrace), and conjugated estrogen (Premarin) creams, Vagisil ointment, Rendell's Cone and Ovule Spermicide, and the sexual lubricant called Elbow Grease.[8]
- For added protection, use a second method of birth control (diaphragm, sponge, spermicidal foam, gel, film, suppository, or birth control pill).
- After intercourse, remove the condom immediately while the penis is still erect, holding on to the base of the condom to prevent spilling.
- Check the condom for tears, then throw it away. Use each condom only once. If tears are detected, immediately insert spermicidal gel or cream into the vagina.

## FEMALE CONDOMS

Two types of female condoms—the Bikini Condom, distributed by International Prophylactics, and the WPC-333 Vaginal Pouch (Reality Female Condom)—are available in the United States.[60–63]

### Bikini Condom

This condom is worn like a pair of panties and made entirely of latex. A rolled up vaginal pouch rests against the vaginal opening. The pouch, shaped like an oversized male condom, serves as a vaginal liner. The Bikini Condom can be worn up to 2 hours prior to intercourse. Just before intercourse, either partner pushes the vaginal pouch one-half inch into the vagina with a finger. A finger or erect penis is used to push the remainder of the pouch into the vagina. After intercourse, the woman grasps the base of the pouch between two fingers, gently pulling the pouch out of the vagina. The entire bikini condom is then removed. It is effective for one act of intercourse, and one size fits most women.[60] The Bikini Condom also can be worn by men and used to cover the penis during intercourse.

### Reality Female Condom

The Reality Female Condom consists of a polyurethane sheath with an outer ring and inner ring. It is inserted vaginally, like a diaphragm and held in place by the pubic bone. The closed upper tip is anchored near the cervix by a flexible inner ring that holds the device in place, preventing expulsion. The condom covers the surfaces of the vaginal wall, allowing the penis to move freely inside the condom. An external ring at the outer opening of the pouch remains outside the vagina and partially covers the labia. It is used for one act of intercourse only. If used correctly with every sex act, it also helps to prevent the spread of STD. This product, distributed by Wisconsin Pharmacal, received FDA approval in 1993.[8,61–65]

### Mechanism of Action

These devices serve as mechanical barriers to prevent sperm from entering the vagina or cervix. Latex or polyurethane female condoms also have the ability to prevent transmission of most STDs, including HIV.[8,60,61,65]

### Effectiveness

Some reports state that female condoms are about as effective as male condoms in preventing pregnancy and exposure to STDs (see Table 6–4). The FDA, however, in reviewing the effectiveness claims of the Reality female condom, stated that its effectiveness rates should not be compared with those of other birth control methods.

### Advantages[8,58–65]

- Use controlled by the woman.
- Available without a prescription or examination.
- Easily reversible.
- Considered medically safe.
- Little danger of systemic effects.
- May provide protection against STDs, cervical neoplasia.
- May be worn prior to intercourse.
- Not dependent on male arousal.
- May be used during lactation.
- May be removed immediately after intercourse.
- Eliminates postcoital drainage of semen.
- Prevents allergic reactions for women sensitive to partner's semen.

### Disadvantages[8,58–65]

- Expensive for frequent use (about three times the price of the male condom).
- For single use only.
- Cumbersome; insertion of Reality can be difficult.
- Can slip or be pushed out of place.
- May make noise during use.
- Unsightly: Reality ring dangles outside the vagina; Bikini has a latex panty.
- Reality Female Condom is made of polyurethane, which is affected by petroleum-based products.

### Contraindications

- Allergy of man or woman to latex or polyurethane.
- Anatomic abnormalities that interfere with proper placement.
- Inability to master insertion technique for Reality female condom.

### Management Considerations[8,58–66]

The following instructions will be helpful to the client:

- Practice wearing and inserting the female condom before depending on it for protection.
- Be careful not to tear the condom with sharp objects such as rings or long fingernails.
- Extra spermicidal lubricant may be used with either the Bikini Condom or Reality Condom.
- Refer to the package inserts for detailed use and insertion instructions.
- After intercourse, remove the female condom carefully to avoid spilling semen.

## SPERMICIDES

*Spermicides* are chemical substances that immobolize and kill sperm. Available in creams, foams, jellies, suppositories, and film, these products are inserted into the vagina prior to intercourse. When used alone, they are inserted vaginally near cervix, forming a chemical barrier. Spermicides are also essential components of vaginal barrier methods of contraception (diaphragm, cervical cap, and sponge). Surfaces of male condoms may be coated with spermicide to enhance the effectiveness of this method as a contraceptive and as protection against STDs.[2,8,52]

When used alone, all spermicidal products provide protection for up to one hour and for one episode of intercourse only. Additional acts of intercourse, or intercourse occurring more than one hour after insertion, require repeated application of the product.

### Foams, Jellies, Creams

These can be used alone or with a condom, diaphragm, or cervical cap. Foams are available in multidose aerosol containers or in small, single use, prefilled cartridges. Creams and jellies come in multidose tubes with reusable applicators. Some jellies are sold in single use packets.

### Suppositories

Referred to as *spermicidal vaginal tablets,* the suppositories are a small ovoid shape. They can be used alone or with a condom but must be inserted 10 to 15 minutes before intercourse in order to melt and disperse the spermicide.

### Vaginal Contraceptive Film (VCF)

VCF, which can be used alone or with a condom or diaphragm, is a paper-thin sheet of film containing nonoxynol-9, measuring 2 × 2 in. The sheet is inserted on or near the cervix (or inside a diaphragm) at least 5 minutes prior to intercourse in order to melt and disperse the spermicide.[2,8,11]

### Mechanism of Action

Spermicides contain a chemical that immobilizes and kills sperm (by destroying sperm cell membrane) and vehicle ingredients to keep the spermicide in place around the cervix. The active ingredient in most spermicidal products sold in the United States is nonoxynol-9. Octoxynol is the active agent in other products and is equally effective as a spermicide. In vitro studies of nonoxynol-9 show that it is lethal to organisms that cause trichomonas, gonorrhea, genital herpes, syphilis, and HIV/AIDS. Clinical studies have shown significant protection against gonorrhea and chlamydia for women who used nonoxynol-9 products alone or with a diaphragm when compared with women who used oral contraceptives or who were surgically sterilized.[8,66,67]

When applying any of these findings, it is important to remember two points.

- The in vitro effect cannot be interpreted to mean absolute protection against transmission of these infections.
- Gonorrhea, chlamydia, and HIV are intracellular organisms. An organism's location inside a cell could shield it from exposure to spermicide.[8]

The presence of spermicide or even a physical barrier contraceptive does not preclude an organism's access to the body via open lesions or through areas beyond which barrier or spermicide is present, such as intracervical or endometrial areas.[8]

### Effectiveness

Spermicides are moderately effective at preventing accidental pregnancy (see Table

6–4). Failures are most frequently attributed to inconsistent use. Proper use, including placement of the product deep inside the vagina against the cervix, is essential. Efficacy is much greater if used with a condom. Data are not available comparing the efficacies of various spermicidal products.[8,21]

## Advantages[8,66–69]

- Widely available without a prescription or examination.
- Relatively inexpensive.
- Medically safe.
- Readily available as a backup method in a variety of circumstances:
  - In the event of condom rupture.
  - To augment other methods during midcycle, when the woman is most fertile.
  - When a woman begins using oral contraceptives.
  - When a woman taking oral contraceptives misses one or more pills.
- Can reduce STD transmission.
- Completely reversible.
- No effect on the return to fertility.
- Women can decide independently to use it.
- Can provide lubrication during intercourse.
- Can be used during lactation.
- Convenient, useful method of contraception after delivery and before the first postpartum visit, and when changing from one method to another.

## Disadvantages[8,11,68,69]

- May interfere with sexual spontaneity (requires forethought and preparedness).
- Must be on hand at or near the time of intercourse.
- Suppositories and film require time to disperse before intercourse can take place.
- Perceived as messy by some individuals (drainage of the substance from the vagina occurs after intercourse).
- Incomplete dissolution of suppositories can cause an uncomfortable, gritty sensation for either partner, and may impair contraceptive effectiveness.
- Some users experience a warm sensation; some feel that the suppository "burns."
- For couples engaging in oral–genital sex, the taste of spermicides is unpleasant. Spermicide may be inserted after this activity, but before penis–vagina contact takes place.
- Skin irritation of the vulva or penis can result from allergy or sensitivity to the spermicide or base ingredients. Another product may be tried.
- A few studies in the early 1980s reported possible adverse effects on the fetus if spermicide was used near or at the time of conception. Subsequent, more carefully designed and controlled studies failed to show adverse effects on the fetus.

## Contraindications[8]

- Allergy of either partner to spermicide or its other ingredients.
- Inability to "remember" to use the product associated with intercourse.
- Inability to learn the proper insertion technique.
- Anatomic abnormalities of the vagina that might interfere with the correct placement or retention of the spermicide.

## Management Considerations[8,11,67]

The following instructions will be helpful to partners using a spermicide.

- The spermicide must be used every time intercourse occurs; must be in place prior to penis–vagina contact.
- Store spermicides in a cool, clean, and dry place.
- Wait the specified time after insertion so that the spermicide is adequately dispersed (for film and suppositories).

- One application is good for one hour after insertion and for one act of intercourse only. Additional application is needed if one hour has passed since insertion or before each additional act of intercourse.
- All spermicides must be left in place for at least 6 hours after the last act of intercourse. Do not douche or rinse the product out for at least six hours.
- Instructions for specific products include the following.
    - *Foam.* Shake vigorously at least 20 times before dispensing. Insert as for jelly or cream, below.
    - *Jelly or Cream.* Fill applicator by squeezing the tube from the bottom. Insert the applicator as far into the vagina as it will go comfortably. Holding the applicator in place, push the plunger to release the product.
    - *Suppository (Vaginal Tablet).* Remove the wrapper and insert as far as possible so that the tablet rests on or near cervix. Wait the specified time before intercourse.
    - *Film.* Fingers must be completely dry. Place one sheet of film on a fingertip and slide it along the back wall of the vagina as far as possible, so that the film rests on or near cervix. Wait at least 5 minutes before intercourse to allow dispersion.
- If burning or irritation occurs, stop use of the product. Changing brands or the form of spermicide may diminish reactions. If a reaction persists, discontinue use.

## VAGINAL BARRIER METHODS: DIAPHRAGMS, CERVICAL CAPS, SPONGES[8,52,70–74]

### Diaphragm

A *diaphragm* is a dome-shaped cup made of latex rubber with a flexible-spring metal rim. It is inserted vaginally prior to intercourse, so that the posterior rim rests in the posterior fornix and the anterior rim fits snugly behind the pubic bone. Spermicidal cream, jelly, or film is applied inside the dome of the diaphragm and around the rim before insertion. Diaphragms are available in a range of sizes and four general styles. Specified sizes refer to millimeters in diameter across the rim, for example, 65 mm, 70 mm, 75 mm.

- *Coil Spring Rim.* This type has a sturdy rim with firm spring strength, which most women with average vaginal musculature and average pubic arch notch can us comfortably. The diaphragm folds flat for insertion and can be used with a plastic introducer. Specific products include Koromex diaphragm (latex), sizes 50–95; Ortho coil spring diaphragm (latex), sizes 50–95; Ramses flexible cushioned diaphragm (gum rubber), sizes 50–95.
- *Flat Spring Rim.* Having a thin, delicate rim with gentle spring strength, this type of diaphragm can be worn comfortably by nulliparous women with firm vaginal musculature or by women with a shallow notch behind the pubic bone. It folds flat for insertion and can be used with introducer. One example of this product is the Ortho-White diaphragm (latex), sizes 55–95.
- *Arcing Spring Rim.* The sturdy rim of this type of diaphragm imparts firm spring strength. Furthermore, the arcing rim facilitates insertion. Most women can use it comfortably, and it can be retained in the presence of cystocele and/or rectocele or relaxed vaginal muscle tone. Specific products include the Koroflex diaphragm (latex), sizes 60–95; Ortho All-Flex diaphragm (latex), sizes 55–95; Ramses Bendex diaphragm (gum rubber), sizes 65–95.
- *Wide-Seal Rim.* This type has a thin, flexible flange approximately 1.5 cm wide attached to the inner edge of the rim to keep

spermicide in place inside the dome and to enhance the seal between the rim and the vaginal wall. It is made in two styles, arcing and coil spring. Specific products include the Milex Wide-Seal arcing diaphragm (latex), sizes 60–95; Milex Wide-Seal Omniflex coil spring diaphragm (latex), sizes 60–95. Milex diaphragms are not available from pharmacies by prescription, but are only distributed to doctors and clinics by the manufacturer.[8,11,70–74]

## Vaginal Contraceptive Sponge

The Today vaginal sponge has been available in the United States since 1983 and is the only such product on the American market at this time. It is a very soft, small, round, disposable polyurethane sponge that is inserted into the vagina. A concave "dimple" in the center of the sponge accommodates the cervix. The sponge measures about 4.5 cm in diameter and is impregnated with spermicide, nonoxynol-9. A woven nylon loop across the bottom facilitates removal. The sponge must be thoroughly wet with tap water prior to insertion to activate the spermicide.[8,11,70–74]

## Cervical Cap

The cervical cap is a soft, rubber, cup-shaped device, resembling a small diaphragm with a deep dome (much like a thimble). It fits over the cervix and is held in place by a seal that forms between its flexible rim and the outer surface of cervix. A small amount of spermicide is placed inside the cap, but not on the rim, which would interfere with the seal that needs to be formed.

The Prentif Cavity Rim Cervical Cap, the only cap currently approved by the FDA for general use in the United States, was first approved for general distribution in 1988 after several years of investigative testing. The Prentif cap is a soft, deep rubber cap with a firm, rounded rim. A groove along the rim's inner circumference enhances the seal that forms between the inner rim and the surface of the cervix. Available in sizes 22–31 mm (inner rim diameter), it is manufactured in England and distributed in the United States by Cervical Cap Ltd., Los Gatos, California.[8,53]

Other specific products (not generally available in the United States at this time) are the Dumas Cap and the Vimule Cap.[8,52,70–74]

## Mechanisms of Action[8,52]

- The contraceptive effect of the diaphragm is related to the barrier effect, which prevents sperm entry into the cervix, and to the sperm-killing action of spermicide used with all diaphragms.
- The vaginal contraceptive sponge forms a barrier to sperm entry, traps sperm within cells of the sponge, and contains spermicide.
- Similar in action to the diaphragm, the cervical cap serves as a barrier to the cervix and holds spermicide within its dome.

## Effectiveness[8,11,53,70–74]

Contraceptive efficacy among these methods is comparable, with the exception of the sponge when it is used by parous women (see Table 6–4). Sponge effectiveness rates differ significantly for parous and nulliparous women. This may be due to more frequent expulsion or dislodgement of the sponge in parous women, secondary to more relaxed pelvic musculature. Some cervical cap failures are attributed to cap dislodgement during intercourse and to deterioration of rubber after prolonged use.[8,21,75]

Vaginal barrier methods depend largely on extremely conscientious use, although individual fertility characteristics are probably equally important. These methods must be used correctly and consistently. They are used with more success by women 30 years of age or older, who have intercourse fewer than four times weekly, and who may have slightly lower fertility than their younger counterparts. Many women who experience accidental pregnancy with these methods report misuse (including inconsistent use). Users must be highly motivated to prevent or delay pregnancy. The role of the clinician can be very significant in assisting women to use these products successfully.

## Advantages[8,70–73]

- Attractive method for women needing contraception on an irregular basis and whose sexual patterns are fairly predictable.
- Does not require partner involvement.
- Considered medically safe.
- Little danger of systemic effects.
- Easily reversible.
- Provides significant protection against STDs.
- Sponge is available without prescription.
- Can be used during lactation.
- Diaphragm and sponge may provide some protection against cervical neoplasia.

## Disadvantages[8,70–77]

- Both the diaphragm and the cervical cap require accurate fitting by a professional clinician, often accompanied by lengthy office visit.
- Properly trained clinicians not widely available, especially for fitting the cervical cap.
- Costs related to use may be high (i.e., professional care, purchase of products).
- May interfere with sexual spontaneity if not readily available.
- Learning insertion and removal techniques may be difficult.
- Sponge can be difficult to remove.
- Perceived as aesthetically objectionable or messy by some individuals.
- Latex, rubber, polyurethane, or spermicide could cause irritation or allergy in either partner.
- Foul odor or vaginal discharge may occur if the product is left in place more than a few days.
- Potential for vaginal trauma associated with difficult insertion or removal of the device.
- Increased risk of urinary tract infection (UTI) in diaphragm users (especially arcing spring).
- Potential for toxic shock syndrome (TSS).
- A few studies have reported Pap smear abnormalities with use of the cervical cap.

## Contraindications[8,54,70–77]

- Allergy to latex, rubber, polyurethane, or spermicide.
- Vaginal bleeding, even menses (because of possible risk of TSS).
- Delivery or abortion in prior 6 weeks (for cap or sponge).
- Anatomic abnormalities that interfere with proper fitting of the cap or diaphragm.
- Inability to master insertion or removal techniques.
- Recurrent UTIs with use of the diaphragm.
- History of TSS.

## Management Considerations[8,53,70–73]

***Fitting the Diaphragm.*** During the pelvic exam, check for a palpable pubic notch behind the symphysis pubis, as well as anatomic abnormalities. Estimate the diagonal length of the vaginal canal from the posterior vaginal fornix to the symphysis pubis, by inserting the middle and index fingers until the middle finger touches the posterior wall of the vagina. Use thumb of the same hand to mark the point that touches the symphysis pubis and withdraw. Select a diaphragm with a diameter that equals the measurement from the tip of the middle finger to the point just in front of the thumb where symphysis pubis contact was made. Select the largest rim size that is comfortable for client. Insert the diaphragm and check its fit. The diaphragm should fit snugly between the posterior fornix and the symphysis pubis, touching lateral vaginal walls and covering the cervix. Check for displacement when the client bears down. Have her walk around the room, sit, and squat. Check again for displacement and client comfort. If the client feels the diaphragm while walking around, it may be too large. If it is easily displaced with a finger or with moving/walking, it can be displaced during intercourse. If in doubt about fit, try the next larger size. Two or three different sizes should be tried before a final decision is made. Instruct the client to practice removal and insertion three times, while you verify proper placement each time.

***Fitting the Cervical Cap.*** The client must be involved in the fitting process. During speculum examination, assist her to visualize her cervix. *Specific teaching sessions for health care professionals who will be fitting caps are strongly recommended.*[71,72,77] Comprehensive training programs for prospective cap pro-viders are available. Information on these programs may be obtained from the National Women's Health Network in Washington, DC.

## Client Teaching and Counseling

The following points should be part of client teaching.

- Devices may be inserted immediately prior to intercourse; however, some experts recommend waiting 30 minutes after cervical cap insertion to be sure that the seal has formed between the rim and the cervix.
- Devices must be left in place for a minimum of 6 hours after the last act of intercourse.
- Diaphragm may not be reliable if coitus is to take place in water because spermicide could wash away.
- Do not use during menses (potential for TSS). Have an alternative method, such as condoms, available.
- The danger signs of TSS include sudden high fever, vomiting, diarrhea, dizziness, faintness, weakness, sore throat, aching muscles or joints, rash.
- The diaphragm or cap should be inspected prior to insertion for cracks, holes, tears, or drying of rubber or latex.
- After using a cap or diaphragm, wash the device with soap and water, dry thoroughly, and store in its container.
- Bring the cap or diaphragm to yearly gynecologic visit so that fit can be reevaluated.

### Specific Instructions for Diaphragm Use

- Place approximately one tablespoon of spermicidal cream or jelly in the dome and around the rim of the diaphragm.
- Insert the diaphragm up to 6 hours prior to intercourse.
- The diaphragm must remain in place for 6 to 8 hours following each coitus. If coitus does not take place within 6 hours of insertion, remove the diaphragm and reapply spermicide. For subsequent acts of coitus, spermicide is added with an inserter.

### Specific Instructions for Cervical Cap Use

- Fill the dome of the cap to one-third with spermicidal cream or jelly. Do *not* apply spermicide to the rim; this might interfere with the seal that must form around the cervix.
- Cap may be left in place up to 48 hours without regard to frequency of intercourse during that period. It is not necessary to insert additional spermicide.
- After inserting, check that the seal has formed around the cervix.

### Specific Instructions for Sponge Use

- Read and follow the package directions carefully.
- Prior to insertion, thoroughly wet the sponge with tap water; work sponge into a lather with fingers to activate spermicide.
- Insert immediately or up to 24 hours prior to intercourse.
- Sponge may remain in place for 24 hours, regardless of frequency of intercourse, but must remain in place at least 6 hours after the last act of intercourse.
- If sponge is expelled accidentally prior to the 6-hour period following last intercourse, immediately wet and insert another sponge for the remaining time.
- Inspect the sponge on removal to make sure it is intact. Any pieces retained in the vagina must be removed.
- With any difficulty removing the sponge, squat deeply, relax, bear down, and attempt to reach sponge with one or two fingers. Partner may assist with removal.
- Discard the sponge after removal.

## INTRAUTERINE DEVICES (IUDs)

Intrauterine devices (IUDs)[4,8,78–82] are small objects, usually plastic, that are placed inside the uterus. They may contain substances such as copper or progesterone that enhance effectiveness. One or more strings are attached that protrude into the vagina so that the presence of the device can be checked by the user and removal facilitated. IUDs are packaged in individual sterile units that include the device, insertion barrel, and manufacturer literature.

Currently in the United States, two IUDs are available, the copper ParaGard-T-380A marketed by GynoPharma, and Progestasert, a progesterone-T device, available through Alza Corporation. By 1986, most U.S. companies had voluntarily withdrawn IUDs from the American market primarily because of decreased popularity, negative consumer perception, increasing litigation costs, and subsequent difficulty obtaining liability insurance.

The Dalkon Shield, associated with a high rate of pelvic infection and septic abortion, was removed from the American market in 1975.

### Paragard-T-380A[8,78,80]

Introduced in the United States in 1988, this is a T-shaped polyurethane device with barium sulphate added (for x-ray visibility). A very fine copper wire is wound around a vertical stem and crossbar. A white polyethylene string attached through a hole in the "T," creates a double string effect that, after insertion, protrudes into the vagina. ParaGard-T-380A is approved for 8 years of use.

### The Progesterone-T (Progestasert)[8,82]

A T-shaped ethylene vinyl acetate copolymer; the vertical stem contains a reservoir holding 38 mg progesterone and barium sulphate in a silicone oil base. This IUD releases 65 μg progesterone per day. It may stay in place one year, then must be removed and/or replaced. Black double string is attached to the hole in the base of the "T," which after insertion, protrudes into the vagina.

### Mechanism of Action[8,81–84]

Precise mechanisms of IUD action are not fully understood. Theories are that IUDs affect fertilization, implantation, and the endometrium.

***Fertilization.*** The IUD produces a foreign body reaction that is toxic to sperm or ova before fertilization occurs (fertilization is found to be rare in IUD users). It inhibits fertilization by increasing the speed of ovum transport through the fallopian tube, by immobilizing sperm, and by interfering with the migration of sperm from the vagina through the tubes.

***Implantation.*** Interference with implantation is *not* the primary antifertility effect. Local foreign body inflammatory response and increased local production of prostaglandins prevent implantation and cause lysis and/or dislodgement of the blastocyte from the endometrium. The progestin-releasing IUD also interferes with the secretory (proliferative) maturation process of the endometrium.

***Endometrium.*** Copper containing IUDs may also inhibit carbonic anhydrase and alkaline phosphatase activity, and interfere with estrogen uptake by uterine mucosa. Hormone-releasing IUDs also produce an atrophic endometrium with long term use.

## Effectiveness[8,21,80,82]

Effectiveness is impacted by IUD characteristics, such as size, shape, expulsion rates, presence of copper or progesterone; and by user characteristics, such as age and parity. Also influential are medical variables, such as experience of the clinician inserting the device, the ease of insertion, placement of the device deep into the uterus, and likelihood that expulsion will be detected (see Table 6–4).

## Advantages[2,8,11,79,80]

- Once inserted, an IUD requires no continuing action, equipment, or motivation on the part of the user.
- Highly effective.
- Continuously effective.
- Allows for sexual spontaneity.
- Consider for women who have difficulty following directions or remembering to use a contraceptive.
- No messy substances needed.
- After initial cost, no additional expense.
- Return to fertility not impaired.
- Progesterone-releasing IUD may decrease menstrual blood flow and dysmenorrhea.
- Can be used during lactation.

## Disadvantages[8,79,80]

Use of an IUD carries potential for some side effects and several serious complications; however, careful screening and counseling of potential users can prevent many of them. *If a contraindication to use arises, or when in doubt about the significance of a symptom or complaint, the recommended action is to remove the IUD immediately.* Always provide the client an alternate method of contraception. IUDs are best suited for parous women not desiring future pregnancy.

GynoPharma, the manufacturer of ParaGard-T-380A, distributes directly to physicians and clinics, provides detailed guidelines about who should use the product, and recommends it only for women who have had at least one child and are in a stable, monogomous relationship.[8]

- Insertion requires a skilled professional.
- May aggravate or initiate menstrual cramping.
- May increase bleeding patterns.
- User may experience pain or nausea during insertion.
- User must regularly check for presence of the IUD string.
- May increase the risk of pelvic infection, which could affect future fertility.
- Provides no protection against HIV or STDs.
- Device can be expelled without the user being aware.
- String may be felt by the partner.
- Progestasert lasts only one year; ParaGard-T-380A for 8 years.

- User may neglect to see a health care professional for several years.

## Contraindications[2,8,80–85]

Carefully screen potential IUD users for contraindications. Include general and focused histories, a physical examination, appropriate current lab work (CBC count, Pap smear, STD testing), and other assessments as indicated.

***Absolute Contraindications (IUD Not Recommended)***

- Past or present history of pelvic inflammatory disease (PID).
- Known or suspected pregnancy.

***Strong Relative Contraindications (Strongly Encourage Choice of Another Contraceptive Method)***

- History of ectopic pregnancy.
- Undiagnosed, abnormal vaginal bleeding.
- Risk factors for PID: multiple sexual partners; past history of STD, especially gonorrhea or chlamydia; postpartum endometritis; infection following abortion in past 3 months; purulent cervicitis.
- Unresolved, abnormal Pap smear.
- Difficult access to medical care.
- Impaired ability (physical or mental) to check for IUD string.
- Known or suspected bleeding disorder.
- Valvular heart disease.
- Anatomic variations that make insertion or retention difficult (e.g., DES exposure, fibroids).
- Severe dysmenorrhea, heavy menses, endometriosis.
- Anemia.
- History of fainting or vasovagal response.
- Allergy to copper.
- History of impaired fertility (in a client desiring future pregnancy).

## Managing Problems and Complications[8,53,82,86]

- Spotting or bleeding may occur at the time of insertion or at any time after. Anemia could result (less likely with Progestasert). Cramping or pain also may occur at the time of insertion or at any time after. If these problems are severe or intolerable, remove the IUD; uterine perforation, pelvic infection, and pregnancy (intrauterine or ectopic) must be ruled out.
- The IUD string may be lost, or the IUD may be expulsed or partially expulsed. In either situation, evaluate for uterine perforation, pregnancy, and infection.
- The IUD can become embedded (less likely with a shorter period of wearing IUDs). If it cannot be removed after reasonable attempts, refer the client to a gynecologist.
- Uterine perforation can occur. Perforation is most common during insertion, but can occur at any time, especially during the postpartum period. Suspect perforation if pain is present; if the string is no longer palpable; if the plastic of the device is felt or visible in the cervix. If perforation is suspected, refer the client to a gynecologist.
- Pregnancy, ectopic pregnancy (low incidence).
- Increased risk of septic abortion if pregnancy occurs. With delayed menses or suspected pregnancy, evaluate for pregnancy and infection. Ectopic pregnancy rates are higher among users of Progestasert than among users of copper IUDs. Of users who become pregnant with IUD in place:
  - One-half will experience spontaneous abortion.
  - Twenty-five percent will abort if the IUD is removed early in pregnancy.
  - If the IUD is left in place, severe pelvic infection resulting in death could occur.

- Five percent will have an ectopic pregnancy.

Inform the client of the above; assist her to determine whether to continue the pregnancy.

- Increased risk of pelvic inflammatory disease (PID). PID is a serious complication that can be life threatening. Infection must be promptly and aggressively treated and the IUD removed. Providers and users of IUDs must be alert to the signs and symptoms suggestive of pelvic infection:
  - Fever of 101°F or higher.
  - Purulent discharge from the vagina/cervix.
  - Abdominal pain.
  - Dyspareunia.
  - Cervicitis.
  - Suprapubic tenderness or guarding.
  - Pain with movement of the cervix on examination.
  - Tenderness on bimanual examination.
  - Adnexal tenderness or mass.

### Management Considerations[8,80–83]

- Women planning to use an IUD must be carefully screened for contraindications. Give each IUD user an identification card with the name and a picture of the IUD, the day of insertion, and the recommended removal date printed on it.
- If the client is not accustomed to following a calendar, inform her about recommended dates for checkups and IUD removal.
- Samples of IUDs should be available so that the client can handle and examine them.
- Insertion may take place at any time during the menstrual cycle (insertion may be more comfortable at midcycle, when the cervix is softer) as long as it is certain that the client is not pregnant. Higher infection and expulsion rates are noted when IUDs are inserted during menses. The IUD may be inserted as soon as 6 weeks postpartum.
- IUD removal may take place at any time during the menstrual cycle, but may be easier at midcycle or at the time of menses.

### Client Teaching and Counseling[8,80–83]

Several points are covered during client teaching and counseling.

- What to expect during and after IUD insertion.
  - How and when to check for the IUD string (frequently during the first few months, then after each period or when abnormal cramping occurs).
  - The signs of infection.
  - The importance of keeping track of periods. Teach the client the IUD early danger signs, using *PAINS*:

    *P*eriod late, abnormal spotting or bleeding.
    *A*bdominal pain, pain with intercourse.
    *I*nfection exposure (especially gonorrhea), abnormal discharge.
    *N*ot feeling well, chills, fever.
    *S*tring missing, shorter, or longer.

## VOLUNTARY STERILIZATION

Sterilization is the surgical interruption or closure of pathways for sperm or ova, preventing fertilization.[8] The method is considered a permanent means of contraception, although some surgical procedures to reverse both vasectomies and tubal ligations have been successful.[8] Sterilization is the most popular method of contraception in the United States and worldwide.

*Female sterilization* is accomplished by bilateral tubal ligation (BTL). The fallopian tubes are ligated and cut, clipped, cauterized, or plugged to prevent ovum from moving toward the uterus. Sterilization is considered a safe operative procedure.[2,3,8,87] A hysterectomy (removal of the organs of reproduction) accomplishes sterilization, but should *never* be performed solely for that purpose.

*Male sterilization* is an operation that blocks the vas deferens to prevent the passage of sperm. Considered a simple procedure, it can be performed quickly, safely, and inexpensively.[8]

## Sterilization Techniques

Sterilization techniques may be performed using general or local anesthesia with sedation. Local anesthesia with light sedation has definite safety advantages over general anesthesia.

***Suprapubic Minilaparotomy.*** Performed at 4 weeks or more postpartum or postabortion (when the uterus is fully involuted). Usually it is performed in lithotomy position. The procedure involves a small (2–5 cm) abdominal incision just above the pubic hairline. The uterus is elevated so that the uterus and tubes are close to the incision. The tubes are lifted, identified, and ligated by any of several occlusion techniques; the incision is sutured.[8,87]

***Laparoscopy.*** A laparoscope consists of a viewing instrument, light source, and operating channel. *Single puncture technique* involves a small subumbilical incision. The abdomen is insufflated with a gaseous combination of nitrous oxide, carbon dioxide, and room air; the laparoscope is inserted, and the tubes are grasped and occluded through the operating channel of the instrument. With *double puncture technique*, a second tiny incision is made in the suprapubic region through which the operating channel is inserted and the procedure performed. Following bilateral tubal occlusion, the organs are inspected, the scope removed, gas gently expelled, and the incisions closed.[8,87]

***Subumbilical Minilaparotomy.*** Most frequently used during the immediate postpartum/postabortion period, when the uterus and tubes remain high in the abdomen. A small (1.5–3.0 cm) incision is made just below the umbilicus. Oviducts are usually easily reached for the occlusion procedure. Lithotomy position is not needed, and organ manipulation and instrumentation are less extensive—facilitating a rapid recovery.[8,87]

***Bilateral Tubal Ligation by Laparotomy.*** BTL using an abdominal incision greater than 5 cm, or vaginal access, or during cesarean section is associated with higher morbidity and complication rates.

***Vasectomy (Male Sterilization).*** Each vas deferens is cut between two ligated sections, preventing sperm from mingling with ejaculate. Local anesthetic (e.g., 1 percent lidocaine without epinephrine) is injected into each side of the scrotum, where a small incision is made to isolate, occlude, and usually resect the vasa. A no-scalpel technique for performing vasectomies is used in other countries and now in the United States. This requires an instrument that "punctures" the scrotal skin and vas sheath. Little bleeding occurs, and no sutures are required. About 20 ejaculations are required for existing sperm in the vasa deferentia to be cleared.[8,88]

## Effectiveness[8,21]

Sterilization includes highly effective, permanent methods of birth control for both sexes. For women who become pregnant following bilateral tubal ligation, failures are usually attributed to errors in surgical technique, equipment failure (laparoscope), fistula formation, and/or spontaneous reanastomosis of a tube. A high percentage of pregnancies run the risk of being ectopic. In some cases, the woman may already have been pregnant at the time of the sterilization procedure.

Vasectomy failures (not including pregnancies resulting from intercourse before the reproductive tract was cleared of sperm) may result from errors in technique or recanalization of the vas. Rarely, congenital duplication of the vas may be present and go unnoticed at the time of the procedure. (See Table 6–4 for failure rates.)

### Advantages[2,8,87]

- One-time decision provides permanent fertility control.
- Highly effective, convenient.
- Considered safe; low complication and morbidity rates.
- Following procedure and recovery, very few or no systemic or side effects occur.
- Short recovery time.
- Certain techniques can be performed immediately after childbirth or abortion.
- BTL immediately effective.
- Low long term risks.
- Low long term cost.
- Can be performed while lactating.
- Vasectomy is equally effective, simpler, safer, much less expensive than BTL.

### Disadvantages[2,8,87,89]

- Carries risks inherent in any surgical procedure (infection, injury to other organs, hemorrhage, complications of anesthesia).
- Procedure is difficult to reverse.
- Initial cost may be high.
- Vasectomy is not immediately effective.
- Some states require a waiting period between time of counseling/consent and actual procedure.
- Provides no protection against HIV or STDs.
- Some individuals may have regrets about having the procedure.
- Uterine perforation is possible.
- Some women report menstrual pattern changes, increased dysmenorrhea, PMS following BTL (research so far has been unable to support any pattern of identifiable changes).
- Vasectomy complications can occur (hematoma formation, congestive epididymitis, sperm granuloma).

### Contraindications[2,8,11]

- Lack of adequately trained personnel to perform the procedure (especially important for laparoscopy techniques).
- Known or suspected pregnancy.
- Existing infection of the reproductive tract.
- Client ambivalence about sterilization.
- Serious uncontrolled health problems.

### Management Considerations[8,19,87]

- A high skill level, involving special training and extensive practice, is needed to perform these procedures (especially for laporoscopy procedures).
- The client must provide informed consent prior to the procedure.
- When federal funds, and in some cases state funds, are used to reimburse for sterilization, the client must have signed informed consent at least 30 days prior to the procedure or before delivery or abortion, if sterilization is planned to immediately follow one of these procedures. The client must also be 21 years of age or older and mentally competent.
- Preoperative assessment includes history (with particular attention to the last menstrual period and most recent use of contraception, to be reasonably confident that the woman is not pregnant) and physical examination (with focus on position and mobility of uterus and detection of possible infection). Minimum lab requirements are hemoglobin and urinalysis.
- The client should have someone accompany her or him home following the procedure.
- The client should rest for a few days following the procedure.

- Sexual activity may be resumed after about one week for women and after 2 to 3 days for men.
- Men must be reminded that they are not sterile initially. Another method of contraception must be used for several weeks or for at least the next 20 ejaculations. Microscopic examination of semen is the best way to ascertain that sterility has been achieved.

## FERTILITY AWARENESS METHODS

Menstrual cycle charting, natural family planning, or periodic abstinence involves making observations of normal physiological changes caused by hormonal fluctuations during the menstrual cycle so that fertile and infertile periods can be identified. Techniques are used in combination with coital abstinence during fertile days. The term *natural family planning* implies exclusive use of these methods and that absolute abstinence from coitus is maintained until "safe days." Charting observed changes is an important component for successful use of these methods. The techniques include the calendar (rhythm) method, basal body temperature (BBT) method, cervical mucus (Billings or ovulation) method, and symptothermal method. At least two of these techniques should be used simultaneously.[2,8,75,76]

### Mechanism of Action

Pregnancy is prevented by avoidance of unprotected intercourse during times that a woman is determined to be fertile.[2,8,90]

***Calendar (Rhythm) Method.***[2,8,90,91] This involves calculation of a woman's fertile period based on three assumptions:

- Ovulation occurs on the 14th day, plus or minus 2 days, prior to next menses.
- Sperm are viable for 3 days.
- The ovum is viable for 24 hours.

The client must chart the length of her menstrual cycles for a minimum of 8 months. The earliest day in the cycle she is likely to be fertile is determined by subtracting 18 days from the length of the shortest cycle occurring during that 8-month period. The latest day of potential fertility is obtained by subtracting 11 days from the longest cycle. These two numbers represent the beginning and end of the fertile period.

For example, if the client's shortest cycle was 27 days, subtract 18 from 27; on the 9th day (27 minus 18) the client must begin to abstain from sexual intercourse. If her longest cycle was 34 days, on the 23rd day (34 minus 11) abstinence may be ended. She must abstain from day 9 through day 23, a total of 14 days, during each cycle. This technique is most effective when menstrual cycles are regular. With less variable cycles, the period of required abstinence is shorter. The abstinent period cannot be less than 7 days.

***Basal Body Temperature (BBT) Method.***[2,8,90–92] BBT usually drops prior to ovulation, then, under the influence of progesterone, rises 1 to 3 days after ovulation and remains elevated for several days or throughout the remainder of cycle. Once temperature rise is maintained for 3 or 4 days, infertility is relatively certain.

*Basal body temperature* refers to the lowest temperature reached by the body of a healthy person during waking hours. Generally, a special BBT thermometer should be used. Temperature is taken daily before rising, eating, or drinking. Based on the patterns observed, one should be able to predict the end of the fertile interval and beginning of the safe, luteal phase of the menstrual cycle. After several months of charting BBT, the client may be able to observe patterns of BBT readings and determine the time when ovulation has passed and the infertile phase has started.

If using BBT method alone, the client should avoid unprotected intercourse from the beginning of the menstrual cycle (or at least from day 4) until after her temperature has been elevated for 3 days. Using other fertility awareness methods along with BBT recording may allow for shortening of the abstinent period.

***Cervical Mucus (Billings or Ovulation) Method.***[2,8,90,91] This method assesses the character of the cervical mucus. The mucus secreted by exocrine glands lining the cervical canal changes in character during the menstrual cycle in response to hormonal levels. The client is taught to assess feelings of wetness or dryness daily and to note changes in the physical properties of the mucus. During a normal menstrual cycle, a woman experiences menses, then a few days of a dry sensation, then early mucus (milky white, translucent, yellow or clear, sticky at first and then smooth). As ovulation approaches, mucus becomes more abundant, clear, slippery, and smooth ("peak" mucus). The mucus can be stretched between two fingers without breaking. This is called *spinnbarkeit* and resembles egg whites. The greatest sensation of smoothness and wetness and longest stretch in mucus corresponds to the peak in estrogen occurring immediately prior to ovulation. This mucus is more permeable to sperm and can prolong the life of sperm. Mucus becomes opaque or sticky again after ovulation, and the sensation of dryness returns. *Conception can result from intercourse on any wet days.* Coital activity should occur only on dry days. Calendar chart must be kept noting observed daily cervical mucus characteristics.

***SymptoThermal Method.***[2,8,11,90,91] This method uses a combination of cervical mucus and BBT to predict ovulation. It may also incorporate other symptoms a woman might observe, such as breast tenderness, changes in libido, and midcycle pain (*mittleshmerz*) or spotting. A combination of techniques is considered the most accurate variation of natural family planning.

### Effectiveness[8,21,91]

Fertility awareness methods are considered moderately effective for preventing pregnancy (see Table 6–4). Effectiveness would be increased if couples limited unprotected intercourse to the postovulatory period only. These techniques require high levels of commitment and participation by both partners. High motivation to prevent pregnancy and ability to learn the necessary concepts are needed. Failures are often related to poor understanding or improper teaching and poor use of methods. Some pregnancies result from couples having trouble coping with periods of abstinence. They may intentionally "break the rules" and take chances.[8] Pregnancy must be an acceptable possible outcome of use of these methods.[91]

### Advantages[2,8,90,91]

- No damaging side effect.
- No interruption of normal body functions.
- No external or internal devices or chemicals.
- Acceptable to most religious groups.
- Low cost.
- Increases awareness of normal female body processes and fertility.
- Encourages communication between partners.
- The concepts and charting skills learned can also be applied to planning conception, diagnosis and treatment of fertility problems, and mapping symptoms of PMS.

### Disadvantages[2,8,90,91]

- Low user effectiveness.
- Interferes with sexual spontaneity.
- Requires copious recordkeeping and intensive, ongoing teaching.
- Couples may have difficulty learning the techniques.
- Periodic abstinence is difficult for some couples.

- Not a reliable method if menstrual periods are irregular.
- No identifiable BBT pattern is seen in some women's cycles, even when ovulating.
- Emotional and physiological stress, shift work, and travel can alter the timing of ovulation.
- No protection provided against HIV or STDs.
- Methods are unreliable during lactation and perimenopausal periods.
- If conception occurs, it may involve the fertilization of an "old" or overripe egg and an increased theoretical risk of fetal abnormalities. Convincing studies are unavailable either to support or negate this concern.[8]

### Contraindications[8,91]

There are no absolute contraindications to fertility awareness methods; however, if unplanned pregnancy would be unacceptable or inadvisable for a client or her family, for any reason, a more reliable contraceptive method should be considered. Relative contraindications include the following.

- Irregular menses.
- History of anovulatory cycles.
- Inability to keep careful records.
- Lack of partner cooperation.

### Management Considerations[2,8,90–92]

Clients must receive intensive and ongoing teaching by a trained fertility awareness counselor. They also will need assistance with interpreting charts. It is recommended that health care professionals be familiar with the available community resources for teaching these techniques and with the philosophy and teaching/learning resources used by the counselor. There should be a philosophical "match" between the needs and beliefs of the client and those of the counselor.

Teaching and counseling involves several aspects.

- Explanation of the normal menstrual cycle.
- Explanation of how the methods work.
- Selection of the methods.
- Techniques involved in the methods selected (e.g., how and when to take BBT, how to evaluate cervical mucus).
- Procedures for charting.
- How to determine fertile periods.
- Alternative sexual activity for fertile periods.

## WITHDRAWAL (COITUS INTERRUPTUS)

Coitus interruptus, or withdrawal, involves a man removing his penis from the vagina before ejaculation, so that ejaculation occurs away from the vagina and external genitalia. Despite being one of the most common methods of preventing pregnancy in many countries and cultures of the world, it is not popular in the United States. Adolescents, however, often use withdrawal.[8,16]

### Mechanism of Action[2,8]

Coitus interruptus theoretically prevents conception by sperm-containing ejaculate being deposited away from the woman's genitalia.

### Effectiveness

Lack of success with this method (see Table 6–4) may be due to the following:

- Presence of sperm in the preejaculate fluid that is emitted without sensation to the man.
- It is often difficult for the man to predict when he will ejaculate.
- Lack of self-control.[8,21]

### Advantages[8,11,93]

Coitus interruptus involves no artificial devices or chemicals, costs nothing, is always available, and can be used during lactation.

### Disadvantages[8,11,93]

- High failure rate.
- Requires considerable self-control by the man.
- Can diminish enjoyment for the couple.
- Depends solely on the cooperation of the man.
- Puts the woman in a dependent role.
- Provides no protection against HIV or STDs.
- Sexual dysfunction and diminished pleasure could develop, as couples must remain alert, concentrate on timing, and interrupt the excitement or plateau phase of sexual response.

### Contraindications[8]

There are no absolute contraindications; however, if unplanned pregnancy is unacceptable or inadvisable, a more reliable method should be used. Relative contraindications include (a) questionable commitment of either partner to the method and (b) lack of effective communication between partners.

### Management Considerations[8,11,93]

The method should be taught as part of contraceptive counseling, especially for those who tend to use this method (i.e., individuals inexperienced with contraceptive use or those who have exhausted all other contraceptive choices). Counseling and instruction should include several topics.

- Before the penis is inserted into the vagina, wipe off any fluid on the tip of the penis; it may contain sperm. This is especially important if the couple intends to have more than one act of intercourse, because semen may be present in clear fluid at the tip of an erect penis.
- When a man feels impending ejaculation, he must immediately remove his penis from the vagina so that ejaculation occurs away from the vagina.
- Condom use with this method would greatly increase its effectiveness and provide protection against HIV and other STDs.
- A supply of spermicide may be kept on hand in case withdrawal is not accomplished in time. An application could be inserted immediately, although this measure probably would not prevent some sperm from entering the uterus.

## LACTATION

Lactation (breastfeeding) is used worldwide to prevent or delay pregnancy for variable periods of time in the postpartum period. Lactation extends the period of ovarian inactivity and delays a return to fertility, but does so in an unpredictable manner.[94]

### Mechanisms of Action[8,94–96]

Theoretically, suckling appears to reduce pulsatile release of gonadotropin-releasing hormone (GnRH), which in turn suppresses release of luteinizing hormone (LH) required for ovarian activity. The small amounts of estrogen secreted are insufficient to stimulate normal follicular development.

Production of prolactin, the hormone essential for milk production, is stimulated by the frequency and duration of suckling. High levels of prolactin have various effects.

- They contribute to lactational amenorrhea and relative infertility.
- They make the ovaries unresponsive to LH.
- They suppress positive feedback effects of estrogen on the midcycle rise of pituitary gonadotropin secretion.
- They interfere directly with ovarian steroid production.

### Effectiveness[96]

Total or nearly-total breastfeeding is associated with longer periods of lactational amenorrhea and infertility. For a woman totally breastfeeding (on-demand feeding over each 24-hour period with no supplements) and who has no vaginal bleeding after the 56th day postpartum, the pregnancy rate is reported to be 2 percent during the first 6 months. The longer a woman breastfeeds, however, the more likely it is that menstruation will return as lactation continues and that ovulation will occur prior to first menses.

### Management Considerations[8,95,96]

Several points need to be considered in client teaching and counseling.

- Emphasize that resumption of ovulation and fertility while lactating cannot be predicted accurately. Women can become pregnant while breastfeeding and before the first menstrual period occurs.
- If the client is totally breastfeeding and wishes to avoid pregnancy, she should begin using a reliable birth control method no later than the time of the 6-week postpartum examination or as soon as the health care professional advises.
- If the client wishes to rely on lactation for contraception, she must breastfeed her infant "on-demand" over each 24-hour period, providing no formula or food supplements. When baby reaches 6 months old or menses return, she must begin using another method of birth control.
- Because U.S. women rarely adhere to such a rigorous breast-feeding pattern, they should be advised not to rely on lactation alone to prevent pregnancy.

## DOUCHING

"Washing" semen out through douching will not prevent sperm from entering uterus. In fact, douching could theoretically enhance movement of sperm up the cervical canal by washing it deeper into the vagina toward the cervix or by washing away protective mucus.[2]

## ELECTIVE TERMINATION OF PREGNANCY: INDUCED ABORTION

Induced abortion is not, strictly speaking, a means of fertility control, but because it is used by some women for family planning or may be recommended for medically therapeutic reasons, some discussion is needed here. Excluding miscarriages, about 30% of all pregnancies in the United States end in abortions.[97] Most abortions (90 percent) are first trimester procedures.

Controversy has been rampant regarding the rights of women to choose abortion since it became legal in 1973 with the landmark U.S. Supreme Court decision *Roe v. Wade.*[98] *Roe v. Wade* allows women to terminate pregnancy in the first trimester; after that, individual state laws become effective.[99] Liberalization of state abortion laws began in the late 1960s and culminated in *Roe v. Wade*. Conflicts related to abortion rights will continue from both sides of the issue in years to come. This section is limited to a discussion of the health needs of women seeking and having abortions, in order to give health professionals information with which to counsel supportively.

Death as a result of induced legal abortion is unusual.[8] After 13 weeks' gestation and with the use of instillation methods, however, the risk increases considerably. For example, for curettage, the mortality rate per 100,000 procedures from 1972 to 1982 was 0.8, as compared with 10.1 for instillation.[100] For gestational age of 12 weeks and under, the mortality rate was 1.8 and less. For gestational age of 13 weeks and more, the rate ranged from 4.3 to 11.8 per 100,000 procedures.[100]

The risk of long term complications is low with legal abortion.[8] Subsequent problems with fertility, spontaneous abortion, premature delivery, and low birthweight infants have not been found to be significantly associated with first trimester abortion.[8]

First trimester abortion, based on the last normal menstrual period, is classified as occurring from conception through weeks 12–13 of gestation, depending on the literature source.[8,101] Second trimester or midtrimester abortion is from weeks 13–14 through week 24.

## CLIENT EVALUATION AND PREPARATION

### Counseling

Counseling prepares a woman to give informed written consent. When a client finds out that she is pregnant with an unplanned conception, it is essential that she (and her partner, if appropriate) be allowed to discuss concerns and needs in an atmosphere that does not promote guilt. Fear, partner conflict, uncertainty, and anger are common responses.[102] Particularly if abortion is chosen because of a serious medical condition, loss and sadness may be prominent.

A rapport based on the health care professional's empathy and listening promotes comfort in making decisions.[103] It permits assessment of the client's emotional and social state and appropriate counseling and support for her decision.[99,101] Explain all options—including routine preparation for the procedures, the procedural techniques and their effects, pain management, and guidance in what to expect—in a thorough, kind, and objective manner. The client must be allowed to make informed choices and to discuss her current and future life status and plans, and their possible impacts. For women who decide against abortion, referral opportunities should be available for prenatal care and adoption.

If the client wishes to consider an abortion, all aspects of the procedure must be carefully reviewed, including the risks. Postabortion contraception options need to be discussed and a method chosen. Furthermore, the client may need assistance in determining community resources. Referrals, for example, for social services or group or individual support resources, may be indicated to assist with coping. In today's volatile environment related to abortion, the woman needs to feel safe.

### History

Historical data are needed.

- Menstrual history, especially last and previous menstrual periods.
- Contraceptive history and what methods the client wants to use in the future.
- Obstetric history.
- Reproductive system disease and/or prior surgery.
- Drug/anesthesia allergies.
- Other illnesses affecting health, past or present.
- Current medications.[8]

### Physical and Reproductive Examination

The *physical exam* may be brief (heart, lungs, breasts, abdomen, vital signs); however, the *reproductive exam* should be thorough to estimate the size and position of the uterus, to estimate the state of the conceptus, and to determine any abnormality, such as a mass.[8]

### Diagnostic Tests

Several diagnostic tests may be done.

- *Pregnancy Test.* A urine test for first screening; if test is negative but pregnancy suspected, a sensitive serum test is done. A wait of 1 to 2 weeks may be needed for more definitive test results if the woman is 6 weeks or less from her last normal menstrual period.
- *Ultrasound Evaluation.* Done for accurate dating when a discrepancy exists be-

tween the size of the uterus and gestational age.

- *Hemoglobin/Hematocrit.*
- *Blood Type.* For Rh negative women with no evidence of isoimmunization, Rh(D) immunoglobulin (RhoGAM), will be needed after the procedure.
- *Vaginitis/STD Screening.* Chlamydia, gonorrhea, saline wet mount, and other if indicated.[8,99]

### Reasons for Elective Termination

A woman may seek to terminate pregnancy for several reasons.

- *Elective reasons* are unrelated to the health of the mother or the fetus, such as pregnancy due to rape or incest or the inability to afford the pregnancy.
- *Maternal indications* are reasons for which the mother's health would be jeopardized if the pregnancy were to continue, such as heart disease, severe depression, or cancer.
- *Fetal indications* most commonly are congenital defects, or exposure to a teratogenic agent.[99,101,104]

## METHODS OF INDUCED ABORTION

### Surgical Abortion Methods

Vacuum (suction) curettage is the most commonly used abortion procedure in the United States.[8] It is an ambulatory care procedure and may be done through week 16 of gestation. The procedure is done under local anesthesia, a paracervical block, and takes about 15 minutes. Prior to surgery, the cervix is dilated by osmotic dilators, which takes about 4 hours. The products of conception are removed by suction evacuation, and completion confirmed by curettage.

Potential complications include incomplete abortion, cervical laceration, seizure, cardiac arrest, allergic reaction, uterine atony, uterine perforation, bleeding, and infection. Advantages of the procedure are that it costs less than procedures performed during later gestation and little time is lost from work. The cost in 1989 for an abortion at 10 weeks' gestation, performed at an abortion clinic with local anesthesia, averaged $245.[105] Private physician costs are generally higher. Dilation with a laminaria may be needed prior to the procedure, thus requiring an additional visit to the office.

Other surgical methods include dilation and curettage (D & C), which is rarely used because it involves more complications; dilation and evacuation (D & E), which is done during weeks 13 to 20 and is more complex with a greater risk of complications; hysterotomy (cesarean section), which is rarely used due to morbidity and mortality; and hysterectomy.[8] Menstrual extraction often fails, especially if done under 8 weeks' gestation; therefore, it is not recommended.[101] Later, after 17 weeks' gestation or more, abortion procedures include D & E, intra-amniotic abortifacient instillation, and extrauterine abortifacient administration.[101]

### Medical Abortion Methods

Substances used to induce medical abortion in the second trimester are prostaglandin $E_2$ suppositories, 12-methyl prostaglandin $F_2$ intramuscular injection, hypertonic saline intra-amniotic infusion, intra-amniotic prostaglandin infusion, or hypertonic urea intra-amniotic infusion.[8] Methods may be combined to ensure evacuation. To ease the procedure, dilation substances such as laminaria, or synthetic osmotic dilators, or prostaglandin suppositories to soften the cervix, are commonly used before the induction is begun. It generally takes about 6 hours for a laminaria to dilate the cervix. To induce abortion, oxytocin may be given alone intravenously to cause uterine contractions, or it may be given in combination with other substances, such as saline.[8] Infusions are inpatient or outpatient procedures; they become more expensive as a hospital stay lengthens. Costs for infusions averaged over $2000 in one report published in 1991.[105] Moreover, the psychological effects on the client may be traumatic.

Induction of early abortion is used outside of the United States. Agents include mifepristone, or RU-486 (used extensively in France), epostane (enzyme inhibitor of progesterone), prostaglandins E and $F_2$ (induce labor), and RU-486 combined with a low-dose prostaglandin analogue.[8] Before their use in the United States is approved, these methods will need to be as safe and effective as first trimester vacuum curettage.

### COMPLICATIONS, SIGNS AND SYMPTOMS, AND PREVENTIVE MEASURES (see Table 6–12)

#### Postabortion Counseling

Clients who undergo vacuum aspiration or suction curettage need to expect menstrual cramping during and after the procedure and some vaginal bleeding that will taper over the next week. Clients undergoing a D & E in the second trimester can expect to enter the hospital, undergo a 30-minute procedure to place the laminaria, then allow about 6 hours for the laminaria's effect. Analgesia may be needed after the abortion for cramping and/or breast engorgement.

Infusions later in pregnancy require hospital stays of 1 to 3 days; severe cramping, necessitating analgesia, can be expected.[20] Instruct all clients not to put anything in the vagina for 7 days after their procedure. They should expect to feel fatigue and breast tenderness for a few days and anticipate feelings of loss, sadness, or relief. Negative feelings are usually short-lived. A return visit should be scheduled for 2 to 4 weeks postoperatively.[106]

## THE OUTLOOK FOR CONTROLLING FERTILITY

Many new contraceptive technologies are being investigated—some targeted for women and some for men.

*Men*

- *Testosterone.* When testosterone is administered by injection or implant, the pituitary is signaled to decrease the levels of testosterone needed for the testes to function. Hence, the production of sperm is temporarily suppressed. Periodic injections are needed.[53]
- *Vaccines.* These block the pituitary hormones that produce sperm and testosterone (immunocontraception).[51,53]
- *Sulfasalazine.* An ulcerative colitis drug, sulfasalazine causes decreased sperm counts and impairs sperm motility and function. The effects of this drug are quickly reversed.[53]
- *Occlusion of the Vas Deferens.* This is accomplished either by injection of a polymer or with flexible silicone plugs. One injectable occlusive technique has been found to be spontaneously reversible after a period of time; that time period is controlled by the dose of substance that is injected.[107]
- *Gossypol.* A constituent of cottonseed oil, gossypol causes reversible infertility by interfering with spermatogenesis. However, several objectionable side effects have been observed, and return to fertility needs to be investigated further.[8,51,53,108]

*Women*

- *Long Acting Progestins.*[8,51,53,108] Long acting progestins in the form of removable and biodegradable implants, injectable microspheres and microcapsules, and vaginal rings are being developed and undergoing clinical trials. They will contain le-

**TABLE 6–12. IMMEDIATE COMPLICATIONS OF INDUCED ABORTION, SIGNS AND SYMPTOMS, AND PREVENTIVE MEASURES**

| Complication | Signs and Symptoms | Preventive Measures |
|---|---|---|
| Excessive or prolonged bleeding | Occurs during or after procedure. Uterus may be atonic; bleeding may be from trauma (see below). | Local anesthesia, I.V. ocytocin or oral or I.M. ergot, uterine massage. Evacuation of placenta within hour of fetal expulsion. May require transfusion and ergotamine treatment if occurs. |
| Infection | Fever, chills, cramps, foul discharge, backache, abdominal pain, abdominal tenderness, muscle aches, tiredness. | Treatment of infections prior to procedure, complete evacuation of products of conception, antibiotic therapy prophylactically. Hospitalization may be indicated for adequate treatment if infection develops. |
| Intrauterine blood clots/ retained products of conception (POC) | Occurs during first 5 days after abortion. Severe pain and cramps; uterus tense, tender, enlarged; no bleeding from cervix. May be accompanied by infection (endometritis). Seen with first trimester abortions. | Vacuum aspiration indicated; oral ergot may decrease occurrence of clots. Complete evacuation of uterus prevents retained POC. |
| Unsuccessful termination | Pregnancy signs/symptoms continue; products of conception not found. | Adequate uterine curettage. |
| Trauma to uterus (perforation) or to cervix (laceration) | Increased risks with younger woman, later gestation, prior delivery. | Preprocedure use of laminaria, osmotic dilators; safe, correct surgical procedure. |

*Source: Adapted from Reference 13.*

vonorgestrel, norethindrone, or any of the newer progestins (desogestrel, gestodene, norgestimate).

- *Removable Implants.* Norplant II, for example, contains two implants that will be effective for 3 to 5 years.
- *Biodegradable Implants.* Capronor (levonorgestrel), effective for 12 to 18 months, may be removed or allowed to degrade. Norethindrone pellets, consisting of 10 percent cholesterol and 90 percent hormone, are effective for 12 to 18 months and disappear by 24 months. Implants containing the newer progestins are undergoing clinical trials.[52]
- *Injectable Microspheres and Microcapsules.* These contain tiny particles of norethindrone attached to a polymer. They are suspended in solution and injected, then slowly dissolve over 1 to 6 months, providing a constant, effective contraceptive dose.[8,52,54]
- *Vaginal Rings.* These may contain only progestin (levonorgestrel, desogestrel) or estrogen and progestin. A natural progesterone ring has also been developed.

- *LH Releasing Hormone Agonists.* These agonists disrupt the pituitary–ovarian axis, preventing ovulation. They may be administered by intranasal spray. Early reports demonstrate high efficacy and no serious short-term side effects.[108]

- *Intrauterine Devices.* IUDs will be more widely used and available. They will contain other forms of progestin and will be longer acting.
- *Vaccines.* Vaccine development is aimed toward disruption of gestation by preventing egg fertilization or implantation (immunocontraception). Problems being addressed with such vaccines include specificity, reversibility, and cytotoxicity. A vaccine for women, developed in India, is currently undergoing clinical trials. Other vaccines for men or women are not at the point where clinical trials can be conducted.[8,53]

## NURSING DIAGNOSES

*Nursing diagnoses reflecting actual or potential concerns or problems related to fertility control:*[11,14,15]

- Powerlessness related to lack of knowledge about fertility control.
- Disturbed self-esteem related to past experience with contraceptive failure.
- Anxiety related to fear of pregnancy.
- Spiritual distress related to conflict between religious beliefs and desire to limit family size.
- Fear of unplanned pregnancy related to unprotected intercourse.
- Potential for sexual dysfunction related to fear of pregnancy.
- Potential for conflict in family (marital) processes related to disagreement about methods of birth control.
- Noncompliance with proper use of contraceptive sponge related to lack of understanding of instructions.
- Others: Altered sexual patterns, ineffective individual coping, knowledge deficit, impaired social interaction, dysfunctional communication patterns (each requires a statement of etiology: related to . . .).

*Nursing diagnoses reflecting functional health patterns for clients seeking family planning services or successfully using a selected birth control method:*

- Positive self-concept related to successful efforts to control fertility.
- Positive health seeking behaviors (evidenced by timely request for fertility control counseling) related to adequate knowledge about contraception.
- Positive sexuality (reproductive) patterns related to successful achievement of desired family size.
- Effective individual coping related to confidence in sexual and reproductive choices.

## REFERENCES


1. McNall, L.K. (1980). *Contemporary obstetrical and gynecologic nursing.* St. Louis: Mosby.
2. Fogel, C.I., & Woods, N.F. (1981). *Health care of women: A nursing perspective.* St. Louis: Mosby.
3. Manisoff, M. (1972). *A teaching guide for nurses* (3rd ed.). New York: Planned Parenthood–World Population.
4. The Boston Women's Health Book Collective. (1984). *The new our bodies, ourselves.* New York: Simon & Schuster.
5. Lynaugh, J. (1991). The death of Sadie Sachs . . . Margaret Sanger. *Nursing Research, 40,* 124–125.
6. Speidel, J.J. (1987, October 20). *Contraceptives: What's new and why isn't there more?.* Paper presented at the annual meeting of the American Public Health Association, New Orleans.

7. Staff. (1991). Product liability and contraceptives. *The Contraceptive Report, 2*(4), 9–11.
8. Hatcher, R.A., Stewart, F., Trussell, J., Kowal, D., Guest, F., Stewart, G.K., Cates, W. (1990). *Contraceptive technology, 1990–92* (15th rev. ed.). New York: Irvington.
9. Forrest, J.D. (1988). Contraceptive needs through stages of women's reproductive lives. *Contemporary Obstetrics & Gynecology Special Issue—Fertility, 32*, 12–22.
10. Lethbridge, D.J. (1991). Choosing and using contraception: Toward a theory of women's contraceptive self-care. *Nursing Research, 40*, 276–280.
11. Fogel, C.I., & Lauver, D. (1990). *Sexual health promotion*. Philadelphia: Saunders.
12. Noble, R.C. (1991, April 1). There is no "safe sex." *Newsweek*, p. 8.
13. Hatcher, R.A., Stewart, F., Trussel, J., Kowal, D., Guest, F., Stewart, G.K., Cates, W. *Contraceptive technology 1990–92* (15th rev. ed.). Expanded from Planned Parenthood memorandum dated August 13, 1987: *New medical standards for HIV testing and counseling*. New York: Irvington.
14. Carpenito, L.J. (1989). *Nursing diagnosis: Application to clinical practice* (3rd ed.). Philadelphia: Lippincott.
15. Iyer, P., Taptich, B., Bernocchi-Losey, D. (1986). *Nursing process and nursing diagnosis*. Philadelphia: Saunders.
16. Committee on Adolescence. (1990). Contraception and adolescents. *Pediatrics, 86*(1), 134–138.
17. Dickey, R.P. (1993). *Management Contraceptive Pills Patients* (7th ed.). Durant, OK: Essential Medical Information Systems.
18. Goldzieher, J.W. (1989). *Hormonal contraception: Pills, injections and implants*. Dallas: Essential Medical Information Systems.
19. Hawkins, J., & Higgins, L. (1982). *Health care of women: Gynecological assessment*. Monterey, CA: Wadsworth Health Sciences.
20. Litchman, R., & Papera, S. (1991). *Gynecology: Well-woman care*. Norwalk, CT: Appleton & Lange.
21. Trussell, J., Hatcher, R.A., Cates, W., Stewart, F.H., Kost, K. (1990). Contraceptive failure in the U.S.: An update. *Studies in Family Planning, 21*(1), 51–54.
22. Rind, P. (1991). Average estrogen and progestin doses in U.S. pill prescriptions have fallen dramatically since 1964. *Family Planning Perspectives, 23*(4), 184–185.
23. Speroff, L., Glass, R.H., & Kase, N.G. (1989). *Clinical gynecologic endocrinology and infertility* (4th ed.). Baltimore/London: Williams & Wilkins.
24. Stergachis, A. (1992). Epidemiology of the non-contraceptive effects of oral contraceptives. *American Journal of Obstetrics & Gynecology, 167*, 1165–1170.
25. Godsland, I.F., Crook, D., & Wynn, V. (1992). Clinical and metabolic considerations of long term oral contraceptive use. *American Journal of Obstetrics & Gynecology, 166*, 1955–1963.
26. Rebar, R.W., & Zeserson, K. (1991). Characteristics of the new progestogens in combined oral contraceptives. *Contraception, 44*(1), 1–9.
27. Blumenthal, P.D., & Huggins, G.R. (1992). A look at the new progestogen OCs. *Medical Aspects of Human Sexuality, 26*(1).
28. Trossarelli, G.F., Bordon, R., Gennarelli, G.L., & Carta, Q. (1991). An open prospective study on the effects of carbohydrate metabolism on an oral monophasic contraceptive containing gestodene. *Contraception, 43*, 423–433.
29. Bringer, J. (1992). Norgestimate: A clinical overview of a new progestin. *American Journal of Obstetrics & Gynecology, 166*, 1969–1977.
30. Runnebaun, B., Grunwald, K., & Rabe, T. (1992). The efficacy and tolerability of norgestimate/ethinyl estradiol: Results of an open, multicenter study of 59,701 women. *American Journal of Obstetrics & Gynecology, 166*, 1963–1968.
31. Phillips, A., Won Hahn, D., McGuire, J.L. (1992). Preclinical evaluation of norgestimate, a progestin with minimal androgenic activity. *American Journal of Obstetrics & Gynecology, 167*, 1991–1996.
32. Kafrissen, M.E. (1992). Norgestimate containing oral contraceptives: Review of clini-

cal studies. *American Journal of Obstetrics & Gynecology, 167*, 1196–1202.

33. Petersen, K.R., Scouby, S., & Pedersen, R. (1991). Desogestrel and gestodene in OCs: Twelve months assessment of carbohydrate and lipoprotein metabolism. *Obstetrics & Gynecology, 78*, 666–672.
34. Staff. (1991, May). Maximizing oral contraceptives effectiveness: Patient compliance, drug interactions, and other factors. *ARHP Clinical Proceedings*, 1–15.
35. Staff. (1992, February). Maximizing oral contraceptive effectiveness: Changing perceptions. *ARHP Clinical Proceedings*, 1–15.
36. Tikkanen, M.J., & Nikkila, E.A. (1980). Oral contraceptives and lipoprotein metabolism. *Journal of Reproductive Medicine, 31*, 898.
37. Krauss, R.M., & Burkman, R.T. (1992). The metabolic impact of oral contraceptives. *American Journal of Obstetrics & Gynecology, 167*, 1177–1183.
38. Utian, W.H. (1989). Oral contraceptives: Safe after 40? *Patient Care, 23*(6), 115–118, 123–124.
39. Spellacy, W.N. (1982). Carbohydrate metabolism during treatment with estrogens, progestogen and low dose oral contraceptives. *American Journal of Obstetrics & Gynecology, 142*, 732–734.
40. Wynn, V., & Godsland, I. (1986). Effects of oral contraceptives on carbohydrate metabolism. *Journal of Reproductive Medicine, 9*, 893–897.
41. Kaunitz, A.M. (1992). Oral contraceptives and gynecologic cancer: An update for the 1990s. *American Journal of Obstetrics & Gynecology, 167*, 1171–1176.
42. Staff. (1990). Current issues in hormonal contraception. *Contraceptive Report, 1*(1), 1–11.
43. Wingo, P.A., Lee, N., Ory, H., Beral, V., Peterson, H., & Rhodes, P. (1991). Age-specific differences in the relationship between OC use and breast cancer. *Obstetrics & Gynecology, 78*, 161–169.
44. Skegg, D. (1991). Oral contraceptives and neoplasia. *Contraception, 43*, 521–530.
45. Kaunitz, A. (1992). Oral contraceptives and gynecological cancer: An update for the 1990s. *American Journal of Obstetrics & Gynecology (suppl.), 167*(4), 1171–1176.
46. Jarrett, M., & Lethbridge, D. (1990). The contraceptive needs of mid-life women. *Nurse Practitioner, 15*(12), 34–39.
47. Youngkin, E., & Miller, L. (1987). The triphasics: Insights for effective clinical use. *Nurse Practitioner, 12*(2), 17–28.
48. Lynn, M.M., & Holdcroft, C. (1992). New concepts in contraception: Norplant subdermal implant. *Nurse Practitioner, 17*(3), 85–89.
49. Bardin, C.W. (1989). Long-acting steroidal contraception: An update. *International Journal of Fertility, 34*(Suppl.), 88–95.
50. Pollack, A. (1991, January). Norplant: What you should know about the new contraceptive. *Medical Aspects of Human Sexuality,* 38–42.
51. Staff. (1989). *Special initiatives in contraceptive development, FY 1986–89*. Washington, DC: National Institute of Child Health and Human Development.
52. Speroff, L., & Darney, P. (1992). *A clinical guide for contraception*. Baltimore: Williams & Wilkins.
53. Franklin, M. (1990). Recently approved and experimental methods of contraception. *Journal of Nurse Midwifery, 35*, 365–375.
54. Konje, J., et al. (1991). Changes in CHO metabolism during 30 months on Norplant. *Contraception, 44*(2), 163–172.
55. Smolowe, J. (1993, June 14). New, improved and ready for battle, the abortion pill. *Time,* pp. 48–51.
56. Glasier, A., Thong, K.J., Dewar, M., Mackie, M., & Baird, D. (1992). Mifepristone (RU-486) compared with high dose estrogen and progestogen for emergency post-coital contraception. *New England Journal of Medicine, 327*, 1041–1044.
57. Couzinet, B., LeStrat, N., Ulman, A., Baulieu, E., & Schaison, G. (1986). Termination of early pregnancy by the progesterone antagonist RU-486 (mefepristone). *New England Journal of Medicine, 315*, 1565–1570.

58. Vinson, R.P., & Epperly, T.D. (1991). Counseling patients on proper use of condoms. *American Family Practice, 43*(6), 2081–2085.
59. Coker, A., Hulka, B.S., & McCann, M.F. (1992). Barrier methods of contraception and cervical intraepithelial neoplasia. *Contraception, 45*(1).
60. International Pharmaceutical. (1991). *Questions and answers about the Bikini Condom.* Princeton, NJ.
61. Two female condoms close to entering U.S. market. (1989). *Contraceptive Technology Update, 10*, 49–50.
62. Staff. (1992, February 10). Approved for a female condom. *U.S. News and World Report.*
63. Staff. (1992, February 10). A condom for women. *Newsweek, 45.*
64. Wisconsin Pharmaceutical Co. (1991). *Reality vaginal pouch.* Product information. Jackson, WI.
65. Jivasak-Apimas, S. (1991). Acceptability of the vaginal sheath (Femshield) in Thai couples. *Contraception, 44*(2), 183–190.
66. Stone, K.M., Grimes, D.A., & Magder, L.S. (1988). Personal protection against STDs. *American Journal of Obstetrics & Gynecology, 155*, 180–188.
67. Feldblum, P.J., & Fortney, J.A. (1988). Condoms, spermicides and the transmission of HIV: A review of the literature. *American Journal of Public Health, 78*, 52–53.
68. Huggins, G.R. (1982). Vaginal spermicides and outcomes of pregnancy: Findings in a large cohort study. *Contraception 25*(3), 219–230.
69. Louik, C., Mitchell, A.A., Werler, M.M., Hanson, J., & Shapiro, S. (1987). Maternal exposure to spermicides in relation to certain birth defects. *New England Journal of Medicine, 317*, 474–478.
70. Pyle, C. (1984). Nursing protocol for diaphragm contraception. *Nurse Practitioner, 9*(3), 35–40.
71. Brokaw, A.K., Baker, N.N., & Haney, S.L. (1988). Fitting the cervical cap. *Nurse Practitioner, 13*(7), 49–55.
72. Chalker, R. (1987). *The complete cervical cap guide.* New York: Harper & Row.
73. Lemberg, E. (1984). The vaginal contraceptive sponge: A new non-prescription barrier contraceptive. *Nurse Practitioner, 9*(10), 24–37.
74. Hastings-Tolsma, M.T. (1982). The cervical cap: A barrier contraceptive. *Maternal Child Nursing, 7*, 382–386.
75. Digest. (1986). The effectiveness of the cervical cap is hampered by problems of dislodgement and rubber erosion. *Family Planning Perspectives, 18*(5), 229–230.
76. Fihn, S.D., Latham, R.H., Roberts, P., Running, K., & Stamm, W.E. (1985). Association between diaphragm use and UTI. *Journal of the American Medical Association, 254*, 240–245.
77. Weiss, B., Bassford, T., & Davis, T. (1991). The cervical cap. *American Family Practice, 43*, 517–523.
78. Staff. (1985, February). Highly effective copper-T 380A IUD earns FDA approval. *Contraceptive Technology Update, 6*(2), 25–27.
79. Klitsch, M. (1988). The return of the IUD. *Family Planning Perspectives, 20*(1), 19, 40.
80. GynoPharma. (1992). Prescribing information for the Copper T-380 A IUD. *Physicians Desk Reference* (46th ed.).
81. Staff. (1990). Compliance with OCs and alternative contraceptive methods. *Contraceptive Report, 1*(4), 1–12.
82. Alza Corporation. (1986). *Progestasert intrauterine progesterone contraceptive system.* Product information.
83. Alvarez, F., Branche, V., Fernandez, F., Guerro, B., Guiloff, E., Hess, R., Salvafierro, A., Zacharias, S. (1988). New insights on the mode of action of IUDs in women. *Fertility & Sterility, 49*, 768–773.
84. Ortiz, M.E., & Croxatto, H.B. (1987). The mode of action of IUDs. *Contraception, 36*(1), 37–53.
85. Centers for Disease Control. (1987). IUDs: Guidelines for informed decision making and uses. Cited in *Contraceptive Technology* (1991).
86. White, M.K., Ory, H.W., Rooks, J.B., & Rochat, R.W. (1980). Intrauterine device termination rates and the menstrual cycle day

of insertion. *Obstetrics & Gynecology, 55*(2), 220–224.

87. Pernoll, M.L. (Ed.). (1991). *Current Obstetrics and Gynecologic Diagnosis and Treatment* (7th ed.). Norwalk, CT: Appleton & Lange.
88. Knox, A. (1990, July 3). Vasectomy innovation. Newark, NJ: Star-Ledgar.
89. Association for Voluntary Sterilization. (1981). Menstrual function following tubal sterilization. *Biomedical Bulletin, 2*(1).
90. Johnson, J.H., & Reich, J. (1980). The new politics of natural family planning. *Family Planning Perspectives, 18*, 277–282.
91. Nofziger, M. (1988). *Signs of fertility: The personal science of natural birth control.* Nashville: MND Publishing.
92. Lewis, J. (Ed.). (1992). Contraception. *NAACOG's Clinical Issues in Perinatal and Women's Health Nursing, 3*(2), 193–290.
93. Lethbridge, D.J. (1991). Coitus interruptus: Considerations as a birth control method. *JOGN Nursing, 20*(1), 80–85.
94. Willson, J.R. (1987). The puerperium. In J.R. Willson & E.R. Carrington (Eds.). *Obstetrics and Gynecology*. St. Louis: Mosby.
95. Neville, M.C., & Neifert, M.R. (Eds.). (1983). *Lactation: Physiology, nutrition and breastfeeding*. New York: Plenum Press.
96. Kennedy, K.I., Rivera, R., & McNeilly, A.S. (1987). Consensus statement on the use of breastfeeding as a family planning method. *Contraception, 39*(5), 477–496.
97. Gold, R.B. (1990). *Abortion and women's health: A turning point for America?* New York: Alan Guttmacher Institute.
98. Rossi, A.S., & Sitaraman, B. (1988). Abortion in context: Historical trends and future changes. *Family Planning Perspectives, 20*(6), 273–281.
99. Brown, J.S., & Crombleholme, W.R. (1993). *Handbook of gynecology and obstetrics.* Norwalk, CT: Appleton & Lange.
100. Atrash, H.K., MacKay, H.T., Binkin, H.J., & Hogue, C.J. (1987). Legal abortion mortality in the United States: 1972–1982. *American Journal of Obstetrics & Gynecology, 156*, 605–612.
101. Hacker, N.F., & Moore, J.G. (1993). *Essentials of obstetrics and gynecology*. Philadelphia: Saunders.
102. Landy U. (1986). Abortion counseling: A new component of medical care. *Clinics in Obstetrics and Gynecology, 13*(1), 33–41.
103. Brown, A.N. (1983, July/August). Adolescents and abortion. *JOGN Nursing*, 241–247.
104. Torres, A., & Forrest, J.D. (1988). Why do women have abortions? *Family Planning Perspectives, 20*(4), 169–176.
105. Henshaw, S.K. (1991). The accessibility of abortion services in the United States. *Family Planning Perspectives, 23*(6), 246–252.
106. Keenan, C. (1986). Unintended pregnancy: Education for choice. In V.M. Littlefield (Ed.), *Health education for women: A guide for nurses and other professionals* (pp. 396–417). Norwalk, CT: Appleton-Century-Crofts.
107. Guha, S.K., Anand, S., Ansari, S., Farroq, A., & Sharma, D.N. (1990). Time controlled injectable occlusion of the vas deferens. *Contraception, 41*(3), 323–331.
108. Atkinson, L.E., Lincoln, R., & Forrest, J.D. (1986). The next contraceptive revolution. *Family Planning Perspectives, 18*(1), 19–26.

## BIBLIOGRAPHY

The Boston Women's Health Book Collective. (1984). *The new our bodies, ourselves.* New York: Simon & Schuster, Inc.

Carpenito, L.J. (1989). *Nursing diagnosis: Application to clinical practice* (3rd ed.). Philadelphia: J.B. Lippincott Co.

Chalker, R. (1983). New-choice birth control: the cap. *Self.* pp. 46–51.

Cupit, L.G. (1984). Contraception: helping patients choose. *JOGN Nursing*, (supplement), 235–295.

Feldblum, P.J., Fortney, J.A. (1988). Condoms, spermicides and the transmission of HIV: a review of the literature. *AJPH. 78*, 52–53.

Gold, R.B. (1983). Depo-provera: the jury still out (special report). *Family Planning Perspectives, 15*(2), 78–81.

Hatcher, R.A., Stewart, F., Trussel, J., Kowal, D.,

Guest, F., Stewart, G.K., Cates, W. (1990). *Contraceptive technology, 1990–92* (15th revised ed.). New York: Irvington Publishers, Inc.

Huggins, G.R. (1982). Vaginal spermicides and outcome of pregnancy: findings in a large cohort study. *Contraception, 25*(3), 219–230.

Jarrett, M.E. & Lethbridge, D.J. (1990). The contraceptive needs of midlife women. *Nurse Practitioner, 15*(12), 34–39.

Johnson, J.H. & Reich, J. (1988). The new politics of natural family planning. *Family Planning Perspectives, 18*(6), 277–282.

Kass-Annesse B. & Danzer, H. (1986). *The fertility awareness workbook.* Atlanta: Printed Matter.

Louik, C., Mitchell, A.A., Werler, M.M. et al. (1987). Maternal exposure to spermicides in relation to certain birth defects. *New Eng. J. of Med.*, 317, 474–478.

Population Crisis Committee. (1987, May). Issues in contraceptive development. *Population*, 1–16.

Speroff, L. & Darney, P. (1992). *A Clinical Guide for Contraception.* Baltimore: Williams & Wilkins.

Staff. (1985, January). Special report: the pill after 25 years. *Contraceptive Technology Update, 6*(1), 1–24.

Staff. (1985, February). Highly effective Copper T-380A IUD earns FDA approval. *Contraceptive Technology Update 6*(2), 25–27.

CHAPTER 7

# INFERTILITY

*Sue C. Wood*

*A couple's ability to admit that they may have a fertility problem is reassuring, but they may also be threatened as potential causes are identified and treatment recommended.*

### *Highlights*

- History, Physical Examination, Diagnostic Studies
- Psychosocial Evaluation
- Female Infertility
  - *Hypothalamic Disorders*
  - *Pituitary Disorders*
  - *Adrenal Disorders*
  - *Ovarian Disorders*
  - *Uterine Disorders*
  - *Pelvic Disorders*
  - *Recurrent Fetal Loss*
- Male Infertility
  - *Endocrine Disorders*
  - *Varicocele*
  - *Genetic Abnormalities, Acquired Obstruction*
  - *Sperm Transport Dysfunction*
- Combined Female and Male Factors
- Treatment: Insemination, Assisted Reproductive Technologies
- Adoption, Surrogacy, Childfree Living

## INTRODUCTION

Infertility is the inability to conceive after a year of regular unprotected intercourse or to carry a pregnancy to a live birth.* Primary infertility means that the couple has never conceived. Secondary infertility occurs when the couple has previously conceived, regardless of the pregnancy outcome.

Today, couples are more aware of specific causes of infertility and of the sophisticated treatments available. Consequently, they increasingly are seeking treatment, as infant adoption resources are becoming depleted. The number of available infertility services also is increasing, as evidenced by increased membership in the American Fertility Society and the creation of the subspecialty Reproductive Endocrinology by the American Board of Obstetrics and Gynecology.[1] The National Certification Corporation (NCC) for the obstetric, gynecologic, and neonatal nursing specialties offers certification for registered nurses in reproductive endocrinology/ infertility. In many cases, however, health care insurance may not share the burden of treatment costs to resolve infertility.

*The author wishes to thank Sanford M. Rosenberg, M.D., for reviewing the manuscript of this chapter.

Infertility is a widespread problem that often is initially identified in the obstetric/gynecologic practice. It may also be identified in the urologic practice. It is imperative that the nurse practitioner recognize infertility and understand its causes and treatment options. Evaluation and treatment may be initiated in the general practice. The necessity of referral to a specialist is determined by the type of setting, credentials of staff, resources to treat, and efficacy of treatment.

The reproductive endocrinologist and nurse practitioner in the reproductive endocrinology/infertility practice collaborate as closely as they would in any medical setting. The health care provider's role is multifaceted: to identify and treat; to understand multiple impacts on the individual, couple, and significant others; to provide information, support, and counseling; and to refer to specialties of internal medicine, endocrinology, urology, and psychiatry. Other roles include research, community education, and advocacy.

Approximately 10 to 20 percent of couples in the United States are infertile,[2] and there is documentation that fertility decreases with age. Couples are postponing marriage and delaying childbearing to pursue advanced education and careers, or to achieve financial stability.[4] In the 1980s, one out of five American women had her first child after age 35.[3] Yet, about one third of women who defer pregnancy until the mid-to-late 30s will have an infertility problem.[1]

#### Causative Factors in Infertility

- *Aging.* Reduced frequency of intercourse, decline in ovarian and uterine function, increase in miscarriages, and increase in diseases of the reproductive tract, in particular, endometriosis.[3]
- *Sexually Transmitted Diseases (STDs).*
- *Exposure to Occupational Hazards.* Chemicals, radiation, noise.
- *Exposure to Environmental Hazards.* Heat, smoking, alcohol, drug abuse.[5]

The cumulative effects of the choice to delay fertility—biologic factors, sexual practices, and exposure to environmental toxins—have resulted in an increase in infertility.

## INFERTILITY EVALUATION

Evaluation must be couple oriented, systematic, thorough, and completed within a reasonable time frame. The nurse practitioner may *begin* the infertility investigation, educate and support the couple, and initiate referral to a specialist. Evaluation is recommended if a couple has not conceived after 1 year of attempting to—or sooner if factors known to affect fertility exist, or if the couple is very anxious.

The etiology of infertility can be identified in 90 percent of couples; 10 percent have unexplained infertility (no abnormality found). Thirty-five percent have male factor infertility, 35 percent have female factor infertility, and 20 percent have a combination of male and female factors.[6] Multiple factors of infertility become more difficult to overcome.

The data considered essential for a thorough evaluation are those gained from a history and physical examination of the couple (see Tables 7–1 through 7–5).

### DIAGNOSTIC TESTS AND METHODS

Numbers 1 through 6 below are the steps of a routine assessment. The order in which they are performed depends on the client's history.

#### 1. Basal Body Temperature (BBT) Chart

The BBT chart helps to determine the time of ovulation (after ovulation, a sustained temperature rise of 0.4–0.6°F occurs) and to plan and interpret fertility tests (see Chapter 6).

**TABLE 7–1. FEMALE HISTORY: SUMMARY OF PERTINENT DATA**

Age of client.

Duration of amenorrhea (if present).

Previous obstetric and gynecologic history.

Time to conceive previous pregnancies.

Previous contraceptive methods and complications.

Menstrual pattern (age at menarche, length of cycle, and duration of menses).

Symptoms of ovulation: molimina (breast tenderness, acne, mood changes, mittelschmerz, increased midcycle discharge, midcycle spotting).

Symptoms of dysmenorrhea.

Symptoms of sexual dysfunction.

Frequency of coitus.

Medical, surgical, social, and sexual history (diethylstilbestrol exposure, multiple partners, sexually transmitted diseases).

History suggestive of endocrine disease (galactorrhea, hirsutism, heat or cold intolerance).

Family history, especially of endocrine disease or reproductive or genetic abnormalities.

Alcohol, drug, or tobacco use.

*Source: From* Ovulation Induction: Clinical Aspects/Practical Applications, A Nursing Perspective, *1988:20, with permission of Serono Laboratories, Inc., Norwell, Massachusetts.*

## 2. Postcoital Test (PCT)

The PCT is performed just before expected ovulation. The couple should refrain from intercourse during the 1 to 2 days before the test; then should have intercourse without the use of lubricants, 2 to 10 hours prior to the appointment. The woman may shower but should not take a tub bath or douche before the appointment. A sample of mucus is taken from the cervix and microscopically assessed for quality of mucus and number of motile sperm.

- A normal test shows clear mucus; spinnbarkeit (SPBK), the elasticity of cervical mucus, is approximately 10 cm. Ferning appears, and 5 to 10 motile sperm per high power field (HPF) are present.
- An abnormal test may suggest improper timing. If the PCT test is well timed, repeat it during the next cycle. Abnormality may be due to coital technique, cervical mucus or sperm factors, or the presence of antisperm antibodies.

**TABLE 7–2. FEMALE PHYSICAL EXAM: SUMMARY OF PERTINENT DATA**

Absence of neurological symptoms.

Normal thyroid gland.

Normal breast development without galactorrhea.

Absence of abdominal masses.

Normal hair distribution.

Normal external genitalia.

Presence of a vagina and cervix on examination.

Estrogenic/hypoestrogenic cervical mucus and vagina.

Normal uterus and ovaries.

*Source: From* Ovulation Induction: Clinical Aspects/Practical Applications, A Nursing Perspective, *1988:20, with permission of Serono Laboratories, Inc., Norwell, Massachusetts.*

## 3. Semen Analysis (S/A)

Early in a woman's evaluation, her partner collects a semen specimen by means of masturbation. The semen is deposited directly into a clean container and evaluated microscopically. Semen analyses vary in different labs.

- Normal semen analysis shows:
  - *Volume.* 2 to 5 mL.
  - *Viscosity.* Liquefaction occurs in 1 hour.
  - *pH*: 7 to 8.
  - *Count.* Equal to or greater than 20 million per mL.
  - *Motility.* Equal to or greater than 50–60 percent.

**TABLE 7–3. MALE HISTORY: SUMMARY OF PERTINENT DATA**

| |
|---|
| Duration of infertility. |
| Prior pregnancies (present partner, different partner). |
| Time to conceive previous pregnancies. |
| Circumcision. |
| Childhood development (cryptorchidism, hypospadias, hernia, testicular torsion/trauma, onset of puberty). |
| Infections (mumps, sexually transmitted diseases). |
| Medical, surgical, social history (illness, recurrent respiratory infection, renal anomalies, surgery, caffeine, nicotine, alcohol, marijuana). |
| Symptoms of sexual dysfunction (libido, ejaculation). |
| Frequency of coitus, sexual practices. |
| Exposure to toxins (chemicals, pesticides, lead, radiation, excessive heat). |
| Drugs (chemotherapy, sulfa drugs, cimetidine, colchicine, nitrofurantoin). |
| Exposure to diethylstilbestrol in utero. |

*Source: Adapted from Ovulation Induction: Clinical Aspects/Practical Applications,* A Nursing Perspective, *1988:32–34, with permission of Serono Laboratories, Inc., Norwell, Massachusetts.*

- *Quality of Motion (Forward Progression).* 3 (good), to 4 (excellent).
- *Morphology.* Greater than 50 percent normal forms.
- *White Blood Cell (WBC) Count.* Less than 1 million per mL.
- *Semen Ureaplasma/Mycoplasma (Semen U/U).* Negative.

■ Abnormal semen analysis requires that the test be repeated in 4 to 6 weeks. Some studies suggest that ureaplasma attaches to sperm and reduces motility. The mycoplasma role in infertility is controversial.

■ With positive ureaplasma/mycoplasma semen culture treatment of both partners is indicated: one coated 100-mg doxycycline hyclate pellet (Doryx) daily, p.o., for 30 days, beginning with the first day of the woman's full menstrual flow. It is necessary to prevent pregnancy by protected intercourse during the cycle of treatment.

**TABLE 7–4. MALE PHYSICAL EXAM: SUMMARY OF PERTINENT DATA**

| |
|---|
| Absence of neurological symptoms (libido, headache, visual impairment, olfactory dysfunction). |
| Normal thyroid gland. |
| Normal breast tissue without galactorrhea. |
| Normal secondary sexual characteristics (hair pattern, body proportions, muscle development). |
| Normal genitalia. |

*Source: Adapted from* Ovulation Induction: Clinical Aspects/Practical Applications, A Nursing Perspective, *1988:32–34, with permission of Serono Laboratories, Inc., Norwell, Massachusetts.*

### 4. Hysterosalpingogram (HSG)

An x-ray test is performed after menses, but before ovulation. Dye is placed in the uterus to outline the uterine cavity and determine the patency of the fallopian tubes. Any cramping will subside quickly. Prior to the test, the client may be given a sedative, midazolam HCL/Roche (Versed), which will virtually eliminate discomfort. Advise the client that someone must accompany her home, and to wear a sanitary pad for fluid leakage and spotting.

### 5. Endometrial Biopsy

The biopsy is performed late in the menstrual cycle, after the 10 or 11 day rise of BBT. It will determine the occurrence of ovulation and the production of adequate hormones after ovulation. Endometrial biopsy is performed only after a negative pregnancy test. The risk of biopsy to an undetected pregnancy is small; however, some couples de-

**TABLE 7–5. COPING WITH INFERTILITY, INDIVIDUALS AND COUPLES**

*Coping with Infertility*
Perception of problem, cause of infertility.
Knowledge of sexual function, anatomy, reproductive cycle.
Meaning of ability or inability to have a child.
Beliefs and values, motivations for pregnancy, responses of significant others to childbearing/childrearing.

*Response to Infertility*
Stage of crisis/grief.
Ability to identify and verbalize feelings; past experiences and effects on feelings, expectations of partner.
Affect on lives and relationship.
Affect on sexual relationship.
Significant others' awareness of infertility, responses to infertility/treatment.

*Coping Strategies*
Problem solving/decision making abilities.
Patterns of communication.
Use of support systems.
Ability to modify stressors in environment.

*Source: Adapted from Eck Menning, B. (1988).* Infertility: A guide for the childless couple *(2nd ed.). Englewood Cliffs, NJ: Prentice-Hall.*

cide to have protected intercourse during this cycle. The client may experience cramping during and shortly after the biopsy. Advise her to wear a sanitary pad home because of the spotting that occurs (see Chapter 5).

### 6. Laser Laparoscopy

The laparoscopy is performed early in the cycle, after menses, as outpatient surgery under general anesthesia. It is recommended when other tests have been completed. The laparoscope is inserted through the navel to visualize the pelvis. Laser can be used to treat endometriosis, pelvic adhesions or scarring, and some tubal diseases, thereby avoiding the need for major abdominal inpatient surgery. Usually the client can return home in several hours (see Chapter 9).

### Hysteroscopy with Laser Laparoscopy

The procedure is performed early during a woman's cycle, after menses, usually when uterine anomalies have been identified (abnormal HSG). Laparoscopy is performed in conjunction with hysteroscopy to delineate the external uterine contour. The laser can be used at hysteroscopy to lyse adhesions, repair septa, or remove polyps or fibroids.

### Additional Diagnostic Tests

A client's history may indicate the need for other tests; urine culture ureaplasma/mycoplasma, Papanicolaou smear, and chlamydia culture are routinely performed.

- Urine culture ureaplasma/mycoplasma (Urine U/U) may be done because some studies suggest an association between the ureaplasma organism and subclinical endometrial inflammation; and between mycoplasma and salpingitis. A positive urine culture is treated with one doxycycline hyclate pellet 100 mg daily, p.o., for 14 days for both the client and her partner, beginning with the client's next full menstrual flow. Repeat the cultures 2 weeks after completion of the doxycycline hyclate regimen. If the repeat culture is positive, treat both partners again for 30 days, beginning with the client's next full menstrual flow. Protected intercourse is necessary to prevent pregnancy during the cycle of treatment. Do not reculture after the 30-day treatment, as the couple cannot be treated further for this condition.
- A Papanicolaou (Pap) smear is done to rule out cervical cancer and inflammatory processes suggestive of infection. The maturation index will detect estrogen defi-

ciency; the procedure may suggest cervical stenosis (see Chapter 3).

- Chlamydia culture will rule out *Chlamydia trachomatis* infection (see Chapters 3 and 8).
- Serum progesterone will confirm the occurrence of ovulation but is not considered a reliable indicator of normal ovulation.
- Serum prolactin test will rule out hyperprolactinemia (see Chapter 5).
- Serum thyroid stimulating hormone (TSH) and triiodothyronine ($T_3$), thyroxine ($T_4$), and $T_7$ (calculation based on $T_3$ + $T_4$) tests will rule out hyperthyroid/hypothyroid disease.

## PSYCHOSOCIAL ASPECTS OF INFERTILITY EVALUATION

Many couples take for granted that they are fertile and hence are not emotionally prepared for the psychological impact of a diagnosis of infertility. Pain and distress may be even greater for couples who experience secondary infertility. A couple's ability to admit that they may have a fertility problem is reassuring, but they may also feel threatened as potential causes are identified and treatment recommended. Infertility is a couple's problem, not an individual's. Both partners need to be involved in diagnostic and treatment choices and to accompany each other to appointments when possible.

### THE RESPONSES AND NEEDS OF PARTNERS

#### Crises of Infertility

Infertility threatens self-esteem, body image, masculinity/femininity, and sexual relations.[7] It may not affect both partners at the same time. Furthermore, one partner may not perceive the problem with the same emotional intensity or have the knowledge or energy to support the other partner. Prior coping strategies may be ineffective.[7]

#### Emotional Responses

Shock and surprise are quickly replaced by denial (expressed as a need to try longer), which helps the couple to deal with intense feelings of loss. As denial subsides, anger emerges and intensifies as the couple loses privacy and undergoes invasive procedures. Often, significant others and health care professionals become targets for anger because the couple feels helpless and has experienced a loss of control. The couple needs to express the anger and receive the concern and empathy of others.[7]

#### Support Systems

Partners may withdraw from each other and significant others in order to avoid uncomfortable sharing. It is often difficult for the couple to identify feelings, verbalize needs, and cope with multiple stressors. Significant persons may recognize the couple's needs but not know how to offer support. Ineffective communication results in increased stress, tension, guilt, and depression. It may even alter relationships and intensify marital dysfunction.

#### Loss

Feelings of loss may be overcome in a positive manner. The couple needs to grieve in order to come to terms with the infertility.

#### Secondary Infertility

Couples who conceived previously with treatment soon remember the multiple impacts of infertility and experience hurt from the wounds that they thought were healed. They also feel guilt because they want another child, and feel pressured to conceive quickly and use the same treatment as when they conceived previously.

## PROFESSIONAL AND PSYCHOLOGICAL SUPPORT

The health care provider can assist the couple experiencing grief by giving accurate information; counseling or making referrals for individual, group, or sex therapy; and encouraging couples to use support services. Couples may contact the American Fertility Society in Birmingham, Alabama, or Resolve in Somerville, Massachusetts, and become involved in self-help groups. Couples may also need to be given permission to stop treatment.

*Counseling is necessary in all cases of infertility, no matter what the cause, to facilitate healthy adaptation/resolution.* The many complex feelings associated with loss and infertility involve self-image, self-esteem, and sexuality. Past experiences and self-concept will affect the couple's understanding of problems and feelings and their problem solving or decision making abilities. Encourage clients to verbalize feelings and help them to strengthen their patterns of communication and support systems. The aim of intervention is to reduce stress, increase coping skills, and enable the couple to regain control and dignity. Referral to appropriate resources is often helpful. Resolution of infertility can be accomplished when one no longer feels imperfect in relation to one's fertility, self-image, self-esteem, and sexuality.

# FEMALE INFERTILITY: CAUSES, DIAGNOSES, AND INTERVENTIONS

Ovulatory disorders, which exist in 30 to 40 percent of infertile women, may be related to hypothalamic, pituitary, adrenal, ovarian, or uterine dysfunction. Ovulation may occur infrequently (oligo-ovulation) or not at all (anovulation) (see Chapter 5).

Figure 7–1 outlines the diagnostic evaluation and treatment of the infertile female client. Table 7–6 describes specific treatment regimens for endocrine disorders and ovulation dysfunction. Drug dosages, common side effects, an evaluation of the therapies, and continued treatment recommendations are included. The *Physicians' Desk Reference (PDR)* or other appropriate pharmacotherapeutic references should be reviewed for drug contraindications and a complete list of effects.

## HYPOTHALAMIC DISORDERS

### Hypothalamic Dysfunction

The dysfunction may result in multisystem disorders requiring that the client be referred to a reproductive endocrinologist. Hypothalamic problems that affect reproduction are diagnosed after pituitary abnormalities are excluded.

The exact cause of hypothalamic dysfunction is unknown; however, extreme weight loss and/or excessive exercise that interfere with estrogen production do impact hypothalamic function. In addition, systemic diseases of the liver or kidney interrupt hormone metabolism and feedback mechanisms.[8] Hormone profiles reveal low serum estradiol ($E^2$ less than 40 pg/mL) and low levels of follicle-stimulating hormone and luteinizing hormone (FSH/LH less than 5 mIU/mL).[9] Idiopathic dysfunction results in lowered gonadotropin-releasing hormone (GnRH) production.

***Subjective Data.*** Subjective data are obtained from an accurate menstrual history and determination of pubertal milestones. Inquire specifically about Crohn's disease, connective tissue disorders, hepatitis, galactorrhea,

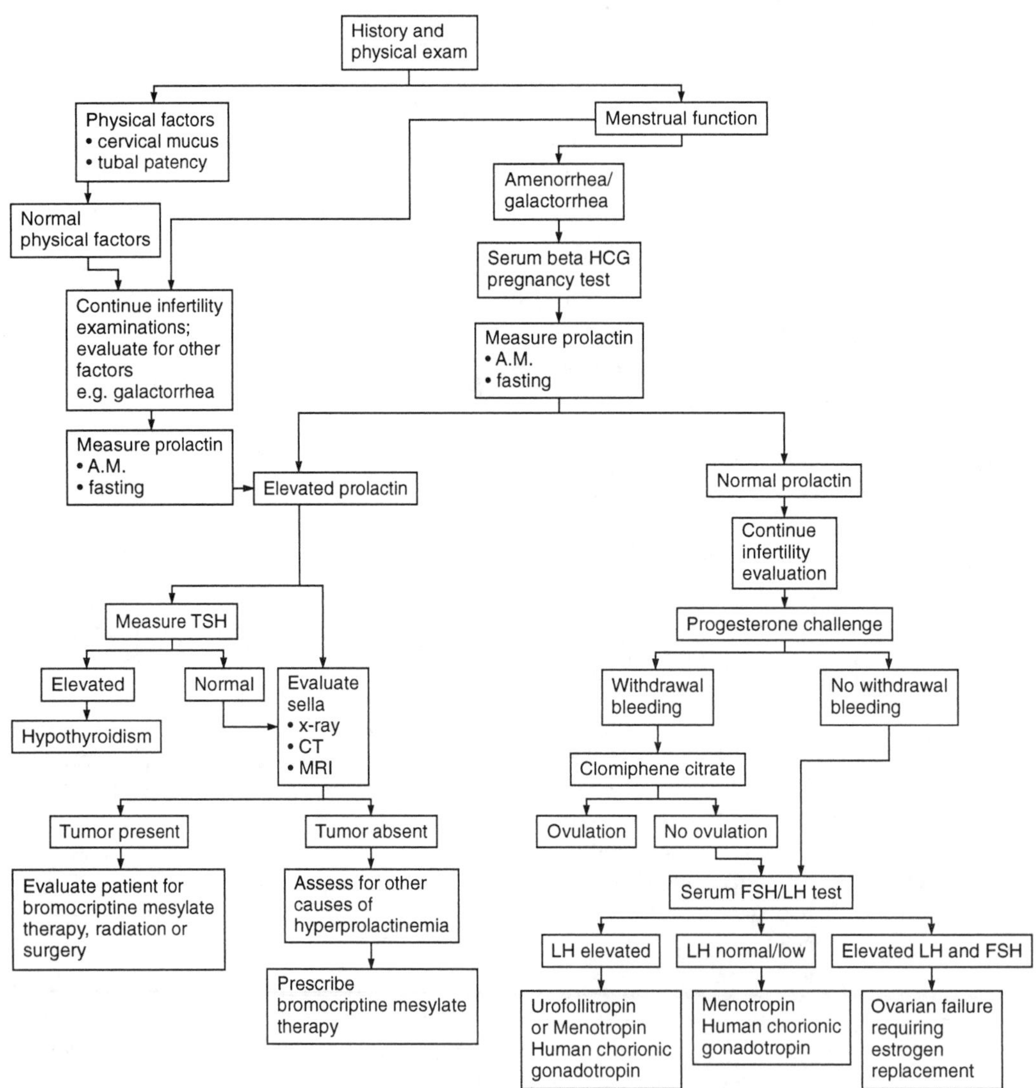


**Figure 7–1.** Suggested management guidelines: Diagnosis and treatment of the infertile female client. (*Used with the permission of Sandoz Pharmaceuticals Corporation.*)

stress, adequacy of nutrition (take a dietary history), exercise, and medications. Clients commonly report absent menses, monophasic basal body temperatures, history of excessive dieting or exercise, and altered eating habits.

### Objective Data

- *Physical Examination.* Includes assessment for low body weight, no fat, little breast tissue, normal secondary sexual characteristics, and hair patterns.
- *Diagnostic Tests and Methods.* The following blood tests are used to diagnose hypothalamic dysfunction (see Appendix C for normal values). For each test, the results usually found with hypothalamic dysfunction are given:
  - *Pregnancy Test.* Negative; radioimmunoassay (RIA) should be used.
  - *Serum Multiphasic Analysis-12 (SMA-12).* Results are evaluated for indications of systemic illnesses that could affect hypothalamic function; may be normal or abnormal.
  - *FSH/LH and $E^2$.* Low.
  - *Thyroid Studies (TSH, $T_3$, $T_4$, $T_7$).* May be abnormally high or low.
  - *Prolactin (PRL).* May be elevated; if so, complete pituitary workup is needed, including computed tomography (CT) scan of the sella turcica.
  - *Gonadotropin Releasing Hormone (GnRH) Test.* Used to stimulate LH/FSH secretion. Two baseline blood samples are obtained at different intervals prior to I.V. infusion of 100 or 150 μg of GnRH. FSH/LH levels are obtained 30 and 60 minutes after infusion. In hypogonadal females, FSH response is greater than LH response. Exaggerated responses may suggest hypothyroidism.

***Differential Medical Diagnoses.*** Anorexia nervosa, bulimia, psychiatric disorders, hyperprolactinemia, androgen excess, polycystic ovarian disease, central nervous system (CNS) infection (meningoencephalitis), neoplasms (craniopharyngioma), anosmia, congenital anomalies, drug ingestion (phenothiazines, oral contraceptives), idiopathic conditions.

### Plan

- Medical therapy as indicated.
- Refer the client to a reproductive endocrinologist for evaluation and ovulation induction.
- Psychosocial interventions are described on page 167. Counseling and evaluation are related to the client's body image, ability to manage stress, and anxiety level.
- Medication commonly includes monthly progesterone or cyclic oral estrogen/progesterone. Clomiphene, urofollitropin (Metrodin), menotropins (Pergonal), or the GnRH pump are used to induce ovulation. Human chorionic gonadotropin (Profasi) I.M. and progesterone vaginal suppositories may be administered to provide luteal phase support (see Table 7–6).
  - *Medroxyprogesterone Acetate (Provera).* To induce cyclic menses or menses prior to ovulation induction, prescribe 10 mg p.o. for 10 days.
  - *Conjugated Estrogens (Premarin).* When the client fails to have withdrawal bleeding after taking progesterone alone, prescribe conjugated estrogen (Premarin) 1.25 mg p.o. for calendar days 1 to 25 *with* medroxyprogesterone acetate (Provera) 10 mg p.o. for days 14 to 25 to induce cyclic menses or menses prior to ovulation induction.
- Anticipated outcome on evaluation is cyclic menses, menses prior to ovulation induction, and normal ovulation induction.
- Teach the client the importance of drug compliance and the characteristics of the drug effects. The client should be provided

**TABLE 7–6. OVULATION INDUCTION[a]**

| Diagnosis | Drug/Action | Dose | Monitor | Side Effects | Continued Treatment |
|---|---|---|---|---|---|
| Increased DHEA-S (dehydroepiandrosterone sulfate). | Dexamethasone.<br>Inhibits corticotropin release; decreases adrenal androgens. | 0.5–0.75 mg p.o. q.h.s. | Serum cortisol.<br>Basal body temperature (BBTs).<br>Endometrial biopsy. | Rare.<br>Decreases resistance to infection, response to medication.<br>Masks symptoms of illness.<br>(Wear ID bracelet.) | Anovulation: Clomiphene + dexamethasone |
| Increased PRL (prolactin). | Bromocriptine (dopamine agonist).<br>Inhibits PRL production by pituitary. 90% attain normal PRL; 80% ovulate and conceive. | 2.5–15 mg p.o. q.d. (Usual dose 2.5–7.5 mg.)<br>Begin 1/2 tablet p.o. q.d.; add 1–2 tablets, p.o. q.d. over 2 weeks.<br>Taper dose when discontinue. | PRL, 4 weeks after begin medication, then as necessary.<br>Visual fields.<br>BBTs.<br>Endometrial biopsy. | Nausea (take with food/milk).<br>Postural hypotension—causes dizziness.<br>Careful operation of machinery.<br>Headache. | Anovulation: Clomiphene + bromocriptine |
| Luteal phase defect. | Progesterone vaginal suppositories or progesterone capsules.<br>Enhances glandular development of endometrium.<br>Conceive in 6–12 cycles. | Suppositories<br>25 mg b.i.d.<br>50 mg q.h.s.<br>Capsules<br>100 mg p.o. t.i.d.<br>Begin after BBT elevated for 2–3 days. | BBTs to assess change in luteal phase.<br>Endometrial biopsy to determine endometrial response to treatment. | Delays onset of menses.<br>Change in menstrual flow.<br>Decrease in vaginal secretions.<br>Vaginal irritation.<br>Capsules may cause drowsiness; can take 1 in am, 2 in pm. | No defect correction: Clomiphene |
| Oligo/anovulation.<br>Polycystic ovarian syndrome (PCO).<br>Normal PRL; increased LH; low to normal FSH. | Clomiphene citrate (CC) (antiestrogen).<br>Binds to estrogen receptor sites.<br>Prevents negative feedback of estrogen. | 50–200 mg p.o.<br>Cycle days 5–9 ($C_{5-9}$).<br>Start at 50-mg dose. In subsequent cycles increase dose by 50-mg incre- | BBTs to assess ovulation; pelvic or ultrasound (U/S) by $C_5$ to determine normal ovaries or presence of cyst. | Mild headache, hot flashes, abdominal tenderness, bloating.<br>With visual disturbances, stop clomiphene citrate. | Clomiphene failure—no conception after 4–6 cycles.<br>With anovulation or abnormal |

| | | | | | |
|---|---|---|---|---|---|
| | Stimulates the pituitary. FSH rises; stimulates follicle development. 50–94% ovulate. 30–61% conceive. Conceive in 4–6 cycles.<br>As indicated, use human chorionic gonadotropin hormone (Profasi). Finishes egg maturation. Triggers LH surge. Assists follicle rupture. Ovulation about 38 h after Profasi. | ments if ovulation abnormal.<br>Ovulation expected $C_{15-21}$.<br>(Increased pregnancy rate occurs at lower doses.)<br>Recommend 100 mg p.o. $C_{5-9}$ + ultrasound (U/S) $C_{15-17}$ and repeat p.r.n. until presence of 19–21-mm size follicle.<br>Administer Profasi 10,000 U I.M. | U/S monitoring of follicle development.<br>Postcoital test (PCT) (to check potential antiestrogen effects on cervical mucus.<br>Intercourse midcycle week.<br>Timed intercourse day of and next 2 days following administration of Profasi. | Multiple pregnancy rate (5%)—twins most often.<br>Abdominal bloating, tenderness at injection site. | ovulation or abnormal cervical mucus, use:<br>Gonadotropins Menotropin (Pergonal–FSH/LH)<br>*or*<br>Urofollitropin (Metrodin—FSH). |
| Hypothalamic disorder.<br>Hypogonadism. | *Priming Cycle*<br>Medroxyprogesterone acetate (Provera) 10 mg p.o. × 10 days.<br>*or*<br>Conjugated estrogens, USP (Premarin) 1.25 mg p.o.—calendar days 1–25.<br>*and*<br>Provera 10 mg p.o. calendar days 14–25. | | Baseline serum estradiol ($E_2$)/FSH/LH.<br>Repeat $E_2$ in 1 week of pump infusion and p.r.n. (Assesses biochemical activity of follicle—midcycle $E_2$ about 300 pg/mL.) Schedule ultrasound and repeat p.r.n. until follicle is about 20 + mm in size. | Provera:<br>Spotting, headache, fluid retention, fatigue, depression.<br>Premarin:<br>Nausea, breast tenderness and fluid retention.<br>GnRH infusion:<br>Headache, hot flashes, abdominal discomfort, irritation at infusion site. | Anovulation or failure to conceive.<br>Candidate for ovum donation IVF (does not respond well to gonadotropins). |

(*continued*)

TABLE 7–6. (CONTINUED)

| Diagnosis | Drug/Action | Dose | Monitor | Side Effects | Continued Treatment |
|---|---|---|---|---|---|
| | GnRH infusion pump: Factrel (subcutaneous)/Lutrepulse (I.V.) Directly stimulates hypothalamus—90–95% ovulate, 30–35% conceive.[b] | Begin continuous infusion pump after menses. Subcutaneous 5–20 μg/dose. I.V. 2.5–5 μg/dose. Pulse q. 90 min. Ovulate within 3 weeks. | BBTs. Use urine LH kit to detect LH surge to assist with timed intercourse. | Ovarian hyperstimulation. Treatment Expensive, multiple blood tests/office visits/adjustment to mechanics of pump. | |
| | *Luteal Phase Support* Progesterone vaginal suppositories. (See Luteal Phase Defect.) | See above. | See Luteal Phase Defect. | See Luteal Phase Defect. | |
| | *or* Profasi Enhances corpus luteum production of progesterone. (See Anovulation.) | 1500–2500 U I.M. × 3 doses. | See Anovulation. | See Anovulation. | |
| Hypothalamic disorder (anorexia). Clomid failure. | Menotropin (Pergonal) *or* Urofollitropin (Metrodin) Directly stimulates ovary. Increases FSH/LH 61–77% ovulate; 20–24% conceive in 6 cycles.[b] *and* | Begin cycle days 2–5 ($C_{2-5}$); 150 IU I.M. q.d. × 5 days, then vary pending $E_2$ and ultrasound results. May need 6–12 day course of daily injections. | Baseline; $E_2$ and U/S results serially p.r.n. ($E_2$ about 300 pg/mL per mature follicle 16–18 mm.) Urine LH kit to detect spontaneous LH surge. BBTs. PCT to determine adequacy of mucus. | Ovarian enlargement, abdominal bloating/tenderness, fatigue, nausea, headache, diarrhea, weight gain; 6% of patients develop severe ovarian hyperstimulation syndrome, 20% have multiple gestation (twins). | Anovulation (poor responder): GnRH pump. Ovum donation/IVF. No conception: Assisted reproductive technologies (IVF/GIFT/ZIFT). |

| | | | | |
|---|---|---|---|---|
| | Profasi<br>Day following last dose of gonadotropin. (See Anovulation.) | When appropriate $E_2$ levels and follicle size attained, administer Profasi 5,000–10,000 IU. | Timed intercourse. (See Anovulation.) | Irritation at injection sites.<br>Painful/bruised arms due to blood tests. |
| | *Luteal Phase Support*<br>Progesterone vaginal suppositories. (See Luteal Phase Defect.)<br>*or* | See Luteal Phase Defect. | | Treatment<br>Expensive, inconvenient due to early am lab and pm ultrasounds; after lab results available, increasingly invasive. |
| | Profasi (See Luteal Phase Anovulation.) | 5000 U I.M. × 1 dose (week after ovulatory dose).<br>*or*<br>1500–2000 U × 2–3 doses. | See Annovulation. | |
| Assisted reproductive technologies. | Leuprolide acetate (Lupron) (GnRh agonist)<br>Suppresses pituitary production of FSH and LH.<br>Helps control ovulation induction.<br>*and* | See Figure 7–3. | See Figure 7–3. | Mild headache, itching, redness, hive at injection site. |
| | Metrodin/Pergonal | See Figure 7–3. | | |

*Note:* See PDR for contraindications and complete list of side effects.

[a] Prior to induction, rule out pregnancy, complete infertility evaluation, and perform semen analysis

[b] Difference in ovulation/and percent who conceive due to multiple factors of infertility.

*Source: Adapted from Rivlin, M. (Ed.). (1990).* Handbook of drug therapy in reproductive endocrinology and infertility. *Boston: Little, Brown.*

with information regarding nutrition, routine exercise, the risks of osteoporosis, cardiovascular disease, endometrial cancer, and ovulation induction.

***Follow-Up.*** Table 7–6 presents guidelines for monitoring and continuing treatment.

## PITUITARY DISORDERS

Hyperprolactinemia is the most common cause of pituitary disorder; it requires extensive evaluation and referral. Hypogonadotropic hypogonadism and Sheehan's syndrome are rare causes of pituitary disorder.[9]

### Hyperprolactinemia

Prolactin (PRL) levels are greater than 20 ng/mL. Elevated PRL interferes with GnRH release, which in turn results in lowered levels of FSH/LH. Elevated PRL may directly inhibit the gonads.[10]

***Subjective Data.*** Take a complete history. Infertility, normal menses or cycle irregularities, milky breast discharge, headache/visual disturbances, and stress are commonly reported.

#### *Objective Data*

- *Physical Examination.* This must be complete and include a thorough neurological exam. Note any milky breast discharge or abnormal neurological findings.
- *Diagnostic Tests and Methods.* The following are indicated:
  - Pregnancy test.
  - PRL level (must be elevated on more than one sample).
  - Slide of breast discharge to determine fat globules that would indicate milk.
  - CT scan of the sella turcica to rule out pituitary adenoma.
  - TSH and $T_3$, total $T_4$, $T_7$ to rule out thyroid disease; elevated TSH and decreased $T_3$ and $T_4$ indicates hypothyroid disease (see Appendix C for normal values).

***Differential Medical Diagnoses.*** Galactorrhea, oligomenorrhea/amenorrhea, ovarian dysfunction (polycystic ovarian disease, luteal phase defect), hypothalamic lesions, pituitary lesions (tumors, acromegaly, Cushing's disease, empty sella syndrome), hypothyroidism, physiological conditions (pregnancy, breast stimulation), pharmacological effects (reserpine, cimetidine, tricyclic antidepressants, estrogens), idiopathic conditions.

#### *Plan*

- Medical therapy as indicated.
- Refer the client to a reproductive endocrinologist for evaluation and ovulation induction.
- Refer the client to a neurologist, ophthalmologist, or surgeon as indicated.
- Psychosocial interventions are described on page 167. Provide the client with information, anticipatory guidance, pain management, stress management, and counseling for anxiety and body image disturbance.
- Medication as indicated:
  - *Bromocriptine.* Indicated for treatment of hyperprolactinemia. For administration and side effects, see Table 7–6. Anticipated outcomes on evaluation are normal PRL levels and thyroid function, decreased galactorrhea, and resumption of ovulatory menstrual cycles. Client teaching is related to drug characteristics (see Table 7–6).
  - *Levothyroxine Sodium.* Indicated for hypothyroid treatment among those few clients with galactorrhea and amenorrhea. The usual starting dose of 50 μg p.o. is taken daily with incremental increases of 25 μg every 2–3 weeks until a

maintenance dosage of 100–200 μg daily is attained. The maintenance dosage is reflected by a normal metabolic state (TSH or $T_3$ levels) and should be achieved within the first month of therapy. Maintenance therapy is continued for an indefinite period. Anticipated outcomes on evaluation are normal prolactin levels, normal thyroid function, a decrease in galactorrhea, and resumption of cyclic menses. Client teaching is related to drug characteristics and the required follow-up evaluation.

- *Bromocriptine with Clomiphene.* Indicated to induce normal ovulation; bromocriptine may correct hyperprolactinemia, but ovulation may not be normal. Combined bromocriptine and clomiphene may be necessary to induce ovulation. For administration, side effects, and client teaching, see Table 7–6 and *Physicians' Desk Reference* or other appropriate pharmacotherapeutic references.
- *Levothyroxine Sodium with Clomiphene.* Levothyroxine sodium therapy may correct hypothyroidism; however, ovulation may not be normal. Levothyroxine sodium and clomiphene may be combined to induce normal ovulation. For administration, side effects, and client teaching, see *Physicians' Desk Reference*, or other appropriate pharmacotherapeutic references.

## Hypogonadotropic Hypogonadism

The hypoestrogenic adolescent has a negative progesterone withdrawal (i.e., no menstrual bleeding after the administration of progesterone) and normal or slightly lower than normal FSH/LH levels.[1] Amenorrhea is caused by GnRH pulse suppression (a decrease in the hypothalamic release of FSH and LH), which in turn inhibits pituitary function.

***Subjective Data.*** Include reports of absent menses, vaginal dryness or perineal sensitivity, stress.

***Objective Data.*** See Objective Data under Hypothalamic Disorders.

- A complete examination should be done. Assess for low body weight, no fat, little breast tissue, normal secondary sex characteristics, and hair patterns. The vagina and uterus are hypoestrogenic.
- Diagnostic tests for FSH/LH reveal normal/low normal values.

***Differential Medical Diagnoses.*** Amenorrhea, anovulation, hyperprolactinemia, psychiatric disorder.

***Plan***

- Medical therapy as indicated.
- Use of oral contraceptives for cyclic menses in the young female.
- Refer the client to a reproductive endocrinologist for evaluation and ovulation induction as indicated.
- Ovulation induction in clients with hypothalamic disorders is best managed with the GnRH pump, although clomiphene, menotropin, or urofollitropin are often used. Pituitary disorders are treated with bromocriptine. If no ovulation results, then clomiphene is used. If this does not result in ovulation, menotropin or urofollitropin is used. Bromocriptine is used to treat hyperprolactinemia; if there is no ovulation, the same steps as for pituitary disorders are used. Medications are given to treat hyperprolactinemia and induce monthly cycles and ovulation. The GnRH pump is used primarily to induce ovulation (see Table 7–6).

## Androgen Excess

Adrenal gland or ovarian dysfunction may result in androgen excess. Androgen excess is a common cause of ovulatory dysfunction and may also be an indicator of adrenal or ovarian tumor. Careful evaluation and referral are required. The three primary female androgens are dehydroepiandrosterone sulfate (DHEA-S), androstenedione (A), and testosterone (T). Androgen excess results in increased FSH/LH levels, which interfere with feedback mechanisms. Adrenal disorders result in the production of sex steroids which interact with GnRH, FSH/LH, and PRL.

Rapid progression of hirsutism, virilization, and changes in menstrual patterns are suggestive of a tumor. An adrenal tumor is suspected if serum DHEA-S levels are greater than 9 ng/mL and are not suppressed with glucocorticoids.[8] Ovarian tumors are suspected if total female serum testosterone is greater than 200–250 ng/mL or greater than male testosterone levels (350–1200 ng/mL).[11]

***Subjective Data.*** Reports of a history of excessive body hair (fine to coarse), oily skin/acne, being overweight, and irregular menses.

***Objective Data***

- *Physical Examination.* A complete physical exam is indicated. Assess the client's face, chin, and abdomen for male hair patterns (fine to coarse); note frontal balding, increased muscle mass, clitoral enlargement, decreased breast size, and voice changes. Assess for ovarian mass.
- *Diagnostic Tests.* Several are indicated:
  - *Testosterone.* Free/weakly bound (normal is 25–95 ng/dL; free T is 1 to 2 percent of total).
  - *DHEA-S.* Normal is less than 250 µg/mL; normal ranges may vary with age.
  - *Androstenedione.* Normal is 65–270 ng/mL.
  - *Dexamethasone Suppression.* Dexamethasone 1.0 mg is given orally at 11 P.M. Plasma cortisol is measured at 8 A.M.; if suppressed to less than 5 µg/mL, Cushing's disease is ruled out.
  - *17-Hydroxyprogesterone (17 OHP)* Screens for androgen excess due to polycystic ovary syndrome (PCO), enzyme deficiency, or congenital adrenal hyperplasia (normal in follicular phase is 80 ng/dL; normal in luteal phase is 30–290 ng/dL). Significant elevation suggests adrenal hyperplasia.
  - *Corticotropin (ACTH) Stimulation Test* During the early morning an I.V. bolus of synthetic ACTH 0.25 mg is administered; blood samples for 17OHP and cortisol are obtained at 30- and 60-minute intervals (normal random cortisol levels are 5–25 µg/dL; normal morning levels are 5–25 µg/dL; normal evening levels are 2–12 µg/dL). Significant elevation suggests enzyme deficiency or adrenal hyperplasia; additional testing is indicated: FSH/LH/$E^2$, PRL, TSH. A vaginal ultrasound may be recommended.

***Differential Medical Diagnoses.*** Ovarian disorders (polycystic ovary syndrome, hyperthecosis, androgen-producing tumors, virilization of pregnancy), adrenal disorders (congenital adrenal hyperplasia, androgen-producing tumors, Cushing's disease, drug related, obesity, postmenopause, incomplete testicular feminization, idiopathic conditions.

***Plan***

- Medical therapy as indicated.
- Refer the client to an endocrinologist and a surgeon as indicated.
- Refer the client to a reproductive endocrinologist for evaluation and management and possible ovulation induction.
- Psychosocial interventions include anticipatory guidance regarding treatment and medications. Offer the client support and referral to a psychologist or licensed counselor for self-esteem and body image dis-

turbance. The client may need instruction to enhance her self-image (see Psychosocial Aspects of Infertility Evaluation).

- *Medication.* For treatment of hirsutism, medications may be used alone or in combination. Consider alternative or combination therapy if there is no clinical improvement in hirsutism after 3 to 6 months of treatment.
  - *Oral Contraceptives.* These are the standard drugs of choice. The usual dosage is ethinyl estradiol 35 µg, norethindrone 1.0 mg, or a similar formulation (see Chapter 6).
  - *Spironolactone (Aldactone).* The usual dosage, if used alone, is 100–200 mg p.o. daily. Begin at 100 mg dose; may increase dose by 50 mg increments. May split dose. Prior to initiating therapy, check serum electrolytes, blood urea nitrogen (BUN), and creatinine. Usual side effects include polyuria/polydipsia (during first few weeks of therapy), menstrual irregularities, and metrorrhagia. Contraindications include anuria, acute renal insufficiency, impaired renal function, and hyperkalemia. Avoid prescribing spironolactone to clients taking a potassium supplement, diuretic, or digoxin. Use care with clients taking antihypertensives. The drug is *not* recommended during pregnancy. The anticipated outcome on evaluation is a positive response from the use of spironolactone alone within 3 months of treatment, as evidenced by clinical improvement of hirsutism. Maintenance therapy may be continued for 1 to 2 years. Lab work to check serum electrolytes (especially potassium), BUN, creatinine, and androgen levels should be performed annually. Therapy should be discontinued to observe the return of ovulatory cycles. Testosterone suppression may continue for 6 months to 2 years after discontinuing treatment. Client teaching is related to drug characteristics and the necessary follow-up evaluation.

    Spironolactone 100–150 mg p.o. daily *plus* contraceptive (ethinyl estradiol 35 µg and norethindrone 1.0 mg). Hirsutism is frequently treated by this combination of medications.

    Spironolactone 100–150 mg p.o. daily *plus* dexamethasone 0.5 mg p.o. q. h.s.
  - *Dexamethasone.* Usual dosage is 0.5 mg p.o. at bedtime. Prior to initiating therapy, a complete medical evaluation should be completed to determine the cause of hyperandrogenism. Serum electrolytes and a complete blood count (CBC) should be performed. A usual side effect is decreased resistance to infection. Dexamethasone may complicate the detection and diagnosis of infection and may impair wound-healing. Contraindications include drug hypersensitivity and systemic fungal infection; use with care during pregnancy or by clients with peptic ulcer disease, hypertension, renal insufficiency, osteoporosis, diverticulitis, hypothyroidism, and psychiatric disorders. Clients taking other medications should be carefully monitored. Maintenance therapy may be continued for 1 to 2 years. Lab work to assess serum electrolytes, CBC count, and androgen levels should be performed annually or sooner if indicated. Morning plasma cortisol levels should be monitored periodically. Reduce the dosage of dexamethasone if the morning basal cortisol level is less than 2.0 µg/dL. When discontinuing the drug, the dosage must be tapered. Client teaching involves describing the drug characteristics and the follow-up evaluation that is necessary.

    Dexamethasone 0.5 mg p.o. q.h.s. *plus* oral contraceptive (ethinyl estradiol 35 µg, norethindrone 1.0 mg).

Dexamethasone, clomiphene citrate (Clomid), urofollitropin (Metrodin), or menotropin (Pergonal) may be indicated for ovulation induction. For implications see Table 7–6 and other pharmacotherapeutic resources.

***Follow-Up.*** Guidelines are presented in Table 7–6.

## OVARIAN DISORDERS

Disorders that can cause infertility include polycystic ovary syndrome (PCO), premature ovarian failure (POF), gonadal dysgenesis, Turner's syndrome, luteinized unruptured follicle (LUF) syndrome, and luteal phase defect (LPD). Another rare disorder is resistant ovary syndrome.[1]

### Polycystic Ovary Syndrome (PCO)

This syndrome results from a combination of androgen excess and anovulation. The symptoms begin during adolescence. LH levels are elevated; FSH levels are low or normal. Increased androgens result in elevated estradiol levels, which further decrease FSH levels. Altered hormone levels interfere with GnRH secretion and follicle development. Increased estradiol levels may stimulate the pituitary and result in hyperprolactinemia.[12]

***Subjective Data.*** Carefully record the client's family history and menstrual history. Ask the client about any use of danazol (Danocrine), progestins, glucocorticoids, anabolic steroids, phenytoin, or minoxidil. The client may reveal concern about a history of excessive body hair, oily skin or acne, being overweight, and having irregular menses.

***Objective Data***

- *Physical Examination.* A complete physical exam is indicated. Assess the client's face, chin, and abdomen for male hair patterns (fine to coarse); note frontal balding, increased muscle mass, clitoral enlargement, decreased breast size, and voice changes. Also note if obesity is present, and evaluate for ovarian mass.
- *Diagnostic Tests.* Several are indicated:
    - *FSH.* Low or normal.
    - *LH.* Elevated.
    - LH–FSH ratio greater than 3.
    - *Serum Testosterone and Free Testosterone.* Mild to moderate elevation.
    - *DHEA-S.* Normal or elevated.
    - *17-Hydroxyprogesterone (17OHP)* Normal or mildly elevated.
    - *PRL.* Normal or mildly elevated.
    - *Basal Body Temperature (BBT).* For indication of ovulation and for scheduling endometrial biopsy.
    - *Endometrial Biopsy.* To diagnose hyperplasia and assess normal ovulation.
    - *Laparoscopy.* To determine and treat pelvic factor infertility.
    - *Vaginal Ultrasound.* May be recommended to assess the ovaries (multiple tiny ovarian follicles present).

***Differential Medical Diagnoses.*** Obesity, anovulation (amenorrhea, dysfunctional uterine bleeding), hyperprolactinemia, congenital adrenal hyperplasia (adult onset), adrenal/ovarian tumors, Cushing's disease, ovarian hyperthecosis, hilar cell hyperplasia, thyroid dysfunction, idiopathic hirsutism.

***Plan***

- Medical therapy as indicated.
- Refer the client to an endocrinologist, or to a reproductive endocrinologist for evaluation alone or evaluation and ovulation induction.
- Psychosocial interventions include anticipatory guidance regarding treatment and medication. Offer the client support and referral to a counselor or psychologist for self-esteem and body image disturbance if

indicated. (See prior section on Psychosocial Aspects of Infertility Evaluation.)

- Prescribe appropriate medication for ovulation induction: clomiphene citrate, dexamethasone, urofollitropin (Metrodin), menotropin (Pergonal) (see Table 7–6 and consult the *Physicians' Desk Reference* or other appropriate pharmacotherapeutic reference).
- Laparoscopy is indicated for clients who have an unsatisfactory response to ovulation induction. Laparoscopy permits laser drilling of multiple ovarian follicles, which decreases androgen production and results in short term ovulation in the majority of clients. Laser drilling has replaced ovarian wedge resection that required laparotomy.

***Follow-Up.*** Guidelines are noted in Table 7–6.

### Premature Ovarian Failure (POF)

In POF, failure of ovarian estrogen production results in elevated FSH/LH levels (greater than 50 mIU/mL) on more than one serum sample. The ovaries do not produce enough estrogen to inhibit hypothalamic release of GnRH. Continued release of GnRH results in elevated FSH/SH levels as ovulation ceases. Failure may occur at any age between menarche and 40 years and requires careful endocrine evaluation. The etiology is unknown.[9]

***Subjective Data.*** These include absent menses, hot flashes/night sweats, vaginal dryness.

***Objective Data.*** A complete physical examination is indicated; assess for signs of hypoestrogenicity. Several diagnostic tests are indicated.

- *Papanicolaou (Pap) Smear Including Maturation Index.* A lack of maturation indicates decreased estrogen activity in the vaginal wall.
- *FSH/LH.* Elevated (on more than one sample).
- *TSH, $T_3$, $T_4$, $T_7$.* Rule out thyroid disease.
- *PRL.* Rule out hyperprolactinemia.

Additional tests to rule out other conditions include CBC with differential and sedimentation rate; total serum protein, albumin–globulin ratio, antinuclear antibodies (ANA), antithyroidglobulin, antimicrosomal antibodies, fasting blood sugar, A.M. cortisol, and serum calcium and phosphorus. If the woman is younger than 30 years, a karyotype is indicated (assessment of normal female versus presence of Y chromosome, which is associated with increased risk of gonadal tumor).

***Differential Medical Diagnoses.*** Chromosome abnormality, autoimmune disease (polyendocrinopathy type I or II, myasthenia gravis, idiopathic thrombocytopenia purpura, hemolytic anemia), thyroid dysfunction (hypoparathyroidism, thyroiditis), adrenal insufficiency/failure, galactosemia, 17-hydroxylase deficiency, gonadal tumor.

***Plan***

- Medical therapy as indicated.
- Hormone replacement as necessary.
- Refer the client to a reproductive endocrinologist.
- Psychosocial interventions involve providing information and anticipatory guidance about the physical and emotional changes that accompany loss of ovarian function, including disturbances in body image, personal identity, self-esteem, the grief process, and sexual dysfunction. The client may need to be referred for individual/marital counseling and possible sex therapy. Review nutrition and exercise as well as the risks of osteoporosis, cardiovascular diseases, and endometrial cancer.
- Medication may include estrogen/progesterone replacement, lubricants, estradiol vaginal cream.
- In vitro fertilization (IVF) or donor oocyte/embryo transfer may be attempted.

***Follow-Up.*** See Table 7–6 and the *Physicians' Desk Reference* or other appropriate pharmacotherapeutic reference. An annual examination is necessary, as well as endometrial biopsy as indicated.

## Gonadal Dysgenesis and Turner's Syndrome (Gonadal Agenesis)

*Dysgenesis* results from oocyte damage prior to the 8th week of embryonic development; the damage leads to abnormal sexual development. Fibrous gonads do not produce hormones. This syndrome is associated with a broad range of mosaic patterns. Women with pure gonadal dysgenesis have an XX chromosome pattern. A majority of clients with dysgenesis have total absence of an X chromosome; others have multiple cell lines of varying sex chromosome composition (mosaicism).[1] Women with XY chromosome patterns (testicular feminization) are at risk for neoplastic changes in the gonads, thus requiring gonad removal.[1]

*Turner's syndrome (gonadal agenesis)* is a condition in which a woman has one X chromosome and is characterized by short stature. The fetus has a normal complement of ova at 20 weeks' gestation; however, they have totally or partially disappeared by birth. The ovaries appear as streak gonads. The incidence of Turner's syndrome is 1 in 10,000 liveborn girls.[1]

***Subjective Data***

- *Gonadal Dysgenesis.* Scant or absent pubic or axillary hair; no history of menses.
- *Turner's Syndrome.* Lack of secondary sexual development; no history of menses.

***Objective Data.*** A complete physical examination is necessary.

***Gonadal Dysgenesis Clients May Have Any of the Following:***

- Normal height or short stature.
- Scant or absent pubic/axillary hair.
- Normal appearing female external genitalia.
- Normal or no breast development.
- Ambiguous genitalia (intra-abdominal testes often found in hernia), blind vaginal pouch, absent uterus and ovaries (testicular feminization); and no secondary sex characteristics.
- Can have no secondary sexual characteristics but normal appearing external female genitalia *or* ambiguous external genitalia.

***Turner's Syndrome***

- Short stature.
- Scant or absent pubic/axillary hair.
- Webbing of the neck.
- Broad "shield-type" chest with laterally placed nipples.
- Lack of breast development.
- Vagina and uterus present but infantile.
- Ovaries absent.

Diagnostic tests include karyotype: abnormal chromosome pattern, abnormally high gonadotropin levels (FSH/LH), normal or elevated testosterone levels. Additional studies to detect cardiac malformations (coarctation of aorta) and renal abnormalities may be indicated in clients with Turner's syndrome.

***Differential Medical Diagnoses.*** Gonadal dysgenesis, Turner's syndrome, testicular feminization, Swyer-James syndrome, coarctation of the aorta, kidney dysfunction.

***Plan***

- Refer the client to a reproductive endocrinologist and for genetic counseling.
- Medical therapy as indicated.
- During psychosocial interventions, information and anticipatory guidance are provided regarding physical differences and the emotional impacts of body stature, impaired sexual development, and lack of reproductive capacity. Refer the client for individual/marital counseling and possible sex therapy.

- Client teaching is related to estrogen deficiencies: Review nutrition, exercise, hormone replacement and risks of osteoporosis, cardiovascular disease, glucose intolerance, and thyroid dysfunction.
- Medication in the management of Turner's syndrome includes oral cyclic administration of estrogen and progesterone.

### Luteinized Unruptured Follicle (LUF) Syndrome

Women with LUF syndrome have an intact graafian follicle containing an oocyte surrounded by luteinized granulosa cells. Dyssynchrony in the events controlling follicle rupture may result in LUF. Traditional tests of ovulation appear normal, although ovulation may occur sporadically. The syndrome should be considered as a possible cause of unexplained infertility.[13]

***Subjective Data.*** These are reported in a menstrual history; in addition, elevated basal body temperatures (BBTs) are reported.

***Objective Data.*** A complete examination should reveal nothing abnormal. Hence, several diagnostic methods are used. The condition is diagnosed by monitoring BBT elevation, using a urine LH ovulation predictor kit, and serial ultrasound monitoring. Ultrasound is performed daily beginning with the LH surge and continued until after BBT elevation (2 to 4 days). Ultrasound demonstrates the continued presence of the ovarian follicle. If LUF is identified, repeat testing in the subsequent cycle.

***Differential Medical Diagnosis.*** Anovulation.

***Plan.*** Provide the client with information and counseling related to ovulation induction, body image disturbance, and anxiety (see Psychosocial Aspects of Infertility).

Medication for ovulation induction is given in conjunction with the diagnostic procedure described above. Ultrasound monitoring is begun the day of the LH surge and continued daily until the follicle reaches 20 to 24 mm, as determined by ultrasound. Human chorionic gonadotropin (Profasi) 10,000 U (2 cc) is then administered I.M. to trigger ovulation (see Table 7–6). Ovulation will occur within 38 hours. Intercourse is recommended the day human chorionic gonadotropin is administered and for the next 2 days. Follow-up ultrasound is performed a week after ovulation is induced to assess the ovaries.

***Follow-Up.*** Refer the client to a reproductive endocrinologist. Instruct her to telephone if menses begins or if no menses occurs after BBT has been elevated for 14 days. Perform a pregnancy test or repeat ovulation induction if warranted.

### Luteal Phase Defect (LPD)

An inadequate luteal phase occurs when progesterone secretion by the corpus luteum is decreased. Also associated with the defect may be abnormal secretion of FSH/LH, hyperprolactinemia, and a lack of normally responsive progesterone receptors in the endometrium.[14] The condition is diagnosed after it has been detected in two cycles. Luteal phase defect is diagnosed in 3 to 4 percent of infertile women.[1]

***Subjective Data.*** Data reported may include a history of irregular (short) cycles and recurrent miscarriage.

***Objective Data***

- A complete physical examination is indicated to rule out other causes of irregular cycles or miscarriage.
- Diagnostic tests and methods are used to detect the defect:
    - BBT rise lasts less than 10 days; abnormal temperature curves are seen.

- Endometrial biopsy is done to diagnose discrepancies in the stroma; biopsy is abnormal if the histology of the endometrium is 2 days or more out of phase. If the biopsy is abnormal, it is repeated before treatment is initiated.
- Never treat LPD on the basis of one abnormal biopsy only. The second may be normal, in which case treatment is not necessary.
- Normal serum progesterone levels are 0.1–1.5 ng/mL in the follicular phase; 2.5–2.8 ng/mL in the luteal phase. Evaluate FHS/LH and prolactin to rule out other abnormalities.

### Differential Medical Diagnoses

Mild hyperprolactinemia, abnormal FSH/LH production.

#### *Plan*

- Refer the client to a reproductive endocrinologist.
- Provide the client with information, support, anticipatory guidance, and counseling.
- Medication includes progesterone vaginal suppositories *or* progesterone capsules to prolong the luteal phase. Bromocriptine may be indicated for mild hyperprolactinemia; clomiphene if FSH/LH are abnormal. Urofollitropin (Methodin) or menotropin (Pergonal) may also be indicated (see Table 7–6).

***Follow-Up.*** BBTs are indicated to monitor the client's cycle (see Table 7–6). Endometrial biopsy is indicated to assess efficacy of progesterone/clomiphene treatment. Ask the client to telephone with the beginning of menses; it is important to evaluate the characteristics of the cycle. A pelvic examination is done after a cycle of ovulation induction to assess ovarian size. Treatment in the subsequent cycle may be delayed if the ovaries remain enlarged. The dosage of medicine may be changed. If menses are late, perform pregnancy testing.

## UTERINE DISORDERS

Uterine causes of infertility are classified in two groups: anatomic abnormality (congenital, diethylstilbestrol [DES] exposure, adhesions, infection, fibroids) and endometrial factor (luteal phase defect). Congenital anomalies result from arrested uterine development, abnormal formation of the uterus, or incomplete fusion of the müllerian ducts.

### Müllerian Anomalies

Such abnormalities result from genetic patterns of inheritance and have been found in 5 to 10 percent of infertile women and in up to 15 percent of women with recurrent abortion.[15] Uterine structural defects, except those caused by DES exposure, are amenable to surgical correction (see Figure 7–2 and Table 7–7).

***Subjective Data.*** May include a history of infertility and/or pregnancy loss, absence of menses, menstrual flow irregularities, dysmenorrhea, dyspareunia.

#### *Objective Data*

- A complete physical with gynecologic examination is indicated to assess for abnormal anatomic structures.
- Diagnostic tests and methods including ultrasound, hysterosalpingogram, and laparoscopy/hysteroscopy are used to detect structural abnormalities. Karyotype is performed to rule out chromosomal abnormalities.

***Differential Medical Diagnoses.*** Congenital anomalies (musculoskeletal deformities, trisomy 13–15), endometriosis, urinary tract anomalies.

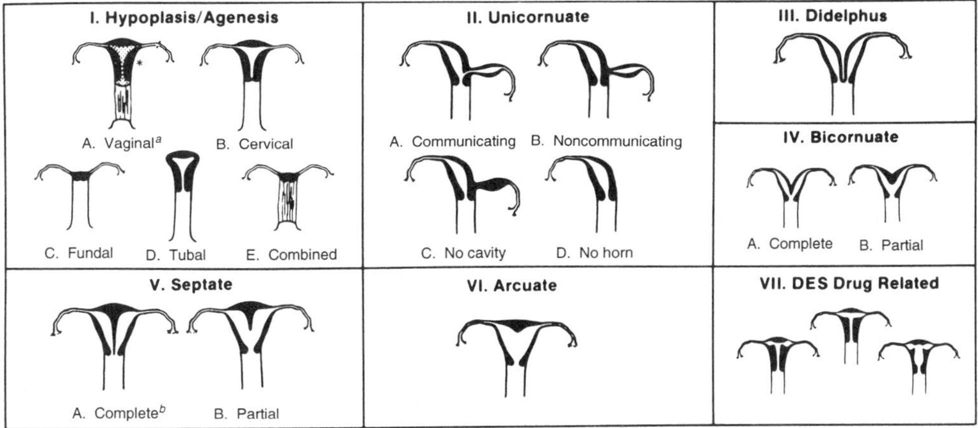


**Figure 7–2.** The American Fertility Society classification of müllerian anomalies. [a]*Uterus may be normal or take a variety of abnormal forms.* [b]*May have two distinct cervices. (Adapted from the American Fertility Society classifications of adnexal adhesion, distal tubal occlusion secondary to tubal ligation, tubal pregnancies, müllerian anomalies and intrauterine adhesions.* Fertil Steril, 49:*6, 1988. Reproduced with permission of The American Fertility Society).*

***Plan***

- Refer the client to a reproductive endocrinologist.
- Psychosocial interventions include providing information, anticipatory guidance, and support.
- If indicated, refer the client to a counselor for individual, group, or sex therapy.
- Pain management includes acetaminophen and nonsteroidal anti-inflammatory agents.
- For management of leiomyomas, see Chapter 9.
- For management of infection, see Chapters 8 and 9.
- No medication is given for müllerian anomalies.
- Laparoscopy/hysteroscopy (metroplasty) is done to correct vaginal and uterine abnormalities, to restore the uterine cavity or endometrium, and to decrease pain.

***Follow-Up.*** Follow-up depends on the extent of the abnormalities and the procedures needed to correct them.

## DES (Diethylstilbestrol) Exposure

Exposure of the female fetus to diethylstilbestrol is associated with uterine cavity abnormalities, including T-shaped uteri, hypoplastic cavities, intrauterine adhesions, and cervical stenosis.[16] In addition, DES exposure in the pregnant woman is linked with ectopic pregnancy, miscarriage, and preterm birth. Abnormalities are thought to be the result of DES-induced disruption of estrogen receptor levels during uterine development.[16] Later cellular abnormalities (adenosis) in vaginal or ectocervical epithelium are associated with DES exposure during fetal life, resulting in susceptibility to carcinogenic effects of endogenous estrogens (clear cell adenocarcinomas).[17]

DES was synthesized in 1948 and used by several million women until 1971 to prevent miscarriage.[17] Research has documented an increased occurrence of clear cell adenocarcinoma in DES-exposed women between 7 and 30 years of age, with a peak incidence at age

**TABLE 7–7. CLASSIFICATION OF MÜLLERIAN ANOMALIES**

*Hypoplasia or Agenesis Malformations*
Varying degrees of uterine development, or lack of development. Vaginal outflow tract obstruction accompanies uterine malformations.

*Unicornuate Uterus*
Varying degrees of developmental arrest of one müllerian duct. Causes abnormal fetal presentations and premature labor. High incidence of miscarriage.

*Didelphus Uterus*
Complete lack of fusion, with duplication of the uterus and cervix. Duplication may extend into the vagina. Vaginal outflow from one uterus may be restricted. High incidence of malpresentations and premature labor: 50 percent survival rate.

*Bicornuate Uterus*
Partial lack of fusion of varying degrees, with a single cervix. Associated with a high rate of second trimester and later fetal loss.

*Septate Uterus*
Partial lack of resorption of the midline septum. Associated with recurrent first trimester loss.

*Arcuate Uterus*
Mild form of septum not associated with pregnancy loss.

*Diethylstilbestrol (DES) Exposure*
Caused by in utero DES exposure. Cavity may be T-shaped with cornual constriction bands and pretubal bulges, lower uterine segment dilation, and small cavities with irregular borders.

*Source: Adapted from Garner, C. (Ed.). (1991).* Principles of infertility nursing. *Boca Raton, FL: CRC Press.*

19.[17] It is unknown whether the incidence will peak again at a later age.

***Subjective Data.*** Data reveal a history of maternal DES treatment; and a client history of menstrual abnormalities, miscarriage, lower fertility rate, ectopic pregnancy, premature delivery, incompetent cervix, or abnormal Pap smears.

***Objective Data.*** A complete physical examination, including speculum and pelvic exam, is indicated to detect abnormalities of anatomic structure. DES-exposed women need to begin having pelvic examinations soon after the onset of menses and to have them at least annually. Common abnormalities include vaginal adenosis (ridge, septum, malformation), cervical adenosis (collar, hood, polyp, malformation, stenosis), and müllerian anomalies.

Diagnostic tests and methods include a Pap smear of the cervix to screen for squamous cell carcinoma, and a colposcopy and biopsy of abnormal tissue. More advanced methods may be indicated to evaluate anatomic abnormalities (ultrasound, hysterosalpingogram, laparoscopy/hysteroscopy).

***Differential Medical Diagnoses.*** Congenital anomalies: musculoskeletal deformities, trisomy 13–15, other chromosomal abnormalities.

***Plan.*** Psychosocial interventions include providing information, anticipatory guidance, and support. No medication is recommended. No treatment is indicated unless complications—such as abnormal Pap smears, pregnancy complication, or infertility—arise.

***Follow-Up.*** Several referrals may be advisable, for example, to a specialist in DES exposure; a counselor for individual, group, or sex therapy; or an infertility specialist if the client is unable to become pregnant or has a history of pregnancy loss. *Careful follow-up for clear cell adenocarcinoma and squamous cell carcinoma is required; immediate referral is made if suspicious findings occur.*

### Intrauterine Adhesions (Asherman's Syndrome)

The syndrome results from damage to the endometrium after excessive curettage, metroplasty, and myomectomy. It interferes with fertility by disrupting sperm migration, mechanically obstructing tubal ostia, and impeding blastocyst implantation.[16] Miscarriage may result from decreased size of the uterine cavity or inadequate endometrium.

***Subjective Data.*** The client may report a history of menstrual abnormalities (scant flow, dysmenorrhea), dyspareunia, uterine infection, pregnancy losses, surgical procedures.

***Objective Data***

- A complete physical examination is indicated. Often, findings are normal. Assess for cervical stenosis; discharge; signs of infection; and abnormal uterine contour, firmness, mobility, tenderness.
- Diagnostic tests and methods include endometrial biopsy to diagnose fibrosis; hysterosalpingogram to determine abnormalities in uterine contour; laparoscopy and hysteroscopy (when indicated). Repeat hysterosalpingogram may be indicated after surgical correction if conception does not occur.

***Differential Medical Diagnoses.*** Amenorrhea, dysmenorrhea, cervical stenosis.

***Plan***

- Provide the client with information, anticipatory guidance, and support.
- Medication may include estrogen/progesterone replacement (see Table 7–6). Cyclic estrogen/progesterone replacement therapy may be given to help restore normal endometrium after surgical correction. Pain is usually managed with acetaminophen or nonsteroidal anti-inflammatory agents.
- Laparoscopy and hysteroscopy may be indicated for lysis of adhesions and cervical dilation.
- Dilatation and curettage may be indicated premenstrually if the client is diagnosed with tuberculosis of the endometrium.

***Follow-Up.*** Refer the client to a reproductive endocrinologist and for counseling.

## Endometritis

Endometritis is an endometrial inflammation due to infection caused by pathogens. It may result from ascending vaginal organisms, use of an intrauterine device (IUD), endometrial trauma, or as a secondary infection associated with cancer. Common pathogens include aerobic/anaerobic bacteria, mycoplasma, chlamydia, viruses, toxoplasmas, parasites, and mycobacterium tuberculosis. Treatment is controversial when no pathogen is identified because resolution may occur spontaneously. Infertility may be associated with an unfavorable endometrial environment that results from infection and interferes with nidation.[16]

Tuberculosis (TB) endometritis is rare. Infertility occurs due to extensive tubal scarring and uterine adhesions. Diagnosis is made by curettage in the premenstrual endometrium. Antituberculosis medications are used until repeat curettage is normal.

***Subjective Data.*** The client may report uterine tenderness and an abnormal vaginal discharge.[16] She may also report a history of infertility.

***Objective Data.*** Physical examination will reveal tenderness on bimanual examination. If discharge is unusually foul and client is elderly, suspect cancer.

Diagnosis of chronic endometritis is accomplished by late luteal phase endometrial biopsy. (See Pelvic Inflammatory Disease in Chapter 9 for tests to diagnose acute infection.)

***Differential Medical Diagnoses.*** Urinary tract infection (UTI), acute pyelonephritis, appendicitis, pelvic abscess, thromboembolism, gastrointestinal disease, endometriosis, uterine adhesions.

***Plan***

- Psychosocial interventions include teaching the client about the causes, treatment, prevention, and effects of infection. Provide support and counseling, and encourage support from significant others.
- Medication is prescribed for recurrent endometrial/pelvic infections because the inflammation, abnormal endometrium, and adhesion formation associated with infection decrease fertility.
- Endometrial biopsy (late luteal phase) is indicated after antibiotic treatment to determine resolution of endometritis.
- Prophylactic antibiotic therapy should be given prior to or at the time of an invasive procedure. Pain management is often indicated.

***Follow-Up.*** Refer the client to a reproductive endocrinologist for evaluation and infertility treatment. Diagnostic evaluation and treatment will be affected by the history of recurrent infection and the degree of pelvic and tubal pathology.

- Other interventions that may be indicated are hysterosalpingogram, laparoscopy, laparoscopy/hysteroscopy, and laparotomy for lysis of adhesions and tubal repair. In vitro fertilization may be necessary if other corrective therapies cannot restore normal tubal function. A client with the diagnosis of TB endometritis who wishes to become pregnant will require in vitro fertilization. After tubal repair, clients are at risk for ectopic pregnancy.
- Referring client for more extensive counseling, relaxation techniques, biofeedback, and pain management may be indicated.

## Leiomyomas (Fibroids)

These tumors, of smooth muscle origin, arise from the myometrium. They may enlarge during pregnancy or when exogenous estrogen is given because of an increase in estrogen receptor levels in the fibroid. Distortion of the pelvic and uterine cavities may interfere with fertility, preventing conception or maintenance of pregnancy.[16] Therapeutic intervention is determined by the size and location of the fibroid and the desire for fertility. Chapter 9 has more information related to condition leiomyomas. Fibroid tumors occur in 20 to 25 percent of women older than 30.[16] They are more prevalent among African American women.

***Plan***

- Refer the client to a gynecologist.
- *Preoperative Medication.* Use of Depot Lupron (leuprolide acetate) or other GnRH analogue may be indicated with large tumors to impose anovulation and thereby decrease tumor size, the risk of hemorrhage, and trauma to the uterus. Drugs similar to Lupron suppress the growth of the fibroid tumor, but also cause osteoporosis, and consequently cannot be given on a long-term basis. When the drug is stopped, the tumor starts to grow again, so usually Lupron is used on a short-term basis to shrink the tumor prior to surgery.
    - Common transient side effects include hot flashes, night sweats, breakthrough bleeding, vaginal dryness.
    - Protected intercourse is indicated during entire course of therapy.
- Laparotomy is required to remove large fibroids; small fibroids may be removed with laparoscopy/hysteroscopy.
- Pain (dysmenorrhea) management includes acetaminophen and nonsteroidal anti-inflammatory agents.

## Luteal Phase Defect

(See Ovarian Disorders.)

### Cervical Factor

Abnormalities in cervical mucus or in mucus–spermatozoa interactions have been identified in 15 to 20 percent of infertile couples.[18] Adequate cervical mucus is critical to sperm transport, storage, and conception. Midcycle mucus increases in quantity and quality (clear, thin) with increased levels of estrogen. Abnormalities may result from female or male causes, poor timing of the postcoital test, or faulty coital technique (performing on demand).

Female causes include ovulatory disorders, cervical surgery or infection, DES exposure, anatomic abnormalities (polyps, severe stenosis), drugs (clomiphene), use of lubricants and douches, and the presence of antisperm antibodies.[18] Male causes include retrograde ejaculation, hypospadias, semen abnormalities, and antisperm antibodies.

- Subjective data may reveal a history of infertility and clear, thin, or absent cervical mucus.
- A complete physical examination is indicated.
- *Diagnostic Tests and Methods*:
    - *Basal Body Temperatures (BBTs).* Sometimes used with a urinary LH predictor kit, BBTs help to schedule the postcoital test appropriately and interpret the test results.
    - *Postcoital Test (PCT).* The PCT must be well timed: performed 1 to 2 days prior to expected ovulation and 2 to 10 hours after coitus. An endocervical mucus sample is needed. *Normal PCT results* are clear, thin, watery mucus; spinnbarkeit 8 to 10 cm; ferning; 5 to 10 motile sperm present per high power field. *Abnormal PCT results* are absent or scant cervical mucus, viscous cellular cervical mucus, thin cervical mucus with few sperm, poorly motile or "shaking" sperm. If PCT results are abnormal, discuss a period of abstinence prior to test, coital technique, and use of lubricants and douches; then repeat the test in subsequent cycle.
    - *Postinsemination Test (PIT).* The PIT is performed after a second abnormal PCT. The client's partner must collect a semen specimen in a sterile container. Cervical insemination is performed in the office and an endocervical mucus sample is obtained 2 to 4 hours later.
    - *Semen Analysis/Penetrak.* Female/male antisperm antibodies test (discussed later in this chapter).

***Differential Medical Diagnoses.*** Ovulatory disorder, cervicitis, cervical anatomic abnormality (polyps, stenosis, surgery, DES exposure), semen abnormalities, female/male antisperm antibodies, sexual dysfunction.

#### *Plan*

- Psychosocial interventions include providing information and support, counseling the client regarding causes of infertility, the diagnostic testing, and treatment.
- Medication as indicated.
    - *Antibiotic Therapy.* Indicated for cervicitis (see Chapter 8).
    - *Conjugated Equine Estrogen.* Premarin 0.3 mg p.o. is given daily, beginning cycle day 6 and continuing until the day of urine LH surge. (Start and stop dates of medication vary depending on day of ovulation; the client may take the medication for 6 to 12 days.) Low dose estrogen may improve the quality of the cervical mucus but may also delay ovulation. The PCT must be repeated on the day of the urine LH surge. If the PCT result is normal while the client is taking

conjugated estrogen, continue treatment for approximately 6 to 9 cycles. If the PCT result is abnormal, discontinue conjugated estrogen and treat with intrauterine insemination (IUI).

- Inseminations are performed to place sperm as close to the egg as possible. Cervical insemination is a simple method of treatment; in vitro fertilization is the most complex (see Infertility Treatment).
  - Artificial insemination–husband (AIH) is done for 6 to 9 cycles if the postinsemination test (PIT) is normal. BBTs are taken and a urine LH predictor kit is used to time insemination. AIH is performed the day of and day after the LH surge.
  - Unstimulated intrauterine insemination (IUI) is done for 3 to 4 cycles. BBTs are taken and a urine LH predictor kit is used to time insemination. IUI, using a washed sperm specimen, is performed the day after the LH surge.
  - Stimulated-ovulation induction IUI is done for 4 cycles, using menotropin (Pergonal), or urofollitropin (Metrodin), and luteal phase support (see Table 7–6). IUIs using washed sperm specimens are performed approximately 24 to 28 and 40 hours after ovulation is induced by administration of human chorionic gonadotropin (Profasi).
  - For in vitro fertilization (IVF), gamete intrafallopian transfer (GIFT), zygote intrafallopian transfer (ZIFT), see Infertility Treatment.

***Follow-Up.*** Referral for more extensive counseling and therapy may be indicated.

## PELVIC DISORDERS

Sequelae of pelvic inflammatory disease, postoperative adhesions, and endometriosis are involved in the pathogenesis of impaired fertility.

### Pelvic Inflammatory Disease (PID)

Tubal pathology is present in 30 to 50 percent of infertile women.[1] Sexually transmitted diseases caused by *Neisseria gonorrhoeae* and *Chlamydia trachomatis* are the major source of tubal disease. Tubal repair may be accomplished by laser laparoscopy or laparotomy (salpingostomy, fimbrioplasty, reanastomosis). The success of tubal repair depends on the extent of disease. Further fertility treatment if repair is unsuccessful may include IVF. (See Uterine Disorders; Endometritis; Chapter 9.)

### Pelvic Adhesions

It is estimated that pelvic adhesions are present in 40 percent of infertility cases.[19] Meticulous surgical technique, minimal tissue handling, stringent hemostasis, constant irrigation, avoidance of abrasion between raw surfaces (adhesion barriers), and microsurgery using unipolar fine wire cautery or the laser will reduce adhesion formation and preserve fertility (laparoscopy/laparotomy).[19]

***Subjective Data.*** The client may report a history of infertility, chronic pelvic pain, dyspareunia, menstrual disorders.

***Objective Data.*** A complete examination is indicated. Tenderness and a fixed uterus on bimanual examination are common. Diagnostic methods are a hysterosalpingogram and laparoscopy to diagnose and treat pelvic pathology.

***Differential Medical Diagnoses.*** Chronic salpingitis, residual inflammatory disease, tubal blockage.

***Plan.*** Psychosocial interventions include providing information and support. Antibiotic and pain therapy may be used prior to invasive procedures. Other possible interventions include laser laparoscopy for lysis of adhesions; tubal repair (salpingostomy, neosalpingostomy, fimbrioplasty) as indicated; laparotomy to treat severe pelvic disease (adhesion lysis; microscopic tubal or cornual reanastomosis); in vitro fertilization if indicated.

Refer the client to a reproductive endocrinologist or, if necessary, for counseling (individual, group, sex therapy). Relaxation techniques, biofeedback, and pain management may also be indicated.

### Endometriosis

Among women with endometriosis, 30 to 40 percent are infertile.[20] Fertility is impaired by mechanical, chemical, and immunologic factors. *Mechanical factors* interfere with ovulation and ovum pick-up; *chemical factors* affect ovulation, tubal motility, and sperm phagocytosis; and *immunologic factors* have cytotoxic effects on the sperm, egg, and embryo.[21] Treatment depends on the severity of symptoms and the desire for fertility. Infertility management may include both laparoscopy and medical management with GnRH agonists. In mild cases, laser laparoscopy may be the only treatment needed. Severe cases, however, may also require either preoperative or postoperative danazol, Depot Lupron, or nafarelin acetate (Synarel).[22] The majority of clients conceive within 6 months of treatment.[23] Further infertility treatment may include stimulated ovulation induction IUI or IVF/GIFT/ZIFT.

## RECURRENT FETAL LOSS

It is not uncommon for a woman to have two or three spontaneous abortions; however, the likelihood that she will have another is approximately 25 to 35 percent.[24] *Recurrent abortion* is defined as three or more consecutive spontaneous pregnancy losses prior to 20 weeks' gestation.

Evaluation of a couple experiencing recurrent abortion should begin after three pregnancy losses, or after two if the couple is over 35 years of age. Pregnancy loss may be caused by anatomic, endocrine, genetic, or immunologic variations; infection; chronic illness; or environmental toxins.

***Subjective Data.*** The client may report a history of recurrent abortion.

***Objective Data.*** A complete physical examination is indicated. During the pelvic examination, special attention is given to detecting anatomic abnormalities. Diagnostic tests include PRL; TSH, $T_3$, $T_4$, $T_7$; systemic lupus screen; lupus anticoagulant; anticardiolipin antibodies; karyotype (both partners); chlamydia, ureaplasma, and mycoplasma cultures; endometrial biopsy; hysterosalpingography; ultrasound; laparoscopy/hysteroscopy.

#### *Differential Medical Diagnoses*

- *Anatomic Abnormalities (Uterus).* Müllerian defects, fibroids, septum defects, Asherman's syndrome, incompetent cervix.
- *Endocrine Abnormalities.* Thyroid (hypothyroid), hyperprolactinemia, ovulatory dysfunction/LPD, endometriosis.
- *Infection.* Chlamydia, TORCH (T, toxoplasmosis; O, other infections (varicella, listeria, tuberculosis); R, rubella; C, cytomegalovirus; H, herpes simplex virus), cytomegalovirus (CMV), ureaplasma/mycoplasma.
- *Chronic Illness.* Wilson's disease, heart/renal disease, blood dyscrasias.
- *Genetic Abnormality.* Trisomy.
- *Immunologic Disorders.* Systemic lupus erythematosus (SLE), parental histocompatibilities.
- *Environmental Toxins.* Radiation, chemotherapy/drugs, smoking, ethyl alcohol abuse.

***Plan.*** Provide the client with information and psychological support; be available for questions and listening. Evaluate the client's stage of crisis and grief, communication patterns, relationships, coping abilities, and use of support systems. Collaborate with medical (reproductive endocrinology) and mental health specialists. Medication is determined by the cause of the recurrent fetal loss.[24]

***Follow-Up.*** As appropriate, provide information about Compassionate Friends, a support group for individuals and couples who have lost pregnancies or children.

## MALE INFERTILITY: CAUSES, DIAGNOSES, AND INTERVENTIONS

Male factor infertility may result from a variety of causes, such as endocrine disorders, varicocele, anatomic (genetic) or obstructive lesions, antisperm antibodies, occupational and environmental practices, and sexual dysfunction. Evaluation of a man's fertility should be coordinated with the evaluation of the woman's. Evaluation may be initiated in the general practice or gynecology office. Frequently medical therapies are unsuccessful; therefore, referral to a urologist may be indicated. Surgery has been successful in treating posttesticular and ductal disorders.

### OBJECTIVE DATA

A detailed history is essential to identify factors that may affect sperm production (see Tables 7–3 and 7–4). For normal spermatogenesis, a delicate balance must exist between the neuroendocrine system and testes.[1,7,25,26]

A thorough physical examination and Doppler evaluation are indicated. Diagnostic tests include semen analysis (performed twice); semen ureaplasma and mycoplasma cultures; Penetrak (bovine mucus penetration) (normal is greater than 30 mm); sperm penetration assay (SPA) (normal is 20 percent penetration); antisperm antibody testing; TSH, $T_3$, $T_4$, $T_7$; FSH (normal is 5–25 mIU/mL); LH (normal is 6–26 mIU/mL); PRL; testosterone (normal is 250–1200 ng/dL); CT scan/MRI sella turcica; karyotyping; PCT (female) (normal is 5 to 10 motile sperm per high power field).

### CAUSES OF MALE INFERTILITY

#### Endocrine Disorders

Such disorders constitute rare causes of male infertility. Measurement of TSH, $T_3$, $T_4$, $T_7$, FSH/LH, PRL, and testosterone may identify abnormalities.[1] Some specific endocrine problems are listed below with usual test results.

- Germ cell aplasia: elevated FSH/LH.
- Testicular failure: elevated FSH/LH.
- Pituitary adenoma/impotence: elevated PRL.
- Thyroid/adrenal dysfunction: rare.
- Hypogonadotropic hypogonadism (Kallmann's syndrome): low FSH/LH, testosterone.[27]

#### Varicocele

This varicosity of the internal spermatic vein is usually on the left side and found in both fertile and infertile men. It impairs infertility by raising testicular temperature. Surgical correction is beneficial in some cases.[1]

#### Anatomic Abnormalities (Genetic) and Obstructive Lesions (Acquired)

Such conditions may be surgically corrected; however, obstructive lesions have a better prognosis than genetic abnormalities. Obstruction is of shorter duration; consequently, the negative effect on testicular and epididymal function is less.[27]

### Sperm Transport Dysfunction

Clients with hypospadias, retrograde ejaculation, or sexual dysfunction are unable to deliver sperm to cervical mucus. Sperm collection by means of masturbation for cervical insemination may be indicated. Sperm may also be retrieved from alkalinized urine and prepared for intrauterine insemination.

### INTERVENTIONS

- Medications:
  - Clomiphene citrate (Clomid) 25 mg, p.o. days 1–25 of the calendar for 6–9 months, to increase sperm count; *or*
  - Human chorionic gonadotropin (Profasi) 2000–2500 IU, I.M. × 3 weekly for 8–10 weeks, to increase sperm motility; *or*
  - Menotropin (Pergonal) 25–75 IU, I.M. × 3 weekly *plus* human chorionic gonadotropin (Profasi) 2000–2500 IU I.M. × 3 weekly for 8–10 weeks, to increase spermatogenesis; *or*
  - GnRH Pump, pulsation q. 2 hours, long term therapy to provide normal gonadotropin pulsation to increase spermatogenesis (see Table 7–6).
- Surgery (varicocelectomy, removal of obstruction, vasectomy reversal).
- Artificial insemination–husband (AIH-cervix).
- Artificial insemination–donor (AID-cervix).
- Stimulated ovulation induction IUI (husband or donor).
- Electroejaculation.
- IVF/ZIFT/GIFT (selected cases).
- Micromanipulation of gametes (zona drilling, subzonal insertion, and direct sperm injection):
  - *Zona Drilling.* A gap is created in the zona pellucida, allowing sperm direct access.[28]
  - *Subzonal Insertion.* Sperm are aspirated in a hollow needle and deposited in the perivitelline space.
  - *Direct Sperm Microinjection.* Sperm are injected into the cytoplasm.[28]

## COMBINED FACTORS OF MALE AND FEMALE INFERTILITY

Combined factors of male and female infertility may be more difficult to overcome. It is critically important to assess each partner's fertility status before the other undergoes corrective surgery. For example, in vitro fertilization (IVF) may be indicated instead of surgical intervention for couples with tubal pathology and a severe male factor. Individual and couple factors determine the choice of therapy. To maximize chances of conception, evaluation and intervention are coordinated, for example, using varicocele repair and endometriosis surgery.[27]

### UNEXPLAINED INFERTILITY

For 10 to 15 percent of infertile couples, no specific cause of infertility can be identified by standard testing.[13] Approximately 60 percent of couples with unexplained infertility will conceive at an unpredictable time. They have multiple needs; although they have the biologic potential to conceive, efforts have been unsuccessful.

***Subjective Data.*** The couple may report a history of infertility.

***Objective Data.*** A complete infertility evaluation is performed using diagnostic studies. Also performed are tests for chlamydia infection; urine and semen ureaplasma and mycoplasma cultures; and sperm penetration assay.

***Differential Medical Diagnoses.*** Luteinized unruptured follicle (LUF) syndrome, immunologic factor; female/male antisperm antibody.

***Plan***

- Refer the couple to a reproductive endocrinologist.
- Psychosocial interventions include providing information and, as treatment becomes more complex, using a variety of educational strategies, such as written information, videotape, demonstration, and individual and group sessions. It is important to be available to answer questions and provide psychosocial support for the individual and couple. Explore all treatment options and allow the couple to regain control by decision making.
- Medication. Stimulation ovulation induction intrauterine insemination (IUI) is accomplished with clomiphene and menotropin, or urofollitropin, and Profasi. (See Table 7–6 and Female Infertility: Causes, Diagnoses, and Interventions.)
- IVF/GIFT/ZIFT.
- Referral may be made for the individual or couple to meet a specialist for counseling.

## FEMALE AND MALE ANTISPERM ANTIBODIES

Female and male antisperm antibodies are found in 5 to 10 percent of infertile couples.[25] The exact cause of female antisperm antibody formation is unknown; an increased incidence of male antisperm antibodies has been noted following vasectomy reversal. Antibodies have been found in serum, cervical mucus, seminal plasma, and the reproductive tracts of fertile and infertile couples. Antibodies decrease sperm motility, transport, and ability to penetrate the egg.[26] Couples with unexplained infertility should have antibody screening performed.

***Subjective Data.*** Clients may report a history of infertility, genital tract infections, surgery, trauma. A man may have cryptorchidism, varicocele, or vasectomy reversal. A genetic influence may be known.

***Objective Data.*** A complete physical examination is indicated. Diagnostic tests and methods include antisperm/antibody testing, semen analysis, and penetrak test.

Antisperm/antibody testing is recommended with a history of vasectomy reversal, unexplained infertility, and two abnormal postcoital tests (PCTs) (normal cervical mucus with no sperm; with poorly motile, shaking, or clumping sperm; and a history of normal semen analysis). Testing of both partners is recommended. The antisperm-antibody screen is performed on serum (indirect immunobead) or semen (direct immunobead) samples.

Immunobead binding determines the presence and location of antibodies. It is used to identify the percentage of sperm coated with antibodies, the area of sperm surface bound to antibodies (head, neck, tail), and type of antibody present (IgG, IgM, IgA). The type of antibody present affects sperm function. The more sperm that are bound and the greater the sperm surface area involved, the greater the risk of impaired fertility.[25] A test result is considered positive if there is greater than 20 percent total binding of any immunoglobulin. Binding greater than 50 percent of the motile sperm by any immunoglobulin is biologically significant.

When semen analyses in the past have been normal, suspect antisperm antibody if "clumping," agglutination of sperm, or decreased motility is seen in the current specimen.

Penetrak (bovine mucus) assesses the ability of sperm to penetrate mucus (normal is greater than 30 mm).

***Differential Medical Diagnosis.*** Unexplained infertility.

#### *Plan*

- Refer the couple to a reproductive endocrinologist.
- Psychosocial interventions include providing information and support.
- Medication indicated for female antisperm antibodies is stimulated ovulation induction IUI (see Table 7–6). In the past, oral steroids were used to decrease antibody titers for male and female antisperm antibodies. This treatment is not recommended today because of the large therapeutic dosage required and the increased side effects (see Table 7–6).
- Stimulated ovulation induction IUI involves the development and ovulation of multiple eggs coupled with timed inseminations. This results in the presence of more than one oocyte (egg) available for sperm penetration. IUI shortens the distance that sperm must travel to reach oocytes and helps to prevent the loss of sperm motility due to antibody binding. A male with positive antibodies should collect the semen specimen in a container with medium. The specimen should be prepared (washed) immediately to decrease agglutination.
- In vitro fertilization (IVF), gamete intrafallopian transfer (GIFT), zygote intrafallopian transfer (ZIFT) (see Infertility Treatment, below).
- Condom use by the male for 6 months was once thought to decrease cervical mucus antibody titers; however, it has limited effectiveness and delays conception.
- Refer the clients for counseling (individual, group, sex therapy).

# INFERTILITY TREATMENT

## THERAPEUTIC INSEMINATION

Therapeutic insemination provides hope of parenthood for many single women and infertile couples. However, it raises many physical, psychosocial, ethical, legal, religious, and financial concerns. Carefully explore all issues before initiating treatment. Establish a rationale for insemination that identifies male and/or female factors of infertility which necessitate the consideration of therapeutic insemination using partner or donor sperm specimens (see Table 7–8). Sperm specimens may be placed in the cervix or into the uterus (IUI). Insemination enables sperm to be deposited closer to the female egg, which may improve the ability to conceive.

### Artificial Insemination

Husband or donor sperm may be used for vaginal, cervical, or intrauterine insemination (IUI). Intrauterine insemination utilizes washed specimens.

#### *Procedures*

- *Artificial Insemination–Husband (AIH).* Requires a fresh specimen for vaginal/cervical insemination. The husband may assist with insemination.
- *Artificial Insemination–Donor (AID).* Must be performed according to American Fertility Society Guidelines for Donor Insemination. Consent forms are signed and donors selected. Female evaluation includes current history and physical examination, including Pap smear, chlamydia culture, rubella titer, cytomegalovirus (CMV) titer, hepatitis profile, and human immunodeficiency virus (HIV) test. Both partners have blood type and group deter-

**TABLE 7–8. RATIONALE FOR THERAPEUTIC INSEMINATION**

| Male Factors | Female Factors | Reasons for Using Donor Eggs or Sperm | Intrauterine Insemination |
|---|---|---|---|
| Low or high semen volume<br>Physical abnormality<br>Retrograde ejaculation<br>Sexual/ejaculatory dysfunction<br>Physical injury<br>Life-threatening physical illness (sperm donated/stored prior to treatment) | Physical abnormality (vagina/cervix)<br>Cervical mucus factor<br>Idiopathic abnormal postcoital test (normal postinsemination test) | Azoospermia<br>Severe oligospermia<br>Decreased motility<br>Vasectomy<br>Genetic disease<br>RH incompatibility<br>Sexual dysfunction<br>Single female | Lack of successful cervical inseminations<br>Male: Abnormal semen, anatomy, antibody<br>Female: Cervical factor, antibody, mild endometriosis, or unexplained infertility |

*Source: Adapted from Table 1: Indications for insemination. In Alexander, N., & Schlaff, W. (1987). Insemination techniques for overcoming infertility.* Contemporary Obstetrics and Gynecology, 30*(Special Issue), 102.*

minations; the female may have an antibody screen as indicated. Donors and specimens are extensively screened, with cryopreserved specimens stored for at least 180 days prior to release for use. Specimens are thawed approximately 20 minutes prior to use. The partner may assist with insemination.

- *Intrauterine Insemination (IUI).* Performed using washed husband specimen or thawed, prewashed cryopreserved donor specimen.

Timing of insemination is determined by using basal body temperature (BBT) readings and urine luteinizing hormone (LH) ovulation predictor kits. Vaginal/cervical insemination is performed the day of the LH surge and may be repeated the next day if the BBT is not elevated. Unstimulated IUI is performed the day after the LH surge. Stimulated ovulation induction IUIs are performed approximately 24 to 28 and 40 hours after ovulation is induced by administration of human chorionic gonadotropin (Profasi).

In continuing treatment, assessment of the proper timing for insemination is critical. The interval during which conception is expected depends on the type of therapeutic insemination; therefore, it is important to evaluate and change the treatment as indicated.

If conception with AIH (fresh specimen) does not occur within 6 to 9 cycles, then treatment proceeds to unstimulated IUI for 3 to 4 cycles, then to stimulated ovulation induction IUI for 4 cycles. With donor insemination (AID) utilizing thawed specimens, conception should occur no later than 12 cycles. Attempt 3 cycles of cervical insemination; then proceed to unstimulated IUI for 3 to 6 cycles; then proceed to stimulated ovulation induction IUI cycles. If conception does not occur after 4 stimulated IUI cycles, assisted reproductive technologies are recommended.

## ASSISTED REPRODUCTIVE TECHNOLOGIES

When other treatment options have been exhausted or when other therapies have a poor

**TABLE 7–9. INDICATIONS FOR IVF, GIFT, ZIFT, DONOR GAMETES, AND EMBRYO CRYOPRESERVATION**

| | |
|---|---|
| *IVF*<br>*Mechanism:*<br>Transfer of embryos into uterus | *Indications for IVF*<br>Tubal disease<br>Male factor<br>Endometriosis<br>Cervical factor<br>Female/male antisperm antibodies<br>Unexplained infertility |
| *GIFT*<br>*Mechanism*<br>Transfer of mature ova/sperm into fallopian tubes<br>*ZIFT*<br>*Mechanism*<br>Transfer of zygotes into fallopian tubes | *Indications for GIFT or ZIFT*<br>Must have one normal fallopian tube<br>Mild male factor<br>Mild endometriosis<br>Cervical factor<br>Female/male antisperm antibodies<br>Unexplained infertility<br>May try instead of repeating IVF after known satisfactory response to stimulation/fertilization of oocytes |
| *Donor Gametes*<br>*Mechanism*<br>Use of oocytes, uterine cavity, or sperm for conception | *Indications for Donor Gametes*<br>Premature ovarian failure<br>Severe endometriosis<br>Surgical removal of partial/entire ovary (cysts, neoplasms)<br>Congenital absence of ovaries, uterus<br>Inaccessible ovaries (adhesions)<br>Failed ovulation induction (poor responders)<br>Uterine anomaly (congenital, distortion of cavity)<br>Medical contraindication to pregnancy<br>Hereditary disorders<br>Severe male factors |
| *Embryo Cryopreservation*<br>*Mechanism*<br>Freezing of excess embryos from original treatment cycle | *Indications for Embryo Cryopreservation*<br>Opportunity to conceive without repeating stimulation and retrieval |

*Source: Adapted from Damewood, M. (Ed.). (1990).* The Johns Hopkins handbook of in vitro fertilization and assisted reproductive technologies. *Boston: Little, Brown.*

prognosis, assisted reproductive technologies are used. The four options are in vitro fertilization (IVF); gamete intrafallopian transfer (GIFT); zygote intrafallopian transfer (ZIFT); and embryo cryopreservation. Assisted reproductive technologies may include the use of donor gametes. The therapy selected will be determined by specific program criteria (see Table 7–9 and Figure 7-3).

## Success Rates

Success rates are variable. Overall, a clinical pregnancy rate of approximately 20 percent is expected with IVF embryo transfer; a slightly higher rate is expected with GIFT retrieval.[29] *Clinical pregnancy* is defined by rising beta human chorionic gonadotropin (beta-HCG) titers and the presence

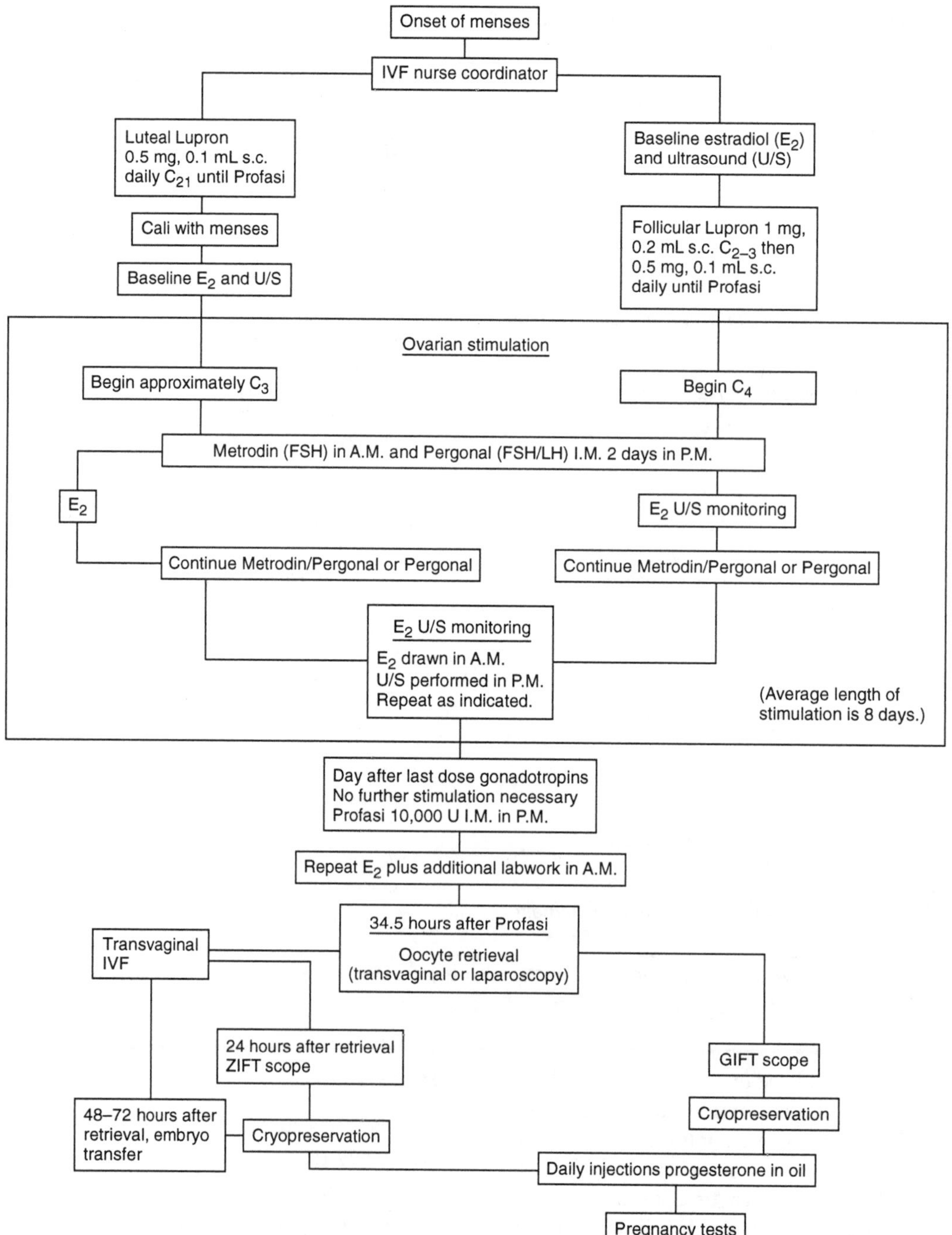


**Figure 7–3.** Treatment cycle. *Note:* Stimulation protocols vary among programs. Cycles may be canceled at different stages pending treatment response. (*Source: Richmond Center for Fertility and Endocrinology, Ltd.*)

of a gestational sac in the uterine cavity, detected by ultrasound monitoring. Multiple gestation and spontaneous abortion may both occur.

### Treatment Consideration

Couples must consider the treatment prognosis and their desire for a biologic child. Grief over the loss of a potential unborn child may be intensified as a couple undergoes treatment. The complex stressors and impacts of infertility may heighten the couple's feelings of loss of control.[30] Additional stressors may include physical, emotional, social, family, religious, ethical, legal, and financial issues. Treatment choice is often dictated by finances and insurance coverage. Both couples and individuals may benefit from counseling, referral, stress management, and assistance with resolving grief.

### Treatment Selection

The specific criteria of each treatment need to be carefully weighed before one is selected. Information about clinics in the United States may be obtained from the American Fertility Society, Birmingham, Alabama, and from Resolve, Somerville, Massachusetts.

### Stress Management

Intensive treatment involving rigorous scheduling and invasive procedures is stressful. During the seemingly long interval between the transfer and pregnancy testing, clients may experience symptoms of pregnancy due to hormone stimulation. Couples may be ambivalent and fearful about the outcome, or feel isolated from the IVF team when daily visits stop.[30]

A positive pregnancy test means heightened anxiety for the couple. Although it is joyous news, the couple fears "something will happen." It is difficult to enjoy pregnancy because of past disappointments.[31]

Failure to conceive is devastating physically, emotionally, and financially. These couples experience tremendous personal loss; they may apologize for "letting the IVF team down." Guilt and self-doubt are often expressed. To conceive, cryopreservation or repeat treatment cycles must be considered.[30]

***Follow-Up.*** Maintain the health of the individuals and the couple, to enable them to cope and eventually resolve their infertility. Education, support, counseling, and referral are part of the intervention.

## ALTERNATIVES TO PREGNANCY

### ADOPTION

The hardest part of adoption is the gradual process of deciding to adopt and how to proceed.[31] During infertility treatment, guide the couple toward adoption resources if they are interested. They may, however, perceive adoption as "giving up on their bodies," and fear that this choice will affect their response to treatment and chance of conceiving. Some couples feel that they can cope only with the stresses of infertility and not with adoption stresses at the same time. Moreover, adoption does not resolve the couple's feelings about infertility, and they must resolve them, with the support of each other, significant others, and professionals.

A couple's concerns relate to their lack of prenatal control and their ability to love and bond to a child not biologically related. In addition, they may have fears related to their parenting abilities. They wonder, too, how they will manage psychologically, financially, and with legal issues, and how they will cope with the potential special needs of an adopted child.[31] The couple must deal with the responses of significant others to adoption, as well as with societal responses.

Options for adoption are by means of a private arrangement or through an agency or international organization. The adoptive child may have special needs or be an older child. The processes can be complicated, time consuming, and costly. The couple may feel that they have lost control.[32]

## SURROGACY

The word *surrogacy* implies a substitution of function.[33] By definition, it encompasses donor insemination, oocyte/embryo donation, and the gestational carrier. Surrogacy may also imply a kind of adoption, as the child may or may not have a biologic connection with his or her parents. Couples considering surrogacy need information, support, and counseling.

### Social and Ethical Concerns

The potential negative effects of surrogacy on the child, the donor, and their families are the focus of concern. Extensive screening must be completed on both donor and recipient, as both parties must be physically and emotionally healthy. Appropriate precautions during pregnancy must be outlined and maintained.[33]

Secrecy versus open conception is a controversial topic. The impact on the child's self-identity is unknown. Secrecy may be regarded as damaging to the child's trusting relationship with his or her parents. Yet, for the child to learn of others' disapproval and that the "mother" was paid to conceive, gestate, and give the child away is considered destructive. Questions arise regarding trauma to donors (bonding in utero and loss of a child) and their families (loss of a sibling). Recipients undergo stress while waiting for the child to be born, fearing the unknown, the loss of a child, or the inability to bond. The long term effects of contact between surrogates and recipients and the potential for shared parenting may create conflict and stress.[34]

Payment for surrogacy is taboo; it is unacceptable to "sell babies" or to discriminate against those who would choose surrogacy if they could afford this option. It is feared that incest may result if surrogacy becomes more widespread.[34]

Legal controversy concerns the rights and responsibilities of donor and recipient, breech of contract, and payment for services. Legislation is needed to regulate but not eliminate surrogacy.[35]

## LIVING WITHOUT CHILDREN

Infertile couples have many difficult decisions to make: How great is their motivation for parenthood? their energy and resources to continue treatment? the value of continuing treatment?[31] Choosing to remain without children is painful, and the couple must come to terms with loss.[36] The decision is made gradually, and it is a mutual decision. It requires close personal examination and intense communication by the couple. This choice indicates that grief regarding infertility has been resolved; it is a positive change.[36]

Finally, the couple feels relieved that their family is complete without children. They no longer feel pressured to "perform on demand," put their "lives on hold," or conform to medical therapies. They are able to regain privacy, control their lives, and focus their energies on themselves, each other, their relationship, and future life goals.[37]

The decision to remain childfree is not easily understood by others. Couples who have resolved their infertility and professionals who work with infertile men and women can help others understand the impact of infertility and the process that occurred in deciding not to have children. Others should be helped to understand that this choice is a positive solution.[36]

## NURSING DIAGNOSES

The following nursing diagnoses are representative of those used in the health care plan of women with an infertility problem. The list, however, is by no means inclusive.

- Altered nutrition, less than body requirements.
- Altered role performance.
- Altered comfort.
- Anxiety.
- Body image disturbance.
- Coping ineffective, individual.
- Grieving.
- Impaired adjustment.
- Knowledge deficit related to
  —disease process and effects.
  —abnormalities.
  —physiological needs and endocrine changes.
  —tests.
  —cause and management of condition, treatment.
  —normal reproductive function.
- Nutrition, less or more than body requirements.
- Pain.
- Personal identity disturbance.
- Role relationship disturbance.
- Self-concept disturbance.
- Self-esteem disturbance.
- Sexual dysfunction.
- Sexuality, reproductive disturbance.
- Spiritual distress.

## REFERENCES


1. Speroff, L., Glass, R., & Kase, N. (1989). *Clinical gynecologic endocrinology and infertility* (4th ed.). Baltimore: Williams & Wilkins.
2. Jaffe, S., & Jewelewicz, R. (1991). The basic infertility investigation. *Fertility & Sterility, 55*(4), 599–613.
3. Nachtigall, R.D. (1991). Assessing fecundity after age 40. *Contemporary Obstetrics & Gynecology, 36*(3), 11–33.
4. Garner, C. (Ed.). (1991). *Principles of infertility nursing.* Boca Raton, FL: CRC Press.
5. Keleher, K.C. (1991). Occupational health: How work environments can affect reproductive capacity and outcome. *Nurse Practitioner, 16*(1), 23–37.
6. Eck Menning, B. (1988). *Infertility: A guide for the childless couple* (2nd ed.). Englewood Cliffs, NJ: Prentice-Hall.
7. Loriaux, T. (1991). Male infertility: A challenge for primary health care providers. *Nurse Practitioner, 16*(3), 38–45.
8. Serono Laboratories. (1988). Ovulation induction: Clinical aspects/practical applications, a nursing perspective. Norwell, MA: Author.
9. Davajan, V., & Kletzky, O. (1991). *Secondary amenorrhea without galactorrhea or androgen excess.* In D. Mishell, Jr., & V. Davajan (Eds.), *Infertility, contraception and reproductive endocrinology* (3rd ed.) (pp. 372–395). Boston: Blackwell Scientific.
10. Kletzky, O., & Davajan, V. (1991). Hyperprolactinemia. In D. Mishell, Jr., & V. Davajan (Eds.), *Infertility, contraception and reproductive endocrinology* (3rd ed.) (pp. 396–421). Boston: Blackwell Scientific.
11. Walter, R., Jr. (1986). Hirsutism. In C. Havens, N. Sullivan, & P. Tilton (Eds.), *Manual of outpatient gynecology* (pp. 173–181). Boston: Little, Brown.
12. Lobo, R. (1991). The syndrome of hyperandrogenic chronic anovulation. In D. Mishell, Jr., & V. Davajan (Eds.), *Infertility, contraception and reproductive endocrinology* (3rd ed.) (pp. 447–487). Boston: Blackwell Scientific.

13. LeMaire, G. (1987). The luteinized unruptured follicle syndrome: Anovulation in disguise. *JOGN Nursing 16*(2), 116–120.
14. McNeeley, M., & Soules, M. (1988). The diagnosis of luteal phase deficiency: A critical review. *Fertility & Sterility, 50*(1), 1–15.
15. March, C.M. (Ed.). (1990). Update: Müllerian anomalies. *Endocrine and Fertility Forum, 13*(1), 1–6.
16. Kelly, A. (1991). The uterine factor and fertility. In D. Barad (Ed.), *Infertility and Reproductive Medicine Clinics of North America, 2*(2) (pp. 391–407). Philadelphia: Saunders.
17. Lichtman, R., & Papera, S. (1990). *Gynecology: Well-woman care* (pp. 313–321). Norwalk, CT: Appleton & Lange.
18. Cohen, B. (1991). The postcoital test. In D. Barad (Ed.), *Infertility and Reproductive Medicine Clinics of North America, 2*(2) (pp. 317–331). Philadelphia: Saunders.
19. Rosenberg, S. (1990). Can we achieve adhesion-free surgery? *Female Patient, 15*, 59–66.
20. Israel, R. (1991). Pelvic endometriosis. In D. Mitchell, Jr., V. Davajan, & R. Lobo (Eds.), *Infertility, contraception and reproductive endocrinology* (3rd ed.) (pp. 723–753). Boston: Blackwell Scientific.
21. Witt, B. (1991). Pelvic factors and infertility. In D. Barad (Ed.), *Infertility and Reproductive Medicine Clinics of North America, 2*(2) (pp. 371–390). Philadelphia: Saunders.
22. Adamson, G.D. (1991). Surgical and medical treatment of endometriosis. *Contemporary Obstetrics & Gynecology, 36*(7), 48–63.
23. Cook, A., & Rock, J. (1991). The role of laparoscopy in the treatment of endometriosis. *Fertility & Sterility, 55*(4), 663–690.
24. Carson, S. (1991). Nongenetic causes of recurrent fetal loss. *Contemporary Obstetrics & Gynecology, 36*(2), 14–26.
25. Bronson, R. (1990, December). Sperm antibodies: Problems in infertility. *Resolve National Newsletter, 15*(5), 1–3.
26. Schulman, S., & Schulman, J. (1991). Immunologic factors as a cause of infertility. In D. Barad (Ed.), *Infertility and Reproductive Medicine Clinics of North America, 2*(2) (pp. 351–369). Philadelphia: Saunders.
27. Jarow, J., & Lipshultz, L. (1987). Urologic evaluation of male infertility. *Contemporary Journal Obstetrics & Gynecology, 30*(Special Issue), 85–96.
28. Cohen, J., Talansky, B., Alikani, M., Adler, A. (1992). Micromanipulation of gametes. In J. Overstreet (Ed.), *Infertility and reproductive medicine clinics of North America 3*(2) (pp. 505–523). Philadelphia: Saunders.
29. Porter, J., Manberg, P., & Hartz, S. (1991). Statistics and results of assisted reproductive technologies. *Assisted reproductive reviews, 1*(1), 28–37. Baltimore: Williams & Wilkins.
30. Cimarusti, L. (1988, May). Coping with IVF cycles. *Resolve Newsletter, Washington Metropolitan Area, 10*(3), 1–16.
31. Glazer, E., & Cooper, S. (1988). *Without child: Experiencing and resolving infertility.* Lexington, MA: Lexington Books.
32. Levy-Shiff, R., Bar, O., & Har-Even, D. (1990). Psychological adjustment of adoptive parents-to-be. *American Journal of Orthopsychiatry, 60*(2), 258–267.
33. Wallach, E. (1990). Ethical aspects of IVF and related assisted reproductive technologies. In M. Damewood (Ed.), *The Johns Hopkins handbook of in vitro fertilization and assisted reproductive technologies* (pp. 151–162). Boston: Little, Brown.
34. Erlen, J., & Holzman, I. (1990). Evolving issues in surrogate motherhood. *Health Care for Women International, 11*(3), 319–329.
35. Charo, R.A. (1988). Legislative approaches to surrogate motherhood. *Law, Medicine, and Health Care, 16*(1–2), 96–110.
36. Carter, J., & Carter, M. (1989). *Sweet grapes: How to stop being infertile and start living again.* Indianapolis: Perspective Press.
37. Salzer, L. (1986). *Infertility: How couples can cope.* Boston: Hall.

## BIBLIOGRAPHY

Alexander, N., & Schlaff, W. (1987). Insemination techniques for overcoming male infertility. *Contemporary Obstetrics & Gynecology, 30*(Special Issue), 99–111.

American Fertility Society. (1988, February). Revised new guidelines for the use of semen-donor insemination. *Fertility & Sterility, 49*(2).

Amuzu, B., Laxova, R., & Shapiro, S. (1990). Pregnancy outcome, health of children, and family adjustment after donor insemination. *Obstetrics & Gynecology, 75*(6), 899–905.

Azziz, R. (1988). Determining the cause of hirsuitism and anovulation. *Contemporary Obstetrics & Gynecology, 33*(5), 126–139.

Barad, D. (Ed.). (1991). Workup of the infertile woman. *Infertility and Reproductive Medicine Clinics of North America, 2*(2), Philadelphia: Saunders.

Baran, A., & Pannor, R. (1989). *Lethal secrets.* New York: Warner Books.

Burden, N. (1988). Nursing care of the patient undergoing laparoscopy in the ambulatory setting. *Journal of Post Anesthesia Nursing, 3*(3), 189–195.

Canape, C. (1986). *Adoption: parenthood without pregnancy.* New York: Avon Books.

Cullins, V., & Huggins, G. (1990). Disorders leading to amenorrhea. *Contemporary Obstetrics & Gynecology, 35*(9), 67–82.

Damewood, M. (Ed.). (1990). *The Johns Hopkins handbook of in vitro fertilization and assisted reproductive technologies.* Boston: Little, Brown.

Davis, D., & Dearman, C. (1991). Coping strategies of infertile women. *JOGN Nursing, 20*(3), 221–225.

Dunnington, R., & Estok, P. (1991). Potential psychological attachments formed by donors involved in fertility technology: Another side to infertility. *Nurse Practitioner, 16*(11), 41–48.

Eck Menning, B. (1981). Donor insemination: The psychological issues. *Contemporary Obstetrics & Gynecology, 18*, 155–172.

Eschenbach, D. (1987). Infertility caused by infection. *Contemporary Obstetrics & Gynecology, 30*(Special Issue), 29–46.

Frank, D. (1990). Factors related to decisions about infertility treatment. *JOGN Nursing, 19*(2), 162–167.

Futterweit, W. (1984). Polycystic ovarian disease. *Clinical perspectives in obstetrics and gynecology.* New York: Springer-Verlag.

Glass, R. (Ed.). (1988). *Office gynecology* (3rd ed.). Baltimore: Williams & Wilkins.

Glazer, E. (1990). *The long-awaited stork: A guide to parenting after infertility.* Lexington, MA: Lexington Books.

Golan, A., & Caspi, E. (1992). Congential anomalies of the müllerian tract. *Contemporary Obstetrics & Gynecology, 37*(2), 39–55.

Gomel, V., & Rowe, T. (1986). Mastering reconstructive tubal microsurgery. *Contemporary Obstetrics & Gynecology, 28*(Special Issue), 31–48.

Grunfeld, L. (Ed.). (1991). Ultrasonography in reproductive medicine. *Infertility and Reproductive Medicine Clinics of North America, 2*(4). Philadelphia: Saunders.

Hammond, M. (1987). Monitoring ovulation. *Contemporary Obstetrics & Gynecology, 30* (Special Issue), 59–68.

Johnston, P. (1984). *An adopter's advocate.* Indianapolis: Perspective Press.

Johnston, P. (1992). *Adopting after infertility.* Indiana: Perspective Press.

Jones, Jr., H., Jones, G., Hodgen, G., & Rosenwaks, Z. (Eds.). (1986). *In vitro fertilization: Norfolk.* Baltimore: Williams & Wilkins.

Keel, B., & Webster, B. (1990). *Handbook of the laboratory diagnosis and treatment of infertility.* Boca Raton, FL: CRC Press.

Milne, B. (1988). Couples' experiences with in vitro fertilization. *JOGN Nursing, 17*(5), 347–352.

Mishell, Jr., D., Davajan, V., & Lobo, R. (Eds.). (1991). *Infertility, contraception and reproductive endocrinology* (3rd ed.). Boston: Blackwell Scientific.

Oehninger, S., & Hodgen, G. (1991). How to evaluate human spermatozoa for assisted reproduction. *Assisted Reproduction Reviews, 1*(1), 15–27. Baltimore: William & Wilkins.

Pittaway, D. (Ed.). (1991). Hyperandrogenism. *Infertility and Reproductive Medicine Clinics of North America, 2*(3). Philadelphia: Saunders.

Reading, A., & Kerin, J. (1989). Psychological aspects of providing infertility services. *Journal of Reproductive Medicine, 34*(11), 861–871.

Rivlin, M. (Ed.). (1990). *Handbook of drug therapy in reproductive endocrinology and infertility.* Boston: Little, Brown.

Rock, J., & Markham, S. (1987). Endometriosis as a cause of infertility. *Contemporary Obstetrics & Gynecology, 30*(Special Issue), 49–55.

Sorosky, A., Baran, A., & Pannor, R. (1989). *The*

*adoption triangle*. San Antonio: Corona.

Stephenson, L. (1987). *Give us a child: Coping with the personal crisis of infertility.* San Francisco: Harper & Row.

Symposium. (1990). New concepts in hysteroscopy. *Contemporary Obstetrics & Gynecology, 35*(10), 84–103.

Symposium. (1990). Who benefits from intrauterine insemination with washed sperm? *Contemporary Obstetrics & Gynecology, 35*(10), 65–77.

Taub, N. (1988). Surrogacy: A preferred treatment for infertility. *Law, Medicine and Health Care, 16*(1–2), 89–95.

Wied, G., Kessel, D., Mishell, D., Ledger, W., & Kaufman, R. (Eds.). (1989). Ovulation induction state of the art. *Journal of Reproduction Medicine, 34*(Suppl.).

Yee, B. (Ed.). (1990). Ovulation induction. *Infertility and Reproductive Medicine Clinics of North America, (1)*1. Philadelphia: Saunders.

Zeevi, D., Younis, J., & Laufer, N. (1991). Ovulation induction: New approaches. *Assisted Reproductive Reviews, 1*(1), 2–8. Baltimore: Williams & Wilkins.

Zoldbrod, A. (1993). *Men, women, and infertility: Intervention and treatment strategies.* New York: Lexington Books.

CHAPTER 8

# VAGINITIS AND SEXUALLY TRANSMITTED DISEASES

*Emily Coogan Bennett*

*Once it enters the body, the herpes virus never leaves, although clinical manifestations disappear as the virus becomes dormant.*

### *Highlights*

- The Centers for Disease Control
- Human Immunodeficiency Virus
- Bacterial Vaginosis
- *Candida albicans*
- Chancroid
- *Chlamydia trachomatis*
- Donovanosis
- Genital Mycoplasmas
- Gonorrhea
- Hepatitis A and B
- Herpes Simplex Virus
- Human Papillomavirus
- Lymphogranuloma Venereum
- Molluscum Contagiosum
- Pediculosis Pubis
- Syphilis
- Trichomoniasis

## INTRODUCTION

Vaginitis and sexually transmitted diseases (STDs) are an almost universal problem among women. The conditions occur most frequently during the reproductive years; in fact, many reach their peak incidence during adolescence and young adulthood. The introduction of acquired immunodeficiency syndrome (AIDS) into the United States has done much to raise our collective consciousness about STDs in general. Sexual activity and direct intimate contact are the mode of transmission in the majority of cases. It is well known that women who are frequently sexually active with multiple partners are at greater risk than women who are sexually inactive or those with stable, mutually monogamous partners. Nevertheless, broad assumptions about women with STDs are inappropriate.

Billions of dollars are expended annually in the United States to diagnose and treat STDs. Many STDs are uncomplicated (e.g., trichomonas); on the other hand, many have serious long term health consequences (e.g., chlamydia), and some are life threatening (e.g., hepatitis B). Prevention should be the primary focus when dealing with all STDs. The effectiveness of latex condoms in reducing the risk of AIDS has had a "spillover" effect in reducing the risk of other STDs.[1] Likewise, the introduction of universal precautions for health care professionals, a direct result of the human immunodeficiency virus (HIV) epidemic, has made the workplace safer against the transmission of all STDs.

Women with vaginitis and sexually transmitted diseases are represented in every socioeconomic class, culture, age group, and workplace. Their story is often one of fear, anxiety, frustration, anger, shame, and guilt. Often, it is also an untold story.

A health care provider giving primary care to women must be able to offer services, education, and counseling. Complete, accurate information conveyed in an open, professional manner is essential. Information rapidly changes and requires constant updating. In providing care, sensitivity and kindness are essential. The emotional impact that

**TABLE 8–1. GENERAL INFORMATION NEEDED IN THE CARE OF WOMEN WITH VAGINITIS AND SEXUALLY TRANSMITTED DISEASES (STDs)**

Provide both written information and verbal explanations to the client.

| | |
|---|---|
| *Disease Process* | Etiology, incubation, risk factors, diagnosis, management, follow-up. |
| *Treatments* | Medications and their side effects; signs of allergic response; discomfort; time commitments; simultaneous partner treatment; the need to keep appointments for treatment and thereby control growth and spread of lesions and worsening of disease and symptoms; avoidance of douching and tampon use (unless medically directed) until healing is complete. |
| *Transmission* | A description of all possible modes; the need to suspend genital and oral sexual relations, foreign body insertion, and manual manipulation until healing is complete; use of lubricated latex condoms until partners are examined and determined disease-free; the dangers of multiple partners and the principles of "safer sex." |
| *Comfort Measures* | Sitz baths and oral analgesics may help some conditions. |
| *Hygiene* | The importance of cleanliness and dryness to enhance healing. Use of a hair dryer on low setting to aid drying. Avoidance of powders, douches (especially perfumed or deodorized), perfumed sprays. Discussion of secondary infection and how it may occur.<br>Wearing clean cotton underwear, loose clothing, and fabrics that "breathe"; washing hands thoroughly before and after touching genitalia; not wearing underwear more than one day; not wearing anyone else's underwear; not allowing anyone other than oneself to wear one's underwear or tight fitting trousers; changing out of moist clothing as soon as possible. |
| *Other Prevention* | Decreasing smoking in infection with human papillomavirus (HPV); self-monitoring of the vulva (HPV); client examination of partner and asking about past exposure; empowerment of client (through role playing) to be motivated and skillful in talking about sensitive issues with her partner; caution in new sexual liaisons; avoidance of alcohol and drugs that limit inhibitions; an agreement ("contract") with her partner that they have a mutually monogamous relationship; for their mutual safety, an agreement between the two partners in the relationship to tell each other if either one has sexual relations with someone else. |

a sexually transmitted disease has on a client is intense; there is no place for judgmental attitudes. Table 8–1 provides an overview of general information that should be provided to women with vaginitis or a sexually transmitted disease.

## SEXUALLY TRANSMITTED DISEASES AND THE CENTERS FOR DISEASE CONTROL

Some STDs, but not all, are reportable to the Centers for Disease Control (CDC) in Atlanta, Georgia. This government agency is part of the U.S. Public Health Service and charged with, among other functions, assisting states to identify and control certain diseases. The actual mandate to report specific diseases comes from individual states through their legislative bodies. The CDC can recommend which diseases should be reported; however, the final decision rests with the states. In 1993 the following STDs are reported to the CDC: AIDS, gonorrhea, hepatitis A, hepatitis B, and syphilis.

Three factors are considered in determining which diseases should be reported.

- *Ability to Test.* If no reasonable test for a condition is readily available (e.g. herpes), then that disease is unlikely to become reportable.
- *Ability to Cure.* Especially important to report are readily curable diseases (e.g., gonorrhea) in order to control epidemics.
- *Public Awareness.* Diseases that gain widespread public attention and represent a public health threat (e.g., AIDS) are usually reportable.

In addition to compiling STD statistics, the CDC recommends treatment for individual diseases. Approximately every 5 years it publishes STD treatment guidelines. The most recent of these, published in 1993, are used throughout this chapter when discussing medication. The conditions described throughout the remainder of the chapter are arranged in alphabetical order.

# ACQUIRED IMMUNODEFICIENCY SYNDROME (AIDS)

AIDS results from a lethal viral infection that renders the immune system incapable of fighting disease. The spectrum of disease ranges from asymptomatic, to moderately affected, to full-blown infection that always results in death. Although AIDS is primarily sexually transmitted, its manifestations are not specific to the reproductive tract. Rather, it is a systemic and devastating disease that can affect virtually every organ system.

## EPIDEMIOLOGY

### Etiology/Risk Factors

The infecting organism is human immunodeficiency virus (HIV). Specific risk behaviors include sharing needles during illicit drug use; anal intercourse; vaginal intercourse or oral sex with someone who uses illicit drugs intravenously; sex with a bisexual male, someone unknown, or someone who has multiple partners; and unprotected sex with an infected individual.[2–4] People with genital ulcer disease (e.g., syphilis and herpes) are at greater risk of contracting and transmitting HIV infection because of a ready viral entry site.

### Transmission

The disease is spread through sexual intercourse with an infected person and through artificial insemination by an infected donor, by sharing needles with an infected person, and from an infected mother to her unborn child, as well as during birth and in the postpartum period while breastfeeding. Risk of transmission from an infected blood transfusion has been dramatically reduced since 1985 when universal testing of donated blood for HIV was initiated. Transmission via casual contacts, fomites, and insect bites does not occur. The incubation period is approximately 3 months. The risk of transmission from deep kissing is unknown but caution is advised.

### Incidence

In 1992, of the approximately 1 million people in the United States estimated in 1992 by the CDC to be infected with the AIDS virus, 10 percent were symptomatic. All 50 states reported cases; most infected persons were younger than 40. The incidence among women was rising; they comprised 14 percent of reported cases in adults.[5,6] A December 1993 report from the National Center of Health Statistics on the results of a nationwide AIDS survey indicates that the CDC estimate may be high. Researchers estimate the national incidence to be about 550,000 in 1994. This is encouraging news, since it means a slower increase than had been expected.

## SUBJECTIVE DATA

HIV positive individuals may be asymptomatic for 10 years or longer. As disease progresses, they may develop fatigue, weight loss, swollen glands, diarrhea, and other nonspecific but persistent symptoms. Women may present with severe, persistent oral or vaginal candidiasis or urinary tract infections (UTIs) unresponsive to standard treatment. Severe dysphagia secondary to candidiasis of the esophagus also has been reported.

## OBJECTIVE DATA

### Physical Examination

As HIV infection progresses to AIDS, mild or rare conditions become severe, then fatal. Opportunistic infections associated with AIDS include *Pneumocystis carinii* pneumonia, Kaposi's sarcoma, *Mycobacterium avium* intracellulare (an avian-type of tuberculosis), systemic cytomegalovirus (CMV), herpes, monilia, and others.

Several gynecologic manifestations may be associated with immunocompromise and, indeed, may clue the health professional to be suspicious of HIV presentation.

- HIV infected women are more likely to present with recurrent vaginal monilia.
- HIV positive status is also associated with pelvic inflammatory disease (PID) that is more fulminant.[8,9]
- Herpesvirus may be shed more readily by HIV positive women, and ulcers may take longer to resolve.
- Chancroid may be more resistant to standard therapy, and syphilis may become more aggressive.[9]
- Finally, genital ulcer disease, which may be unique to women with HIV, has been mentioned in the literature.[9]

### Diagnostic Tests and Methods

HIV-antibody tests reliably diagnose HIV infection. Antibodies are usually detected within 3 months of exposure. A confirmed positive test means that an individual is infected with HIV and infectious to others. A negative antibody test, if related to a specific exposure, should be repeated 3 to 6 months after the exposure.[4]

***Enzyme-Linked Immunosorbent Assay (ELISA) and Western Blot Assay.*** Diagnostic evaluation includes a screening test for HIV antibody (ELISA) and a confirmatory test (Western blot) if ELISA is positive. Anyone who tests HIV positive should have a complete medical evaluation, including physical examination, complete blood cell (CBC) count, purified protein derivative (PPD) test for tuberculosis, lymphocyte subset analysis, and syphilis serology.

The test procedure is venipuncture and collection of blood sample. As with all blood collection, gloves should be worn.

Advise the client that a positive screening test must be confirmed with a more specific and definitive test. HIV testing should be voluntary, confidential, and carried out with both pretest and posttest counseling. Encourage clients with any STD to undergo HIV testing because they have exhibited risk behaviors. Pretest counseling should include assessment of the client's risk of HIV infection and education about ways to reduce risk.

If the client tests negative, posttest counseling should explain ways to modify sexual behavior to reduce risk. If the client tests positive, posttest counseling must be done by someone qualified to discuss the medical, emotional, and social impact of HIV infection. Routes of transmission and methods to prevent further transmission must be emphasized.[4]

***Papanicolaou (Pap) Smear.*** The Centers for Disease Control (CDC) recommend annual Pap smears if cytological specimens are adequate for interpretation and the results show normal cytology.[10] The American College of Obstetricians and Gynecologists, however, suggests more aggressive surveillance due to a fulminant course of cervical disease and greater incidence of false negative cytologic findings in HIV infected women. Semiannual Pap smears may be indicated. Colposcopy may be used if the Pap is uninterpretable or abnormal, even with findings of koilocytes or inflammation.[8]

In addition, a link has been reported between HIV disease and human papillomavirus infections, and between HIV and cervical neoplasia. Moreover, an increased incidence of abnormal Pap smears is reported among HIV infected women. Further study is necessary.[8]

## DIFFERENTIAL MEDICAL DIAGNOSES

The list of possible differential diagnoses is as vast as the list of opportunistic infections associated with HIV disease. A complete list is beyond the scope of this book.

## PLAN

*Health professionals must use universal precautions with all clients and in all settings.*

### Psychosocial Interventions

Advise illicit I.V. drug users to stop using drugs, or at least not to share needles and to clean equipment with bleach after each use. Consistent condom and spermicide use reduces risk of transmission.

Infected prenatal clients, although asymptomatic, may pass HIV to their child; the perinatal transmission rate is 30 to 40 percent.[5] HIV infection in newborns may not become evident until 12 to 18 months after birth. A recent study of HIV-IgA (immunoglobulin A) assays offers promise of diagnosing perinatally acquired HIV infection just after the third month of age. Early diagnosis would aid in the implementation of antiviral therapy.[11] AZT dramatically decreases mother-to-child HIV transmission.[11a]

Psychological counseling and support are essential. Multiple community resources should be identified as referral sites for AIDS clients.[4]

Counseling about "safer sex" is important. A mutually monogamous relationship between two uninfected individuals is safest. Specific "safer sex" practices include using a condom with vaginal, anal, and oral intercourse; using spermicide containing nonoxynol-9 with vaginal or anal intercourse; reducing the number of sex partners; avoiding sex when open sores are present; and practicing nonpenetrative sex practices such as hugging, kissing, and masturbation.[3]

### Medication

Clients must be cared for by physicians knowledgeable about AIDS. Therapy with zidovudine (Retrovir), previously known as azidothymidine (AZT), is of benefit in late stage disease. Its use in all stages of disease, including asymptomatic HIV positive status, is being studied. Serious side effects, especially anemias and cytopenias, are common. Drug use requires careful management and follow-up by specialists.

In addition to zidovudine, many other drugs may be used in the treatment of AIDS, and these are usually site dependent. For example, oral fluconazole is used for esophageal candidiasis. Much research is being conducted on various anti-HIV drugs.

Other interventions are indicated by the course of the disease.

# BACTERIAL VAGINOSIS (BV)

This form of vaginitis is the most prevalent among childbearing women. The causative organism is *Gardnerella vaginalis*. Traditionally thought to be sexually transmitted, BV is now known to result from homeostatic disruption in the vagina. Recent research suggests that BV is associated with preterm labor, chorioamnionitis, postpartum endometritis, and PID.[4,12] These studies need further validation. Other names for this condition are gardnerella vaginalis, hemophilus vaginalis, nonspecific vaginitis, and bacterial vaginitis.

## EPIDEMIOLOGY

### Etiology/Risk Factors

*G. vaginalis* interacts with anaerobic bacteria (e.g., the *Bacteroids* and *Mobiluncus* species) and genital mycoplasmas to produce vaginal symptoms. Concurrently, normal *Lactobacillus* is markedly decreased.[8]

### Transmission

Recent research suggests a nonsexual mode of transmission, although BV occurs in sexually active women.[4,12] The treatment of male partners does not reduce the risk of recurrence. BV-associated bacteria can be recovered from the urethra of male partners, but the disease entity is not known in men.

### Incidence

BV is not a reportable disease; hence, there are no accurate incidence figures.

## SUBJECTIVE DATA

Clients with BV may be asymptomatic, or have malodorous vaginal discharge. Often clients report foul odor after intercourse. Symptoms such as pruritus, abdominal pain, dyspareunia, and dysuria do not reliably correlate with BV.

## OBJECTIVE DATA

### Physical Examination

***Genitalia/Reproductive.*** Homogeneous, whitish vaginal discharge often is adherent to the vaginal mucosa. A foul odor is apparent.

### Diagnostic Tests and Methods

***Saline Wet Mount.*** Diagnostic evaluation for clue cells: characteristic epithelial cells with bacteria adherent to the cell wall, giving it a stippled, granular appearance. Cell margins become blurred, and few white blood cells are noted.

The test procedure is to mix a sample of vaginal secretions (obtained from the vaginal pool or posterior blade of the speculum) with normal saline, place on a slide, and cover with a coverslip. Examine microscopically under low and high power.

Explain the procedure to the client. Advise her that an immediate diagnosis is possible.

***"Whiff Test."*** Diagnostic evaluation for a "fishy" amine odor. The test procedure is to mix vaginal secretions with 10 percent potassium hydroxide; the characteristic odor is readily emitted. Advise the client of the test purpose.

***Vaginal pH.*** Diagnostic evaluation for acidity of vaginal secretions. In BV, pH is greater than or equal to 4.5, but this acidity is not specific for BV alone. The test procedure is to dip appropriate pH paper (pH range 4.0 to 6.0) into vaginal secretions and observe the color change. The sample may be obtained by swabbing the lateral and posterior fornix and applying directly to pH paper, or by dipping pH paper into the posterior blade of the speculum after removal from the vagina. Advise the client of the purpose of the test.

## DIFFERENTIAL MEDICAL DIAGNOSES

Trichomonas vaginitis, foreign body vaginitis, monilia.

## PLAN

### Psychosocial Interventions

Because the etiology of BV is uncertain and changing, a client's confusion is understandable. Counsel clients about what is currently known and what is being suggested. It is reasonable to allay fear that BV is an STD. Male partners need not be treated unless the infection is recurrent. Routine treatment is not recommended for asymptomatic women who are not planning pregnancy or not at high risk for pregnancy. Recurrence rates are high. Over-the-counter remedies such as lactobacillus products are not therapeutic. Symptomatic pregnant clients can be treated after the first trimester.

### Medication

#### *Metronidazole/Metronidazole Vaginal Gel*

- *Indications.* Recommended treatment for BV in females and males.
- *Administration.* Oral tablets: 500 mg b.i.d. for 7 days or 2 g single dose stat.[4,13] Vaginal gel 0.75 percent: one applicator full intravaginally b.i.d. for 5 days.
- *Side Effects and Adverse Reactions.* Occur with the use of alcohol when taking metronidazole; vomiting and flushing may result. Transient nausea and a metallic taste have also been reported. Because metronidazole has a broad antimicrobial spectrum, normal vaginal flora may be suppressed with subsequent monilial infection. Vaginal gel: vaginal candidiasis, occasional genitourinary-perineal itching, irritation, swelling; gastrointestinal complaints.
- *Contraindications.* Known allergy to metronidazole. Do not use during the first trimester of pregnancy.
- *Anticipated Outcomes on Evaluation.* Symptoms clear rapidly after treatment. A test for cure is not routinely indicated.
- *Client Teaching and Counseling.* Stress the need to avoid alcohol. If symptoms return, reexamination is indicated. Treatment of the sexual partner with recurrent infection is recommended. For vaginal gel, advise the client about side effects.

#### *Clindamycin*

- *Indications.* Alternative treatment of BV; may be useful in recurrent cases and for pregnant clients.

- *Administration.* Orally 300 mg b.i.d. for 7 days or 2 percent clindamycin cream intravaginally daily (usually at bedtime) for 7 days.[4,14]
- *Side Effects and Adverse Reactions.* Colitis, may be severe.
- *Contraindications.* Known sensitivity to clindamycin. Clindamycin cream is as or more effective than metronidazole, thus the indicated choice in pregnancy.[15] Vaginitis from *Candida albicans* is more common with clindamycin use, however.
- *Anticipated Outcome on Evaluation.* Symptoms resolve rapidly. Test for cure is not necessary.
- *Client Teaching and Counseling.* The regimen of medication must be completed.
- *Follow-Up and Referral.* No follow-up is necessary.

# CANDIDIASIS

*Candida albicans* is a common cause of vaginitis that is not sexually transmitted. An upset in the homeostatic balance in the vagina leads to an overgrowth of the organism and infection. Predisposing factors include antibiotic use, diabetes, and pregnancy. Other names for the condition are fungus, yeast, and candidasis.

## EPIDEMIOLOGY

*C. albicans* is a fungal species. The organism gains access to the vaginal mucosa primarily from the perianal area.

The mode of acquisition of infection is nonsexual. Data are conflicting about whether *C. albicans* is pathogen or part of normal vaginal flora; however, most agree that the host environment must be altered for symptomatic infection to occur. *C. albicans* can be transmitted from infected mother to newborn at delivery. Neonates develop an oral infection known as thrush.

Accurate incidence figures are unavailable because this is not a reportable disease. Some authors have suggested a 20 percent prevalence among women of childbearing age.[12]

## SUBJECTIVE DATA

Vaginal itching, burning, and irritation. Dysuria (burning when urine hits the involved tissue) is common. Vaginal discharge, which may be scanty or profuse, is white and thick. Symptoms frequently worsen prior to menses. Most clients report an acute onset of symptoms that rapidly clear with treatment. A small subset of women experience persistent chronic infection that does not respond well to classic treatment.

## OBJECTIVE DATA

### Physical Examination

The vulva may be red and inflamed or appear normal. Scratches may be present. Typically a white discharge with the consistency of cottage cheese is adherent to the vaginal mucosa. Odor is absent.

### Diagnostic Tests and Methods

***Wet Mount, Saline or 10 Percent Potassium Hydroxide.*** Diagnostic evaluation for yeast cells and mycelia. The test procedure involves mixing a sample of vaginal secretions with saline, covering with coverslip, and viewing under microscope. May prepare wet mount with 10 percent potassium hydroxide, which will obliterate everything but yeast from the slide.

Focus client teaching on explaining that immediate diagnosis is possible.

***Vaginal Culture.*** Diagnostic evaluation for *C. albicans*. A culture may be useful if the wet mount is negative but symptoms suggest *Candida*.

The test procedure is to obtain a sample of

vaginal secretions and place it on Nickerson's medium or Sabouraud's agar. Accurate culture is only possible using the appropriate medium.

Advise the client that the yeast culture is the most sensitive test but results take up to 72 hours to obtain. Culture is imperative when documenting chronic infection.

## DIFFERENTIAL MEDICAL DIAGNOSES

Bacterial vaginosis, trichomonas, allergic contact dermatitis, pediculosis pubis.

## PLAN

### Psychosocial Interventions

Advise the client that infection is not sexually transmitted and treatment of her partner is unnecessary. Rigorous, immediate treatment in pregnancy is recommended to avoid neonatal thrush. Women with chronic moniliasis need intensive counseling to cope with discomfort and long term medication regimens. Often chronic infection leads to chronic dyspareunia, which can stress relationships. Advise clients to wear cotton underwear, avoid tight fitting nylons and slacks, wipe the perineum from front to back, and use mild soaps. Douching should be avoided.

### Medication

A wide variety of effective antimycotic topical agents are available. The more commonly prescribed medications are discussed here.

***Miconazole (Monistat).*** 2 percent cream, 100 mg vaginal suppository, 200 mg vaginal suppository. Now available over the counter.

- *Indications.* Acute and chronic infections. Safe during pregnancy.
- *Administration.* One applicator of cream in vagina q.h.s. for 7 nights, *or* one 100-mg vaginal suppository q.h.s. for 7 nights, *or* one 200 mg suppository q.h.s. for 3 nights. Clients who are diagnosed soon after the onset of symptoms may be treated with a 3-day regimen. Those with longstanding symptoms should use a 7-day treatment.
- *Side Effects and Adverse Reactions.* Few reactions are reported. Occasional burning after application may occur.
- *Contraindications.* Known hypersensitivity to miconazole.
- *Anticipated Outcomes on Evaluation.* Symptoms will rapidly resolve. Routine test for cure (wet mount) is not recommended for acute infection but is advised with chronic recurrent vaginitis.
- *Client Teaching and Counseling.* Advise the client that medication is to be completed as prescribed. Symptoms often will abate before medication is finished, but it must be completed to avoid recurrence. Cream or suppositories should be inserted immediately before retiring or lying down. Some may leak out on arising. Panty liners are helpful during the daytime to prevent moist underwear. Avoid tampon use with cream or suppository because tampons absorb medication, interfering with delivery of the therapeutic dose.

***Clotrimazole (Gyne-Lotrimin, Mycelex).*** 1 percent cream, 100 mg vaginal tablet. Now available over the counter; 500 mg vaginal tablet.[4]

- *Indications.* Acute and chronic infections. Safe during pregnancy.
- *Administration.* One applicator of cream in vagina q.h.s. for 7 to 14 nights, *or* one vaginal suppository q.h.s. for 7 nights, *or* two vaginal suppositories q.h.s. for 3 nights, *or* 1 single 500 mg vaginal suppository once.[4]
- *Side Effects and Adverse Reactions.* Same as miconazole/clotrimazole.
- *Contraindications.* Known hypersensitivity to miconazole.

- *Anticipated Outcomes on Evaluation.* Symptoms will rapidly resolve. Routine test for cure (wet mount) is not recommended for acute infection but is advised with chronic recurrent vaginitis.
- *Client Teaching and Counseling.* Advise the client that medication is to be completed as prescribed. Symptoms often will abate before medication is finished, but it must be completed to avoid recurrence. Cream or suppositories should be inserted immediately before retiring or lying down. Some may leak out on arising. Panty liners are helpful during the daytime to prevent moist underwear. Avoid tampon use with cream or suppository because tampons absorb medication, interfering with delivery of the therapeutic doses.

***Terconazole (Terazol).*** 0.4 or 0.8 percent vaginal cream; 80 mg vaginal tablets.

- *Indications.* Acute infection; other forms of candidiasis may respond better to terconazole than to miconazole or clotrimazole.
- *Administration.* One applicator of 0.4% cream intravaginally q.h.s. for 7 days; or 1 application of 0.8% cream intravaginally q.h.s. for 3 days; or 1 vaginal suppository q.h.s. for 3 days.[4]
- *Side Effects and Adverse Reactions.* Same as miconazole.
- *Contraindications.* Same as miconazole.
- *Anticipated Outcomes on Evaluation.* Same as miconazole.
- *Client Teaching and Counseling.* Same as miconazole.

***Ketoconazole (Nizoral).*** 200 mg oral tablets.

- *Indications.* Effective for acute infection but very expensive. Should be reserved for long term suppression of chronic infection with *C. albicans.*
- *Administration.* Acute infection: one tablet p.o. b.i.d. for 5 days. Suppressive therapy: 1/2 tablet p.o. daily for 6 months.
- *Side Effects and Adverse Reactions.* Liver toxicity has been reported; therefore, liver function studies should be obtained with long term therapy.
- *Contraindications.* Known sensitivity to ketoconazole.
- *Anticipated Outcomes on Evaluation.* Symptoms will improve.
- *Client Teaching and Counseling.* Once long term therapy is completed, rebound infection may result.

***Other Medications***

- Other intravaginal formulations that may be used include butoconazole 2% cream q.d. for 3 days or tioconazole 6.5% ointment once intravaginally in one single dose.[4]

## Nontraditional Interventions

Other therapies have been used for *C. albicans* infections, including boric acid suppositories and intravaginal instillation of plain yogurt or ingestion of yogurt. In one study, boric acid capsules, 600 mg nightly for 2 weeks, were effective and acceptable.[16] Boric acid has not gained widespread acceptance, perhaps because so many other preparations are readily available. The use of intravaginal yogurt has not been scientifically studied, and reports of its efficacy are only anecdotal; however, a recent study compared the rates of infection among women who ate yogurt containing *Lactobacillus acidophilus* for 6 months and women who did not. The yogurt group had significantly fewer infections.[17]

Nystatin was, for many years, a mainstay of treatment for *C. albicans* infection, but its use has been eclipsed by newer, more effective drugs that require shorter use.

## Follow-Up and Referral

Clients with simple, acute candidiasis do not require a follow-up visit. Those with chronic infection must be seen 1 to 2 weeks after treatment. A test for cure, preferably via culture, should be done.

# CHANCROID

Chancroid is an ulcerative bacterial infection that is primarily sexually transmitted. Lesions are usually confined to the genitals and accompanied by inguinal lymphadenopathy. Systemic illness does not occur.

## EPIDEMIOLOGY

*Haemophilus ducreyi*, a gram negative bacillus, is the causative agent. The condition occurs most commonly in uncircumcised males; incidence among women is low. Transmission is by direct contact with an infected individual. Autoinoculation has been reported occasionally. Fomite transmission does not occur. The incubation period is 4 to 7 days.

Although a major public health problem in some less developed countries, chancroid is rare in the United States: approximately 3000 reported cases per year.[12] Its association with increased rates of HIV infection makes it a significant infection.[18]

## SUBJECTIVE DATA

Ragged, painful ulcers that occur especially in men. Most ulcers occur around the prepuce, on the frenulum, or in the coronal sulcus. Inguinal tenderness also occurs. Women may have nonspecific symptoms such as dysuria, vaginal discharge, and dyspareunia; or they may be asymptomatic.

## OBJECTIVE DATA

### Physical Examination

A characteristic ulcerative lesion is seen on the genitalia and, in over 50 percent of the cases, a bubo will be present. This unilateral inguinal adenitis is tender and the overlying skin is inflamed. Bubos may spontaneously rupture. One or two lesions are the norm, although more may occur.

### Diagnostic Tests and Methods

***Culture of Ulcers.*** Diagnostic evaluation to isolate *H. ducreyi*. The test procedure is to swab the base of the ulcerative lesion with a cotton or calcium alginate swab. Transport the specimen to a laboratory within 4 hours (refrigerate the swab if transportation time is longer). Do not culture a bubo unless it has ruptured; unruptured bubos are usually sterile.

Explain to the client that a culture is the best test. (A gram stain may be inaccurate, and newer enzyme immunoassay tests are still being developed.) Culture results take up to 1 week.

## DIFFERENTIAL MEDICAL DIAGNOSES

Genital herpes, syphilis, donovanosis.

## PLAN

### Psychosocial Interventions

Chancroid may increase the risk of HIV infection. Advise the client that her sexual partners within the past 10 days need examination and treatment. Symptoms improve within 3 days; ulcers heal within 7 days. Bubos resolve more slowly and may require aspiration.

### Medication

***Erythromycin***

- *Indications.* Suspected or culture-proven chancroid. A presumptive diagnosis is made if the clinical picture is clear.
- *Administration.* 500 mg p.o., q.i.d. for 7 days.

- *Side Effects and Adverse Reactions.* Gastrointestinal distress.
- *Contraindications.* Known hypersensitivity to erythromycin.
- *Anticipated Outcomes on Evaluation.* Ulcerative lesions resolve.
- *Client Teaching and Counseling.* Advise the client to complete the entire course of medication. If no improvement occurs within 7 days, diagnosis must be reconsidered. Infection with other STDs, including HIV, may also exist.

#### *Ceftriaxone*

- *Indications.* A good alternative to erythromycin, especially if client compliance is a concern.
- *Administration.* 250 mg I.M. stat.
- *Side Effects and Adverse Reactions.* Although usually well tolerated, ceftriaxone is occasionally associated with pain at the injection site, diarrhea, rash, and headache.
- *Contraindications.* Known sensitivity to cephalosporins. Use with caution for clients sensitive to penicillin.
- *Anticipated Outcomes on Evaluation.* Treatment failure is rare. Test for cure with this regimen is not essential.
- *Client Teaching and Counseling.* Advise the client to complete all oral medication and report any drug intolerance. If symptoms recur, retesting is necessary. Stress the need for the client's partner to be treated.

#### *Other Medications*

- Azithromycin 1 g orally in a single dose is now suggested as an alternative for ceftriaxone or erythromycin.
- Two other possible alternatives are amoxicillin 500 mg plus clavulanic acid 125 mg p.o. t.i.d. for 7 days or ciprofloxacin 500 mg p.o. b.i.d. for 3 days.
- However, these last two regimens have not been studied in the United States. Amoxicillin plus clavulanic acid may not be used for pregnant or lactating women, children, and adolescents age 17 years and under.[4]

### Follow-Up/Referral

Only if nonresponsive to drug treatment.

## CHLAMYDIA TRACHOMATIS INFECTIONS

The infections associated with *Chlamydia trachomatis* are extremely prevalent among the STDs. The disease spectrum is very similar to that of gonorrhea. Men and women may be asymptomatic or symptomatic. Men primarily develop nonspecific urethritis. In women, chlamydia is associated with cervicitis, salpingitis, and subsequent infertility, acute urethral syndrome, and perihepatitis. Newborns delivered to infected mothers may develop conjunctivitis or pneumonitis. In the adult population worldwide, chlamydia is the etiologic agent of trachoma, the leading cause of preventable blindness. Trachoma is not endemic to the United States, however.

### EPIDEMIOLOGY

*Chlamydia trachomatis* is an obligate intracellular parasite that displays some bacterial properties and some viral properties. Unable to produce its own energy, it depends on the host for survival. Risk factors parallel those of gonorrhea.

Transmission may be *sexual*, requiring direct contact with an infected individual; or *congenital*, acquired at birth when delivery occurs through an infected birth canal. Transplacental transmission does not occur. The incubation period is 10 to 30 days.

Chlamydial infection is not reportable to the CDC; therefore, figures of the exact incidence are unavailable. They are known to be high, however: from 3 to 5 percent among asymptomatic women and 20 percent among women attending STD clinics. The highest rates are among the 15- to 21-year-old age group. Studies indicate that 45 percent of clients with gonorrhea have concurrent chlamydia.[4,12] The estimated number of acute infections annually in the United States is 4 million.

## SUBJECTIVE DATA

Women may be asymptomatic. Subjective symptoms are similar to those seen with gonorrhea and relate to the site of infection. They include vaginal discharge, pelvic pain (dull or severe), fever, dysuria (frequency and urgency). Men report a penile discharge and burning with urination.

## OBJECTIVE DATA

### Physical Examination

Because the majority of women with chlamydial infection are asymptomatic, the physical examination may reveal nothing abnormal. The cervix, however, may show mucopurulent discharge, hypertrophic ectopy, and friability.

### Diagnostic Tests and Methods

A wet mount of the discharge shows numerous white blood cells. Urine culture may be sterile in the presence of urinary symptoms.

***Culture.*** Diagnostic evaluation for symptomatic or asymptomatic chlamydial infection. A culture is the "gold standard" for identification of infection.

The test procedure involves collection of a sample that contains many epithelial cells. This is essential. Cleanse the ectocervix of excessive secretions. Insert a cytologic brush or sterile Dacron-tipped swab 1 to 2 cm into the endocervix. Rotate it and withdraw it. Place the swab in transport media. Refrigerate and transport the swab on ice to a laboratory within 24 hours.

Explain to the client the minor discomfort that may occur with endocervical sampling. Test results take 1 to 2 weeks or more to obtain and are costly. Because of the complex laboratory methods required and their cost, the chlamydial culture test is not widely available.

***Antigen Detection Tests.*** Diagnostic evaluation for symptomatic or asymptomatic infection. This nonculture, rapid detection method uses enzyme linked immunoassay (e.g., Chlamydiazyme) or direct immunofluorescent staining (e.g., Microtrak).

First obtain an adequate sample, as noted above for Culture. Many commercial kits are available. Follow the manufacturer's directions exactly.

Prepare the client for the minor discomfort that may occur with sampling. Advise her that results are available in 1 to 2 days, depending on the method used and laboratory access.

The *direct smear* is best suited to labs that handle a small number of samples. It requires a high quality fluorescent microscope and a well trained technician, and it is labor intensive. The *enzyme linked immunoassay* is better suited to labs that run a large number of samples. They are automated and labor saving. Both are good for screening high-risk populations. If the availability of chlamydial testing is limited, priority should be given to screening adolescents, high-risk pregnant women, and those with multiple sexual partners.

***Papanicolaou (Pap) Smear.*** Diagnostic evaluation is nonspecific for chlamydia but may show a characteristic inflammatory pattern that suggests the need for definitive testing.[19] For test procedure and nursing implications/client teaching, see Chapters 3 and 9.

## DIFFERENTIAL MEDICAL DIAGNOSES

Gonorrhea, salpingitis, urethritis.

## PLAN

### Psychosocial Interventions

Encourage clients to have chlamydia screening if they are in a risk group. Those with multiple partners or a new sexual partner are especially at risk. Partners of individuals diagnosed with chlamydia should be tested and treated; if testing is unavailable, the partners should be treated presumptively. High-risk pregnant women need screening and treatment to prevent congenital transmission. Individuals with chlamydia should be tested for other STDs because of the high rate of concurrent disease.

### Medication

#### *Doxycycline*

- *Indications.* Treatment of uncomplicated urethral, endocervical, and rectal infections in women and men.
- *Administration.* Doxycycline 100 mg p.o., b.i.d. for 7 days.
- *Side Effects and Adverse Reactions.* Gastrointestinal (GI) upset, rash, photosensitivity. Overgrowth of vaginal candida.
- *Contraindications.* Known pregnancy; sensitivity to tetracyclines.
- *Anticipated Outcomes on Evaluation.* Antimicrobial resistance to this treatment has not been observed. Provided that treatment is completed, test for cure is not recommended.
- *Client Teaching and Counseling.* Instruct the client that all medication must be taken. Doxycycline is taken 2 hours after meals and before dairy products are consumed. Use of antacids must be avoided during treatment. Doxycycline is preferable to tetracycline because fewer pills are needed and less GI distress is reported. In addition compliance may be more accurate with doxycycline. Partners should be treated concurrently and should abstain from intercourse until the treatment is completed.

#### *Erythromycin*

- *Indications.* Chlamydial infection during pregnancy.
- *Administration.* 500 mg p.o., q.i.d. for 7 days.
- *Side Effects and Adverse Reactions.* Gastrointestinal distress.
- *Contraindications.* Sensitivity to erythromycin. Pregnant clients who cannot tolerate erythromycin may be treated with sulfisoxazole 500 mg p.o., q.i.d. for 10 days.
- *Anticipated Outcomes on Evaluation.* Because experience in treating with erythromycin and sulfisoxazole is limited, a test for cure 7 days after completion of medication is recommended.[4]
- *Follow-Up and Referral.* Necessary only if the client was nonresponsive to the medication.

#### *Azithromycin*

- *Indications.* Treatment of uncomplicated urethral, endocervical, and rectal infections in women and men.
- *Administration.* 1 gm once p.o.[4,20]
- *Side Effects and Adverse Reactions.* GI side effects are most common; hepatic changes, renal changes, headache, dizziness, rash are less common. Also photosensitivity; overgrowth of vaginal candida.
- *Contraindications.* Known pregnancy; sensitivity to tetracyclines.
- *Anticipated Outcomes on Evaluation.* Similar cure rates as with doxycycline; azithromycin may be indicated if compliance is a concern. Expense must be considered.

#### *Other Medications*

- Alternative regimens are ofloxacin 300 mg p.o., b.i.d. for 7 days *or* erythromycin ethylsuccinate 800 mg p.o., q.i.d. for 7 days *or* sulfisoxazole 500 mg p.o., q.i.d. for 10 days.[4]
- Ofloxacin is more expensive than doxycycline. It cannot be used in pregnancy or with adolescents age 17 years and under. The efficacy of sulfisoxazole is poorer than other regimens.[4]

# DONOVANOSIS

A chronic, progressive bacterial infection of the genitals, donovanosis presents with large, unsightly ulcers of the genitalia, inguinal region, and anus. Other names for the condition are granuloma inguinale and granuloma venereum.

## EPIDEMIOLOGY

*Calymmatobacterium granulomatis*, a gram negative bacterium, is the causative agent. Anal intercourse, often associated with homosexuality, is a particular risk factor. Transmission is by sexual or nonsexual trauma to infected sites, primarily the anus and penis. The disease is mildly contagious; repeated exposures are needed in order for clinical manifestations to develop. The incubation period is not clearly known but is thought to be long.

Rarely reported in the United States, donovanosis is epidemic in parts of Australia and common in India and many tropical and subtropical environments.[12]

## SUBJECTIVE DATA

Single or multiple subcutaneous nodules erode through the skin to form granulomatous lesions; they appear beefy, and are friable, slow growing, and usually painless.

## OBJECTIVE DATA

### Physical Examination

An examination reveals the characteristic lesions, as noted above.

### Diagnostic Tests and Methods

***Wright's or Giemsa Stain.*** Diagnostic evaluation for pathognomonic Donovan bodies (common name for causative organism). The test procedure is to crush/smear a clean piece of granulation tissue on a slide. Air dry, then stain using appropriate Wright's or Giemsa staining technique. Explain to the client that the test procedure is simple and reliable.

## DIFFERENTIAL MEDICAL DIAGNOSES

Chancroid, carcinoma, secondary syphilis, amebiasis.

## PLAN

### Medication

A variety of antibiotics are useful. The first line treatment is tetracycline.

#### *Tetracycline*

- *Indications.* Positive diagnosis of donovanosis.
- *Administration.* Tetracycline 500 mg p.o., q.6h. until lesions have healed.
- *Side Effects and Adverse Reactions.* GI upset, rash, photosensitivity. Overgrowth of vaginal candida.
- *Contraindications.* Pregnancy; allergy to tetracycline.
- *Anticipated Outcomes on Evaluation.* Lesions will heal and Donovan bodies will disappear from the smears.
- *Client Teaching and Counseling.* Advise the client that compliance with treatment is

critical. Medication must be continued until all lesions are healed. This may take 3 to 5 weeks. Discontinuing therapy early results in high recurrence rates.

### Follow-Up and Referral

The client should be seen 1 to 2 months after the initial diagnosis to ensure resolution.

# GENITAL MYCOPLASMA INFECTIONS

These ubiquitous organisms (genital mycoplasmas) are associated with widespread disease among men and women. Mycoplasmas are also frequently found in the absence of disease.

## EPIDEMIOLOGY

Primarily *Mycoplasma hominis* and *Ureaplasma urealyticum.* Sexual contact transmits the disease in adults. Colonization in infants may occur through an infected birth canal, although the disease rarely results and colonization does not persist. The incidence of genital microplasma infections is unknown, but it is very high. Infection is more common among low socioeconomic groups and minorities.

## SUBJECTIVE DATA

Genital mycoplasmas among women have been associated with Bartholin's abscess, vaginitis, pelvic inflammatory disease (PID), postabortion and postpartum sepsis, urinary tract infections (UTIs), infertility, stillbirths, habitual abortion, chorioamnionitis, and low birthweight infants.[12]

## OBJECTIVE DATA

### Physical Examination

Examination depends on the particular disease entity, as noted above. Most individuals who are colonized with genital mycoplasmas are asymptomatic.

### Diagnostic Tests and Methods

***Culture.*** Diagnostic evaluation is done for genital mycoplasmas when the index of suspicion is high (i.e., when the client has one of the conditions associated with mycoplasmas). The test procedure is to do a vaginal culture, which is better than an endocervical culture. An adequate sample from the vagina is necessary to enhance the yield. Obtain the specimens, place them immediately in medium, and transport them to the lab as soon as possible. Keep specimens refrigerated. Mycoplasma culture facilities are not widely available.

Explain the procedure to the client.

## DIFFERENTIAL MEDICAL DIAGNOSES

*Chlamydia trachomatis;* gonorrhea.

## PLAN

### Psychosocial Interventions

Explain to the client the widespread, nonspecific nature of genital mycoplasmas. Also important is providing information that the regular use of barrier contraceptives may reduce colonization with the organism. Reassure the client that the organism may be identified in the absence of a disease process.

### Medication

Clinical syndromes associated with the organism (see Subjective Data) should be kept in mind and treated empirically, because often culture facilities are not available. Standard treatment for gonorrhea and chlamydia as well as pelvic inflammatory disease (PID) and nongonococcal urethritis (NGU) are effective.

## GONORRHEA

Gonorrhea is a classic bacterial STD that can be symptomatic or asymptomatic in both men and women. In women, gonorrhea primarily infects the cervix and fallopian tubes and is a leading cause of PID. Rectal transmission is common with anal intercourse, and pharyngeal transmission with oral sex is possible but rare. Gonorrhea (GC) can be transmitted during birth and cause conjunctivitis and blindness in neonates. Other rare manifestations of gonorrhea include arthritis, meningitis, perihepatitis, and disseminated gonococcal infection. In pregnancy, gonorrhea has been associated with chorioamnionitis, premature labor, premature rupture of membranes, and postpartum endometritis.

### EPIDEMIOLOGY

The causative agent is *Neisseria gonorrhoeae*, a gram-negative intracellular diplococcus. Risk factors include low socioeconomic status, urban residency, nonmarried status, and multiple sexual partners. Women who use oral contraceptives have a higher rate of gonorrhea; women who use spermicides have lower rates. Often, gonorrhea and chlamydia coexist.[20]

Direct sexual contact with mucosal surfaces of an infected individual is required for the transmission of gonorrhea. Although the organism has been recovered from inanimate objects artificially inoculated with the bacteria, there is no evidence that natural transmission occurs this way. The incubation period is 3 to 7 days.

Just under 1 million cases are reported annually in the United States. More than 80 percent are among individuals younger than age 30. Nonwhites with gonorrhea outnumber whites by 10 to 1. The incidence is seasonal, with peaks during late summer.[12]

### SUBJECTIVE DATA

Among women, asymptomatic infection can be present in the urethra, endocervix, rectum, or pharynx. Symptoms may include vaginal discharge, pelvic pain, fever, menstrual irregularities, and dysuria.

### OBJECTIVE DATA

#### Physical Examination

The examination may be normal. Some women exhibit mucopurulent cervicitis, erythema, and friability of the endocervix. Bartholin's abscess is infrequent. Other STDs, among them chlamydia, trichomonas, monilia, and herpes, are frequently seen with gonorrhea and may confound the clinical picture.

#### Diagnostic Tests and Methods

***Culture Using Modified Thayer Martin Medium.*** Diagnostic evaluation for asymptomatic and symptomatic infection. A specimen for culture can be obtained from the urethra, endocervix, rectum, pharynx, or conjunctivae.

The test procedure is to use culture plates that have been stored in the refrigerator and brought to room temperature before inoculation. Use a sterile cotton-tipped swab. For cervical culture, place the swab in the endocervix and rotate for 30 seconds. Transfer the specimen to medium using zigzag technique. Store in a carbon dioxide rich environment, such as a candle extinction jar. Care must be taken in obtaining and storing the specimen.

In addition, advise the client that results are available in 1 week.

***Culture Using Transgrow Medium.*** Diagnostic evaluation for asymptomatic or symptomatic infection. The test procedure is to use a sterile cotton-tipped swab. Place the swab in the endocervix and rotate for 30 seconds. Transfer the specimen to medium. Transgrow bottles are filled with carbon dioxide and must be held upright when uncapped. Swab along the side of the bottle containing medium. Recap and transport to lab.

***Gram Stain.*** Diagnostic evaluation is highly predictive when used for a symptomatic client. The test procedure includes obtaining an endocervical or urethral specimen with a sterile swab and using Gram stain according to standard technique. The presence of typical gram-negative intracellular diplococci is diagnostic of gonorrhea.

Advise the client that immediate results are available.

## DIFFERENTIAL MEDICAL DIAGNOSIS

*Chlamydia trachomatis* infection.

## PLAN

### Psychosocial Interventions

Advise the client that the risk of untreated gonorrhea is the development of PID and subsequent infertility. Sexual partners must be treated concurrently and abstain from intercourse during their treatment. With proper treatment gonorrhea is curable. Check for other STDs, especially syphilis, as multiple infections are common. Pregnant clients should be screened at the first prenatal visit, and those at high risk should be rescreened late in the third trimester.

### Medication

#### *Ceftriaxone*

- *Indications.* Uncomplicated urethral, endocervical, and rectal infection.
- *Administration.* Ceftriaxone 125 *or* 250 mg I.M. once *plus* doxycycline 100 mg p.o., b.i.d. for 7 days. For pregnant clients, substitute erythromycin 500 mg p.o., q.i.d. for 7 days in place of doxycycline.
- *Side Effects and Adverse Reactions.* Although usually well tolerated, ceftriaxone has occasionally been associated with pain at injection site, diarrhea, rash, and headache. Doxycycline is also well tolerated but may occasionally produce GI upset, rash, and overgrowth of fungi in both the vagina and intestines. Photosensitivity has been reported. May be taken with food or milk; avoid antacids.
- *Contraindications.* Known sensitivity to cephalosporins or tetracyclines. In pregnancy and lactation, tetracyclines are not used. Ceftriaxone should be used with caution in clients sensitive to penicillin.
- *Anticipated Outcomes on Evaluation.* Treatment failure is rare. Test for cure with this regimen is not essential. Antibiotic resistant organisms, however, increase significantly; therefore, if a follow-up culture is done, it is indicated at 3 to 7 days posttherapy.[20]
- *Client Teaching and Counseling.* Advise the client to complete all oral medication and report any drug intolerance. If symptoms recur, retesting is needed. Stress the need for the partner's treatment.

#### *Other Medications*

- Other recommended regimens for uncomplicated gonococcal infections among adolescents and adults include cefixime 400 mg p.o. in a single dose *or* Ciprofloxacin 500 mg p.o. in a single dose *or* Ofloxacin 400 mg p.o. in a single dose. All of these drugs must be given with 7 days of doxycycline 100 mg p.o., b.i.d.[4]

Recommended treatment schedules for special circumstances and complications are available from the CDC.[4,20]

## HEPATITIS A

Hepatitis A, or infectious hepatitis, is a viral inflammation of the liver resulting in a clinical syndrome of jaundice, malaise, nausea, vomiting, and fever.

### EPIDEMIOLOGY

*Hepatitis A virus* (HAV) is the causative organism. At particular risk are parents of children in diapers, daycare workers, residents and staff of institutions for the mentally handicapped, and travelers to developing nations.

Transmission is by any practice that allows fecal–oral spread. The virus is transmitted by hand after touching the diapers or linens of infected individuals or using common household items such as glasses and eating utensils of infected individuals, via contaminated water, and by ingesting raw shellfish. Sexual practices that include oral–anal contact favor transmission of HAV. Daycare centers provide a significant reservoir of HAV. Because infants often do not have the jaundice associated with HAV, the disease goes unrecognized and is passed to other infants in the daycare setting and to adult caretakers, parents, and siblings. The average incubation period is 4 weeks. An infected individual is contagious 2 weeks prior to the onset of symptoms and up to 1 week after their onset.[12]

Annual incidence in the United States is low, ranging from 4 to 30 per 100,000. Less than 10 percent of hepatitis cases are due to HAV. Improved sanitation has led to a declining prevalence.[8]

### SUBJECTIVE DATA

Children under 3 years of age rarely develop symptoms; adults almost always do. Symptoms include malaise, low grade fever, diarrhea, nausea and vomiting, and loss of appetite. Symptoms have rapid onset and usually last about 1 week.

### OBJECTIVE DATA

#### Physical Examination

Examination reveals jaundice, fever, and possibly right upper-quadrant abdominal pain. Chronic hepatitis and carrier states do not occur with HAV infection.

#### Diagnostic Tests and Methods

***Serologic Immunoassay.*** Diagnostic evaluation for antibodies to the hepatitis A antigen (anti-HAV). IgM anti-HAV occurs with early acute and acute infections, and total (IgG and IgM) anti-HAV persists for life. The test procedure is to obtain a blood sample. Advise the client that the test is highly accurate when symptoms are present.

***Liver Enzymes.*** Diagnostic evaluation to determine abnormal liver function. The test procedure is to collect a blood sample. Advise the client that enzymes may be elevated.

### DIFFERENTIAL MEDICAL DIAGNOSES

Hepatitis B, C, or D; cirrhosis.

### PLAN

#### Psychosocial Interventions

Advise the client to rest and eat a balanced diet. Hands should be washed well after using the toilet. Educate the client not to prepare or handle food for others; to avoid ingesting substances that require primary liver metabolism, such as alcohol and large doses of vitamins; and to take only essential medications. In addition, inform the client that hepatitis A virus confers lifelong immunity.[12]

### Medication

#### *Immune Globulin (IG)*

- *Indications.* If administered within 2 weeks of exposure, immune globulin is very effective against contracting HAV.
- *Administration.* Intramuscular injection, 0.02 mL/kg.
- *Side Effects and Adverse Reactions.* Side effects are minimal. Some local inflammation occurs at the injection site.
- *Contraindications.* None are known.
- *Anticipated Outcomes on Evaluation.* Exposed individuals will not contract the disease.
- *Client Teaching and Counseling.* Postexposure prophylaxis is recommended for all household and sexual contacts of clients with HAV. Prophylaxis is also recommended for daycare and institution workers where HAV transmission has been documented. It is required for travel to some foreign countries. Local health departments can advise concerning requirements.

***Hepatitis A Vaccine.*** This is currently being studied for anticipated public use in the near future.

# HEPATITIS B

Hepatitis B, or serum hepatitis, is a viral inflammation of the liver that results in a broad spectrum of disease: from mild illness and chronic carrier state to cirrhosis, liver cancer, and death secondary to liver failure. An important implication of hepatitis B is its transmission from a pregnant woman to her newborn at birth.

## EPIDEMIOLOGY

*Hepatitis B virus* (HBV) is the causative organism. Those at special risk include intravenous drug users, heterosexuals and homosexuals with multiple partners, contacts of HBV carriers, infants of HBV-infected mothers, health workers who have contact with blood, and people born in areas where HBV is endemic. Hepatitis B may be transmitted parenterally, sexually, or perinatally. The incubation period ranges from 6 weeks to 8 months.

Annually, 300,000 cases are reported; the majority are adults. More than half are symptomatic and 10,000 require hospitalization. In addition, 350 deaths occur due to fulminant disease. The CDC estimates that there are 1 million HBV carriers in the United States.[12]

## SUBJECTIVE DATA

Many persons have asymptomatic infection and develop lifelong immunity. The symptoms, which may be mild or severe, include fatigue, loss of appetite, nausea/vomiting, diarrhea, malaise, and myalgias. The onset of symptoms is usually gradual, and resolution is slow.

## OBJECTIVE DATA

### Physical Examination

Examination reveals jaundice, low grade fever, dark urine, light-colored bowel movements.

### Diagnostic Tests and Methods

***Serologic Immunoassay (Radioimmunoassay or Enzyme Immunoassay).*** Diagnostic evaluation for anti-HBc (antibody to HBV core antigen, lifetime marker for past or active/acute or chronic infection). One marker for hepatitis B is HBsAg (HBV surface antigen), the earliest marker for acute infection. It can, however, indicate chronicity. Another marker, HBeAg (HBV early antigen), indicates an extremely infectious phase in the disease process. If HBeAg persists more than 10 weeks, it may indicate chronicity or liver disease. Anti-HBc IgM (IgM specific antibody to HBV core antigen) and anti-HBc (total IgM and IgG antibody to core antigen) indicate that an acute phase with a seroconversion process is occurring. A negative HBsAg with continuance of positive anti-HBc IgM, anti-HBc, and anti-Hbe indicates a convalescent state; however, the client is still considered infectious. In early recovery, anti-HBc, anti-HBe, and anti-HBs remain positive, but infectiousness is unclear. Recovery finds the latter markers still positive and immune status is conferred at this time.

The test procedure is to obtain blood sample. Advise the client that blood testing is highly accurate and can determine active infection, chronic infection, and immune status.[21]

## DIFFERENTIAL MEDICAL DIAGNOSES

Hepatitis A, C, and D.

## PLAN

### Psychosocial Interventions

Advise the client to rest and eat a nutritious diet. Activity restrictions are based on how the individual feels. Sexual partners and household contacts should be tested and immunized as appropriate. In addition to vaccination, general counseling to prevent HBV includes information about using latex condoms and spermicides, limiting sexual partners, and not sharing needles, razors, toothbrushes, and other personal items.

### Medication

#### Hepatitis B Immune Globulin (HBIG)

- *Indications.* Sexual contacts of clients with acute HBV, those who have sexual contact with HBV carriers, and newborns of mothers with HBV.
- *Administration.* Intramuscular injection, 0.06 mL/kg. In neonates, 0.5 cc I.M. is given at birth, followed by HBV vaccination.
- *Side Effects and Adverse Reactions.* Minimal, local irritation at the injection site.
- *Contraindications.* None known.
- *Anticipated Outcomes on Evaluation.* Highly effective, immediate immunity, although temporary.
- *Client Teaching and Counseling.* HBIG should be given within 24 to 48 hours of HBV exposure.[4]

#### Hepatitis B Vaccination

- *Indications.* Persons with multiple sexual partners, homosexual/bisexual men, illicit intravenous drug users, prison inmates and other institutionalized individuals, prostitutes, health care workers with exposure to blood products, infants of HBV infected mothers, clients attending STD clinics, and household or sexual contacts of HBV carriers. Universal vaccination of newborns is now recommended.[4]
- *Administration.* Requires three intramuscular injections: an initial injection, another 1 month later, and the third at 6 months. The deltoid muscle should be used.
- *Side Effects and Adverse Reactions.* Minimal, local soreness at injection site.
- *Contraindications.* None.
- *Anticipated Outcomes on Evaluation.* Active immunity to HBV has occurred, lasting 5 years or longer. Postvaccination testing to confirm immunity is not routinely recommended.[11]
- *Client Teaching and Counseling.* Educate the client that prevaccination HBV

testing is recommended only for very high risk groups where the presence of HBV antibodies would negate the necessity of vaccination. The cost effectiveness of such testing in moderate risk groups must be considered. HBsAg positive individuals who receive the vaccine are unharmed.

## HERPES SIMPLEX VIRUS (HSV)

No cure is known for this acute, recurring viral disease. Characteristic painful lesions can occur in the mouth and genitalia, of men and women, although virtually any skin or mucous membrane is vulnerable. Children develop oral lesions as well. Neonates who contract the virus congenitally develop infection of the central nervous system (CNS) and eyes. Significant perinatal morbidity and mortality are associated with congenital herpes simplex. Once it enters the body, the herpes virus never leaves, although clinical manifestations disappear as the virus becomes dormant (it is believed in neural ganglia). When recurrence is triggered, the virus travels from nerve roots to the skin surface, where lesions develop. Many clients with HSV infection are asymptomatic.

### EPIDEMIOLOGY

Herpes simplex virus type 1 (HSV-1) produces oral lesions, and herpes simplex virus type 2 (HSV-2) produces genital lesions. Differentiation of the two types is academic because they are transmitted identically, their symptomatology is the same, and the procedures for diagnosis and treatment are the same.

Herpes simplex virus is transmitted by direct contact with an infected individual who is shedding the virus. Kissing, sexual contact, and vaginal delivery are means of transmission. Primary herpes in pregnancy may be passed to the neonate transplacentally. Autoinoculation is possible.

The transmission rate of primary HSV in pregnancy may be as high as 50 percent, whereas neonatal transmission of recurrent HSV is estimated to be only 3 to 5 percent. The incubation period of HSV is 7 to 10 days.

Nationwide statistics on the incidence of HSV are not available in the United States. Prevalence of both genital and neonatal herpes increased markedly from 1960 to 1980. The rate is slightly higher for nonwhites than whites, and higher for women than men.[12] A total prevalence of 20 to 30 million cases with 500,000 new cases per year is estimated.[22]

### SUBJECTIVE DATA

*Primary herpes* is a systemic disease characterized by multiple painful vesicular lesions, fever, chills, malaise, and severe dysuria if the lesions are genital. Symptoms peak 4 to 5 days after onset and may last 2 to 3 weeks. *Recurrent herpes*, on the other hand, is a localized disease characterized by typical HSV lesions at the site of initial viral entry. Recurrent herpes lesions usually are fewer, are less sensitive, and resolve more rapidly than primary herpes lesions. Recurrent HSV lasts an average of 5 to 7 days, preceded by a prodromal symptom—frequently a burning, itching or swelling sensation. Lesions will appear within 24 hours of prodrome.

### OBJECTIVE DATA

#### Physical Examination

Characteristic lesions are visible. They are vesicular, usually multiple, and exquisitely painful to touch. The vesicles will open and weep and finally crust over, dry, and disappear without scar formation. Clients with primary HSV may have low grade fever and tender lymphadenopathy.

### Diagnostic Tests and Methods

***Viral Culture.*** Diagnostic evaluation for primary and recurrent HSV infections, which are often diagnosed by clinical signs and symptoms. The culture yield is best if the specimen is taken during the vesicular stage of disease; viral isolation is markedly reduced as lesions resolve. In primary episodes, viral shedding is prolonged and HSV more easily isolated.

The test procedure involves vigorously rubbing the lesion with a cotton- or Dacron-tipped swab. Vesicular fluid is obtained whenever possible; it is high in viral particles. When lesions are large, vesicu-lar fluid can be aspirated. Once obtained, place the sample in appropriate transport medium. Do not allow the swab to dry. When performing a cervical culture, a cotton or Dacron swab should be inserted in the endocervix and rotated. The same swab should then be rubbed over the ectocervix.

Advise the client that obtaining the culture will be painful because vigorous sampling is essential to collect adequate cells. A preliminary report will be available within 48 hours, but final results may take 1 to 2 weeks.

***Pap Smear.*** Diagnostic evaluation for multinucleated giant cells with intranuclear inclusions. Cytology is a specific but not sensitive test.

The test procedure is to identify giant cells, which are highly reliable for diagnosis if identified. When sending a specimen from a genital lesion for cytological examination, use the same technique as described above in Viral Culture. The swab should be transferred to a glass slide and fixed immediately.

Cytology is inexpensive, and the procedure is readily carried out. Inform the client that discomfort is likely when obtaining the sample.

***Serologic Testing for HSV Antibodies.*** Diagnostic evaluation may be accomplished by antibody testing to document past infection with HSV-1 and HSV-2. In addition, it may be useful to differentiate seronegative individuals from seropositive individuals and asymptomatic carriers. Many widely used serological assays, however, do not differentiate HSV-1 and HSV-2 antibodies and do not reliably predict recurrent infection. Furthermore, serological testing is not always reliable. Hence, it should be used with caution.

## DIFFERENTIAL MEDICAL DIAGNOSES

Primary syphilis, mucocutaneous manifestations of Crohn's disease, Behçet's syndrome, chancroid, lymphogranuloma venereum (LGV).

## PLAN

### Psychosocial Interventions

Clients diagnosed with herpes require extensive counseling to understand the complex nature of the disease and its ramifications. Support groups may be helpful. Advise clients to abstain from intercourse during the prodrome and when lesions are present in any stage. Consistent condom use may reduce transmission rates. In addition, clients must know to wash their hands to avoid autoinoculation. Risk of acquiring HIV may be enhanced while genital lesions are present.

There is no evidence that HSV causes cervical cancer. Earlier suspicions that implicated it as an etiologic agent of cervical malignancy have been laid to rest.[12] Annual Pap smears, however, are recommended for women with HSV infection—as they are with all sexually transmitted diseases (STDs), because STD is an epidemiological risk factor for cervical cancer development. Undoubtedly this relates to beginning sexual intercourse at an early age and having multiple sexual partners.

Client with genital HSV, both primary and recurrent, will benefit from such comfort measures as nonconstricting clothes, lukewarm sitz baths, and air drying of lesions with a hand-held hair dryer on medium setting. Clients with severe dysuria may benefit by urinating in water. Extremes of temperature such as ice packs or heating pads should be avoided, as should steroid creams, anesthetic sprays, and any type of lotion or gel (e.g., petroleum jelly).

#### Management of Recurrent HSV in Pregnancy

- Culture recurrent lesions to document HSV.
- Know that routine viral cultures do not predict viral shedding at delivery and are not recommended.
- Examine the client carefully at onset of labor for evidence of signs, symptoms, or prodrome (if none are present, vaginal delivery is indicated).
- Take a specimen for culture at delivery, which may be helpful to determine neonatal management.
- Know that evidence of active infection at the onset of labor will necessitate a cesarean section.[22]

### Medication

#### Acyclovir (Zovirax)

- *Indications.* Primary herpes infection and severe recurrent disease. Clients with frequent recurrences (more than six per year) may benefit from daily suppressive therapy. The safety and effectiveness for up to 3 years of acyclovir use have been documented.
- *Administration. For primary HSV:* 200 mg p.o., 5 times daily for 7 to 10 days or until symptoms resolve. *For recurrent HSV:* 200 mg p.o., 5 times daily for 5 days, *or* 800 mg p.o., 2 times daily for 5 days. *Daily suppression:* 200 mg p.o., 2 to 5 times daily. Dosage may be individualized.
- *Side Effects and Adverse Reactions.* These are minimal, even with long term use. Nausea, vomiting, and headache have been reported, however. Clients on long term suppression can expect a rebound recurrence when therapy is stopped.
- *Contraindications.* Known hypersensitivity to acyclovir.
- *Anticipated Outcomes on Evaluation.* Accelerated healing and shortened course of the disease.
- *Client Teaching and Counseling.* Advise the client that acyclovir neither eradicates HSV nor has an impact on the subsequent risk and frequency of recurrences. Clients on daily suppressive therapy should stop after 1 year and reevaluate the recurrence rate. Topical therapy with acyclovir ointment is substantially less effective than oral medications.[4,12] Safe use during pregnancy has *not* been established and should be used only for life-threatening maternal HSV. Advise the client not to exceed recommended doses and not to share acyclovir with others.[4]

## HUMAN PAPILLOMAVIRUS (HPV) INFECTION

Clinically visible or subclinically invisible lesions on the external genitalia, perineum, anus, vaginal mucosa, and/or cervix occur in this infectious viral disease. Both sexes may exhibit the lesions. Sometimes they are a precursor to vulvar and cervical dysplasia. Other names for the condition are condylomata acuminata, venereal warts, and genital warts.

### EPIDEMIOLOGY

Human papillomavirus (HPV) is a slow growing DNA virus of the papovavirus family; more than 60 strains are identified. Strains 16, 18, 31, 33, 35, 39, 51, and 56 are known to be oncogenic with a propensity for the reproductive tract, especially the cervix; 16 and 18 are more often associated with invasive cervical cancer[23]; 6 and 11 with benign lesions or mild dysplasia. More than one type may be present at one time.

HPV is most commonly spread by means of sexual or other intimate contact. The organism may have limited survival on fomites, but nonsexual transmission is rare and difficult to document. Autoinoculation and mother–child transfer at birth can occur. The incubation period is 1 to 6 months or longer; the virus may remain latent for decades.

An estimated 3 million people are infected annually. Human papillomavirus infection is thought to be the most common viral sexually transmitted disease (STD) in the United States. Incidence has increased markedly in the past decade; 10 to 15 million are thought to be infected. Among cases of abnormal cervical cytology, 80 to 96 percent are associated with HPV.[24]

## SUBJECTIVE DATA

The infection is usually visible as wartlike growths or "bumps," usually painless. Less commonly, malodorous vaginal discharge, pain and burning with urination, pruritis, and bleeding during and after coitus occur. The lack of visible lesions or complaints is not uncommon, however. A woman may have a history of an infected partner, but have no evidence of infection. Lesions may grow so large in pregnancy as to affect urination, defecation, mobility, and descent of the fetus, although rarely is cesarean delivery necessitated.[25]

## OBJECTIVE DATA

### Physical Examination

Genitalia/reproductive tract shows one or more soft, pale, pink or flesh-colored, dry, irregular lesions on the external genitalia, perineum, or anus. The lesions, 1 mm or larger, may be flat vulvar or bowenoid papules, hairlike papillae, or pedunculated papules on the vulva, introitus, vagina, cervix, perineum, urethra, and/or anus. Large lesions may be cauliflower-like in appearance, exist in coalesced clusters, and be friable. Areas most often traumatized during coitus are common sites.

### Diagnostic Tests and Methods

No one test alone is advocated.

***Pap Smear (Cytology).*** Screening evaluation to identify koilocytosis, dyskaryosis, keratinizing atypia on traditional reports, or cellular changes associated with HPV on Bethesda System reports. A Pap smear is diagnostic; the sample can miss the lesion. Hence, it is useful for screening only. Be suspicious of HPV infection if Pap results show squamous atypia, atypical inflammation, parakeratosis, koilocytosis, or other terms that suggest HPV. Refer for colposcopy if Pap is suspicious.

For test procedure and implications, see Chapters 3 and 9.

***Colposcopy with Directed Biopsy (Histology).*** Diagnostic evaluation for subclinical lesions, dysplasia, and malignancy, performed by trained, experienced colposcopist using colposcope. The procedure provides a magnified view of direct biopsy sites. An abnormal Pap report, cervical lesions, or extensive lesions warrant referral for colposcopy. Some professionals advise colposcopy with any visible lesion. Endocervical curettage should not be performed if the client is pregnant.

The test procedure includes the application of 3 to 5 percent acetic acid to the tissue of the vulva or cervix. After several seconds, abnormal areas turn white. The tissue is then examined under magnification with the colposcope. Directed biopsy is done on the most abnormal sites (e.g., acetowhite with punctation and mosaic pattern).

Explain the procedure to the client: no anesthesia required; lithotomy position; instrument introduced through wide speculum opening; uncomfortable stinging from acetic acid; pinching, cramping sensation when tissue is removed. Tell the client that no excessive bleeding should occur, although a blood-tinged discharge may continue for 2 to 3 days; no coitus, douching, tampon use, or putting other objects in the vagina for 3 days.

***DNA Typing (Nucleic Acid Hybridization Tests).*** Diagnostic evaluation to determine the specific HPV strain; may be useful to identify latent infection. The test procedure includes the use of Virapap and ViraType HPV detection kits, which are commercially available but limited in the number of HPV strains they are able to detect. Other DNA probes are being researched. Obtaining an adequate sample is critical; the cytologic brush method appears to be most effective.

Explain to the client that HPV typing may identify particularly virulent strains of the virus. Explain the procedure and that its cost may be high. In addition, results take a long time and false negatives do occur. (DNA typing is not considered cost effective for mass screening.)

## DIFFERENTIAL MEDICAL DIAGNOSES

Condyloma lata, molluscum contagiosum; carcinoma; concomitant sexually transmitted diseases.

## PLAN

Considerable disagreement exists regarding protocols and recommendations for diagnosis and treatments. The goal of treatment is to eliminate lesions and dysplasia, not annihilate the virus.

### Psychosocial Interventions

Implications for counseling include relationship dissatisfaction, depression, and fear regarding secondary diagnosis (dysplasia leading to cancer). Referral may be indicated. Discuss treatment options with the client (and partner, if appropriate); fully involve her in the therapy plans.

Emotionally, HPV infection may affect self-esteem, body image, feelings (shame, guilt, or blame), satisfaction with intimate relationships, and overall mental health. Anxiety associated with knowing one has a potentially malignant disease and lack of a definitive cure may necessitate referral for psychological counseling and support. Partners should also be counseled. A client's concerns may relate to sharing with future partners the fact that she has the disease. Through education about HPV, anxiety may be reduced. Involvement in controlling decisions empowers the client by decreasing her dependency.[25]

### Medication

***Trichloracetic Acid (TCA)—80 to 90 percent.***

- *Indications.* To decrease external genital and vaginal lesions, therefore, viral shedding.
- *Administration.* Application of an 85 percent TCA or BCA solution to lesions, using a cotton swab and avoiding the surrounding tissue. Area will turn white. A mixture of baking soda and water may be applied to neutralize the acid after application. Applications are repeated once weekly; may be repeated twice weekly if the client can tolerate it.
- *Side Effects and Adverse Reactions.* Burning sensation on application should resolve quickly. There may be erythema, tenderness, swelling, and sloughing of tissue in the area for a few days after application. No systemic effects.

- *Contraindications.* TCA and BCA are contraindicated with severely irritated tissues. The medication has been used safely in pregnancy.
- *Anticipated Outcomes on Evaluation.* Lesions will become smaller and finally disappear after a few applications. If no visible improvement occurs after three treatments, use another method. If lesions persist or are multiple or internal, refer the client to a specialist.
- *Client Teaching and Counseling.* Tell the client that it is not necessary to wash off the acid. Persistent leukorrhea, increased pain, and redness may indicate infection. Spotting or bleeding may occur if the healing tissue is jarred. Nonoxynol-9 cream applied to treated areas at bedtime may help healing. In addition, lidocaine (Xylocaine) ointment may be given, or warm sitz baths and a baking soda/water mixture may soothe.

***Podophyllin.*** 10 to 25 percent in tincture of benzoin compound.

- *Indications.* For external lesions only.
- *Administration.* Compound is applied to the lesion using a cotton swab and avoiding normal tissue. Unaffected areas may be protected by applying petroleum or lubricant jelly to them. Podophyllin must be washed off 4 hours after application. Applications are repeated weekly; more frequent use may result in burning.
- *Side Effects and Adverse Reactions.* Erythema, burning, swelling, tissue damage. Lesions may become tender several days after treatment.
- *Contraindications.* Pregnancy or presence of large warts. Absorption may cause toxicity.
- *Anticipated Outcomes on Evaluation.* The same as for trichloracetic acid (TCA), above. Do not exceed four application times if no significant improvement results.
- *Client Teaching and Counseling.* Provide the client with information about the signs of toxicity: nausea, vomiting, lethargy, coma, paralysis. Repeated use may be carcinogenic. Instruct the client to wash off podophyllin 4 hours after application with mild soap and water; sooner if irritation causes discomfort.

***Other Medications***

- Podofilox 0.5%, a self-treatment, may be prescribed.[4] Advise the client to apply it twice a day only to the warts for 3 days with a cotton swab. The treatment may be repeated after 4 days of no therapy for a total of 4 cycles. The healthcare provider must teach wart identification, proper medicine application, and avoidance of getting any solution on other areas. The total treatment area should be 10 cm or less. No more than 0.5 mL of solution should be used daily. It is not used in pregnancy.[4]
- Podophyllin and TCA, in combination or alternated. These two agents may be alternated on a weekly basis (see above). Either podophyllin or TCA is used initially. The other drug is used the next week; the initial drug the third week. After three treatments, some other treatment is indicated.

***Liquid Nitrogen Cryotherapy***

- *Indications.* External warts. For internal lesions, the client is referred to a gynecologist.
- *Administration.* Application may be accomplished with a finely twisted cotton tip, or the wooden end of a cotton-tipped applicator, or a special applicator jet. The lesion will turn white. Cryotherapy, 10 to 20 seconds. May be followed by application of podophyllin or TCA.
- *Side Effects and Adverse Reactions.* The same as for TCA and podophyllin.
- *Contraindications.* None.
- *Anticipated Outcomes on Evaluation.* The lesions will disappear in 1 to 2 weeks.

- *Client Teaching and Counseling.* Inform the client that the application of the drug may burn. For the discomfort, the same teaching and counseling as used for application of TCA or podophyllin are appropriate.

***5-Fluorouracil 5 % Cream (Efudex)***

- *Indications.* To treat widespread vaginal warts and biopsy-proven subclinical vaginal disease. It is a cytotoxic agent and not useful for external warts, because side effects are too severe.
- *Administration.* Treatment protocols vary widely. *Treatment*: 1/3 to 1/2 applicator deep in the vagina at bedtime once a week for 10 weeks. *Prophylaxis*: 1/2 applicator deep in the vagina once every 2 weeks at bedtime for 6 months. Insert a tampon just inside the introitus and protect the vulva with zinc oxide.[26]
- *Side Effects and Adverse Reactions.* Watery vaginal discharge. Applications that are more frequent than once weekly cause much irritation and pain in the surrounding tissues.
- *Contraindications.* Pregnancy: During pregnancy the drug is teratogenic. No systemic toxicity is usual.
- *Anticipated Outcomes on Evaluation.* Vaginal warts will disappear and the Pap smear return to normal. The client should be reevaluated in 3 months.
- *Client Teaching and Counseling.* Include information about inflammation, discharge, and local discomfort caused by 5-fluorouracil. Severe pain and burning are *not* usual. A vaginal tampon may be inserted after application to reduce irritation to other tissues. Effective contraception is essential.

## Surgery and Other Interventions

Indications are internal lesions, large lesions, or external lesions unresponsive to prior therapy. The client is referred to a trained, experienced specialist.

***Laser Carbon Dioxide Vaporization.*** This outpatient procedure is done with the client under general or regional anesthesia or heavy sedation. A laser beam vaporizes large areas of lesions without scarring. Small lesions are done under local anesthesia.

During the procedure, warmth and menstrual-like cramps are felt. Pain after treatment is mild to moderate; profuse, watery discharge occurs for up to 2 weeks. Healing takes 3 to 4 weeks. For pregnant women, trichloracetic acid (TCA) is used with laser vaporization to decrease time of treatment. For nonpregnant women, 5-F cream may be used as a follow-up. This may improve the cure rate. The secondary infection rate is higher with large treatment areas.

***Cryosurgery (Nitrous Oxide).*** Cryosurgery is performed as an office procedure for cervical disease (dysplasia). Nitrous oxide is the freezing agent of choice. The cryoprobe is applied to the cervix using a 3–5–3 minute technique. Mild to moderate cramping during the procedure usually subsides once freezing is complete. A profuse, watery, foul-smelling vaginal discharge continues for 2 to 3 weeks. Nothing is to be put into the vagina for 3 weeks. The client may shower or bathe in a clean tub.

***Surgical Excision.*** Performed on an outpatient or inpatient basis, depending on the extent of disease. Healing varies with the degree of trauma, but generally takes 2 to 3 weeks for smaller lesions.

***Interferon.*** Interferon is an antiviral agent thought to reduce human papillomavirus (HPV) lesions by improving the immune system. It is injected directly into lesions three times per week for 1 month. Useful for recalcitrant cases or immunosuppressed clients. This expensive treatment is available primarily in medical centers. Side effects include fever, flu-like symptoms, and malaise.

### Long Term Follow-Up

Requirements for screening Pap smears and/or colposcopy are at the discretion of the health care provider. A normal Pap smear is to be followed by another smear every 6 months. Routine pelvic examinations are indicated annually. Self-examination of external genitalia is recommended.

# LYMPHOGRANULOMA VENEREUM (LGV)

The most common manifestation of this chronic bacterial STD is inguinal lymphadenopathy. It is rarely seen in the United States but endemic to parts of Africa, Asia, and South America.[12]

## EPIDEMIOLOGY

The causative organism is *Chlamydia trachomatis* serovars: L1, L2, and L3. In the United States, LGV is more common in urban settings, in lower socioeconomic classes, and among the sexually promiscuous.[27] Men with the disease outnumber women by 5 to 1. The incubation period is 3 to 12 days or longer.

## SUBJECTIVE DATA

Clients are usually asymptomatic, however, may report genital ulcers and painful groin nodes. A wide variety of nonspecific symptoms may be present.

## OBJECTIVE DATA

### Physical Examination

Tender inguinal lymphadenopathy is the most common sign. A spectrum of other clinical symptoms may occur, including papules, ulcers, herpetic-type lesions of the groin, nongonococcal urethritis, cervicitis, proctitis, bubo formation (tender lymphadenitis), and genital edema.

### Diagnostic Tests and Methods

Serological tests using fixation, neutralizing antibody, or immunofluorescents are available. Because LGV is so rare in the United States, specific information should be obtained from the local laboratory when testing is required.

## DIFFERENTIAL MEDICAL DIAGNOSES

Chancroid, genital herpes, syphilis.

## PLAN

### Psychosocial Interventions

Prevention is critical. When LGV is diagnosed, all sexual contacts must be identified and treated to eliminate a reservoir of continued transmission.[4]

### Medication

*Clients should be referred to an infectious disease specialist if LGV is suspected.* Antibiotic therapy is indicated, and adequate treatment and follow-up are essential.

***Tetracyclines***

- *Administration.* Doxycycline 100 mg p.o., b.i.d. for 21 days. Tetracycline 500 mg p.o., q.i.d. for 21 days.
- *Side Effects and Contraindications.* The same as those discussed in the section on tetracycline therapy for chlamydia.
- *Anticipated Outcomes on Evaluation.* Resolution of symptoms. Relapse is common, as is spontaneous remission. No test of cure is available.
- *Client Teaching and Counseling.* Assist the client to complete the medication regimen, which is difficult because it lasts 21 days.

#### *Other Medications*

- Alternative treatment regimens include erythromycin 500 mg p.o., q.i.d. for 21 days *or* sulfisoxazole 500 mg p.o., q.i.d. for 21 days.[4]

## MOLLUSCUM CONTAGIOSUM

This benign, viral, papular infection occurs on the abdomen, thighs, and genitals of adults and on the face, trunk, and extremities of children. The infection is often minor and self-limited. Another name for the condition is seed wart.

### EPIDEMIOLOGY

Molluscum contagiosum virus (MCV), a member of the pox virus family, is the causative organism. In adults, transmission is primarily sexual; in children, it is nonsexual and via fomites. Autoinoculation may also occur. The incubation period ranges from 1 week to 6 months (2 to 3 month average). The exact incidence is unknown, but is thought to be low.

### SUBJECTIVE DATA

The client is asymptomatic, and diagnosis is often made when treatment is sought for some other reason.

### OBJECTIVE DATA

#### Physical Examination

A firm, smooth, nontender dome-shaped papule with a central umbilication is seen (may be single or multiple). Diagnosis is often made upon sight of a characteristic lesion.[12]

#### Diagnostic Tests and Methods

***Punch Biopsy.*** A diagnostic evaluation for the characteristic histological changes if visual diagnosis is uncertain. The test procedure is to apply topical anesthetic ointment to the lesion, infiltrate with lidocaine, and obtain tissue with a punch biopsy instrument. Apply pressure to the area. Monsel's solution will stop excessive bleeding if needed. Apply an adhesive bandage. Check with the client about allergy to procaine hydrochloride (Novocain). Advise her that something like a "bee sting" may be felt when the anesthetic is injected. The biopsy site should be kept clean and dry. Test results are available in 1 week.

### DIFFERENTIAL MEDICAL DIAGNOSES

Genital warts, genital herpes, dermatologic folliculitis.

### PLAN

#### Psychosocial Interventions

Reassure the client that MCV is benign, self-limiting, and grows slowly. Many cases spontaneously resolve over time. Bacterial superinfection may require a systemic antibiotic, but such a condition is rare. Advocate good handwashing.

#### Medication

No medication is very effective against MCV. Podophyllin, trichloracetic acid, and silver nitrate applications have been tried but are often unsuccessful and require multiple applications.[12]

#### Surgical Interventions

Unroofing the lesion with a fine gauge needle to remove the central core is effective and practical if there are only a few lesions. Multiple lesions have been successfully treated using cryotherapy with liquid nitrogen; direct destruction is achieved.

## PEDICULOSIS PUBIS

A species of human lice causes this common sexually transmitted disease. Another name for this condition is pubic lice or crabs. Body and head lice also occur in humans, but do not infect the pubic area. Pubic lice, however, have been found in axillae, beards, eyebrows, and eyelashes.

### EPIDEMIOLOGY

*Phthirus pubis* is the crab louse. It requires human blood to survive. Off the host, pubic lice will die within 24 hours. Sexual or other direct contact must occur for transmission. Some cases of fomite transmission have been documented. The examination table and toilet used by the client will need to be washed with an appropriate disinfectant, or the rooms may be closed for the life span of the lice (24 hours) if this is feasible.

Estimates are that 3 million cases of pediculosis are treated annually, including both pubic and head lice. Young adults have the highest incidence of pubic lice; prevalence declines after age 35.[12]

### SUBJECTIVE DATA

Itching is the primary symptom. It leads to scratching, erythema, and skin irritation. The client may be asymptomatic. Some clients report small dark red or black "dots" (excrement of the pubic lice) in their panties.

### OBJECTIVE DATA

#### Physical Examination

Adult lice may be viewed moving along pubic hairs. Eggs (nits) appear as minute white dots adherent to pubic hair. Occasionally small scabs (crab bites) are noted on underlying skin.

#### Diagnostic Tests and Methods

Characteristic lice and nits may be observed.

### DIFFERENTIAL MEDICAL DIAGNOSIS

If small white flakes are noted in the pubic hair, seborrheic dermatitis must be considered.

### PLAN

#### Psychosocial Interventions

Assist the client to deal with the anxiety and embarrassment that diagnosis causes. Assure her that pubic lice are curable and have no long term consequences. In addition, advise her that contacts need to be checked and treated if they are infected. Clothing and household items require disinfection. Washable items may be laundered in hot water or dry cleaned. Nonwashable items can be treated with products that contain pyrethrin (Black Flag or Raid). These should be used only on inanimate objects.

#### Medication

A variety of prescription and over-the-counter medications are available. Ideally, medication should be lethal to both adult lice and eggs.

***Pyrethrins and Piperonyl Butoxide (RID, Triple X)***

- *Indications.* For treatment of pubic lice and eggs. These are over-the-counter preparations.
- *Administration.* Application is as a shampoo or liquid. Manufacturer's directions for application must be followed exactly.

Repeat application is usually unnecessary but may be done 7 to 10 days after initial treatment. Do not exceed two applications within 24 hours.

- *Side Effects and Adverse Reactions.* Minimal, but minor skin irritation may occur. Avoid contact with mucous membranes. Safe during pregnancy.
- *Contraindications.* Sensitivity to ragweed; for these individuals the solutions should be used with caution.
- *Anticipated Outcomes on Evaluation.* Destruction of pubic lice and eggs. Reexamination is needed 1 week after initial treatment to confirm positive outcome.
- *Client Teaching and Counseling.* Encourage the client to follow the directions exactly. Instruct her in the use of the finetooth comb usually provided with the medication; dead nits are combed out of the pubic hair.

#### *Lindane 1 % (Kwell)*

- *Indications.* This prescription solution is used in the treatment of pubic lice. It kills both adult lice and eggs.
- *Administration.* Application is as a shampoo. Apply exactly according to the manufacturer's directions. One application is usually adequate, but the treatment may be repeated in 7 days.
- *Side Effects and Adverse Reactions.* May include skin irritation, but it is usually minor. Lindane permeates human skin and has potential central nervous system (CNS) toxicity. Care must be taken to avoid contact with the eyes.
- *Contraindications.* Known seizure disorders and known sensitivity to lindane. Do not use during pregnancy and lactation; use RID.
- *Anticipated Outcomes on Evaluation.* The same as that achieved with the use of pyrethrins and piperonyl butoxide.
- *Client Teaching and Counseling.* Includes the measures described for pyrethrins and piperonyl butoxide. In addition, clients who telephone to say they have pubic lice can be believed and given treatment over the telephone. No office visit is needed to confirm the diagnosis.

## SYPHILIS

Syphilis is a classic sexually transmitted disease that occurs in distinct stages with diverse clinical manifestations. Its natural history begins with *primary syphilis*, which is characterized by a chancre at the site of bacterial entry. *Secondary syphilis* is recognized by flulike symptoms and a maculopapular rash of the palms and soles. Following secondary syphilis, *latency* occurs. Ultimately *tertiary (late) syphilis* overtakes the body, resulting in systemic disease.

### EPIDEMIOLOGY

*Treponema pallidum*, a bacterium in the spirochete family, is the causative organism. Direct sexual contact with an infected individual transmits the disease. Transplacental transmission of an infected mother to her fetus is also possible. Transmission requires exposure to lesions. Longstanding untreated disease is less contagious than the primary or secondary stage. The incubation period is from 10 to 90 days (3 weeks average).

Before penicillin, syphilis affected upwards of 25 percent of the population. Widespread use of antibiotics dramatically decreased incidence. Since 1985, however, a steady upward climb has occurred in the reported cases of primary, secondary, and congenital syphilis. In 1990, more than 50,000 cases were reported in the United States, the highest incidence since 1949. Rates are highest among African Americans in urban areas, and in the southern states. A substantial portion of the current syphilis epidemic is directly attributable to crack cocaine use.[28,29]

## SUBJECTIVE DATA

- *Primary Syphilis.* Client is asymptomatic or may report a lesion.
- *Secondary Syphilis.* Low-grade fever, headache, sore throat, rash on the palms and soles.
- *Tertiary Syphilis.* Primarily neurological symptoms, somewhat site dependent.
- *Congenital Syphilis.* See Objective Data.

## OBJECTIVE DATA

### Physical Examination

- *Primary Syphilis.* Classic chancre is a painless, rounded, indurated ulcer with serous exudate. It may be genital or extragenital. Usually a single chancre occurs, but multiple chancres may be present. An extragenital chancre is likely to be atypical in appearance. Lymphadenopathy, which may accompany the chancre, will heal spontaneously in 3 to 6 weeks.
- *Secondary Syphilis.* Classic maculopapular rash that gradually covers the body, including the palms and the soles. Less common signs include patchy alopecia, generalized nontender lymphadenopathy, mucosal ulcers, and condyloma lata (flat broad wartlike papules on warm, moist skin surfaces). Spontaneous healing of all secondary manifestations occurs.
- *Tertiary Syphilis.* Manifestations are dependent on whether the client has neurosyphilis, cardiovascular syphilis, or other expressions of the disease.
- *Congenital Syphilis.* Premature birth, intrauterine growth retardation, mucocutaneous lesions, snuffles (serous nasal discharge), hepatosplenomegaly, condyloma lata, skeletal lesions, CNS involvement, ocular lesions, and others. Symptomatology is diverse and usually divided into early congenital syphilis (up to 2 years of age) and late congenital syphilis (older than 2 years).[12]

### Diagnostic Tests and Methods

Diagnosis is largely dependent on microscopic examination of primary and secondary lesion tissue and serology during latency and late infection.

***Dark Field Examination.*** Diagnostic evaluation for definitive identification of *T. pallidum* is possible when lesions (e.g., chancre, rash) are present. If antibiotics have been taken, the test is not useful.

The test procedure is first to cleanse the lesion with sterile saline. Then gently abrade to produce oozing of serous fluid. Avoid active bleeding. Collect serous fluid on a slide, cover with coverslip, and examine using dark field microscope. Specimens for dark field examination cannot be transported.

Advise the client that the testing procedure is not uncomfortable and that immediate results will be available.

***Serological Tests, Nontreponemal.*** Diagnostic evaluation for antilipid antibodies produced by the host exposed to *T. pallidum.* Examples are Venereal Disease Research Laboratory (VDRL) and Rapid Plasma Reagent (RPR). Ideal for syphilis screening and follow-up after treatment.

The test procedure is to collect a blood sample in a dry tube without anticoagulant.

Advise the client that venipuncture is required. Results are reported as either reactive (positive) or nonreactive (negative). *Reactive results* are quantitated in the form of a titer. The false positive rate is 1 to 2 percent in the general population, higher in low risk groups. All reactive results require confirmation by the treponemal test (description follows). Tests become reactive 14 days after the chancre appears. If results are equivocal, repeat testing is indicated. A rising titer is evidence of primary syphilis. If syphilis is suspected and the initial nontreponemal test is nonreactive, repeat in 1 week, 1 month, and 3 months.

*Nonreactive results* after 3 months exclude the diagnosis of syphilis.[12] A fourfold titer increase of a 1:1 or greater titer indicates infection, reinfection, or failure of treatment.[30]

***Serological Tests, Treponemal.*** Diagnostic evaluation to detect *T. pallidum* specific antibodies. This test is designed to confirm the diagnosis of a reactive nontreponemal test. One example is fluorescent treponemal antibody absorption (FTA-ABS). The test procedure is to collect a blood sample in a dry tube without anticoagulant.

A venipuncture is required. The treponemal test should only be used *after* the nontreponemal test is reactive—never as the initial screen. It is also used if symptoms of tertiary syphilis are present. The results are reported as reactive or nonreactive. Once reactive, the client usually will remain so for life, even with adequate treatment. The false positive rate is 1 percent.[12]

## DIFFERENTIAL MEDICAL DIAGNOSES

Other conditions with genital lesions, such as herpes, are considered when a chancre is present. Numerous medical conditions may be indistinguishable from early secondary syphilis, but appearance of the characteristic rash is highly suggestive.

## PLAN

### Psychosocial Interventions

Extensive counseling and support are needed. Explain the complex nature of the disease and its ramifications. Case finding and treatment of sexual partners are essential to epidemic control but difficult when the relationship is associated with crack or cocaine use. The need must be stressed for follow-up testing to ensure adequate treatment. Explain the meaning of test results, especially rising or falling titers and persistent reactive results. Clients with serological evidence of syphilis in any stage are best treated by practitioners experienced in the management of this complex disease. Suggest HIV counseling and testing.

### Medication

Penicillin is the treatment of choice for all clients with syphilis and the only proven therapy for syphilis during pregnancy and for congenital syphilis. Current dual-drug therapy for gonorrhea will probably cure incubating syphilis.[4]

#### *Benzathine Penicillin G*

- *Indications.* Primary and secondary syphilis and early latent syphilis of less than 1 year's duration.
- *Administration.* 2.4 million units I.M. in one dose.
- *Side Effects and Adverse Reactions.* Penicillin adverse effects include wheezing, weakness, abdominal pain, nausea or vomiting, diarrhea, rash, fever, increased thirst, and seizures. In addition, Jarisch-Herxheimer reaction, an acute febrile illness with headache and flu-like symptoms, may occur a few hours after antibiotic administration. It subsides within 24 hours. It may be severe.
- *Contraindications.* A known sensitivity to penicillin.
- *Anticipated Outcomes on Evaluation.* Includes a follow-up with a nontreponemal test at 3 and 6 months. Titers should fall fourfold to eightfold, indicating adequate therapy. Titer should become nonexistent within 1 year.
- *Client Teaching and Counseling.* Provide the client with information about the possibility of the Jarisch-Herxheimer reaction and its treatment: rest, fluids, and antipyretics. Stress the importance of follow-up testing. Clients allergic to penicillin may be treated with doxycycline/tetracy-

cline/erythromycin. Specific protocols are recommended by the Centers for Disease Control (CDC).[4]

## TRICHOMONIASIS

In this common form of sexually transmitted vaginitis, women may be markedly symptomatic or asymptomatic. Men are asymptomatic carriers.

### EPIDEMIOLOGY

*Trichomonas vaginalis*, a flagellated, anaerobic protozoon, is the causative organism.

Sexual contact is the means of transmission. Although nonsexual transmission via fomites is theoretically possible, clinically it is rare. The organism lives in the vagina and urethra of women and the urethra and prostate gland of men. It is transmitted during vaginal–penile intercourse, and transmission rates are high. There is no finite incubation period. Detection of trichomonas in young, premenarchal girls can indicate child abuse.[12]

No accurate incidence figures are available because it is not required that trichomoniasis be reported to the CDC. Conservative estimates suggest that 6 million women and their partners are infected annually. Prevalence is highest in STD clinics and lowest in the private sector. Use of oral contraceptives and barrier methods decreases prevalence.[12,31]

### SUBJECTIVE DATA

Foul-smelling, yellow-green, frothy vaginal discharge may be profuse or scanty. Vaginal odor is the primary presenting symptom. Infrequently, women report dyspareunia and dysuria. Infrequently, men have symptoms of urethritis or prostatitis.

### OBJECTIVE DATA

Infection is often detected on routine examination in the absence of subjective complaints.

#### Physical Examination

The vulva may be red and irritated; the vagina shows typical discharge and an odor that is apparent to the examiner. Cervicitis is sometimes noted with friability and "strawberry spots."

#### Diagnostic Tests and Methods

- A culture is the most sensitive and specific diagnostic method, but it is expensive and not widely available.
- Wet mount using saline is the most clinically useful test. Diagnosis is made when a motile flagellated trichomonad is visualized. In addition, an increased number of white blood cells may be evident in the wet mount.
- Pap smear results often include reporting of trichomonads, but the sensitivity of the method is low. Clients should be reexamined and a wet mount performed to confirm diagnosis.

### DIFFERENTIAL MEDICAL DIAGNOSES

Bacterial vaginosis, candidiasis, foreign body vaginitis.

### PLAN

#### Psychosocial Interventions

The client may experience anxiety and fear with the knowledge that trichomoniasis is sexually transmitted. Reassure her that the infection is minor and its relationship to the development of cervical cancer is not significant. Infection does not affect pregnancy, except that vaginal discharge and odor may be unpleasant. Counseling should include the need to treat male partners.

## Medication

### *Metronidazole*

- *Indications.* Symptomatic and asymptomatic clients and partners; it is the drug of choice for *Trichomonas* infection.[4]
- *Administration.* Metronidazole 2 g p.o., in a single dose for both partners. If treatment fails, clients should be retreated with metronidazole 500 mg b.i.d. for 7 days. Another alternative is 2 g p.o., daily for 3 to 5 days.
- *Side Effects and Adverse Reactions.* Occur with the use of alcohol when taking metronidazole; vomiting and flushing may result. Transient nausea and a metallic taste have also been reported. Because metronidazole has a broad antimicrobial spectrum, normal vaginal flora may be suppressed with subsequent candidiasis infection.
- *Contraindications.* Known allergy to metronidazole. Do not use during the first trimester of pregnancy.
- *Anticipated Outcomes on Evaluation.* Symptoms clear rapidly after treatment. A test for cure is not routinely indicated.
- *Client Teaching and Counseling.* Stress the need to avoid alcohol. If symptoms return, reexamination is indicated. Routine treatment of the sexual partner is recommended.

## NURSING DIAGNOSES

The following nursing diagnoses are representative of those used in the health care plan of women with general vaginitis and sexually transmitted diseases. The list, however, is by no means inclusive.

- Anxiety.
- Body image disturbance.
- Disruption in skin integrity.
- Discomfort.
- Fatigue.
- Fear.
- Lowered self-esteem.
- Pain.
- Sexual dysfunction.
- Social isolation.

## REFERENCES


1. Condoms for prevention of sexually transmitted diseases. (1988). *Morbidity and Mortality Weekly Report, 37*, 133–137.
2. *Understanding AIDS: A message from the surgeon general.* (1988). Atlanta, GA: Centers for Disease Control.
3. AIDS education: A beginning. (1989). *Population Reports, L*(8).
4. Morbidity and Mortality Weekly Report. (September 24, 1993). *1993 Sexually Transmitted Diseases Treatment Guidelines* Vol. 42, No. RR-14, Atlanta, GA: U.S. Department of Health and Human Services, PHS, Centers for Disease Control and Prevention.
5. AIDS in women. (1990). *Morbidity and Mortality Weekly Report, 39*, 845–846.
6. Update: Acquired immunodeficiency syndrome—United States, 1992. (1993). *Morbidity and Mortality Weekly Report, 42*, 547–557.
7. Associated Press (December 14, 1993). Survey puts HIV figure at 550,000. *Richmond Times Dispatch*, A2.
8. American College of Obstetricians and Gynecologists (ACOG). (1992 March). Human immunodeficiency virus infections. *ACOG Technical Bulletin, 165*, 1–11.
9. Minkoff, H. (1990). Care of women infected with the HIV virus. *Journal of the American Medical Association, 266*(16), 2253–2258.
10. Centers for Disease Control (CDC). (1990). Risks for cervical disease in HIV-infected women—New York City, *Morbidity and Mortality Weekly Report, 39*, 846–849.

11. Quinn, T.C., Kline, R., Halsey, N., Hutton, N., Ruff, Butz, A., Boulos, R., Modlin, J. et al. (1991). Early diagnosis of perinatal HIV infection by detection of viral specific IgA antibodies. *Journal of the American Medical Association, 266*(24), 3439–3442.

11a. AZT found to reduce HIV in newborns. (February 21, 1994). *Richmond Times Dispatch*, A2.

12. Holmes, K.K., Mard, H.P., Sparling, P.F., Wiesner, P.J., Cates, W., Jr., Lemon, S.M., & Stamm, W.E. (1990). *Sexually transmitted diseases* (2nd ed.). New York: McGraw-Hill.

13. Lugo-Miro, V.I., Green, M., Mazur, L. et al. (1992). Comparison of different metronidazole therapeutic regimes for bacterial vaginosis. *Journal of the American Medical Association, 268*, 92–95.

14. Hillier, S., Krohn, M.A., Watts, H., Wolner-Hanssen, P., & Eschenbach, D. (1990). Microbiologic efficacy of intravaginal clindamycin cream for the treatment of bacterial vaginosis. *Obstetrics & Gynecology, 76*, 407–413.

15. Fischbach, F., Peterson, E., Weissenbacher, E., Martius, J., Hosmann, J., & Mayer, H. (1993). Efficacy of clindamycin vaginal cream versus oral metronidazole in the treatment of bacterial vaginosis. *Obstetrics & Gynecology, 82*, 405–410.

16. Van Slyke, K.K., Michel, V.P., & Rein, M.F. (1981). Treatment of vulvovaginal candidiasis with boric acid powder. *American Journal of Obstetrics & Gynecology, 141*, 145–148.

17. Hilton, E., Isenberg, H., Alperstein, P., France, K., Borenstein, M. et al. (1992). Ingestion of yogurt containing lactobacillus acidophilus as prophylaxis for candidal vaginitis. *Annals of Internal Medicine, 116*, 353–357.

18. Alexander, L. (1992). Sexually transmitted diseases: Perspectives on this growing epidemic. *Nurse Practitioner, 17*, 31–42.

19. Chlamydia trachomatis infections. (1985). *Morbidity and Mortality Weekly Report, 34*, 53S–74S.

20. Martin, D.H., Mroczkowski, T., Dalu, Z., McCarty, J., Jones, R., Hopkins, S., Johnson, R. et al. (1992). A controlled trial of a single dose of azithromycin for the treatment of chlamydial urethritis and cervicitis. *New England Journal of Medicine, 327*, 921–925.

21. Public Health Service inter-agency guidelines for screening donors of blood, plasma, organs, tissues, and semen for evidence of hepatitis B and hepatitis C. (1991). *Morbidity and Mortality Weekly Report, 40*, 1–6.

22. Davies, K. (1990, September/October). Genital herpes. *JOGN Nursing*, 401–406.

23. Macnab, J.C., Walkinshaw, S.A., Cordiner, J.W., & Clements, J.B. (1986). Human papillomavirus in clinically and histologically normal tissue of clients with genital cancer. *New England Journal of Medicine, 315*, 1052–1058.

24. Bourcier, K.M., & Seidler, A.J. (1987, January/February). Chlamydia and condyloma acuminata: An update for the nurse practitioner. *JOGN Nursing*, 17–21.

25. Enterline, J., & Leonardo, J. (1989). Condyloma acuminata. *Nurse Practitioner, 14*,8–16.

26. Krebs, H.B. (1986). Prophylactic topical 5-fluorouracil following treatment of human papilloma virus-associated lesions of the vulva and vagina. *Obstetrics & Gynecology, 68*, 837–841.

27. Nettina, S.L., & Kauffman, F.H. (1990). Diagnosis and management of sexually transmitted genital lesions. *Nurse Practitioner, 15*, 20–39.

28. Primary and secondary syphilis—United States, 1981–1990. (1991). *Morbidity and Mortality Weekly Report, 40*, 314–323.

29. Relationship of syphilis to drug use and prostitution. (1988). *Morbidity and Mortality Weekly Report, 37*, 755–758.

30. Buckley, H.B. (1992). Syphilis: A review and update of this "new" infection of the '90s. *Nurse Practitioner, 17*, 25–32.

31. Thomason, J.L., & Gelbart, S.M. (1989). Trichomonas vaginitis. *Obstetrics & Gynecology, 74*, 536–541.

## BIBLIOGRAPHY

Alexander, L.L. (1992). Sexually transmitted diseases: Perspectives on this growing epidemic. *Nurse Practitioner, 17*, 31–42.

Carlone, J.P., & Schenk, C.P. (1990). Genital HPV infections in the nonpregnant woman: Diagnosis and management options. *Nurse Practitioner Forum, 1*, 16-24.

Fiumara, N.J. (1987). *Pictorial guide to sexually transmitted diseases*. Secaucus, NJ: Hospital Publications.

Pagana, K.D., & Pagana, T.J. (1990). *Diagnostic testing and nursing implications*. (3rd ed.). St. Louis: Mosby.

Shapiro, C.N., Schulz, S.L., Lee, N.C., & Dondero, T.J. (1989). Review of human immunodeficiency virus infection in women in the United States. *Obstetrics & Gynecology, 74*, 800–808.

CHAPTER 9

# COMMON GYNECOLOGIC PELVIC DISORDERS

*Donna E. Forrest*

*Many times an etiology for chronic pain cannot be found or treatment of the presumed etiology fails; hence pain becomes the illness.*

### *Highlights*

- Endometriosis
- Adenomyosis
- Pelvic Inflammatory Disease
- Adnexal Masses: Functional, Inflammatory, Metaplastic, and Neoplastic Ovarian Tumors
- Dyspareunia
- Leiomyomas
- Pelvic Relaxation Syndrome
- Chronic Pelvic Pain
- Bartholinitis
- Cervical Polyps
- Cancers: Cervical, Uterine, Ovarian, and Vulvar
- Diethylstilbestrol Exposure

## INTRODUCTION

The health care provider needs to be familiar with the diagnosis, management, and follow-up of the more common gynecologic pelvic disorders encountered in practice, and must recognize when a client should be referred for further evaluation and management. The evaluation of any complaint of pelvic pain or discomfort begins with a thorough client history that includes the following.

- The onset and a description of the pelvic symptoms and any associated abdominal symptoms.
- A description of the character, nature, location, and timing of any pain.
- A detailed menstrual and sexual history.
- A history of previous related surgeries or hospitalizations.
- An obstetric history.
- A thorough psychosocial history.

Screening for gynecologic cancers and referral of clients with gynecologic cancers are also important responsibilities of the health care provider.

Frustrating for all health care providers, including the gynecologist, is the client who presents with chronic pelvic pain, because in most cases, a specific etiology cannot be determined and care is very difficult. For these clients, a thorough history, physical examination, and diagnostic evaluation are critical. Consultation with a gynecologist is necessary, and in most situations, consultation with a psychotherapist is beneficial.

Although a goal is to prevent unnecessary medical and surgical intervention, the fact remains that surgical intervention often is necessary to evaluate and manage pelvic disorders. The health care provider has a responsibility to the client to review alternative therapies, to evaluate the severity of her symptoms and their impact on her lifestyle, to discuss the potential benefits of proposed surgery, and to assist the client in seeking consultation with a qualified, reputable surgeon.

## ENDOMETRIOSIS

*Endometriosis* is the presence of endometrial tissue, composed of glands and stroma, at sites outside the endometrial cavity. The most common sites include the ovary, broad ligament, cul-de-sac, and rectovaginal septum; however, endometrial implants can occur in any organ. Endometrial tissue responds cyclically to estrogen by swelling and producing local inflammation. The severity of pain appears unrelated to the extent of the disease, so that clients with small implants of endometriosis may experience the severest pain. The condition commonly occurs in women in their twenties and thirties; it does not occur before menarche or after menopause. Endometriosis is a major cause of infertility[1,2] (see Figures 9–1 and 9–2).

### EPIDEMIOLOGY

A specific etiology for endometriosis is unknown, although three major theories have been put forth.

- Sampson's theory of retrograde menstruation describes menstrual or endometrial tissue flowing backward through the fallopian tubes and into the abdominal cavity.
- Halban's lymphatic spread theory describes endometrial tissue spreading to distant sites through the lymphatic system.
- Meyer's müllerian metaplasia theory describes the metaplasia of mesothelial cells into endometrial epithelium under some unidentified influence, such as repeated inflammation.[2]
- Dioxin theory is one of the newest theories that strongly links the environmental contaminant, dioxin, to the development of endometriosis in female rhesus monkeys.[3] Other researchers are investigating human females with endometriosis for similar chemicals, including dioxin.

Endometriosis is found equally among all races and socioeconomic groups.[4] It is more likely to occur and progress in women with early menarche, and in those with menstrual flow exceeding seven days, cycles of less than 27 days, years of menstruation uninterrupted by pregnancy, and a family history of endometriosis.[5,6]

Endometriosis occurs in 10 to 15 percent of women of reproductive age;[6] it is found in 40 to 50 percent of women undergoing surgery for evaluation of infertility; and the average age at diagnosis is 28.[7]

### SUBJECTIVE DATA

Dysmenorrhea, dyspareunia (especially on deep penetration), perimenstrual back pain, and infertility are the most frequently reported symptoms. The client may also complain of dyschezia, abdominal pain, or irregular bleeding patterns, especially premenstrual spotting. Less commonly, clients describe urgency in urination, hematuria, or rectal bleeding.[1,2,8]

### OBJECTIVE DATA

#### Physical Examination

The genitalia and reproductive tract may appear completely normal if lesions are small

Patient's Name ______________________ Date ______________________

Stage I (Minimal) - 1-5
Stage II (Mild) - 6-15
Stage III (Moderate) - 16-40
Stage IV (Severe) - >40
Total ____________

Laparoscopy ________ Laparotomy ________ Photography ________
Recommended Treatment ______________________

Prognosis ______________

| | ENDOMETRIOSIS | <1cm | 1-3cm | >3cm |
|---|---|---|---|---|
| PERITONEUM | Superficial | 1 | 2 | 4 |
| | Deep | 2 | 4 | 6 |
| OVARY | R Superficial | 1 | 2 | 4 |
| | Deep | 4 | 16 | 20 |
| | L Superficial | 1 | 2 | 4 |
| | Deep | 4 | 16 | 20 |

| | POSTERIOR CULDESAC OBLITERATION | Partial | Complete |
|---|---|---|---|
| | | 4 | 40 |

| | ADHESIONS | <1/3 Enclosure | 1/3-2/3 Enclosure | >2/3 Enclosure |
|---|---|---|---|---|
| OVARY | R Filmy | 1 | 2 | 4 |
| | Dense | 4 | 8 | 16 |
| | L Filmy | 1 | 2 | 4 |
| | Dense | 4 | 8 | 16 |
| TUBE | R Filmy | 1 | 2 | 4 |
| | Dense | 4* | 8* | 16 |
| | L Filmy | 1 | 2 | 4 |
| | Dense | 4* | 8* | 16 |

*If the fimbriated end of the fallopian tube is completely enclosed, change the point assignment to 16.

Additional Endometriosis: ______________________

Associated Pathology: ______________________

To Be Used with Normal Tubes and Ovaries

L R

To Be Used with Abnormal Tubes and/or Ovaries

L R

**Figure 9–1.** Classification of endometriosis. (*From Fertil Steril 43:352, 1985. Reproduced with permission from The American Fertility Society.*)

and few. In more advanced disease, a speculum exam reveals cervical displacement of 1 cm or more to the left or right of midline; with bimanual exam tenderness and nodularity of the uterosacral ligaments and posterior cul-de-sac are detected. Also seen are fixed retroversion of the uterus, and adnexal masses that vary in size, shape, and consistency and may be asymmetric, fixed, cystic, or indurated.[1,9,10]

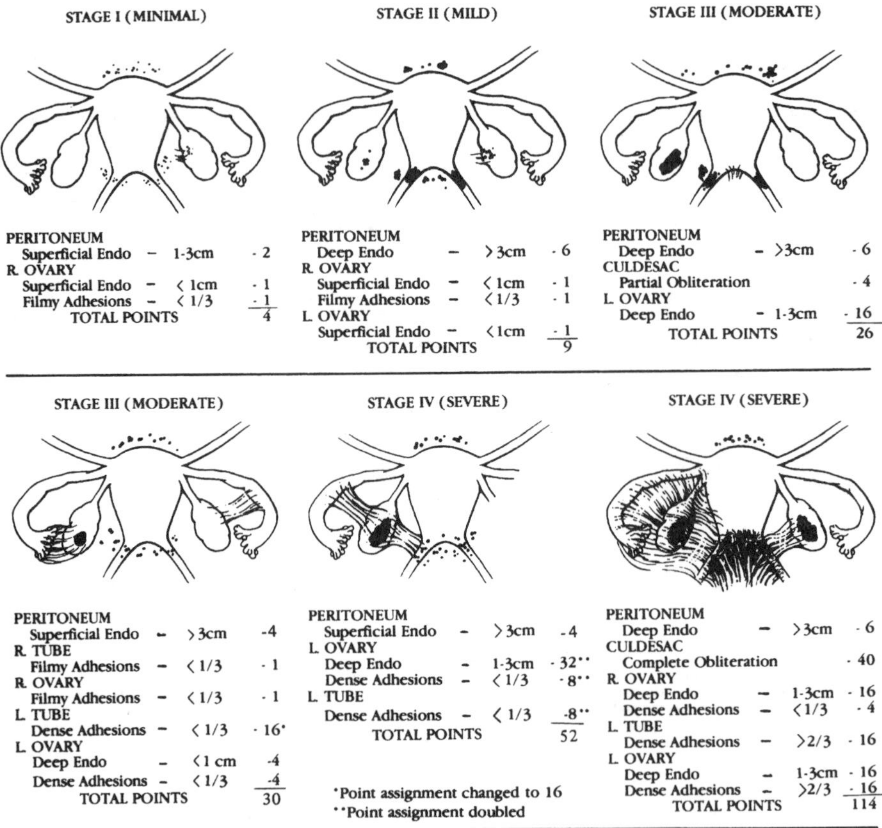


Determination of the stage or degree of endometrial involvement is based on a weighted point system. Distribution of points has been arbitrarily determined and may require further revision or refinement as knowledge of the disease increases.

To ensure complete evaluation, inspection of the pelvis in a clockwise or counterclockwise fashion is encouraged. Number, size and location of endometrial implants, plaques, endometriomas and/or adhesions are noted. For example, five separate 0.5cm superficial implants on the peritoneum (2.5 cm total) would be assigned 2 points. (The surface of the uterus should be considered peritoneum.) The severity of the endometriosis or adhesions should be assigned the highest score only for peritoneum, ovary, tube or culdesac. For example, a 4cm superficial and a 2cm deep implant of the peritoneum should be given a score of 6 (not 8). A 4cm deep endometrioma of the ovary associated with more than 3cm of superficial disease should be scored 20 (not 24).

In those patients with only one adenexa, points applied to disease of the remaining tube and ovary should be multipled by two. **Points assigned may be circled and totaled. Aggregation of points indicates stage of disease (minimal, mild, moderate, or severe).

The presence of endometriosis of the bowel, urinary tract, fallopian tube, vagina, cervix, skin etc., should be documented under "additional endometriosis." Other pathology such as tubal occlusion, leiomyomata, uterine anomaly, etc., should be documented under "associated pathology." All pathology should be depicted as specifically as possible on the sketch of pelvic organs, and means of observation (laparoscopy or laparotomy) should be noted.

**Figure 9–2.** Classification of endometriosis—examples and guidelines. (*From Fertil Steril 43:352, 1985. Reproduced with permission from The American Fertility Society.*)

## Diagnostic Tests and Methods

***CA-125 Assay.*** Diagnostic evaluation to determine the degree of a disease and a woman's response to treatment. The levels of cell surface antigen found on derivatives of the coelomic epithelium (includes endometrium) are elevated in clients with endometriosis. This test can be used to differentiate between endometriotic adnexal cysts and nonendometriotic benign adnexal cysts.[10] If the erythrocyte sedimentation rate and the leukocyte count are normal, but the CA-125 level is elevated, endometriosis is a likely diagnosis.[2]

The test procedure is to obtain a blood sample and send it to a laboratory with experience in analyzing CA-125.

Tell the client that the assay is very expensive to perform, and is not covered by many insurance companies. Providing such information will facilitate decisions related to the necessity of the assay. (Its low sensitivity makes it an inappropriate screening tool.) In addition, advise the client that the test's overall purpose is to evaluate the response to therapy. Use the test in consultation with a physician.

***Diagnostic Laparoscopy.*** Diagnostic evaluation through direct visualization of endometriosis. Positive findings include "powder burns" (flat, brownish discolorations of the peritoneal surface due to adherent endometrial implants), "mulberry spots" (raised, bluish implants of endometriosis), and adhesions.[9,10,11] The American Fertility Society has developed a classification system for disease severity (see Figure 9–2).

The test procedure requires that the client be referred to a gynecologic surgeon with special training and experience using the laparoscope. Laparoscopy is usually performed as an outpatient procedure, with the client under general anesthesia. The laparoscope is inserted through a small incision just above the navel after the abdomen has been inflated with carbon dioxide gas. The surgeon is able to visualize the pelvic organs directly.

Explain the procedure to the client in detail. In addition, discuss the risks. Complications, which are rare, may include bleeding or injuries to nearby organs. Anesthesia complications are also a possibility. Discuss the recovery process. Usually, the client may return home the same day. Common discomforts are neck and shoulder pain from the gas used to inflate the abdomen, mild nausea, pelvic discomfort at the incision site, mild cramps, and mild vaginal discharge. Instruct the client that she may shower or bathe in 24 hours and return to normal activities as soon as she feels able. Review the signs and symptoms of infection and explain how to keep the incision site clean and dry. To reinforce this discussion, provide the client with written information about the procedure and recovery.

## DIFFERENTIAL MEDICAL DIAGNOSES

Chronic pelvic inflammatory disease (PID), recurrent acute salpingitis, hemorrhagic corpus luteum, benign or malignant ovarian neoplasm, ectopic pregnancy, adenomyosis.[2]

## PLAN

### Psychosocial Interventions

Encourage active participation by the client and her significant other in treatment decisions. Assess the client's lifestyle and future plans, such as childbearing, marriage, education, and career. Discuss the impact of the disease on her life and which treatment option will best suit her lifestyle. Sexual therapy should be offered if the disease has significantly impacted sexual relations.[12,13]

### Medication

The goal of medication is to interrupt cycles of stimulation and bleeding.[10]

#### *Danazol*

- *Indications.* Mild to moderate endometriosis in women who desire fertility but not in the immediate future.[2] It is the medication of choice and may be used alone or in conjunction with conservative surgery.[9,15]

- *Administration.* Danazol, 100–800 mg daily, may be needed to suppress symptoms.[2] An 800-mg dose is given as two 200-mg tablets twice daily for 6 to 9 months beginning on the fifth day of menses.
- *Side Effects and Adverse Reactions.* Possible weight gain, fluid retention, fatigue, decreased breast size, acne, oily skin, hirsutism, atrophic vaginitis, hot flushes, muscle cramps, emotional lability, voice changes, spotting.
- *Contraindications.* A history of liver disease, hypertension, congestive heart failure, or renal impairment; or pregnancy.
- *Anticipated Outcomes on Evaluation.* The relief of pain, resorption of endometrial implants, return to fertility, and pregnancy if desired; few side effects.
- *Client Teaching and Counseling.* Tell the client about the high cost of danazol therapy and the length of treatment. Review the side effects, and stress the importance of following the administration regimen correctly. Barrier contraception is recommended during therapy with danazol and during the first menstrual cycle after treatment.[10,15]

#### Progestogens

- *Indications.* Suppression of the cyclic hormonal response of endometrial implants, and resorption of tissue. Indicated in mild to moderate endometriosis.[2,10,14] Progestogens are better tolerated than combination oral contraceptives, having fewer estrogen-related side effects. However, progestogens are considered as the first choice medication only if danazol is poorly tolerated or contraindicated.
- *Administration.* Medroxyprogesterone acetate (Depo-Provera), 100 mg I.M. every 2 weeks for 4 doses, followed by 200 mg I.M. monthly for 4 additional months, or MPA (Provera), 30 mg p.o. every day for 6 months.
- *Side Effects and Adverse Reactions.* Breakthrough bleeding, depression, delayed fertility, headache, dizziness, weight gain.
- *Contraindications.* Traditionally, contraindications for progestin-only medication have been the same as those for combination oral contraceptives. Progestin-only is also contraindicated for women with undiagnosed abnormal genital bleeding. A relative contraindication is for women who desire fertility immediately after completing therapy.
- *Anticipated Outcomes on Evaluation.* The relief of pain and the resorption of endometrial implants.
- *Client Teaching and Counseling.* Review with the client the instructions for selected regimens, their possible side effects, and the danger signs (see Combined Oral Contraceptives).[10,14]

#### Combined Oral Contraceptives (OCs)

- *Indications.* Suppression of the cyclic hormonal response of endometrial implants and eventual resorption of the tissue. Oral contraceptives (OCs) induce a "pseudopregnancy." The combination of estrogen and progestin causes endometrial tissue to become decidual and necrotic, leading to resorption. The therapy may be useful for mild to moderate endometriosis associated with clinical symptoms of pain or infertility. OCs are best considered if other therapeutic alternatives are contraindicated or not advisable.[14]
- *Administration.* Escalating doses of combined OCs or progestins alone may be indicated for severe symptoms but minimal disease.[2] Continuous progestin may be the most helpful (see previous section on Progestogens).

  One pill daily, taken continuously for 6 to 12 months. Consult with the gynecologist regarding dosages of OC to use. If breakthrough bleeding occurs, add conjugated estrogen, 2.5 mg per day for 1 week. Alternatively, the OC dosage may be increased to two tablets or more per day if breakthrough bleeding occurs.

- *Side Effects and Adverse Reactions.* Possible weight gain, breast pain and tenderness, abdominal bloating, nausea, increased appetite, breast secretion, superficial vein varicosities, and increased risk of deep vein thrombosis.
- *Contraindications.* In addition to those usually listed for OCs are known or suspected pregnancy, history of thromboembolic disease, liver disease (see Chapter 6 and the *Physicians' Desk Reference*).
- *Anticipated Outcomes on Evaluation.* The relief of pain, resorption of endometrial implants, return to fertility, and pregnancy if desired.
- *Client Teaching and Counseling.* Review with the client the instructions for taking OCs continuously, stressing the importance of not skipping pills. Warn her of the possible side effects and danger signs, for example, abdominal pain, severe headache, and leg pain. Explain the purpose of the therapy.[14]

#### *Gonadotropin-Releasing Hormone Agonists (GnRH-a)*

- *Indications.* Suppression of endometriosis and as an alternative to danazol or progesterone. Newly approved, these agonists are for mild to moderate endometriosis.
- *Administration.* Leuprolide acetate (Lupron) 0.5–1.0 mg s.c. daily for 6 months or 3.75–7.5 mg I.M. every 28 to 60 days. Nafarelin acetate (Synarel) nasal spray may be used instead; one spray (200 μg/spray) into one nostril in the morning and one into the other nostril at night for 6 months.[2,9]
- *Side Effects and Adverse Reactions.* Hot flushes, vaginal dryness, mood swings, depression, weight gain, decreased breast size, decreased libido, fatigue, and insomnia. In addition, GnRH-a may interfere with calcium and bone metabolism.
- *Contraindications.* Known or suspected pregnancy, hypersensitivity to GnRH, undiagnosed abnormal vaginal bleeding, breastfeeding.
- *Anticipated Outcomes on Evaluation.* The relief of pain, resorption of endometrial implants, return to fertility, and pregnancy if desired; few side effects.
- *Client Teaching and Counseling.* Provide instructions for the drug's proper administration, and tell the client that the therapy is costly and would continue for 6 months. Review the side effects. A supplement of calcium carbonate may be necessary: 1000–1500 mg q.d. Barrier contraception is recommended during therapy and for the first menstrual cycle.[10,16]

### Surgical Interventions

***Conservative Surgery.*** One surgical option is to destroy and dissect endometriomas and endometriotic implants while preserving reproductive function. The procedure may be performed by a specially trained gynecologic surgeon directly after laparoscopic diagnosis, while the client is still under anesthesia. Conservative methods include fulguration, excision and resection, and/or laser vaporization. Conservative surgery is indicated for adnexal masses, symptoms unresponsive to medical therapy, severe endometriosis in a client who desires future fertility, and concomitant conditions such as leiomyomas or adhesions.

The possible adverse effects are few: a reaction to anesthesia, incisional infection, bleeding, or injury to nearby organs. The anticipated outcomes on evaluation are the relief of pain and return of fertility.

When explaining the procedure to the client, point out that conservative surgery is not curative. Review the postoperative instructions, addressing the client's return to activity, resumption of sexual relations, and signs and symptoms of infection.[11]

***Definitive Surgery.*** Abdominal hysterectomy, with or without bilateral salpingo-oophorectomy, is indicated for clients with severe disease. These are women who either have completed their families or have no desire for future fertility, or whose disease has not responded to medical therapy or conservative surgery, or whose disease involves other organs, such as the bowel or bladder. Referral is made to a board-certified gynecologic surgeon. The procedure, performed under general anesthesia, involves removal of the uterus through an abdominal incision. The ovaries and fallopian tubes may or may not be removed; among the determining factors are the age of the client and the extent of endometriosis.

There are possible adverse effects, namely, bleeding, infection, wound infection, or damage to nearby organs. The anticipated outcome on evaluation is complete resolution of the disease, including relief of dysmenorrhea, dyspareunia, dyschezia and/or dysuria.

Prepare the client by giving her a thorough explanation of the anatomy and physiology, surgical procedure, and risks and benefits. Reassure her that femininity remains unchanged by the surgery. Hormonal replacement therapy may be needed. Full recovery us-ually takes about 6 weeks. Review the postoperative instructions, including topics such as the return to activity, the expectation that vaginal bleeding will change to clear discharge, signs of infection, return to sexual activity, and dietary needs.[11]

### Follow-Up and Referral

Endometriosis tends to recur at a rate of 5 to 20 percent per year when definitive surgery is not performed.[10] Appropriate follow-up intervals depend on the choice of therapy and the client's needs. An initial evaluation, made after 6 months of therapy, should report the incidence, severity, and cyclicity of pain, dysmenorrhea, and dyspareunia. Review the side effects and their impact on the client. Inquire about the issue of pregnancy and provide emotional support and encouragement.[13]

# ADENOMYOSIS

Adenomyosis occurs when the endometrial glands and stroma within the endometrium have grown into the uterine wall. The cause is believed to be disruption of the uterine wall during pregnancy, labor, and postpartum involution.[2] It occurs in 10 to 20 percent of multiparous women in their thirties and forties, but it does not occur in postmenopausal women.[8]

## SUBJECTIVE DATA

Clients are often asymptomatic but may report severe dysmenorrhea and menorrhagia.[2,8]

## OBJECTIVE DATA

### Physical Examination

Bimanual examination of the genitalia and reproductive organs reveals a large, globular, soft uterus, but rarely larger than a 10 weeks pregnant uterus. It is symmetrical and softer than a leiomyoma.[8]

### Diagnostic Tests and Methods

***Endometrial Biopsy.*** Diagnostic evaluation of any abnormal bleeding; requires referral to a gynecologist. Explain the procedure to the client: The test is performed with a biopsy curette, or a suction catheter, or other instrument passed through the cervical canal into the uterus. The client will be an outpatient, and, generally, no anesthesia will be necessary. Obtain the client's menstrual history. Explain that she may return to normal activities immediately.

***Ultrasound.*** Diagnostic evaluation to rule out leiomyomas or other tumors. The procedure should be performed by a trained professional with expertise in obstetrics and gynecology. The method, performed abdominally or vaginally, employs sound waves to provide detailed images of the pelvic structures.

Explain the procedure to the client and assure her that it is painless. In the *abdominal method*, the lower abdomen is covered with a water soluble gel, a probe is moved slowly across the abdomen, and images are projected onto a video display monitor. In the *vaginal method*, a probe with ultrasound is inserted into the vagina. The client remains awake. In order to obtain clearer images, a client may be required to undergo a 24-hour bowel preparation (i.e., laxative, enema, clear liquid diet).

### DIFFERENTIAL MEDICAL DIAGNOSES

Leiomyomas, endometriosis.

### PLAN

#### Psychosocial Interventions

Discuss the condition with the client and determine the impact of her symptoms. The severity of symptoms will determine therapy, which should be described to the client. Reassure her if necessary.

#### Medication

No specific medications are given for treatment or resolution of adenomyosis. However, if symptoms are mild, palliative management with nonsteroidal anti-inflammatory drugs (NSAIDs) is helpful (see Chronic Pelvic Pain).

#### Surgical Interventions

Hysterectomy is indicated for severe, symptomatic adenomyosis, including severe dysmenorrhea, menorrhagia, or enlarged uterus greater than 10 weeks size. (For procedure, see Definitive Surgery, under Endometriosis, page 248).[8]

#### Follow-Up and Referral

If medical therapy is the initial treatment of choice, then the client is evaluated in 3 to 6 months. Increasing pain or bleeding may necessitate referral to a gynecologic surgeon for possible hysterectomy. Sarcoma can be a complication.

## PELVIC INFLAMMATORY DISEASE (PID)

In pelvic inflammatory disease (PID), infection and inflammation develop in the pelvic organs—namely the uterus, fallopian tubes, and ovaries. Most often, the condition is localized in the tubes. Complications include ectopic pregnancy, pelvic abscess, infertility, recurrent or chronic episodes of the disease, chronic abdominal pain, pelvic adhesions, premature hysterectomy, and depression.[8,17]

### EPIDEMIOLOGY

*Neisseria gonorrhoeae* and *Chlamydia trachomatis* are the two major causative organisms; however, PID is usually a mixed infection caused by both aerobic and anaerobic organisms.[18] Adolescents and young women are three times more likely to develop the infection. Nonwhite women are at higher risk.

Other risk factors include multiple sex partners; a history of PID or sexually transmitted disease (STD); intercourse with a partner who has untreated urethritis; recent intrauterine device (IUD) insertion; and nulliparity. PID is more likely to occur during the first 5 days of the menstrual cycle.[7,19–21]

The causative organisms are transmitted through sexual intercourse with an infected partner. One million new episodes are diagnosed annually in the United States, requiring 300,000 hospitalizations. One in seven women of reproductive age reports having been treated for pelvic inflammatory disease.[1,7,20,21]

## SUBJECTIVE DATA

A client may report one or all of the following symptoms: pain and tenderness of the lower abdomen, fever, chills, nausea, vomiting, increased vaginal discharge, symptoms of urinary tract infection (UTI), and irregular bleeding. The severity of symptoms may be mild or severe. Abdominal pain is usually present. If Fitz–Hugh–Curtis syndrome is present, upper abdominal pain will occur due to liver capsule inflammation. A client may also report experiencing any of the aforementioned risk factors.[1,7,21] Consultation with a gynecologist is advised due to the seriousness of this condition.

## OBJECTIVE DATA

### Physical Examination

- Determination of vital signs may show an elevated body temperature (≥38°C).[7]
- The abdomen may be distended with rebound tenderness, guarding, and hypoactive bowel sounds.
- The genital and reproductive exam is positive for cervical motion tenderness (pain upon movement of the cervix), purulent cervical discharge, uterine tenderness, adnexal pain and fullness, or the presence of an adnexal mass.[1,18]

### Diagnostic Tests and Methods

***Complete Blood Count (CBC) and Erythrocyte Sedimentation Rate (ESR).*** Diagnostic evaluation to detect any inflammatory process. The white blood cell (WBC) count is above 10,000, and erythrocyte sedimentation rate (ESR) is elevated in PID. A venous blood sample is obtained according to laboratory protocol after the procedure and its purpose have been explained to the client.

***Pregnancy Test.*** Diagnostic evaluation (urine or blood level of human chorionic gonadotropin [hCG]) for unsuspected intrauterine pregnancy or suspected ectopic pregnancy. A urine pregnancy test is done, or if ectopic pregnancy is suspected, blood quantitative radioimmunoassay of hCG.

Explain the procedure to the client and determine her last normal menstrual period. If the client is pregnant, ultrasound should be ordered to rule out ectopic pregnancy or missed abortion. Whether a treatment regimen is contraindicated during pregnancy must be determined.

***C-Reactive Protein.*** Diagnostic evaluation to detect inflammation; the test is highly sensitive for detecting PID. A venous blood sample is obtained according to laboratory protocol after the procedure and its purpose have been explained to the client.

***Vaginal Smears/Cervical Cultures.*** Diagnostic evaluation to detect the causative organisms of infection. Wet mount with saline can detect bacterial vaginosis or trichomoniasis. Cervical tests will detect *N. gonorrhoeae* and *C. trachomatis*. PID is usually due to polymicrobial, ascending infection (see Chapter 8 for the test procedures).

***Ultrasound.*** Diagnostic evaluation to identify fluid in the cul-de-sac, distended tubes, masses or a pelvic abscess, and to rule out intrauterine and ectopic pregnancy (see Adenomyosis for a description of the test procedure).

***Laparoscopy.*** Diagnostic evaluation to identify fluid in the cul-de-sac, distended tubes, masses or pelvic abscess. Laparoscopy is also done to rule out ectopic pregnancy (see Diagnostic Laparoscopy, under Endometriosis for the test procedure.)[1,18,19,22,23] Although laparoscopy provides more definitive diagnosis of PID, it is expensive. Laboratory and physical findings are usually accurate for diagnosis.[7]

## DIFFERENTIAL MEDICAL DIAGNOSES

Ectopic pregnancy, appendicitis, ruptured corpus luteum cyst, septic abortion, torsion of an adnexal mass, pyelonephritis, degeneration of a leiomyoma, endometriosis, endometritis, ulcerative colitis.[1,8]

## PLAN

### Psychosocial Interventions

Thoroughly discuss with the client the disease, its implications, and risk factors. If possible, the client's partner should participate. Review the serious sequelae that may occur if the disease is not treated, or if the client does not comply with treatment. *Refer partners for evaluation and treatment of any sexually transmitted disease that is diagnosed.* Discuss the use of condoms, especially if the client has multiple sexual partners. Provide emotional support. Stress the importance of follow-up care and evaluation.[1,8,17]

### Medication[1,7,18,24–27]

The client is treated on an ambulatory basis or admitted for hospitalization, and the medication regimen is determined by this choice. *The following factors will contribute to the decision to refer a client to a physician for hospital admission and care.*

- Questionable diagnosis.
- Possible ectopic pregnancy or appendicitis.
- Suspected pelvic abscess.
- Severe illness (nausea, vomiting, fever ≥38.0°C, severe pain, dehydration).
- Pregnancy.
- Inability to tolerate or follow an outpatient regimen.
- Lack of response to outpatient treatment after 48 to 72 hours.
- Prepubertal client.
- Inability of the client to seek follow-up evaluation in 48 to 72 hours.[1,19]

***In-Hospital Medication.*** Doxycycline, 100 mg I.V., b.i.d., *plus* one of the following: cefoxitin, 2.0 g I.V., q.i.d., *or* cefotetan, 2.0 g I.V., b.i.d. Continue at least 2 days after the client begins to show clinical improvement. Following discharge, the client continues doxycycline 100 mg p.o., b.i.d., for 10–14 days of treatment.

Explain to the client the necessity of hospitalization. Make sure that the client understands all discharge instructions and the need to return for evaluation after discharge.

***Alternative In-Hospital Medication.*** Clindamycin 900 mg I.V., t.i.d., *plus loading dose* of gentamicin 2 mg/kg I.V. *with maintenance dosage* of 1.5 mg/kg I.V., t.i.d.

Explain to the client the necessity of hospitalization. Make sure the client understands all discharge instructions and the need to return for evaluation after discharge.

***Side Effects and Adverse Reactions***

- *Cefoxitan, Cefotetan, Ceftriaxone (Cephalosporins).* Few; most serious is pseudomembranous colitis.
- *Doxycycline.* Gastrointestinal (GI) distress, fetal teeth discoloration if given during pregnancy, photosensitivity.

- *Gentamicin.* Nephrotoxicity, ototoxicity.
- *Clindamycin.* Diarrhea, pseudomembranous enterocolitis.

***Contraindications***

- *Cefoxitin, Cefotetan, Ceftriaxone (Cephalosporins).* Known allergy to cephalosporins.
- *Doxycycline.* Pregnancy, or hypersensitivity to tetracyclines.
- *Gentamicin.* Hypersensitivity to aminoglycosides.
- *Clindamycin.* Hypersensitivity to aminoglycosides.

Anticipated outcomes on evaluation are the resolution of symptoms of pelvic inflammatory disease and the prevention of serious sequelae.

***Ambulatory Medication.*** This regimen is followed when a client with PID can be managed safely on an outpatient basis at home. Cefoxitin, 2.0 g I.M. stat., *plus* probenecid, 1.0 g p.o. stat.; *or* ceftriaxone, 250 mg, I.M. stat., *plus* doxycycline, 100 mg p.o., b.i.d. for 10–14 days; *or* tetracycline, 500 mg p.o. q.i.d. for 10–14 days. Stress to the client the importance of taking the complete medication prescription to help prevent complications; review all medication-related instructions. Convey the importance of returning for a follow-up evaluation 48 to 72 hours after the medication is started and again in 7 to 10 days. Instruct the client that if symptoms worsen during outpatient treatment, she must call the health professional immediately because hospitalization will probably be necessary.

## Surgical Interventions

***Conservative Surgery.*** This involves removal of grossly abnormal tissue only. The uterus and at least one ovary are preserved to allow for possible later in vitro fertilization.

Conservative surgery is indicated when the hospitalized client with acute PID or a pelvic mass does not respond after 72 hours of appropriate therapy, or when a ruptured tubo-ovarian abscess is suspected.[19] An experienced gynecologic surgeon should perform the surgery.

The potential adverse effects are few: the usual potential anesthesia complications and the risk of excessive bleeding or postoperative infection. The anticipated outcomes on evaluation are the resolution of pelvic infection with the preservation of reproductive capability.

Explain the procedure to the client and inform her that it will be carried out using general anesthesia. Informed consent forms must be signed. Provide postoperative instructions regarding the return to activity, signs and symptoms of infection, and return to sexual activity.[19]

***Colpotomy.*** Colpotomy permits drainage of abscesses located in Douglas' cul-de-sac. It is performed transvaginally by an experienced gynecologic surgeon using direct ultrasonographic or radiographic guidance.

The possible adverse effects include the usual anesthesia complications and the risk of excessive bleeding or postoperative complications. The anticipated outcomes on evaluation are the resolution of the pelvic abscess and the prevention of chronic pelvic infection and chronic pelvic pain.

Explain the procedure to the client and inform her that it will be carried out using general anesthesia. Informed consent forms must be signed. Provide postoperative instructions regarding the return to activity, signs and symptoms of infection, and return to sexual activity.[19]

***Unilateral/Bilateral Salpingo-Oophorectomy.*** One or both fallopian tubes and ovaries are removed, depending on the location and extent of a tubo-ovarian abscess. Indications for the surgery are extensive involvement of the tubes or ovaries by the inflammatory process, including scarring and abscess.

The possible adverse effects are few; the most severe is loss of reproductive capability with a bilateral salpingo-oophorectomy. The usual potential for anesthesia complications and postoperative infection also exists. The anticipated outcomes on evaluation are the complete resolution of infection and symptoms and the prevention of chronic pelvic pain and chronic pelvic infections.

Discuss with the client the impact of the surgery on her reproductive function. Provide emotional support, and refer the client for counseling if her reproductive function is lost.

### Follow-Up and Referral

Any woman with PID who is being treated on an outpatient basis should be seen again in 48–72 hours after therapy is initiated. Marked improvement in symptoms should be exhibited by then. If no or less improvement than is deemed acceptable has occurred, the client must be referred to a specialist or hospitalized. If ambulatory care is progressing acceptably, reevaluate again in 1 week. If tenderness or any mass persists, refer immediately to a specialist. Advise immediate treatment for any sexual partner who has not received evaluation and treatment.

## ADNEXAL MASSES (OVARIAN TUMORS)

The word *adnexal* pertains to the appendages of the uterus: the ovaries, fallopian tubes, and ligaments of the uterus. The adnexal masses discussed here are ovarian tumors.

### CATEGORIES OF OVARIAN TUMORS

Four major categories of ovarian tumors have been identified: functional, inflammatory, metaplastic, and neoplastic.[2]

#### Functional Ovarian Tumors

- *Follicular cyst* is caused by the failure of the ovarian follicle to rupture in the course of follicular development and ovulation. The cyst formed is lined by one or more layers of granulosa cells.
- *Lutein cyst* forms when the corpus luteum becomes cystic or hemorrhagic and fails to degenerate after 14 days.
- *Theca-lutein cyst* development is accompanied by abnormally high blood levels of human chorionic gonadotropin (hCG). The cyst occurs in clients with hydatidiform mole, or with choriocarcinoma, or who are undergoing ovulation induction with gonadotropins or clomiphene.
- *Polycystic ovary syndrome* (Stein-Leventhal syndrome) is characterized by the presence of multiple inactive follicle cysts within the ovary. The syndrome is associated with androgen excess and chronic anovulation.[2]

#### Inflammatory Ovarian Tumors

- *Salpingo-oophoritis* is inflammation of a fallopian tube and ovary. (Salpingo-oophorectomy is discussed in the preceding section on Pelvic Inflammatory Disease, page 252.)
- *Tubo-ovarian abscess* is the tumor that develops in direct response to acute or chronic salpingo-oophoritis.

#### Metaplastic Ovarian Tumor

- *Endometriosis* is the presence of endometrial tissue, composed of glands and stroma, at sites outside the endometrial cavity (see Endometriosis, page 242).

#### Neoplastic Ovarian Tumors

- *Epithelial tumors*, the most common type of tumor, include serous tumors, mucinous tumors, and endometrioid tumors. Epithelial tumors are derived from mesothelial cells lining the peritoneal cavity. They have the highest potential for malignancy.

- *Stromal tumors* are derived from the sex cords and specialized stroma of developing gonads. They include fibromas, granulosa-theca cell tumors, and Sertoli-Leydig cell tumors.
- *Germ cell tumor* is a benign cystic teratoma or dermoid cyst, derived from early embryonic germ cells. It may contain calcifications; the majority are benign.[2]

## EPIDEMIOLOGY

The etiology of adnexal masses is unclear. However, it is known that the risk of ovarian malignancy increases significantly with age. Benign cystic teratoma (germ cell tumor) is the most common *ovarian* neoplasm; epithelial neoplasm is the most common *malignant* neoplasm. Stromal neoplasms, on the other hand, are uncommon. During the reproductive years, 70 percent of all noninflammatory tumors are functional; 20 percent are neoplastic; 10 percent are endometriomas. After menopause, half of all ovarian tumors are malignant; however, before puberty, only 10 percent are malignant.[2,28]

## SUBJECTIVE DATA

- *Functional Ovarian Tumors.* A *follicular cyst* is usually asymptomatic but can cause minor lower abdominal discomfort, pelvic pain, or dyspareunia. A *lutein cyst* causes pain or signs of peritoneal irritation, delayed menses. The rupture of a cyst may produce acute lower abdominal pain and tenderness.
- *Inflammatory Ovarian Tumors.* A client may report symptoms that are similar to those of pelvic inflammatory disease (discussed earlier in this chapter): pain and tenderness of the lower abdomen, fever, chills, nausea, vomiting, increased vaginal discharge, irregular bleeding patterns.
- *Metaplastic Ovarian Tumors.* A client may report symptoms that are similar to those of endometriosis (discussed earlier in this chapter): dysmenorrhea, dyspareunia, perimenstrual back pain, infertility, dyschezia, abdominal pain, irregular bleeding patterns.
- *Neoplastic Ovarian Tumors.* Subjective data are nonspecific. The client may be asymptomatic unless torsion or rupture occurs. Abdominal enlargement or bloating may occur, usually later in the tumor development. With rupture or torsion of the tumor, mild, intermittent pelvic pain or severe pelvic pain may be reported, as well as peritoneal irritation.

## OBJECTIVE DATA

### Physical Examination

Physical examination, including bimanual gynecologic exam, is done to detect the following.

- Functional ovarian tumor is 4 to 8 cm, noted on bimanual examination. It regresses following the next menstrual cycle, is mobile, is unilateral, and may be tender.
- Inflammatory ovarian tumor (see Pelvic Inflammatory Disease).
- Metaplastic ovarian tumor (see Endometriosis).
- Neoplastic ovarian tumor may be palpable by an abdominal exam; percussion may reveal dullness anteriorly with tympany toward the flanks as a result of bowel displacement. Bimanual exam is usually positive for an adnexal mass.

### Diagnostic Tests and Methods

In some situations, it may be appropriate to begin an initial diagnostic work-up as described below; however, *if the client is premenarcheal or postmenopausal and a palpable adnexal mass is discovered, then refer her immediately to a gynecologist for further evaluation and management.*[29]

***Pregnancy Test.*** Diagnostic evaluation to rule out pregnancy (uterine enlargement may be mistaken for an adnexal mass) and ectopic pregnancy. A urine or blood sample is obtained and measured for quantitative human chorionic gonadotropin (hCG).

Explain the procedure to the client and determine her last normal menstrual period.

***Pelvic Ultrasound.*** Diagnostic evaluation to confirm the suspicion of an adnexal mass, especially in an obese client or uncooperative client. With ultrasound it is possible to exclude intrauterine or extrauterine pregnancy, distinguish between solid or cystic masses, or identify calcification associated with a teratoma. Ultrasound is also helpful in measuring the mass.[2,29] Explain to the client the various aspects of the ultrasound procedure (see Adenomyosis).

***Barium Enema.*** Diagnostic evaluation to determine whether the mass may be of a gastrointestinal source, especially if abdominal signs and symptoms are present (ascites, bloating). The test procedure requires that the client fast for 1 day, ingesting clear liquids only, taking magnesium citrate orally, and using bisacodyl suppositories. The test itself begins with rectal instillation of barium. As the progress of the barium flow is traced by fluoroscope, obstructions are noted. X-ray films are taken. Explain the procedure to the client and review the preparation instructions carefully. Explain that she may resume her regular diet after the procedure and increase fluids.

***Intravenous Pyelogram.*** Diagnostic evaluation to determine the size of the mass by evaluating ureteral displacement and distortion of the bladder contour. Kidney position and function and ureteral obstruction are also evaluated, especially before diagnostic laparoscopy.

It is necessary to evacuate the bowels using bisacodyl suppositories the night before the pyelogram. On the day of the test, a contrast dye is infused intravenously, and x-rays are taken at set intervals. The dye is traced through the glomeruli, renal tubules, renal pelvis, ureters, and bladder.

Before beginning, ask the client if she is allergic to iodine. Explain the procedure. Tell client to expect flushing of her face, a feeling of warmth, and a salty taste.

***Laparotomy/Laparoscopy.*** Diagnostic evaluation of any adnexal mass larger than 8 cm or any adnexal mass in a premenarcheal or postmenopausal client (see Endometriosis for the test procedure). These procedures make it possible to distinguish between a uterine myoma, hydrosalpinx, and an ovarian tumor. However, functional cysts, benign neoplasms, and encapsulated malignant ovarian neoplasms cannot be differentiated.[29]

## DIFFERENTIAL MEDICAL DIAGNOSES

Pelvic inflammatory disease (PID), endometriosis, uterine leiomyomas, nongynecologic masses (e.g., neoplastic colon mass), pelvic kidney, pregnancy. If rupture or torsion of the mass occurs and pain is present, rule out ectopic pregnancy and acute PID.

## PLAN

If the mass is smaller than 8 cm, unilateral, mobile, smooth, and suspected to be a functional ovarian cyst, then wait and reevaluate the mass after the next menstrual period. If the mass does not meet these criteria, or if it does not regress after the next menstrual period, then the health care provider must consult with a gynecologist and refer the client for further evaluation and management. In addition, refer all premenarcheal and postmenopausal clients with a palpable adnexal mass immediately.

### Psychosocial Interventions

The client surely will experience major fear and anxiety with any suspicion of malignancy. Therefore, it is particularly important to provide support, encouragement, and reassurance during any period of observation or evaluation. Stress the importance of compliance with diagnostic testing requirements and of keeping scheduled appointments. Make certain that she understands that early diagnosis and treatment provide the best prognosis.

### Medication

An oral contraceptive (OC) is indicated in the management of a functional ovarian cyst. By suppressing gonadotropin levels, the OC increases resolution of the cyst.[29]

Details about OC administration, side effects, and contraindications are discussed in Chapter 6. The anticipated outcome on evaluation is complete resolution of the adnexal mass (functional cyst).

Provide the client with detailed instructions about taking OCs; stress the importance of not skipping any pills. Warn her that pregnancy is possible during the first cycle of pills, and urge use of a barrier method of contraception; and emphasize the importance of returning for the follow-up visit immediately after the first menstrual cycle.

### Surgical Interventions

Surgical exploration and management of adnexal masses is headed by a board-certified surgeon specializing in gynecology. The surgical procedure varies with the type of ovarian tumor, but the health care provider should be aware of the possibilities in order to provide counseling and support to the client. Definitive treatment will depend on the client's age and her desire for reproductive capability.

*Epithelial ovarian neoplasms* may be managed with unilateral salpingo-oophorectomy, including appendectomy. If the client is older than 40, then total abdominal hysterectomy and bilateral salpingo-oophorectomy may be indicated. On the other hand, if the client is young and nulliparous and the ovarian neoplasm is unilocular with no excrescences within the cyst, an ovarian cystectomy, which preserves the ovary, is performed.[30,31]

*Stromal neoplasms* may be managed with unilateral salpingo-oophorectomy and appendectomy. If the client is older than 40, then a total abdominal hysterectomy and bilateral salpingo-oophorectomy may be indicated.[30,31]

*Germ cell tumors* are managed with an ovarian cystectomy if future childbearing is desired.[30,31] If it is not desired, then total abdominal hysterectomy and bilateral salpingo-oophorectomy are indicated.

### Follow-Up and Referral

If a functional ovarian mass is suspected, follow-up examination should occur in 4 to 6 weeks, or immediately after the next menstrual period. If the mass persists, referral to a gynecologist for further evaluation and management is necessary.

## DYSPAREUNIA

Dyspareunia is painful sexual intercourse occurring either on intromission or on deep penetration of the penis. Pain results from inflammation, anatomic abnormalities, pelvic pathology, atrophy or failure of lubrication, or psychological conflicts.[32]

## EPIDEMIOLOGY

Pain on intromission may be caused by vulvovaginitis, atrophic vulvovaginitis, hymenal strands, scar tissue, recent episiotomy, or vaginismus (involuntary perineal muscle contractions). Pain on deep penetration may be caused by uterine prolapse, pelvic inflammatory disease (PID), endometriosis, adhesions, or pelvic masses.[33]

Risk factors for dyspareunia include menopause, psychological factors (including restrictive sexual attitudes), relationship difficulties and history of sexual trauma, history of sexually transmitted disease (STD), recurrent infection (candidiasis), and poor hygiene.[34]

The incidence is unclear because clients tend not to report dyspareunia to health professionals. Of the reported cases, the most common cause is vulvovaginitis/infection. In one 1990 study of 313 women,[35] over 60 percent had experienced dyspareunia at some point in their lives. The average age of women in this study was the early 30s.

## SUBJECTIVE DATA

A client's history is crucial to determining the etiology of dyspareunia. Pain may occur on intromission or on deep penetration; it may occur after long pain-free intervals or with first intercourse. Vaginal discharge or irritation may be present. The client's history may reveal recent surgery, pregnancy and childbirth, trauma, or unrelated pelvic pain. Relationship difficulties may be reported. The client may have been unable to use tampons previously or may have had difficult pelvic exams. Menopausal symptoms may be beginning.[7,33]

## OBJECTIVE DATA

### Physical Examination

Examination includes the genitalia and reproductive tract. The vulvar/vaginal mucosa may reveal irritation, inflammation, lesions, discharge, atrophy, hymenal remnants, Bartholin's cyst/abscess or vestibulitis (focal irritation/inflammation of the vestibular glands). Involuntary contraction of the perineal muscles (vaginismus) may occur during a speculum or digital exam, prohibiting examination. In this situation, proceed carefully and allow the client control during pelvic exam. Bimanual exam may reveal uterine prolapse, pelvic mass, nodularity of endometriosis, cervical motion tenderness of pelvic inflammatory disease, or loss of pelvic support (cystocele, rectocele).[8]

### Diagnostic Tests and Methods

Select tests discriminately as indicated by the findings of the history and physical examination. Review previous test results in order to avoid unnecessary and repetitive diagnostic testing.

***Complete Blood Count (CBC) and Erythrocyte Sedimentation Rate (ESR).*** Diagnostic evaluation to detect any inflammatory process (see Pelvic Inflammatory Disease for test procedure). The white blood cell (WBC) count and ESR are elevated in pelvic inflammatory disease.

***Urinalysis.*** Diagnostic evaluation to identify any urinary tract conditions that might be a source of pain. White blood cells, bacteria, or red blood cells in the urine may indicate chronic or recurrent urinary tract infection (UTI).

To enhance test accuracy, explain to the client how to obtain a clean-catch urine sample in a sterile container.

***Pregnancy Test (Urine or Blood Level of beta-hCG).*** Diagnostic evaluation to detect unsuspected intrauterine pregnancy or suspected ectopic pregnancy (see Pelvic Inflammatory Disease for procedure).

***Vaginal Smears/Cervical Cultures.*** Diagnostic evaluation to determine whether infection is present. Wet mount with normal saline is used to detect bacterial vaginosis or trichomoniasis; potassium hydroxide (KOH) preparation is used to detect candidiasis; and cervical tests can detect *N. gonorrhoeae* and *C. trachomatis*. (See Chapter 8 for the test procedures.)

***Ultrasound.*** Diagnostic evaluation using ultrasound may be useful if a bimanual exam is difficult, as with clients who are obese or unable to tolerate the exam. The procedure is most useful in diagnosing acute pelvic pain conditions, such as ruptured ovarian cyst, adnexal masses, or ectopic pregnancy; it should not be performed in clients with a clearly negative pelvic examination. (See Adenomyosis for the test procedure.)

***Diagnostic Laparoscopy.*** Diagnostic evaluation is accomplished by directly visualizing the pelvic pathology that may be causing dyspareunia (see Endometriosis for the test procedure).

## DIFFERENTIAL MEDICAL DIAGNOSES

Vulvovaginitis, atrophic vulvovaginitis, hymenal strands, scar tissue, episiotomy, vaginismus, pelvic relaxation, uterine prolapse, PID, endometriosis, adhesions, pelvic masses, Bartholin's cyst. Consider possible contributing psychological factors, such as previous sexual trauma, conflictual relationships, stress, or restrictive sexual attitudes. Also consider inappropriate sexual technique, including lack of foreplay, or low estrogen in the oral contraceptive.[34]

## PLAN

The management of dyspareunia depends on the symptoms and etiology.

### Psychosocial Interventions

Refer the client for psychotherapy if her history reveals the possibility of a psychological component to the dyspareunia. Select a therapist with special training in sexual problems. Discuss fully with the client the findings of the physical examination and diagnostic testing, and include her partner whenever possible. Address and discuss all client fears, concerns, and anxieties. Sexual attitudes may need to be addressed.[31,34]

### Medication

The etiology of the dyspareunia determines whether medication is prescribed.

- *Vaginitis/Sexually Transmitted Disease.* See Chapter 8.
- *Atrophic Vaginitis*
  - Hormonal replacement therapy (HRT) (see Chapter 11). HRT may be the treatment of choice for perimenopausal or menopausal women with atrophic vaginitis. Estrogen revitalizes atrophic tissues.
  - A water-based lubricant (K-Y jelly or Replens), available over the counter, is indicated for poor vaginal lubrication. The lubricant may be administered prior to or during intercourse to improve vaginal lubrication and enhance foreplay. Vaginal suppositories may be inserted three times weekly, without regard to intercourse. Instructing the client in the use of a lubricant is important.
  - Anticipated outcomes on evaluation are improved vaginal lubrication and relief of dyspareunia secondary to vaginal dryness. However, local allergic irritation is

a potential adverse reaction that would contraindicate lubricant use.

- *Pelvic Inflammatory Disease, Endometriosis, Adnexal Mass, and Leiomyoma.* Medications for these causes of dyspareunia are described in other sections of this chapter.

### Surgical Intervention

The cause of dyspareunia is what determines whether surgery is necessary. In cases where surgical evaluation is needed, referral should be made to a board-certified gynecologist. For descriptions of specific surgical interventions, see the appropriate section in this chapter: Endometriosis, Pelvic Inflammatory Disease, Adnexal Masses, Leiomyomas, or Pelvic Relaxation Syndrome. Other surgical interventions would depend on the specific cause, such as marsupialization of a Bartholin's cyst.

### Progressive Dilation and Muscle Awareness Exercise

This procedure, with appropriate counseling, is indicated for clients with vaginismus, an anatomically narrow introitus, hymenal remnants or scar tissue, or psychogenic factors.

Begin by reviewing the anatomy and physiology of the sexual organs and sexual response, stressing the normalcy of vulvar tissue. Using a mirror, have the client become familiar with her genitalia. Instruct the client on how to perform Kegel's exercises to increase her awareness of the muscles involved. Involve the client's partner whenever possible.

For progressive dilation, the client or health care provider inserts progressively larger objects into the vagina, beginning with a single finger, then a medium Pederson's speculum, two fingers, and finally a medium Graves' speculum. Measured vaginal dilators are also available. Allow the client to stop at any point that pain occurs. Have her bear down on insertion and use water-soluble lubricant to alleviate discomfort. Progressive digital dilation may be practiced by the client at home in order to familiarize her with her tissue, sensitization, and muscular control.[34]

Support and reassure the client. Reinforce her normalcy and that dyspareunia commonly occurs. Proceed at the client's pace, and never force an exam. Encourage her partner to participate, and try to correct any myths or knowledge deficits.

### Follow-Up and Referral

As with the entire evaluation and plan of care for clients with dyspareunia, follow-up will depend on the cause and the therapy selected. Follow-up evaluation is important, especially when dyspareunia is multifactorial. Stress to the client the importance of keeping follow-up appointments. Reassess the client frequently to determine whether psychological intervention is needed.

## LEIOMYOMAS

Leiomyomas are benign smooth muscle tumors of the uterus, commonly called "fibroids." They are classified according to their location within the uterus.

- *Submucous*, protruding into the uterine cavity.
- *Intramural*, within the myometrial wall.
- *Subserous*, growing toward the serous surface of the uterus.
- *Intraligamentous*, located in the cervix or in between the folds of the broad ligament.

Leiomyomas are estrogen dependent; they rarely occur before menarche or after menopause. They grow larger during pregnancy. Rarely malignant, leiomyomas may be small and asymptomatic or may grow very large and extend up into the abdomen. Because they interfere with fetal growth and nutrition, they increase the risk of spontaneous abortion during the first and second trimesters and the risk of preterm labor.[1,2] They are the most common indication for pelvic surgery in women.[36]

## EPIDEMIOLOGY

Leiomyomas develop from smooth muscle cells by means of metaplasia. What influences their growth is unknown. The condition occurs most often among African American women, and it is seen among nulliparous women, women older than 35, nonsmokers, and oral contraceptive or IUD users. Leiomyomas occur in 20 percent of women of reproductive age.[37]

## SUBJECTIVE DATA

Usually clients are asymptomatic. Symptoms increase, however, as the tumors grow. Common symptoms are pelvic pressure, bloating, pelvic congestion, a feeling of "heaviness," urinary frequency, dysmenorrhea, dyspareunia, menorrhagia, and less commonly, pain. Clients may report infertility. Pregnant women complain more frequently of pain.[1,2,37]

## OBJECTIVE DATA

### Physical Examination

An abdominal exam may reveal a large mass if the leiomyoma has grown larger than a 12- to 14-week pregnant uterus. The absence of ascites and presence of rebound tenderness and normal bowel sounds should be noted.

The genitalia and reproductive tract are also examined. Prior to the pelvic exam, ask the client to empty her bladder so that the examiner avoids confusing the tumor with the bladder. A pelvic exam may reveal an enlarged uterus that is firm and irregular but not tender. Usually palpated at midline, a leiomyoma may feel very firm or soft and cystic. If it is situated laterally, it may be mistaken for an adnexal mass. If the mass moves with the cervix, then it is likely to be a leiomyoma.[2]

### Diagnostic Tests and Methods

***Complete Blood Count (CBC).*** Diagnostic evaluation to determine whether the client is anemic, especially if she has experienced menometrorrhagia, and to detect any inflammatory process. (For procedure, see Pelvic Inflammatory Disease.)

***Urinalysis.*** Diagnostic evaluation to identify urinary tract conditions that might account for any urinary tract symptom. White blood cells, bacteria, or red blood cells in the urine may indicate chronic or recurrent urinary tract infection (UTI). Hematuria may indicate the presence of renal stones or a tumor of the urinary tract. Further diagnostic testing may be indicated, specifically cystoscopy or intravenous pyelogram.

Explain to the client how to obtain a clean-catch urine sample.

***Pregnancy Test (Urine or Blood Level of beta-hCG).*** Diagnostic evaluation for unsuspected intrauterine pregnancy (see Pelvic Inflammatory Disease for procedure).

***Stool Guaiac (Colocare or Hemoccult).*** Diagnostic evaluation to detect gastrointestinal (GI) pathology that may be the source of a palpable abdominal mass, for example, an inflammatory diverticulum or an intestinal mass. A stool found to be positive for occult blood suggests GI polyps or malignancy, but that result alone is insufficient for a definitive diagnosis. If the test is positive, or if the client's history and physical exam are suggestive, then refer her for gastroenterology consultation and further diagnostic testing, such as an upper GI series, barium enema, sigmoidoscopy, and/or colonoscopy.

With the Colocare method, the client floats a special card in the toilet after a bowel movement. A specific color change represents a positive result. The test should be repeated for three bowel movements at home. Alternatively, the older guaiac test (Hemoccult) requires the client to smear a stool sample onto a card and return the card to the health care professional, who subsequently applies solution to it; bluish discoloration represents a positive result. This test also should be repeated three times.

Provide instructions that will prepare the client for the test. Tell her that for 2 days before the test and during the testing period she is not to eat red or rare meats and is not to take vitamin C supplements, laxatives, or medications such as aspirin, corticosteroids, reserpine, indomethacin, or phenylbutazone. A high fiber diet is advised.

***Ultrasound.*** Diagnostic evaluation to identify the leiomyoma and confirm its location. Ultrasound helps to distinguish between uterine leiomyoma and an adnexal mass, and helps in assessing obese clients or others for whom the exam is not well tolerated (see Adenomyosis for the test procedure).

***Barium Enema.*** See Adnexal Masses.

***Intravenous Pyelogram.*** See Adnexal Masses.

***Fractional Curettage.*** Diagnostic evaluation to determine the etiology for menorrhagia or metrorrhagia, especially in women older than 35. *Fractional curettage is necessary to rule out endometrial carcinoma and should be done prior to any planned surgery.*[2]

The procedure is performed by a board-certified gynecologist. The uterus is dilated and sounded; endometrial tissue is either gently scraped or suctioned and then sent to a pathologist for evaluation.

When referring the client to a gynecologist for fractional curettage, explain the procedure to her. The procedure may be done on an outpatient basis, and depending on its extent and whether it is therapeutic or diagnostic, general anesthesia may or may not be necessary. Usually general anesthesia is not necessary for a simple diagnostic endometrial biopsy. Light vaginal bleeding may occur afterward. Stress to the client that she should immediately report any fever or pain. Instruct her to abstain from sexual intercourse and tub baths until vaginal bleeding and discharge ceases.[1,2,38] Bleeding and discharge should last less than 7 days.

## DIFFERENTIAL MEDICAL DIAGNOSES

Ovarian neoplasm, tubo-ovarian inflammatory mass, diverticular inflammatory mass, pregnancy, ectopic pregnancy, adenomyosis, pelvic kidney, malignancy.[1,2]

## PLAN

### Psychosocial Interventions

Provide the client with explanations and printed information about leiomyomas (fibroids). Reassure her that leiomyomas occur commonly, that they are rarely malignant, and that if she is asymptomatic or if symptoms are mild, treatment will be unnecessary. Assess her future reproductive plans and the extent of her symptoms. Stress the importance of regular monitoring and follow-up examinations. If the client is taking oral contraceptives, encourage her to select an alternative method of birth control and provide the necessary information and assistance.[1]

If the client is or becomes pregnant, provide reassurance and support. Inform her of her increased risks of miscarriage and preterm labor associated with fibroids, and allow her to express her fear and anxiety. Discuss the signs and symptoms of miscarriage, and later in her pregnancy, discuss the signs and symptoms of preterm labor.

## Medication

### *Medroxyprogesterone Acetate (MPA)*

- *Indications.* To suppress menorrhagia and inhibit tumor growth.
- *Administration.* MPA, 20 to 30 mg p.o., q.d. for several weeks.
- *Side Effects and Adverse Reactions.* Breakthrough bleeding, depression, delayed fertility, headache, dizziness, weight gain.
- *Contraindications.* MPA should not be used if there is a history of thromboembolic disease or thrombophlebitis, cerebrovascular accident, ischemic heart disease, reproductive organ or breast cancer, undiagnosed vaginal bleeding, pregnancy, liver tumor, impaired liver function, or cholestasis.
- *Anticipated Outcomes on Evaluation.* Cessation of bleeding, decrease in the size of the leiomyoma, absence of anemia.
- *Client Teaching and Counseling.* Review the instructions for taking the medication, list the possible side effects and danger signs, and tell the client what actions to take. If the effects are severe, she must call her provider and stop the medication. Advise the client to keep a record of her bleeding pattern and the amount.[37]

### *Gonadotropin-Releasing Hormone Agonist (GnRH-a) (Leuprorelin, Nafarelin)*

- *Indications.* To suppress growth of leiomyomas and promote possible shrinkage. GnRH-a is useful for reducing the size of the leiomyoma prior to surgery; it may permit vaginal hysterectomy rather than abdominal hysterectomy. It also may prevent the need for surgery in the perimenopausal client.
- *Administration. Leuprorelin (Lupron),* 0.5 mg s.c., q.d. for 8–12 weeks *or* 3.75–7.5 mg Depot Lupron once every 28 days. *Nafarelin (Synarel),* one spray (200 μg/spray) into one nostril q.a.m. and one spray into the other nostril q.h.s. 8–12 weeks.[2,7]
- *Side Effects and Adverse Reactions.* Hot flashes, vaginal dryness, mood swings, depression, weight gain, reduced breast size, decreased libido, fatigue, and insomnia. In the event of interference with calcium and bone metabolism, supplement with calcium carbonate: 1000–1500 mg/day.
- *Contraindications.* Known or suspected pregnancy, hypersensitivity to GnRH agonists, undiagnosed abnormal vaginal bleeding, breastfeeding.
- *Anticipated Outcomes on Evaluation.* A reduction in uterine and leiomyoma size.
- *Client Teaching and Counseling.* Instruct the client about proper drug administration and inform her that the GnRH agonists are very expensive. The length of therapy (8 to 12 weeks) needs to be discussed. Review the side effects and the possible need for calcium carbonate supplementation. Barrier contraception is recommended during therapy and for the first menstrual cycle. Explain that it is likely that within 6 months following treatment the leiomyomas will recur.[39,40]

### *Oral Iron Preparation*

- *Indications.* The client who is experiencing significant menorrhagia or metrorrhagia and whose hemoglobin and hematocrit are falling below normal levels.
- *Administration.* Select one of many commercially available preparations. Begin with one tablet (300 mg ferrous sulfate or the equivalent) daily; increase to two daily if hemoglobin falls below 10.0 g/dL. Follow with reticulocyte counts to monitor response to the therapy.
- *Side Effects and Adverse Reactions.* Constipation and other gastrointestinal symp-

toms, such as indigestion, nausea, loss of appetite.

- *Contraindication.* Known allergy to oral iron preparations.
- *Anticipated Outcome on Evaluation.* Anemia secondary to menometrorrhagia is prevented.
- *Client Teaching and Counseling.* Provide information about foods that are rich in iron (leafy green vegetables, enriched flour products, raisins, prunes, dried apricots). Instruct the client that for better absorption of the iron, she should take the preparation with a citrus juice and avoid eating or drinking dairy products for 1 hour before and 1 hour after.

### Surgery

***Myomectomy.*** The procedure is indicated for the client with leiomyoma who is symptomatic and wishes to maintain her reproductive capability. The uterus is 12 weeks size or larger; a solitary pedunculated myoma is present; the nature or location of the myoma appears to be interfering with fertility; the myoma is causing pregnancy loss; the rapid growth of the myoma carries the possibility of malignant sarcoma transformation.

Refer the client to a board-certified gynecologist. The size and location of the myomas will determine the site of abdominal incision. Some surgeons are skilled at removing small myomas through the laparoscope or hysteroscope. Smaller tumors may be destroyed with the laser. The goal of surgery is to remove all leiomyomas, relieve symptoms, and increase fertility. Adverse effects may develop as a result of a difficult, demanding procedure with the potential for increased blood loss, increased operating time, increased postoperative risks of infection, ileus, anemia, and increased pain. Among women who undergo myomectomy, 20 to 25 percent must have repeated surgery due to recurrence. Most myomectomy clients who subsequently become pregnant will require delivery by cesarean section.

Discuss the difficult surgery and its potential complications with the client. Inform her about the high rate of myoma recurrence and the possible later need for a hysterectomy. Warn her not to attempt pregnancy until 4 to 6 months after the procedure. Review the postoperative/discharge instructions.[41,42]

***Hysterectomy.*** The procedure is indicated when rapid enlargement of the uterus signals possible malignancy. In addition, hysterectomy may be done to resolve any of the following: abnormal uterine bleeding that may lead to anemia, pelvic pain and secondary dysmenorrhea, urinary symptoms, or uterine growth after menopause.[37] The surgery is indicated if the client has completed childbearing or if the health care provider is unable to evaluate the adnexa because the uterus has become an abdominal organ. The route of hysterectomy depends on the size of the leiomyoma: if less than 12 weeks size, vaginal hysterectomy is possible.

Surgery should accomplish complete relief of symptoms. Few adverse effects occur; however, bleeding, infection, and damage to nearby organs is possible.

Client teaching and counseling include discussion of the alternatives to hysterectomy, especially if there is indecision regarding future childbearing. Provide the client with a thorough explanation of hysterectomy, including descriptions of anatomy, physiology, and the surgical procedure, its risks and benefits. Reassure the client that femininity remains unchanged. Hormonal replacement therapy may need to be initiated if salpingo-oophorectomy is done. Full recovery usually occurs within 6 weeks. Review the postoperative instructions, including the return to activity, expectation that vaginal bleeding will change to clear discharge, signs of infection, resumption of sexual activity when bleeding ceases (usually in about 14 days), and dietary counseling (including information about preventing constipation and weight gain).[37]

### Follow-Up and Referral

For the client who is asymptomatic or has mild symptoms, the treatment of choice is conservative (expectant) management.[2,37] During pregnancy, rest and analgesics are appropriate if pain is present. Stress the importance of keeping appointments for close follow-up. If expectant management, medical therapy, or myomectomy is chosen as a treatment option, the client should be reexamined at 3- to 6-month intervals. Uterine size and the leiomyoma should be evaluated carefully by pelvic exam and if necessary, ultrasound should be used. Discuss with the client any new or worsening symptomatology. Alter the plan of care as necessary. Monitor hemoglobin and hematocrit frequently if menorrhagia or metrorrhagia is present.[1,2,37]

## PELVIC RELAXATION SYNDROME

Pelvic relaxation syndrome is the failure of the pelvic musculature to maintain support and position of the pelvic organs. When supporting pelvic ligaments, muscles, and fascia can no longer withstand constant increased intra-abdominal pressure, such as that which occurs with obstetric damage, chronic coughing or straining, surgery, or aging, the vaginal wall weakens, descends, and the pelvic organs protrude into the vaginal canal. Five major types of genital prolapse may occur: cystocele, urethrocele, rectocele, enterocele, and uterine prolapse.[2,7] The vagina can also prolapse to or beyond the introitus but this generally occurs only when the uterus has been removed.[7]

*Types of Genital Prolapse*

- *Cystocele.* Prolapse of the posterior bladder wall through the anterior vaginal wall.
- *Urethrocele.* Bulging of the urethra through the anterior vaginal wall; usually not a single entity, occurs with cystocele.
- *Rectocele.* Bulging of the bowel through the posterior vaginal wall; involves loss of support of the fascia and levator ani muscles.
- *Enterocele.* Bulging of the bowel through the posterior cul-de-sac and vaginal wall; may be part of a high rectocele.
- *Uterine Prolapse.* Descent of the uterus through the pelvic floor and into the vaginal canal.

The extent of genital organ prolapse is described in terms of degree: *first degree*, prolapse of an organ into the vaginal canal; *second degree*, presence of an organ at the introitus; *third degree*, an organ has completely prolapsed outside the introitus.[43]

### EPIDEMIOLOGY

- Weakening of the pelvic supports through the stretching and trauma of childbirth.
- Increased intra-abdominal pressure secondary to chronic respiratory problems, heavy lifting, ascites, obesity, and habitual straining due to constipation.
- Normal downward pressure because the human posture is erect.
- Atrophy of the supporting tissues with aging, especially after menopause.
- Congenital weakness.

Risk factors include obesity, Caucasian race, multiparity, and menopause with lack of estrogen replacement.[2]

Pelvic relaxation occurs with increasing frequency during the postreproductive years; in fact, the majority of parous women show some evidence of pelvic relaxation. Approximately 10 to 15 percent will require surgery.[2]

## SUBJECTIVE DATA

Clients frequently state, "Something feels like it is falling out." Other symptoms include backache; pelvic pressure or heaviness; bearing-down sensation; urinary frequency, urgency, or incontinence; dyspareunia; discomfort walking or sitting; difficult defecation; or protrusion of an organ through the introitus.[1,2,43]

## OBJECTIVE DATA

### Physical Examination

Physical examination, including complete gynecologic inspection, is the most important step in diagnosing pelvic relaxation. Examine the external genitalia for atrophy and any obvious protrusion of the uterus, bladder, urethra, or vaginal wall. Use lithotomy position and Sims's speculum (Graves' speculum may be used if the anterior blade is removed). Ask the client to perform the Valsalva maneuver; note which organ prolapses first and the degree to which it occurs.

Systematically examine the anterior and posterior walls of the vagina. Ask the client to contract the pubococcygeal muscles (Kegel's exercise); with two fingers in the vagina, note the strength and symmetry of the contraction. Note any ulcerations of the cervix and uterus if third degree prolapse is present. Note bladder leakage during the exam.

Perform a rectal exam; observe any bleeding, and determine muscle tone and the presence of any rectocele.[43]

## DIFFERENTIAL MEDICAL DIAGNOSES

Pelvic or abdominal tumors, tumors of the rectovaginal septum, cervical hypertrophy, Gartner's cyst, urethral diverticulum.

## PLAN

### Psychosocial Interventions

Describe the normal anatomy and the etiologies for pelvic prolapse to the client. Determine the impact of the prolapse on the client's daily functioning and ask whether she has future reproductive desires. Reassure the client that she can achieve relief of symptoms, restoration or partial restoration of anatomy, and return to normal functioning.

### Medication

***Estrogen Replacement Therapy.*** Indicated to improve tone and vascularity of the supporting tissue in perimenopausal and menopausal women.

***Nonnarcotic Analgesics.*** Indicated for temporary relief of associated discomfort, especially back pain. The desired outcome of treatment is partial or complete pain relief. Over-the-counter analgesics, such as acetaminophen, should be tried first, but more potent nonsteroidal anti-inflammatory drugs (NSAIDs) may be needed.

- *Administration.* Continuous use is most effective. Several types of NSAIDs are available, and their dosages vary.
  - Ibuprofen (Motrin), 400–800 mg q.i.d.
  - Naproxen (Naprosyn or Anaprox), 275 mg q.i.d., *or* 550 mg b.i.d.
  - Ketoprofen (Orudis), 50–100 mg b.i.d.
  - Flurbiprofen (Ansaid), 50–100 mg b.i.d.
- *Side Effects and Adverse Reactions.* Most often reported is GI irritation. If GI irritation occurs, sucralfate (a GI antiulcerative) may be added to the regimen. Sucralfate dosage is one 1 g tablet p.o. 1 hour before or 2 hours after meals and at bedtime.
- *Contraindications.* Previous allergy to NSAIDs and a history of ulcer disease.

- *Client Teaching and Counseling.* Stress the need to follow the NSAID regimen carefully and to take the drug with food. *Counsel the client to report immediately any signs of indigestion, epigastric pain, or hematochezia.*

### Dietary Interventions

Dietary habits can exacerbate the prolapse by causing constipation and consequently chronic straining. Dietary modifications will help to establish regular bowel movements without discomfort and eliminate excessive gas or bloating.

Teach the client about increasing dietary fiber and fluids to prevent constipation. Explain how constipation can contribute to straining and pelvic prolapse. Provide the client with instruction, materials, and support.[2,43]

### Respiratory Interventions

Correction or improvement of respiratory problems that cause chronic cough will decrease intra-abdominal pressure and thereby prevent worsening of pelvic prolapse. Intervention is indicated for clients who smoke, have asthma, or have chronic bronchitis. Anticipated outcomes on evaluation are that the client has stopped smoking, coughs less, and has less shortness of breath.

Counseling of a client who is not receiving care for a respiratory problem should include referral for evaluation and management. Encourage her to follow prescribed regimens, to stop smoking, and possibly to join a support group. Discuss with the client how reducing respiratory symptoms will help improve the symptoms of prolapse and prevent them from worsening.[43] Reinforce the discussion by providing written information.

### Surgery

Procedures that are frequently done include the following.

- Anterior colporrhaphy (plication of the pubocervical fascia) to correct cystocele/urethrocele.
- Posterior colporrhaphy (midline approximation of the endopelvic fascia and perineal muscles) to correct rectocele/enterocele.
- Enterocele repair (approximation of the uterosacral ligaments and levator ani muscles after reduction of the bowel).
- Manchester operation (involves anterior colporrhaphy, posterior colporrhaphy, amputation of the cervix, and suturing of the cardinal ligaments in front of the stump) to preserve, support, and antevert the uterus.
- Vaginal hysterectomy, done for any degree of uterine prolapse.
- Le Fort's partial colpocleisis (suturing of the anterior and posterior vaginal walls so that the uterus is supported above), performed in elderly clients with substantial prolapse.

Indications for surgery are when childbearing is completed and/or symptoms begin to interfere with the client's daily living patterns and do not respond to nonsurgical treatment. The procedure chosen depends on the type and severity of pelvic prolapse. The client is referred to a board-certified gynecologic surgeon for evaluation.

Potential adverse effects depend on the surgical procedure performed. For example, with preservation of the uterus and closure of the vaginal canal, abnormal uterine bleeding could occur undetected. Coitus is also affected. A major adverse effect is recurrence of the prolapse; other effects include urinary retention, chronic urinary tract infection (UTI), incontinence, and difficult defecation.

Anticipated outcomes on evaluation are a return to optimal function; cessation or significantly fewer and less severe symptoms; normal patterns of elimination; and prevention of prolapse of other organs and of recurrence of the prolapse that was repaired.

Provide in-depth discussions of the procedure to be performed, emphasizing anatomy and postoperative instructions. Allow the client to express her fears and anxieties. Stress that femininity will be preserved; however, discuss how sexual function may be altered.[1,2,43]

### Pessaries

A *pessary* is a hard rubber or plastic ring used to maintain the normal position of the uterus or bladder by exerting pressure and providing support. It is placed in the vagina behind the pubic arch and the posterior fornix. An indication for pessary use is uterine prolapse or cystocele especially among elderly clients for whom surgery is contraindicated.

Adverse effects include chronic vaginal infection and recurrent UTI. Anticipated outcomes on evaluation are that the uterus and bladder are supported, symptoms are decreased, and no interference occurs with intercourse. Client teaching must include instruction for removing and cleaning the pessary every 2 to 3 months. Review the symptoms associated with pessary use: leukorrhea; vaginal burning or itching; loss of the pessary; urinary retention, frequency, urgency; and dysuria.[43,44] Instruct the client to report any symptoms.

### Kegel's Exercises

The exercises strengthen pelvic muscles, which prevents further prolapse. They can be performed at any time and are very easy to learn. They have no adverse effect.

Help the client to identify the pubococcygeus muscle by having her stop and start her urinary flow. Have her tighten the muscle for a count of 3, then relax it. The client should repeat the exercise 10 times. Then, instruct the client to contract and relax the muscle rapidly 10 times. In addition, have her try to bring up the entire pelvic floor and bear down 10 times. This movement may be repeated 5 times daily.

### Lifestyle Changes

Several changes in lifestyle may help to prevent pelvic relaxation. For example, the client should attempt to achieve her ideal weight; wear a girdle or abdominal support belt; avoid or reduce heavy lifting; avoid high impact aerobics and jogging.

### Follow-Up and Referral

Emphasize to all clients that worsening or recurrence of any symptoms should be reported immediately. If nonsurgical therapies are employed, regular follow-up visits at least every 6 months are necessary to assess the degree of prolapse and any worsening symptomatology. If a pessary is used, the client should be seen every 2 to 3 months to remove the device for inspection and cleaning. After surgery, the client should be seen at least annually to assess any recurrent prolapse.

## CHRONIC PELVIC PAIN

Chronic pain persists for longer than 6 months and significantly impacts a woman's daily functioning and relationships. It can be *episodic* (i.e., cyclic, recurrent pain that is interspersed with pain-free intervals) or *continuous* (i.e., noncyclic pain). Chronic pelvic pain frustrates both the client and her health care providers. Many times an etiology for chronic pain cannot be found or treatment of the presumed etiology fails; hence pain becomes the illness.[45]

## EPIDEMIOLOGY

One-third of clients with chronic pelvic pain have no obvious pelvic pathology.[2,46] Since the 1920s, researchers have attempted to discover etiologies for chronic pelvic pain syndrome. At various times, different theories gained popularity, but the studies on which they were based were problematic (e.g., small samples, observer bias). Among the more popular theories that lack definite diagnostic criteria and management protocol are Allen-Masters Syndrome (universal joint syndrome), pelvic congestion syndrome, and retrodisplacement of the uterus.[47] The more common etiologies of chronic pelvic pain are as follows.

- *Episodic.* Dyspareunia, midcycle pelvic pain (mittelschmerz), dysmenorrhea.
- *Continuous.* Endometriosis, adenomyosis, chronic salpingitis, adhesions, loss of pelvic support.[48]

Risk factors include the following.

- History of childhood or adult sexual abuse or trauma.
- Previous pelvic surgery.
- Personal or family history of depression.
- History of other chronic pain syndromes.
- History of alcohol and drug abuse.
- Sexual dysfunction.
- Tendency toward somatization.[45,49]

Chronic pelvic pain comprises up to 10 percent of outpatient gynecologic visits and is the reason for 20 percent of laparoscopies and 12 percent of hysterectomies. Approximately 70,000 hysterectomies are performed annually because of chronic pelvic pain.[49]

## SUBJECTIVE DATA

The client may report pain duration of 6 months or longer; incomplete relief by most previous treatments, including surgery and nonnarcotic analgesics; significantly impaired functioning at home or work; signs of depression such as early morning awakening, weight loss, and anorexia; pain out of proportion to pathology; and altered family roles. The client may also have a history of childhood abuse, incest, rape or other sexual trauma, substance abuse, or current sexual dysfunction. A client usually reports previous consultation with one or more health care providers and dissatisfaction with their management of her condition.[45,50]

## OBJECTIVE DATA

### Physical Examination

Perform a systematic physical examination of the abdominal, pelvic, and rectal areas, focusing on the location and intensity of the pain. Attempt to reproduce the pain. The use of relaxation/breathing techniques will facilitate examination for both client and health professional.[44,49] *Check the client's vital signs; fever indicates an acute process.*

Note the client's general appearance, demeanor, and gait; these may suggest the severity of pain and possible neuromuscular etiology. Vomiting may indicate an acute process.

Abdominal symptoms of a more acute process are rebound tenderness (peritoneal irritation) and decreased abdominal pain on palpation with tension of the rectus muscles. Ask the client to perform a straight leg raise; with the client's legs slightly raised and rectus muscles taut, pain on deep palpation will decrease if it is of pelvic origin and increase if it is of abdominal wall or myofascial origin. Inspect and note any well healed scars. Palpate scars for incisional hernias, and palpate for any unsuspected masses. To help identify femoral or inguinal hernias, palpate the groin while the client performs the Valsalva maneuver.

During the speculum exam, note any cervicitis, which may be a source of parametrial irritation. With bimanual/rectal exam, a tender pelvic or adnexal mass, abnormal bleeding, tender uterine fundus, or cervical motion tenderness may indicate an acute process, such as pelvic inflammatory disease (PID), ectopic pregnancy, or a ruptured ovarian cyst.

Nonmobility of the uterus may indicate the presence of pelvic adhesions. Note existence of any adnexal mass, fullness, or tenderness. Cul-de-sac nodularities are palpable with endometriosis. Identify any areas that reproduce deep dyspareunia.

Palpate the coccyx, both internally and externally, for tenderness of coccydynia.[48]

### Diagnostic Test and Methods

Diagnostic tests should be selected discriminately as indicated by the findings of the history and physical examination. Review previous test results in order to avoid unnecessary and repetitive diagnostic testing.[45,50]

***Complete Blood Count (CBC) and Erythrocyte Sedimentation Rate (ESR).*** See Pelvic Inflammatory Disease.

***Urinalysis.*** Diagnostic evaluation to identify any urinary tract conditions that might represent the source of pain. White blood cells, bacteria, or red blood cells may indicate either chronic or recurrent urinary tract infections (UTI). Hematuria may indicate renal stones or a tumor of the urinary tract. Further diagnostic testing, specifically cystoscopy or intravenous pyelogram, may be indicated.

Teach the client how to obtain a clean-catch urine sample in a sterile container.

***Pregnancy Test (Urine or Blood Level of hCG).*** See Pelvic Inflammatory Disease.

***Vaginal Smears/Cervical Cultures.*** Diagnostic evaluation to detect existing pelvic infection as the etiology of acute or chronic pelvic pain. Wet mount with saline can detect bacterial vaginosis or trichomoniasis. Cervical tests can detect *N. gonorrhoeae* and *C. trachomatis*. (See Chapter 8 for the test procedures.)

***Stool Guaiac (Colocare or Hemoccult).*** Diagnostic evaluation to detect gastrointestinal (GI) pathology as a possible source of pain (see Leiomyomas for the test procedure). The stool may be positive for occult blood in cases of ulcerative colitis, irritable bowel syndrome, GI polyps, or malignancy, although this test is not definitive. If the result is positive, or if history and physical exam suggest, then refer the client for gastroenterology consultation and further diagnostic testing, such as upper GI series, barium enema, sigmoidoscopy, and/or colonoscopy.

***Ultrasound.*** Diagnostic evaluation to identify and locate potential causes of pelvic pain (see Adenomyosis for the test procedure).

***Laparoscopy.*** Diagnostic evaluation accomplished by direct visualization, performed when pelvic pathology is not detectable by pelvic exam or other diagnostic testing (see Endometriosis for the test procedure). Laparoscopy is useful in the diagnosis of acute or chronic salpingitis, ectopic pregnancy, hydrosalpinx, endometriosis, ovarian tumors and cysts, torsion, appendicitis, and adhesions. (Researchers have been unable to demonstrate a direct correlation between laparoscopic findings and the severity of pelvic pain.[51,52])

## DIFFERENTIAL MEDICAL DIAGNOSES

Common medical conditions that are not gynecologic but may present as chronic pelvic pain include GI conditions, such as irritable bowel syndrome, ulcerative colitis, and diverticulosis; urinary tract disease; and neuromuscular/musculoskeletal disorders, such as disc problems.[2,48]

## PLAN

Specific management of a client with chronic pelvic pain depends on the pain's etiology. Therefore, careful physical, psychosocial, and diagnostic evaluations represent the most important steps in providing care for these clients. Many clients, however, either fail to respond to therapy or do not demonstrate any known pathology.

The goal of care is to alleviate pain so that the client is able to maintain optimal daily functioning. The emotional, psychological, and physical aspects of the pain should be managed simultaneously.

### Psychosocial Interventions

If the client has one or more of the following indications, then refer her for skilled psychological evaluation and therapy.

- No apparent etiology for pain found during a thorough evaluation, including diagnostic laparoscopy.
- History of psychosexual trauma.
- History of consultation and therapy for multiple, unrelated somatic symptoms.

Review all findings with the client and involve her in decisions about care. If appropriate, involve the client's partner in planning care. Set realistic goals for evaluating therapy, stressing that a "cure" may not be possible. Refer the client for sexual counseling and therapy if indicated. Encourage her to keep a diary of the timing, location, and severity of the pain and the significant circumstances surrounding it.[53,54]

### Medication

The goal of treatment with medication is to ameliorate pain, not eliminate it. Long term narcotic use has been proved ineffective in the management of chronic pelvic pain and may lead to abuse and dependency behaviors.[45,48]

***Nonsteroidal Anti-inflammatory Drugs (NSAIDs)***

- *Indication.* Partial or complete relief of episodic or continuous pain.
- *Administration.* Continuous use is most effective. Several types of NSAIDs are available, and their dosage varies.
  - Ibuprofen (Motrin), 400–800 mg q.i.d.
  - Naproxen (Naprosyn or Anaprox), 275 mg q.i.d. *or* 550 mg b.i.d.
  - Ketoprofen (Orudis), 50–100 mg b.i.d.
  - Flurbiprofen (Ansaid), 50–100 mg b.i.d.
- *Side Effects and Adverse Reactions.* The major side effect is GI irritation. If it occurs, sucralfate may be added to the regimen.
- *Contraindications.* Previous allergy to NSAIDs and previous history of ulcer disease.
- *Client Teaching and Counseling.* Advise the client to take the NSAID continuously, on schedule, and with food. Stress that she should immediately report any signs of indigestion, epigastric pain, or hematochezia.

***Antidepressants.*** Antidepressants are used to enhance the effectiveness of NSAIDs, manage simultaneous depression, and improve sleep patterns. Many different types are available, with varying side effects and actions. The lowest possible dose is given and then increased if necessary. Administration follows consultation with a gynecologist concerning use.

- Side effects and contraindications vary greatly among the different antidepressants. The anticipated outcomes on evaluation are perception of decreased pain and less interference with the activities of daily living.
- Instruct the client to monitor her response to the drug and its side effects. Help ensure that the client takes the proper dose and understands the possible side effects.

***Oral Contraceptives.*** Indicated for the management of cyclic, chronic pain, specifically that associated with dysmenorrhea, mild endometriosis, and recurrent functional ovarian cysts (see Endometriosis and Chapter 5, Dysmenorrhea).

## Dietary Interventions

Modifications in diet may be indicated when the client is experiencing constipation, bloating, edema, excessive fatigue, irritability, or lethargy, or is overweight. Dietary habits may contribute to the pain pattern, although not directly cause it.

Anticipated outcomes on evaluation are regular bowel movements without discomfort; decreased gas, bloating, and edema; improved energy level and stability of mood; and attainment and maintenance of ideal body weight.

Provide the client with information about the need for a high fiber diet and increased fluids to prevent constipation; explain how constipation can contribute to the pain pattern. In addition, less sodium, caffeine, and carbonated beverages reduce edema and abdominal bloating. Discuss with the client alternative cooking and seasoning methods, explain pertinent information on food labels, and suggest alternatives to soft drinks, coffee, and tea in order to limit intake of caffeine and carbonated beverages. Instruction may also include information about achieving stable blood sugar levels and weight loss by reducing refined carbohydrates and sugar in the diet, and eating low-fat foods with fewer calories. Reinforce the information with printed materials.

## Surgical Interventions

***Laparoscopy.*** Indications are for therapeutic as well as diagnostic purposes. Therapeutically, laparoscopy may be used for lysis of pelvic adhesions and ablation of endometrial implants.

***Hysterectomy.*** This type of surgery is indicated when a known pathology is suspected to represent the source of pain, for example, leiomyomas, endometriosis, chronic PID, adenomyosis, or suspected malignancy. Pain that does not have a known or suspected etiology is not an indication for a hysterectomy; however, chronic pelvic pain is listed as the indication for 10 to 15 percent of the hysterectomies performed in the United States.[49] (See the discussion of hysterectomy under Endometriosis.)

***Presacral Neurectomy.*** Previously performed to alleviate severe, intractable chronic pelvic pain caused by dysmenorrhea and edometriosis, presacral neurectomy is no longer advocated now that NSAIDs are available. In clients who previously underwent the surgery, it may have failed to relieve the pain. Counseling of these clients should include an explanation of why the procedure is no longer performed.[55]

## Alternative Interventions

Other interventions for the management of chronic pelvic pain include biofeedback, stress management techniques, self-hypnosis, relaxation therapy, transcutaneous nerve stimulation (TNS), trigger-point injections, spinal anesthesia, and nerve blocks. For many of these alternative interventions, referral to a chronic pelvic pain clinic is recommended.[45]

## Follow-Up and Referral

Regularly scheduled client appointments are crucial to the management of chronic pelvic pain. Visits are scheduled at intervals unrelated to specific pain episodes. Maintain consistent communication with the client, coordinate results of other providers' evaluations and therapies, and review this information with the client.[45]

## BARTHOLINITIS

Bartholinitis is the inflammation of one or both of the Bartholin's glands, two pea-sized glands located bilaterally beneath the vaginal vestibule. Their function, it is thought, is to lubricate the vestibule.[56]

### EPIDEMIOLOGY

Mechanical obstruction of the duct leading to the gland occurs with secondary infection, most commonly caused by *Neisseria gonococcus, Staphylococcus, Streptococcus, Escherichia coli, Trichomonas,* and *Bacteroides.*[7,56] Secondary infection may be sexually transmitted.

Approximately 2 percent of adult women develop bartholinitis.[56]

### SUBJECTIVE DATA

Unilateral swelling of the labia; extreme tenderness, pain, and throbbing; dyspareunia; pain when walking or sitting; history of recurrent abscess.[8]

### OBJECTIVE DATA

Examination of the genitalia/reproductive tract may reveal erythema, acute tenderness, edema, a fluctuant mass located laterally to the vestibule, purulent drainage, tender and enlarged inguinal nodes.[7,56]

A culture and sensitivity test is done to identify the source of infection, especially with recurrent infection. Drainage from the gland is collected on a sterile swab. If gonorrhea is suspected, Thayer-Martin medium may be used for the culture. Explain the procedure to the client.[8]

### DIFFERENTIAL MEDICAL DIAGNOSES

Inclusion cyst, sebaceous cyst, primary cancer of Bartholin's gland or duct (especially among women older than 40), secondary metastatic malignancy, lipoma, fibroma, hernia, hydrocele.[2,56]

### PLAN

#### Psychosocial Interventions

Describe for the client how the infection occurs, and explain the treatment in detail. Allow time for questions and concerns to be expressed.

#### Medication

**Broad Spectrum Antibiotics *(Erythromycin, Doxycycline, Cephalosporins).*** Indicated when gonorrhea is suspected or identified (see Chapter 8). Administer erythromycin, 250 mg p.o., q.i.d. for 10 days; *or* doxycycline, 100 mg p.o., b.i.d. for 10 days; *or* cephalexin, 250 mg p.o., q.i.d. for 10 days.

A side effect is GI upset; contraindications include previous sensitivity to any of the aforementioned antibiotics. Doxycycline/tetracycline is contraindicated during pregnancy.

Anticipated outcomes on evaluation are relief of symptoms and resolution of infection/abscess. Instruct the client to take the medication with food (meal or snack) but not with milk, to complete the entire course of medication, and if taking doxycycline, to stay out of the sun or use sunscreen.

***Analgesics.*** Used to relieve pain.

#### Surgical Interventions

***Incision and Drainage/Insertion of Word Catheter.***[56] This procedure is done by a gynecologist in cases of abscess formation and when response to antibiotic therapy is inadequate. The procedure involves cleansing the area with povidone iodine (Betadine) and using local anesthetic, such as lidocaine (1 percent). A small incision is made approximately at the opening of the duct, and as much purulent drainage as possible is expressed. The cavity is explored for other pockets of infection. Finally, a Word catheter (a bulb-tipped inflatable catheter that remains in the cyst) is inserted and 2 to 4 mL of sterile water is injected to hold the catheter in place for 4 to 6 weeks. The plugged end of the catheter is tucked into the vagina.

An adverse effect of overinflation of the bulb is pressure necrosis of the cyst wall with chronic defect.

The anticipated outcome on evaluation is complete resolution of the abscess and infection.

Provide the client with instructions to follow during the 4 to 6 weeks that the catheter is in place. The catheter is checked weekly and deflated as the abscess becomes smaller and drainage slows. The client may take sitz baths and warm soaks for comfort. Sexual intercourse is permitted as soon as tenderness subsides; care must be taken not to dislodge the catheter.

***Marsupialization.*** Creation of a pouch is performed in cases of recurrent abscess formation. Referral is made to a gynecologic surgeon, who performs the procedure on an outpatient basis using local, regional, or general anesthesia. After an incision is made over the cyst, exploration and drainage is performed if necessary, and the wall of the cyst is everted and fixed to the surrounding skin. Adverse effects, although rare, may include postoperative infection and pain.

The anticipated outcomes on evaluation are permanent drainage and no further cyst/abscess recurrences.[1,56,57]

Explain the procedure to the client and tell her that it is curative.

### Alternative Interventions

Rest, heat, and sitz baths may also be used to treat barthinolitis.

### Follow-Up and Referral

Follow-up for conservative treatment (antibiotics, rest, heat) should occur 7 to 10 days after the treatment is begun. Swelling, pain, erythema, and tenderness or throbbing should be resolved or resolving. If a Word catheter is inserted, follow up weekly. A 4 to 6 week follow-up is appropriate for marsupialization.[7,57]

## CERVICAL POLYPS

Cervical polyps are benign, pedunculated growths of varying size that extend from the ectocervix or endocervical canal. Polyps may occur singularly or they may be multiple.[1]

### EPIDEMIOLOGY

The etiology is unknown—however, polyps are believed to result from chronic inflammation; they may be associated with hyperestrogen states; and they are found commonly with endometrial hyperplasia. Polyps are most common among multiparous women in their thirties and forties.[56]

Cervical polyps are the most common benign neoplastic growth of the cervix and occur in 4 percent of all gynecologic clients.[56]

### SUBJECTIVE DATA

The client is usually asymptomatic, although thick leukorrhea, postcoital bleeding, intermenstrual bleeding, menorrhagia, postmenopausal bleeding, or mucopurulent or blood-tinged vaginal discharge may occur.[56]

### OBJECTIVE DATA

#### Physical Examination

Single or multiple pear-shaped growths may protrude from the cervix into the vaginal canal. They are usually smooth, soft, reddish purple to cherry red, and readily bleed when touched. They may be small or very large.[56]

### Diagnostic Tests and Methods

***Pathology.*** A diagnostic microscopic evaluation of all polyps should be done by a pathologist; diagnosis is confirmed during evaluation.[1] This requires collection of a specimen to be labeled and sent in preservative medium to a pathology laboratory. (See Surgical Interventions, below, for a description of the procedure.)

Explain the procedure to the client and tell her when she can expect test results. Reassure her that the majority of polyps are benign.

***Papanicolaou (Pap) Smear.*** (See Chapter 3.)

## DIFFERENTIAL MEDICAL DIAGNOSES

Endometrial polyps, small prolapsed myomas, cervical malignancy.[1,56]

## PLAN

### Psychosocial Interventions

Explain to the client what polyps are and that they are usually benign; encourage her to express her concerns.

### Surgical Interventions

Cervical polyps should be removed and sent to a pathology laboratory. The procedure can be performed in an office without anesthesia by any appropriately trained health care provider. Paint the cervix with povidone-iodine (Betadine); using ring forceps, grasp and twist the polyp at the base. Apply silver nitrate or Monsel's solution to the site of removal to control bleeding. Excessive bleeding is a potential adverse effect.

Client teaching includes the need for pelvic rest for 24 hours to ensure that bleeding does not occur at the removal site. If excessive bleeding or excessive vaginal discharge does occur, the client must return for evaluation and possible endometrial sampling.

### Treatment of Vaginal Infections

Accompanying vaginal infections must be treated appropriately (see Chapter 8).

### Follow-Up and Referral

Regular Pap smears and gynecologic exams are important, and this needs to be stressed to the client.

# GYNECOLOGIC CANCERS: SCREENING AND REFERRAL

## CERVICAL CANCER

Human papillomavirus (HPV) has been linked with cervical cancer; HPV 16 and HPV 18 are the most prevalent types.[58] Risk factors for cervical cancer include early age at first coitus, multiple sexual partners, first child prior to age 20, lower socioeconomic status, history of sexually transmitted diseases (STDs) (especially HPV), exposure to diethylstilbestrol (DES) in utero, and cigarette smoking.[59,60]

Cervical cancer is the third most common malignancy in women[59] and accounts for 18 percent of all gynecologic cancers in the United States. In the past 45 years, its incidence has decreased from 45 to 15 per 100,000 women. An increase, however, has occurred in the prevalence of dysplasia and preinvasive lesions.[58,59]

### Screening

The screening technique is the Pap smear (see Chapter 3). The cytology brush is now recommended to obtain better endocervical samples in nonpregnant women.[58,61] Screening should begin when a woman becomes sexually active, requests contraceptive advice, or reaches age 18. The American College of Obstetricians and Gynecologists and the American Cancer Society recommend annual Pap smears thereafter.[58,61]

### Follow-Up and Referral

The most commonly employed system of reporting Pap smear results is the cervical intraepithelial neoplasia (CIN) system. The National Cancer Institute (NCI) in Bethesda, Maryland, however, proposed an alternative classification system describing squamous intraepithelial lesion (SIL).[60,62] The systems are compared in Chapter 3, Table 3–7, Pap Smear Report Findings, Interpretation, and Action.

Follow-up of Pap smear results is somewhat controversial, and protocols may differ from one provider or institution to another. Current recommendations, however, are generally as follows.

- With normal findings, repeat screening once per year.
- With inflammatory atypia, gynecologic evaluation employs wet mount, gonorrhea culture, and/or chlamydia culture. Treat any infection. Repeat Pap smear 8 to 12 weeks after treatment. Colposcopy is indicated for suspicious atypia or SIL.
- With CIN of any grade, refer the client to an experienced colposcopist for biopsy and endocervical curettage.[60,63,64]

## UTERINE CANCER

Uterine cancer may occur with exposure of the endometrium to high levels of exogenous and/or endogenous estrogen.[1,58] Unopposed estrogen replacement, obesity, nulliparity or low parity, history of diabetes, history of hypertension, and menopause are risk factors for uterine cancer.[2,58,65] This cancer is responsible for 7 percent of all cancers in women; 1 in 45 women will develop invasive cancer of the uterine corpus.[58] It is the most common cancer of the reproductive organs.[2]

### Screening

The incidence of endometrial carcinoma in women younger than 40 is low; hence, routine screening of these women is not recommended. Screening of all women over age 40 is neither practical nor cost effective. The criteria used in performing endometrial sampling include the following.

- Any postmenopausal bleeding.
- Premenopausal clients with polycystic ovarian syndrome.
- Postmenopausal clients taking exogenous estrogen, especially if unopposed.
- Obese, nulliparous clients with diabetes or hypertension.[58,65]

Techniques for endometrial sampling vary. Screening is performed by an experienced gynecologist, usually in an office without anesthesia. Fractional dilation and curettage (D & C) in a hospital may be required in some circumstances.

### Follow-Up and Referral

Any high risk client (see criteria for endometrial sampling) should be followed by a gynecologist with regular biopsies. Positive findings warrant intervention based on the clinical stage of the disease. A gynecological oncologist should be consulted.

## OVARIAN CANCER

Risk factors include aging (especially in 45–60 year old women); postmenopause; periods of prolonged ovulation without pregnancy; having a mother or sister with ovarian, colon, or breast cancer; having a father or brother with colon cancer; and being Caucasian.[1,2] Some association with using talc contaminated with asbestos has been suggested as a risk factor, as has a prior history of mumps infection.[2] Postmenopausal estrogen use is not associated with a higher incidence of ovarian cancer.[2] Prior hysterectomy decreases the risk.[1]

Annually, 20,000 cases occur.[2] The incidence increases with age: from 1.4 per 100,000 among women younger than 40, to 38 per 100,000 among women older than 60.[58] Late diagnosis and early metastasis usually signify a poor prognosis and low survival rate.[58]

### Screening

No effective method of mass screening has yet been developed. Publicity has increased the public's awareness of the difficulty of early detection. Clients may ask about routine ultrasound and CA-125, although neither method is currently recommended for routine screening due to expense and poor sensitivity and reliability. An annual bimanual examination is currently recommended. Symptoms of ovarian cancer are not specific, i.e., abdominal fullness and bloating, pain, or intestinal complaints.[7]

### Follow-Up and Referral

Any postmenopausal client with a palpable ovary or mass should be referred for laparoscopic evaluation.[7] Any woman who has completed childbearing and who has a first-degree relative with ovarian cancer should be considered for a prophylactic bilateral oophorectomy.

## VULVAR CANCER/VULVAR INTRAEPITHELIAL NEOPLASIA (VIN)

The etiology and pathophysiology of vulvar cancer are largely unknown; however, human papillomavirus (HPV) is closely associated with the development of vulvar carcinoma.[58,66] The majority of vulvar cancers occurs among women age 55 or older.

Vulvar cancer is responsible for only 1 to 4 percent of all gynecologic cancers.[1] Invasive squamous cell carcinoma accounts for 90 percent of vulvar cancers. Approximately 500 deaths per year are attributed to vulvar carcinoma. The incidence is increasing among younger women.[58]

### Screening

Physical examination may reveal some of the various lesions.

- *Paget disease* presents with extreme pruritus and soreness, usually of long duration. Red or bright pink, desquamated, eczematoid areas among scattered, raised, white patches of hyperkeratosis. The borders are well demarcated and raised.
- *Basal cell carcinoma* is very rare and is associated with a long history of pruritus. The carcinoma occurs over the anterior two-thirds of the labia majora, with slightly elevated margins.
- *Verrucous carcinoma* appears as condyloma, but does not respond to treatment.
- *Invasive squamous cell carcinoma* occurs when a woman is in her 60s and 70s. It presents with ulceration, friability, or induration of surrounding tissues.
- *A melanoma of the vulva* involves the labia minora and clitoris. It is a darkly pigmented lesion, rare among African American women. Any recent growths, changes in appearance of existing moles, or bleeding of growths should be investigated.
- *Sarcoma* occurs in women of all ages. The vulvar sarcoma is a rapidly expanding, painful mass.[58]

### Follow-Up and Referral

Any client with a persistent, suspicious lesion of the vulva should be referred to a gynecologist for colposcopy, biopsy, and further evaluation and treatment.[66]

## DIETHYLSTILBESTROL (DES) EXPOSURE

DES was used extensively in the United States during the 1940s and early 1950s to prevent miscarriage and premature births. Although studies during the late 1950s proved its ineffectiveness, DES use continued through 1971. An estimated 2 million women were exposed in utero.[67]

### DES Exposure Sequelae

- Structural changes include transverse vaginal and cervical ridges (cocks combs, collars, and pseudopolyps), abnormally shaped uterine cavity, uterine hypoplasia.
- Vaginal adenosis shows columnar epithelium on or beneath the vaginal mucosa; it is self-limiting and gradually disappears.
- Clear-cell adenocarcinoma of the cervix or vagina may develop (incidence rises at age 15, and median age at diagnosis is 19 years).[67]
- Increased incidences of spontaneous abortion, ectopic pregnancy, premature cervical dilation, and premature rupture of membranes are reported.[68,69]

### Screening

All women born between 1940 and 1971 should be questioned about possible exposure to DES. If history suggests exposure, the following screening techniques may be employed.

- *An initial examination* is recommended following menarche or at age 14 if no menarche; routine examination is every 6 to 12 months thereafter and includes inspection, palpation, and cytology.[2,58]
- *Cytology* requires vaginal scrapings taken from all four quadrants of the fornix and fixed on slides for cytological review.
- *Colposcopy* is performed by an experienced colposcopist if the Pap smear is abnormal. Appropriate biopsies are done for evaluation.[2,58]

### Follow-Up and Referral

Any abnormal cytology or undiagnosed lesion requires referral to a gynecologist.

Provide the client with information about DES and its possible effects. Stress the importance of having a regular examination and cytology. Allow time for the client to express her concerns. In addition, stress that DES exposure is not known to interfere with fertility, although there may be some risk of premature delivery. There is no known contraindication to oral contraceptive use.[67]

### NURSING DIAGNOSES

The following nursing diagnoses are representative of those used in the health care plan of women with common gynecologic pelvic disorders. The list, however, is by no means inclusive.

- Activity intolerance, potential for.
- Altered patterns of urination.
- Altered patterns of sexuality.
- Altered family processes.
- Altered comfort: pain, chronic pain.
- Altered bowel elimination: dyschezia, constipation.
- Altered role performance.
- Anxiety.
- Disturbance in self-concept, self-esteem, body image.
- Fear.
- Hopelessness.
- Hyperthermia.
- Impaired mobility.
- Incontinence.

- Ineffective coping: family, individual.
- Knowledge deficit concerning sexual function, technique, etiology of pain.
- Posttrauma response.
- Potential for infection.
- Potential for decreased tissue perfusion secondary to anemia.
- Potential activity intolerance.
- Potential fluid volume deficit.
- Powerlessness.
- Rape trauma syndrome.
- Sensory alterations.
- Sexual dysfunction or altered sexual patterns.
- Sleep pattern disturbance.
- Social isolation.

## REFERENCES


1. Lichtman, R., & Papera, S. (1990). *Gynecology: Well woman care*. Norwalk, CT: Appleton & Lange.
2. Hacker, N.F., & Moore, J.G. (1992). *Essentials of obstetrics and gynecology*. Philadelphia: Saunders.
3. Gibbons, A. (1993). Dioxin tied to endometriosis. *Science, 262*, 1373.
4. Houston, D.E., Noller, K.L., Melton, L.J., & Selwin, B.J. (1988). The epidemiology of pelvic endometriosis. *Clinical Obstetrics & Gynecology, 31*, 787–800.
5. Gerbie, A.B., & Merrill, J.A. (1988). Pathology of endometriosis. *Clinical Obstetrics & Gynecology, 31*, 779–786.
6. Metzger, D.A., & Haney, A.F. (1988). Endometriosis: Etiology and pathophysiology of infertility. *Clinical Obstetrics & Gynecology, 31*, 801–812.
7. Brown, J., & Crombleholme, W.R. (1993). *Handbook of gynecology and obstetrics*. Norwalk, CT: Appleton & Lange.
8. Havens, C., Sullivan, N.D., & Tilton, P. (1986). *Manual of outpatient gynecology*. Boston: Little, Brown.
9. Batt, R.E., & Severino, M.F. (1990). Endometriosis: A comprehensive approach. *Female Patient, 15*, 77–84.
10. Speroff, L., Glass, R.H., & Kase, N.G. (1989). *Clinical gynecologic endocrinology and infertility* (4th ed.). Baltimore: Williams & Wilkins.
11. Wilson, E.A. (1988). Surgical therapy for endometriosis. *Clinical Obstetrics & Gynecology, 31*, 857–865.
12. Weinstein, L. (1988). The emotional aspects of endometriosis: What the patient expects from her doctor. *Clinical Obstetrics & Gynecology, 31*, 866–882.
13. Miller, M.M., & Pelvar, R.W. (1988). An approach to patients with endometriosis. *Clinical Obstetrics & Gynecology, 31*, 883–889.
14. Moghissi, K.S. (1988). Treatment of endometriosis with estrogen and progestin combination and progestogens alone. *Clinical Obstetrics & Gynecology, 31*, 823–828.
15. Dmowski, W.P. (1988). Danazol-induced pseudomenopause in the management of endometriosis. *Clinical Obstetrics & Gynecology, 31*, 829–839.
16. Muse, K. (1988). Clinical manifestations and classification of endometriosis. *Clinical Obstetrics & Gynecology, 31*, 813–822.
17. NAACOG. (1989). PID: painful for the patient, puzzling for the nurse. *NAACOG Newsletter, 16*, 1–4.
18. American College of Obstetricians and Gynecologists. (1990). Pelvic infections. *Precis IV*, 42–44.
19. Apuzzio, J.J., & Pelosi, M.A. (1989). The "new" salpingitis: Subtle symptoms, aggressive management. *Female Patient, 14*, 25–66.
20. Washington, A.E., Arral, S.D., Wolner-Hanssen, P., Grimes, D.A., & Holmes, K.A. (1991). Assessing risk for pelvic inflammatory disease and its sequelae. *Journal of the American Medical Association, 266*, 2581–2586.
21. Holner-Hanssen, P. (1991). Incidence and diagnosis of acute salpingitis. *Contemporary Obstetrics & Gynecology, 36*, 67–75.
22. Sellors, J., Mahoney, J., Goldsmith, C., Rath, D., Rajinder, M., Hunter, B., Taylor, C.,

Groves, D., Richardson, H., & Chernesky, M. (1991). The accuracy of clinical findings and laparoscopy in pelvic inflammatory disease. *American Journal of Obstetrics & Gynecology, 164*, 113–120.

23. Kahn, J.G., Walker, C.K., Washington, A.E., Landers, D.V., & Sweet, R.L. (1991). Diagnosing pelvic inflammatory disease. *Journal of the American Medical Association, 266*, 2594–2604.
24. American College of Obstetricians and Gynecologists. (1986). Antimicrobial therapy for gynecologic infections. *ACOG Technical Bulletin, 97.*
25. Landers, D.V., Wolner-Hanssen P., Paavonen, J., Thorpe, E., Kiviat, N., Ohm, A., Smith, M., Green, J.R., Schachter, J., Holmes, K.K., Eschenbach, D., & Sweet, R.L. (1991). Combination antimicrobial therapy in the treatment of acute pelvic inflammatory disease. *American Journal of Obstetrics & Gynecology, 164*, 849–858.
26. (1990). Treatment of sexually transmitted diseases. *Medical Letter, 32*, 5–10.
27. Paavonen, J., Roberts, P.L., Stevens, C.E., Wolner-Hanssen, P., Brunham, R.C., Hiller, S., Stamm, W.E., Kuo, C.C., DeRouen, T., Holmes, K.K., & Eschenbach, D.A. (1989). Randomized treatment of mucopurulent cervicitis with doxycycline or amoxicillin. *American Journal of Obstetrics & Gynecology, 161*, 128–135.
28. Koonings, P.P., Campbell, K., Mishell, D., & Grimes, D. (1989). Relative frequency of primary ovarian neoplasms: A 10 year review. *Obstetrics & Gynecology, 74*, 921–925.
29. American College of Obstetricians and Gynecologists. (1990). Disorders of the ovaries. *Precis IV*, 202–204.
30. Berek, J.S., & Hacker, N.F. (1989). Practical gynecologic oncology. Baltimore: Williams & Wilkins.
31. Disaia, P.J., & Creesman, W.T. (1989). *Clinical gynecologic oncology* (3rd ed.). St. Louis: Mosby.
32. Sandberg, G., & Quevillon, R.P. (1987). Dyspareunia: An integrated approach to assessment and diagnosis. *Journal of Family Practice, 24*, 66–69.
33. Sarazin, S.K., & Seymour, S.F. (1991). Causes and treatment options for women with dyspareunia. *Nurse Practitioner, 16*, 30–41.
34. American College of Obstetricians and Gynecologists. (1990). Sexuality and sexual dysfunction. *Precis IV*, 50–56.
35. Glatt, A.E., Zinner, S.H., & McCormack, W.M. (1990). The prevalence of dyspareunia. *Obstetrics & Gynecology, 75*, 433–436.
36. Parazzini, F., La Vecchia, C., Negri, E., Ceccheti, G., & Fedele, L. (1988). Epidemiologic characteristics of women with uterine fibroids: A case-control study. *Obstetrics & Gynecology, 72*, 853–857.
37. American College of Obstetricians and Gynecologists. (1990). Disorders of the uterus. *Precis IV*, 193–198.
38. Mishell, D.R., & Brenner, P.F. (1988). Management of common problems in obstetrics and gynecology. Oradell, IL: Medical Economics Books.
39. Friedman, A.J., Barbieri, R.L., Benacerraf, B.R., & Schiff, I. (1987). Treatment of leiomyomata with intranasal or subcutaneous leuprolide, a gonadotropin-releasing hormone agonist. *Fertility & Sterility, 48*, 560–564.
40. Schlaff, W.D. (1990). Treating myomas and endometriosis with GnRH analogs. *Contemporary Obstetrics & Gynecology, 33*, 26–34.
41. Wallach, E.E. (1988). Myomectomy: A guide to indications and technique. *Contemporary Obstetrics & Gynecology, 31*, 74–88.
42. Ben-Baruch, G., Schiff, E., Menashe, Y., Menczer, J. (1988). Immediate and late outcome of vaginal myomectomy for prolapsed pedunculated submucous myoma. *Obstetrics & Gynecology, 72*, 858–860.
43. American College of Obstetricians and Gynecologists. (1990). Pelvic support defects. *Precis IV*, 189–193.
44. Bump, R.C., Fantyl, J.A., Hurt, W.G. (1988). The mechanism of urinary incontinence in women with severe uterovaginal prolapse: Results of barrier studies. *Obstetrics & Gynecology, 72*, 291–295.
45. American College of Obstetricians and Gynecologists. (1989). Chronic pelvic pain. *ACOG Technical Bulletin, 129.*

46. Reiter, R.C. (1990). Occult somatic pathology in women with chronic pelvic pain. *Clinical Obstetrics & Gynecology, 33,* 154–160.
47. Stenchever, M.A. (1990). Symptomatic retrodisplacement, pelvic congestion, universal joint, and peritoneal defects: Fact or fiction? *Clinical Obstetrics & Gynecology, 33*, 161–176.
48. American College of Obstetricians and Gynecologists. (1990). Low abdominal and pelvic pain. *Precis IV*, 12–21.
49. Reiter, R.C. (1990). A profile of women with chronic pelvic pain. *Clinical Obstetrics & Gynecology, 33*, 130–136.
50. Julian, T.M. (1989). Chronic pelvic pain: Workup and diagnosis. *Female Patient, 14*, 28–47.
51. Roseff, S.J., & Murphy, A.A. (1990). Laparoscopy in the diagnosis and therapy of chronic pelvic pain. *Clinical Obstetrics & Gynecology, 33,* 137–144.
52. Kresch, A.J., Seifer, D.B., Sachs, L.B., & Barrese, I. (1984). Laparoscopy in 100 women with chronic pelvic pain. *Obstetrics & Gynecology, 64*, 672–674.
53. Wood, D.P., Weisner, M.G., & Reiter, R.C. (1990). Psychogenic chronic pelvic pain: Diagnosis and management. *Clinical Obstetrics & Gynecology, 33*, 179–175.
54. Kresch, A.J., Seifer, D.B., & Steege, J.F. (1985). How to manage patients with chronic pelvic pain. *Contemporary Obstetrics & Gynecology, 26*, 213–220.
55. Slocumb, J.C. (1990). Operative management of chronic abdominal pelvic pain. *Clinical Obstetrics & Gynecology, 33*, 196–204.
56. Doegemuller, W., Herbst, A.L., Mishell, D.R., & Stenchever, M.A. (1987). Comprehensive gynecology. St. Louis: Mosby.
57. Cho, J.Y., Ahn, M.O., & Cha, K.S. (1990). Window operation: An alternative treatment method for Bartholin gland cysts and abscesses. *Obstetrics & Gynecology, 76*, 886–888.
58. American College of Obstetricians and Gynecologists. (1990). Oncology. *Precis IV*, 237–282.
59. Moore, M.D. (1990). Precursor lesions of the cervix. *Clinical Issues in Perinatal and Women's Health Nursing, 1*, 513–523.
60. Beal, M.W. (1990). Cervical cytology. *Clinical Issues in Perinatal and Women's Health Nursing, 1*, 470–478.
61. Taylor, P.T., Andersen, W.A., Barber, S.R., Covell, J.L., Smith, E.B., & Underwood, P.B. (1987). The screening Papinicolaou smear: Contribution of the endocervical brush. *Obstetrics & Gynecology, 70*, 734–737.
62. National Cancer Institute. (1988). The 1988 Bethesda system for reporting cervical/vaginal cytologic diagnosis. *Journal of the American Medical Association, 262*, 931–934.
63. Koss, G. (1989). The Papanicolaou test for cervical cancer detection: A triumph and a tragedy. *Journal of the American Medical Association, 261*, 737–743.
64. Beal, M.W. (1987). Understanding cervical cytology. *Nurse Practitioner, 12*, 8–22.
65. Parazzini, F., La Vecchia, C., Negri, E., Fedele, L., & Balotta, F. (1991). Reproductive factors and risk of endometrial cancer. *American Journal of Obstetrics & Gynecology, 164*, 522–527.
66. Roy, M. (1988). VIN: Latest management approaches. *Contemporary Obstetrics & Gynecology, 30*, 170–179.
67. Vieivalves-Wiltgen, C., & Engle, V.F. (1988). Identification and management of DES-exposed women. *Nurse Practitioner, 13*, 15–27.
68. Richart, R.M., Habst, A.L., Kaufman, R., & Robboy, S.J. (1985). DES daughters: The risks in their childbearing years. *Contemporary Obstetrics & Gynecology, 26*, 204–233.
69. Eisenberg, E. (1987). Diethylstilbestrol's effect on fertility. *Contemporary Obstetrics & Gynecology, 29*, 35–48.

CHAPTER 10

# BREAST HEALTH

*Lynette Galloway Branch*

*Breast cancer is rare among women younger than 30 years. The incidence, however, rises among women in their early 40s, levels off at about 45 years, and increases again after age 55.*

### *Highlights*

- Breast Examination: Professional, Self-Exam, and Mammography
- Benign Breast Disorders
  - *Fibrocystic Changes*
  - *Fibroadenoma*
  - *Nipple Discharge*
- Malignant Neoplasms
- Breast Reconstruction
  - *Tissue Transfer*
  - *Augmentation Mammoplasty*
  - *Mastopexy*
  - *Breast Reduction*

## INTRODUCTION

The female breast is closely linked with womanhood in the American culture. The more amply endowed the female bosom, the "sexier" and more womanly one is perceived. Although the primary function of the breasts is lactation, breasts are perceived as erotic. They are attractive and alluring to men and a source of sensual pleasure for women as well. Thus, the loss or injury of these important anatomic structures is potentially psychologically devastating to both sexes.

For women in their childbearing years, breast injury or loss threatens the ability to nourish and nurture offspring by means of breastfeeding. This intimate, interactional process may be perceived as the ultimate way of connecting and communicating with a newborn. Middle-age women, who have begun to observe the effects of aging on their bodies, may perceive breast loss or injury as an additional change to their once youthful bodies. Elderly women, who are living longer, desire to maintain their fitness, which entails keeping their bodies healthy and intact. Hence, maintaining breast health is conducive to maintaining optimal physical and psychological health.

Concerns about breasts and breast symptoms are among the most common complaints of women who seek medical attention. Although most concerns have no disease or have benign changes as their underlying condition, the fear of cancer and malignancy causes great anxiety and stress for most women who have any breast symptoms. This anxiety is indeed warranted: Breast cancer now occurs in one of every nine women.[1]

Because concerns about breast health are common in primary care settings, health care providers must have substantial knowledge about breast related disorders and diseases. A basic understanding of the most severe form of breast disease—cancer—is paramount, so that immediate referral can be made and mortality reduced.

## BREAST EXAMINATION AND ASSESSMENT

Breast examination may be carried out by a health professional, the client herself, or by means of mammography. Breast self-examination (BSE) is practiced today by many women, which is evidenced by the fact that approximately 70 percent of all breast masses are self-detected.[2] Yet many more women fail to carry out this valuable monthly exercise. Why is not clear. It is speculated, however, that motivating factors are health beliefs, fear and anxiety of discovering a lump, hence, a cancer; lack of knowledge or self-confidence regarding the technique of BSE; denial; discomfort with body manipulation; lack of perceived susceptibility to or risk of breast cancer; lack of perceived benefits; and apathy.[2,3] If the 10-minute routine is not incorporated into a woman's lifestyle, breast cancer may not be detected early and the risk of death due to breast cancer may increase. The American Cancer Society recommends the following examination schedule to detect breast cancer in asymptomatic women[1]:

- *Breast Self-Exam.* Monthly BSE for all women older than 20 years.
- *Breast Exam by a Health Professional.* Every 3 years for women 20 to 40 years of age and annually for women older than 40. Annual breast exam performed by a health professional may enhance the detection of masses in all age groups, and it provides the opportunity for client teaching and review of the BSE.
- *Mammography.* Baseline mammogram between ages 35 and 39; mammogram every 1 to 2 years between ages 40 and 49; annual mammogram thereafter.[1]

Some controversy exists over the usefulness of mammography under age 50 on a routine basis. The National Cancer Institute suggests that it is unnecessary, not detecting enough cancer to warrant the exposure to even a small amount of radiation. However, some physicians feel that an annual mammography from ages 40 to 50, especially for women in high risk groups, could increase detection of early cancers, because existing tumor growth is more rapid during this time.[4]

### TECHNIQUE FOR BREAST SELF-EXAMINATION (BSE)

BSE follows a specific technique (see Figure 10–1).[5] The exam should be done each month, after the menstrual period; day 4, 5, 6, or 7 is optimal. Menopausal and pregnant women should perform the exam on the first day of each month.

1. While standing in front of a mirror, observe both breasts for symmetry, dimpling, scaling, redness, bruising, and nipple irritation, discharge, or retraction (Figure 10–1A).
2. Continue observations with hands elevated above the head (Figure 10–1B).
3. Continue observations with hands placed firmly on the hips, and body bowed slightly forward (Figure 10–1C).
4. Place one arm above the head and palpate the breast closest to that arm for lumps, masses, and tenderness. Use the fingers (not fingertips) of the opposite hand to glide over the breast in a circular fashion,

starting in the upper outer quadrant of the breast and continuing until the entire breast, including the areola and nipple, has been examined (Figure 10–1D).

Observe the nipple for discharge during this examination. Next, thoroughly palpate the axillary region for enlarged or tender nodes. Repeat the procedure for the other breast. (*Note*: Right hand examines the left breast, and left hand examines the right breast.)

5. Finally, lie supine with a pillow or towel behind the chest wall of one breast; examine the breast as in step 4 (Figure 10–1E). Move the pillow or towel to the opposite side and repeat the procedure for the other breast.

## BREAST ASSESSMENT BY THE HEALTH CARE PROVIDER

Thorough breast assessment, including history-taking for risk factors and education regarding BSE, should be standard protocol for the health provider during a client's annual exam.

### History

Obtain the client's history and her family history of breast disease and breast cancer (focus on the maternal family, especially the mother and female siblings), since breast cancer in the family increases client's risk of cancer. Also inquire about the client's menstrual and reproductive history, including information about menarche, onset of menopause, number of pregnancies and deliveries and age at both, as well as lactation or breastfeeding.[5] Ask the client about her current medication usage—specifically, psychotropic drugs, hormonal therapy (estrogen, progesterone), and oral contraceptives, which could induce breast changes—and her dietary habits, including fat and caffeine intake.

### Breast Examination

Devote ample time to examining the breasts, teaching the proper technique for BSE, and encouraging monthly BSE. Then ask the client to demonstrate BSE. Breast models that allow clients to practice on normal and abnormal breasts often help to increase client confidence in BSE. The breast exam by the health care provider should be systematic[5]:

1. Observe the client while she is sitting with her hands resting in her lap, with hands overhead and chest wall forward, and with her hands placed firmly on her hips (which contracts the pectoral muscles). Observe the breasts for dimpling, retraction, asymmetry, skin thickening, spontaneous nipple discharge, and color changes.
2. If the client has large, pendulous breasts, ask her to lean over while placing her hands on your shoulders. In this position, observe the breasts for symmetry, retraction, and dimpling.
3. Allow the client's arm to rest diagonally on your arm (positioned from the client's right to your right) as you palpate the axillary nodes. Repeat this procedure for the opposite axilla. Then palpate the supraclavicular and infraclavicular lymph nodes. If the breasts are pendulous, palpate them while the client is seated.
4. Ask the client to lie supine and extend the arm on the side of the breast to be examined overhead. Place a pillow beneath the same shoulder.
5. Then palpate the client's breast from the upper outer quadrant to the nipple in a circular fashion, taking care to cover each breast quadrant. Give careful attention to the tail of Spence.
6. Observe the nipple for discharge.
7. Perform steps 3 through 6 on the opposite breast.

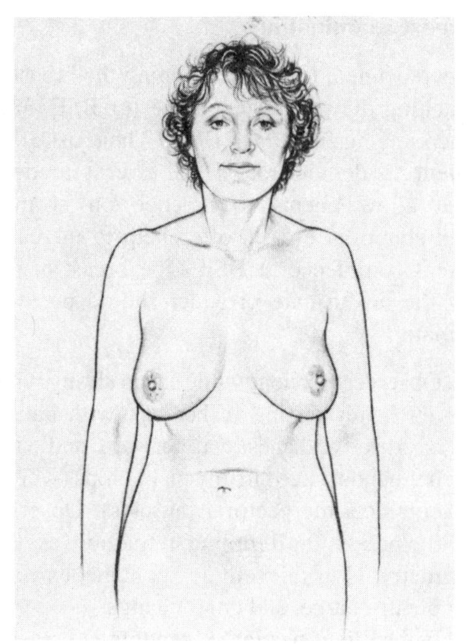

A

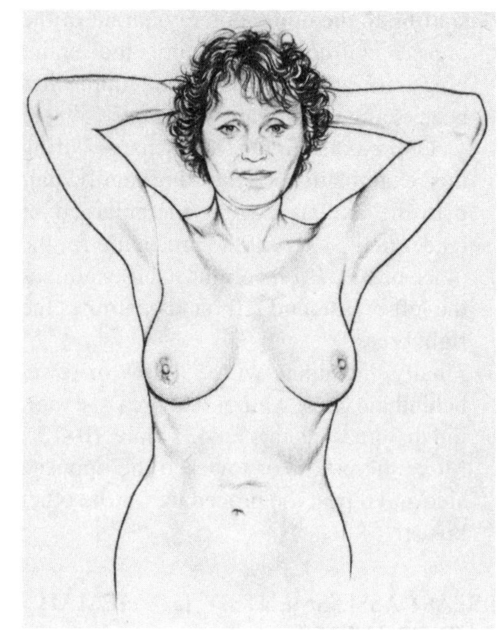

B

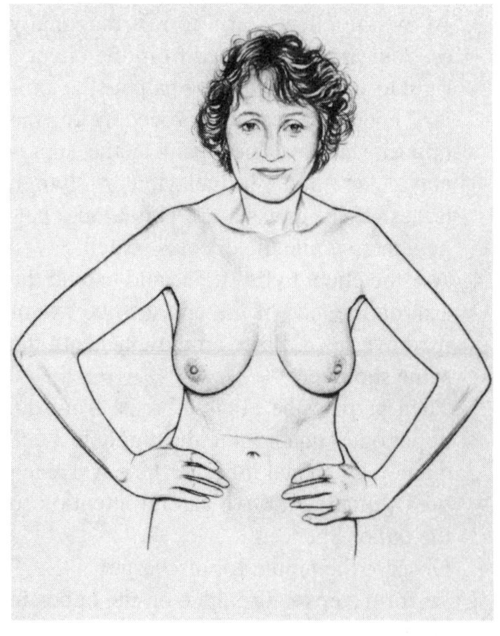

C

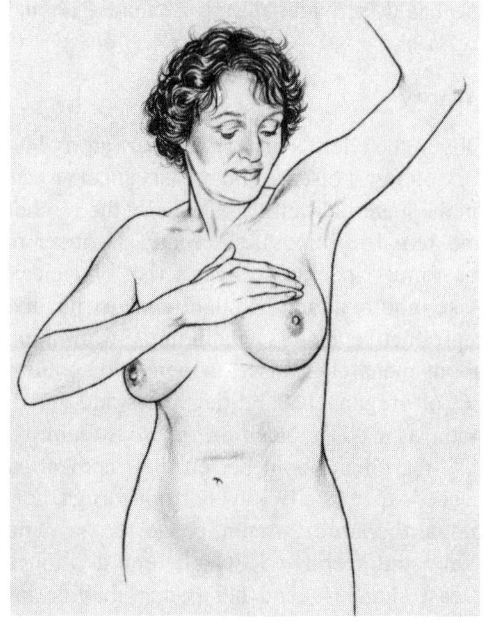

D

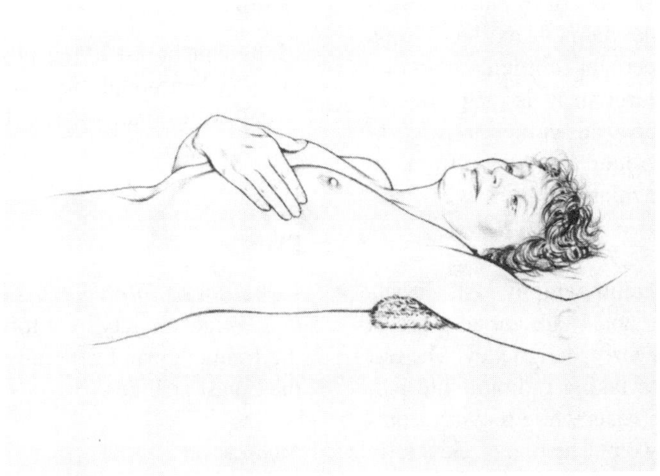

E

**Figure 10–1**. Breast self-examination (BSE) (perform procedure each month). See pages 282–283. *From National Cancer Institute (March, 1984).* Breast Exams—What You Should Know. *(NIH pub. no. 84-2000.) Bethesda, MD: National Institutes of Health.*

## BENIGN BREAST DISORDERS

### FIBROCYSTIC CHANGES

Fibrocystic changes are poorly delineated thicknesses or palpable nodularity of the breast that is accompanied by pain. Cyst formation, stromal fibrosis, ductal epithelial hyperplasia, duct ectasia, and sclerosing adenosis are all fibrocystic changes. An atypical occurrence of fibrocystic change may be a precursor of cancer. Pain is thought to be due to stromal edema, ductal dilation, and inflammation.[6–9]

#### Epidemiology

The etiology is unknown. Nodularity and tenderness may be physiological and due to hormone stimulation, or they may be secondary to estrogen excess. Another theory is that the breast tissue becomes extra sensitive to estrogen and proliferates.[7–9] Fibrocystic changes occur among at least 50 percent of all women.[9] These changes, however, are most often found in the premenopausal woman and occur in approximately 10 percent of women under age 21.

#### Subjective Data

The client reports bilateral or unilateral breast pain and tenderness (the symptom is usually bilateral).[7] Pain frequently begins 7 to 14 days prior to the menses and resolves as the menses progresses. Sometimes, however, pain is present at all times.[7] The client may also report that the breasts feel thick and lumpy.

#### Objective Data

***Physical Examination.*** Examination of the breasts reveals thickening fibrosis and lumpiness (usually bilateral), palpated primarily in the outer quadrants. Usually no discharge from the nipples is seen; however, some clear discharge may be present. Lymphatic examination reveals tender palpable axillary lymph nodes among 20 percent of clients.[7] No clavicular nodal enlargement is palpable. In older or postmenopausal women, a ridge of nodularity may be found along the inframammary margin, particularly in the lower quadrant of the breast.[10]

***Mammography.*** Mammography is performed to identify and characterize a breast mass and to detect early malignancy. The test procedure involves taking radiographic pictures of the bare breasts while they are compressed between two plastic plates. Generally two views of the compressed breasts are taken. Most women find the 10-minute procedure temporarily uncomfortable but not painful. To decrease discomfort, advise routine mammography for the week after menses. Mammography in clients younger than 35 years of age is controversial. Although a mammograph may detect cancer in younger women, it should not be a standard method of evaluation.[11] Also a woman should be advised that 10 percent of breast cancers can be missed by mammography.[12]

Inform the client that breast compression may cause tenderness for 1 to 2 days. Acetaminophen, ibuprofen, or aspirin may relieve discomfort. The procedure may be scheduled for a time of the menstrual cycle when breasts are less tender. Deodorant and powder can cause a mammogram to appear abnormal (because of opacity); therefore, they should be removed with soap and water before x-ray or they should be avoided the day of the exam.

Help the client to choose a mammography facility that is accredited by the American College of Radiology (ACR) and ascertain that machines are designed specifically for mammography. Try to ensure that the mammogram is performed by a registered technologist and that the radiologist is trained to read mammography.[13]

## Differential Medical Diagnoses

Malignant breast mass, physiological nodularity (when nodularity varies with the menstrual cycle). Pain—costochondritis, respiratory infection.

## Plan

***Psychosocial Intervention.*** Focus on helping to alleviate anxiety by informing the client of the frequency and generally benign nature of the breast changes.

### *Medication*

*Oral Contraceptives (OCs)*

- *Indications.* To prevent or slow the development of new fibrocystic changes and to minimize symptoms of existing changes.[7,9] Symptoms are suppressed in 70 to 90 percent of clients with fibrocystic changes.[7] An OC is especially appropriate if the client needs a birth control method and OC use is not contraindicated. The effectiveness of oral contraceptives is based on the reduction of ovarian estradiol production and on the modulation of breast estrogen receptors by progestin.[7]
- *Administration.* Low-dose estrogen (e.g., ethinyl estradiol, 0.02 mg) and relatively high-dose progesterone (e.g., norethindrone, 1.0 mg) pill daily for 3–6 months. If contraception is needed, 0.030 to 0.035 mg of ethinyl estradiol with progestin is used. Medroxyprogesterone acetate, 5–10 mg, improved breast symptoms in 80 to 85 percent of the clients.[6]
- *Side Effects and Adverse Reactions.* Possible water retention, weight gain, hypertension, cardiovascular changes, and breakthrough bleeding (see Chapter 6).
- *Contraindications.* See Chapter 6.
- *Anticipated Outcomes on Evaluation.* A decrease in symptoms associated with fi-

brocystic changes. If improvement is noted, oral contraceptives are continued. Symptoms will probably recur when therapy is discontinued.[6]

- *Client Teaching and Counseling.* Explain to the client that her menstrual cycle may change and that breakthrough bleeding is possible when the pill is not taken as prescribed. Counsel her about the side effects and danger signs associated with pill use (see Chapter 6). Caution the client about expecting immediate results; it may take several months for improvement. Inform the client that symptoms may return when therapy is discontinued.

*Vitamin E (Effectiveness Controversial)*

- *Indications.* To decrease pain and tenderness associated with fibrocystic changes and decrease the proliferation of breast tissue.[7,9] Even though the use of vitamin E is controversial, it has been proven effective in relieving the symptoms of fibrocystic disease in some women.[14,15]
- *Administration.* Oral vitamin E, 150 to 600 IU daily.
- *Side Effects and Adverse Reactions.* Vitamin E's fat solubility and slow excretion may cause it to build up to a toxic level. Blood vessels may become constricted; therefore, the vitamin should be used cautiously for individuals with hypertension, diabetes mellitus, or cardiovascular disease.
- *Contraindications.* Hypertension, diabetes mellitus, or cardiovascular disease.
- *Anticipated Outcomes on Evaluation.* Decrease in pain, lumpiness, and thickness.
- *Client Teaching and Counseling.* Explain that vitamin E is given on a trial basis and should be discontinued in 2–3 months if no improvement occurs. Caution the client about the dangers of overusing this fat soluble vitamin that may result in vitamin toxicity.

*Danazol*

- *Indications.* To reduce pain, tenderness, and nodularity caused by fibrocystic changes.[16] Because of its possible side effects, this drug should be used only after other methods have failed.[6]
- *Administration.* Danazol, 100 to 400 mg p.o., daily in two divided doses.[6] Therapy should begin during menstruation or after a negative pregnancy test. Length of therapy is usually 3 to 6 months.
- *Side Effects and Adverse Reactions.* Weight gain, menstrual irregularity (including amenorrhea), acne, increased cholesterol levels, decreased breast size, oily skin, growth of facial hair, deepening voice, liver dysfunction, nervousness, depression, vaginitis, and prolonged prothrombin time.[17]
- *Contraindications.* Undiagnosed abnormal genital bleeding; markedly impaired hepatic, renal, or cardiac function; pregnancy; breastfeeding; and clients whose symptoms occur only during the premenstrual period or who experience mild fibrocystic changes.
- *Anticipated Outcomes on Evaluation.* A decrease in breast tenderness and nodularity, and a decrease in the size of the breast cyst if present.
- *Client Teaching and Counseling.* Advise the client that improvement normally occurs within the first month of therapy but may require 3 to 6 months. Also inform her that 50 percent of clients notice the return of some symptoms when danazol is discontinued. High cholesterol foods should be decreased in the diet, and a lipid profile drawn 3 months after therapy is initiated.

**Dietary Intervention.** *Caffeine* consumption should be reduced, as that may alleviate breast tenderness and reduce nodularity. This treatment, although controversial, may be tried in conjunction with other treatment modalities.[18,19] Other nonprescriptive or lifestyle interventions that may help reduce fibrocystic discomfort include low-salt diet, warm compresses, supportive bra for sleep, and mild analgesics.[2] The anticipated outcomes on evaluation by the client include decreased breast pain, tenderness, and nodularity.

Advise the client to decrease her intake of coffee, tea, cola drinks, chocolate, and drugs containing caffeine. Explain that 3 to 6 months may be required for symptoms to improve. Encourage perseverance, as many clients find it difficult to eliminate such foods as cola, coffee, and chocolate from their diet. Caffeine should be gradually reduced to prevent withdrawal symptoms.

***Surgical Intervention: Bilateral Total Mastectomy (Prophylactic).*** Indications for the surgery are to decrease the likelihood of developing cancer in clients who have a strong family history of cancer or who have progressive fibrocystic disease or who request the procedure because they are tired of the constant pain caused by fibrocystic changes.[20] The procedure is usually considered too aggressive an approach in treating precancerous changes.[9] All breast tissue is removed, including the nipple–areolar complex and some axillary nodes. A subcutaneous mastectomy in which the nipple remains attached to the skin envelope and the nipple–areola complex remains intact may be performed.[20] Possible adverse effects include mild lymphedema, disfigurement, and anesthesia reactions.

The anticipated outcomes on evaluation include decreased anxiety related to developing cancer. Survivability may improve in high risk clients. High risk clients who undergo bilateral total mastectomy have a 2.5 to 5 percent chance of developing invasive cancer and a 5 to 10 percent chance of developing cancer in situ.[9]

When counseling the client, carefully convey the risks and advantages of the voluntary procedure. Advise the client that breast cancer may not be prevented, even if mastectomy is performed, however, the risk will be decreased. Cancer may develop in subcutaneous tissue that may be left after surgery.[20] Professional counseling is strongly advised prior to this extreme surgery. Significant others of the client's choosing should be involved in decision making. Refer the client to at least three qualified surgeons for their opinions about the surgery.

***Follow-Up.*** Clients who receive oral contraceptives for fibrocystic breast changes as well as for contraception should have a physical examination and evaluation every 3 months for the first 6 months of therapy, and every 6 months thereafter (see Chapter 6).

Clients who receive danazol will require a lipid profile after 3 months of therapy. Normally symptoms associated with fibrocystic breast changes resolve in 3 to 6 months, and danazol can be terminated. A lipid profile should be repeated at the termination of therapy.

Clients who have surgery should be followed per the recommendations of the surgeon.

Advise all clients to try caffeine reduction for 3 to 6 months to ascertain if pain and nodularity decrease. Continue reduced intake indefinitely if improvements are noticed.

## FIBROADENOMA

A fibroadenoma is a solid, firm, or rubbery, well-defined mobile mass which is usually painless. The mass is usually found unilaterally as a single breast mass but may be multiple and bilateral.[21–23]

### Epidemiology

The cause of a fibroadenoma is thought to be hormonal.[22] The mass, considered a disorder of normal breast development—not a neoplasm—presumably arises from the lobules and terminal ducts of the breast. It is basically an overgrowth of elements thought to be found in these ducts.[21] Usually a mass will grow to 1 to 3 cm in diameter and remain that size. A small number, however, grow to be larger than 5 cm; these are called giant fibroadenoma.[24] The occurrence of a unilateral discrete breast mass is most common after puberty and before age 35.[22] Peak incidence is between ages 15 and 25. A mass may also be detected more frequently in women older than 65 years—perhaps as a result of the loss of fatty breast tissue that occurs with involution in this age group. The disorder is twice as common among African American women as among Caucasian women.[22] Rapid growth of these tumors often occurs during pregnancy and just prior to menopause. In 15 to 20 percent of cases, fibroadenoma are multiple and in both breasts.[22] The risk of developing fibroadenoma is *not* increased by age, weight, parity, age at first pregnancy, socioeconomic status, or a family history of breast cancer.

## Subjective Data

The client reports a "seed-like" or "marble-like," discrete, mobile, painless lump in one breast. Less often, she will find a lump in both breasts. It may be observed in any area of the breast, but is most frequently found in the upper outer quadrant. No nipple discharge or retraction, dimpling, or other breast symptoms are reported.

## Objective Data

Physical examination of the breasts reveals a firm, well delineated, freely mobile, nontender mass, best palpated with the client in the dorsal recumbent position with hand behind her head. Usually the mass is palpable unilaterally, but it also may be bilateral.

### *Diagnostic Tests and Methods*

Fine Needle Aspiration. Diagnostic evaluation using fine needle aspiration is done to identify a solid tumor, cyst, or malignancy. The procedure should be done by a trained health care provider, usually an obstetrics/gynecology specialist or a surgeon. The test procedure involves first cleaning the breast with an antiseptic solution (usually ethyl alcohol). Then the mass is stabilized between the fingers of one hand and compressed downward. A needle (25 gauge or smaller) is inserted into the mass. A 21-gauge needle is the largest that should be used.[25] As the needle is moved around in the mass, suction is applied to remove the contents.[25] The needle is gently withdrawn, and pressure is applied to the puncture site.

Place the specimen on a clean glass slide and spread gently using a second slide at a 10° angle. Fix the slide with alcohol. Prepare a second slide and allow it to air dry. Send both slides to a cytology lab.[26,27] If the fluid withdrawn is straw colored, the diagnosis is usually fibroadenoma; in this case the fluid may be discarded. If, however, there is doubt, send the remaining fluid to the lab in a sterile glass tube. Absence of fluid may indicate a solid mass, which is suspicious of malignancy, necessitating open biopsy.

Provide the client with an explanation of fine needle aspiration and a rationale for it. If referral is necessary, allow the client to participate in the selection of the care provider. If the client wishes to have the mass removed, refer her to a surgeon. Encourage BSE.

Mammography. (See Benign Breast Disorders, Fibrocystic Changes.) A mammogram may be used to evaluate any mass. However, since fibroadenoma are most common in young adult women who have dense breast tissue, fibroadenoma may not be visualized accurately in this age group.

### Differential Medical Diagnosis

Breast macrocyst, cystosarcoma phyllodes, tubular adenoma, and mucinous carcinoma.

### Plan

Psychosocial interventions include helping the client to alleviate anxiety by informing her of the benign status of this mass. In addition, literature should be provided about common benign breast lesions.

Medication is not warranted.

***Surgical Intervention: Excisional (Open) Biopsy.*** This procedure is done to remove and diagnose a breast lesion. The fibroadenoma is surgically excised under local anesthesia, and Steri-strips are used to close the incision. The specimen is sent to a pathology lab. This type of biopsy is done when a suspicious mass persists beyond menses; if a cystic mass retains fluid after aspiration; if the fluid in a cyst is bloody; if nipple discharge is serous or serosanguineous with no mass but a trigger point is present; or when a suspicious mammogram occurs without clinical findings.[28] Adverse effects are virtually nonexistent. The client, however, may react to the local anesthesia, and bleeding and infection are possible with virtually any surgical procedure.

The anticipated outcomes on evaluation include reduced anxiety because the lesion has been removed. Greater accuracy is achieved in diagnosis because the lesion is sent to a pathology lab.

Explain to the client that the surgery may be done in an ambulatory setting under local anesthesia. A small dressing will be required. The pain is usually mild, and time lost from work is usually minimal. No heavy lifting or strenuous work should be done until the site is healed.

The procedure should be performed soon after diagnosis. Although adolescents may delay surgery because malignancy is rare in this age group, removal should be scheduled before lesion growth occurs. Excision of a larger lesion causes more unsightly cosmetic changes.

***Follow-Up.*** After fine needle aspiration and surgery, follow-up should be done at the physician's discretion. Routine breast exams should be done every year by a health professional, and breast self-examination (BSE) should be carried out monthly.

## NIPPLE DISCHARGE

Fluid emission from the mammary nipple is the third most common symptom of breast disease,[29] and may occur in 5 to 8 percent of all women with breast symptoms. Although discharge is symptomatic of serious disease in only 8 to 10 percent of women evaluated,[29] it may represent malignancy in 50 percent of women 60 years and older.[22] Discharge may be caused by factors outside the breasts, primarily neuroendocrine or drug induced; by pathology of the ductal system; or by disease of the nipple.[24]

At least seven types of nipple discharge have been identified: serous (yellow), serosanguineous, bloody, clear (watery), milky, purulent, and multicolored.[30] All discharge is abnormal when it occurs spontaneously; however, 21 percent of watery discharge and 25 percent of bloody discharge are associated with carcinoma.[26]

## NIPPLE DISCHARGE CAUSED BY FACTORS OUTSIDE THE BREASTS

### Galactorrhea

Galactorrhea is a spontaneous milky nipple discharge that is unrelated to lactation. It is usually bilateral. The etiology of galactorrhea may involve medications or other disorders. For example, it can be induced by oral contraceptives (OCs), antihypertensive medications (e.g., reserpine, methyldopa), or psychotropic medications (e.g., imipramine).[31] Galactorrhea can also be caused by thyroid disorders, brain tumors, benign pituitary adenomas, or prolactinomas.[32] It is often associated with menstrual abnormalities. Details about the incidence of galactorrhea are unknown.

***Subjective Data.*** The client reports a milky white discharge from both nipples and says that she is not pregnant or lactating. She also indicates that she neither has experienced trauma nor has pain. She may, however, acknowledge ammenorrhea or irregular menses. Visual complaints of spots, whiteness, glowing, or progressive blurring may be given by a client suspected of having a pituitary tumor.[32,33]

***Objective Data.*** Physical examination of the breasts reveals a milky nipple discharge that occurs spontaneously and with manual stimulation. It is not expressed from any particular areolar quadrant or duct. No redness or tenderness is visible. Fundoscopic may be normal. Papilledema may be present and is suggestive of a parapituitary tumor.[34]

## Diagnostic Tests and Methods

***Serum Prolactin Test.*** Diagnostic evaluation to identify elevated prolactin, which may be indicative of a pituitary tumor or thyroid disorder. A level of greater than 200 ng/mL is essentially diagnostic of a prolactin secreting tumor.[34] If the blood level is elevated, the test may be repeated to ensure accuracy. When hyperprolactinemia exists, the presence of a prolactinoma is assumed until otherwise proven.[35]

The test procedure is to draw 3 to 5 mL of blood in a red-top tube and send it to a lab for evaluation. Use universal precautions when procuring blood.

Explain to the client the rationale for the laboratory test and help her to allay her anxiety about the diagnosis.

***Thyroid Function Test.*** Diagnostic evaluation to identify an elevated level of thyrotropin (TSH), which may be indicative of thyroid disease (hypothyroidism).[32] The test should also be done if the serum prolactin test results show an elevated prolactin level.

The test procedure is to draw 3 to 5 mL of blood in a red-top tube and send it to a lab for evaluation. Use universal precautions when procuring blood.

Explain the rationale for the laboratory test and help to allay the client's anxiety.

***Computed Tomography (CT) Scan of the Pituitary Fossa.*** Diagnostic evaluation to identify pituitary tumors, performed if the client has hyperprolactinemia.[35]

The test procedure involves the use of narrow x-ray beams to reveal the differences in radiation absorption among different kinds of tissue. Intravenous dye (usually Renografin) is used to enhance the x-ray contrast of vascular lesions.[36]

Explain to the client the rationale for the test and refer her for financial screening if the test is not covered by medical insurance. Determine if the client is allergic to dyes. Support the client and help to allay her anxiety. Explain that the test is painless, but the client may be required to remain still for long periods during testing.

***Visual Fields Measurement.*** Diagnostic evaluation to determine visual field defects caused by a pituitary tumor or mass. It is performed if the CT scan result is abnormal or if the client has visual complaints. Referral to an ophthalmologist is warranted for precise testing to evaluate peripheral vision; gross screening and a fundoscopic exam should be performed by the primary care provider.

Explain the reason for referral and the rationale for the exam. Involve the client in the selection of an ophthalmologist.

Differential Medical Diagnoses. Drug-induced galactorrhea, pituitary tumor, prolactinoma, hypothyroidism.

## Plan

PSYCHOSOCIAL INTERVENTIONS. Help to allay the client's anxiety through teaching and providing literature about galactorrhea. Encourage significant persons in the client's life to be supportive. Discuss sexuality and body image issues as appropriate. Refer the client for professional counseling if needed. *Consult closely with the physician while managing a client with galactorrhea.*

***Medication: Bromocriptine***

- *Indications.* Bromocriptine is a dopamine receptor agonist that inhibits the secretion of prolactin. It is used to lower prolactin levels, end galactorrhea, and restore the menses to normal if they have been irregular. Bromocriptine is used after a tumor or another cause of galactorrhea is ruled out. It may be used successfully when a microadenoma is identified.
- *Administration.* Individualized. Start with 1.5 to 2.5 bromocriptine daily and increase to 2.5 mg two to three times a day.[32]
- *Side Effects and Adverse Reactions.* Nausea, vomiting, dizziness, fatigue, headache, abdominal cramps, diarrhea, constipation, nasal congestion, drowsiness. Hypertension may also occur when the drug is initiated.
- *Contraindications.* Uncontrolled hypertension, pregnancy, and sensitivity to ergot alkaloids.
- *Anticipated Outcome on Evaluation.* Cessation of nipple discharge.
- *Client Teaching and Counseling.* Advise the client to practice safe, effective birth control to avoid pregnancy while taking bromocriptine and to notify her care provider of any side effects.

***Surgical Intervention: Transsphenoidal Excision of Pituitary Tumor.*** The purpose of this surgery is to remove the causative pathology and consequently abate the symptom. The tumor is excised through the nasal cavity. Adverse effects are virtually unknown; however, tumor recurrence is possible.37 The anticipated outcome on evaluation is cessation of nipple discharge.

Refer the client to a qualified surgeon, encouraging client participation in the selection of a surgeon.

***Follow-Up.*** Consultation with a physician is recommended. If the galactorrhea is being managed with bromocriptine, the client should be evaluated in 2 to 3 months. The medication may be discontinued if the symptom resolves in 2 to 3 months; thereafter, the client may be evaluated in 6 months and yearly. If, however, the symptom does not abate in 2 to 3 months, bromocriptine may be continued and the client evaluated 1 month later. If at that time galactorrhea is unresolved, the client should be referred to a physician or managed with frequent consultation with a physician.

If hypothyroidism is the cause of galactorrhea, then the disorder may be managed with thyroid hormone. The client may be referred to an internist for management if desired. Evaluate the client every 6 months once hypothyroidism is stabilized.

If surgery is required for tumor removal, then follow-up is per the surgeon's recommendations.

# NIPPLE DISCHARGE CAUSED BY DUCTAL SYSTEM DISORDERS

## Intraductal Papilloma

The intraductal papilloma is a small, usually nonpalpable benign tumor located in the mammary duct that produces a spontaneous serous or serosanguineous nipple discharge.[23] The tumor is usually solitary and affects only one duct, but occasionally it affects multiple ducts.

***Epidemiology.*** It is thought that intraductal papilloma is caused by a proliferation and overgrowth of ductal epithelial tissue. On rare occasions the papilloma may be intracystic rather than intraductal; however, in these cases, discharge will occur only if the cyst communes with a duct. Although a papilloma is usually millimeters in size and nonpalpable, it can grow large enough to obstruct the duct and thereby become palpable. A nodule is usually located close to the areola.[7]

Intraductal papilloma occurs most frequently among women 35 to 55 years of age. Usually the tumor occurs just prior to menopause, but it may occur at any time from adolescence to old age.

***Subjective Data.*** The client reports yellow or bloody discharge on her clothing. The discharge may occur spontaneously or with nipple stimulation. If the papilloma is large, the client may be able to observe a nonpainful, mobile mass. On rare occasions, the client may only be able to palpate the mass. She may complain of an associated feeling of fullness or pain beneath the areola.[22]

***Objective Data.*** Physical examination of the breasts reveals serous or serosanguineous discharge, which is expressed manually from the affected duct when the nipple is systematically massaged in quadrants. The tumor, if palpable, may be a 1- to 3-cm mass, soft and poorly delineated. Occasionally, skin dimpling is observed.

***Diagnostic Tests and Methods***

Test for Occult Blood of Breast Fluids. Diagnostic evaluation to identify the presence of blood in nipple discharge. The procedure involves placing a small amount of nipple discharge on the designated area of a Hemoccult card (front side). Use a gloved finger to transfer the specimen from the nipple (use universal precautions). Apply 2 drops of developer on the designated area on the reverse side of the card. Blue coloration indicates the presence of blood.

Explain the purpose of the test to the client.

Cytology of Breast Fluid (Papanicolaou Smear). Diagnostic evaluation to screen for cancerous cells. Usually, on microscopic examination, an intraductal papilloma shows scattered macrophages and tight clusters of epithelial cells with minimal atypia.[26] Test results should be treated with caution because negative results are not diagnostic of intraductal papilloma. False negative results may occur in 12 to 35 percent of cases, and false positive results occur in 3 to 4 percent of cases.[26]

The test procedure requires that a drop of breast fluid be expressed onto a clean glass slide. Spread the specimen gently with a second glass slide at approximately a 10° angle. Then fix the slide with alcohol, label it to indicate which breast the sample was taken from, and send it to a lab.

Explain the procedure and its purpose to the client; caution that the results are inconclusive.

Ductography (Controversial). Diagnostic evaluation to identify, by means of radiography, the ductal orifice that drains the pathological ductal system. The test is considered unnecessary by some because the affected ductal quadrant can be identified by manual examination of the nipple and surgery is required whether or not this radiological procedure is done.[24] Some specialists, however, find the test valuable for a more precise diagnosis.

The test procedure requires introducing radiographic dye through a cannulated duct, followed by x-rays.

Discuss the pros and cons of this procedure with the client and assist her in choosing a qualified radiologist.

Mammography. See Benign Breast Disorders, Fibrocystic Changes.

***Differential Medical Diagnoses.*** Intraductal carcinoma, multiple papillomatosis. (Intraductal carcinoma and Paget's disease, a disease of the nipple, are included in the section Malignant Neoplasms of the Breast.)

### *Plan*

Psychosocial Interventions. Counseling the client regarding the benign etiology of this diagnosis. Encourage her to verbalize her feelings and emotions. Discuss sexuality issues as appropriate.

Medication. Not given for intraductal papilloma.

Surgical Intervention: Wedge Excision. Wedge excision of the affected duct is the removal of the pathological ductal system and papilloma. (If the diseased duct is not removed, the nipple discharge will continue.) Local anesthesia is used. The excised papilloma and duct are sent to a pathology lab to rule out cancer.

Adverse effects may include a reaction to the anesthetic or possibly infection. The anticipated outcomes on evaluation include cessation of the discharge. In addition, anxiety is relieved if pathology results show a benign lesion.

Client counseling includes information that the procedure can be performed in an outpatient surgical setting under local or general anesthesia. Tell the client that usually only a small areolar incision is required, thus major alteration in the cosmetics of the breast is averted. Only a small surgical dressing is necessary. More extensive surgery is required if the lesion is hard to access. Referral to a surgeon who specializes in the treatment of the breast is required; and client participation in the selection of a surgeon is appropriate.

Follow-up to see whether postoperative visits are kept with the surgeon as directed. Advise the client to continue with annual breast exams performed by the health care provider and monthly breast self-examination (BSE).

## Duct Ectasia

Duct ectasia is dilation and inflammation of the major mammary ducts resulting in noncyclic breast pain and pasty nipple discharge that may be straw-colored, cream-colored, green, or brown.

***Epidemiology.*** The etiology of duct ectasia is unclear. Mammary ducts are thought to become distended with cellular debris and lipid-containing material, which causes a subareolar duct obstruction.[7] Anaerobic organisms or ductal irritation from debris cause inflammation, which in turn produces symptoms.[38]

Duct ectasia is most common among women in their fifth decade.[28] It tends to affect perimenopausal women in their fifties and is the most common cause of nipple discharge in women over age 55.[39] Clients are usually parous and have lactated, but may have experienced difficult lactation because of inverted nipples.[39]

***Subjective Data.*** Clients report a bilateral, pasty discharge that may be green, cream, brown, or straw-color. In addition, dull nipple pain, a "drawing" sensation, subareolar swelling, and burning and nipple itching frequently occur.[38,39] When the condition is advanced, the client may report a breast mass and nipple retractions; young women will most likely have pain, older women nipple retraction.[39]

***Objective Data.*** Physical examination of the breasts may reveal subareolar redness and swelling. Nipple retraction and dimpling may also be present. There is mild to moderate tenderness on palpation. Nipple discharge, manually expressed, is green, brown, straw-colored, or cream-colored with the consistency of toothpaste. Discharge is usually observed from one ductal quadrant of the nipple when the breast is palpated in a systematic fashion. In advanced cases, a round, firm, and somewhat fixed tumor may be palpable. Also in advanced cases, axillary lymphadenopathy is observed.

***Diagnostic Tests and Methods.*** Test for occult blood of breast fluid (see page 293); *mammography* (performed most often for clients with a palpable mass; see page 286); ductography (see page 293).

Differential Medical Diagnosis. Intraductal carcinoma.

***Plan***

Psychosocial Interventions. Include providing information on the benign status of the disease to help alleviate the client's anxiety. Use the opportunity to promote breast self-examination (BSE). Encourage support by significant others in the client's life. Encourage the client to express her feelings and emotions. Discuss sexuality issues if problematic, and refer the client for professional counseling if indicated.

Surgical Intervention: Wedge Excision. The affected duct, including any mass that is present, is surgically removed by wedge excision and sent to pathology for evaluation (see page 294).

Follow-Up. Follow-up care is directed by the surgeon. In addition, routine breast exams are carried out by the primary care provider; monthly BSE is done by the client.

## Galactocele

A galactocele is a discrete, cystic or firm mass in the breast of a lactating or recently lactating woman. It may or may not be painful.

***Epidemiology.*** The galactocele is thought to arise from dilation and obstruction of the lactiferous duct with retained milk and desquamated epithelial cells.39 It is most often found in the upper quadrants beyond the areolar border and may be singular or multiple.

***Subjective Data.*** The client may report a lump, knot, or cyst in her breast that may or may not be painful. Usually no bloody or purulent nipple discharge is reported, but occasionally pain may be described.

***Objective Data.*** Physical examination usually reveals a visible, palpable, firm, round mass in one or both breasts. Milk may be manually expressed from the nipple.

*Fine Needle Aspiration.* Performed to identify and eradicate the lesion (see page 289 for the procedure). If the fluid is milky, it may be discarded; cytology is not required. No further treatment is needed if the mass disappears with aspiration. If the fluid is other than milky or if the galactocele does not disappear with aspiration, an excisional biopsy is indicated.[28]

*Mammography.* Described on page 286.

***Differential Medical Diagnosis.*** Microcyst.

***Plan***

Psychosocial Interventions. Once a definitive diagnosis is made, reassure the client that galactocele is a benign condition that rarely interferes with lactation. In addition, discuss issues related to self-concept or sexuality. Encourage the client to express her feelings and concerns. If necessary, refer her to a breastfeeding support group, for example, La Leche League.

Surgical Intervention: Excision of the Affected Duct. This surgery is indicated if the lesion recurs frequently. An incision is made in the quadrant of the areola where the affected duct is located. The duct is then removed and sent to a pathology lab.

Adverse effects, or complications, may include infection and a possible reaction to the local anesthetic. The anticipated outcome on evaluation is total obliteration of the mass.

Help the client to choose a surgeon with expertise in this type of breast surgery. In addition, explain that the procedure is most often performed in ambulatory surgery under local anesthesia. Usually a periareolar incision is made and a small bandage is required. Minor cosmetic change may result. Mild to moderate pain is associated with the procedure, but there are virtually no complications.

Follow-up visits should be made to the surgeon. Routine breast exams should be continued by the health care provider; a monthly BSE is advocated for the client during and following lactation.

## MALIGNANT BREAST NEOPLASMS (BREAST CANCER)

Breast cancer, an overgrowth of neoplastic cells of the breast, is a life threatening disease.

### EPIDEMIOLOGY

The precise etiology of breast cancer is unknown; however, the disease is thought to develop in response to a number of related factors: increasing age, positive family history, previous breast cancer, high fat diet, late menopause, hormonal factors, and nulliparity.[40]

Breast cancer is primarily a disease of women in the Western Hemisphere.[41] It occurs second only to lung cancer in American women; one of every nine women in the United States will develop breast cancer.[1] Approximately 46,000 deaths from breast cancer and diagnosis of approximately 182,000 new cases among American women were estimated for 1993.[1] Breast cancer is rare among women younger than 30 years. The incidence, however, rises among women in their early 40s, levels off at about 45 years, and increases again after age 55.[25]

Two-thirds of all cancer patients are older than 50 years. Breast cancer is two to three times more likely to develop in women whose mothers or sisters have had breast cancer,[40,41] and its incidence is higher among nulliparous women and women whose first full-term pregnancy occurred after age 30.[41,42] The incidence may be higher among women having estrogen replacement therapy (specifically unopposed estrogen) and among stocky or obese women.[42] Ten to 15 percent of women who have had cancer in one breast will develop cancer in the other. Like many cancers, the incidence of breast cancer death is higher among African American women, and it is more likely to cause death in that population.[1,40,42] Accordingly, these women should be strongly advised to perform BSE, have regular examinations by health professionals, and have mammography. Common sites of metastasis are the lungs, liver, bone, soft tissues, and brain.[43,44]

### Profile of Specific Malignant Tumors[23,45]

***Invasive Ductal Carcinoma.*** Represents about 70 percent of all breast cancers. It can spread rapidly to lymph nodes even while small. Breast hardness, dimpling, and nipple retraction develops. The 5-year survival rate is 80 to 90 percent if lymph nodes are negative and hormone receptors are positive (see Hormone Receptor Assays, pages 298–299.)

***Medullary Carcinoma.*** Represents 7 percent of breast cancers and is most often found among women younger than 50 years. Because it grows in a capsule with a duct, it does not metastasize as frequently as other cancers. Signs include a large palpable tumor that is fixed to the chest wall or skin and ulceration. The survival rate is approximately 80 percent.

***Comedocarcinoma.*** Accounts for about 5 percent of breast cancers. It originates in the lining of the mammary duct, and as it grows, fills the duct. The tumor is sometimes large but is not likely to spread beyond the breast or into the skin. The prognosis is usually good.

***Mucinous Carcinoma.*** A ductal cancer that accounts for about 3 percent of breast cancers. Usually it grows slowly and contains large amounts of extracellular mucin. Mucinous carcinoma may have sharp borders and may be confused with a fibroadenoma. It usually presents as a mass but may be accompanied by nipple discharge, fixation, and skin ulceration. Less often, it is associated with metastasis; thus prognosis is usually good.

***Tubular Ductal Carcinoma.*** Rare cancer, representing about 2 percent of breast cancers. It is an invasive cancer whose cells are arranged in regular, well defined tubules typically lined by one epithelial layer and accompanied by fibrous stroma. Axillary metastases are uncommon (6 percent). The presenting symptom, a palpable mass, is occasionally accompanied by skin retraction or fixation. The prognosis is better than for invasive carcinoma.

***Invasive Lobular Carcinoma.*** Accounts for approximately 3 percent of breast cancers. It originates in the lobules of the breast and is invasive. The presenting tumor is frequently located in the upper-outer breast quadrant. Skin retraction and fixation accompany large lesions. The prognosis is poor.

***Inflammatory Breast Cancer.*** Represents 1 percent of all breast cancers and is usually widespread when it is diagnosed. Inflammatory breast cancer is not actually a distinct cancer, but represents an extension of tumor into the intradermal lymphatics. It metastasizes rapidly. The breast may appear inflamed, thickened with peau d'orange skin, and may have an accompanying breast mass. The prognosis is very poor.

***Paget's Disease.*** A cancer of the nipple, occurs in 1 to 4 percent of all women with breast cancer. It is almost always associated with an underlying intraductal carcinoma and frequently with a long history of eczema of the nipple with itching, burning, oozing, or bleeding.

## Subjective Data[23]

A client may report one or more of the following conditions.

- A fixed, poorly defined lump or mass may be noted in one breast. Rarely is it painful. The lump is usually located in the upper-outer quadrant of the breast. (*Note*: A lump can be palpated when it reaches a size of approximately 1 cm; it has possibly been present for 7 to 8 years when palpable at that size.)
- Spontaneous nipple discharge that is clear, yellow, or bloody may appear unilaterally.
- Persistent nipple irritation is reported.
- Dimpling or redness of the skin, nipple retraction, change in breast contour, and swelling (advanced malignancy) may occur.
- Axillary adenopathy, or supraclavicular/intraclavicular adenopathy (advanced malignancy) is described.

## Objective Data

Physical examination of the breast requires observation and palpation of the subjective symptoms. Peau d'orange skin of the breast may also be observed, and in advanced malignancies, a mass fixed to the chest wall may be palpated.[23]

Lymphatic palpation is done to determine supraclavicular and infraclavicular axillary nodal involvement.

## Diagnostic Tests and Methods

***Mammography.*** See page 286.

***Fine Needle Aspiration.*** See page 289. *Note: The procedure for fine needle aspiration is altered for a solid mass.*[26,46]

- The plunger of the syringe should not be pulled back while the needle is inserted in the mass. The needle should be withdrawn from the mass and the plunger gently pulled back.
- Air is used to expel the cellular sample onto a clean glass slide.
- A second clean slide is used to gently spread the sample.
- The sample is fixed with ethyl alcohol.
- A second smear is air dried.
- Both samples are sent to the lab.

***Ultrasound.*** Diagnostic evaluation to detect lesions that are not clearly identified by mammography. The procedure also helps to differentiate a cystic mass from a solid one found on mammogram.[47] Ultrasound is usually performed after mammography in the patient older than 30 years with a palpable mass and may be the only modality employed in women younger than age 30.[48] Images of the breasts are produced via sound waves that travel through a gel medium that is applied to the breasts.

Explain the procedure to the client and offer support. The test must be performed by a qualified radiologist. It is not contraindicated during pregnancy.

***Excisional Biopsy (Surgical Procedure).*** Diagnostic evaluation to identify small lesions of the breast that can be completely excised.[27] The procedure requires cleansing the breast with an antiseptic solution. The mass is then surgically excised under local anesthesia, and the biopsied lesion is sent to the pathology lab. The incision is sutured or held together with Steri-strips.[27]

Explain the procedure to the client and refer her to a qualified surgeon. The client should participate in selecting the surgeon. Review the possible complications of the procedure: hematoma, stitch abscess, malignant tumor remaining partially intact, reaction to local anesthetic, and infection.[27] Provide client support.

***Incisional Biopsy.*** A rarely used surgical procedure in which a majority of the tumor, which is possibly malignant, is left in the client.[27] This diagnostic evaluation is done to determine quickly, prior to surgical intervention, whether a tumor is malignant. It is rarely used but can confirm the diagnosis of advanced cancer.[27]

The procedure requires skin preparation with an antiseptic solution. Under local anesthesia, a small wedge of tissue is excised from the diseased area and the incision is closed. Steri-strips may be used. The specimen is sent to the pathology lab.

Explain the procedure to the client and offer support. Teach her about possible complications: bleeding, infection, reaction to local anesthetic. In explaining, reinforce for the client that only a small wedge of the lesion will be taken, and that the remaining, possibly malignant, tumor will be left intact. Referral to a qualified surgeon is required. Encourage the client to participate in selecting a surgeon.

***Hormone Receptor Assays (Surgical Procedure).*** This procedure is done to determine a tumor's dependency on female hormone. The assay predicts metastatic disease response to hormone manipulation.[23] If the estrogen receptor (ER) is negative, the client is less likely to benefit from hormonal therapy.[49] In contrast, if the estrogen receptor is positive, the client is likely to respond to hormonal therapy. Positive ER levels are those greater than or equal to 10 fm/mg protein. Negative levels are those less than 10 fm/mg protein.[50]

The tumor is excised, put in a sterile container, and immediately chilled. If necessary, the specimen can be frozen and stored until it is sent to a lab for analysis.[49] The procedure is done under local anesthesia.

Explain the procedure to the client and provide support. Also explain the possible complications: bleeding, infection, and reaction to local anesthetic. Referral to a qualified surgeon is required; encourage the client to participate in the selection of a surgeon.

## Differential Medical Diagnoses

Fibroadenoma, intraductal papilloma.

## Plan

***Psychosocial Interventions.*** Help the client to cope with her fear, anxiety, and lowered self-image, and encourage family support. Referral to a support group, for example, Reach to Recovery, or to a counselor or religious counselor may be appropriate. (The client's family usually needs support as well.) A cooperative/interactive team approach with this client is vital.

### *Medication*

Chemotherapy. Any of 50 or more chemotherapy agents may be used.[23,51,52] Often used drugs include doxorubicin, cyclophosphamide (Cytoxan), methotrexate, 5-FU, and vincristine. Usually combinations of two to five drugs are used.

An indication for chemotherapy is systemic malignancy. Frequently, however, it is used concomitantly with local treatment and surgery for women whose cancer has spread to axillary nodes.

- *Administration.* Administration of the therapy depends on the agent, disease stage (see Table 10–1), and site of metastasis if present. It is given intravenously, orally, or possibly intrathecally.[23]
- *Side Effects.* Side effects include nausea, vomiting, alopecia, stomatitis, leukopenia, and destruction of healthy cells.[51]
- *Anticipated Outcomes on Evaluation.* Regression in the dissemination of cancer and improved survival.[23]
- *Client Teaching and Counseling.* Refer the client to a qualified oncologist for treatment, and advise her to consult with more than one. Provide literature about chemotherapies. Discuss possible adverse reactions to the drugs and other possible drug effects on body image, self-perception, or self-esteem. Inform the client that medications may be prescribed to treat some symptoms and that a cap is available to help reduce hair loss. Refer her to a local support group such as Reach to Recovery.

**TABLE 10-1. STAGING OF BREAST CANCER**

| Stage | Characteristics |
|---|---|
| I | Small tumor, less than 2 cm, or 0.78 in, negative lymph nodes; no detectable metastases. |
| II | Tumor greater than 2 cm across, but less than 5 cm, and negative lymph nodes; *or* tumor less than 5 cm, positive lymph nodes, and no detectable distant metastases. |
| III | Large tumor greater than 5 cm; *or* tumor of any size with invasion of skin or chest wall or associated with positive lymph nodes in clavicular area. |
| IV | Tumor of any size; lymph nodes either positive or negative with distant metastases. |

*Note:* Cancer staging is used to determine the extent of local, regional, or distant cancer involvement.[14]
*Source: American Cancer Society (1991). Cancer Response System. Atlanta: Author.*

#### Hormonal Therapy

- *Indications.* To promote tumor regression and to delay recurrence, postmastectomy, among women who have cancer that is sensitive to estrogen and progesterone.[23,53] Tamoxifen is the drug most frequently used. Tamoxifen, now widely used as an adjuvant therapy in the treatment of breast cancer, is currently being used in clinical trials in the National Surgical Adjuvant Breast and Bowel Project (NSABP). This project, funded in part by the National Cancer Institute was begun in 1992. The NSABP Breast Cancer Prevention Trial is a randomized, double-blinded, placebo-controlled, clinical trial of tamoxifen. Sixteen thousand women age 35 and over who are considered at high risk for breast cancer will be recruited for the trial. Treatment will continue for at least 5 years. Equal numbers of women will be assigned to a placebo and tamoxifen group. All women 60 years of age and older are eligible to participate in the trial. Women who are 35–59 years of age are eligible if their 5-year risk of breast cancer is equal to or greater than that of a 60-year-old woman.[54] It is projected that 62 breast cancers and 52 myocardial infarctions will be prevented with tamoxifen during the 5-year trial.[55]
- *Administration.* Tamoxifen, one to two 10-mg tablets, p.o., b.i.d.
- *Side Effects and Adverse Reactions.* Hot flashes, nausea, depression, vomiting, vaginal bleeding and discharge, unintended pregnancy, menstrual irregularities, and bone pain. More serious side effects are endometrial cancer, liver cancer, thromboembolitic disease, and retinopathy.[53]
- *Contraindications.* None are known.
- *Anticipated Outcomes on Evaluation.* Tumor regression and increased likelihood of survival. Additional benefit of reduction in cardiovascular death is anticipated because tamoxifen lowers the cholesterol level. This effect occurs within the first 3 to 6 months and is sustained during the treatment.[55]
- *Client Teaching and Counseling.* Refer the client to a qualified oncologist; the client should consult with more than one oncologist. Inform the client that therapy is most effective in cancers sensitive to estrogen and progesterone. Discuss the side effects/risk factors in detail. Discuss data related to the tamoxifen trials.

***Radiation Therapy.*** Radiation therapy is used to treat early stage breast cancer. It is generally used in combination with a lumpectomy (breast conservation surgery) to destroy or suppress cells that are not removed by surgery.[23,56] External radiation (x-rays) is directed to the breast and possibly the axillary lymph nodes. Sometimes a booster or concentrated dose of radiation is given in the area where cancer is located.[23] Radiation may be administered by electron beam or internal radioactive implant.[56]

- *Adverse Effects.* Fatigue, temporary discoloration of the skin, itching or peeling, leukopenia, retraction of the breast, breast fibrosis, cancer secondary to radiation therapy, and pleural effusion.[56]
- *Anticipated Outcomes on Evaluation.* Eradication of the pathology, maintenance of breast integrity, and improved chances for survival.
- *Client Teaching and Counseling.* Provide the client with information about the course of radiation therapies: It usually requires 5 to 6 weeks and daily trips to the treatment site, where a qualified radiologist administers therapy. Refer the client to a support group, such as Reach to Recovery. Discuss need for annual mammography.

#### Surgical Interventions[57–59]

Radical Mastectomy. Radical mastectomy is indicated for the removal of cancers with large bulky tumors involving the pectoralis major or fascia, bulky axillary lymph involvement, or grossly involved interpectoral nodes. With improvements in early detection, radical mastectomy is done less frequently. The surgery involves removal of the breast, pectoralis major and pectoralis minor muscles, skin overlying the tumor, and all axillary nodes. Adverse effects include extensive scarring, hollow chest, lymphedema, infection, skin necrosis, and disfigurement.[60] Breast reconstruction is difficult if possible at all.

The anticipated outcomes on evaluation are the removal of the pathology and improved chances for survival.

Center client teaching on the procedure and its possible adverse effects. Hospitalization and general anesthesia are required. In addition to a qualified surgeon, a physical and/or occupational therapist will be needed. A team approach is preferable for rehabilitation. Discuss the difficulty of breast reconstruction, and inform the client that breast prostheses are available. A visit by a specialist in fitting breast forms or foundations may be arranged. The management of lymphedema and other side effects must also be taught, and exercises to reduce lymphedema or arm stiffness should begin 24 hours after surgery.[61] Encourage ROM exercises and encourage the client to avoid restrictive clothing such as tight sleeves. The client should avoid underarm creams, depilatories, and deodorants. Reinforce importance of BSE. Refer the client to a support group such as Reach to Recovery for preoperative and postoperative support. If indicated, suggest professional counseling.

Modified Radical Mastectomy. Modified radical mastectomy is indicated when tumors are not large or bulky, when axillary adenopathy is not bulky, and when interpectoral nodes are not grossly involved.[57,58] The surgery involves removal of the breast, axillary nodes, and often the pectoralis minor. Adverse effects include lymphedema, infection, and hematoma.

The anticipated outcomes on evaluation are the removal of the pathology and improved chances for survival.

Provide the client with information about the procedure (e.g., surgeon qualifications, general anesthesia, and managing lymphedema and other adverse effects). (See the preceding section on radical mastectomy.) Referral to physical and occupational therapists is imperative. Counsel the client about breast reconstruction and inform her that breast prostheses are available. Refer her to a support group for preoperative and postoperative support. In addition, a professional counselor may be needed. A team approach is helpful for the client's rehabilitation. Reinforce practice of BSE.

Total, or Simple, Mastectomy. This surgery is indicated for women with in situ carcinoma (ductal or lobular) with no suspicious axillary involvement;[60] or for women whose tumor recurred after partial mastectomy and axillary dissection.[57] The surgery involves removal of the breast and pectoralis major muscle fascia.

Adverse effects may arise because the axillary chain is left intact and not checked for cancer. If cancer is later detected in the axillary lymph nodes, further surgery will be necessary.[59] Nodal involvement may be microscopic and nonpalpable, which frequently necessitates radiation therapy. Postoperative infection is possible.

The anticipated outcomes on evaluation are the removal of the pathology and improved chances for survival.

In client teaching, contrast and compare total mastectomy with modified radical mastectomy and include a discussion of reconstructive surgery. Inform the client that breast prostheses are available. Radiation therapy may be recommended to destroy cancer cells that may be in the lymph nodes. Refer the client to a support group such as Reach to Recovery for preoperative and postoperative support. Reinforce practice of BSE.

Partial, or Segmental, Mastectomy. Partial mastectomy is indicated for small tumors with negative axillary nodes. The procedure is also selected if the client wishes to preserve her breast. The surgery involves removal of the tumor. A wedge of normal-appearing tissue surrounding the tumor is also removed and tested to ensure that the pathology has not invaded it. In addition, some lymph nodes may be removed. Radiation therapy follows to eradicate other cancer cells that may be present. Further surgery may be necessary if microscopic nodal involvement was overlooked.

The procedure may be cosmetically unappealing for women with small breasts if a large portion of breast is removed.

The anticipated outcomes on evaluation are the removal of the pathology and improved chances for survival while preserving the majority of breast tissue.

Provide the client with information about qualified surgeons who perform the procedure. Teach her about the management of lymphedema. A radiologist will be required for radiation therapy, and professional counseling may be helpful. In addition, refer the client to a support group such as Reach to Recovery for preoperative and postoperative counseling. Encourage BSE.

Lumpectomy. Lumpectomy is indicated for the removal of small tumors from a client who has clinically negative nodes. The surgery involves the gross removal of the tumor with no attention to breast margins. Radiation therapy follows. (Undetectable microscopic nodal involvement may be present, necessitating later surgery.) An adverse effect is the possibility of infection.

The anticipated outcomes on evaluation are that the pathology is removed, the majority of breast tissue preserved, and the chances for survival are improved.

Client teaching includes providing reasons for referral to a qualified surgeon and radiologist. Explain that local anesthesia will be used. The client should also know that a greater risk of cancer recurrence exists following a lumpectomy if follow-up radiation is not used after surgery. Refer the client to a support group for preoperative and postoperative support and, if necessary, to a professional counselor.

Autologous Bone Marrow Transplant.[62,63] Transplant is indicated for the treatment of extremely aggressive breast cancer or cancers that have metastasized.[62] Bone marrow is withdrawn from the client to protect it. Extremely high doses of chemotherapy are then administered to the client to destroy cancerous cells. The bone marrow is reinjected or transplanted after chemotherapeutic agents have been absorbed.[62,63] Adverse effects include nausea, vomiting, alopecia, leukopenia, and fatigue. The anticipated outcome on evaluation is regression of the spread of cancer.

Advise the client that several weeks of hospitalization will be required. A hospital with the facilities and staff capable of performing transplant will need to be selected. Advise the client that most insurance companies do not cover the cost of this high risk therapy.

***Follow-Up.*** The follow-up of clients who have had chemotherapy is variable, and depends on their response to the drugs and the oncologist's recommendations. Clients may receive tamoxifen for 2 to 5 years, with follow-up every 6 months or per the care provider's preference.

Clients who undergo a mastectomy are evaluated postoperatively at the discretion of the surgeon. Complications, if encountered, may require more frequent evaluation or may necessitate rehospitalization. Clients undergoing autologous bone marrow transplants are followed closely by the oncologist and may require weekly visits upon leaving the hospital.

## BREAST RECONSTRUCTION

Breast reconstruction, a voluntary procedure, is available to many women who have undergone mastectomy. In addition to being an option following mastectomy, breast reconstruction and augmentation may also be chosen for cosmetic reasons that are unrelated to cancer surgery.[57–59]

### TISSUE TRANSFER (TRANSVERSE RECTUS ABDOMINIS MYOCUTANEOUS—TRAM—FLAP)[58,62]

Tissue transfer is recommended when breast reconstruction is desired and the client chooses not to risk the possible side effects of breast implants (which requires the implanting of foreign materials). A similar procedure, the latissimus dorsi musculocutaneous flap, may be performed as well when the client does not desire breast implants.[58,64] The rectus abdominis muscle is transferred from the abdomen via a tunnel under the skin and extended through a new incision in the breast area. The flap is sutured into position and, along with fat, is contoured to form a breast.[58,62] Sufficient abdominal girth is required to perform the procedure. The procedure can be very painful, and may require 6 to 8 weeks for recuperation. Untoward responses to anesthesia and postoperative infection and bleeding are possible.

The anticipated outcome on evaluation is a favorable body image.

Explain to the client that the recovery period required is often long and that appropriate pain management will be necessary. Inform her that tissue transfer is not recommended for women who smoke or who have chronic disease. In addition, further surgery will be necessary for nipple formation.

### AUGMENTATION MAMMOPLASTY (BREAST ENLARGEMENT)

Augmentation mammoplasty is performed to improve the cosmetic appearance of the breast by increasing its size, and to reconstruct the breast following a mastectomy.[65,66] An implant (saline or saline and gel with a polyurethane foam cover, or saline or viscous silicone with a silicone rubber outer shell) is placed behind the breast through a surgical incision. The implant is most often placed between the breast and chest wall but may be placed beneath the pectoral muscles to decrease scarring around the implant.[65] The procedure is performed under general anesthesia.

There is a 2 to 5 percent risk of infection, and infection may persist until the implant is removed.[65] The risk of hematoma is 5 to 10 percent; this complication requires removal of the implant and evacuation of the hematoma.[65] Scar formation around the implant usually causes the breast to be firm or hard. Nipple numbness and asymmetry rarely occur.[65,66] Leakage of silicone gel is also possible and has been alleged to cause connective tissue diseases, unexplained immune disorders, persistent flu-like symptoms, cancer, and other health problems[67] (see Appendix, page 307). Mammography screening may be complicated by the presence of implants because the implants obscure breast tissue.[68,69] Ultrasound may be used in conjunction with mammography to characterize lesions.

The anticipated outcomes on evaluation are improved self-esteem and a favorable body image.

Inform the client of the controversies surrounding breast implants and the possible leakage of silicone gel. Discuss the possibility of decreased sexual pleasure associated with nipple numbness and breast firmness. Clients with a history of or a propensity for keloid (common among African Americans) should consider the possibility of unsightly keloid scarring. Encourage the client to continue BSE and provide her with the instruction she needs (see Figure 10–1). Inform the client about the American Cancer Society guidelines for mammography screening. Discuss the difficulties associated with imaging breast tissue when breast implants are present,[67] and help the client to find a mammography facility that uses specialized techniques for women with breast implants.[13]

## MASTOPEXY (CORRECTION OF PTOSIS)

Mastopexy is performed to improve the appearance of sagging breasts, which may be caused by gravity, hormone regression (postpartum, menopausal) or weight loss.[66] Surgical resection of the breasts is done, with elevation of the breast mount, areola, and nipple to a new (usually higher) location.[65] General anesthesia is used. Infection, hematoma, nipple numbness (usually temporary), asymmetry, and scarring of the breast may develop.[65] A reaction to the anesthesia is possible.

The anticipated outcomes on evaluation are a favorable body image and improved self-esteem.

Encourage the client to weigh very carefully the risks and advantages of the procedure. Clients with a history of or a propensity to develop keloid (particularly common in African Americans) should consider possible formation of unsightly keloid scarring. Inform the client that breast ptosis may recur and that sensation in the breast and nipple may be lost, which may decrease sexual gratification.[66] Include significant others of the client's choosing in decision making and advise them to seek the opinions of at least two surgeons. Encourage BSE and mammography if age appropriate.

## BREAST REDUCTION

Breast reduction surgery is performed to reduce breast size and relieve back and shoulder pain caused by heavy pendulous breasts. During the surgery, the breasts are surgically restructured and made smaller. The potential adverse effects and complications are asymmetry, infection, hematoma, nipple numbness, and extensive scarring.[65]

The anticipated outcomes on evaluation are reduced back and shoulder pain, reduced pressure on skin and irritation from brassiere straps, and improved self-esteem.

Encourage the client to weigh the advantages and risks of this elective surgical procedure. Clients with a history of or propensity to develop keloid (common among African Americans) should consider the possibility of extensive and unsightly keloid scarring. Include significant others of the client's choosing in decision making. Discuss the possible relationship between nipple numbness and decreased sexual gratification. Encourage BSE and mammography if appropriate. Advise the client to seek the opinions of at least two surgeons. Inform her that the procedure generally is covered by insurance because it is not performed for cosmetic reasons alone. The client, however, should consult with her insurance company.

## FOLLOW-UP

Follow the postoperative care guidelines provided by the surgeon. Immediate evaluation is especially important if signs or symptoms of infection occur in a client who has had the TRAM flap procedure, because abdominal and chest wounds are present.

## NURSING DIAGNOSES

The following nursing diagnoses are representative of those used in the health care plan of women with breast problems. The list, however, is by no means inclusive.

- Altered role performance.
- Anticipatory grieving.
- Anxiety.
- Body image disturbance.
- Fear.
- Hopelessness.
- Impaired skin integrity.
- Ineffective individual or family coping.
- Ineffective breastfeeding.
- Knowledge deficit.
- Low self-esteem.
- Pain.
- Powerlessness.
- Sexual dysfunction.
- Situational low self-esteem.
- Sleep pattern disturbance.

## REFERENCES

1. American Cancer Society. (1992). *Cancer facts and figures*. Atlanta: Author.
2. Dondero, T., & Lichtman, R. (1990). The breasts. In R. Lichtman & S. Papera (Eds.), Gynecology: Well-woman care (pp. 141–171). Norwalk, CT: Appleton & Lange.
3. Jacob, T., Penn, N., & Brown, M. (1989). Breast self examination: Knowledge, attitudes, and performance among black women. *Journal of the National Medical Association, 81*, 769–776.
4. Knaysi, G. (1991, May). *You found a breast mass—Now what?* Paper presented at the meeting of the Annual Mid-Atlantic Nurse Practitioner Conference, Richmond, VA.
5. Drukker, B. (1990). Examination of the breasts by the patient and by the physician. In W. Hindle (Ed.), *Breast disease for gynecologists* (pp. 47–54). Norwalk, CT: Appleton & Lange.
6. ACOG Technical Bulletin #156 (1991). Nonmalignant conditions of the breast. *International Journal of Gynecology and Obstetrics, 39*, 53–58.
7. Drukker, B., & de Mendonca, W. (1987, September). Fibrocystic change and fibrocystic disease of the breast. *Obstetrics and Gynecology Clinics of North America, 14*, 685–702.
8. Haagensen, M. (1986). *Diseases of the breast*. Philadelphia: Saunders.
9. Jones, R., & Hendler, F. (1990). Fibrocystic changes of the breast. In W. Hindle (Ed.), *Breast disease for gynecologists* (pp. 155–165). Norwalk, CT: Appleton & Lange.
10. Devitt, J. (1989). Benign breast disease in postmenopausal women. *World Journal of Surgery, 13*, 731–735.
11. Kopans, D. (1993). Evaluation of breast mass. *New England Journal of Medicine, 328*, 810–811.
12. Winchester, D. (1990). Evaluation and management of breast abnormalities. *Cancer, 66*, 1345–1347.
13. U.S. Department of Health and Human Services. (1991, February). *Mammography Screening Update #2*. Rockville, MD: Food & Drug Administration.
14. London, R., Sundaram, S., Murphey, L., et al. (1985). The effect of vitamin E on mammary dysplasia; A double blind study. *Obstetrics and Gynecology, 65*, 104–106.
15. Ernstr, B., Goodson, W., Hunt, T., et al. (1985). Vitamin E and benign breast disease. A double blind randomized. *Clinical Trial Surgery, 97*, 490–494.
16. Souba, W. (1991). Evaluation and treatment of benign breast disorders. In K. Bland & E. Copeland (Eds.), *The breast* (pp. 715–727). Philadelphia: Saunders.
17. Issacs, J. (Ed.). (1992). Clinical diagnosis and management of benign breast disorders. *Textbook of breast disease* (p. 194), Chicago: Mosby Year Book.

18. Lewison, W., Dunn, P. (1986). Nonassociation of caffeine and fibrocystic disease. *Archives in Internal Medicine, 146*, 1773.
19. Heyden, S., Muhlbaier, L. (1984). Prospective study of fibrocystic disease. *Surgery, 96*, 479.
20. McInnis, W. (1990). Plastic surgery of the breast. In G. Mitchell & L. Bassett (Eds.), *The female breast and its disorders* (pp. 196–217). Baltimore: Williams & Wilkins.
21. Dent, D., & Pant, P. (1989, November/December). Fibroadenoma. *World Journal of Surgery, 13*, 706–710.
22. Stehman, F. (1990). Benign neoplasms of the breast. In W. Hindle (Ed.), *Breast disease for gynecologists* (pp. 167–172). Norwalk, CT: Appleton & Lange.
23. American Cancer Society. (1991). *Cancer response system.* Atlanta: Author.
24. Smallwood, J., & Taylor, I. (1990). *Benign breast disease.* Baltimore: Urban & Schwarzenberg.
25. Oertel, Y. (1987). Fine needle aspiration of the breast (pp. 20–25). Boston: Butterworths.
26. Hindle, W. (1990). Fine needle aspiration. In W. Hindle (Ed.), *Breast disease for gynecologists* (pp. 67–118). Norwalk: CT: Appleton & Lange.
27. Isaacs, J. (1987, September). Breast biopsy and surgical treatment of early carcinoma. *Obstetrics and Gynecology Clinics of North America, 14*, 710–732.
28. Hackner, N., & Moore, J. (1992). *Essentials of obstetrics and gynecology* (2nd ed.). Philadelphia: Saunders.
29. Wertheimer, M. (1990). Diagnosis of malignant breast disease. In W. Hindle (Ed.), *Breast Disease for Gynecologists* (pp. 173–181). Norwalk, CT: Appleton & Lange.
30. Leis, A. (1989). Management of nipple discharge. *World Journal of Surgery, 13*, 736–742.
31. Brumsted, J., & Riddick, D. (1990). The endocrinology of the mammary gland. In W. Hindle (Ed.), *Breast disease for gynecologists* (pp. 21–28). Norwalk, CT: Appleton & Lange.
32. Edge, D., Segatore, M. (1993). Assessment and management of galactorrhea. *Nurse Practitioner, 18(6)*, 35–36, 38, 43–44, 47–49.
33. Katz, E., Adashi, E. (1990). Hyperprolactinemic disorders. *Clinical Obstetrics and Gynecology, 33(3)*, 622–639.
34. Cooper, P., Martin, J. (1991). Neuroendocrinology. In Rosenberg, R. (Ed.). *Comprehensive neurology* (pp. 605–621). New York: Raven Press.
35. Hughes, L., Mansel, R., & Webster, D. (1989). *Benign disorders and diseases of the breast: Concepts and clinical management.* London: Bailliere Tindall.
36. Bleeker, M., & Gordon, B. (1986). Evaluation of the patient with neurological symptoms. In L. Barker, J. Burton, & P. Zieve (Eds.), *Principles of ambulatory medicine* (pp. 1105–1118). Baltimore: Williams & Wilkins.
37. Molitch, M. (1989). Management of prolactinomas. *Annual Review of Medicine, 40*, 225–232.
38. Dixon, J. (1989). Periductal mastitis/Duct ectasia. *World Journal of Surgery, 13*, 715–720.
39. Stehman, F. (1990). Infections and inflammations of the breast. In W. Hindle (Ed.), *Breast disease for gynecologists* (pp. 151–154). Norwalk, CT: Appleton & Lange.
40. Colditz, G. (1993). Epidemiology of breast cancer. *Cancer 71(4)*, 1480–1487.
41. Jones, R. (1990). Epidemiology-risk factors. In W. Hindle (Ed.), *Breast disease for gynecologists* (pp. 29–37). Norwalk, CT: Appleton & Lange.
42. Berkowitz, G. (1986). Risk factors. In D. Marchant (Ed.), *Breast disease* (pp. 13–43). New York: Churchill Livingstone.
43. Price, J. (1990). The biology of metastatic breast cancer. *Cancer, 66,* 1113—1320.
44. Bassett, L., Guiliano, A., & Gold, R. (1990). Diagnostic imaging for staging and follow-up of breast cancer patients. In G. Mitchell & L. Bassett (Eds.). *The female breast and its disorders*, p. 173. Baltimore: Williams &Wilkins.
45. Rosen, P. (1991). The pathology of breast carcinoma. In J. Harris, S. Hellman, I. Henderson, & D. Kinne (Eds.), *Breast diseases* (pp. 247, 254, 256, 257). Philadelphia: Lippincott.
46. Glant, M. (1990). Fine needle aspiration cytology: A cytopathologist's perspective. In W. Hindle (Ed.), *Breast disease for gynecologists* (pp. 121–140). Norwalk, CT: Appleton & Lange.

47. Schoenberger, S., Sutherland, C., & Robinson, A. (1988). Breast neoplasms: Duplex sonographic imaging is an adjunct in diagnoses. *Radiology, 168*, 665.
48. Jokich, P., Monticciolo, D., & Adler, Y. (1992). Breast ultrasonography. *Radiologic Clinics of North America, 30(5)*, 993–1009.
49. Osborne, C. (1991). Receptors. In J. Harris, S. Hellman, I. Henderson, & D. Kinne (Eds.), *Breast diseases* (pp. 304, 314). Philadelphia: Lippincott.
50. Carbone, P. (1990). Breast cancer adjuvant therapy. *Cancer, 66*, 1378–1386.
51. Plotkin, D. (1990). Chemotherapy of breast cancer. In W. Hindle (Ed.), *Breast disease for gynecologists* (pp. 227–235). Norwalk, CT: Appleton & Lange.
52. Wertheimer, M. (1990). Primary treatment of early breast cancer. In W. Hindle (Ed.), *Breast Disease for Gynecologists*, pp. 203–214. Norwalk, CT: Appleton & Lange.
53. Bush, T., & Helzlsouer, K. (1993). Tamoxifen for the primary prevention of breast cancer: A review and critique of the concept and trial. *The Johns Hopkins University School of Hygiene and Public Health, 15(1)*, 223–243.
54. Morrow, M., & Jordan, V. (1992). The tamoxifen trial for breast cancer: Clinical issues. *Cancer prevention* (pp. 1–10). Philadelphia: Lippincott.
55. Nayfield, S., Karp, J., Ford, L., Door, A., & Kramer, B. (1991). Potential role of tamoxifen in prevention of breast cancer. *Journal of the National Cancer Institute, 83(20)*, 1450–1459.
56. Ratanatharathorn, V., & Powers, W. (1987). Primary radiation therapy as an alternative to mastectomy for early-stage breast cancer. *Obstetrics and Gynecological Clinics of North America, 14(3)*, 733–758.
57. Kinne, D. (1991). Primary treatment of breast cancer. In J. Harris, S. Hellman, I. Henderson, & D. Kenne (Eds.), *Breast Diseases*, pp. 354–358. Philadelphia: Lippincott.
58. Lanigan, E. (1987, September). Plastic surgical procedures related to breast disease. *Obstetrics and Gynecology Clinics of North America, 14*, 761–781.
59. U.S. Department of Health and Human Services. (1990). *Breast cancer, understanding treatment options*. Washington, D.C.: Author.
60. Marchant, D. (1990). Surgery for breast cancer. In G. Mitchell & L. Bassett (Eds.), *The female breast and its disorders* (p. 233). Baltimore: Williams & Wilkins.
61. Knobf, M. (1990). Symptoms and rehabilitation needs of patients with early stage breast cancer during primary therapy. *Cancer, 66*, 1392–1401.
62. Billingsly, A.B. (1991, July 2). Victims can fight back with an array of options. *The Richmond News Leader* (pp. 1, 8–9).
63. McKenzie, R. (1992). Metastatic breast cancers and medical emergencies. In J. Isaacs (Ed.), *Textbook of breast disease* (pp. 331–339). Chicago: Mosby Year Book.
64. McGibbon, B. (1984). Latissimus dorsi musculocutaneous flap. In *Atlas of breast reconstruction following mastectomy*. Baltimore: University Park Press.
65. Penoff, J. (1990). Plastic surgery for the female breast. In W. Hindle (Ed.), *Breast disease for gynecologists* (pp. 237–250). Norwalk, CT: Appleton & Lange.
66. Carlson, G., & Bostwick, J. (1989). Aesthetic surgery for benign disorders of the breast. *World Journal of Surgery, 13*, 761–764.
67. Silver, R.M., et al. (1993). Demonstration of silicone in sites of connective tissue disease in patients with silicone-gel breast implants. *Archives in Dermatology, 129(1)*, 63–68.
68. Steinbach, B.G. (1993). Mammography: breast implants—types, complications and adjacent breast pathology. *Current Problems in Diagnostic Radiology, 22(2)*, 39–86.
69. Shestak, K., Ganott, M., Harris, K., & Losken, H. (1993). Breast masses in the augmentation mammoplasty patient: The role of ultrasound. *Plastic and Reconstructive Surgery, 92*, 209–216.

## APPENDIX: SILICONE GEL IMPLANTS

On January 6, 1992, following complaints of unexplained immune disorders, connective tissue diseases, persistent flu-like symptoms, cancer, and other health problems, the U.S.

Food and Drug Administration (FDA) called for a moratorium on the use of silicone gel implants in reconstructive breast surgery until further study on the safety of these implants could be conducted by an advisory panel.

On February 20, 1992, after hearing intense testimony regarding the use of silicone gel implants, the advisory panel unanimously urged the FDA to make silicone gel implants available. They recommended, however, that the use of these implants be strictly limited for females seeking breast augmentation for cosmetic reasons, but that women seeking breast reconstruction following breast cancer surgery be given the easiest access to these implants. (To date, 80 percent of all silicone gel implants have been used in women requesting breast enlargement.) Moreover, the panel advised that all breast implant patients be enrolled in clinical trials to enable their health to be closely monitored for years following the surgical procedure.

Even though the panel concluded that there is no credible evidence that silicone gel implants cause disease, it acknowledged that strong anecdotal evidence warranted further study. They also advised that women should expect that the silicone gel implants will fail at some point in their lives.

Dow Corning, maker of the silicone gel implant, voluntarily discontinued marketing the implant in late 1991, pending further study of its safety. On February 10, 1992, the company released documents that revealed its knowledge of implant problems for 2 decades. Dow Corning officials insisted, however, that the implants posed no threat of cancer or other life-threatening diseases. They did acknowledge that persistent tissue inflammation could occur if leaking silicone gel worked its way beyond the scar tissue that normally forms around breast implants.

## SOURCES

Associated Press. (1992, February 12). Dow Corning aims: Damage control. *Richmond News Leader*, p. 4.

Associated Press. (1992, February 11). Dow Corning names new chief after admission. *Richmond News Leader*, p. 2.

Associated Press. (1992, February 21). Panel suggests limits to breast implants. *Richmond News Leader*, p. 2.

CHAPTER 11

# THE CLIMACTERIC, MENOPAUSE, AND THE PROCESS OF AGING

*Catherine H. Garner*

*Women today can expect to live one-third of their lives after their reproductive years.*

*Highlights*

- Physiology of Menopause
- Physical Changes of Aging: Body Systems
- Sexuality and Aging
- Hypoestrogenic Changes
  - *Vasomotor*
  - *Vaginal*
  - *Urinary*
  - *Menstrual*
- Alterations in Mood
- Sleep Disorders
- Hormone Replacement Therapy
  - *Counseling, Assessment*
  - *Treatment Considerations: Preparations, Contraindications, Follow-up*
- Midlife Education, Evaluation, Screening
- Osteoporosis
- Hirsutism
- Nonreproductive Health Concerns
  - *Social Security*
  - *Abuse*
  - *Chronic Illness, Depression*
  - *Health Status*
  - *Access to Care*

## INTRODUCTION

In 1900, the average life expectancy was 48.7 years for white American women and 33.5 years for African American women. By 1987, however, average life expectancy had reached 75 years for American women generally. Today, a woman in the United States who reaches age 65 can expect to live to be 84.[1] Only recently, then, has society been faced with the issues of aging beyond menopause. Research is now focusing on factors that positively impact physical and psychological aging. Women today can expect to live one-third of their lives after their reproductive years,[2] and preventive health care and healthy lifestyle habits can greatly improve the quality of life in those later years.

As women age they face numerous transitions that require adaptation, new coping strategies, and assimilation of new information and skills.[3] The primary task of the midlife and later years is *reappraisal*, which includes a review of past and present accomplishments; reassessment of goals and life direction; and redirection of energies or rededication to life's goals.

*Life Changes in Middle and Later Years*

- Roles—parent, spouse, partner, breadwinner, child.
- Relationships—parenting older adults, losses, remarriage, children leaving home, parenting grandchildren.
- Routine—caring for grandchildren, an aging parent, or a retiring spouse; change from home to career or from career to home.
- Assumptions about oneself—finality of infertility, physical signs of aging, changing sexuality.

## THE CLIMACTERIC AND MENOPAUSE

*Menopause* is medically defined as ovarian failure evidenced by the cessation of menses for 6 months or by a serum follicle-stimulating hormone (FSH) level of over 40 mIU per mL on two occasions 1 week apart, outside a normal FSH surge. It is possible to induce menopause surgically by bilateral oophorectomy.

The *climacteric* refers to the 7 to 10 years of physiological change in the reproductive system that culminates in the last menstrual period. The Greek *climacteric* means "rungs on a ladder"—a rather appropriate and positive way to view maturation.

The average age of menopause in the United States is 50 years. Despite consistent lowering of the age of puberty, the age of natural menopause has remained consistent.[2] Ovarian failure prior to 30 is premature and requires chromosomal analysis to rule out gonadal dysgenesis. Menopause between ages 31 and 40 is considered early and, because of the increased incidence of autoimmune disorders, requires referral for medical endocrine evaluation. Menopause after age 40 is considered normal.

The only consistent predisposing factor for earlier menopause is cigarette smoking. Other factors that have been suggested are low socioeconomic status, multiparity, and never having used oral contraceptives.[2]

### THE PHYSIOLOGY OF MENOPAUSE

Menopause results from a series of changes initiated in the ovary. General atresia of ovarian follicles begins with the onset of puberty and becomes more significant after age 35 when the ovary contains fewer follicles that are responsive to FSH. Eventually the atresia leads to a decline in ovarian production of estrogen and progesterone.

#### Loss of Estrogen Feedback

In the normal menstrual cycle, estrogen secreted by the ovarian follicles exerts primarily negative feedback due to absent folliculogenesis, as does inhibin from the granulosa cells on the hypothalamus. In the absence of negative feedback, gonadotropin production is no longer inhibited; large quantities of FSH and luteinizing hormone (LH) are secreted. Thus, an increased level of FSH (greater than 40 mIU per mL) is the classic determinant for ovarian failure.[2]

This change in ovarian steroid production is often gradual, resulting in anovulatory bleeding patterns. Eventually, the ovaries are completely unable to respond to FSH and LH, and the level of gonadotropin hyperactivity stabilizes. Gonadotropin levels never return to premenopausal levels.

### Postmenopausal Estrogen Sources

The major source of estradiol prior to menopause is the ovarian follicle. Estradiol is produced cyclically, and the ovary accounts for over 90 percent of total body production. Relatively constant production of estrone by adrenal glandular secretion and peripheral conversion of androstenedione also occurs. Postmenopause, little estradiol is produced in the ovarian follicles. Ovarian stroma, under stimulation by LH, continues to produce androstenedione and testosterone, which along with androstenedione produced by adrenal glands, are converted to estrone in peripheral adipose tissue. Thus, the body weight of the woman contributes to her overall postmenopausal level of circulating estrogen.

Initially, both the ovary and the adrenal glands are major sources of androstenedione. With advanced age, however, the ovarian stroma ceases production of androstenedione and is unable to maintain sufficient estrone production. Specific target deficiencies may then be noted. The degree of deficiency will vary with the individual woman. During the climacteric, ovarian secretion of androgens decreases markedly; however, most postmenopausal women maintain ovarian testosterone at about the levels found in younger women (see Hirsutism).

## THE PHYSICAL CHANGES OF AGING

The changes that occur as a woman ages are the culmination of heredity, the effects of living and lifestyle, and hormonal changes.

### DERMAL CHANGES

With aging, the skin undergoes progressive changes: The epidermis becomes thinner and flatter; the density of scalp and body hair follicles decreases; and the sebaceous glands and sweat glands have reduced function and become less responsive to stimuli.[4] The dermis becomes less elastic, collagen is lost, and a wrinkling of the epidermis results. Decreases in resilience, protection, and moisture occur. The incidence of skin cancer increases markedly after age 50. Hair grays as functioning melanocytes in hair decrease.[4]

### SENSORY CHANGES

*Visual disorders* (i.e. decreased visual acuity, excessive tearing, dry eyes), increase with age. Nearly 13 percent of Americans age 65 and older have some form of visual impairment, and glaucoma is more prevalent among people over age 65.[4,5]

*Hearing loss* that occurs with aging becomes more prevalent after age 50. Hearing impairment is reported by 23 percent of persons 65 to 74 years old, 33 percent of persons 75 to 84, and 48 percent of persons 85 and older.[4,6]

### CARDIOVASCULAR CHANGES

Cardiovascular disease (CVD) is responsible for more than 50 percent of the deaths in women in the United States. More women die of heart disease than endometrial, breast, and ovarian carcinomas combined.[7] CVD affects women primarily during the seventh and eighth decades of life. The changes in lipid components that accompany postmenopausal estrogen deficiency (see Table 11–1) favor the slow formation of atherosclerosis.[8] These changes are compounded by elevated blood

**TABLE 11-1. LABORATORY VALUES WITH OLDER ADULTS**

| Test | Unchanged/Same as Younger Reference | Decrease with Older Subjects | Increase with Older Subjects |
|---|---|---|---|
| CBC | | | |
| RBC | unchanged | or slight decrease | |
| Hgb | unchanged | or slight decrease | |
| Hct | unchanged | or slight decrease | |
| RBC indices | unchanged | | |
| WBC count | unchanged | | |
| Differential | | | |
| Basophils | unchanged | | |
| Eosinophils | unchanged | | |
| Myelocytes | unchanged | | |
| Bands | unchanged | | |
| Monocytes | unchanged | | |
| Lymphocytes | unchanged | or slight decrease | |
| Platelets | unchanged | | |
| ESR | | | slight increase |
| $B_{12}$ | | decrease | |
| Folate/folic acid | | decrease | |
| TIBC/transferrin | unchanged | | |
| Serum Fe | unchanged | | |
| Blood chemistry electrolytes | | | |
| Na | unchanged | or slight decrease | |
| K | unchanged | | or slight increase |
| Cl | unchanged | | |
| Ca | unchanged | or slight decrease | |
| P | unchanged | | |
| Mg | | decrease | |
| Glucose | | | |
| FBS | unchanged | | or slight increase |
| PPBS | | | increase |
| OGTT | | | increase |
| $HgA_{1c}$ | | | increase |
| End products of metabolism | | | |
| BUN | unchanged | | or slight increase |
| Creatinine | unchanged | | or slight increase |
| Creatinine clearance | | decrease | |
| Bilirubin | unchanged | | |
| Uric acid | | | slight increase |
| Liver function tests | | | |
| ALAT (SGPT) | unchanged | | |
| AST (SGOT) | unchanged | | |
| LDH | unchanged | | or slight increase |
| Alkaline phosphatase | | | gradual increase |

**TABLE 11-1. CONTINUED**

| Test | Unchanged/Same as Younger Reference | Decrease with Older Subjects | Increase with Older Subjects |
|---|---|---|---|
| Total protein | unchanged | or slight decrease | |
| Albumin | | decrease | |
| Globulin | unchanged | | |
| Lipoproteins | | | gradual increase |
| Total cholesterol | | | gradual increase |
| LDL | | | increase |
| HDL | unchanged | or slight decrease in women | or slight increase in men |
| Triglycerides | | | increase |
| Thyroid function tests | | | |
| $T_4$ | unchanged | or slight decrease | |
| $T_3$ | | decrease | |
| TSH | | | slight increase |

*Source: Reprinted by permission of the publisher from Interpretation of Laboratory Values in Older Adults, by K.D. Melillo, in* Nurse Practitioner 18*(7) 59–67. Copyright 1993 by Elsevier Science Publishing Co., Inc.*

pressure, smoking, obesity, and heredity. The usual postmenopausal lipid changes are as follows.

- A gradual increase in low-density lipoproteins (LDL).
- A very slight decrease over time in high-density lipoproteins (HDL).
- A gradual increase in total cholesterol (TCHO). For every 1 percent rise in a person's LDL cholesterol, there is a 2 percent rise in the risk of coronary heart disease.[8] The efficiency and muscle contractility of the heart decrease with aging, causing reduced cardiac output. This decreased output is tolerable under conditions of low stress.

## PULMONARY CHANGES

Lung expansion decreases gradually with aging, as the thorax becomes more rigid and tissues less elastic. Reductions occur in pulmonary reserve and in vital capacity, and there is a decline over time in arterial oxygen concentration.[9]

## GASTROINTESTINAL (GI) CHANGES

The GI system can handle food that is chewed properly, albeit more sluggishly with aging. For proper chewing, gums and teeth must be in good condition. Estrogen deficiency can cause atrophic changes in the gums and influence mastication, as can poor dental hygiene and gum disease. Generally, the amount of hydrochloric acid in the stomach decreases with time, as does pepsin. Peristaltic action and emptying times decrease, and absorption of certain substances, such as the B vitamins, iron, and calcium, is affected.

## REPRODUCTIVE CHANGES

- *Vulva.* With the loss of estrogen, the vulva undergoes atrophy and subcutaneous tissues diminish.[9] The labia majora become small and the labia minora almost nonexistent. The skin becomes thinner, and pubic hair loss is progressive. Dystrophies and pruritus are more frequent.

- *Vagina.* Epithelial maturation decreases. The failure to produce glycogen-containing superficial cells causes an increase in the vaginal pH to between 6.5 and 7.5,[9] and resistance to pyogenic organisms is thereby lowered. The vagina becomes shorter and narrower, with obliteration of the vaginal fornices and eventual loss of vaginal rugae. Changes may be prevented or slowed by the continuation of regular intercourse.
- *Uterus.* Over time, the uterus decreases in size and weight.[10] The cervix pales and shrinks with loss of the fornices, so that the external os is nearly flush with the vaginal wall. The endocervix becomes atrophic and the cervical canal stenotic. The endometrium glands and stroma atrophy.[4,10]
- *Pelvic Floor.* The muscular tissue loses tone after menopause, causing increases in uterine prolapse, cystocele, and rectocele.[4,9] This loss of tone may be heightened by past pregnancy and vaginal delivery.
- *Breasts.* Glandular breast tissue decreases before menopause, and after menopause it becomes atrophic.[4,10] Along with some erectile properties' loss, the nipples become smaller and flatter.[4]

## URINARY CHANGES

Atrophy of the bladder and urethral structure causes an increase in urinary incontinence, urgency, frequency, and dribbling.[9] Cystocele with loss of pelvic floor integrity is common. Urinary tract changes are secondary to estrogen deficiency, aging, and past trauma from childbearing. Renal clearance diminishes, but the kidneys are able to maintain a proper fluid balance in the body.

## ENDOCRINE CHANGES

- *Thyroid.* Irregularity and nodularity of the thyroid increase with age.[4] Thyroid function appears to remain stable after menopause, although hyperthyroidism and hypothyroidism are more common in women, in general, and in the elderly.[11] See Table 11–1 for normal changes in thyroid values with aging.
- *Adrenal.* The production of epinephrine, corticotropin, and cortisol decrease with aging (see Hirsutism).[9]
- *Pituitary.* Adequate hormonal secretion continues despite decreased pituitary size.

## MUSCULOSKELETAL CHANGES

Muscle tone is related to exercise. In the sedentary woman, normal tone and strength diminish. Atrophy occurs more rapidly with aging if muscles are not used (see Osteoporosis). The proportion of fat and water change with aging: Fat increases and water decreases.

## NEUROLOGICAL CHANGES

Forgetfulness is not uncommon and may be related to neuron loss that begins when a woman is in her twenties. Some brain and spinal cord efficiency is lost, which is evident, for example, in slowed pupillary response. Sleep may be more easily disrupted. *Memory loss* is reported by many women in the perimenopausal years.[12] The incidence of Alzheimer's disease increases with age.

The third leading cause of death in the United States is *cerebrovascular accident* (CVA). The principal risk factors are age, hypertension, smoking, coronary artery disease, and diabetes.

## SEXUALITY AND AGING

Sexuality continues as an important component of a woman's life until her death. It represents a need to be accepted, a need for intimacy and companionship. Sexuality is influenced by many factors.

Although most older adults continue to be sexually active, physical changes associated with aging, illness, and opportunity have major influence on the frequency and satisfaction of sexual behaviors. Physical changes in women that may have a negative impact on sexuality include the following.

- Thinning of vaginal walls.
- Decrease in vaginal lubrication.
- Lessening of desire and frequency.
- Slower response.
- Shorter duration of orgasm.
- Decrease in clitoral hood/body.
- Loss of elasticity, length, and width of vagina.
- Decrease in strength of muscular contractions occurring with orgasm.

Changes caused by hormonal deficiency may be lessened with estrogen or testosterone therapy.

Other factors that affect sexuality, either positively or negatively, include longer life span; issues surrounding aging, such as physical and social losses and transitions; an increase in chronic illness; body image changes; effects of medications on libido; more time for intimacy; and freedom from worry about contraception/pregnancy.

Sexuality is seldom considered in the counseling of midlife and aging women, yet women in this age group have a variety of concerns and information needs. A widowed or divorced woman who is new to dating may need information about sexually transmitted diseases and "safer sex." Whether single or married, women may desire information about common sexuality concerns, such as masturbation. They may also want information about male sexuality and aging, and may need help adapting sexual practices to accommodate physical and emotional changes.

## HYPOESTROGENIC CHANGES

The loss of estradiol with decreasing ovarian function results in a host of changes among postmenopausal women. The incidence and severity of complaints vary greatly, but most frequently, they involve vasomotor instability, vaginal changes, urinary incontinence, and menstrual irregularity.

### VASOMOTOR INSTABILITY

Vasomotor instability involves rapid rises in core body temperature with resultant perspiration, often profuse. Hot flushes usually start at the waist and progress upward to the head and face. They tend to increase at night. Serum LH rises a few minutes after the symptoms start to subside and then drops before the next episode.

#### Epidemiology

Hot flushes may be aggravated by emotional stress, warm weather, and alcohol ingestion. They last for 3 to 4 minutes. As many as 85 percent of women experience hot flushes in the perimenopausal years.[2] Surveys have found that in the absence of hormone replacement therapy (HRT), 85 percent of affected women will have symptoms for more than 1 year, and 25 to 50 percent will have symptoms for more than 5 years.[12] The symptoms of vasomotor instability can begin 2 to 3 years prior to last menses;[2] their severity varies with the individual.

## Subjective Data

Evaluate the client's menstrual history for changes suggestive of perimenopause, such as decreasing or increasing intervals between menses and dysfunctional/anovulatory bleeding patterns. The client will report episodes of feeling extreme warmth rising from the chest up to the face and head, followed by perspiration and sometimes chills. If these vasomotor symptoms occur at night, they disrupt sleep—causing insomnia, exhaustion, and irritability. Flushes can occur frequently during a 24-hour period; hence the client may report the need to change clothing and bed linens often.

## Objective Data

***Physical Examination.*** Findings include vasodilation of peripheral blood vessels in the skin coupled with mild increase in pulse, but without alteration in blood pressure; increased digital temperature; and decreased intracore temperature with chills.

### *Diagnostic Tests and Methods*

- *Serum FSH Level.* A level greater than 40 mIU per mL is diagnostic of menopause.
- *Client Diary of Episodes.* Confirms verbal history.

## Differential Medical Diagnoses

Hypothalamic/pituitary tumor, infection (viral illness, tuberculosis, systemic infection with fever, human immunodeficiency virus [HIV] infection), alcoholism, thyroid disease.

## Plan

***Psychosocial Interventions.*** Reassure the client that vasomotor instability is normal during the perimenopause. In addition, explain the physiology of menopause. Offer adaptive measures as follows.

- Adjust the room temperature; leave a window open; use a portable fan to accommodate an office environment.
- Wear clothing in layers for ease of removal; wear more cotton.
- Try stress management techniques such as relaxation exercises, meditation, and yoga.

### *Medication*

Hormone Replacement Therapy (HRT). Estrogen replacement therapy (ERT) is effective in greater than 90 percent of women. Adjust the dosage to accommodate client symptoms. (See Hormone Replacement Therapy, later in this chapter, for a complete description of administration, side effects, contraindications, evaluation outcomes, and teaching/counseling.)

Alternative Therapies. Alternative therapy is indicated if ERT is contraindicated. The following drugs may be offered to decrease vasomotor instability if ERT cannot be used.

- *Medroxyprogesterone Acetate (MPA).* Prescribe 10 to 30 mg q.d. Side effects include weight gain, depression, and breast tenderness. MPA treatment is moderately effective (see Hormone Replacement Therapy for more information about MPA).
- *Bellergal.* Prescribe three times daily (one tablet morning and noon, and two at bedtime). *Warning: The phenobarbital component of this drug can be habit forming.* Bellergal is a combination of belladonna, phenobarbital, and ergotamine. Prescribe it for a short period only, withdraw it gradu-

ally, and advise the client about the drug's side effects (drowsiness, dry mouth, tachycardia, constipation, flushing, or blurred vision). The therapeutic effect relates to relaxation of smooth muscle.

- *Clonidine*. Prescribe 0.1 mg b.i.d. Side effects include severe hypotensive episodes, dizziness, nausea, nasal stuffiness, and mood swings.[2] Treatment is moderately effective.

***Other Interventions.*** Advise the client to limit her caffeine and alcohol intake and not to smoke. Drinking 8 to 10 glasses of water daily is also advised; drinking cold water at the beginning of a flush may help to alleviate the discomfort. Hot drinks and foods should be avoided. Separate bed sheets and blankets can be used, then taken off without disturbing the bed partner. Regular exercise every day may improve sleep; however, heavy exercise must be avoided immediately before bedtime.

***Follow-Up.*** Call the client to evaluate the effectiveness of therapy in relieving the signs and symptoms of perimenopause. (See Hormone Replacement Therapy for follow-up related to that therapy.) If therapy is ineffective, suggest referral to a gynecologist.

## VAGINAL CHANGES

The vagina, composed of thick tissue with accordion-like folds (rugae) during the childbearing years, thins dramatically in the absence of estrogen. It becomes atrophic and easily traumatized, predisposing the woman to vaginal infection.[9]

### Epidemiology

Decreased estrogen, whether because of natural or surgical menopause, contributes to vaginal atrophy. Infection aggravates the atrophic changes, often causing vaginal bleeding with intercourse. Vaginal changes are common among postmenopausal women and often occur during perimenopause.

### Subjective Data

A menstrual history will reveal symptoms of vaginal change, possibly including vaginal dryness, loss of lubrication with intercourse, pain or soreness with penile thrusting during intercourse, unusual vaginal discharge, infection, and postcoital bleeding.

### Objective Data

***Physical Examination.*** Findings include thinning and paleness of vaginal epithelia, bloody vaginal discharge, brittle pubic hair, disappearance of rugae, and infection.

***Diagnostic Tests and Methods***

- *Serum FSH.* A level of greater than 40 mIU per mL is diagnostic of menopause.
- *Papanicolaou (Pap) Smear*. Maturation index for indication of estrogen deficiency (test is optional: not as diagnostic as FSH level is).
- *Gonorrhea Culture, Wet Mount, and Chlamydia Test.* Performed if appropriate.

### Differential Medical Diagnoses

Vaginitis and sexually transmitted diseases (bacterial, viral, fungal infection), leukoplakia, lichen sclerosis, malignancy, postmenopausal uterine bleeding, diabetes mellitus.

### Plan

***Psychosocial Interventions.*** Teach the client about the normal physiological changes of menopause, aging, and sexuality that may occur.

***Medication.*** *Estrogen cream* (Premarin Vaginal Cream) is indicated to reverse vaginal atrophic changes (see Hormone Replacement Therapy for a general description of hormone use).

Apply 1 g estrogen cream or the equivalent intravaginally daily, for 2–4 weeks; then decrease to 1 g, 2–3 times weekly when symptom relief is achieved. Then decrease to one application per week or eliminate altogether based on symptoms. Vaginal absorption into the bloodstream is very efficient; therefore, the client is at risk for endometrial hyperplasia due to unopposed estrogen stimulation of the endometrium. Medroxyprogesterone acetate (Provera), 10 mg for 10–12 days every 3 months, is recommended if the uterus is intact.[2]

*Oral hormone replacement therapy* (HRT) is described later in this chapter.

***Other Interventions.*** Treat any vaginal infection as indicated, and educate the client about "safer sex" (see Chapters 6 and 8). Teach her Kegel's exercises, as these may help with arousal (see next section, Urinary Incontinence, Pelvic Muscle Exercises, for more detail).[13] Offer the client suggestions or readings on sexual pleasuring to increase arousal (see Chapter 4). Advise her to use a water-soluble vaginal lubricant with intercourse to prevent trauma from penile thrusting and alleviate the discomfort of friction (lubricants will not reverse epithelial changes). Lubricant jellies, creams, and suppositories are available over the counter (without prescription). Vegetable oils or lotions without perfume may be suggested. Advise the client to wash her hands thoroughly before and after applying any vaginal lubricant.

- *Lubrin Vaginal Suppositories.* Insert one suppository 5 to 20 minutes prior to intercourse as needed.
- *K-Y Jelly.* Apply as needed.
- *Replens Vaginal Suppositories or Cream.* Insert cream or suppository 5 to 20 minutes prior to intercourse. May be used as needed.
- *Astroglide.* Apply intravaginally as-needed.

***Follow-Up.*** Advise the client to return to the health care provider if no relief occurs. Referral for sexual therapy may be indicated if the problem seems unrelated to physical changes in the vagina.

## URINARY INCONTINENCE

Urinary incontinence means loss of normal urinary control. It occurs when pressure in any part of the urethra is the same as or exceeds that of the bladder. Factors that contribute to the maintenance of a normal pressure differential include an intact urethral sphincteric mechanism and proper anatomic support of the urethra and urethrovesicular junction.[14] Mild urinary incontinence may be the result of relaxed bladder neck support by tissues. With aging, tissues may lose some elasticity and the bladder may decrease in size. In addition, urinary frequency and urgency are often related to hypoestrogenism. The female urethra contains estrogen receptors in high concentration.[15] Thinning of the urethral mucosa in postmenopausal women decreases their total urethral resistance by as much as 30 percent, leading to stress incontinence (see below).[16]

*Types of Incontinence*

- *Detrusor instability (unstable bladder)* is uncontrolled bladder activity. The unstable detrusor muscle in the bladder contracts spontaneously or on provocation during bladder filling while the woman is attempting to inhibit micturition.[16] The majority of cases are idiopathic.
- *Detrusor hyperreflexia* describes detrusor instability secondary to a known neurological abnormality. Only a small percentage of clients have an underlying neurological pathology.[14]

- *Stress urinary incontinence* (SUI) is the most common diagnosis in incontinent women. Diagnosis is made if urinary leakage is observed when intraabdominal pressure is raised and no detrusor contraction occurs, for example, when laughing or coughing.[17]

## Epidemiology

Temporary incontinence may be caused by problems common in aging clients, such as impacted stools with constipation, bed rest, or certain drugs (diuretics, sedatives, antidepressants, phenothiazine derivatives, certain antihistamines, as well as excessive amounts of estrogens and progestins).[14] Other causes of incontinence include damage to urogenital structures from childbearing, nerve damage from disease or other conditions (diabetes mellitus, spinal damage from protruding disks), bladder neoplasms, infection, or fistula. Fifteen to 20 percent of healthy women aged 30 to 50 years—and as many as 57 percent of women over 64—have urinary incontinence. Eighty-seven percent of exercisers have noticed incontinence during at least one form of exercise.[14]

## Subjective Data

The client's history may include urinary frequency; urinary urgency; leakage of urine on sneezing, coughing, or exercising; unexpected loss of urine at intervals; and nocturia. A review of drug intake is indicated.[14]

## Objective Data

***Physical Examination.*** Findings include leakage of urine with an increase in abdominal pressure on a command to bear down during examination; cystocele; relaxation of pelvic floor musculature; perineal irritation; and vaginal atrophy. A thorough examination is indicated to rule out systemic and neurological disease.

***Diagnostic Tests and Methods***

- *Urinalysis and Culture.* Clean-catch or catheterized specimen to rule out infection.
- *STD/Vaginitis Tests.* Rule out infection (see Chapter 8).
- *Diary of Intake and Output.* Should include notations of activity when incontinence occurs.
- *Urodynamic Testing.* The details of this type of testing are beyond the scope of this book. For other than mild stress incontinence, refer the client to a urogynecologic specialist for testing. Dynamic cystourethroscopy may be done to delineate functional and anatomic abnormalities. Testing may also include a cystometrogram.

## Differential Medical Diagnoses

Urinary tract infection, bladder prolapse, uterine fibroids or other tumors compressing the bladder.

## Plan

***Psychosocial Interventions.*** Educate the client about causes, diagnostic measures, and treatments. Acknowledge that this is a disturbing problem that does affect the quality of life, but that methods of treatment may help. Suggest that the client contact a support group (e.g., Help For Incontinent People [HIP], Inc., P.O. Box 544, Union, SC 29379) for information, or call the local urogynecologic department of her hospital.

***Medication.*** Refer the client to a urogynecologic specialist.

- *Hormone Replacement Therapy (HRT).* Evidence suggests that estrogen administration improves stress incontinence[16] (see Hormone Replacement Therapy).

- *Drugs Inhibiting the Parasympathetic Nervous System.* The detrusor has primarily β-adrenergic innervation; the urethra primarily has α-adrenergic innervation. One of two drugs is commonly used: imipramine timed release capsule, 75–200 mg q.d.; *or* oxybutynin (Ditropan), 5 mg b.i.d. or t.i.d.
- *Calcium Channel Blockers.* By inhibiting the intracellular movement of calcium, these drugs decrease the number of detrusor contractions and increase bladder capacity. Side effects include dizziness, nausea, flushing, and headaches. Commonly used drugs are nifedipine, 10 mg t.i.d.; *or* terodidine, 25 mg b.i.d.[14]

***Pelvic Muscle Exercises (PME).*** Also called Kegel's exercises. Important muscle groups to exercise to alleviate stress urinary incontinence include the pelvic and urogenital diaphragms. Insert a gloved finger into the vagina and instruct the client to tighten muscles around the finger. Instruct the client to practice tightening that muscle regularly. Another way to identify the muscle group is to remember that the same muscles are used to stop urinary flow. Advise the client to choose set intervals each day to concentrate on the exercise (e.g., five times per half hour throughout the day).[13] Some women prefer short periods (10 minutes) at the end and beginning of each day. Others practice with each voiding. Regular, repeated contraction of the pubococcygeal muscle will help to alleviate incontinence.[18]

***Bladder Training.*** The client may extend the interval between urinations in an attempt to retain reflux responses. Bladder training exercises include a scheduled series of exercises that combine Kegel's exercises and timed voiding; relaxation techniques can help in this training.[19,20]

***Perineal Hygiene.*** Instruct the client to wipe the perineal area from front to back, bathe or shower regularly, and avoid douching.

***Follow-Up.*** If mild incontinence does not respond to initial therapies, refer the client to a urogynecologic specialist for urodynamic testing, in-depth diagnosis, and treatment.

## MENSTRUAL IRREGULARITY

As the number of ovarian follicles capable of producing estrogen decreases, a woman experiences irregularities of the menstrual cycle. Ideally her periods are shorter and less frequent, but often they are a mix of heavy, longer bleeding episodes that are closer together due to anovulation. With anovulation, the epithelium builds from unopposed estrogen stimulation with no progesterone to transpose it to a secretory state. Breakthrough bleeding is common, and the woman experiences distressing irregularity and an increased risk of endometrial hyperplasia.

### Subjective Data

The client's history indicates a change in the regularity of cycles and characteristics of menses (waxing and waning menses) or the absence of menses, and, often, other symptoms of hypoestrogenism.

### Objective Data

***Physical Examination.*** The physical and pelvic exam should be normal, and may or may not reveal changes suggestive of approaching menopause (see Chapter 5 for causes of abnormal menstrual bleeding and physical findings).

***Diagnostic Tests and Methods.*** A pregnancy test must be used to rule out pregnancy as a cause of the bleeding. A serum FSH level of greater than 40 mIU per mL is diagnostic of menopause; often, the level rises as ovarian failure progresses. Endometrial abnormalities (hyperplasia and carcinoma) may be ruled out with an endometrial biopsy.

### Differential Medical Diagnoses

Pregnancy, spontaneous abortion, anovulation, hyperplasia, carcinoma, infection, abnormalities of the uterus such as fibroids or polyps, endometriosis, adenomyosis, injury, ovarian abnormalities such as tumors or cysts.

### Plan

***Psychosocial Interventions.*** Reassure the client that bodily changes are normal; explain the physiology of menopause; and educate regarding methods of treatment, if indicated.

***Medication.*** Medroxyprogesterone acetate (Provera) or comparable progestogen therapy may be used alone during the perimenopausal period to regulate cycles and protect the client from hyperplasia (see Hormone Replacement Therapy). These women are not quite ready for HRT, which employs estrogen and progesterone (discussed later in this chapter).

***Dilation and Curettage (D & C).*** D & C or surgery may be needed. D & C is employed if bleeding does not respond to medical therapy. A hysterectomy or other, newer surgical interventions, such as ablation, may also be considered.

***Follow-Up.*** Refer the client to a gynecologist for evaluation of suspected abnormalities, especially carcinoma. Any bleeding that does not respond to therapy also requires that the client be referred.

## ALTERATIONS IN MOOD

A significant number of women report that changes in mood and overall lifestyle occur between ages 40 and 60. The relationships between hormonal changes and anxiety and depression in the perimenopausal woman remain to be clarified, however. Both the central and peripheral nervous systems contain 17 β-estradiol sensitive cells, and even the brain responds to withdrawal or absence of ovarian steroids. Research has shown direct effects of estrogen and progesterone on neurotransmitters that regulate mood, appetite, sleep, and pain perception.[21] Very few clinical correlations are available.

### EPIDEMIOLOGY

No single cause for mood alterations has been identified. Hormonal deficiency may play a role, but consideration must be given to other factors in the client's life, such as aging and how she feels about it. American society reveres youth, and the reality of lost youth and changes in body image may upset some women. Other major life changes that are common for a woman of perimenopausal and menopausal age include one's children leaving home; death or illness of a parent, which necessitates that one become the "parent"; realization that one may not have achieved all of one's life goals, loss of childbearing capacity; and concerns about retirement and finances.

Incidence reports vary. In one study, perimenopausal women reported mood swings (80 percent), depression (86 percent), irritability (93 percent), loss of memory (75 percent), and inability to concentrate (82 percent).[12]

## SUBJECTIVE DATA

The client's history may reveal periods of crying, anger, sadness, irritability, depression, anxiety attacks, family members' reports of mood swings, and expressions of suicide. If a psychological disorder is suspected, an extensive social history is indicated.

## OBJECTIVE DATA

### Physical Examination

Findings on physical examination may include decreased affect, lethargy, inappropriate responses, and crying. A complete examination is indicated to rule out systemic diseases, drug use, or other conditions that could affect physiological function and cause symptoms.

### Diagnostic Tests and Methods

General diagnostic tests, such as complete blood cell (CBC) count, thyroid studies, FSH/LH, urinalysis, and blood chemistry analysis are indicated to determine normal baselines and deviations. Drug testing may also be indicated. Other tests that may be done are psychological scales and questionnaires, such as CAGE, MAST, and T-ACE alcoholism questionnaires,[22–24] and Zung or Beck depression scales.[25,26]

## DIFFERENTIAL MEDICAL DIAGNOSES

Depression, anxiety disorders, neurological impairment, sexual dysfunction, psychiatric disorder.

## PLAN

- *Psychosocial Interventions.* Less serious mood alterations may respond to lifestyle alterations or hormone replacement therapy (HRT). Refer the client for psychological evaluation as appropriate; protect if the client is suicidal. Life transitions, grief work, and affective and physical changes associated with perimenopausal transitions may require individual or group therapy and support. Education about physical changes may reassure the client.
- *Medication.* *Hormone replacement therapy* (discussed later in this chapter) is moderately effective in reducing mood symptoms, if they are related to estrogen deficiency. Certain progestins, especially medroxyprogesterone acetate may exacerbate depression.[27] See antianxiety and antidepressant therapy in Chapter 18 or other reference texts.
- *Exercise.* Advise the client to engage in regular aerobic exercise and resistance training to improve muscle strength, unless contraindicated. Exercise may improve the client's psychological outlook and reduce mood swings.
- *Balanced Diet.* Advise the client to maintain a nutritionally balanced diet and to avoid simple carbohydrates, which can induce hypoglycemic reactions.
- *Stress Reduction Techniques.* Relaxation exercises, yoga, meditation, and regular physical exercise may reduce stress.
- *Follow-Up.* If the client does not respond to lifestyle changes and/or medication therapy, she should be referred to a psychiatrist or psychologist after consultation with a gynecologist or other primary care physician.

# SLEEP DISORDERS

Rapid eye movement (REM) sleep decreases with age and the hypoestrogenic state.[28] Alterations in sleep pattern may be the result of hot flushes and night sweats. The need for overall sleep diminishes slightly with age; the average adult needs 7 to 8 hours of sleep each day.

## EPIDEMIOLOGY

Any number of factors may contribute to sleep disturbances in addition to estrogen deficiency: lack of exercise, excessive napping during the day, stress, depression, anxiety, illness, restless sleep partner, uncomfortable sleeping accommodations, excessive activity prior to bedtime, and stimulant drugs.

Sleep disorders are common among the general population and increase in the perimenopausal and postmenopausal years. The exact incidence is unknown.

## SUBJECTIVE DATA

The client reports signs and symptoms of menopause, as well as irritability, interrupted sleep, and feelings of tiredness.

## OBJECTIVE DATA

Findings on physical examination include lethargy, dark circles under the eyes, and possible altered response time. Diagnostic tests are used to rule out other diseases that cause lethargy, fatigue, and insomnia, such as anemia or hypothyroidism. An elevated FSH level would indicate menopause.

## DIFFERENTIAL MEDICAL DIAGNOSES

Neurological disorders, psychological disturbances.

## PLAN

Reassure and educate the client about causes and remedies of sleep disorders. Referral to a sleep therapy specialist may be indicated. Consult current pharmacological therapy references for information on sedatives and sleeping medications, but only after giving nonpharmacological interventions a fair trial of several months.

### *Nonpharmacological Interventions*

- *Evaluate naps.* Encourage 10 to 30 minute naps during the daytime if the client is severely sleep deprived. However, if napping is interfering with night sleep, urge decreasing naps if possible.
- *Avoid caffeine.* Foods and beverages containing caffeine should be decreased or eliminated, especially after 5 P.M. Evaluate prescription and over-the-counter medications that might contain caffeine, for example, some cold remedies.
- *Limit alcohol intake.* Alcohol consumption should be less than 4 oz per day or, preferably, eliminated altogether.
- *Avoid smoking.* Encourage the client to stop smoking. Offer literature and referral to a group for support.
- *Exercise before or in the early evening.* Exercising should occur no later than 7 P.M. (Aerobic exercise in late evening increases wakefulness).
- *Arrange for a comfortable sleep environment.* Make suggestions concerning mattress comfort, soundproofing or earplugs, room darkening, sleeping clothes, room temperature, elimination of distractions.
- *Arrange quiet activity prior to bedtime.* Reading or listening to soothing music or environmental sounds may encourage sleep.
- *Avoid sleeping medications.* If the client is unable to sleep, advise her to get up and read or watch television, then try again in 30 to 60 minutes. Learning relaxation techniques, such as slow breathing from the diaphragm or playing mental games, and using them at bedtime may be beneficial. By setting aside a time to review concerns and activities of the day and coming up with so-

lutions to problems before going to bed, the client may succeed in separating worries from the act of going to bed. (The bed should not be used as an office.) Taking warm baths, drinking milk (but not too much), and eating light (non-sugar) snacks before bedtime may also be helpful.

### Follow-Up

The client may require referral to a sleep disorder program.

## HORMONE REPLACEMENT THERAPY (HRT)

Women now have the option, unless medically contraindicated, of hormone replacement therapy (HRT) during the perimenopause and after. The concerns related to an increased risk of endometrial cancer, which peaked during the 1970s, have been tempered by the realization that the addition of a progestogen to estrogen replacement therapy (ERT) offers significant protection against progressive hyperplasia. This benefit of the progestogen, however, must be weighed against its possible negative effects, such as lipid alterations, symptoms similar to premenstrual syndrome (PMS), or breast pathology. Thus, the decision to use HRT must be made by the informed client.

### CLIENT EDUCATION AND COUNSELING

The health care provider must provide the client with accurate, current information about the positive and negative aspects of HRT. Generally, the following areas are included in discussion with the client.

- *Signs and Symptoms of Hypoestrogenism.* HRT provides varying levels of effectiveness in alleviating signs and symptoms associated with hypoestrogen.[2] The dosage is individualized for relief of hot flushes, urinary symptoms, vaginal dryness, and subjective symptoms of anxiety or distress.
- *Osteoporosis.* HRT is effective in the prevention and treatment of osteoporosis (osteoporosis is discussed more fully later in this chapter).[29,30]
- *Endometrial Cancer.* Estrogen with a progestin added for at least 12 days per month protects against endometrial cancer.[31] The addition of a progestin, recommended for the client who still has a uterus, does not detract from the favorable estrogen effects on bone density or most other hypoestrogen complaints.
- *Lipid Changes.* Although estrogen alone positively impacts lipid fractions, conflicting studies exist on the impact of estrogen-progestin combination on the lipid profile. Several reports do show comparably favorable lipid profiles with estrogen alone and estrogen-progestin combination.[32]
- *Breast Cancer.* Study results are mixed on the relationship of the estrogen-progestin combination on breast cancer. Although meta-analytic studies have been done on HRT and breast cancer,[33] further research is needed to clarify the issue.
- *Blood Pressure.* ERT and HRT do not negatively impact blood pressure; indeed, there may be a positive impact.[34,35] The "natural estrogens" and their more potent synthetic counterparts, however, may be different. For example, ethinyl estradiol stimulates renin substrate and may pose a risk.[36] Progestins can produce a dose-related elevation in blood pressure, possibly by elevating selected liver globulins.[37]
- *Stroke.* A reduction in the incidence of mortality from stroke has been reported among estrogen replacement users, with and without history of hypertension.[38]

- *Cardiovascular Disease.* Most studies show at least a 50 percent reduction in coronary heart disease and related mortality with oral estrogen use.[39] Clinical trials have not shown any increase in thromboembolism in postmenopausal women on ERT, despite elevation of clotting factors with synthetic estrogens.[39] Elevations in clotting factors are not observed with estrogen patches.[40] Estrogen increases local production of prostacyclin, a vasodilatory prostaglandin that opposes platelet aggregation.[39] Variations in dosages, types of estrogen, and modes of delivery produce somewhat different results. Oral ERT increases HDL, lowers LDL, and lowers total cholesterol; transdermal ERT does not alter HDL, LDL, and total cholesterol levels. (Oral and transdermal ERTs are discussed later in this chapter.) The use of progestins may modify beneficial changes.
- *Gallbladder Disease.* ERT/HRT may increase the risk of gallbladder disease. Estrogen may increase the risk of gallstones in obese women and women with a personal or family history of the condition. The primary cause of gallstones in women is obesity; cholesterol gallstones occur when cholesterol in the bile exceeds the normal range and precipitates out. The precipitate creates seeds, or crystals, that form stones. In women who are not obese, gallstones are caused by a reduced rate of production of bile salts and other substances. In evaluating, each client, family history, current risk factors, and the need for preventive health measures are assessed. Dosages are modified for each individual, as well as the type of estrogen/progestin preparation.
- *Mood and Sleep.* Many women report improved overall psychological well-being while taking estrogen.[41]
- *Rheumatoid Arthritis.* Evidence exists that ERT use before the onset of joint disease is associated with protection against rheumatoid arthritis.[42]
- *Glucose Tolerance.* The use of estrogen and medroxyprogesterone acetate (MPA) is not associated with impaired glucose tolerance.[43]

## REQUIRED ASSESSMENT BEFORE INITIATING HRT

Take a complete client history with special emphasis on symptoms of hypoestrogenism, and note any family history of osteoporosis, heart disease, or hypertension. During the required complete physical examination, note signs of hypoestrogenism in the presence or absence of menses.

### Diagnostic Tests and Methods

- Complete evaluation per midlife protocol includes determination of baseline values for common tests. The basic testing/evaluations done initially include cholesterol and lipid profile, urinalysis, complete blood count, blood chemistry profile, a screen for colorectal cancer, cervical screening, and mammogram. Time intervals for testing are provided in the subsequent section on Midlife Women's Health Care Program.
- Serum FSH level of greater than 40 mIU per mL is diagnostic of ovarian failure.
- Bone density evaluation is indicated if the reason for initiating therapy is to prevent or inhibit osteoporosis.
- Endometrial biopsy is indicated if dysfunctional bleeding is present, if the client is at high risk for endometrial cancer (obese, family history of endometrial or breast cancer, long history of amenorrhea or oligomenorrhea during the reproductive years), or if the client has a history of alcoholism or hepatic disease.
- A menstrual diary and an accurate record of other bleeding episodes over several

months may provide insights for diagnosis and treatment. The diary may also be helpful after HRT is begun.
- Ovarian/pelvic ultrasound is indicated if the ovaries are nonpalpable due to obesity or if there is a suspected enlarged ovary or pelvic mass, or if there is a family history of ovarian cancer.

## TREATMENT CONSIDERATIONS

Hormone dosages, preparations, and schedules are individualized according to symptoms and client choice. Table 11–2 lists some of the more widely used preparations of estrogen and progestin and their dosages.

***Absolute Contraindications to Estrogen Use***
- Known or suspected cancer of the breast.
- Known or suspected estrogen-dependent neoplasia.
- Undiagnosed abnormal genital bleeding.
- Active thrombophlebitis.
- Pregnancy.
- Otosclerosis.
- Malignant melanoma.[2]

***Absolute Contraindications to Progestin Use***
- Past or present history of thrombophlebitis.
- Liver dysfunction or disease.
- Known or suspected cancer of the breast.
- Undiagnosed abnormal vaginal bleeding.
- Pregnancy.

### Breast Cancer and Hormone Replacement Therapy

Evidence is conflicting at this time about the effect of estrogen and the risk of breast cancer. Data are not conclusive regarding more than 20 years of using unopposed estrogen.[44] Some authorities suggest estrogen may be used after breast cancer if the tumor was nonestrogen dependent.[45] In addition, progestogens are being given increasing attention in relation to breast cancer.

## POSTMENOPAUSAL HORMONE REPLACEMENT THERAPY

Hormone replacement therapy (estrogen, progestin, and/or testosterone) is given orally, transdermally, and vaginally. Oral estrogens include natural, conjugated, and synthetic estrogens. Natural estrogens, such as micronized estradiol (Estrace) and estropipate (Ogen), are converted in the liver to estrone, which becomes the primary circulating estrogen. Conjugated estrogens (Premarin) and synthetic estrogens, such as ethinyl estradiol (Estinyl) and diethylstibestrol, all have a 30 percent reduction in bioavailability because of the first-pass effect through the liver.[46]

The most commonly used progestin is medroxyprogesterone acetate (Provera). Norethindrone is also frequently used. The most commonly used testosterone is methyltestosterone.

Side effects of the hormonal components are estrogen or progestin or androgen related. Estrogen related side effects include breast tenderness, nausea (usually subsides in 3 to 6 months), and headaches. Progestin related side effects include nausea, acne, headaches, and PMS-like symptoms, such as irritability. Androgen related side effects include acne, hirsutism, and clitoromegaly.

### Oral Regimens

***Cyclic Estrogen/Progestin Therapy.*** Start with continuous daily conjugated estrogens (Premarin) 0.625 mg, or an equivalent. If hypoestrogenic symptoms persist after 30 days of Premarin, increase the daily dosage incrementally to 0.9 mg or 1.25 mg. If the client has an intact uterus, add medroxyprogesterone acetate (Provera) 10 mg daily, on days 1 to 12 or days 13 to 25 of the month. It is well established that 10 mg daily for 12 days is protective against endometrial cancer;[31] however, the side effects of progestin at this dosage may

**TABLE 11-2. ESTROGEN EQUIVALENCIES, VAGINAL ESTROGEN CREAMS, AND PROGESTIN EQUIVALENCIES**

| Trademark | Generic Name | Dosages | Manufacturer | Method |
|---|---|---|---|---|
| *Equivalencies of Commonly Used Estrogens* | | | | |
| Premarin | Conjugated estrogens | 0.3 mg<br>0.625 mg<br>0.9 mg<br>1.25 mg<br>2.5 mg | Ayerst | Oral |
| Estrace | Micronized estradiol | 1.0 mg<br>2.0 mg | Mead Johnson | Oral |
| Ogen | Estropipate | 0.625 mg<br>1.25 mg<br>2.5 mg | Abbott | Oral |
| Estratab | Esterified estrogens | 0.3 mg<br>0.625 mg<br>1.25 mg<br>2.5 mg | Reid-Rowell | Oral |
| Estraderm | Transdermal estradiol | 0.05 mg<br>0.1 mg | Ciba-Geigy | Transdermal patch |
| Estratest | Esterified estrogens with methyltestosterone | 0.625 mg estrified estrogens plus 1.25 mg methyl-testosterone<br>1.25 mg estrified estrogens plus 2.5 mg methyl-testosterone | Reid-Rowell | Oral |
| Orthoest | Estropipate | 0.625 mg<br>1.25 mg | Ortho | Oral |
| *Vaginal Estrogen Creams* | | | | |
| Premarin Vaginal Cream | Conjugated estrogens | 0.625 mg/gm | Ayerst | Vaginal |
| Estrace Vaginal Cream | 17 beta-estradiol | 0.1 mg/gm | Mead Johnson | Vaginal |
| Ogen Vaginal Cream | Estropipate | 1.5 mg/gm | Abbott | Vaginal |
| *Equivalencies of Commonly Used Oral Progestins* | | | | |
| Provera | Medroxyprogesterone acetate | 2.5 mg<br>5.0 mg<br>10 mg | Upjohn | Oral |
| Curretabs | Medroxyprogestone | 10 mg | Reid-Rowell | Oral |
| Aygestin | Norethindrone acetate | 5 mg | Ayerst | Oral |
| Micronor | Norethindrone | 0.35 mg | Ortho | Oral |

*Source: Adapted from Cutler, W.B. (1988).* Hysterectomy *(pp. 148–152). New York: Harper & Row.*

not be acceptable to the client. Equivalent dosages of other progestins may be tried. Some clinicians reduce the Provera to 5 mg and carefully observe the effects, as this dosage may not offer the endometrial protection of 10 mg. Prolonged withdrawal bleeding may indicate the need for more estrogen.

- *Advantages.* Cyclic therapy is effective for relief of hypoestrogenic symptoms and prevention of osteoporosis. Conflicting data, however, exist on changes in the lipid profile when adding progestins.
- *Disadvantages.* Withdrawal bleeding after the progestin is stopped may lead to decreased client compliance. Data are inconclusive regarding effects on lipid levels of Provera;[47] and dosing every 3 months may be less problematic (10 mg per day for 12 to 14 days). However, whether this type of regimen protects the endometrium is unproved by research at this time. Effects of the cyclic regimen on the breast are not well-established.

***Continuous Daily Estrogen/Progestin Therapy.*** Start with conjugated estrogens (Premarin) 0.625 mg, once a day, or an equivalent. If the uterus is intact, continuous medroxyprogesterone acetate (Provera) 2.5 mg is added daily. If hypoestrogenic symptoms persist after 30 days of Premarin, increase the dosage incrementally to 0.9 mg or 1.25 mg daily. If Premarin is increased, also increase Provera to 5 to 10 mg daily.

- *Advantages.* No cyclic bleeding occurs with the continuous therapy, and therapy is effective in preventing osteoporosis.
- *Disadvantages.* If the client has been menstruating during the 6 months prior to therapy, she may have frequent dysfunctional bleeding during the first few months; this usually resolves by 9 to 12 months. The client may find the unpredictable bleeding pattern unacceptable; if so, switch to the cyclic option.

Lipid profile data, although inconclusive, suggest the same beneficial effects of continuous HRT as intermittent progestin therapy.[46] The most exhaustive data on efficacy have been collected on Premarin, but Table 11–2 also lists substitutes. *Generic estrogens are not recommended because of quality control issues.*

### Transdermal Estrogen

Transdermal estradiol (Estraderm) 0.05 mg, continuously, starts this regimen. The patch is changed every 3 to 4 days according to the schedule printed on the package; for example, Friday and Monday or Saturday and Tuesday. If hypoestrogenic symptoms persist after 30 days, increase the dosage to 0.1 mg. If the uterus is intact, add medroxyprogesterone acetate (Provera) 10 mg for 12 days per month or Provera 2.5 mg continuously as presented in the continuous daily estrogen/progestin therapy discussion (above).

- *Advantages.* Among the advantages of transdermal estrogen are prompt relief of hypoestrogenic symptoms and delivery of natural 17β-estradiol directly to target cells. Continuous levels are delivered without fluctuation. Improved compliance is noted among women who do not desire oral medication. Short term data suggest that the patch is equal to oral estrogens in the prevention of osteoporosis. The patch does not significantly affect clotting factors.[48]
- *Disadvantages.* Skin irritation from the patch may occur; however, preventive measures can be taken.
  - Make sure that the application area is clean, dry, and free of oil, powder, perfume, and soap.
  - Leave the system open to the air (with protective covering off) for 10 to 15 minutes prior to application to allow some of the alcohol to evaporate.
  - Rotate the patch with each change.

- Apply to upper outer quadrants of buttocks (less sensitive).[40] Do not use on breasts or thighs.

Lipid profile data in transdermal estrogen use are inclusive; to date, no significant changes in lipids are seen with use of the patch.

### Testosterone Therapy

Esterified estrogens with methyltestosterone (Estratest tablets) or conjugated estrogens (Premarin) with methyltestosterone may be used when a client's primary complaint is loss of libido, in the absence of other medical and psychosocial factors.[48] Progestins must be added if the client has an intact uterus.

- *Advantages.* Improvement in libido with some women; prevention of osteoporosis, relief of hypoestrogenic symptoms.
- *Disadvantages.* Androgenic side effects: acne, hirsutism, clitoromegaly.

Lipid profile data for testosterone therapy are inclusive, although suggestive of a beneficial effect.[48]

## PERIMENOPAUSAL HORMONE REPLACEMENT THERAPY

Clients who are still ovulating may need contraception as they approach menopause, yet have indications for supplemental estrogen therapy as their estrogen level declines. The points to consider in continuing or initiating low dose contraceptive therapy are many.

- Estrogen may be necessary as the aging ovary begins to secrete lower levels of estradiol several years prior to the last menstrual period. The client may have some beginning signs or symptoms of deficiency but continue to have regular menses. *Reference point:* Postmenopausal estrogens are about 1 percent as potent as ethinyl estradiol. Thus, 10 μg of ethinyl estradiol (EE) is about equivalent to 1 mg of conjugated estrogen.
- Control of irregular or breakthrough bleeding may be required. The bleeding may occur because of inadequate production of luteal phase hormone or because of an estradiol peak without subsequent ovulation.
- HRT does not provide contraception. The incidence of elective abortion is highest among women who are between the ages of 40 and 50, with the exception of girls younger than 15 years.[49] Postmenopausal estrogens will not provide contraception, although they will ameliorate symptoms.
- No data suggest an increased risk of heart disease. Studies indicate no increased risk in women over age 35 using low dose ethinyl estradiol (less than 30 μg) oral contraceptives, provided they do not smoke.[49]
- Oral contraceptive (OC) users are half as likely to develop endometrial cancer as women who do not take OCs. Protection persists at least 10 years after discontinuation.[49]
- Risk of epithelial cancer of the ovary is reduced by 40 percent in short term OC users and by 80 percent in long term OC users.[49]
- Data from formal studies regarding the effect of OCs on cervical neoplasia lack consistency.[49] OC users are likely to be sexually active, often not using a barrier method, a risk factor for cervical cancer.
- The incidence of benign breast disease is lower among OC users (after 2 years of OC use). Breast cancer data, however, are inconclusive.[49]
- The incidence of fibroids is 30 percent lower among OC users.[49]
- Pelvic inflammatory disease (PID) and ectopic pregnancy are less common among OC users.[49]
- OC users have slightly more bone density at menopause, which may reflect a degree

of protection from normal hypoestrogenic bone loss.[50]

Therapy options for perimenopausal women include oral contraceptives containing less than 30 μg of estrogen. These may be used if no contraindications to estrogen exist. Low dose oral conjugated estrogen (0.3–0.625 mg Premarin) or an estrogen patch are options if contraception is not an issue. Progestin is added when the uterus is intact. Management includes annual screening exams—Pap smear, colorectal cancer screen, and FSH level evaluation. Begin annual FSH evaluation when the client is 50 years old: When the FSH level exceeds 40 mIU per mL on days 6 to 7 of a pill-free week, switch the client to ERT/HRT.[51] (See subsequent section on the Midlife Women's Health Care Program for other tests/diagnostic methods that may be indicated based on age and assessment findings.) Allay the fears of older clients about the increased risks of heart disease and stroke. Communicate to the client the contraindications to OC use: smoking, hypertension, diabetes[49] (see Chapter 6).

## OPTIONS AFTER HYSTERECTOMY/OOPHORECTOMY

### Post-Hysterectomy (without Oophorectomy)

Monitor all post-hysterectomy clients for ovarian failure, which occurs in 50 percent of women within 5 years of their hysterectomy,[52] and for hypoestrogenic symptoms. Measure the FSH level every 1 to 2 years.

### Post-Oophorectomy

An abrupt, drastic fall in estradiol occurs following oophorectomy (no gradual adaptation is possible, as with natural menopause). The symptoms are often severe, particularly hot flushes and intestinal symptoms. ERT is generally begun immediately postoperatively; high doses, such as 1.25 mg of Premarin, may be needed for up to a year postoperatively.

## INITIATING HORMONE REPLACEMENT THERAPY AND FOLLOW-UP

Provide the client with written and verbal information about HRT. Explain the risks and benefits as they apply to the client's own situation. Request that the client keep a menstrual calendar; educate her concerning what constitutes abnormal bleeding. Advise the client to telephone the health care provider immediately if she experiences any of the following:

- Unexpected bleeding.
- Abdominal pains, bloating.
- An increase in headaches.
- Symptoms not relieved or that increase.
- Visual disturbances.
- Shortness of breath or chest pain.
- Calf pain.

Obtaining written consent for HRT from the client is optional, but advised because consumers continue to be confused about estrogen and its risks and benefits.

Telephone the client 1 month and 3 months after therapy is initiated to evaluate the response to medications, side effects, and need for a physical exam. Schedule a 6-month visit to evaluate the client's response to medication, including a vaginal exam if dryness was an initial complaint. Review the menstrual calendar for abnormal bleeding patterns.

Stress to the client that even if she experiences no problems, annual exams, routine tests, and communication are important.

## CHANGING DOSAGE OR DISCONTINUATION OF THERAPY

Adjustment of ERT dosage may be needed to provide symptom relief. The dosage is increased gradually to find the minimum level needed for symptom relief. After 6 months of adequate relief at a dosage higher than 0.625 mg Premarin or equivalent, gradually decrease doses to 0.625 mg (see Table 11–2). (*Example:* 1.25 mg for 3 weeks, 0.9 mg for 1 week; if tolerated, 1.25 mg for 2 weeks, 0.9 mg for 1 week; 1.25 mg for 1 week, 0.9 mg for 1 week; stabilize at 0.9 mg for 2 weeks, then 0.9 mg for 3 weeks, 6.25 mg for 1 week, and so on.)

Hormone replacement therapy (HRT) should be discontinued gradually. (*Example:* 7 tablets per week for 1 month; 6 tablets per week for 1 month; 5 tablets per week for 1 month, and so on until zero.)

## WOMEN'S MIDLIFE HEALTH CARE PROGRAM

Comprehensive, planned, convenient health evaluations should be available for women during their midlife years. Emphasis is on health education, appropriate screenings for early detection of disease, and discussion of positive health behaviors, particularly balanced nutrition.[53] A holistic health care program includes education and appropriate evaluation and testing.

### EDUCATION

Many women lack knowledge of the emotional, sexual, social, and medical aspects of the perimenopause/postmenopause; hence, client education must be comprehensive.

- *Anatomy and Physiology.* Explain the changes expected with the perimenopausal transition, including the most common signs and symptoms and usual nonmedical and medical methods of management.
- *Nutrition.* Explain the dietary need to decrease fat, especially saturated fats (Table 11–3); increase complex carbohydrates; have a moderate protein intake; and increase dietary calcium or add a calcium supplement.
- *Exercise.* Encourage weightbearing, aerobic, flexibility, and joint mobility activities (Table 11–4).
- *Smoking, Alcohol and Drug Use.* Communicate the need to stop all untoward substance use. Refer the client to a smoking cessation program, Alcoholics Anonymous, or drug treatment program as appropriate. Stress the need for caution with prescription drug use also (see Chapter 18).
- *Relaxation and Stress Reduction.* Emphasize the need for awareness of one's stress level and the contributing factors. Promote the use of relaxation techniques and behavior modification, rather than alcohol or drugs.
- *Contraception.* Give information about effective, safe birth control methods if the client desires protection during the transition before menopause (see Chapter 6).
- *Hormone Replacement Therapy.* Tell the client about the risks, benefits, and side effects of HRT.
- *Sexuality.* Discuss how the transition to menopause will affect sexuality, particularly the frequent vaginal changes and ways to counter them satisfactorily (e.g., lubrication and Kegel's exercises).

### ROUTINE EVALUATION AND TESTING

Women between the ages of 40 and 60 years will benefit from specific tests and evaluations.[53,54] A comprehensive health history that specifically addresses midlife issues is invaluable. A complete physical examination, also necessary, includes height, weight, integumentary, oral cavity, thyroid, cardiovascular and thoracic systems, breasts (including instruction in breast self-examination [BSE]), abdomen, extremities, and pelvic and rectal components.

**TABLE 11-3. RECOMMENDED DIETARY MODIFICATIONS TO LOWER BLOOD CHOLESTEROL: THE STEP-ONE DIET**

| | Choose | Decrease |
|---|---|---|
| Fish, chicken, turkey, and lean meats. | Fish, poultry without skin, lean cuts of beef, lamb, pork, veal, shellfish. | Fatty cuts of beef, lamb, pork; spare ribs, organ meats, regular cold cuts, sausage, hot dogs, bacon, sardines, roe. |
| Skim and low-fat milk, cheese, yogurt, and dairy substitutes. | Skim, or 1 percent fat milk (liquid, powdered, evaporated), buttermilk. | Whole milk (4 percent fat): regular, evaporated, condensed; cream, half and half, 2 percent milk, imitation milk products, most nondairy creamers, whipped toppings. |
| | Nonfat (0 percent fat) or low-fat yogurt. | Whole-milk yogurt. |
| | Low-fat cottage cheese ( 1 percent or 2 percent fat). | Whole-milk cottage cheese (4 percent fat). |
| | Low-fat cheeses, farmer or pot cheeses (all of these should be labeled no more than 2 to 6 g of fat per oz). | All natural cheeses (eg., blue, roquefort, camembert, cheddar, Swiss), low-fat or "light" cream cheese, low-fat or "light" sour cream, cream cheeses, sour cream. |
| | Sherbet, sorbet. | Ice cream. |
| Eggs. | Egg whites (2 whites equal 1 whole egg in recipes), cholesterol-free egg substitutes. | Egg yolks. |
| Fruits and vegetables. | Fresh, frozen, canned, or dried fruits and vegetables. | Vegetables prepared in butter, cream, or other sauces. |
| Breads and cereals. | Homemade baked goods using unsaturated oils sparingly, angel food cake, low-fat crackers, low-fat cookies. | Commercial baked goods: pies, cakes, doughnuts, croissants, pastries, muffins, biscuits, high-fat crackers, high-fat cookies. |
| | Rice, pasta. | Egg noodles. |
| | Whole-grain breads and cereals (oatmeal, whole wheat, rye, bran, multigrain, etc.). | Breads in which eggs are a major ingredient. |
| Fats and oils. | Baking cocoa. | Chocolate. |
| | Unsaturated vegetable oils: corn, olive, rapeseed (canola oil), safflower, sesame, soybean, sunflower. | Butter, coconut oil, palm oil, palm kernel oil, lard, bacon fat.<br>Margarine or shortenings made from one of the unsaturated oils listed here, diet margarine. |
| | Mayonnaise, salad dressings made with unsaturated oils listed above, low-fat dressings. | Dressings made with egg yolk. |
| | Seeds and nuts. | Coconut. |

*Source: Expert Panel. (1988). Report on the National Cholesterol Education Program, Expert Panel on Detection, Evaluation, and Treatment of High Blood Cholesterol in Adults.* Arch Internal Med, 148, *49.*

**TABLE 11-4. EXERCISES FOR MIDLIFE WOMEN**

Run in place, or around a room. (This is just as beneficial as running, or jogging, outdoors.)

Lie on your back, knees slightly bent. Catch your feet securely under a bed, couch, cabinet, or heavy chair. Clasp your hands behind your head. Rise to a sitting position, then return to a reclining position.

Lie flat, with knees slightly bent and arms at your sides. Raise your left leg straight up. Lower it. Repeat with your right leg.

Repeat the exercise above, but when leg is raised, swing it slowly to one side and back up, then lower it to the floor.

Stand, placing your hands flat against each other as if in prayer. Push them together as hard as you can.

Lie down, knees flexed, soles on the floor. Extend your left leg as far as you can, pointing your toe. Return to a flexed position, then relax it. Repeat with your right leg.

Kneel and put hands on floor. Raise your back the way a cat stretches, then lower your abdomen in a reverse movement. Repeat several times.

Sit on the floor cross-legged. Reach as high as you can with your right hand, then with your left hand. Repeat. Do the same thing, reaching forward with each hand.

Stand on your tiptoes. Rock back and forth from heels to toes.

Stand straight. Keeping your knees slightly bent, bend to touch the floor with your fingertips.

Stand straight. Reach for the ceiling with both hands.

*Note:* These exercises emphasize strength and stretching, and they are suitable for women who have not been very active.

Source: *Fogel, C.I. (1991). Nutrition and health patterns in midlife women. In C.H. Garner (Ed.),* NAACOG's Clinical Issues in Perinatal and Women's Health Nursing: Mid-Life Women's Health 2*(4), 523. Used with permission.*

## Diagnostic Tests and Methods

- *Cholesterol and/or Lipid Profile.* (See Chapter 3 for general screening guidelines.) If no prior testing has been done, obtain baseline data at age 40 or when HRT is initiated. Draw a lipid profile if cholesterol is over 200 mg per dL; if normal, repeat every 5 years to age 50. If cholesterol is 200 mg per dL or above, advise a low cholesterol, low fat, high fiber diet and regular exercise for 3 months and then repeat the test. If cholesterol is still elevated, referral to a primary care physician is appropriate.
- *Urinalysis.* Perform every 2 years.
- *Complete Blood Cell (CBC) Count.* Perform every 2 to 5 years.
- *Blood Chemistry Profile.* Establish at age 40, then repeat every 5 years.
- *Colorectal Cancer Screening.* Begin when the client is 40 years old. The annual screening includes a digital rectal exam and fecal occult blood test. For women 50 or older, a sigmoidoscopy is recommended every 3 to 5 years following two consecutive annual negative exams.
- *Cervical Screening.* Annual Pap smear and pelvic exam are recommended for all women age 18 and older. If a client has three or more consecutive normal Pap smears, then the test may be done less frequently, at the discretion of the health care professional. However, annual pelvic exams are warranted to evaluate other areas, for example, the ovaries. If the client has had a hysterectomy for benign disease, then repeat the Pap smear 1 year after surgery; if negative, then every 2 years. If the cervix was not removed, or if the client has ever had an abnormal Pap, then continue Pap smears annually.
- *Ovarian Cancer Screening.* Perform routinely during bimanual exams. No other techniques are suitable for routine screening,[55] although a pelvic sonogram or CA125 may be considered if there is a family history of ovarian cancer. To date, however, neither test has been proved cost effective.[55]

- *Endometrial Cancer Screening.* Screening of the total population is neither cost effective nor warranted.[56] A biopsy is indicated if abnormal uterine bleeding occurs.
- *Lung Cancer Screening.* No suitable techniques are available, although some clinicians support annual chest x-rays for women 50 years and older who smoke more than a pack of cigarettes daily. The American Cancer Institute and National Cancer Institute have not adopted this guideline. Advise the client to stop smoking, because of the increased risks of breast disease, hypertension, osteoporosis, cervical cancer, early menopause, and lung cancer.
- *Breast Cancer Screening.* Teaching and reinforcing BSE, and encouraging an annual exam by a health care provider are important. A baseline mammogram is needed between ages 35 and 40 years, every 1 to 2 years from ages 41 to 50, and annually after age 50. Recommendations vary for women with a family history of breast cancer (see Chapter 10).
- *Cardiovascular Screening.* No good data support the effectiveness of routine screening electrocardiograms (ECGs) for women. The risk of cardiovascular disease does increase with age, however, and the health professional may want to consider more regular ECG use in the later decades of a client's life.
- *Hearing Examinations.* The optimal frequency of hearing screening has not been determined; hence, examinations are at the discretion of the health provider. An otoscopic exam and audiometric testing should be performed on all persons with evidence of impaired hearing.
- *Vision Screening.* Ophthalmoscopy and tonometry are indicated for all clients over age 40. A complete ocular examination by an ophthalmologist at least once between ages 35 and 45 years and every 5 years after 50 is suggested.
- *Immunizations.* Updated diphtheria and tetanus immunizations are needed every 10 years. Annual influenza immunization beginning at age 65 and Pneumovax (pneumonia vaccine) at age 65 are recommended.
- *Bone Density Screening.* Routine screening is not currently recommended due to the expense, limited availability, and inability to correlate various methods (e.g., dual photon, single photon, computed tomographic [CT] scan). It may be used to monitor the need for HRT, however. Osteoporosis is better observed in the trabecular bone of the hips and spine.
    - Dual photon absorptiometry (DPA) uses the radioisotope gadolinium to project gamma rays through the body. They are measured by computer to calculate the quantity of minerals present.
    - CT densitometry—modified quantitative computerized tomography of the lumbar spine—calculates bone mass. The method uses a higher dosage of radiation.
    - Dual-energy ray absorptiometry, or dual x-ray absorptiometry (DXA), is a relatively new method that uses a dual-energy ray source; resolution is superior to DPA, with comparable radiation.[57]
    - Single photon absorptiometry measures the density of cortical bone of the distal radius, different from the trabecular bone of the spine and hip. It has limited usefulness in identifying women at high risk for fractures.
- *Diabetic Screening.* Screening is indicated if there is a history of gestational diabetes, or an immediate family history of diabetes; if the client is symptomatic, more than 50 percent overweight, or has glycosuria (see Chapter 17).

- *Endometrial Biopsy*
  - *With Hormone Replacement Therapy.* In the absence of risk factors causing endometrial alterations associated with unopposed estrogen exposure, such as alcoholism, liver disease, thyroid disease, ovulation, and anovulation, routine endometrial biopsy is not indicated.[2] (See also DUB, below).
  - *With Dysfunctional Uterine Bleeding (DUB).* DUB is defined as any bleeding that occurs a year or more after a previous episode of perimenopausal bleeding (single episodes of spotting or blood-tinged discharge are significant), heavy or frequent bleeding episodes, or bleeding at inappropriate times with hormone replacement therapy (HRT). Initially, the health care provider must rule out endometrial carcinoma; refer the client to a gynecologist for evaluation (see Chapter 5).

# OSTEOPOROSIS

Osteoporosis is a disorder characterized by a reduction of bone mass, which compromises the structural integrity of the skeleton. Bone mass peaks at age 30, is reduced slightly prior to ovarian failure, then is reduced rapidly during postmeno-pausal years. Critical sites of hypoestrogenic loss are the trabecular bone of the spine and hip, predisposing to fracture. A long, silent, asymptomatic period (10 to 20 years postmenopause) is typical.

The costs of treating osteoporosis and related skeletal fractures are estimated to be 10 billion dollars or more annually.[57,58]

## EPIDEMIOLOGY

Seventy-five percent or more of the bone loss that occurs in the first 20 years postmenopause is attributed to estrogen deficiency.[2] The risk factors for osteoporosis are listed in Table 11–5. Approximately 12 to 20 percent of women with hip fractures die of complications within 6 months,[57] and many others are permanently disabled. Osteoporosis is preventable in most women with estrogen replacement therapy (ERT).

## SUBJECTIVE DATA

The client may report a history of back pain. The pain may be localized at site of vertebral compression and radiate from midline to the flank, may worsen with movement, and may be severe with muscle spasm. The client may also report some of the risk factors listed in Table 11–5; for example, smoking or a sedentary lifestyle.

## OBJECTIVE DATA

### Physical Examination

Findings include loss of height, frequent fractures, and "dowager's hump" (curvature of the cervical and upper thoracic spine). Maintain a careful record of the client's height in centimeters, in order to detect any decrease.

**TABLE 11-5. RISK FACTORS FOR OSTEOPOROSIS**

| |
|---|
| Early female menopause or oophorectomy. |
| Family history of osteoporosis. |
| European or Asian descent. |
| Small boned and/or underweight. |
| Low consumpton of calcium, high consumption of caffeine, and high consumption of alcohol. |
| Sedentary lifestyle. |
| Smoking. |

### Diagnostic Tests and Methods

- Bone density tests, including bone densitometry (dual photon) or quantitative CT of the spine, may be indicated to determine decreased bone mass.
- Erythrocyte sedimentation rate (ESR) is determined to rule out rheumatoid arthritis.

## DIFFERENTIAL MEDICAL DIAGNOSES

Multiple myeloma, Cushing's syndrome, rheumatoid arthritis, hyperparathyroidism, corticosteroid use.

## PLAN

### Psychosocial Interventions

Discuss with the client the importance of preventing or inhibiting further bone loss during the perimenopausal and postmenopausal years. Stress diet, exercise, health, and medication regimens. Advise the client to eliminate or decrease her alcohol intake, and to improve ERT effectiveness, eliminate smoking.

### Medication

Among the therapies are estrogen, calcium, calcitonin, fluoride, and vitamin D:

- *Estrogen Replacement Therapy (ERT).* ERT is the most significant therapy for the prevention and treatment of postmenopausal osteoporosis. The minimum dose without supplemental calcium is Premarin 0.625 mg or the equivalent. One study found that Premarin 0.3 mg in combination with calcium 1000 mg daily also prevented loss of bone density.[59] Smokers may require higher dosages of estrogen, as smoking increases liver metabolism of estrogen.[2,9]
- *Calcium.* By itself, calcium does not significantly influence bone resorption;[2] however, adequate intake is necessary for a positive calcium balance. A negative balance pulls calcium stores from the bone. In combination with regular exercise, calcium may slow bone loss.
  - *Dietary Calcium.* Optimal dietary calcium comes from dairy products and tofu (bean curd), derived from soy bean milk. Factors that interfere with absorption include being older than 35, taking aluminum-containing antacids, consuming caffeine, and a high-protein diet. Generally, about 500 mg of calcium can be gained through the diet.
  - *Calcium Supplements.* The recommended daily calcium dosage is 1000 mg per day prior to menopause; 1000 to 1500 mg per day postmenopause if not on ERT; and 500 mg per day if on ERT (500 mg is gained through diet).[2] When dietary intake is insufficient, a supplement is indicated. Products with calcium carbonate, for example Tums, provide the most calcium for the money. Possible side effects to the calcium supplements include constipation, flatulence, and gastric distress. Advise the client to consult a pharmacist and try several brands to determine the best option for her. Calcium supplementation is contraindicated in women who have a history of renal stones.
- *Calcitonin.* May be used with hormone replacement therapy to decrease bone resorption. The recommended dosage is 50 units subcutaneously 3 times per week (may be increased to 100 units). Bone density should be monitored with scanning, but it is expensive.[60]
- *Fluoride.* In 40 to 60 percent of women, fluoride increases bone density and decreases fractures. Sodium fluoride 40 to 60 mg q.d. in divided doses is suggested.[61] Side effects include GI toxicity, arthritis, joint pain, and fascitis.

- *Vitamin D.* Vitamin D supplementation has no place in prophylaxis because women are rarely Vitamin D deficient.[2] It may be indicated, however, if osteoporosis is present and progressing.

### Weightbearing Exercise

Walking about 1.5 to 2 miles three times per week or other weightbearing exercises for 30 minutes three times per week will increase the mineral content of the bone. Ambulation during at least 4 hours out of 24 is recommended. The vertebrae require ERT, calcium, and exercise to decrease fracture risk.

### Follow-Up

Consultation with or referral to a gynecologic and/or orthopedic specialist is indicated for progressing disease. Preventive measures in childbearing clients include adequate dietary or supplemental calcium, weightbearing exercise several times per week for at least 30 minutes, and evaluation for estrogen deficiency during periods of amenorrhea longer than 6 months, particularly during adolescence.

# HIRSUTISM

Hirsutism (increased hair in unusual amounts and places) is one sign of benign hyperandrogynism (the appearance of testosterone stimulated characteristics). The signs include excess facial and abdominal hair of a coarse nature, oily skin, and hoarseness. Hirsutism often causes extreme distress in women.

## EPIDEMIOLOGY

Androgens enter the blood from the adrenal glands, ovaries, and peripheral tissues. Benign rises in testosterone are caused by ovarian stromal hyperplasia that sometimes develops under the influence of high luteinizing hormone (LH) levels. Testosterone levels, however, decrease in all women between the fourth and fifth postmenopausal year. Obesity may be correlated with hirsutism because the amount of androgen that the peripheral tissues release into the circulation is primarily a function of how much androgen precursor the tissue extracts from blood, and the inherent ability of that tissue to convert a precursor to an active androgen.[2]

## SUBJECTIVE DATA

The client may report an increase in facial, areolar, abdominal, and chest hair, and acne.

## OBJECTIVE DATA

During the physical examination note any increase in facial, areolar, chest, and abdominal hair and acne. On pelvic examination, check for clitoral enlargement and abnormal ovarian size (ovaries should not be palpable in postmenopausal women).

Diagnostic tests include serum testosterone level, to rule out ovarian and adrenal tumors; and dehydroepiandrosterone sulfate (DHEA-S) level, to rule out adrenal tumor. If either serum testosterone or DHEA-S is elevated, refer the client immediately to a gynecologist to rule out an androgen-producing tumor.

## DIFFERENTIAL MEDICAL DIAGNOSES

Ovarian or adrenal androgen-producing tumors.

## PLAN

Reassure the client that the increased hair growth is not abnormal and that it may abate as testosterone levels decrease in a few years. If hair growth is excessive, offer suggestions for its removal (e.g., electrolysis).

Spironolactone (aldosterone antagonist) 25 mg q.i.d. *or* 50 mg b.i.d. may help to decrease androgen production and block the effect of testosterone on hair follicles. Cimetidine, generally used to treat ulcers and excess gastric acid, may also provide an antiandrogenic effect. Dexamethasone (corticosteroid) 0.5 mg q.h.s. has been used to suppress adrenal hyperfunction, but this drug can cause osteoporosis, so it should be used with caution. Consult the *Physicians' Desk Reference* (*PDR*) or another current pharmacotherapeutics reference before prescribing drugs to treat hirsutism, and confer with a gynecologist who specializes in endocrinology.

### Follow-Up

Immediate referral to a gynecologic specialist is required whenever androgen-producing tumors are suspected.

## NONREPRODUCTIVE HEALTH CONCERNS OF AGING WOMEN

More women are taking a proactive role in health maintenance and the prevention of disease. Preventive health care is a major area that the health care provider must focus on with women, especially as they age. The menopause provides a unique opportunity for the provider to assist the woman in maintaining ongoing cost-effective health care that includes appropriate referrals if necessary.[9] Many risk factors can be modified by adapting positive health measures, such as not smoking, eating a low fat, low cholesterol diet (Table 11–3), and exercising (Table 11–4). However, the aging process is affected by biologic, social, economic, and psychological influences. Assessment of all these factors is critical to the development of an effective health care strategy for older women. Certain areas posing more serious problems for the aging woman that may negatively affect her health include the following.

### HEALTH CARE INSURANCE AND SOCIAL SECURITY

Ninety-five percent of American women over age 65 have Medicare coverage.[62] Women who have lost spouses through death, divorce, or separation are more likely to have only public health care coverage or no insurance. Making co-payments, payment for services not covered by Medicare, or payment of insurance deductible is often a hardship for elderly women. Elderly women who live alone or who are of ethnic minority tend to be poorer than elderly men. White women are more likely to have private insurance than nonwhite women. Women are more likely to have health insurance than men are, except in the 45- to 64-year-old group. Research shows that if people cannot pay, they are unable to get needed health care, which clearly affects their health status and longevity.[62]

Out-of-pocket costs of health care, including medications, often increase with acute and chronic illness as the woman ages; and if a choice between rent, food, and medicine confronts the elderly woman, she may forgo her medication. More serious illness is a likely consequence.

Under Social Security, women's benefits are expected to be two-thirds of men's through the year 2055, yet 33 percent of single elderly women depend on Social Security for more than 90 percent of their income.[63]

It is essential that the health care provider be aware of resources in her/his locale to use for referral that can aid the woman in maintaining her finances in health or illness.

## SOCIAL SUPPORT

Social support in life is a need of all human beings. The lack of social support can be a source of serious concern and increasing health risks in the aging woman.

With a life expectancy of over 75 years, most American women will live half of their adult lives after their last child has left home.[63] Statistical research indicates that women who live to the age of 65 can expect to live to be 84.[9] Nearly one-quarter of women over age 70 have no surviving children.[62] Only 39 percent of women are married at age 65, and because the proportion of women to men increases after age 65, the likelihood of finding male partners is decreased. By age 85, there are only 45 men for every 100 women.[9]

Of the almost 10 million older women without spouses, approximately 70 percent live alone or with people unrelated to them. The lack of social support can be a source of serious concern and increasing health risks in the elderly. It also necessitates changing patterns of sexual activity: a decline in intercourse and an increase in masturbation.

The health care provider must be sensitive to the social living conditions of the woman, and work with her to find ways to enhance her support systems.

## RISK OF ABUSE

In assessing the older woman, the health care provider should always evaluate for signs of abuse. Dependency and increasing longevity put the elderly woman at risk for abuse and crime. Although the reported risk of abuse is 4 percent, it is likely to be underreported.[62] Assisting the woman to seek appropriate avenues for support, as well as reporting suspected abuse, are inherent in providing holistic health care.

## CHRONIC ILLNESS

Chronic illnesses increase in women over age 60.[63] Elderly women are likely to have three or more chronic conditions.[62]

### *Common Chronic Problems*

- Visual and hearing impairments.
- Arthritis.
- Hypertensive disease.
- Coronary heart disease.
- Diabetes.
- Impairments of lower extremities.
- Chronic respiratory disease.
- Urinary tract disorders.
- Upper gastrointestinal disorders.
- Constipation.
- Anemia.
- Cirrhosis.

Heart disease, cancer, and stroke continue to be the leading causes of death among older women.[62]

Although there is a fixed life span, the decline of vigor and onset of chronic illness can be slowed by preventive health behaviors.[9]

## CHRONIC DEPRESSION AND SUICIDE RISK

As well as assessing for physical changes, the provider must be alert to emotional depression in the aging woman. Chronic depression and suicide are increasing among the elderly.

### *Risk Factors for Depression and Suicide*

- Unrecognized or untreated affective disorders.
- Physical illness.
- General stresses of aging.
- Bereavement.
- Isolation.

The major risk factor is bereavement. The risk of suicide is increased in surviving spouses for 4 years after the death of a partner.[61] Alcohol use plays an important role. The interaction of multiple medications must be considered also.

Prompt treatment can alleviate depression in the elderly and prevent serious consequences.

## LIMITED ACCESS TO CARE

Decreasing vision and other physical impairments may limit an older woman's driving ability and access to care. Alternative transportation may create a financial burden, particularly if multiple health services at multiple sites are needed.

There may be a shortage of health care providers who are trained and interested in holistic care of perimenopausal and postmenopausal women, or who will accept Medicare and Medicaid.

When family members and other caretakers are lacking, elders become dependent on the health care system, particularly nursing homes. But for the women of midlife who are the caretakers for elderly parents, stress is increased during the perimenopausal transition. Women's health providers must emphasize preventive measures and appropriate use of early detection in order to address the problems of morbidity and chronic illness in the elderly. Health and social services for older women are often interdependent, providing a comprehensive, holistic approach.

## NURSING DIAGNOSES

The following nursing diagnoses are representative of those used in the health care plan of women experiencing problems during the climacteric and menopause, and with the process of aging. The list, however, is by no means inclusive.

- Altered body image.
- Altered mobility.
- Altered sexuality.
- Anxiety.
- Body image disturbance.
- Children leaving home.
- Discomfort.
- Fear.
- Grief, secondary to losses such as childbearing capabilities.
- Grief, anticipatory.
- Individual coping, ineffective.
- Pain.
- Thermoregulation, ineffective.

## REFERENCES


1. Speroff, L. (1989). The woman over 50: A new challenge for the gynecologist. *Contemporary obstetrics & gynecology, S,* 22–29.
2. Speroff, L., Glass, R.H., & Kase, N.G. (1989). *Clinical gynecologic endocrinology and infertility* (4th ed.) (pp. 34–36). Baltimore: Williams & Wilkins.
3. Sheehy G. (1977). *Passages.* New York: Bantam.
4. Seidel, H.M., Ball, J.W., Dains, J.E., & Benedict, G.W. (1991). *Mosby's guide to physical examination.* St. Louis: C.V. Mosby.
5. Nelson, K.A. (1987). Visual impairment among elderly Americans: Statistics in transition. *Journal of Visual Impairment and Blindness, 81,* 331–334.
6. Havlik, R.J. (1986). *Aging in the eighties: Impaired senses for sound and light in persons age 65 and over* (DHHS Publication No. PHS 86-1250). Washington, DC: National Center for Health Statistics.
7. Pereman, J., Wolf, P., Finucan, F., & Madans, J. (1989). Menopause and the epidemiology of cardiovascular disease in women. In C.V. Hammond, F.P. Haseltine, & I. Schiff (Eds.), *Menopause: Evaluation, treatment*

*and health concerns* (p. 283). New York: Alan R. Liss.

8. Stampfer, M.J., Colditz, G.A., Willett, W.C., Manson, J.E., Rosner, B., Speizer, F.E., & Hennekens, C.H. (1991). Postmenopausal estrogen therapy and cardiovascular disease. *New England Journal of Medicine, 325*, 765–772.
9. Byyny, R.L. & Speroff, L. (1990), *A clinical guide for the care of older women.* Baltimore: Williams & Wilkins.
10. Maddox, M.A. (1992). Women at midlife: Hormone replacement therapy. *Nursing Clinics of North America, 24*(4), 959–969.
11. Kane, R.L., Ouslander, J.G., & Abrass, I.B. (1994). *Essentials of clinical geriatrics* (3rd ed.). New York: McGraw-Hill, Inc.
12. Anderson, E., Hamburger, S., Lin, J.H., et al. (1987). Characteristics of women seeking assistance. *American Journal of Obstetrics & Gynecology, 156*, 428–433.
13. U.S. Department of Health and Human Services. (1992). *Urinary incontinence in adults.* (AHCR Publication No. 92-0038). Rockville, MD: PHS.
14. Ostergood, D.R., & Bent, A.E. (Eds.). (1991). *Urogynecology and urodynamics* (3rd ed.). Baltimore: Williams & Wilkins.
15. Ingelman-Sunberg, A., Rosen, J., Gustafesson, S.A., & Charstron K. (1981). Cytosol estrogen receptors in the urogenital tissues in stress incontinence women. *Acta Obsetricia et Gynecologia Scandinavica, 60*, 585–586.
16. German, A., Karram, M.M., & Bhatia, N.M. (1990). Changes in urethral cytology following estrogen administration. *Gynecology & Obstetrics Investigation, 29*, 211–213.
17. Wise, B., & Cardozo, L. (1991). Urge incontinence and stress incontinence. *Current Opinion in Obstetrics & Gynecology, 3*, 520–527.
18. Fergusson, K.L., McKey, P.L., & Bishop, K.R., et al. (1990). Stress urinary incontinence: Effective pelvic muscle exercise. *Obstetrics & Gynecology, 75*, 671–675.
19. Hadley, E.C. (1986). Bladder training and related therapies for urinary incontinence in older people. *Journal of the American Medical Association, 256*, 327–379.
20. Burgio, K.L., Pearce, K.L., & Lucco, A.J. (1989). *Staying dry: A practical guide to bladder control.* Baltimore: Johns Hopkins University Press.
21. McEwen, B.S. (1976). Ovarian hormone action in the brain: Implications for the menopause. In M. Notelvotiz & P.A. Jankeep (Eds.), *The climacteric in perspective* (pp. 207–209). Lancaster, England: MPT Press.
22. Mayfield, D., McLeod, G., & Hall, P. (1984). The CAGE questionnaire. *American Journal of Psychiatry, 131*, 1121.
23. Selzer, M.L. (1980). The Michigan Alcoholism Screening Test (MAST). *American Journal of Psychology* (revised 25), *3*, 176–181, 197.
24. Sokol, R.J., Martier, S.S., & Agee, J. (1989). The T-ACE questions: Practical prenatal detection of risk-drinking. *American Journal of Obstetrics & Gynecology, 160*, 863.
25. Beck, A.P. (1967). *Depression: Clinical, experimental, and therapeutic aspects.* New York: Harper & Row.
26. Zung, W.W.K. (1989). *The measurement of depression.* Indianapolis: Dista Products.
27. Whitehead, M.I., Hillard, T.C., & Crook, D. (1990). Role and use of progestins. *Obstetrics & Gynecology, 75*(4 suppl): 59S–76S.
28. Czeisler, C. (1982). Rotating shift work schedules that disrupt sleep are improved by circadian principles. *Science, 217*, 460–463.
29. Stevenson, J.C. (1990). Pathogenesis, prevention and treatment of osteoporosis. *Obstetrics & Gynecology, 75*(4 suppl): 36S–41S.
30. Lindsay, R., & Tohme, J.F. (199). Estrogen treatment of patients with established postmenopausal osteoporosis. *Obstetrics & Gynecology, 76*, 290–291.
31. Gibbons, W.E., Moyer, D.L., Lobo, R.A., Roy, S., Mishell, D.R. (1986). Biochemical and histologic effects of sequential estrogen/progestin therapy on the endometrium of postmenopausal women. *American Journal of Obstetrics & Gynecology, 154*, 454–460.
32. Clisham, P.R., deZiegleo, D., Loza, O.K., & Judd, H.L. (1991). Comparison of continuous versus sequential estrogen and progestin

therapy in postmenopausal women. *Obstetrics & Gynecology, 77,* 241–246.

33. Speroff, L. (1992). The risk of breast cancer associated with oral contraception and hormone replacement therapy. *Women's Health Issues, 2,* 63–74.
34. Wren, B.G., & Routledge, D.A. (1983). The effect of type and dose of oestrogen on the blood pressure of postmenopausal women. *Maturitas, 5,* 135–142.
35. Kay, C.R. (1982). Progestogens and arterial disease: Evidence from the Royal College of General Practitioners study. *American Journal of Obstetrics & Gynecology, 142,* 762–765.
36. Lobo, R.A. (1987). Absorption and metabolic effects of different types of estrogens and progesterones. *Obstetrics & Gynecology Clinics of North America,* 143–167.
37. Luotola, H. (1983). Blood pressure and hemodynamics in postmenopausal women during estradiol-17-beta substitution. *American Clinical Research, 15*(Suppl. 18), 9–21.
38. Paginini-Hill, A., Ross, R.K., & Henderson, B.E. (1988). Postmenopausal oestrogen therapy and stroke: A perspective study. *British Medical Journal, 297,* 519–522.
39. Lobo, R.A. (1990). Cardiovascular implications of estrogen replacement therapy. *Obstetrics & Gynecology, 75,* 18–25.
40. Youngkin, E.Q. (1990). Estrogen replacement therapy and estraderm transdermal system. *Nurse Practitioner, 15,* 19–31.
41. Ditkoff, E.C., Crary, W.A., Cristo, M., & Lobo, R.A. (1991). Estrogen improves psychological function in asymptomatic postmenopausal women. *Obstetrics & Gynecology, 78,* 991–995.
42. Vanden Brouchke, J.P., Witteman, J.C.M., Valkenburg, H.A., Boersma, J.W., Cats, A., Hartman, A.P., Humber-Bruning, O., Rasker, J.J., & Weber, J. (1986). Non-contraceptive hormones and rheumatoid arthritis in perimenopausal and postmenopausal women. *Journal of the American Medical Association, 255,* 1299–1304.
43. Barrett-Connor, E., & Laasko, M. (1990). Ischemic heart disease in postmenopausal women: Effects of estrogen use on glucose and insulin levels. *Arteriosclerosis, 10,* 531–534.
44. Speroff, L. (1990). Breast cancer and postmenopausal hormone therapy. *Contemporary Obstetrics & Gynecology,* 71–82.
45. Creaseman, W.T. (1991). Estrogen replacement therapy: Is previously treated cancer a contradiction? *Obstetrics & Gynecology, 77,* 308–312.
46. Notelovitz, M. (1989). Estrogen replacement therapy: Indications, contraindications, agent selection. *American Journal of Obstetrics & Gynecology, 161,* 1832–1841.
47. Barrett-Connor, E., Wingard, D.L., & Criqui, M.H. (1989). Postmenopausal estrogen use and heart disease risk factors in the 1980's. *Journal of the America Medical Association, 261,* 2095–2099.
48. Speroff, L., Grambrell, R.D., Sherwin, B.B., et al. (1988). Androgens in the menopause. New York: McGraw-Hill.
49. Mishell, D.R. (1990). Oral contraception for women in their 40's. *Journal of Reproductive Medicine, 35,* 447–481.
50. Lindsay, R., Tobme, J., & Kanders, B. (1986). The effect of oral contraceptive use on vertebral bone mass in pre- and postmenopausal women. *Contraception, 34,* 333.
51. Speroff, L. (1991). A clinician's approach to therapy during a woman's transited years. *Contemporary Obstetrics & Gynecology, 86,* 65–68.
52. Cutler, W.B. (1988). *Hysterectomy: Before and after* (pp. 104–105). New York: Harper & Row.
53. Garner, C. (1992). *Mid-life women's health* (pp 473–482). Philadelphia: Lippincott.
54. Fisher, M. (Ed). (1989). *U.S. Preventive Services Task Force: Guide to clinical preventive services.* Baltimore: Williams & Wilkins.
55. American College of Obstetrics and Gynecology. (1990). Cancer of the ovary (Tech. Bull. No. 141). Washington, DC.
56. American College of Obstetrics and Gynecology. (1990). *Estrogen replacement therapy and endometrial cancer.* (ACOG Comm. Opinion No. 80). Washington, DC.
57. Wahner, H.W., Dunn, W.L., Brown, M.L., Morin, R.L., Riggs, B.L. (1988). Comparison

of dual-energy x-ray absorptiometry for bone mineral measurements of lumbar spine. *Mayo Clinic Proceedings*, *63*, 1075.

58. Hacker, N.F. & Moore, J.G (1992). *Essentials of Obstetrics and Gynecology,* 2nd Ed. Philadelphia: W.B. Saunders Co.
59. Ettinger, B., Genant, H.K., & Cann, C.E. (1987). Postmenopausal bone loss is prevented by treatment with low-dosage estrogen with calcium. *American Internal Medicine*, *106*, 40.
60. MacIntyre, I., Stevenson, J.C., Whitehead, M.I., Wimala Warsa, S.J., Banks, L.M., & Healy, M.J.R. (1988). Calcitonin for prevention of postmenopausal bone loss. *Lancet*, *i*, 900–902.
61. Briancon, P., & Meunier, P.J. (1981). Treatment of osteoporosis with fluoride, calcium, and vitamin D. *Orthopedic Clinics of North America*, *12*, 629.
62. Horton, J.A. (1992). *The women's health data book: A profile of women's health in the United States*. Washington, DC: Jacobs Institute of Women's Health, Elsevier.
63. U.S. Department of Health and Human Services. (1985). *Women's Health: Report of the PHS task force on women's health issues* (DHHS Publication No. PHS 85-5026).

# PROMOTION OF HEALTH CARE DURING PREGNANCY

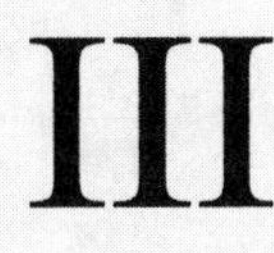

III

CHAPTER 12

# ASSESSING HEALTH DURING PREGNANCY

*Valerie Johnson South • Cynthia W. Bailey*

*A National Institutes of Health and Human Services expert panel . . . recommended that prenatal care begin prior to conception, preferably within 1 year of a planned pregnancy.*

### *Highlights*

- Barriers to Prenatal Care
- Preconception Counseling, Assessment
- Presumptive, Probable, and Positive Signs and Symptoms
- Sexuality During Pregnancy
- Initial Prenatal Visit, Subsequent Visits
- Progressing Physical Changes
- Commonly Recommended Tests
- Risk Assessment
  - *Genetic and Preterm Assessments*
  - *Attachment*
  - *Environmental, Occupational Hazards*
- Psychosocial Assessment
- Nutrition
- Major Theories of Maternal Role Development
- Preparation for Childbirth: Counseling and Classes
- Adolescent Pregnancy
- Delayed Pregnancy
- Nontraditional Families
- Substance Abuse Screening

## INTRODUCTION

Prior to the early 1900s few women received prenatal care or evaluation. The advent of consistent and comprehensive prenatal care, begun in early pregnancy, has markedly decreased both maternal and infant morbidity and mortality in the United States. Today prenatal care encompasses risk assessment, social services, client education, and medical care. Ideally this care should begin prior to conception.[1]

Despite advances in prenatal care, several barriers to initiating care exist.[2]

*Barriers to Prenatal Care*

- *Unrecognized Pregnancy.* Pregnancy may go unrecognized because of lack of knowledge about the signs and symptoms of pregnancy, limited body awareness, a history of irregular menses, or obesity.
- *Denied Pregnancy.* Pregnancy may be denied, particularly if unplanned, because of the woman's ambivalence regarding motherhood.

- *Limited Finances.* Financial constraints or limited health insurance may discourage a woman from securing prenatal care.
- *Inaccessibility of the Health Care System.* An inconvenient location of the health care facility, lack of transportation, or fear of the health care system may make it difficult for a woman to obtain prenatal care.

Today many women have jobs outside the home both for financial reasons and for professional accomplishment. In two income families, partners share childrearing responsibilities, and the male partner is expected to be active in the care and nurturing of offspring. Our concept of *family* has expanded to include nontraditional households, such as same sex relationships, single parent families, and cohabitation.

The advent of consumerism in health care also has influenced our concept of pregnancy.[2] Current biostatistics indicate that the typical American couple will have one or two children. Many women/couples make a conscientious effort to have a healthy pregnancy, and therefore couples with the availability of modern medical technology have greater expectations for a healthy pregnancy and infant. Ultimately, this raises legal and ethical demands on health care providers, particularly in obstetrics and gynecology.[3]

Clients as consumers have come to expect an optimal outcome in pregnancy, and preconception counseling has become common. Throughout pregnancy, women may question the safety of various activities and the effects of substances on the developing fetus. Women and their partners are also increasingly included in the decision-making process, and frequently they participate in community prenatal classes. All of these changes make for a different experience of pregnancy and parenthood for today's women.

## PLANNING FOR A HEALTHY PREGNANCY

### PRECONCEPTION COUNSELING

Interest in preconception education and counseling began in the 1980s in the United States. In evaluating new information and reconsidering older data, many health care providers became convinced that pregnancy may be too late for expectant parents to correct unhealthy habits. A National Institutes of Health and Human Services expert panel reviewed the factors that contribute to good pregnancy outcomes for women and infants, and subsequently recommended that prenatal care begin prior to conception, preferably within 1 year of a planned pregnancy.[2] The status of a woman's health can influence not only her ability to conceive, but also her ability to maintain the pregnancy.[4]

At the time of conception, a woman should be in an optimal state of emotional and physical health. Health educators and health care providers have concluded that this directly improves pregnancy outcomes.[1] The goal of preconception care and counseling is to maximize the health of the woman and the health of her potential infant.[1] Ideally, preconception counseling is accompanied by a complete gynecologic evaluation. Prior to conception, prospective parents have an opportunity to make informed decisions and ultimately to make lifestyle adjustments to maximize their chances of a successful outcome in pregnancy.[5]

#### Counseling/Learning Methods

A healthy lifestyle can be promoted through individual counseling during routine gynecologic examinations, community adult health education programs, or traditional classes with content directed toward prospective parents. Although current studies do not demonstrate that preconception education in the classroom directly influences perinatal outcomes, new information can be acquired during these sessions.[6] Demonstrated statistical changes in the ultimate outcome for pregnancy may not be available for several generations of infants, thus long term goals such as parental behavior changes and improved health status in someday parents needs to be the guiding philosophy for marketing these classes.[3]

Reva Rubin investigated the relationship between social support and pregnancy outcomes and found that the mother's ability to identify with the developing fetus fostered attachment to the child. Hence, the quality of the social support given to a woman during pregnancy correlates positively with maternal–fetal attachment.[3] In addition, enhancing a parent's knowledge about fetal growth and development promotes intrauterine bonding and subsequent parenting skills. These concepts reinforce the importance of programs directed toward preconception health promotion.[7]

Nonpregnant couples may not feel compelled to attend preparation classes; therefore, tools must convey the importance of preconception education and the potential for improved perinatal outcomes. Information should focus strongly on maternal and fetal health and the timing of pregnancy, and how these factors influence a couple's life plan.[2] The normal physiological changes associated with pregnancy and their affect on the woman's body and self-image, and legal/ethical issues, such as genetic and diagnostic testing, are other subjects that need to be covered in these classes. Moreover, pertinent information about commun-ity agencies and family services should be provided for those in need of follow-up support.[8]

## PRECONCEPTION ASSESSMENT DATA

Preconception care and counseling are valuable in identifying risks in the client's medical history and current health status, and their potential impact on a pregnancy. Assessment includes history-taking and a physical examination, often augmented by laboratory/diagnostic testing.[5]

### Subjective Data

During the gynecologic evaluation, obtain a detailed medical, social, reproductive, and family history. By identifying problems early, it is sometimes possible to resolve them prior to conception and ultimately improve the obstetric outcome.[2]

A comprehensive screening tool, such as the Preconceptional Health Appraisal, can facilitate risk assessment with prospective parents.[9] This appraisal includes a checklist of 53 items that assess the health status of the prospective mother. Through it, information specific to the client's family, medical, reproductive, and drug histories can be obtained. Nutrition and lifestyle choices also can be evaluated.

In addition, it is important to assess human immunodeficiency virus (HIV) risk factors. These factors include history of homosexual activity, intravenous drug use, multiple sexual contacts, blood or blood product transfusion, or close contact with bodily fluids.

### Objective Data

***Physical Examination.*** A complete physical examination is needed, with special emphasis on the systems identified during the risk appraisal. A thorough pelvic examination should also be performed, including a Papanicolaou (Pap) smear, cultures for gonorrhea and chlamydia, and a wet smear evaluation.[2]

***Diagnostic Tests and Methods.*** These include rubella titer and antibody screen, serology for syphilis, complete blood cell (CBC) count with indices, blood type/Rh, random blood sugar, and urinalysis.[5] Hemoglobin electrophoresis may be performed if sickle cell or thalassemia status is of concern. Screening for viral disease, such as HIV, hepatitis, cytomegalovirus (CMV), or toxoplasmosis, can be offered.[5]

Provide instruction in basal body temperature (BBT) assessment and charting to interested couples (see Chapter 7).

## CLIENT EDUCATION AND COUNSELING

Preconception counseling and intervention for the client and her partner should focus on the following areas.[2]

- *Menstrual Cycles.* Advise the client to keep an accurate record of her menstrual cycles in order to help establish gestational dating.
- *Adequate Exercise and Nutrition.* A vitamin/mineral supplement is often recommended to increase maternal nutrition stores. In September 1992 the U.S. Public Health Service Centers for Disease Control announced new recommendations regarding folic acid supplementation in the periconceptional period. These advise all women of childbearing age to consume 0.4 mg of folic acid per day for the purpose of reducing the risk of a neural-tube-defect affected pregnancy. Women with a history of an affected pregnancy are at particular risk in each subsequent pregnancy, and thus may also benefit from supplementation during the periconceptional period.[10] Encourage overweight or underweight clients to attain an ideal weight prior to conception. Beginning an exercise program prior to pregnancy will hopefully improve cardiovascular status and impart a feeling of overall well-being into the pregnancy as well. Exercise may also help the overweight woman attain close to ideal and ideal weight, thus lessening the potential for problems, such as diabetes and hypertension, in the pregnancy.
- *Avoidance of Teratogens.* Warn the client that potential teratogens can be related to occupation and lifestyle, for example, cleaning solutions, hair colors/perms, photography solutions, radiation, and chemicals used in processing food and textiles.
- *Affirmation of Pregnancy Decision.* Stress that the couple needs time to affirm the decision to attempt pregnancy.
- *Readiness for Parenthood.* Assess the couple's social, financial, and psychological readiness for pregnancy and commitment to parenthood.
- *Identification of Unhealthy Behaviors.* Assist the couple to identify and alter unhealthy behaviors, such as smoking, alcohol consumption, and drug use (i.e., prescription, over-the-counter, and illegal drugs).
- *Treatment of Jeopardizing Conditions.* Ensure that medical conditions which may jeopardize the pregnancy outcome are evaluated. Refer the couple to a specialist as needed.
- *Identify Genetic Risk.* When risks are identified, refer the couple for genetic counseling and laboratory testing to determine carrier status (see Figure 12–1).
- *Effective Professional Relationship.* To encourage the client's early entry into prenatal care, initiate and nurture a positive professional relationship.
- *Preconception Classes.* Where appropriate, refer the couple to community adult educational resources for preconception classes (e.g., March of Dimes).
- *Laboratory Tests.* Order all appropriate laboratory tests, evaluate the results, and

Name ____________________ Patient # ____________________ Date ____________

1. Will you be 35 years or older when the baby is due? Yes ___ No___

2. Have you, the baby's father, or anyone in either of your families ever had any of the following disorders?
   - Down syndrome (mongolism) Yes ___ No___
   - Other chromosomal abnormality Yes ___ No___
   - Neural tube defect, spina bifida (meningomyelocele or open spine), anencephaly Yes ___ No___
   - Hemophilia Yes ___ No___
   - Muscular dystrophy Yes ___ No___
   - Cystic fibrosis Yes ___ No___

   If yes, indicate the relationship of the affected person to you or to the baby's father: ____________

3. Do you or the baby's father have a birth defect? Yes ___ No___
   If yes, who has the defect and what is it? ____________________

4. In any previous marriages, have you or the baby's father had a child, born dead or alive, with a birth defect not listed in question 2 above? Yes ___ No___
   If yes, what was the defect and who had it? ____________________

5. Do you or the baby's father have any close relatives with mental retardation? Yes ___ No___
   If yes, indicate the relationship of the affected person to you or to the baby's father: ____________
   Indicate the cause, if known: ____________________

6. Do you, the baby's father, or a close relative in either of your families have a birth defect, any familial disorder, or a chromosomal abnormality not listed above? Yes ___ No___
   If yes, indicate the condition and the relationship of the affected person to you or to the baby's father: ____________________

7. In any previous marriages, have you or the baby's father had a stillborn child or three or more first trimester spontaneous pregnancy losses? Yes ___ No___
   Have either of you had a chromosomal study? Yes ___ No___
   If yes, indicate who and the results: ____________________

8. If you or the baby's father is of Jewish ancestry, have either of you been screened for Tay-Sachs disease? Yes ___ No___
   If yes, indicate who and the results: ____________________

9. If you or the baby's father is black, have either of you been screened for sickle cell trait? Yes ___ No___
   If yes, indicate who and the results: ____________________

10. If you or the baby's father is of Italian, Greek, or Mediterranean background, have either of you been tested for ß-thalassemia? Yes ___ No___
    If yes, indicate who and the results: ____________________

11. If you or the baby's father is of Philippine or Southeast Asian ancestry, have either of you been tested for $\alpha$-thalassemia? Yes ___ No___
    If yes, indicate who and the results: ____________________

12. Excluding iron and vitamins, have you taken any medications or recreational drugs since being pregnant or since your last menstrual period? (Include nonprescription drugs.) Yes ___ No___
    If yes, give name of medication and time taken during pregnancy: ____________________

*Note:* Any patient replying "YES" to questions should be offered appropriate counseling. If the patient declines further counseling or testing, this should be noted in the chart. Given that genetics is a field in a state of flux, alterations or updates to this form will be required periodically.

**Figure 12–1.** Sample prenatal genetic screen. *(Source: The American College of Obstetricians and Gynecologists.* Antenatal Diagnosis of Genetic Disorders. *ACOG Technical Bulletin #108. Washington, DC ©1987.)*

discuss the findings and their implications with the client.

- *Appropriate Vaccinations.* If the client is not immune to rubella, administer the vaccine and advise the client to wait 3 months before attempting conception. Also vaccinate for tetanus and hepatitis when indicated.
- *Special Dietary Needs.* If the client has special dietary needs (e.g., vegetarian, cultural, overweight, underweight), refer her to a dietician.

## ASSESSMENT DURING PREGNANCY

Well woman's health care during pregnancy begins with a complete history and thorough physical examination during the initial visit. The initial visit is the ideal time to screen for particular risk factors suggesting preterm delivery or other poor outcomes (see Risk Assessment, later in this chapter).

The health care provider and the client establish the foundation of a trusting relationship by jointly developing a plan of care for the pregnancy. This plan is tailored to the client's lifestyle preferences as much as possible and focuses primarily on education for overall wellness during pregnancy. The ultimate goal is early detection and prevention of potential problems in the pregnancy.

Return office visits include physical evaluation of the client and her fetus, client education, and the continuation of a holistic approach to pregnancy care. (Nursing diagnoses that might be established during this period are listed at the end of this chapter.)

### SIGNS AND SYMPTOMS OF PREGNANCY

Signs and symptoms that may be reported by the pregnant client are traditionally categorized into three groups, defined below and summarized in Table 12–1.

- *Presumptive.* Signs or symptoms frequently reported with pregnancy, although not conclusive for pregnancy.
- *Probable.* Signs or symptoms that are more reliable indicators of pregnancy, often noted on the physical examination or with laboratory testing.
- *Positive.* Signs or symptoms noted when absolute confirmation of pregnancy is made.

Although these signs and symptoms assist in confirming pregnancy, they *cannot* enable the health care provider to differentiate an intrauterine pregnancy from an ectopic pregnancy.

### OVERVIEW OF INITIAL PRENATAL VISIT

During the initial visit, the health care provider performs a complete assessment and counsels the client about risk factors and prenatal care. Several components are included.[12]

- *Confirmation of Pregnancy.* Perform a beta-human chorionic gonadotropin (β-hCG) urine test; if negative, retest using a radioimmunoassay (RIA) β-hCG serum test (see Table 12–5 on page 358).
- *History.* Obtain a complete medical, psychosocial, family, and reproductive history (see Chapter 3). Several areas require more in-depth evaluation during pregnancy.[13]
  - Menstrual history.
  - Contraceptive history.
  - Gynecologic history.
  - Sexual history.
  - Surgical history.
- *Physical Examination.* (See Chapter 3.) Assess the client's vital signs and perform a complete head-to-toe examination with

**TABLE 12-1. SIGNS AND SYMPTOMS OF PREGNANCY**

| Presumptive | Probable | Positive |
|---|---|---|
| Amenorrhea. | Abdominal enlargement. | Auscultation of fetal heart sounds. |
| Breast tenderness and enlargement. | Ballottement. | Palpation of fetal movements. |
| Chadwick's sign. | Braxton-Hicks contractions. | Radiological and/or ultrasonic verification of gestation. |
| Fatigue. | Goodell's sign. | |
| Hyperpigmentation. | Hegar's sign. | |
| Chloasma. | Palpation of fetal contours. | |
| Linea nigra. | Positive pregnancy test. | |
| Fetal movements (quickening). | Uterine enlargement. | |
| Urinary frequency. | | |
| Nausea/vomiting. | | |

*Source: Adapted from reference 11.*

particular attention to the pelvic evaluation. Establish the client's baseline cervical status and perform clinical pelvimetry if it is part of the protocol in a particular setting. Testing the adequacy of the pelvis, if unproven by previous vaginal delivery, includes measurement of the diagonal conjugate from the posterior inferior edge of the symphysis pubis to the sacral promontory (normally 12.5 cm or greater), which estimates the inlet; the transverse diameter of the midpelvis includes evaluation of the ischial spines (sharp or blunt and degree of prominence) and of the anteroposterior diameter by the shape of the sacrum (curved or flat). The ischial tuberosities should be 8 cm or more apart.[13]

- *Laboratory Tests.* Perform routine laboratory tests (Table 12–2) and additional testing as needed (Table 12–3).
- *Risk Assessment.* Refer the client for a thorough risk assessment test as indicated (see pages 357–362).
- *Prenatal Educational Materials.* Provide and review information about prenatal classes, nutrition, exercise, teratogens, sexuality, and choices in infant feeding.
- *Sexuality During Pregnancy.* See discussion below.
- *Schedule Follow-Up Visits.* Discuss the importance of continued prenatal care and work out a schedule for follow-up visits.

## SEXUALITY DURING PREGNANCY

### Physiological Changes

Table 12–4 gives a summary of physiological changes that may enhance pleasure or diminish a woman's sexual response during pregnancy. Opportunities arise to review the physiological changes that influence sexuality both during the initial prenatal visit and during subsequent visits.

### Psychosocial Changes

Pregnancy is often a time of profound emotional and developmental upheaval and can present a developmental crisis for both partners. Sexuality during pregnancy can be affected directly. The health care provider's role involves providing anticipatory guidance through sexuality education and assessment,

**TABLE 12-2. ROUTINE TESTS TO BE PERFORMED ON ALL PREGNANCY CLIENTS[a]**

| |
|---|
| ABO blood group/Rh factor identification. |
| Complete blood cell count with indices (Hb, Hct, MCV, MCH, MCHC). |
| Rubella titer. |
| Syphilis screening/VDRL, RPR. |
| Hepatitis screening. |
| Urinalysis. |
| Chlamydia screening. |
| Gonorrhea screening. |
| HIV screening (based on risk identification). |

[a]Values may vary according to the laboratory used.
*Note*: Hb = hemoglobin; Hct = hematocrit; MCV = mean corpuscular volume; MCH = mean corpuscular hemoglobin; MCHC = mean corpuscular hemoglobin concentration; VDRL = Venereal Disease Research Laboratories test; RPR = rapid plasma reagin; HIV = human immunodeficiency virus.
*Source: References 12, 13.*

both at the initial prenatal evaluation and during subsequent visits. Several concerns are often reported.[14,15]

- Fear of causing miscarriage or harm to the developing fetus.
- Need for modifications in positioning for coitus with advancing gestation.
- Fluctuating libido by both partners and the resulting effect on coital desire.
- The woman's perceived loss of attractiveness to her sexual partner.
- Misinformation and misconception regarding sexuality, safety; the impact of religious taboos.
- A declining desire for intimacy as the woman withdraws or focuses on infant preparation.

### Guidelines for Intervention

Take a sexual history early in the pregnancy to establish baseline information about both partners. To the extents that medical findings allow, give permission for the couple to be sexually active during and after pregnancy.

### Contraindications to Sexual Intercourse

The following conditions may preclude sexual relations during a portion of the pregnancy.[14,15]

- History of repeated miscarriage.
- History of cervical incompetence, without cerclage.
- Current possibility of threatened abortion.
- Placenta previa.
- Undiagnosed vaginal bleeding.
- Premature rupture of membranes, preterm labor.
- Severe vulvar varicosities.

## SUBSEQUENT PRENATAL VISITS

At each subsequent prenatal visit, measure the client's weight and blood pressure; assess fetal movement; evaluate the client's urine

**TABLE 12-3. ADDITIONAL TESTS PERFORMED ON THE BASIS OF THE PREGNANT CLIENT'S HISTORY[a]**

| |
|---|
| α-fetoprotein. |
| Antibody screening. |
| Blood chemistry. |
| Cytomegalovirus titer. |
| Fifth disease titer. |
| Glucose tolerance tests. |
| Group beta strep culture. |
| Hemoglobin A1C. |
| Hemoglobin electrophoresis. |
| Herpes culture. |
| Serum iron studies. |
| Toxoplasmosis titer. |
| Thyroid studies. |
| Urine culture. |
| Tuberculin skin test. |

[a]Values may vary according to the laboratory used.
*Source: References 12, 13.*

**TABLE 12-4. PHYSIOLOGICAL CHANGES IN PREGNANCY THAT INFLUENCE SEXUALITY**

| First Trimester | Second Trimester | Third Trimester |
|---|---|---|
| Fatigue and lethargy. | Increased pelvic congestion. | Physical discomfort, backache. |
| Nausea and vomiting. | Increased vaginal moisture. | Increasing uterine irritability. |
| Breast tenderness. | | Excessive pelvic congestion. |
| Abdominal bloating. | | Vulvar/femoral varicosities. |
| Increased urination. | | |

*Source: References 14, 15.*

for blood, protein, ketones, nitrites, and glucose; determine fundal height; and assess fetal heart tones. Also at each visit, evaluate any client complaints and answer questions appropriately. Later in pregnancy, Leopold's maneuvers should be performed to determine fetal presentation and position.[1] Include the partner when possible in auscultation of fetal heart tones and palpation of fundal height changes. Review with the couple the common discomforts of pregnancy and how they may influence sexuality. Encourage the partner's participation in the labor and delivery process to improve his ability to empathize during the postpartum period. As appropriate, offer the couple suggestions about coital positioning and frequency, foreplay, and alternate forms of intimacy.

### Weeks 12 to 16

Review laboratory findings with the client and her partner. If appropriate order genetic testing, such as amniocentesis or α-fetoprotein serum.

### Weeks 16 to 20

Assess for fetal movements (quickening). Ultrasound evaluation may be performed to confirm gestational age and assess fetal well-being. Encourage the couple to enroll in prenatal classes.

### Weeks 24 to 28

Reevaluate the antibody screen titer. Perform glucose screening for gestational diabetes. Administer RhoGAM immune globulin as indicated. Reactions to RhoGAM [$Rh_o$(D) immune globulin] are infrequent, mild, and primarily at the injection site. An occasional person may react more strongly. A few women may experience a slight temperature elevation. Retest hemoglobin and hematocrit. Evaluate the client for risk of preterm labor and perform a cervical assessment including cervical position, consistency, length and dilation.

### Weeks 28 to 32

Offer the client counseling regarding the choice of a pediatrician. Assess the client's breasts and discuss preparation for breastfeeding. Discuss the importance of daily fetal movement as an indicator of fetal well-being.

### Weeks 32 to 34

Reassess the client for risk of preterm labor; assess the cervix as indicated.

### Weeks 34 to 36

Review with the client the signs and symptoms of labor; provide a handout listing them.

### Weeks 36 to 40

Assess fetal position and presentation. Review and negotiate the client's birth expectations. Forward a copy of the client's prenatal records to the hospital labor area for future reference. Document the client's final choice of a pediatrician. Initiate fetal surveillance as indicated. A cervical examination may be performed per the protocol of the institution.

### Week 40 and Beyond

Prepare the client for postdate pregnancy protocol. Perform a cervical assessment. Institute fetal surveillance, such as ultrasound, nonstress testing, and biweekly office visits.

## PROGRESSING PHYSICAL CHANGE

Several changes commonly occur during pregnancy.[1]

- *Skin.* Increased vascularity; increased pigmentation of face (chloasma), areola, abdomen (linea nigra), and genitalia; striae of breasts and abdomen.
- *Head.* Mild changes in scalp; excessive oiliness or dryness.
- *Eyes.* Vessel dilation in the sclera.
- *Mouth.* Edematous, friable gums.
- *Chest/Cardiovascular.* Increased respiratory effort and rate; progressive elevation of the diaphragm; hand/pedal edema by third trimester.
- *Breasts.* Increased fullness, tenderness, and enlargement; and excretion of colostrum are common by the third trimester.
- *Heart.* Exaggerated heart sounds, particularly functional murmurs in systole.
- *Abdomen.* Distention secondary to flatus and increased uterine size; diminished bowel sounds as peristaltic movements are slowed; enlarging uterus, which displaces abdominal organs.
- *Genitalia/Reproductive*
  - *External.* Increased pigmentation; pubic hair may lengthen. Near term, pelvic congestion and overall swelling of labia majora are common; vulvar varicosities may be noted.
  - *Vagina.* Increased pelvic congestion and hypertrophy; rugation of vaginal mucosa is prominent.
  - *Cervix.* Positive Chadwick's sign (bluish/purple color) is noted; may soften, dilate, and efface close to term. Positive Goodell's sign (softening with growth of cervical glands) may be noted.
  - *Uterus.* Positive Hegar's sign (softening of the lower uterine segment) often present by 6 weeks' gestation. Uterine enlargement occurs in linear fashion (1 cm per week). At 12 weeks' gestation the fundus is noted at the symphysis pubis; at 16 weeks' gestation the fundus is midway between the symphysis and the umbilicus. By the 36th week the fundus is just below the ensiform cartilage; the fundal height drops slightly near term (lightening). The uterus maintains a globular/ovoid shape throughout pregnancy.
  - *Adnexa.* Discomfort may be noted with exam due to stretching of the round ligaments throughout pregnancy. The ovaries are not palpable once the uterus fills the pelvic cavity at 12 to 14 weeks' gestation.
  - *Urinary.* The bladder may be palpable; incontinence is common, particularly with multiparity.
  - *Rectal.* Increased vascular congestion with resulting hemorrhoids is often noted.
- *Musculoskeletal.* Increased relaxation of pelvic structures; lordosis; sciatica (common).
- *Endocrine.* May have mildly enlarged

thyroid; however, diffusely enlarged thyroid nodularity or increased firmness is abnormal.

## DIAGNOSTIC TESTS AND METHODS

To assess the development of the fetus and the well-being of the mother, the health care provider may use a variety of invasive and noninvasive tests.

### Pregnancy Tests[16,17]

It is important to diagnose pregnancy as early as possible to maximize the benefits from health care and minimize risks to the developing fetus. (See Table 12–5 for a description of pregnancy tests.)[16,18]

*Human chorionic gonadotropin (hCG)* is detected in pregnancy at about the time of implantation. Levels in normal pregnancy usually double every 48 to 72 hours; by the first missed period, serum values reach 50 to 250 mIU per mL. Levels peak at approximately 60 to 70 days postfertilization, then decrease to plateau at 100 to 130 days of pregnancy. Tests vary in sensitivity, specificity, and accuracy—influenced by the length of gestation, concentration of specimen, proteins or blood present, and some drugs. Human chorionic gonadotropin is composed of alpha and beta subunits. The alpha subunit of hCG reacts with the alpha subunits of luteinizing hormone (LH), follicle-stimulating hormone (FSH), and thyrotropin (TSH) due to similar molecular structure. Tests that are specific for beta subunit are more accurate; serum tests are generally more sensitive and specific than urine tests.

Quantitative, serial measurements of serum *beta-human chorionic gonadotropin (β-hCG)* are valuable in documenting the viability of the gestation. Serum and urine tests specific for β-hCG have accuracy rates of 99 percent, with few false positives. With urine testing, early gestational age and decreased specimen concentration often yield false negatives (Table 12–5).

Technological advances in *ultrasonic imaging* (see Chapter 15) have enabled accurate evaluation or monitoring of several aspects of pregnancy.[1]

- Early identification of intrauterine pregnancy and or multiple pregnancy.
- Demonstration of growth and viability of the embryo.
- Identification and evaluation of uterine, fetal, and placental anomalies.
- Serial measurements to evaluate fetal growth.
- Evaluation of amniotic fluid levels.

Commonly recommended tests are described in Tables 12–6 and 12–7.[1,13,16,19,20]

## ASSESSMENT OF COMMON CONCERNS

The pregnant client may report common concerns in a multitude of areas. These concerns are mainly physical (see Chapter 13) and may include nausea and vomiting, fatigue, backache, constipation, and edema. Psychological/developmental concerns (see Chapter 13) may include changes in libido, emotional lability, and nightmares.

## RISK ASSESSMENT

Assessment of an obstetric client for risk factors encompasses physical, historical, and psychosocial aspects. The client at risk is identified, evaluated, and observed, with special consideration given to the course and outcome of pregnancy. Screening is done to detect genetic defects, to determine the risk of preterm labor and delivery, and to assess parental–fetal attachment and hazards in the environment and workplace. Screening should ideally be done at the initial visit, dur-

**TABLE 12-5. PREGNANCY TESTS**

| Type | Specimen Source | Sensitivity (mIU/mL) | Example | Comments |
|---|---|---|---|---|
| Beta Subunit Radioimmuno-assay (RIA). | Serum | 5 | Used mainly in hospitals and large outpatient laboratories. | Radioisotopes.<br>*Uses:* Quantifies β-hCG. Serial measurements useful in determination of pregnancy viability, trophoblastic disease, ectopic pregnancy.<br>*Specificity:* For β-hCG. No cross-reaction with LH, FSH, TSH.<br>*Reliable:* 7 days post-conception.<br>*Time:* 1 to 2 hours, usually run in batches. |
| Enzyme-linked immunosorbent assay (ELISA); immunometric test. | Serum urine | 25–100 | Tandem Icon QSR (Hybritech), cards (Pacific Biotech), First Response (Tambrands). | Monoclonal antibodies; enzyme coupling.<br>*Uses:* Serum tests quantify β-hCG and hCG. Same as RIA if β-hCG specific; urine tests qualify β-hCG.<br>*Specificity:* No cross-reaction with LH, FSH, TSH if β-hCG specific.<br>*Reliable:* 7 to 10 days post-conception.<br>*Time:* 3 to 80 minutes. |
| Agglutination inhibition test. | Urine | 150–2500 | Pregnospia (Organon), UCG-Beta Slide (Wampole), β-hCG (Ortho), Pregnosticon (Organon.) | Agglutination of coated latex particles and hCG antibodies. Positive if no agglutination occurs.<br>*Uses:* Qualifies pregnancy.<br>*Specificity:* Varies; if β-HCG specific, no cross-reaction to LH, FSH, TSH. Sensitivity set at higher levels to decrease cross-reaction in test to whole hCG molecule.<br>*Reliable:* 14 to 21 days post-conception.<br>*Test:* 2 to 60 minutes. |

*Source: References 16–18.*

**TABLE 12-6. LABORATORY AND DIAGNOSTIC TESTS OFTEN PERFORMED DURING PREGNANCY**

| Test | Nonpregnant Values | Pregnant Values | Implications for Mother/Fetus |
|---|---|---|---|
| *Cervix-Vagina* | | | |
| Chlamydia | Negative | Negative | Culture remains gold standard for diagnosis; neonatal infection; implicated preterm labor. |
| Gonorrhea | Negative | Negative | Culture remains gold standard for diagnosis; neonatal infection; implicated in preterm labor. |
| Group beta strep | Negative | Negative | May be considered normal vaginal flora in a client who is not pregnant; however, neonatal infection can be fatal; implicated in preterm labor. |
| Herpes simplex genitalis | Negative | Negative | Neonatal infection can be fatal. Implicated in preterm labor and spontaneous abortions. |
| Listeria | Negative | Negative | Strong association with intrauterine fetal demise (IUFD); preterm delivery. Congenital defects not widely noted. Found in unpasteurized dairy products. |
| Mycoplasma | Negative | Negative | May be considered normal vaginal flora in a client who is not pregnant; however, implicated in spontaneous abortions; controversial rare cause of anencephaly. |
| *Serology* | | | |
| Antibody | Negative | Negative | Positive screen indicates sensitization; done at initial and 28th week visits, and after maternal fetal blood exchange in Rh-negative woman. |
| Cytomegalovirus | Negative | Stable titer | Majority demonstrate immunity; maternal immunity does not prevent congenital infection; primary infection is more severe for fetus; cytomegalic inclusion disease is evident in 10 percent of those affected; overall fetal morbidity, cost factors, predictability of occurrence/recurrence limit use of this testing. |
| Hepatitis | Negative | Negative | If positive screen to $HB_sAg$ or $HB_cAg$, IgM titer to assess active, chronic, convalescent states; the presence of anti-$HB_c$ IgG indicates previous infection; anti-$HB_s$ is positive only in those with successful vaccination; transplacental transmission is rare; neonatal infection can occur. |
| Rubella | Immunity greater than 1:10 | Stable titer | If nonimmune, vaccinate postpartum, delay if breastfeeding; infection during first trimester associated with high rates of spontaneous abortion and congenital malformation. |
| Syphilis | Nonreactive | Nonreactive | If reactive, perform FTA-ABS test or MHA-TP to confirm presence of *Treponema pallidum* organism; if woman is untreated, approximately 25 percent of offspring die in utero, 25 percent perinatally/neonatally, 40 percent develop syphilis; long-term sequelae beginning in newborn. |
| Toxoplasmosis (IgG titer) | Negative | Stable titer | If positive, repeat titer in 2 weeks; more virulent if new infection during first trimester, but less frequent; less than 10 percent of infected infants display disease; for woman with risk of exposure to seropositive cats or uncooked meat and eggs. |

(*continued*)

**TABLE 12-6. CONTINUED**

| Test | Nonpregnant Values | Pregnant Values | Implications for Mother/Fetus |
|---|---|---|---|
| *Serology (cont.)* | | | |
| Type/Rh | A+ A-<br>B+ B-<br>O+ O-<br>AB+ AB- | | If Rh negative, screen for antibodies; ABO incompatibility usually result of O woman carrying an A or B fetus; degree of hemolysis is usually mild. |
| Fifth disease (erythema infectiosum) | Immune | Stable titer | Parvovirus B19; controversial rare cause of nonimmune hydrops; 50 percent of women are immune. |
| *Hematology* | | | |
| Red blood cell count | 3.5–5.5/mm$^3$ | | Stable during pregnancy. |
| White blood cell count | 4.5–11/mm$^3$ | 5–12/mm$^3$; may increase | Values of up to 25 mm$^3$ have been noted during labor. |
| Hematocrit | 37–47 percent | 28.6–38.4 percent | Decreased values reflect overall 50 percent increase in plasma volume—physiological anemia. |
| Hemoglobin | 12–16 g/dL | 11–16 g/dL | Increased oxygen carrying capacity of red blood cells compensates for volume expansion. |
| Platelets | 250,000–500,000/mm$^3$ | | May decrease with severe preeclampsia. Rule out immune thrombocytopenic purpura (ITP). |
| Hemoglobin A1c | 4.0–8.2 percent | 6.5 percent | Measure of long term glucose control in identified gestational diabetic; changes are seen in 3–5 weeks after optimal diet and insulin control; not accurate in diabetics with chronic renal failure or disease that impairs erythrocytes. |
| Hemoglobin electrophoresis | HgbA1 96–98.5 percent;<br>HgbA2 1.5–4.0 percent;<br>HgbF 0–2.0 percent | | Detects amounts of hemoglobin normally found and presence of HgbS HgbC; diagnosis of trait and disease is dependent on percentage of types to HgbA; screen all African American, Mediterranean, Asian women; occasionally noted in white population. |
| *Blood Chemistry* | | | |
| Alkaline phosphatase | 12–63 IU/L | May double | Elevated in liver conditions; increases due to placental involvement; in diseases involving connective tissue. |
| Blood urea nitrogen (BUN) | 10–15 mg/dL | 8–10 mg/dL | Pregnant values are lower due to increased glomerular filtration rate. In pregnancy induced hypertension (PIH), values increase to nonpregnant levels due to pathological arterial spasm and vasoconstriction. |
| Cholesterol | 130–200 mg/dL | 243–305 mg/dL | Accurate levels not reflected in pregnancy. |
| Creatinine | 0.8 mg/dL | 0.5–0.7 mg/dL | Pregnant values are lower due to increased glomerular filtration rate. In PIH, values increase to nonpregnant levels due to pathological arterial spasm and vasoconstriction. |

**TABLE 12-6. CONTINUED**

| Test | Nonpregnant Values | Pregnant Values | Implications for Mother/Fetus |
|---|---|---|---|
| *Blood Chemistry (cont.)* | | | |
| Iron—serum | 60—160 μg/dL | Decrease | Iron demands increase during pregnancy. |
| Lactate dehydrogenase (LDH) | 30–200 IU/L | | Elevated in various conditions, especially those with tissue destruction, hypoxia, or an inflammatory process; seen in heparin therapy. |
| Serum alanine aminotransferase | 3–35 IU/L | | Used primarily to monitor the liver; may increase in severe preeclampsia. |
| Serum aspartate aminotransferase | 5–40 IU/L | May decrease | Elevated in conditions where cardiac or hepatic damage occurs; also elevated post IM injections; may also be depressed in diabetic ketoacidosis (DKA) and beriberi. |
| Thyroid panel: triiodothyronine ($T_3$) | 24–35 percent | Decrease | Due to increase of thyroid binding globulins by estrogen. |
| Thyroxine ($T_4$) | 5.3–14.5 μg/dL | Increase | Basal metabolic rate increases by 25 percent; increased thyroid binding globulins. |
| Thyrotropin (TSH) | 0.5–10 μU/mL | | Most sensitive indicator for hypothyroid/hyperthyroid states in pregnancy. |
| Total iron binding capacity (TIBC) | 250–460 μg/dL | Increase | Estrogen increases ability for iron to bind to transferrin, which regulates transport in the body. |
| Uric Acid | 4.2–6.0 mg/dL | 3.0–4.2 mg/dL | Pregnant values are lower due to increased glomerular filtration rate. In PIH, values increase to nonpregnant levels due to pathological arterial spasm and vasoconstriction. |
| *Urinalysis* | | | |
| Albumin | Negative | Less than 100 mg/24 h | Elevations seen in preeclampsia and urinary tract infections. |
| Chloride | 170–250 mEg/24 h | Slight increase | Due to increased glomerular filtration rate. |
| Creatinine | 1.0–1.8 g/24 h | Elevated | Due to increased glomerular filtration rate. |
| Glucose | 120 g/24 h | Elevated | Due to decreased renal threshold and increased glomerular filtration rate. |
| Ketones | Negative | Same | Presence may indicate dehydration; starvation states; ketoacidosis in insulin-dependent diabetic. |
| White blood cells | Less than 1–3 per high power field | Same | Often vaginal contamination, urinary tract infection if other indicators. |
| Red blood cells | Less than 2–3 per high power field | Same | May be due to violent exercise kidney trauma, systemic or renal disease. |
| Bacteria | Greater than 100,000 colonies/mL | Greater than 10,000 colonies/mL | Infection if same species. |

*Note*: $HB_sAg$ = hepatitis B surface antigen; $HB_cAg$ = hepatitis B core antigen; Ig = immunoglobulin; FTA-ABS = fluorescent treponemal antibody absorption; MHA-TP = microhemagglutination assay for antibody to *Treponema pallidium*.
*Source: References 13, 16, 19, 20.*

**TABLE 12-7. ADDITIONAL TESTS OFTEN CARRIED OUT DURING PREGNANCY**

| Test | Values | Significance | Implications |
|---|---|---|---|
| α-fetoprotein (AFP) | Less than 0.4 MOM (multiples of the mean) | At risk for Down syndrome (experimentally) | Relative to maternal weight, age, race, gestational dating, diabetic status. |
| | 0.4–2.5 MOM | Normal range is 85–95 percent | Margin of error is 5–15 percent. |
| | Greater than 2.5 MOM | At risk for neural tube defect | All abnormal values should be evaluated selectively by ultrasound, fetal scan, and amniocentesis; identified strong family/maternal history of neural tube defect. |
| Fasting blood sugar (FBS) | 70–105 mg/dL | ≥105 mg/dL elevated | Not valuable in healthy pregnancy. |
| 1-hour glucose tolerance test (GTT) | 135–140 mg/dL | ≥140 mg/dL elevated | Suspicious for diagnosis of gestation diabetes. Screening done at 24–28 weeks' gestation; screen earlier if H/O[a] 4000-g infant, history of gestational diabetes, or previous fetal death. Diagnostic of gestational diabetes. |
| 3-hour GTT | | | |
| FBS | 70–105 mg/dL | ≥105 mg/dL elevated | Requires fasting prior to testing. |
| 1 h | 120–190 mg/dL | ≥190 mg/dL elevated | Elevated FBS is indicator of probable need for insulin therapy. |
| 2 h | 120–165 mg/dL | ≥165 mg/dL elevated | Criterion: Requires treatment if 2 of the 4 values are elevated. |
| 3 h | 70–145 mg/dL | ≥145 mg/dL elevated | |

[a]H/O = history of.
*Source: References 1, 13, 16, 20.*

ing each remaining trimester, and whenever necessary.

## Genetic Screening

The purpose of genetic screening is to identify those at risk for an inherited or acquired defect and to identify unrecognized defects in healthy individuals.[16] It is estimated that 3 to 5 percent of infants in the United States have recognizable defects present at birth. Another 4 to 5 percent will reveal defects by 1 year of age, and 6 to 7 percent by age 7.[16,21] Approximately 25 percent of birth defects are attributed to genetic factors, 15 percent to environmental factors, 30 percents to a combination of these—leaving 30 percent unaccountable. It is estimated that 50 percent of spontaneous abortions and 5 to 7 percent of intrauterine fetal deaths are caused by chromosomal abnormalities.[16,21] Clients with potential risks (Figure 12–1) should receive further counseling, testing, education, and guidance in decision making.[22]

***Tools for the Detection and Diagnosis of Genetic Defects (Also See Chapter 15)***

- *Family Pedigree.* A graphic record of family medical history may reveal an inheritance pattern and help to identify whether further laboratory testing and clinical evaluation are needed.[23]
- *Alpha-fetoprotein.* Levels of α-fetoprotein circulating in maternal serum or amniotic fluid are reflective of gestational age, maternal age, weight, race, presence of diabetes, or previous history of neural tube defects.[23]
- *Amniocentesis.* Fluid aspirated from the amniotic sac has multiple test applications such as chromosome analysis, karyotype, α-fetoprotein, deoxyribonucleic acid (DNA) markers, viral studies, biochemical linkage assays, and inborn errors of metabolism.[23]
- *Chorionic Villus Sampling.* Transcervical aspiration of chorionic villi permits results for the same test as does amniocentesis, with the exception of α-fetoprotein results.[23]
- *Level 2 Ultrasound/Fetal Scan.* Indirect visualization of the fetus enables evaluation of overt, structural changes; it is usually performed in a tertiary setting.[23]
- *Fetoscopy.* Direct visualization of the fetus and placenta allows for tissue sampling or limited interventions with the fetus in life threatening situations. Fetoscopy has become rarely used since the advent of recombinant DNA techniques and amniocentesis. The risk of miscarriage with fetoscopy is 3 to 5 percent higher than with amniocentesis or chorionic villus sampling.[13]

## Preterm Labor Screening

The demographic, historical, and psychosocial factors associated with increased incidence of preterm labor and delivery are assessed with preterm screening. *Preterm labor* is the presence of regular uterine contractions causing cervical dilation and effacement prior to 37 completed weeks' gestation. The etiology of preterm labor is unknown. Current estimates are that preterm labor occurs in 7 to 15 percent of women.[13] Perinatal morbidity/mortality increase as length of gestation decreases. Even with the most advanced technology, outcomes are poor for gestations of less than 26 weeks.[24] Long term sequelae such as chronic respiratory and neurological handicaps, blindness, learning disabilities, and financial strain are often reported.[16] Parental emotional and financial strain may be significant.

The incidence of preterm labor and delivery may be reduced by early identification of risk factors, continuous assessment of physical changes, education, and treatment that reduces controllable risk factors. A screening tool is illustrated in Table 12–8.[25] If one or more major factors, or two or more minor factors, are present, the client is identified as belonging to a high risk group. (For further information on diagnosis and treatment, see Chapter 14.)

## Assessment of Parental–Fetal Attachment

Assessing parental–fetal attachment may help to identify a family at risk for maladaptive behaviors in relation to the developmental tasks of pregnancy. The major developmental task for the family is achieving a strong sense of self (differentiation), while maintaining psychological and physical closeness (attachment). Another task is establishing a safe environment for the family unit.[26]

Major risk factors for maladaptive behaviors are unplanned pregnancy, marital discord or family violence, sexually transmitted disease, limited finances, substance abuse, positive HIV status, and adolescence. Other risk factors include poor social support system and educational background, compli-

**TABLE 12-8. MAJOR AND MINOR RISK FACTORS IN THE PREDICTION OF SPONTANEOUS PRETERM LABOR**

| Major | Minor |
|---|---|
| Multiple gestation. | Febrile illness. |
| Diethylstilbestrol (DES) exposure. | Bleeding after 12 weeks' gestation. |
| Hydramnios. | History of pylonephritis. |
| Uterine anomaly. | Cigarette smoking—more than 10 per day. |
| Cervix dilated more than 1 cm at 32 weeks' gestation. | Second trimester abortion. |
| 2 second-trimester abortions. | More than 2 first-trimester abortions. |
| Previous preterm delivery. | |
| Previous preterm labor. | |
| Abdominal surgery during pregnancy. | |
| History of cone biopsy. | |
| Cervical shortening of less than 1 cm at 32 weeks' gestation. | |
| Uterine irritability. | |

*Note:* Presence of one or more major factors and/or two or more minor factors places client in high risk group.
*Source: Creasy, R., & Resnick, R. (1989).* Maternal–fetal medicine: Principles and practice. *(2nd ed.). Philadelphia: Saunders. Printed with permission.*

cated pregnancy, or conditions that interfere with the ability to reason effectively.[16,27,28] *All* women have the potential for maladaptive behaviors during pregnancy; therefore, interventions are directed toward reducing the effect of situations that lead to maladjustment.

Family assessment tools may provide a means for identifying women at risk for less than optimal maternal–fetal and maternal–infant attachment.[26]

- *The Family Environment Scale* uses self-reporting to assess the internal family milieu.
- *The Card Sort Procedure* measures how family members relate to one another through a group problem-solving task.
- *The Support System Questionnaire* assesses the support system within the family, assesses outside influences on the family, and identifies family members at perinatal risk.[26]

## Assessment of Environmental and Occupational Hazards

The environmental and occupational factors that place mother and fetus at risk for injury or death need to be identified. Women of childbearing age comprise a significant proportion of the U.S. work force. Women are exposed to chemicals and infectious agents, demanding labor, and often less than ideal working conditions. Assessment should be made of the possible exposure to teratogens, physical demands of employment, and the workplace environment.[16,29]

*Teratogens* are substances or disorders with the potential to alter the fetus permanently in form or function.[23] Strongly suspected teratogens include various drugs, chemicals, infectious agents, and selected maternal disorders. Often the effect is dose related; the effect is greatest during fetal organogenesis (see Chapter 13).

Physically intensive employment increases the likelihood of low birthweight and preterm labor and delivery. Standing for long periods; increased pulling, pushing, or lifting of more than 10–25 pounds; and decreased rest periods also increase these risks.[16,29] The physical setting needs to be assessed for risks of falling or being crushed; exposure to temperature extremes; and exposure to teratogens such as radiation, chemicals, or infectious agents.[30]

Recommended favorable working conditions for pregnant women[30] include:

- Work only 8-hour shifts: no more than 48 hours per week, ideally less than 40 hours per week.
- Limit hours of work to between 6 A.M. and midnight.
- Take at least two 10-minute rest periods and one nutrition break per shift, with adequate rest facilities available.
- Avoid occupations that involve heavy lifting, hard physical labor, continuous standing, or constant moving about.
- Do not work in places where a good sense of balance is required for job safety, or where there is exposure to toxic substances.
- Be aware that substances permissible by state codes for a nonpregnant individual may be *unsafe* for a pregnant woman and a developing fetus. The Occupational Safety and Health Administration (OSHA) can answer questions about specific substances and situations (see Chapter 13).

## PSYCHOSOCIAL ASSESSMENT AND INTERVENTIONS[31]

During the first trimester, assess the meaning of pregnancy to the client and the positive, negative, or ambivalent feelings she may have, particularly if her pregnancy is unplanned. Explore her feelings about this pregnancy, her economic concerns, and her level of anxiety. Validate the pregnancy with and help her to identify her support systems. Suggest childbirth education classes; begin anticipatory guidance counseling (see Chapter 13).

During the second trimester, assess the client's adaptation to pregnancy and to the body changes she has experienced. Explain how fetal growth/development and the client's own body/emotional changes will facilitate adaptation.

During the third trimester, determine how well the client is prepared for birth, delivery, and the physical needs of a newborn. Explore her expectations about labor, birth, and the newborn—and her fears concerning motherhood, pain of labor, loss of control, and harm to herself or the fetus. Begin planning for postpartal contraception.

## DIETARY ASSESSMENT

A well balanced diet is essential to optimal nutrition for maternal well-being and fetal growth (see also Chapter 13.) Requirements during pregnancy include daily servings of dairy products, meat products, fruits/vegetables, and grains/bread. Routine dietary supplements also are required during pregnancy.

It is always desirable that maternal weight gain and fetal growth be adequate; that appropriate weight be achieved by the neonate, depending on gestation age; that labor and delivery do not occur preterm; and that the mother be normotensive with stable hemoglobin. However, inadequate nutrition may place the client at risk for having a low birthweight infant, preterm labor, pregnancy induced hypertension, and anemia with resulting sequelae.[1]

### Nutrition Counseling

The pregnant woman's diet should include 1800 to 2400 kcal and 75 to 100 g protein per day. A woman who is of ideal weight at conception should gain 24 to 28 pounds; a woman who is 20 percent over ideal weight should gain 15 to 20 pounds; and a woman who is 10 percent under weight should gain 30 to 35 pounds. Teach the client about how to maintain a balanced diet from the basic food groups. Advise her to limit nonnutritional foods and snacks, especially those high in sodium. Explain the rationale for good nutrition in terms of maternal/fetal growth demands and the results of poor nutrition. Clients maintaining special diets due to a medical condition or a religious, cultural, or taste preference require special counseling.

## PREPARATION FOR SURGICAL INTERVENTION

Complications related to fetal distress and failure for labor to progress at delivery are the primary reasons for surgical intervention. Surgical options include cesarean section, episiotomy, and forceps delivery.[13,16] Maternal medical conditions unrelated to pregnancy, such as appendicitis, also may necessitate surgery. Counsel clients at risk about the reasons for an episiotomy at delivery and the care involved; and discuss cesarean birth with clients whose medical conditions predispose them to this type of delivery. For those needing forceps delivery, instruction is given at the time of delivery. *Providing in-depth education concerning surgical intervention to clients not at risk may add to their anxiety level.*

### Cesarean Birth

Any condition that prevents the safe passage of the fetus through the birth canal or that seriously compromises maternal–fetal well-being may be an indication for cesarean birth.[16] Examples include breech and transverse presentations, maternal–fetal hemorrhage, fetal distress, severely impaired maternal cardiac status, cephalopelvic disproportion, and placenta previa.

***Implications.*** It is estimated that 1 out of 5 deliveries in the United States is by cesarean section. Several factors may explain the increase that has occurred.[16]

- Reduced parity with greater numbers of nulliparous women.
- Electronic fetal monitoring (EFM), which facilitates detection of fetal distress.
- Repeat cesarean deliveries, usually with prior classical incision.
- Fewer forceps deliveries.
- More advanced-age pregnancies.
- Greater threat and incidence of legal malpractice suits.

Surgery is done under regional or general anesthesia with combination cold-knife, electrocautery techniques.[16] Vaginal birth after cesarean section (VBAC) is common today, as most surgeons employ a low transverse uterine incision to deliver the infant. The vertical, or classical, incision requires that cesarean section be done for subsequent births, as it is more likely to rupture during active labor.[16]

***Side Effects and Adverse Reactions.*** The side effects of a cesarean section are related to infection, hemorrhage, embolus, injury to proximal organs, and anesthesia. Studies in maternal mortality statistics vary, with approximately 5 per 100,000 cesarean births.[16] Select studies show substantially lower rates of maternal mortality related to the cesarean section itself.[16]

***Contraindications.*** Vaginal delivery is preferred in cases of maternal coagulopathies, or when the fetus has died or is too premature to survive outside the uterus.[16]

***Counseling.*** Inform the client about the procedure and its rationale, anesthesia, recovery, and postoperative care. Explain how the surgery will affect the newborn, breastfeeding, and activities of daily living. Also explain that signs of infection/complication will be monitored.

## THE DEVELOPMENTAL STAGES OF PREGNANCY

Maternal role attainment is not an inevitable, instinctive event initiated by the act of birth; instead it is an active process requiring personal motivation.[26] It is believed that the "roots" of this role develop during childhood. During pregnancy a woman actively works on assuming the behaviors she believes encompass the "ideal" mother.[26]

### MAJOR THEORIES OF MATERNAL ROLE DEVELOPMENT

Two leading theorists in maternal role development are Reva Rubin and Regina Lederman.

Reva Rubin's contributions to maternity nursing provide valuable insights into the biopsychosocial experience of childbearing. Rubin developed a framework for the process of maternal role assumption in 1967, although she published from 1961 to 1984. Her early publications "Basic Maternal Behaviors" and "Maternal Touch" are considered classics in maternity nursing.[33]

Rubin's writings include concepts about body image, self-esteem, and thought process during pregnancy, as well as assumption of the maternal role prior to and after delivery.[33] Without the desire for children, there is no active motivation to assume a maternal role. Rubin identified maternal tasks and behaviors normally seen during the antepartum and postpartum periods. Assessment of those behaviors can be used to evaluate the mother's progress toward assumption of a maternal role (see Table 12–9).[26,33,34] Rubin concluded that if the mother perceived a threat to her pregnancy, such as HIV infection or miscarriage, then she was less likely to bond with her infant and therefore was at risk for poor attachment.

When Rubin made her initial observations of maternal behaviors, strong consumer participation in childbirth education and health care was in its infancy. Today, childbearing couples have the option of knowing the gender of their fetus, see their fetus through the technology of ultrasound, and are more knowledgeable and less passive than parents of previous generations. Ultimately, some of Rubin's observations may have less relevance for contemporary women, but they are a timeless framework for family-centered maternity care. Using Reva Rubin's three postpartum developmental phases, a mother's progress during the postpartum period may be assessed. (The three phases and their characteristic behaviors are described in Table 12–10.[26,33,35])

Regina Lederman views maternal role assumption as identification with motherhood; namely, as part of the larger process of psychosocial development in pregnancy that includes taking the developmental step from being a woman without child to being a woman with child.[36] This process is a progressive change in thinking for the mother, away from concerns about self and more toward concern for the mother–infant unit. Two important factors come into play to achieve this goal: motivation and the degree of preparation for the mothering role.

According to Lederman, motivation for motherhood is reflected by the degree to which one expresses the interest and the ability to nurture and empathize with a child. This encompasses the perception of motherhood as a life-fulfilling event.[36] The woman's motivation for pregnancy is questioned if her

**TABLE 12-9. REVA RUBIN THEORY: THE ANTEPARTUM PHASE**

| Trimester | Maternal Task/Behavior | Nursing Significance |
|---|---|---|
| First | "Who me?"<br>"Pregnant?"<br>"Now?" | Question of identity—conception thought to be a surprise—resulting ambivalence related to the reality of pregnancy. |
| | | Incorporation of concept of fetus into self. |
| | | Acceptance of pregnancy/fetus by self and significant others. |
| Second | Seeking safe passage for self and child. | Acceptance of growing fetus by self, others. |
| | Ensuring the acceptance of the child. | Willingness to "house" fetus even with body/role/ego changes. |
| | Protective behaviors by the mother for the child. | Passage of socially accepted values, behaviors, attitudes, skills from mother to child. |
| Third | Mother's binding-in to her unknown child.<br>Learning to give of self. | "Binding-in" developed from initial maternal–fetal bonds to adult–child companionship. These bonds include fetal movements, maternal anatomic changes. |
| | | Nurturant behaviors given from mother to child. |

*Source: References 26, 34, 35.*

thoughts toward the child (fetus) are infrequent, aversive, avoided or denied, or if the woman desires the pregnancy but not the child.

Preparation for motherhood involves acquiring the ability to see oneself as a mother.[36] This is accomplished through *fantasizing/dreaming*, which is an arena for rehearsing motherhood skills. The woman relies on her life experiences of being nurtured, and on her ability to identify with other women in their positive role as mothers. According to Lederman, all women bring conflicts to a pregnancy. But if the conflicts are not resolved through preparation and bargaining during pregnancy, then the woman may find the motherhood role unrewarding, thereby increasing her feelings of inadequacy.

Lederman describes a woman's relationship with her own mother as the final aspect of maternal role development. The availability of the client's own mother, her acceptance of that pregnancy, her respect for the daughter's autonomy, and her willingness to share her previous childbearing/childrearing experiences all impact the outcome of preparation.[36]

Rubin's and Lederman's frameworks are generally considered compatible, although they use different names for similar concepts. Absence of these processes or inability to pass through them satisfactorily may impede the progress of maternal role development.[26,33,35] This recognition is fundamental for nursing assessment during pregnancy and the postpartum period.

*Implications of Rubin's and Lederman's Theories*

- Identify whether the client is at higher risk for maladaptation at initial and ongoing prenatal visits.
- Monitor the client's progress by observing for expected role behaviors.
- When maladaptive behaviors are identified, refer the client for appropriate counseling.

**TABLE 12-10. REVA RUBIN THEORY: THE POSTPARTUM PHASE**

| Phase | Behaviors |
|---|---|
| Taking in | Passive, receptive, dependent infant mode; sleep, food are paramount. Often thought to be a process of regeneration. Mother spends time claiming her infant, bringing the infant into her social fabric. Mother begins with initial touching activities: first fingertips then to whole-hand touching within days 1 to 5 postdelivery. |
| Taking hold | Increased autonomy, independence usually begin on third day postpartum. Characterized by accomplishing what *must* be done over the next 2 to 3 weeks of the postpartum period. Mother demonstrates mastery of her own body's functioning, readiness to master some of her many tasks of motherhood. |
| Letting go | Starts during second and third weeks postdelivery. Mother begins to separate herself from the symbiotic relationship she and her infant enjoyed during pregnancy/delivery. Prior to this point, guilt was predominate feeling for the mother when separated from her infant. |

## PREPARATION FOR CHILDBIRTH: COUNSELING AND CLASSES

The prospect of having a problem-free pregnancy and healthy baby is aided by early and complete prenatal education. Maternal expectations of labor and delivery based on prenatal experience/knowledge are predictive of postpartum maternal–infant attachment. The primary goal of childbirth education classes is to reduce the fear–pain–tension cycle and make the childbirth experience a positive one—and thereby facilitate maternal–infant attachment.[12]

Prior to the 19th century, childbirth was a social event, centered in the home with family members and friends. That changed, but by the 1960s women began to question the extensive procedures and strong medications often used for hospital managed labor and delivery. Women began to change the rigid structure of medical practice.

Society was finally ready for the 1944 classic by Grantley Dick-Read, *Childbirth without Fear*, which espoused that the pain of labor could be eliminated by reducing the fear, apprehension, and tension associated with childbirth. The underlying principle behind childbirth education is that the woman can use skills and intellect to control her body during childbirth.[36]

### STRATEGIES FOR PREPARATION

In *childbirth preparation classes*, accurate information is provided about the physiological and psychological adaptations that occur during parturition. Only information pertinent to managing labor and delivery process is included. In *prenatal parenting classes*, on the other hand, discussions may include a variety of topics surrounding parenting. In addition, comprehensive formats may be presented as refresher courses. How many clients pursue some form of prenatal education with their first baby is not known.

The education may be sought in a traditional classroom, from a resource book at the library, or from group sessions organized by local health departments. Programs are also offered by hospitals, community agencies and groups, or individuals qualified to teach childbirth education. The participation of health care providers and obstetric staff nurses as educators is desirable to ensure con-

**TABLE 12-11. SUBJECTS COMMONLY COVERED IN PRENATAL CLASSES**

| |
|---|
| Anatomy and physiology of reproduction. |
| Physiological and psychological changes during pregnancy. |
| Sexuality during pregnancy. |
| Nutritional needs. |
| Teratogens and their impact on the fetus. |
| Danger signs in pregnancy. |
| Fetal growth and development. |
| Role of the father and siblings. |
| Prenatal exercise. |
| Signs and stages of labor. |
| Preparation for labor and delivery. |
| Cesarean delivery. |
| Postpartum support groups/parenting skills. |
| Infant care. |
| Infant safety/first aid/cardiopulmonary resuscitation (CPR). |
| Postpartum family planning. |

tinuity of care and consistency of childbirth preparation instruction (see Table 12–11).[12] To help ensure that a client is adequately prepared for childbirth, the health care provider may implement various strategies.[12]

- During the initial prenatal evaluation, encourage enrollment in a prenatal class.
- Provide the client with resources according to her assessed knowledge level and financial ability.
- Provide prenatal counseling on an individual basis during ongoing prenatal visits.
- Supply pertinent pamphlets regarding pregnancy concerns throughout antepartum care.
- Act as role model and client advocate to encourage the client's educational responsibility.
- Periodically evaluate the client's knowledge deficits and intervene when appropriate.

## CHILDBIRTH METHODS

Some couples will need help choosing birth preparation classes; they may be confronted with many alternatives. Childbirth education classes, such as Bradley (partner coached) and Lamaze (psychoprophylactic) techniques serve the dual purpose of explaining the birth process and dispelling fears concerning labor and delivery.

### The Lamaze Method

Classes in the Lamaze method or "prepared childbirth classes" are the most popular. This method uses techniques that focus the mother's attention on breathing and relaxation exercises as well as massage.[12] Consequently, the perception of pain is lessened, as is the amount of medication needed for pain relief. The father's presence and active support during the birthing process can heighten the sense of family at the moment of birth, thereby increasing the perception of a positive birthing experience. Partner or coach involvement is a fundamental cornerstone of both methods.

### The Bradley Method

The primary goal of the Bradley method is a completely unmedicated labor and delivery. The training techniques are directed toward the coach, not the mother. The coach is educated in massage/comfort techniques to use during labor and delivery.[39]

### Other Options

The Read method, or "natural" childbirth, is also based on relaxation and breathing technique; the Wright method, based on psychoprophylaxis but with less active breathing than that in the Lamaze method, is also called "new childbirth." Sheila Kitzinger's psychosexual method includes chest breathing and simultaneous abdominal release. Yoga and hypnosis are other techniques that are used.

In counseling the client regarding the many approaches to childbirth education, it is paramount to consider her readiness to learn, knowledge base, attitudes and fears about pregnancy, and the support systems available to her. It is an ongoing process, begun at the initial prenatal evaluation.

## Adolescent Pregnancy

Adolescent pregnancy is usually defined as pregnancy occurring between the age of menarche and 19 years of age, but it also can be viewed in relation to emotional maturity and financial independence. Most adolescent pregnancy is unplanned. Often adolescent mothers and their babies form a nontraditional family (nontraditional families are discussed later in this chapter). Perinatal/maternal morbidity is significantly higher in pregnancies of adolescent mothers, which is in part due to incomplete maternal growth and the increased psychological needs of adolescent women. "Magical" thinking, feelings of invincibility, and limited abstract thought processes contribute significantly to the incidence of unplanned pregnancy.[16,27,28]

*Facts about Adolescent Pregnancy*[27,28]

- Adolescent pregnancy can be related to cultural norms, peer interaction, immature cognitive abilities, psychological needs, increasing societal acceptance, unprotected coitus, birth control failure or misuse.
- It is estimated that 23 percent of females are sexually active by age 15; 71.4 percent by age 19.
- Less than 40 percent of sexually active adolescents attempt some form of birth control; use is often sporadic.
- Adolescents are typically sexually active for 6 to 12 months prior to seeking birth control services or choosing a method of contraception.
- Among 15- to 19-year-old women, 1 of 10 will become pregnant during a calendar year; among that group (estimated at 1 million), 29 percent will end their pregnancies in abortion. A significant number will conceive again shortly thereafter.
- Many young women deny signs and symptoms of pregnancy, or feel embarrassed to admit their inability to use birth control.

### OBJECTIVE DATA

A physical exam will reveal changes similar to those seen during an adult physical exam, particularly during the breast, abdominal, and pelvic evaluations. Evaluate Tanner staging (see Chapter 3), as young adolescents may be physically immature, which would significantly impact growth and development in pregnancy. A final area of evaluation would be for evidence of eating disorders, substance abuse, or depression.[16,27,28]

### DIFFERENTIAL MEDICAL DIAGNOSIS

Ectopic pregnancy, postpill amenorrhea, polycystic ovary disease, immature hypothalamic–pituitary–gonadal axis with primary amenorrhea, secondary amenorrhea, pseudocyesis, anorexia/eating disorders, ovarian tumors.[1,13]

### NURSING DIAGNOSES

Potential nursing diagnoses include those related to adult pregnancy (see list at the end of the chapter) as well as high risk for altered parenting.[37]

### PLAN

Pregnant adolescents, especially those younger than 16 years, are at risk for having low birthweight infants and preterm births. Moreover, they are at increased risk for cesarean births, in part because of immature skeletal development of the pelvis. Cephalopelvic disproportion results. It remains the primary goal of the health care provider to promote the best possible pregnancy outcome through client evaluation and education. Therefore, focus education on general health maintenance and how pregnancy needs will change health status. The cognitive abilities of adolescents vary, however, as do their abilities to assimilate information. Foster behaviors that will promote independence in adolescent development.[27,28]

Encourage the client to maintain peer interactions and continue to meet educational needs. Help her to clarify the father's role, make use of family support systems, and set realistic goals. Assess the client's cognitive abilities (e.g., concrete versus abstract). Be aware of the increased rate of suicide among adolescents, the risk of substance abuse, and the need to promote a nonjudgmental atmosphere in which the client may express views about the pregnancy.

Health care providers need to assess their own value system, particularly to avoid stereotyping. The foundation for a trusting relationship is based on mutual acceptance, caring, and a nonjudgmental approach. Assisting the client to achieve the developmental tasks of adolescence, such as financial, emotional, and physical independence, is the underlying task for the health provider.[27,28] Remember that despite increasing public awareness and concern, adolescents continue to need support from the community in the areas of wellness, education, finance, and family planning.

## Medication

Stress the importance of *no* medication use without the consent of a health care provider.

## Diet

The adolescent diet is notoriously inadequate. Because of the increased risk for inadequate nutrition, it is imperative to stress the value of daily prenatal vitamins and iron supplementation. Changing body image and the increased demands of fetal growth and development place adolescent mothers at further risk for eating disorders. Careful periodic assessment during prenatal care will aid the health care provider in early detection of inadequate nutrition.

Adolescent dietary needs include 50 kcal/per kg of body weight and 90 to 100 g of protein per day, and a 25- to 30-pound weight gain depending on prepregnant weight.[27,28] Encourage a balanced diet from the food pyramid, and limit nonnutritional foods or snacks. Instruction in good nutrition is related to maternal/fetal growth needs and should reinforce the need for compliance on the part of the adolescent mother.

## Smoking

Although the harmful effects of smoking cigarettes are well documented, adolescents continue to smoke at alarming rates; adolescent females smoke more than adolescent males. Cigarette smoking is highly correlated to early sexual activity; it is often seen as a display of "adult" behavior, rebellion, or peer pressure.

Smoking increases the risk of spontaneous abortion, preterm labor and birth, hypertension, placenta previa/abruptio, low birthweight infants, perinatal death, and long term developmental delays in offspring.[27,28] Direct counseling strategies toward decreasing or cessation of smoking and investigating support groups for that purpose. Education must be appropriate for the client's knowledge level and address both the immediate and long term impact of tobacco on the client and her offspring. Another strategy to help a client stop smoking is to encourage other outlets, such as chewing gum, sugarless candy, handiwork, and exercise.

### Self-Care

Emphasize proper hygiene techniques. Advise the client to avoid contact sports but maintain physical activity by walking, swimming, and participating in prenatal exercise classes. Stress the importance of not consuming chemical substances during pregnancy without knowledge or direction of a health care provider.

### Education

Encourage the client to remain in school during pregnancy or to obtain her general equivalency diploma. Home tutoring and schools for pregnant adolescents are also viable options, although peer interaction is decreased.

### Finances

Financial concerns are heightened if education is interrupted as a result of pregnancy. Three areas of assessment may be helpful: insurance coverage; government assistance through such programs as Women/Infant/Children (WIC) or Aid to Dependent Children (ADC); job benefits (if employed).

### Family Planning

Frequent conception is common with adolescent mothers; as many as 40 to 50 percent conceive again within 24 months. Discuss motivation, maturity, and physical and financial practicality of contraceptive methods. Advise the client to choose a reliable method prior to completion of pregnancy. Explore the client's options for contraception, sexual responsibility, and risk behaviors for sexually transmitted disease.

### Follow-Up

Adolescent mothers are at higher risk for inflicting child abuse, being victims of domestic violence, conceiving frequently, contracting sexually transmitted disease (including HIV), having education disrupted, and having maladaptive peer interaction. Evaluate such situations when they become evident and initiate intervention in areas of greatest concern.

## DELAYED PREGNANCY

Any woman who completes her pregnancy on or after her 35th birthday is referred to as a mother of advanced maternal age.[40] Extensive literature in medicine and genetics has debated whether any significant risks are associated with childbearing after age 35. These risks generally stem from preexisting medical conditions, infertility, chromosomal abnormalities, or nutritional deficits.[41] With proper control of underlying medical conditions, most women can have successful pregnancy outcomes.

Women may delay childbearing for medical or economic reasons, or because of career or personal relationship choices. By postponing childbearing, women have increased their life experiences and psychological stability.[42] This may better equip them to rear children. A major influence on a woman's parenting behavior is the type and number of roles she has undertaken in life. Taking on multiple roles is thought to be either self-enhancing (promoting self-esteem and personal fulfillment) or personally divisive (increasing stress and anxiety).[42] Older mothers may particularly cherish the ability to have children, and if these mothers have higher salaries they may be better able to provide for their children financially.[42] Society encourages increased paternal involvement; consequently, the financial and emotional needs of parenting are shared more by both partners. Furthermore, postponing parenthood or choosing not to have children has gained acceptance.

Delayed parenting is probably influenced to the greatest degree by the increasing availability of effective contraception. Advances in contraceptive techniques have enabled greater freedom to time the birth of the first child. An additional reason for delayed childbearing may be the steady increase in late or second marriages.[41] Moreover, for women who previously suffered from infertility, the prospect of bearing a child has improved with advances in reproductive technology.

### HISTORY AND PHYSICAL EXAMINATION

For women whose pregnancy occurs later in life, the history and physical examination are the same as for other pregnant clients. Pay particular attention to nutritional and immunization status; reproductive, medical, occupational, and social histories; chemical substance use; and genetic concerns. Offer the client referral for genetic counseling and a review of available genetic testing. Identify any occupational hazards.

### DIAGNOSTIC TESTS AND METHODS

The minimum standard tests are needed; medical conditions may require additional individual assessment. The American College of Obstetricians and Gynecologists (ACOG) recommends genetic testing for all women who are 35 years of age or older at the time of delivery. If the client elects genetic testing after counseling has been completed, scheduling for amniocentesis or chorionic villus sampling follows.

### PLAN

Initiate discussions of pregnancy and encourage the client's questions. Several subjects may require review and counseling.[42]

- Normal physiology of pregnancy.
- Pertinent medical history findings.
- Genetic concerns and the testing available.
- Occupational hazards; exposure to teratogens.
- Nutrition and weight control.
- Warning signs in pregnancy; client do's and don'ts.
- Substance use/abuse.
- Exercise, travel, and leisure activities.
- Sexuality.

Make referrals where appropriate and encourage the client to explore educational resources within the community (e.g., prenatal classes). Tailor follow-up visits to pertinent medical findings and individual needs.

## NONTRADITIONAL FAMILIES

The American family has made several remarkable changes in the past 25 years. Today's American families include the "typical" nuclear family and nontraditional families, including one parent households, same sex parents, single-by-choice parents, unmarried heterosexual couples living together, and those choosing to remain childfree. These patterns are the result of profound social and demographic changes in the United States and are becoming increasingly accepted. The contraceptive revolution of the 1960s greatly influenced family structure by changing the role of women. Selective fertility has played a fundamental role in economic shifts within households.

### THE RISKS

Increased stress and maladaptive behaviors are reported among many nontraditional families. For health care providers, particular attention to the client's lifestyle choices may help in identifying her particular needs prior to pregnancy. Often women in nontraditional families have greater financial, education, and legal concerns. They may make many requests of their health care provider or they may feel reluctant to share their private lives. As always, the establishment of a trusting relationship is vital for both health care provider and client.

A higher incidence of the following maladaptive behaviors has been reported among certain nontraditional mothers.[17,43]

- Suicide (adolescents).
- Alcoholism/chemical abuse (lesbians, adolescents).
- Greater dependency on welfare monies (adolescents).
- Domestic violence (nontraditional families).
- Higher incidence of noncompliance with health care advice due to mistrust of "the system" (lesbians, adolescents).

### HISTORY AND PHYSICAL EXAMINATION

History taking during the initial workup is important in identifying nontraditional family units. Several areas need to be explored.

- Sexual preference/practices.
- Legal status of relationship (i.e., paternity).
- Length of relationship and overall support systems for pregnancy.
- Employment setting, income, and how loss of income would impact pregnancy.
- Social ramifications of role modeling as a parent in a nontraditional household.
- Dietary practices (provide nutritional counseling and referral where appropriate).[17,44]

During the initial prenatal examination, carefully observe for signals of physical or chemical abuse (e.g., bruises, unusual marks, history of numerous bone fractures or excessive "accidents"), because women in nontraditional lifestyles are often at risk for maladaptive behaviors.

### DIFFERENTIAL MEDICAL DIAGNOSES

Intrauterine pregnancy, substance abuse, dysfunctional adolescence, battering.[43]

### PLAN

Counseling, support, anticipatory guidance, and education are among the psychosocial interventions.[17]

- Counsel the client about feelings of anger, hostility, fear, anxiety, aversion, and ambivalence throughout the pregnancy.
- Provide a calm, supportive, nonjudgmental environment for improved communication.
- Give anticipatory guidance regarding common stressors of pregnancy, both physical and emotional.
- Counsel about general wellness issues such as hygiene and breast self-exam (BSE), anatomy and physiology, and prevention of sexually transmitted diseases and HIV infection.
- Provide resource/referral information when domestic violence or substance abuse is a potential or identified risk, or when financial concerns are great.

#### Follow-Up

Periodically throughout pregnancy and postpartum, reevaluate the client for continued risk. In addition, periodically evaluate the strength of the client's support systems.

## SUBSTANCE ABUSE SCREENING IN PREGNANCY*

Screening is done to detect the use or misuse of any substance known or suspected to exert a deleterious effect on the client or her fetus.[45] The effects of specific drugs are difficult to assign, because often multiple drugs are used and nutritional status is poor. The use of multiple drugs is associated with intrauterine growth retardation (IUGR) and increased

*The authors wish to acknowledge the contributions of Marion Fuqua, RNC, MS, OGNP to this section.

anomalies. Factors that may impact a drug's effects are duration of use, dosage, timing in gestation, and use of other drugs.[46,47] Ideally, counseling a client concerning substance abuse begins prior to conception. Open discussions may make a client aware of the need to prevent pregnancy and to obtain counseling if necessary. Clients who use substances only occasionally need to be aware of the potential teratogenic effect of one exposure.

Ascertain whether the mother and fetus have been exposed to harmful substances, assess the mother's need for counseling, and design intervention that targets and eliminates the abuse and decreases potential harm to mother and fetus. Being nonjudgmental is a key to success; a client is more apt to trust and reveal patterns of abuse if the health provider does not display dismay or disgust.

Initially the goal of the health care provider is to prevent complications of pregnancy and in utero exposure, thereby minimizing permanent sequelae. Behavioral problems, learning disabilities, and physical anomalies may be present in the newborn. If multigenerational drug use is to be prevented, a link in the chain of addiction must be broken. Getting the client into treatment may help to identify her needs as an individual, teach her how to cope with the stresses that lead to drug use, and perhaps introduce skills for coping and potential parenting. In turn, these measures may enhance parent–child bonding and reduce the incidence of emotional, physical, or sexual abuse and neglect, which are often a common experience among children of substance abusers.[48]

It is important to stop drug abuse during pregnancy to prevent the potential for parents to give their infant or child drugs in food or a bottle as a means of consoling, or for a mother to breastfeed her infant while continuing to use illicit drugs. Accidental ingestion of drugs may occur if drugs are in the house.[48]

## SCREENING QUESTIONS

We have developed questions that may aid the health care provider evaluating a client who is at risk for substance abuse during pregnancy.

1. Have you ever used illegal/recreational drugs? If so, what, when, and how much?
2. Have you ever taken a prescription drug other than as intended? If so, what, when, and how much?
3. Have you used any legal or illegal drugs during this pregnancy? If so, what, when, and how much?
4. What are your feelings about drug use during pregnancy?

## ASSESSMENT

The following overview briefly describes only a few side effects of specific drug use. Further reading is encouraged concerning other substances and sequelae documented in research.

### Smoking

Smoking increases the risk of spontaneous abortion, preterm labor and delivery, maternal hypertension, placenta previa, abruptio placenta, low birthweight infant, perinatal death, and possibly long term developmental delays in offspring.[16,49] Moreover, the perinatal death rate among infants of smoking mothers is 34 percent higher.[50] Central apnea, intrauterine growth retardation, and increased incidence of childhood respiratory infections have been noted.[50] Nicotine reduces fetal blood flow, and this may be related to the transient decrease in fetal movement associated with maternal smoking.[51] The risk of a low birthweight infant appears to be increased if the pregnant woman both smokes and ingests large amounts of caffeine.[52,53] Prenatal exposure and passive exposure after birth may be risk factors for the development of childhood cancers, such as acute lymphocytic leukemia and lymphomas, and sudden infant death syndrome (SIDS).[54,55]

In counseling a client, present measures to decrease smoking cues and behaviors; provide information about support groups for smoking cessation; stress the immediate and long term impact of tobacco use on her and her fetus; encourage her to seek appropriate outlets to replace smoking, such as chewing gum, eating sugarless candy, doing handiwork or exercise.

### Cocaine

Fifteen percent of infants exposed to cocaine in utero later develop SIDS. Genitourinary, gastrointestinal, and cardiac anomalies; intracranial hemorrhage; and neurobehavioral dysfunction are also reported. General growth retardation has been documented.[46,50,56,57] Also associated with cocaine use are abruptio placentae, possibly premature labor and precipitate delivery,[46,57] a higher incidence of first trimester spontaneous abortions, premature rupture of membranes, and meconium passage from the infant. A possible link is also seen between cocaine use and uterine rupture during pregnancy.[58,59] Women who use cocaine may have nearly twice the number of abruptions. Damage done by cocaine to the placenta in the first trimester may continue throughout pregnancy; women who stopped using cocaine after the first trimester had the same rate of abruptio placentae as women who continued to use cocaine throughout pregnancy.[60]

### Alcohol

The leading known cause of mental retardation in the United States is fetal alcohol syndrome (FAS).[62-64] Long term sequelae of in utero exposure to alcohol extends into adulthood with varying degrees of severity. Characteristics of the syndrome include structural anomalies (facial, height and/or weight lags, microcephaly), behavioral problems (hyperactivity, attention deficit disorder, maladaptive behavior), neurological changes (below average intellectual functioning), and growth retardation.[48,64] The most severe complications of FAS during pregnancy are abortion, stillbirth, and abruption.[63,64]

Consuming 1 to 1.5 ounces pure alcohol per day greatly increases the incidence of alcohol related effects; however, no safe amount of alcohol has been established.[63,64]

### Opiates

An increased incidence of SIDS has been found among infants who were exposed to opiates in utero.[50] Intrauterine growth retardation, increased fetal distress, and persistently small fetal head circumference have also been noted.[48,50] Additional teratogenic effects may result if an opiate is "cut" with other substances. When compared with drug-free children, opiate-exposed children had deficits ranging from poor motor performance to hyperactivity and impulsiveness.[48]

A woman's withdrawal from opiates has been associated with fetal demise.[65] Methadone substitution has been successful during pregnancy, but must be used in a closely supervised treatment program.[65]

### Methamphetamines

Methamphetamines produce some of the same effects as cocaine, such as increased risk for abruption, hemorrhage, preterm labor, fetal distress, and intrauterine growth retardation. Evidence exists that exposure may also increase the incidence of cerebral hemorrhage, infarction, or cavitation.[48]

### Marijuana

Among women who use marijuana, a higher risk exists for having a small-for-gestational-age infant (SGA) or a preterm infant, and there is a potential for the child to exhibit anomalies similar to those of a child with FAS.[48] One study reports an increase in acute nonlymphoblastic leukemia if a mother has used marijuana prior to conception and during pregnancy.[48] Mild neurobehavioral changes similar to those of infants with opiate withdrawal have also been noted.[48]

### Toluene

Women who are exposed to toluene have an increased risk for premature delivery and renal tubular acidosis, which results in newborn acidosis. Fetuses have a greater risk for perinatal death and growth retardation.[65] Because toluene crosses the placenta, teratogenicity has been suggested.[66,67] Developmental delays have been noted in children exposed to toluene in utero. They have dysmorphology similar to that seen in children with FAS.[66] Toluene based products, such as glue and spray paint, are easily accessible and inexpensive.

## PHYSICAL EXAMINATION

The physical examination of a woman abusing a chemical substance may reveal fresh needle or track marks, a dazed appearance, inappropriate behavior or affect, extreme agitation or stupor, frequent conjunctivitis, tremors, fetal/maternal tachycardia, or poor maternal weight gain (or weight loss) not attributed to underlying maternal disease.[27] (See Chapters 14 and 18 for evaluation, diagnosis, and treatment.)

## PLAN

Client counseling must continue into the postpartum period. During that time, her problem may worsen if the infant is not feeding, sleeping only for short intervals, crying shrilly, difficult to console, and avoiding eye contact.[48] For some women addicts, fear of legal action may deter them from getting any form of prenatal care, and they may choose to forgo hospital delivery.

A drug screen should be done to identify all drugs that a client is using. Assist the client to enroll in a drug rehabilitation program that offers her ease of accessibility and provides optimum social support. (Be aware that resources for treating pregnant substances abusers are often limited and have long waiting lists.) Management includes dietary counseling, ideally by a nutritionist. The client should be seen perhaps every one to two weeks and begin non-stress tests by 30 weeks' gestation. Serial ultrasounds are indicated to assess fetal growth patterns.[56]

Constant encouragement and motivation are required to reinforce the need for compliance. Be honest about drug effects, but do not humiliate the client. Some women do not see their infant as part of themselves, nor do they care to. Most, however, genuinely do not want to harm their child. Consequently, discussing long term effects may heighten compliance and promote a sense of maternal responsibility for the fetus and infant. Most importantly, clients need to understand and value consistent prenatal care.

## NURSING DIAGNOSES

The following nursing diagnoses are representative of those used in the health care plan of some pregnant women. This list, however, is by no means inclusive.

- Activity intolerance.
- Anxiety.
- Body image disturbance.
- Constipation.
- Decisional conflict.
- Denial, ineffective.

- Family coping compromised, disabling, ineffective.
- Family processes altered.
- Family coping, potential for growth.
- Fatigue.
- Fear.
- Grieving, anticipatory.
- Health seeking behaviors.
- Hopelessness.
- Incontinence.
- Individual coping ineffective.
- Knowledge deficit.
- Noncompliance.
- Nutrition altered, less or more than body requirements.
- Parenting role conflict.
- Parenting altered.
- Personal identity disturbance.
- Physical mobility impairment.
- Powerlessness.
- Protection altered.
- Role performance altered.
- Self-esteem disturbance.
- Sexual performance altered.
- Sleep pattern disturbance.
- Social interaction impaired.
- Social isolation.
- Stress.
- Violence, high risk for, self-directed or directed at others.

## REFERENCES


1. Scott, J., DiSaio, P., Hammond, C., & Spellacy, W. (1990). *Danforth's obstetrics and gynecology*. Philadelphia: Lippincott.
2. Editors. (1989, Summer). Care before conception. *Childbirth Educator, 8*, 16–19.
3. Bushy, A. (1992). Preconception health promotion: Another approach to improve pregnancy outcomes. *Public Health Nursing, 9*, 10–14.
4. Moos, M., & Cefalo, R. (1987). Preconceptional education: A focus for obstetric care. *American Journal of Perinatology, 4*, 63.
5. Jones, T., Johnson, M., Drugan, A., & Evans, M. (1990). Preconceptional planning. *Obstetrics and Gynecology Clinics of North America, 17*, 801–815.
6. Littlefield, V.M. (1986). *Health education for women: A guide for nurses and other health professionals*. Norwalk, CT: Appleton-Century-Crofts.
7. Davis, M., & Akridge, K. (1987). The effects of promoting intrauterine attachment in primiparas on post delivery attachment. *Journal of Obstetric, Gynecologic and Neonatal Nursing, 16*, 430–437.
8. Bushy, A., & Graner, R. (1990). Preconceptional education: A program of community health nurses. *Family and Community Health, 13*, 82–84.
9. Moos, M. (1989). Preconception health promotion: A health education opportunity for all women. *Women and Health, 15*, 55–68.
10. Murphy, P. (1992). Periconceptional supplementation with folic acid: Does it prevent neural tube defects? *Journal of Nurse Midwifery, 37*, 25–32.
11. Holmes, J., & Magiera, L. (1987). *Maternity nursing*. New York: Macmillan.
12. American College of Obstetrics and Gynecology. (1992). *Guidelines for perinatal care*. Washington, DC: Author.
13. Niswander, K. (1992). *Manual of obstetrics: Diagnosis and therapy* (3rd ed.). Boston: Little, Brown.
14. Zalar, M. (1976). Sexual counseling for pregnant couples. *Maternal Child Nursing, 2*, 176–181.
15. Mims, F., & Swenson, M. (1980). *Sexuality: A nursing perspective*. New York: McGraw-Hill.
16. Cunningham, G., MacDonald, P., & Gant, N. (1993). *Williams obstetrics* (19th ed.). Norwalk, CT: Appleton & Lange.
17. Mishell, D., & Brenner, P. (1988). *Common*

*problems in ob/gyn* (2nd ed.). Oradell, NJ: Medical Economics Books.
18. Hatcher, R., Stewart, F., & Trussell, J., Kowal, D., Guest, F., Stewart, G., & Cates, W. (1990–1992). *Contraceptive technology* (15th ed.). New York: Irvington.
19. Pagana, K., & Pagana, T. (1986). *Diagnostic testing and nursing implications: A case study approach*. St. Louis: Mosby.
20. Bakerman, S. (1984). *ABC's of interpretive laboratory data*. (2nd ed.). Greenville: Interpretive Laboratory.
21. Cohen, F. (1984). *Clinical genetics in nursing practice*. Philadelphia: Lippincott.
22. Simpson, J. (1987). *ACOG technical bulletin: Antenatal diagnosis of genetic disorder* (No. 108). Washington, DC: American College of Obstetrics and Gynecology.
23. Berini, R. & Kahn, E. (1987). *Clinical genetics handbook*. Oradell, NJ: Medical Economics Books.
24. Gabbe, S., Niebyl, J., & Simpson, J. (1986). *Obstetrics: Normal and problem pregnancies*. New York: Churchill Livingstone.
25. Creasy, R., & Resnick, R. (1989). *Maternal–fetal medicine: Principles and practice* (2nd ed.). Philadelphia: Saunders.
26. Sherwen, L. (1987). *Psychosocial dimensions of the pregnant family*. New York: Springer.
27. Corbett, M., & Meyer, J. (1987). *The adolescent pregnancy*. Boston: Blackwell Scientific.
28. Goldstein, P., (1990). *ACOG technical bulletin: Adolescent obstetric-gynecologic client* (No. 145). Washington, DC: American College of Obstetrics and Gynecology.
29. Keleher, K. (1991). Occupational health: How work environments can affect reproductive capacity and outcome. *Nurse Practitioner, 16*, 23–37.
30. Jones, J.M., Cox, A.R., Levy, E.Y., & Thompson, C.E. (1984). *Women's health management: Guidelines for nurse practitioners*. Englewood Cliffs, NJ: Prentice-Hall.
31. Perez, R.H. (1987). *Protocols for perinatal nursing practice*. St. Louis: Mosby.
32. Winick, M. (1989). *Nutrition in pregnancy and early infancy*. Baltimore: Williams & Wilkins.
33. Gay, J., Edgil, A., & Douglas, A. (1988). Reva Rubin revisited. *Journal of Obstetric Gynecologic and Neonatal Nursing, 17*, 394–399.
34. Rubin, R. (1984). *Maternal identity and the maternal experience*. New York: Springer.
35. Ament, L. (1990). Maternal task of the puerperium reidentified. *Journal of Obstetric Gynecologic and Neonatal Nursing, 19*, 330–335.
36. Lederman, R. (1984). *Psychosocial adaptation in pregnancy*. Englewood Cliffs, NJ: Prentice-Hall.
37. Carpenito, L.J. (1991). *Handbook of nursing diagnosis* (4th ed.). Philadelphia: Lippincott Company.
38. Lindell, S. (1988). Education for childbirth: A time for change. *Journal of Obstetric Gynecologic and Neonatal Nursing, 17*, 108–112.
39. American College of Obstetrics and Gynecology. (1990). *Guide to planning for pregnancy, birth and beyond*. Washington, DC: Author.
40. Winslow, W. (1987). First pregnancy after 35: What is the experience? *MCN, 12*, 92–96.
41. Barnes, L. (1991). Pregnancy over 35: Special needs. *American Journal of Maternal Child Nursing, 16*, 272.
42. Harker, L., & Thorpe, K. (1992). The last egg in the basket? Elderly primiparity: A review of findings. *Birth, 19*, 23–29.
43. Sanford, N. (1989). Providing sensitive health care to gay and lesbian youth. *Nurse Practitioner, 14*, 30–36.
44. Ziedenstein, L. (1990). Gynecological and childbearing needs of lesbians. *Journal of Nurse Midwifery, 35*, 10–18.
45. Koren, G. (1990). *Maternal-fetal toxicology*. New York: Marcel Dekker.
46. Chasnoff, I. (1991). Cocaine and pregnancy: Clinical and methodologic issues. *Clinics in Perinatology, 18*, 113–123.
47. Little, B., Snell, L., Gilstrap, L., & Johnston, W. (1990). Patterns of multiple substance abuse during pregnancy: Implications of mother and fetus. *Southern Medical Journal, 83*, 507–510.
48. Bays, J. (1990). Substance abuse and child abuse. *Pediatric Clinics of North America, 37*, 881-891.

49. Larson, J. (1987). *Teratology: ACOG bulletin.* Washington, DC: American College of Obstetrics and Gynecology.
50. Hogerman, G., Wilson, C., Thurmond, E., & Schnoll, S. (1990). Drug exposed neonates. *Western Journal of Medicine, 152*, 559–564.
51. Baskett, T., & Liston, R. (1989). Fetal movement monitoring: Clinical application. *Clinics in Perinatology, 16*, 613–625.
52. Alcohol and caffeine use appears to compound LBW risk in smokers. (1991, December). *Ob-Gyn News, 26*, 38.
53. McKim, E. (1991). Caffeine and its effects on pregnancy and the neonate. *Journal of Nurse-Midwifery, 36*, 221-226.
54. John, E., Savitz, D., & Sandler, D. (1991). Prenatal exposure to parents' smoking and childhood cancer. *American Journal of Epidemiology*, 133:123–132.
55. SIDS susceptibility seems to be established in utero, could be tied to maternal smoking. (1991, February). *Ob-Gyn News, 26*, 2–12.
56. Chasnoff, I. (1987). Perinatal effects of cocaine. *Contemporary Obstetrics & Gynecology, 29*, 163–179.
57. Janke, J. (1990). Prenatal cocaine use: Effects on perinatal outcome. *Journal of Nurse-Midwifery, 35*, 74–77.
58. Lynch, M., & McKeon, V. (1990). Cocaine use during pregnancy. *Journal of Obstetric Gynecologic and Neonatal Nursing, 19*, 285–292.
59. Gonsoulin, W., Borge, D., & Moise, K. (1990). Rupture of unscarred uterus in primigravid woman in association with cocaine use. *American Journal of Obstetrics and Gynecology, 163*, 526–527.
60. Dombrowski, M., Wolfe, H., Welch, R., & Evans, M. (1991). Cocaine abuse is associated with abruptio placentae and decreased birth weight, but not shorter labor. *Obstetrics and Gynecology, 77*, 139–141.
61. Chasnoff, I., Griffith, D., MacGregor, S., et al. (1989). Temporal patterns of cocaine use in pregnancy. *Journal of the American Medical Association, 261*, 1741–1744.
62. Streissguth, A., Aase, J., Clarren, S., Randels, S., LaDue, R., & Smith, D. (1991). Fetal alcohol syndrome in adolescents and adults. *Journal of the American Medical Association, 265*, 1961–1967.
63. Welch, R., & Sokol, R. (1991). Detecting risk-drinking. *Contemporary Obstetrics & Gynecology, 4*, 30–40.
64. Piertrantoni, M., & Knuppel, R. (1991). Alcohol use in pregnancy. *Clinics in Perinatology, 18*, 93–111.
65. Hogerman, G., & Schnoll, S. (1991). Narcotic use in pregnancy. *Clinics in Perinatology, 18*, 51–74.
66. Wilkins-Haug, L., & Gabow, P. (1991). Toluene abuse during pregnancy: Obstetric and perinatal outcomes. *Obstetrics and Gynecology, 77*, 504–509.
67. Hersh, J. (1989). Toluene embryopathy: Two new cases. *Journal of Medical Genetics, 26*, 333–337.

CHAPTER 13

# PROMOTING A HEALTHY PREGNANCY

*Maryellen Remich*

*The issues of concern to pregnant women involve safety, comfort, and uncertainty about what to expect during pregnancy, labor, and delivery.*

*Highlights*

- Nutrition and Weight Gain
- Immunization
- Common Complaints
- Anticipatory Guidance
    - *Chemical Use, Radiation*
    - *The Workplace*
    - *Sexual Activity*
    - *Exercise*
    - *Dental Care, Bathing*
    - *Travel*
    - *Accidents, Blows to the Abdomen*
    - *Infant Care*
    - *Sibling Rivalry*
    - *Family Planning*
- Danger Signs: First, Second, and Third Trimesters
- Initial Assessment in Labor

## INTRODUCTION

The ultimate goal of pregnancy is the birth of a healthy infant into a healthy and nurturing family who can provide for his or her physical, psychological, emotional, and spiritual needs. During pregnancy, many normal physiological changes lead to discomfort or concern for the mother. Health care providers must differentiate between normal and pathological changes, educate clients about changes, and help them to recognize and respond appropriately to signs of pathology and labor. In addition, health care providers need to individualize client education about prenatal nutrition and weight gain.

## NUTRITION AND WEIGHT GAIN

Good nutrition before and during pregnancy decreases the risks of significant infant health problems, such as premature birth, low birthweight, malformations, and inadequate cell development. Pregnant women with poor dietary habits are at increased risk for anemia, preeclampsia, obesity, and osteoporosis with associated morbidity and mortality. Women who are underweight or who gain little weight during pregnancy are more likely to have a small-for-gestational-age infant. Women who are obese or whose weight gain is excessive are at risk for hypertension and diabetes. Ideally, issues of nutrition and weight gain should be addressed during preconception counseling (see Chapter 12). Because most women are highly motivated to eat properly during pregnancy, the nutrition instruction that they receive during pregnancy could result in positive lifestyle changes for the entire family.

## SUBJECTIVE DATA

Several points are assessed during the first prenatal interview and reassessed as necessary at subsequent visits.

- Nutrition knowledge
- A 24-hour recall of the client's diet
- Food storage and preparation capacities
- Portion of income spent for food
- Food buying practices
- Cultural and religious preferences
- Food aversions or allergies (e.g., lactose intolerance)
- Prepregnancy weight; percentage of desirable body weight (see Table 13–1)
- Activity level and any change since pregnancy
- Lactation during pregnancy
- Reproductive age (number of years menstruating)
- Gravity and parity (two or more pregnancies within 2 years or five or more total deliveries increase risk of perinatal problems and of maternal health problems, e.g., anemia)
- Megavitamin use
- Nicotine, alcohol, or drug use
- Psychosocial disorders (e.g., depression, bulimia) that may affect food intake
- Discomforts from pregnancy (e.g., dyspepsia) that may affect food intake
- Complications during past pregnancies (e.g., small-for-gestational-age neonate, preterm delivery, perinatal loss, gestational diabetes)[1]

## OBJECTIVE DATA

### Physical Examination

Several findings may indicate nutritional risk.

- Being overweight or underweight
- An abnormal pattern of weight gain (see Figure 13–1).
- An increase in blood pressure (may indicate pregnancy-induced hypertension)
- Nondependent edema (may indicate pregnancy-induced hypertension)
- Angular fissures and cheilosis of the lips (may indicate a riboflavin deficiency)
- Diffusely swollen, red interdental papillae of the gums (may indicate a vitamin C deficiency)
- Filiform papillary atrophy of the tongue (may indicate an iron or folate deficiency)
- Diffusely enlarged thyroid (may indicate an iodine deficiency)
- Follicular hyperkeratosis of upper arms (may indicate a vitamin A deficiency)[1]

### Diagnostic Tests and Methods

- Complete blood cell count (CBC) to screen for anemia
- One-hour 50-g Glucola to rule out gestational diabetes
- Urine dipstick to detect proteinuria (indicative of pregnancy-induced hypertension), glycosuria (indicative of gestational diabetes), and ketonuria (indicative of hyperemesis gravidarum)
- Other less commonly used laboratory assays available to diagnose other nutritional deficiencies (normal values in pregnancy

TABLE 13–1. DESIRABLE WEIGHT FOR HEIGHT: WOMEN 25 YEARS OR OLDER

| Height[a] (in.) | Desirable Weight Range[b] (lb) | Midpoint of Desirable Weight Range (lb) | Less than 90% of Midpoint of Desirable Weight Range (lb) | Greater than 120% of Midpoint of Desirable Weight Range (lb) | Greater than 135% of Midpoint of Desirable Weight Range (lb) |
|---|---|---|---|---|---|
| 58 | 92–121 | 106 | 94 | 128 | 144 |
| 59 | 95–124 | 109 | 97 | 132 | 148 |
| 60 | 98–127 | 112 | 100 | 136 | 152 |
| 61 | 101–130 | 115 | 102 | 139 | 156 |
| 62 | 104–134 | 119 | 106 | 144 | 162 |
| 63 | 107–138 | 122 | 109 | 148 | 166 |
| 64 | 110–142 | 126 | 112 | 152 | 171 |
| 65 | 114–146 | 130 | 116 | 157 | 177 |
| 66 | 118–150 | 134 | 119 | 162 | 182 |
| 67 | 122–154 | 138 | 123 | 167 | 188 |
| 68 | 126–159 | 142 | 126 | 172 | 193 |
| 69 | 130–164 | 147 | 131 | 178 | 200 |
| 70 | 134–169 | 151 | 134 | 183 | 205 |

[a]Height without shoes.
[b]Weight without clothes.
*Source: Reprinted with permission from Gutierrez, Y. (1990). Nutrition protocol. In W.L. Star, M.T. Shannon, L.N. Sammons, L.L. Lommel, & Y. Gutierrez (Eds.),* Ambulatory obstetrics: Protocols for nurse practitioners/nurse-midwives *(2nd ed., pp. 361–377). San Francisco: The Regents, University of California.*

differ from nonpregnant values) (see Table 13–2)[2]

## DIFFERENTIAL MEDICAL DIAGNOSIS

Normal nutrition in pregnancy, ruling out overweight or underweight; anemia; gestational diabetes; drug, alcohol, or nicotine abuse; and complications of pregnancy requiring dietary intervention.

## PLAN

### Psychosocial Interventions

Encourage the client to verbalize any physical and psychosocial problems and explore interventions with her. Interventions for the normal physiological changes that may interfere with a woman's ability to eat an adequate diet are described later in the chapter (see Common Complaints).

### Dietary Interventions

Ask the client to recall her diet during the previous 24 hours; assess its adequacy (see Table 13–3). Assuming the client's dietary intake was adequate before conception and her weight is within a normal range, protein intake should increase by 10 g per day and total kilocalories (kcal) by 200 to 300. Normal weight gain is 24 to 32 pounds (see Figure 13–1).[1,3] Educate the client about the dietary adjustments needed to supply nutrients, tak-

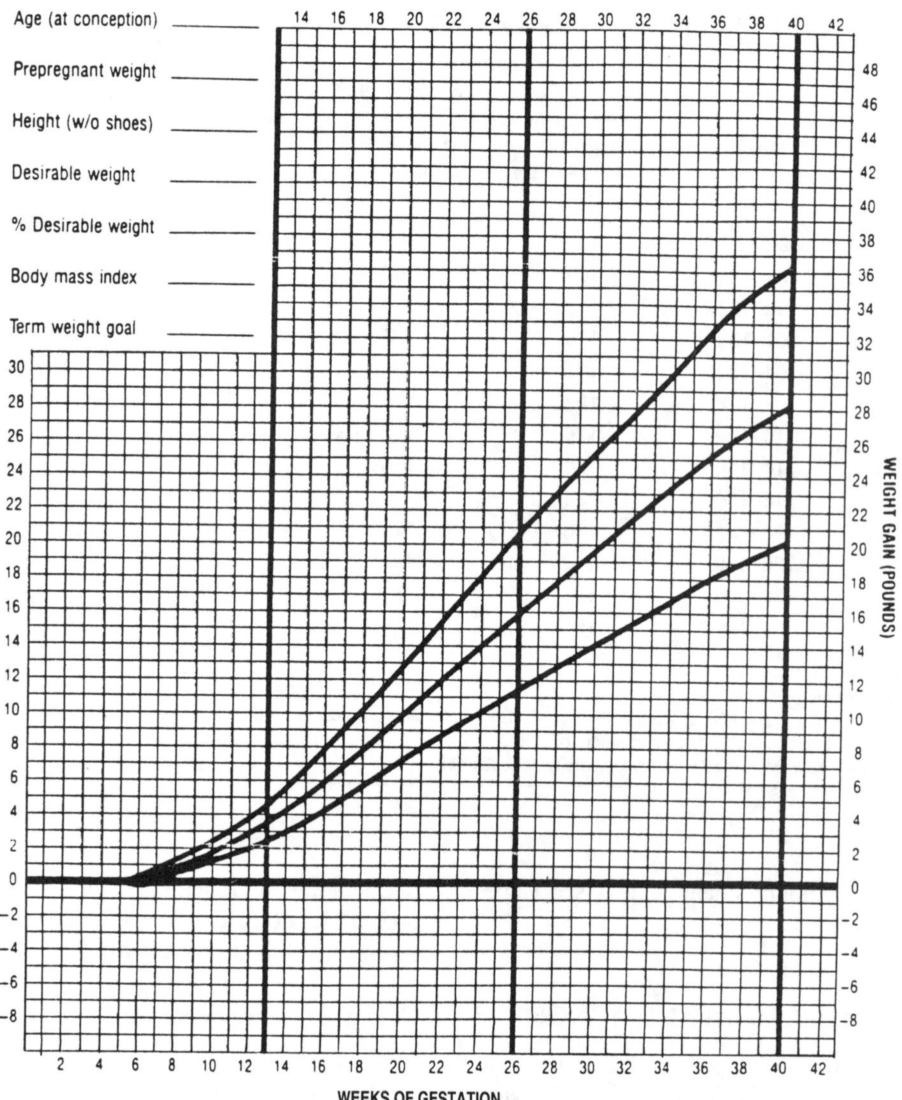


**Figure 13–1.** Prenatal weight gain grid. Total weight gain should be to the top line for underweight clients, about the middle line for normal and overweight clients, and between the bottom and middle lines for obese clients. *(Source: California Department of Health Services. (1989).* Nutrition during pregnancy and the postpartum period: A manual for health care professionals. *Sacramento, CA: Author.)*

**TABLE 13–2. LABORATORY VALUES REFLECTING NUTRITIONAL STATUS DURING PREGNANCY**

| | Normal Range | | |
|---|---|---|---|
| **Laboratory Test** | *Nonpregnant* | *Pregnant* | **Findings in Deficiency** |
| Hemoglobin/hematocrit | >12/36 | >11/33[a] | <11/33[a] |
| Serum folic acid | 5–21 ng/mL | 3–15 ng/mL | <3 ng/mL |
| Serum iron/iron binding capacity | >50/250–400 ng/100 mL | >40/300–450 ng/100 mL | <40/450 ng/100 mL |
| Urinary acetone | Negative | Faint positive in AM | Positive |
| Fasting blood sugar | 70–100 mg/100 mL | 65–100 mg/100 mL | <65 mg/100 mL |
| 2-Hour postprandial blood sugar | <110 mg/100 mL | <120 mg/100 mL | — |
| Serum protein, total | 6.5–8.5 g/100 mL | 6–8 g/100 mL | <6 g/100 mL[a] |
| Serum albumin | 3.5–5 g/100 mL | 3–4.5 g/100 mL | <3.5 g/100 mL[a] |
| Blood urea nitrogen (BUN) | 10–25 mg/100 mL | 5–15 mg/100 mL | <5 mg/100 mL |
| Urine urea nitrogen/total nitrogen ratio | >60 | >60 | <60 |
| Cholesterol | 120–220 mg/100 mL | 200–335 mg/100 mL | — |
| Serum vitamin A | 20–60 ng/100 mL[a] | 20–60 ng/100 mL | <20 ng/100 mL |
| Serum carotene | 50–300 ng/100 mL | 80–325 ng/100 mL | <80 ng/100 mL[a] |
| Serum calcium | 4.6–5.5 mEq/L | 4.2–5.2 mEq/L | <4.2 mEq/L or normal |
| Serum phosphate | 2.5–4.8 mg/100 mL | 2.3–4.6 mg/100 mL | No change |
| Alkaline phosphatase | 35–48 IU/L | 35–150 IU/L | No change |
| Serum ascorbic acid | 0.2–2.0 mg/100 mL[a] | 0.2–1.5 mg/100 mL[a] | <0.2 mg/100 mL[a] |
| Prothrombin time | 12–15 s | 12–15 s | Prolonged |
| Blood thiamine | 1.6–4.0 ng/100 mL | — | Decreased |
| Urinary thiamine | >55 ng/g creatinine | — | <50 |
| Blood lactic acid | 5–20 mg/100 mL | — | Increased |
| Urinary riboflavin | >80 mg/g creatinine | — | <90[a] |
| *N*-Methyl nicotinamide | 1.6–4.3 mg/g creatinine | 2.5–6 mg/g creatinine | <2.5 mg/g creatinine[a] |
| Kynurenic acid excretion | 3 mg/24 h | — | Increased |
| Xanthurenic acid excretion | 3 mg/24 hr | — | Increased |
| Formiminoglutamic acid (FIGLU) | <3 mg/24 h | — | Increased |
| excretion (after 15 g L-histidine) | 1–4 mg/24 h | — | Increased |
| Serum vitamin $B_{12}$ | 330—1025 pg/mL | Decreased | Decreased |
| Methylmalonic acid | <10 mg/24 h | — | Increased |
| Serum calcium | 4.6–5.5 mEq/L | 4.2–5.2 mEq/L | Normal |
| Serum thyroxine ($T_4$) | 4.6–10.7 ng/mL | 6–12.5 ng/mL | Decreased or normal |

[a]Criteria from the Centers for Disease Control. (1972). *Ten state nutrition survey, 1968–1970.* DHEW Publication No. (HSM) 72-8134:72-8133. Washington, DC: U.S.Government Printing Office.

*Source: Reprinted with permission from Aubry, R.H., Roberts, A., & Cuenca, V.G. (1975). The assessment of maternal nutrition.* Clinics in Perinatology, 2*(2), 207.*

**TABLE 13–3. DIETARY PLAN FOR PREGNANCY**

| Food and Serving Size | Servings per Day | Rationale |
|---|---|---|
| *Protein Food* | | |
| Meat, poultry, fish (2 oz)<br>Beans (1 cup cooked)<br>Nut butters (¼ cup)<br>Nuts or seeds (½ cup)<br>Tofu (1 cup)<br>Cottage cheese (½ cup)<br>Eggs (2) | 4 | To build tissues in mother and fetus. These foods contain iron, protein, zinc, and other nutrients. |
| *Milk/Dairy Foods** | | |
| Milk, *all types* (1 cup)<br>Tofu (1 cup)<br>Yogurt (1 cup)<br>Cheese (1.5–2 oz)<br>Nonfat milk powder (⅓ cup) | 4 | To build bones and teeth in fetus. These foods are a major source of calcium, vitamins A & D. (Clients wishing to limit their saturated fat/cholesterol intake should use skim milk products.) |
| *Whole Grains* | | |
| Bread (1 slice)<br>Roll (1)<br>Macaroni, rice, noodles, hot cereal (½ cup)<br>Cold cereal (1 oz)<br>Wheat germ (1tbsp) | 6 | To provide B vitamins, iron, and trace minerals for blood and fetal nerve growth; fiber for bowel function. |
| *Vitamin C Rich Fruits and Vegetables* | | |
| Orange/grapefruit juice (½ cup)<br>Orange (1)<br>Grapefruit (½)<br>Bell pepper (½ cup)<br>Tomato (2)<br>Cantaloupe (½)<br>Broccoli (½ cup)<br>Cabbage (½ cup)<br>Cauliflower (½ cup) | 2 | To provide vitamin C for connective tissue development and resistance to disease. (Avoid juice with added sugar. Smokers have particular need for vitamin C.) |
| *Green Leafy Vegetables* | | |
| Broccoli, brussel sprouts, greens, asparagus, red leaf/romaine lettuce, bok choy, watercress (1 cup raw or ¾ cup cooked) | 1–2 | To provide folacin, iron, fiber, and vitamins E, C, and K. Needed for good eyesight and soft skin. |
| *Other Fruits & Vegetables, Including Those Rich in Vitamin A* | | |
| All fruits and vegetables not listed above and their juices; apples, carrots, green beans, bananas, sweet potatoes (½ cup) | 3 | To promote general health. They contain many nutrients and fiber. Orange and yellow vegetables and fruits are rich in vitamin A. |
| *Fats and Oils* | | |
| Butter, margarine, salad dressing, cream cheese, cooking fats, fatty cheeses | 3 tsp | For energy and healthy skin. They should be used in moderation. |

*Source: Adapted from May, K.A., & Mahmeister, L.R. (1990).* Comprehensive maternity nursing: Nursing process and the childbearing family *(2nd ed.). Philadelphia: Lippincott; and California Department of Health Services (1989).* Nutrition during pregnancy and the postpartum period: A manual for health care professionals. *Sacramento, CA: Author.*

ing into account the client's cultural, religious, and personal preferences, as well as lifestyle and food intolerances and aversions.

High or low activity levels require adjustment of calorie and protein intake. Encourage an ideal weight gain pattern.

Advise clients with lower than optimal intake of calcium to increase their dietary calcium with dairy products, green leafy vegetables, tofu, canned salmon, egg yolks, whole grains, legumes, and nuts. Juices and bread with calcium supplementation have recently become available. A calcium supplement may be necessary. Clients with lactose intolerance may benefit from taking lactose-reducing supplements (e.g., Lactaid), eating lactose-reduced dairy products (yogurt, cheese, milk, or cottage cheese), or eating dairy products in small quantities.

Vegans (strict vegetarians who do not consume egg or dairy products) should eat two to four servings of whole grains and starches, one to two 4-oz servings of legumes, three 4-oz servings of green and yellow vegetables, and three to six pieces of fruit daily; three servings of sea vegetables (e.g., kelp, seaweed, dulse, laver) per week; plus vitamin $B_{12}$ fortified cereals, soy milk, or soy meat products.[4] Although all pregnant women are advised to take prenatal vitamin/mineral supplements, this is even more important for the vegetarian client.

If the client's body weight at conception is above or below her normal range, counsel her to adjust her caloric intake appropriately. Table 13–1 lists the desirable weight range (normal weight), weights that are less than 90 percent of the midpoint of the desirable weight range (underweight), weights that are greater than 120 percent of the midpoint (overweight), and weights that are greater than 135 percent of the midpoint (obese). Recommended weight gain is 28 to 36 pounds if underweight, 24 to 32 pounds if of normal weight or overweight, or 20 to 24 pounds if obese (Figure 13–1 and Table 13–1).[1,3]

Adolescents have nutritional needs not only of the pregnancy but also of their own growth. Pregnant teens 11 to 15 years old require 50 kcal and 1.7 g of protein per kilogram of pregnant body weight and 1600 mg of calcium each day. Pregnant teens 15 to 18 years old require 40 kcal and 1.5 g of protein per kilogram of pregnant body weight and 1600 mg of calcium each day.[3]

For clients with multiple gestations, data indicate that a weight gain of 35 to 45 pounds is ideal.[3] Although recommendations for calorie, protein, or calcium intake are lacking, prudence suggests that increases in these nutrients are needed.

For the client with five or more pregnancies or with pregnancies that are closely spaced, emphasize optimal nutrition in all areas but particularly protein, calcium, iron, and folic acid.

Risk factors for anemia include menorrhagia, vegetarian diet (particularly with the exclusion of eggs), diets lacking red meat or low in vitamin C, multiple gestation, more than three blood donations per year, and chronic aspirin use. Encourage a diet that includes foods high in iron (e.g., liver, lean red meats, oysters, dark green vegetables, peas, iron-fortified cereals, dried beans, and blackstrap molasses). Use of iron pans or skillets to prepare food adds iron to the food.[1,3] Iron supplementation is often recommended.

If the client has been diagnosed with hyperemesis gravidarum, optimal nutrition is essential for the remainder of pregnancy. Weight gains in the second and third trimesters have the greatest impact on fetal growth.[3] In one study, impaired fetal growth was reported if more than 8 pounds of prepregnant weight was lost.[3]

If the client has been diagnosed with intrauterine growth retardation or pregnancy-induced hypertension in the current or a previous pregnancy, optimal protein and caloric intake is essential. Some studies show a possible link between pregnancy-induced hypertension and low calcium intake. Additional investigation is needed.[3]

There are many substances that are very deleterious to both the mother and her fetus/infant. Every effort should be made to assist the woman to stop use of these substances. Referral to appropriate counseling services is warranted. Ideally these interventions should be initiated prior to pregnancy.

Smoking increases one's need for vitamins $B_{12}$ and C, zinc, folate, and amino acids. It has also been suggested that smoking increases metabolic needs. Encourage pregnant clients to stop smoking. For clients who refuse to quit, the diet will need adjustment to compensate for the increased energy and nutrient needs of pregnancy. A prenatal vitamin/mineral supplement is recommended.[3]

Alcoholics frequently have histories of poor dietary intake. Alcohol may also alter the metabolism, absorption, and activation of nutrients. Whether it is the excessive intake of alcohol, or the associated changes in nutrient metabolism, or a combination of these and other factors, the cause of fetal alcohol syndrome (FAS) has not been determined. Unfortunately, if a client has liver disease, vitamin and mineral supplementation may be detrimental. The health care provider must advise the client of the detrimental effects of alcohol intake during pregnancy, encourage her to stop alcohol use, and counsel her to correct nutritional deficits.[3]

Some illegal drugs are appetite stimulants (e.g., marijuana), and others are appetite depressants (e.g., cocaine and crack). Studies are inconclusive as to the effects of drug use on nutrient metabolism, absorption, and activation. Advise the client of the detrimental effects of drug use on the fetus and encourage her to stop the abuse and correct any nutritional deficits.[3]

## Medication

***Prenatal Vitamin/Mineral Supplements.*** Although needed only by those whose diet is inadequate, supplements are usually prescribed for all pregnant women.

- *Administration.* One tablet by mouth each day. The supplement should contain 30 to 60 mg elemental iron, 15 to 20 mg zinc, 2 mg copper, 250 mg calcium (*not* in the form of calcium phosphate), 4 to 10 mg vitamin $B_6$, 20 mg vitamin E, 0.8 to 1.0 mg folic acid, 1 mg vitamin C, and 400 I.U. vitamin D.[1,3]
- *Side Effects and Adverse Reactions.* Gastric upset, constipation, diarrhea.
- *Contraindications.* None are known.
- *Anticipated Outcomes on Evaluation.* The client's hemoglobin level is within normal range, and neither the client nor the infant develops pathology related to vitamin or mineral deficiencies.
- *Client Teaching and Counseling.* Inform the client of the need for a healthy, balanced diet even when taking a prenatal supplement. To maximize the absorption of iron in the supplement, the tablet should be taken when the stomach is empty, with a drink that is high in vitamin C content, not with coffee, tea, or milk.[3] The client should discontinue megavitamin doses. Some (e.g., vitamin A in doses greater than 4000 IU per day) have been documented as teratogenic.[5] This exceeds amounts found in routine supplementation.

***Iron Supplementation.*** If the client is not anemic, a supplement of 30 mg elemental iron is recommended during the second and third trimesters. If the client is anemic (i.e., a hemoglobin level of less than 11.5 g/dL during the first and third trimesters and 10.5 g/dL during the second trimester), then supplementation of 60 to 120 elemental mg iron is recommended.[3]

Owing to the physiologic anemia which develops in most pregnancies secondary to a rapid increase in plasma volume, it is impossible for most women to have enough iron in their diet to keep up with their needs during pregnancy. An iron supplement, in addition to the iron already contained in prenatal vitamins, is commonly prescribed.

- *Administration.* One tablet (30 mg elemental iron) each day. If more than 30 mg is required, give in divided doses.
- *Side Effects and Adverse Reactions.* Gastric upset, constipation, diarrhea.
- *Contraindications.* Some hemoglobinopathies (e.g., ß-thalassemia without a dietary deficiency in iron; see Chapter 14).[1]
- *Anticipated Outcomes on Evaluation.* Hemoglobin levels above 11.5 g/dL during the first and third trimesters and above 10.5 g/dL during the second trimester.
- *Client Teaching and Counseling.* Address the fact that the amount of elemental iron available for absorption depends on the solubility of the particular iron supplement compound. Generally, ferrous sulfate contains 20 percent iron by weight, ferrous gluconate contains 12 percent, and ferrous fumarate contains 32 percent; that is, a 300-mg tablet of ferrous sulfate contains 60 mg of elemental iron.[3] If the client is anemic as a result of low dietary iron intake, supplemental iron should be increased to 60 to 120 mg per day in divided doses. Advise the client to take the iron supplement on an empty stomach and with liquids containing vitamin C (e.g., orange, cranberry or tomato juice), not with milk, tea, or coffee. When hemoglobin levels return to normal, the dosage may be returned to 30 mg each day.[3] The addition of 15 mg of zinc and 2 mg copper is recommended because high levels of iron interfere with absorption of those minerals.[3]

***Calcium Supplement.*** A calcium supplement is recommended in some circumstances. One source recommends that women younger than 25 years whose calcium intake is less than 600 mg receive 600 mg of supplemental calcium per day.[3] Another source recommends calcium supplementation for all clients with inadequate intake, but no more than 1000 mg per day.[1]

- *Administration.* The concentration of elemental calcium varies among common calcium supplements: Calcium carbonate supplies 40 percent elemental calcium; calcium citrate supplies 24 percent; calcium lactate supplies 14 percent; and calcium gluconate supplies 9 percent. Because calcium phosphate is poorly absorbed and interferes with iron absorption, it is not recommended.[1] Other calcium sources (e.g., dolomite, oyster shell calcium) are not recommended. Calcium will be better absorbed if given in divided doses.
- *Side Effects and Adverse Reactions.* Increased intestinal gas.
- *Contraindications.* History of kidney stones. Do not take calcium at the same time as an iron supplement.
- *Anticipated Outcome on Evaluation.* Neither the client nor the infant develops pathology related to inadequate calcium intake.
- *Client Teaching and Counseling.* Advise the client to split the calcium supplement into 250- to 300-mg doses and take with a light meal or snack to enhance absorption. Calcium should not be taken at same time as an iron supplement.[1]

## Follow-Up

Refer to a dietitian any client with a drug or alcohol abuse problem, a chronic medical problem that requires a therapeutic diet, gestational diabetes, or a vegetarian diet. If psychosocial problems are affecting the client's diet or appetite, refer her to a mental health care provider. If the client has inadequate financial resources, refer her to a social worker for advice about government and private programs (e.g., Women, Infants, and Children [WIC]).[13] If needed, ensure that client is linked with appropriate resources to help with cessation of smoking, alcohol consumption, or use of drugs.

## IMMUNIZATION

### BEFORE PREGNANCY

Clients should have all childhood immunizations before conception to protect the fetus from an illness that could produce congenital anomalies and from the theoretical risk of exposure to immunizations. The health care provider should be aware of recent changes in the measles, mumps, and rubella (MMR) immunization schedule, which may require that the client receive an additional MMR immunization. Diphtheria/tetanus boosters are required every 10 years.[6] These issues should be addressed at the preconception checkup.

### DURING PREGNANCY

#### Rubella

Despite large-scale immunization of preschool-age children, a resurgence of rubella and congenital rubella syndrome occurred between 1988 and 1990. Among women of reproductive age, 6 to 11 percent remain seronegative. The risk of congenital rubella syndrome is related to the gestational age of the fetus at the time of maternal infection. One study showed a fetal infection rate of 90 percent before 11 weeks, 33 percent at 11 to 12 weeks, 11 percent at 13 to 14 weeks, 24 percent at 15 to 16 weeks, and 0 percent after 16 weeks.[7]

Administering serum immunoglobulin to a pregnant client with rubella reduces her symptoms but does not alter the risk or severity of congenital rubella syndrome in the fetus.[7] The theoretical risk of congenital rubella syndrome from immunization just prior to pregnancy or during the first trimester is as high as 1.7 percent, but the observed risk is 0 percent.[8]

If the client has a positive serological test, then there is no risk to the fetus if she is exposed to rubella. *All prenatal clients should be tested.* If seronegative, they should be cautioned to avoid anyone with a rash or viral illness.

All nonimmune clients should be immunized postpartum. Breastfeeding is not a contraindication. If Rho(D) immune globulin (human) (RhoGAM) is given, seroconversion should be checked at the postpartum visit. Theoretically, RhoGAM could block antibody development.

All preschool children should be immunized even if a pregnant woman is in the household. Furthermore, all nonpregnant persons of unknown immunity status should be immunized, particularly health care providers. Because of theoretical risk, women of childbearing age should not become pregnant for 3 months following immunization.[7]

#### Hepatitis B Virus

Infection with hepatitis B virus (HBV) carries significant sequelae if the client becomes a chronic carrier. Infection can lead to chronic hepatitis, cirrhosis, or primary hepatocellular carcinoma. Infants whose mothers test positive for hepatitis B surface antigen (HBsAg) may become infected and are at 25 percent risk for the same serious sequelae.

Certain populations are at high risk for HBV infection, but limiting screening to persons in those groups results in failure to identify 50 percent of women who are HBV carriers.[9]

*All clients should be screened for HBsAg prenatally or, if not then, when they are admitted to the hospital.* If HBsAg is positive, further testing of the client, her children, and her sexual partner is advised. The pediatrician should be advised of the mother's positive status and is responsible for appropriate care of the infant.

If a client is HBsAg and HBsAb (antibody to HBsAg) negative and at risk for infection, serious consideration should be given to immunization during pregnancy; pregnancy is not a contraindication. Groups at risk include women of Asian, Pacific Island, or Eskimo descent, no matter where they were born; women born in Haiti or sub-Saharan Africa; women with work histories in public safety or health care (especially those exposed to blood); women who live with HBV carriers or hemodialysis clients; or women who have a history of intravenous drug use or sexual partners who have used intravenous drugs. Others at risk are women with a history of acute or chronic liver disease, women who work or live in institutions for the mentally disabled, women who have been rejected as a blood donor, women with a history of blood transfusion, or women with multiple sexually transmitted disease (STD) episodes or multiple sexual partners.[9]

### Other Immunizations

Other immunizations (e.g., influenza) are usually not indicated during pregnancy. The decision to immunize should be made only after the risk of disease has been weighed against the risk of vaccination and after several factors have been taken into account.

Determination of susceptibility should include a history of prior illness, previous vaccinations, and, most important, serological tests. Other information is helpful, but *only serological tests can prove immunity.* The Centers for Disease Control (CDC) have developed definitions of susceptibility, which may be obtained through the Immunization Practices Advisory Committee.

Risk of exposure is reduced by avoiding travel to endemic areas, practicing appropriate hygiene, and avoiding infected persons. This strategy is preferred to immunization.

Pregnancy may alter the rate of maternal complications in some diseases and cause special health problems.

In general, live vaccines are to be avoided; killed vaccines are safer.[10]

### New Vaccines

Varicella–zoster immunoglobulin is recommended for susceptible, exposed pregnant women within 96 hours of exposure.[11] Two cytomegalovirus (CMV) vaccines have reached clinical trials.[12]

## COMMON COMPLAINTS

Many symptoms that are frequently reported to health care providers are most often attributable to pregnancy but must be evaluated to rule out other pathology.

### FIRST TRIMESTER

### Nausea and Vomiting

***Etiology.*** Physiological changes that cause nausea and vomiting during pregnancy are unknown; however, unusually high levels of estrogen and progesterone and the introduction of human chorionic gonadotropin (hCG) have been studied. Smooth muscle relaxation in the gastrointestinal (GI) tract causing delayed emptying of the stomach has been implicated. Also explored have been relative hyponatremia caused by first-trimester vascular changes, fatigue of early pregnancy, emotional factors, and dietary factors, including vitamin $B_6$ deficiency. Multiple gestation and molar pregnancies are associated with higher incidences of nausea and vomiting. Sixty to eighty percent of Western women experience nausea and vomiting, but women in other cultures experience those symptoms less frequently.[1,2,13] They generally last 14 to 16 weeks into pregnancy and are associated with a positive pregnancy outcome.[14]

***Subjective Data.*** Nausea and/or vomiting are reported by the client between the 4th and 16th weeks of pregnancy. It may or may not be limited to certain times of the day. The client may have had nausea while taking oral contraceptives. The history should *not* include fever, lethargy, muscle aches, abdominal pain, cramping, diarrhea, jaundice, dark urine, changes in the shape or color of bowel movements, vaginal bleeding, head injury, headache, projectile vomiting, vomiting blood, neurological signs, ataxia, chest pain, ear pain, or psychosocial distress, as these symptoms/signs indicate other conditions that may require medical or other appropriate follow-up.[15]

***Objective Data.*** Physical examination and vital signs are within normal limits. Significant negatives include the absence of signs of dehydration and vaginal bleeding. A hydatidiform gestation may present with hyperemesis and vaginal bleeding.

Uterine size should be appropriate for dates. Fetal heart tones should be audible at 12 weeks' gestation.

Weight changes may depend on the severity of the vomiting. If greater than 5 percent of the client's total body weight is lost, hyperemesis gravidarum should be suspected.[14]

*Urine ketone* and *specific gravity tests* are used to rule out dehydration.

***Differential Medical Diagnoses.*** Nausea and vomiting related to pregnancy ruling out hyperemesis gravidarum, multiple gestation, hydatidiform gestation, gastroenteritis, cholecystitis, hepatitis, inner ear infection, sinusitis, hiatal hernia, diabetes, thyroid dysfunction, increased intracranial pressure, migraine headache, pica, food poisoning, vitamin deficiencies, emotional problems, eating disorders.

### *Plan*

Psychosocial Interventions. Explain to the client that nausea and vomiting usually are limited to the first trimester and related to positive pregnancy outcomes. Advise her to notify the health care provider if any symptoms ruled out during history-taking occur in the future.

Medication

- Vitamin $B_6$ Supplement
  - *Indications.* Nausea and vomiting in pregnancy.
  - *Administration.* Vitamin $B_6$ 50 mg p.o. t.i.d. or q.i.d.
  - *Side Effects and Adverse Reactions.* None are known.
  - *Contraindications.* None are known.
  - *Anticipated Outcome on Evaluation.* Decreased nausea and vomiting.
  - *Client Teaching and Counseling.* Instruct the client not to exceed 200 mg per day, as vitamin $B_6$ dependency has been documented.[1]
- Phosphorated Carbohydrate Solution (Emetrol)
  - *Indications.* To reduce smooth muscle contractions of hyperactive gastric muscles.
  - *Administration.* Emetrol 1 to 2 tablespoons. Repeat every 15 minutes up to 5 times until nausea and vomiting are relieved.

- *Side Effects and Adverse Reactions.* None are known.
- *Contraindications.* Diabetes or hereditary fructose intolerance.
- *Anticipated Outcome on Evaluation.* Decreased nausea and vomiting.
- *Client Teaching and Counseling.* Instruct the client never to dilute this medication[16] or drink fluids of any kind immediately before or after taking a dose.

- Diphenhydramine
  - *Indications.* Nausea, vomiting, and/or postnasal drip.
  - *Administration.* Diphenhydramine 25 to 50 mg p.o., every 4 to 6 hours, not to exceed 400 mg per day.
  - *Side Effects and Adverse Reactions.* May cause drowsiness.
  - *Contraindications.* Asthma, emphysema, chronic pulmonary disease, sensitivity to diphenhydramine. Sources conflict on antihistamine use in pregnancy.
  - *Anticipated Outcomes.* Decreased nausea, vomiting, and/or postnasal drip.
  - *Client Teaching and Counseling.* Instruct the client not to drive a car, operate dangerous machinery, or do any activity that requires alertness while taking this medication.[16]

Lifestyle Changes

- Ask the client to keep a diary listing when and for how long nausea and vomiting occur and what activities, associated factors, or foods trigger or improve symptoms. Interventions suggested by this diary are most likely to succeed.
- Advise the client to rest when the nausea occurs, avoid stress, avoid sights and smells that trigger nausea, refrain from wearing clothing that is tight and constricting about the abdomen, and reduce work loads. Support and assistance from the client's partner may also improve symptoms.
- Suggest hypnosis, acupressure (e.g., Sea-bands), cold compresses to the throat, or acupuncture as a possible intervention. To reduce the risk of human immunodeficiency virus (HIV) or hepatitis B infection, acupuncture should be performed only by a specially trained physician.
- Describe relaxation techniques that may help: progressive relaxation (systematic tensing and relaxing of muscle groups), autogenic training (using suggestions such as, "My right arm is heavy"), meditation (repeating a sound or gazing at an object while clearing the mind of all distractions), visual imagery (visualizing self in a relaxing place), and touching/massage.[1]

Dietary Interventions

- Symptoms may be relieved by eating small, frequent meals that do not allow the stomach to become too empty or full, including high-carbohydrate or high-protein meals and snacks, sipping carbonated drinks, including foods that tend to neutralize stomach acid (e.g., apples, milk, bread, potatoes, calcium carbonate tablets), eating crackers on arising, drinking fluids between meals instead of with meals, and avoiding foods that may irritate the stomach (e.g., spicy or fatty foods).
- If a vitamin/mineral supplement is causing nausea, it may be discontinued until the client is less nauseated, often after about 14 to 16 weeks of pregnancy. A balanced diet would provide all necessary vitamins and minerals, except iron (see Nutrition and Weight Gain).
- Remind the client of the need for adequate hydration (6 to 8 glasses per day). Sipping lukewarm fluids every 5 minutes is tolerated better than drinking an entire glass of fluid at one time.

Follow-Up. Refer to a physician any client who is unable to hold down liquids for more than 12 hours, who loses 5 pounds or more, or who has ketonuria or any symptoms of pathology.

### Constipation

***Etiology.*** Large amounts of circulating progesterone cause decreased contractility of the GI tract, resulting in slow movement of chyme and increased water reabsorption from the bowel. The large bowel is also mechanically compressed by the enlarging uterus, most noticeably in the first and third trimesters. The client may have changed her food and fluid intake or exercise level in response to nausea and vomiting, culturally prescribed expectations of pregnant women, or medically prescribed treatment. Prenatal vitamins with iron or calcium can also be constipating.[1,2,13]

***Subjective Data.*** The client may report abdominal cramping, flatulence, or increasing difficulty with bowel movements or intervals between them. Stools may be small, hard, round, and dark. Often the client has a history of constipation before pregnancy. Her diet may be low in bulk and fluids, and she may rarely exercise. The client may have taken antacids, calcium, iron supplements, anticholinergics, tricyclic antidepressants, or codeine medications; these can constipate. The history should *not* include change in stool (i.e., color, shape, or pattern), diarrhea, abdominal pain, fever, anorexia, periumbilical pain, rectal bleeding, emotional distress, or excessive laxative use for weight control (purging), as these symptoms/signs may indicate other conditions requiring medical or other appropriate follow-up.[15]

***Objective Data.*** Physical examination and vital signs are within normal limits, although hyperactive bowel sounds, constipated stool in the rectum, a sausage-shaped mass in the lower left quadrant that disappears after bowel movements, hemorrhoids, or hemorrhoidal tags may be revealed.

The *stool for occult blood* test is used to detect the presence of blood in the stool. A stool sample is collected during a digital rectal examination. The stool is applied to the card provided, and a drop of developer is placed on the card. If the card turns bright blue, blood is present.

*Client teaching* in preparation for the test includes diet information. For the most accurate results, the client should eliminate meats, fish, poultry, and green leafy vegetables for 3 days prior to the test. Aspirin should not be consumed during that same 3-day period. Hemorrhoids, anal fissures, and vaginal bleeding may also result in positive readings.

***Differential Medical Diagnosis.*** Constipation related to pregnancy ruling out preterm labor, irritable bowel syndrome, appendicitis, intestinal obstruction, or fecal impaction.

***Plan***

Psychosocial Interventions. Explain to the client how pregnancy exacerbates the symptoms of constipation and that symptoms should improve after delivery. Advise her to notify the health care provider if any symptoms ruled out during history-taking occur in the future.

Medication. Advise the client to avoid mineral oil, as it will decrease the absorption of fat-soluble vitamins.[1] Cathartics are contraindicated if the client is at risk for preterm labor.

Review with client what other medication (e.g., codeine, iron) she is taking to determine whether constipation is a side effect—then help her to reduce their use if possible.

- Bulk-forming, nonnutritive laxatives (e.g., Metamucil, Fibercon)
  - *Indications.* Constipation caused by low dietary bulk.
  - *Administration.* Available in tablets or granules. Take per package instructions.
  - *Side Effects and Adverse Reactions.* None are known.

- *Contraindications.* Fecal impaction or intestinal obstruction.
- *Anticipated Outcome on Evaluation.* Decreased constipation.
- *Client Teaching and Counseling.* Instruct the client to drink 8 oz of water or more with each dose. She may need to continue treatment for 2 to 3 days before maximum effect is noted.[16]

▪ Docusate sodium (e.g., Colace), a stool softener
  - *Indications:* Can be used to prevent constipation.
  - *Administration.* 50 to 200 mg per day.
  - *Side Effects and Adverse Reactions.* Bitter taste, throat irritation, nausea.
  - *Contraindications.* Sensitivity to docusate sodium.
  - *Anticipated Outcome on Evaluation.* Formation of softer, less constipating stools.
  - *Client Teaching and Counseling.* Instruct the client to take docusate sodium with milk or juice to mask its bitter taste.[16]

Lifestyle Changes. It may be helpful to encourage the client to exercise regularly (according to ACOG guidelines), to establish a time of day to defecate, to avoid prolonged attempts to defecate, and to elevate her feet on a stool while defecating to avoid straining.

Dietary Interventions. Advise the client to eat foods high in bulk (e.g., fresh fruits and vegetables, whole-grain breads and cereals) and to drink fluids (6 to 8 glasses of water per day above that drunk with meals) and to drink warm fluids on arising to stimulate bowel motility. Explain that if she drinks prune juice with her vitamin/mineral supplement every second or third day or changes to a supplement without iron and calcium temporarily, then constipation may be less of a problem.

Follow-Up. If prenatal vitamins or iron are discontinued, monitor the client for anemia. If purging or psychosocial stress is causing constipation, refer the client to a mental health care provider. If symptoms of a pathological condition develop, refer the client to a physician.

### Hemorrhoids

***Etiology.*** Hemorrhoids occur when the vascular submucosa in the rectoanal canal bulges and becomes congested with varicosities. They become significant only when they become symptomatic. Hemorrhoids are exacerbated during pregnancy by increased intravascular pressure in veins below the uterus, constipation, and straining at stool.

***Subjective Data.*** The client may report a history of constipation, hemorrhoids before pregnancy, multiparity, increased age, or a family history of hemorrhoids. She may notice swelling, fullness, or a lump at her anus; bright red, painless bleeding on the stool surface during defecation; or increased mucus with defecation.

***Objective Data.*** Physical examination and vital signs may be within normal limits, or hemorrhoids may be visible externally or palpated internally. Anal fissures or hemorrhoidal tags may be noted. Thrombosed hemorrhoids are a painful, shiny, bluish or purple clot-containing mass near the anus.

Diagnostic tests and methods include evaluation of the *hemoglobin level* in the blood. The hemoglobin level may be decreased if bleeding is extensive or prolonged.

Stool for occult blood is the other diagnostic tool (see Constipation).

***Differential Medical Diagnosis.*** Hemorrhoids exacerbated by pregnancy; rule out abscessed or thrombosed hemorrhoids, cancerous lesions, idiopathic pruritus ani, condyloma acuminata, all of which may require more extensive medical referral and intervention.

### *Plan*

Psychosocial Interventions. Explain to the client the underlying changes that created or exacerbated the hemorrhoids, and assure her that the condition will improve or resolve after pregnancy. Encourage her to contact a health care provider if any symptoms occur in the future.

Medication

- Topical Anesthetics (e.g., Preparation H, Anusol)
  - *Indications.* To shrink the swelling of hemorrhoids and reduce itching.
  - *Administration.* Free application of cream, as needed, to hemorrhoids up to three to five times per day: in the morning, at night, and after each bowel movement. If a suppository is used, insert it into the rectum after cleaning and drying the anal area, three to five times per day as needed.
  - *Side Effects and Adverse Reactions.* Occasional burning of irritated tissues.
  - *Contraindications.* Client sensitivity to components of the medication. Heart disease, thyroid disease, and diabetes are contraindications to suppository use.
  - *Anticipated Outcomes on Evaluation.* Decreased swelling, pain, or itching of hemorrhoids.
  - *Client Teaching and Counseling.* Instruct the client in cream or suppository use. With the suppository, remove the foil wrapper before insertion. With the cream, use a dispensing cap: Attach the cap to the tube and fill it by squeezing the tube. Lubricate the tip, gently insert it into the anus, and squeeze the tube to deliver cream into the rectum. Clean the cap with soap and water after use.[16]

Lifestyle Changes. Advise the client to try to avoid constipation by following the measures described in the preceding section (see Constipation). Encourage her to use warm or cool sitz baths (Epsom salts may be added), witch hazel pads (e.g., Tucks), and ice packs or cold compresses to reduce the size of the hemorrhoids. Furthermore, advise her to avoid straining by elevating her feet on a stool while attempting to defecate. Applying petroleum jelly around the anus before defecating will help reduce pain and bleeding.

Advise the client to sleep and rest on her side. Moreover, Kegel's exercises will improve circulation. They should be done 50 to 100 times per day. Self-digital replacement of hemorrhoids if possible and careful perineal cleansing habits are also helpful.

Refer the client to a physician if she has symptoms of thrombosed hemorrhoids, does not respond to interventions, or has symptoms of other pathology.

## Flatulence

***Etiology.*** The physiological changes that result in constipation also may result in increased flatulence.[2]

***Subjective Data.*** A client may report increased passage of rectal gas, abdominal bloating, epigastric pain, constipation, or belching.

***Objective Data.*** Often, hyperactive bowel sounds or abdominal distention is detected on physical exam.

***Differential Medical Diagnoses.*** Flatulence; rule out irritable bowel syndrome, lactose intolerance, medication side effects, hyperventilation.

### *Plan*

Psychosocial Interventions. Reassure the client that increased flatulence is related to pregnancy and should resolve afterward.

Lifestyle Changes. Teach the client measures to avoid constipation. Help her to recognize the symptoms of hyperventilation or air swallowing in order to alleviate flatulence. The client may find that she is breathing fast, sighing, or feeling the need for frequent deep breaths. She may feel tingling in her fingers, toes, or lips, dizziness, or confusion. Rebreathing air that is exhaled into a paper bag or cupped hands may help decrease symptoms. Because stress often causes hyperventilation, becoming aware of areas in her life that cause stress may be helpful for the client. Avoiding gum chewing, large meals, and smoking also will reduce flatulence.

Dietary Interventions. Advise the client to limit gas-forming foods (e.g., carbonated beverages, cruciferous vegetables, baking soda, cheese, beans, bananas, peanuts, calcium carbonate supplements).

Follow-Up. Refer her to a mental health care provider if symptoms of psychosocial stress are evident.

## Fatigue

***Etiology.*** Fatigue during pregnancy occurs primarily during the first and third trimesters (the highest energy levels often occur during the second trimester). First-trimester fatigue may be caused by physical changes (e.g., increased oxygen consumption, progesterone levels, and fetal demands) and psychosocial changes (e.g., reexamination of roles). Third-trimester fatigue is usually caused by sleep disturbances that result from increased weight, physical discomforts, and decreased exercise. Fatigue, in particular, can be a symptom in most pathological problems—emotional, physical, or dietary.[1,2,17]

***Subjective Data.*** The client may report fatigue despite normal amounts of sleep or insomnia due to difficulty in getting comfortable. Fetal movements, urinary frequency, vivid dreams, increased stress, or emotional problems may interfere with sleep. Her family or work situation may not allow her to rest during the day. The history should *not* include depression, anxiety, difficulty with concentration, anorexia, anemia, exercise intolerance, chest pain or discomfort, change in bowel habits, flulike symptoms, sore throat, coughing, or dyspnea, or other symptoms/signs indicating other conditions requiring medical or other appropriate follow-up.[15]

***Objective Data.*** The physical examination and vital signs are within normal limits.

A *complete blood count* (CBC) is used to evaluate the client for signs of anemia, infection, or blood dyscrasias. The procedure involves venipuncture and withdrawal of blood which is sent to laboratory for evaluation. The client may apply pressure to the venipuncture site until bleeding stops. Hematoma formation at the site is common and will resolve.

***Differential Medical Diagnosis.*** Fatigue due to pregnancy ruling out other pathological states.

### *Plan*

Psychosocial Interventions. Explain to the client that increased fatigue is expected in the first trimester and insomnia is common in the third. Encourage her to contact the health care provider if she develops other symptoms.

Encourage verbalization of psychosocial problems and explore appropriate interventions. Encourage the client to accept offers of help. Advise the client to avoid, if possible, major life stresses (e.g., moving) during pregnancy.

Medication. Supplemental iron may be appropriate if anemic. No sleeping medications are prescribed.

Lifestyle Changes. Encourage adequate sleep and rest periods; help the client to arrange work, child care, and other activities to permit additional rest.

Encourage good posture, wearing of low-heeled shoes, and pelvic rock exercises to ease backaches. Pelvic rock exercises are taught to the client by having her stand against a wall and insert her hand behind the small of her back. By moving so as to roll her uterus up toward her chest and push her buttocks toward the floor, the client rocks her pelvis. Encourage her to do this while standing, walking, and sitting.

Suggest ways to increase comfort and reduce insomnia (e.g., placing pillows behind her back, raising the head of the bed up on blocks).

Demonstrate exercises that consume less energy (isometric instead of aerobic exercises). Have the client avoid exercise during the 2 hours prior to sleep.

Recommend exercise for sedentary clients (see Exercise later).

Relaxation techniques may help.

Dietary Interventions. Correct nutritional inadequacies, paying attention to total nutrient intake and distribution of those nutrients throughout the day (see Nutrition). Advise client to avoid caffeine and heavy meals at the end of the day. Suggest that warm milk may induce sleep.

Follow-Up. Refer the client to a physician if symptoms of pathology are evident. When severe psychosocial stress is noted, referral to a mental health care provider is appropriate.

### Urinary Frequency or Incontinence

***Etiology.*** A physiologic change during the first trimester that causes urinary difficulty is the enlargement of the uterus, which compresses the bladder. In the second trimester, however, as the uterus becomes an abdominal organ, these symptoms improve. In the third trimester, fetal presenting parts often compress the bladder. This, in addition to hyperplasia and hyperemia of the pelvic organs and increased kidney output, leads to urinary frequency and incontinence.[1,2,13]

***Subjective Data.*** The client may report increased urination, nocturia, or involuntary loss of urine. The history should *not* include back pain, fever, flulike symptoms, hematuria, dysuria, urgency, dribbling, suprapubic pain, as these symptoms/signs indicate other conditions requiring more thorough follow-up and possible medical referral. She may report use of alcohol or caffeine.

To differentiate urine loss from rupture of membranes (ROM), know that ROM may be described as fluid from her vagina that cannot be controlled with Kegel exercises or as fluid that does not smell of urine and that may increase while she is lying down and decrease after standing.

Polyuria may indicate hypokalemia, which may be caused by chronic vomiting or diarrhea. Other symptoms accompanying hypokalemia are neuromuscular weakness, irregular heartbeats, constipation, and orthostatic hypotension. Polyurea can be seen with diabetes,[18] and clients with such symptoms should be referred to a physician.

***Objective Data.*** Physical examination and vital signs are within normal limits. The costal vertebral angle and suprapubic area are not tender. Vaginal exam does not reveal pooling of amniotic fluid but may reveal a cystocele. Abdominal exam does not reveal contractions or uterine irritability.

*Urinalysis and culture and sensitivity tests* are used to detect urinary tract infection and renal and metabolic diseases. The test procedure first involves obtaining the best specimen. Instruct the client to wash her hands, then separate her labia. Provide three cleansing wipes and have her wipe from front to back once with each wipe, on the right side, then the left side, and then the middle. She should start to urinate in the commode, then catch a small amount of urine midstream in a sterile cup, and finish urinating in the commode. She should replace the lid on the cup tightly without touching the inside or top edge. Client teaching should stress that failing to follow this procedure jeopardizes the accuracy of the test.

The *nitrazine test* discriminates between vaginal discharge and amniotic fluid. Use of a sterile speculum reduces the possibility of introducing infection if the membranes have ruptured. A sterile cotton-tipped applicator is used to remove discharge from the vaginal pool. It is placed on nitrazine paper and the color change is compared with the chart. If the pH is 3.5 to 5, the fluid is normal vaginal discharge. If the pH is 7, the discharge may be amniotic fluid. Note that blood and vaginal discharge associated with certain vaginal infections (e.g., bacterial vaginosis and trichomonas vaginitis) may give a pH reading of 7.

The *fern test* also discriminates between vaginal discharge and amniotic fluid. Again, a sterile speculum is used. The sample of vaginal discharge is placed on a clean slide and allowed to dry. Amniotic fluid forms a fernlike pattern under microscopic examination. Inform the client that the nitrazine and fern tests are the best way to discriminate between vaginal discharge and amniotic fluid. Differentiation is important because premature rupture of membranes can cause amniotitis or preterm labor. The practitioner may also look for fluid leaking from the cervix, which may not necessarily be amniotic fluid, but would certainly raise suspicion.

The screening 50-g glucola test is negative (see Chapter 12) reducing the likelihood of diabetes.

***Differential Medical Diagnosis.*** Urinary frequency/incontinence due to pregnancy ruling out urinary tract infection, pyelonephritis, gestational diabetes, preexisting diabetes mellitus, hypokalemia, and spontaneous rupture of membranes.

***Plan***

Psychosocial Interventions. Show the client diagrams of female anatomy. Often when a client can view the anatomical changes that occur during pregnancy, she understands the reason for urinary frequency and incontinence. Reassure her that these symptoms should improve after delivery. Advise the client to notify the health care provider if any symptoms ruled out during history-taking occur in the future.

Lifestyle Changes. Resting and sleeping in the lateral recumbent position enhance kidney function. Kegel exercises increase perineal muscle tone.

Crede's method of bladder emptying may decrease frequency if a client with a cystocele has difficulty completely emptying her bladder. Instruct the client to apply pressure down and in above pubic bone over the bladder after voiding. This completely empties the bladder. Refer client if there are persistent problems related to cystocele, such as incontinence or urinary tract infections.

Dietary Interventions. Advise the client to maintain an adequate fluid intake (6 to 8 glasses of water) to decrease the incidence of urinary tract infections. Water intake should decrease 2 to 3 hours before bedtime. In addition, advise the client to discontinue drinking beverages that contain alcohol or caffeine.

Follow-Up. A client with urinary tract infection (UTI) must be treated appropriately. Refer clients with symptoms of pathology, such as frequently repeated UTIs, to a urologist.

## Varicosities of Vulva and Legs

***Etiology.*** Physiologic changes during pregnancy that exacerbate varicosities are the increased venous stasis caused by the pressure of the gravid uterus and the vasodilation resulting from hormonal changes.[1,2,13] Women who develop varicosities often have a congenital predisposition, are inactive, are obese, and have poor muscle tone. Prolonged standing or sitting aggravates the condition.

***Subjective Data.*** The client may report aching, throbbing, swelling, or heaviness in the legs or vulvar area. The client may also report multiparity, prolonged standing or sitting, or decreased activity. She may note increased symptoms as she becomes older. A family history of varicosities may be reported. The history should *not* include clotting; swelling, redness, or tenderness; or a white, cold, numb leg, as these symptoms/signs indicate other conditions requiring immediate medical follow-up.

***Objective Data.*** Diagnostic tests are not necessary. Physical examination and vital signs are within normal limits. Knotted, twisted, and swollen veins, however, are visible in the legs or vulva with possible edema below the varicosities. Peripheral pulses are normal. Significant negatives include no inflammation over the varicosities; no firm, cordlike feel; no dependent cyanosis; no positive Homan's sign; no deep pain on palpation; no distention of veins on the dorsal side of the foot after it is elevated 45 degrees; no positive Louvel's sign (pain in calf with coughing or sneezing that decreases with compression above varicosities); and no restlessness, fever, or tachycardia.[1]

***Differential Medical Diagnosis.*** Varicosities of legs and/or vulva exacerbated by pregnancy ruling out venous thrombosis, thrombophlebitis, phlebothrombosis, edema from pregnancy-induced hypertension, and physiologic edema of pregnancy.

#### *Plan*

Psychological Interventions. Explain to the client the reasons for the varicosities and inform her that the varicosities will not resolve until after delivery. Advise the client to notify the health care provider if any symptoms ruled out during the history-taking occur in the future.

Any surgical intervention would be delayed until after delivery or, optimally, until after childbearing is complete.

Lifestyle Changes. Some lifestyle changes may help to relieve discomfort. Teach the client proper application of support hose and compression stockings: Have her lie flat and raise her legs to drain the veins. While her legs are elevated, have her roll the stockings on. Advise the client to do this before she rises in the morning and to leave the stockings on until she goes to bed at night.

Instruct the client to avoid crossing her legs and not to wear knee-high stockings or a constrictive band around the legs.

Because orthostatic hypotension is common, tell the client to change position gradually when rising to avoid dizziness.

Explain the importance of elevating the legs above the level of the heart at least twice a day. Advise the client to wear comfortable shoes, to avoid prolonged standing or sitting, and to alter position frequently.

Instruct the client in the use of perineal pads with a sanitary belt to compress vulvar varicosities.

Explain to the client the need to avoid leg injury, as hemorrhage may result.

Dietary Interventions. Warn the client to avoid excess weight gain during pregnancy, and encourage weight loss during the postpartum period.

Follow-Up. Refer a client with symptoms of pathology to a physician.

### Headache

***Etiology.*** Physiologic changes during pregnancy that cause headaches include increased circulatory volume, vasodilation caused by high levels of circulating progesterone, tissue edema resulting from vascular congestion, stress, fatigue, and low blood sugar. Headaches not caused by pathology are very common in pregnancy. Women who had headaches prior to pregnancy improve 60 percent of the time, worsen 13 percent of the time, and remain unchanged 27 percent of the time. Headache can be a symptom of serious illness, which must be ruled out.[1,2]

***Subjective Data.*** Focus on the nature, frequency, intensity, location, and description of the pain; factors that trigger the pain and those that alleviate it; and changes that have occurred during pregnancy in the quality of the headaches. The client may report a past or family history of headaches or increased stress. The history should *not* include injury to the head, neck, or back; occupational exposure to chemicals; consumption of alcohol, chocolate, or aged cheese; unbalanced intake of calories; or fatigue, as these symptoms/signs may indicate other conditions requiring medical or other appropriate follow-up. Pathology may also be present if there is a history of facial edema; changes in the level of consciousness; memory changes; motor, visual, or sensory changes; nausea; vomiting; stiff neck; fever; ear or eye pain; rhinitis; flulike symptoms; injury; or prodomata (i.e., visual, auditory, or sensory changes preceding a headache).[15]

***Objective Data.*** Physical examination and vital signs, particularly blood pressure, weight gain pattern, ophthalmoscopic examination, and ear, nose, throat, neurological, musculoskeletal, and upper respiratory exams, are within normal limits.

A *urine dipstick test* that is negative for protein and ketones reduces the possibility of pregnancy-induced hypertension and dehydration from vomiting.

The *serum glucose test* procedure begins with venipuncture; blood is withdrawn into a tube containing chemicals that stabilize the glucose. The tube is sent to a laboratory. Another method involves performing a fingerstick to withdraw a drop of blood that is then placed on a reagent strip. The strip is then analyzed in a machine or read against a scale (least accurate method).

Teach the client that a hematoma is common at the venipuncture site and will resolve. Tenderness at the fingerstick is common. Accurate interpretation of the results depends on obtaining an accurate history of food intake during the time preceding the test. This test is often performed after the client fasts or ingests a measured amount of glucose.

A complete blood count is another diagnostic test used (see Fatigue).

***Differential Medical Diagnosis.*** Tension, migraine, cluster, sinus, or benign vascular headache of pregnancy ruling out pregnancy-induced hypertension, upper respiratory or sinus infection, fever, cardiovascular disease, cervical arthritis, muscle tension headache, cerebral mass or hemorrhage, central nervous system infections, or hypoglycemia.

***Plan***

Psychosocial Interventions. Explain to the client the physiologic changes that are causing the headache and that it may improve in the second trimester. Advise the client to notify the health care provider if any symptoms ruled out during the history-taking occur in the future.

Ask the client to keep a diary of activities, foods, and environmental stimuli that occur around the time of the headache. This may reveal triggering factors.

Teach the client symptoms of pregnancy-induced hypertension (headache that is different in nature, visual changes, photophobia, confusion, swelling in the face or hands, severe swelling in the feet, epigastric pain) and encourage immediate contact with a physician.

Medication. Acetaminophen is indicated for headache and other pain.

- *Administration.* 325 to 650 mg every 4 hours as needed for pain.
- *Side Effects and Adverse Reactions.* None are known.
- *Contraindication.* Sensitivity to acetaminophen.
- *Anticipated Outcome on Evaluation.* Reduced headache pain.
- *Client Counseling.* Instruct the client to notify the health care provider if headache pain continues. Overdose of acetaminophen has been associated with liver damage.[16]

Lifestyle Changes. Advise the client to avoid activities and situations that may trigger headaches (stress, smoking, smoke-filled rooms, blinking lights, sleeping late). Advise her to reduce stress as much as possible, get adequate sleep, have her neck and shoulders massaged with heat or coolness applied.

Encourage the client to practice relaxation techniques (see Nausea and Vomiting).

Dietary Interventions. Advise the client to eat a regular, balanced diet and to avoid intake of food that triggers headaches (e.g., caffeine, chocolate, nitrites, hard aged cheese, alcohol—especially red wine).

Refer the client to a physician if the headache is severe, does not respond to interventions, requires strong pain killers, or demonstrates other signs of pregnancy-induced hypertension, pathology, or eye strain. If signs of severe psychosocial stress are present, refer the client to a mental health care provider. Referral to a pain center may help severe headache that is not due to pathology.

## Breast Pain, Enlargement, and Changes in Pigmentation

***Etiology.*** Physiologic changes that underlie these complaints are the increased levels of estrogen and progesterone, which cause the fat layer of breasts to thicken and the numbers and development of milk ducts and glands to increase. As a result, the breasts, especially the area around the areola, increase in size, weight, and tenderness, and bluish veins appear on the chest. The nipples become erect, melatonin causes the areolae to darken, the Montgomery tubercles enlarge, and there is a slight colostrum discharge.[2,13]

***Subjective Data.*** The client may report increasing tenderness, weight, and size of the breasts, darkening of the areolae, leakage of colostrum from the nipples. The client should *not* report pain and redness localized in one area of the breast, fever, flulike symptoms, injury, masses, dimples, bloody discharge, changes in skin texture, or changes in breast or nipple size, shape, symmetry, as these symptoms/signs may indicate other conditions requiring medical follow-up.

***Objective Data.*** No diagnostic tests are necessary. Physical examination and vital signs are within normal limits. Areas of induration, inflammation, or heat; masses; skin dimpling; skin changes; enlarged nodes; or unilateral or bloody nipple discharge should not be present.

***Differential Medical Diagnosis.*** Breast tenderness, enlargement, and pigment changes due to pregnancy ruling out mastitis, breast injury, and breast cancer.

### *Plan*

Psychosocial Interventions. Explain to the client the reasons for the breast changes. Inform her that pain often improves in the second trimester but the other changes will remain until after lactation. Advise the client to notify the health care provider if any symptoms ruled out during the history-taking occur in the future.

Lifestyle Changes. Advise the client to examine her breasts in the same way as before pregnancy, except that no special time of month is indicated. If instruction is necessary, provide it (see Chapter 10).

In addition, the client may need to constantly wear a supportive bra. She may find wearing a bra while sleeping more comfortable.

Dietary Interventions. Advise the client to avoid the use of caffeine.

Follow-Up. Clients with symptoms of mastitis must be treated appropriately (see Chapter 10). Refer the client with symptoms of pathology to a physician.

## Menstrual-like Cramping

***Etiology.*** The physiologic changes underlying the sensation of cramping may be the increased vascular congestion in the pelvis, the pressure exerted by the presenting fetal part, or stretching of the round ligaments.[2,13] Many women report such cramping during the first 1 or 2 months of pregnancy and again at the end of pregnancy.

***Subjective Data.*** The client reports sensations similar to those she experienced just prior to her menses, before she was pregnant. The client should *not,* however, report severe cramping, unilateral or suprapubic abdominal pain, contractions, vaginal bleeding, rupture of membranes, or urinary tract symptoms (see Urinary Frequency or Incontinence), as these symptoms/signs may indicate other conditions which may require medical follow-up.

***Objective Data.*** Physical examination and vital signs are within normal limits. There is no vaginal bleeding, cervical dilatation, adnexal masses, tenderness, or vaginal pooling of amniotic fluid. Uterine size equals dates. There is no suprapubic tenderness.

*Serum β human chorionic gonadotropin* (hCG) is evaluated to identify and monitor pregnancy and to diagnose certain pregnancy-related complications (e.g., abortion, ectopic pregnancy, hydatidiform gestation). A blood sample is withdrawn by venipuncture and sent to a laboratory. In normal pregnancies, the hCG level is expected to double every other day. A deviation could indicate a complication of pregnancy and requires further testing.

*Nitrazine* and *fern tests* and *urinalysis and culture and sensitivity* may also be indicated (see Urinary Frequency and Incontinence).

***Differential Medical Diagnosis.*** Normal menstrual-like cramping in pelvis ruling out ectopic pregnancy, abortion, premature labor, and urinary tract infection.

***Plan***

Psychosocial Interventions. Explain to the client the physiologic changes that underlie the sensations. In addition, inform the client that no signs of imminent abortion or labor exist and that the sensations should decrease in the second trimester but may return again in the third. Advise the client to notify the health care provider if any symptoms ruled out during the history-taking occur in the future.

Follow-Up. Refer the client with symptoms of pathology to a physician.

# SECOND TRIMESTER

## Backache

***Etiology.*** Physiologic change underlying a backache is the shift in the center of gravity caused by the enlarging uterus. Muscle strain results. In addition, a high level of circulating progesterone softens cartilage and loosens once stable joints, thereby increasing discomfort. Upper back pain can also be caused by increased breast size.[1,2,13]

***Subjective Data.*** The client reports dull, aching pain in the upper or lower back that increases as the day goes on. Ask the client to describe the location, nature, and duration of the pain, exacerbating and relieving factors, the changes in pain that occur with movement. She may wear improperly fitting or high-heeled shoes. The client may have gained excessive weight, report being obese before pregnancy, or be fatigued. She may be large-busted and wear an improperly fitting or poorly supporting bra. Many clients lift heavy objects by bending from the waist rather than bending the knees; low back muscles are strained as a result of this movement. There should be *no* history of back injury or other problems, surgery, or symptoms of urinary tract infection, ruptured membranes, uterine contractions, or neurologic deficit.

***Objective Data.*** No diagnostic tests are done. Physical examination and vital signs are within normal limits; however, lordosis, abnormal gait, or tenderness along paraspinous muscles may be revealed. Significant negatives include no costal vertebral angle tenderness; no pain with straight-leg raises; normal patellar, deep tendon, and plantar reflexes; and a normal neurologic exam. No urinary tract symptoms (see Urinary Frequency and Incontinence), no abnormal vaginal discharge (see Leukorrhea), and no uterine contractions are detected.

***Differential Medical Diagnosis.*** Backache related to pregnancy ruling out uterine contractions, genital infections, urinary tract infections, sciatica, herniated disk, vertebral tumor, muscle sprain, or strain.

***Plan***

Psychosocial Interventions. Explain to the client the changes underlying the backache, and inform her that it should decrease or resolve after pregnancy. Advise the client to notify the health care provider if any symptoms ruled out during the history-taking occur in the future.

Medication. Acetaminophen (see Headache).

Lifestyle Changes. Instruct client in the pelvic tilt exercise (see Fatigue) and proper body mechanics, particularly when lifting something. Instruct her to keep her back straight when lifting and to bend her knees, keeping the object close to her body; if she must hold her breath to lift an object, it is too heavy. Advise her to avoid excessive twisting, bending, and stretching.[13]

Inform the client that an exercise program encourages general fitness.

Advise the client, when standing for long periods, to rest one foot on a low stool, and when sitting for long periods, to rest her feet on a low stool, to raise her knees above the waist, and to sit with her back firmly against the back of the chair. While driving, she should sit straight and position the seat so that her knees are slightly bent when using the pedals.

Advise the client to avoid excessive walking or standing.

Inform the client that a firm, supportive mattress may be helpful. Advise her to assume a lateral recumbent position while sleeping, with pillows supporting the back and legs; sleeping in this position promotes comfort.

Advise the client with upper back pain to wear a good, supportive bra, and the client with lower back pain, to wear a maternity support girdle.

Warm tub baths may be soothing. Advise the client to be careful when rising from the tub, as she may experience dizziness; she should have someone's help or hold on to some other support. Do not recommend tub baths for clients in whom rupture of membranes is suspected.

Inform the client that massage and relaxation techniques, as well as use of a heating pad for short periods, but not during sleep (to avoid a burn) may promote comfort.

Dietary Interventions. Advise the client to avoid gaining excessive weight.

Follow-Up. If severe pain does not respond to intervention, refer the client to a physical therapist. Refer any client who requires strong pain medication or who has symptoms of pathology to a physician.

## Syncope

***Etiology.*** The physiologic changes underlying syncope (fainting) are related to pooling of blood in the lower extremities, expansion of blood volume, and compression of the vena cava and lungs by the gravid uterus. True vertigo is often described as the room spinning or disorientation in relation to space. Syncope is also caused by nausea and vomiting, low blood sugar, substance abuse, hyperventilation, and illness.

***Subjective Data.*** The client reports lightheadedness or dizziness that lasts a minute or less when she is standing, lying on her back, or changing position. She may report low or sporadic intake of calories. There should be *no* history of exposure to toxic agents, reports of substance abuse, sinus or ear problems, numbness or tingling in the digits or around the mouth, nausea or vomiting, melena, heart palpitations, shortness of breath, double vision, loss of strength or sensation, incoordination, or anxiety or depression, as these symptoms/signs may indicate other conditions that may require medical or other appropriate follow-up.[15]

***Objective Data.*** Physical examination and vital signs are within normal limits. *Hemoglobin* tests may reveal anemia.

***Differential Medical Diagnosis.*** Syncope related to the hemodynamic changes in pregnancy ruling out orthostatic hypotension, compression of vena cava, hyperventilation, anemia, hypoglycemia, substance abuse, exposure to a toxic agent, psychosocial stress, or central nervous system, cardiac, respiratory, endocrine, eye, ear, or sinus pathology.

***Plan***

Psychosocial Interventions. Explain to the client the physiologic changes causing syncope. Advise the client to notify the health care provider if any symptoms ruled out during the history-taking occur in the future.

Advise the client to avoid stressful situations. Teach her to recognize hyperventilation. Encourage her to verbalize problems and explore appropriate responses.

Lifestyle Changes. Advise the client to rest in the lateral recumbent position; to change position gradually, holding on to something when rising; or to lower her head below the level of the heart if feeling faint.

To reduce blood pooling in the extremities, instruct the client to apply compression stockings before getting out of bed and to perform leg pumping exercises (flexing and extending the ankle several times).

If being in a crowd induces symptoms, advise the client to move to an open window or go outside and loosen or remove layers of clothing.

Dietary Interventions. Advise the client to eat regularly throughout the day. Assess her diet for adequate calorie and fluid intake.

Follow-Up. Refer a client with symptoms of pathology to a physician.

## Leukorrhea

***Etiology.*** The physiologic changes underlying leukorrhea arise from the high levels of estrogen that cause increased vascularity and hypertrophy of cervical glands as well as vaginal cells. As a consequence, leukorrhea production increases; the discharge is white or yellow, thin, and more acidic than normal vaginal discharge.[1,2]

***Subjective Data.*** The client reports increased vaginal discharge. She should *not,* however, report green, watery, bloody, itchy, or irritating discharge that smells foul or fishy; fever; flulike symptoms; abdominal pain; bleeding after intercourse; or dyspareunia. Ask the client if she has multiple or new sexual partners, has recently resumed sexual activity or douching, has had abnormal Pap smears in the past, or has recently used antibiotics.

***Objective Data.*** Physical examination and vital signs are within normal limits; however, the pelvic exam may show increased but normal-appearing vaginal discharge.

A *normal saline and potassium hydroxide test* (wet mount) is used to determine whether candida, trichomonads, clue cells, white or red blood cells, or bacteria are present in the vaginal discharge. A Q-tip is used to withdraw some vaginal discharge which is placed on two clean, dry microscope slides. A drop of normal saline is placed on one and a drop of potassium hydroxide on the other. Coverslips are used and the specimens are examined under the microscope. Candida, trichomonads, clue cells, and abnormal numbers of coccal bacteria, red cells, and white blood cells all indicate a vaginal infection.

A *Papanicolaou smear* is done to detect changes in the cervical or endocervical cells that could indicate dysplasia, carcinoma, human papillomavirus, or herpes simplex. Signs of vaginal infection may also be noted.

Both tests are speculum exams; that is, cervical and endocervical cells are collected using a wooden or preferably plastic spatula and cytobrush (though during pregnancy, a Q-tip is preferred to reduce cervical bleeding from the collection procedure), placed on a microscope slide, sprayed with a fixative, and sent to a pathology laboratory for examination.

Inform the client that the Pap smear is a screening test used to determine which clients require additional testing. Advise the client that she should not douche, use vaginal medications, or have intercourse for 24 hours before the test. The procedure may cause slight spotting up to 24 hours afterward.

The *nitrazine* and *fern tests* are also used (see Urinary Frequency and Incontinence).

***Differential Medical Diagnosis.*** Physiologic leukorrhea of pregnancy ruling out ruptured membranes, vaginitis, cervicitis, condyloma acuminatum, genital herpes, sexually transmitted diseases, and cervical dysplasia or neoplasia.

#### *Plan*

Psychosocial Interventions. Reassure the client that increased leukorrhea is normal and will decrease postpartum. Advise the client to notify the health care provider if any symptoms ruled out during the history-taking occur in the future.

Lifestyle Changes. Advise the client to keep the vulva clean and dry; to avoid pantyhose and other tight or layered clothing; to wear cotton underwear and a nightgown without underwear at night; and if using panty liners to use uncented/nondeordorant ones, changing them frequently. Also, advise her to avoid douching and tampon use unless otherwise instructed by the health care provider.

Dietary Interventions. Some clients have recurrent monilia during pregnancy. Instruct these clients to avoid large amounts of simple sugar in their diets. If an antibiotic has been prescribed, advise any client to eat yogurt containing active cultures (sugar-free yogurt unless the client has phenylketonuria or sensitivity to sugar substitutes) to reduce the risk of candida infection. Inform the client that adding lactobacillus, in tablet or granular form, to food may also help; it may be purchased at a pharmacy, where it is kept refrigerated.

Follow-Up. Refer all clients with abnormal Pap smears or symptoms of pathology to a physician. Clients with symptoms of vaginitis require appropriate treatment (see Chapter 8).

## Epistaxis and Epulis

***Etiology.*** The physiologic change underlying epistaxis and epulis is the high level of circulating estrogen. The nasal mucosa and gums become hypertrophic and hyperemic and, as a result, bleed more easily.[1,2]

***Subjective Data.*** The client reports that her nose or gums bleed easily, but she is able to control a nosebleed within 15 minutes. Nosebleeds are usually preceded by blowing the nose, picking at the nose, or overexertion. Gums bleed after teeth brushing or flossing, but the bleeding stops quickly. The client reports continuing her dental care during pregnancy. She has no history of hypertension, bleeding problems, sinus symptoms, fever, trauma, or cocaine use. She may report a history of nasal stuffiness, postnasal drip, or hay fever.

***Objective Data.*** Physical examination and vital signs, particularly blood pressure, are within normal limits. The nasal mucosa may be swollen and dull red or pink, and clotted blood may be observed. Increased vascularization may be evident as may postnasal drip. The gums may show evidence of trauma caused by a toothbrush or floss. Nasal polyps, growths, and evidence of cocaine use should not be observed. A *complete blood count* is the diagnostic test performed (see Fatigue).

***Differential Medical Diagnosis.*** Epistaxis and/or epulis of pregnancy ruling out sinusitis, polyps, or ulcerative disease of the nasal mucosa, hypertension, anemia, bleeding disorders, cocaine use, gingivitis, and other dental disease.

***Plan***

Psychosocial Interventions. Explain to the client the underlying physiologic changes that cause the problem and inform her that the condition should resolve after pregnancy. Advise the client to notify the health care provider if any symptoms ruled out during the history-taking occur in the future.

Lifestyle Changes. Advise the client, when nosebleeds occur, to loosen clothing around the neck, sit with her head tilted forward, pinch her nostrils for 10 to 15 minutes, and apply ice packs to her nose. Light packing of the nose with sterile gauze may help. Inform her that applying petroleum jelly to the nostrils will lubricate and protect the mucosa. Advise the client to avoid overheated air, excessive exertion, and nasal sprays.

Inform the client that the reduced air pressure at high altitudes may precipitate nosebleeds. Instruct the client to blow her nose gently, one nostril at a time and not to pick at her nose.

Advise clients with epulis to practice good oral hygiene, using a soft toothbrush and flossing regularly and gently, and to have regular dental care. Instruct clients that warm saline mouthwashes relieve discomfort.

Dietary Interventions. Advise the client to maintain a healthy diet; to avoid decay-causing, sugary, starchy food; and to cut food that is difficult to chew into small pieces to reduce gum trauma.

Follow-Up. Refer clients with gum disease to a dentist. Clients whose nose bleeds cannot be controlled within 15 minutes or who have high blood pressure or symptoms of pathology should be referred to a physician.

## Muscle Cramps in the Calf, Thigh, or Buttocks

***Etiology.*** The physiologic change underlying muscle cramps in pregnancy is uncertain. An imbalance in the phosphorus/calcium ratio has been postulated, but a correlation with calcium intake has not been established. Cramps occur primarily in the second and third trimesters and could be related to the pressure of the gravid uterus on pelvic nerves and blood vessels.[1,2]

***Subjective Data.*** The client reports calf, thigh, or buttocks cramps that occur mostly at night or in the early morning. She may report a similar history with previous pregnancies, excessive exercise or walking, wearing of high-heeled shoes, or consumption of foods very high or low in calcium. There should be *no* history of deep-vein thromboembolytic disease.

***Objective Data.*** Physical examination and vital signs, particularly Homan's sign, and pulses are within normal limits. No redness, tenderness, heat, swelling, coldness, numbness, or whiteness appears in a calf or leg.

Diagnostic tests are not done unless pathology is suspected.

***Differential Medical Diagnosis.*** Calf, thigh, or buttocks cramps, ruling out thromboembolytic disease, varicosities, dehydration, and nerve root compression.

### *Plan*

Psychosocial Interventions. Explain to the client the physiologic changes that could possibly cause cramping and inform her that the condition should improve after delivery. Advise the client to notify the health care provider if any symptoms ruled out during the history-taking occur in the future.

Lifestyle Changes. Advise the client to avoid stretching her legs, pointing toes, walking excessively, and lying on her back, and to wear low-heeled shoes.

Instruct the client in calf stretching: Have the client stand 3 ft from a wall and lean toward it to rest the lower arms against the wall, keeping her heels on the floor. Advise her that performing this exercise 10 to 12 times before going to bed may reduce cramping.

Dietary Interventions. Correct excessive or inadequate intake of dairy and calcium products.

Follow-Up. Refer a client with symptoms of pathology to the physician.

## Round Ligament Pain

***Etiology.*** The physiologic change underlying round ligament pain is the growth of the uterus, which causes the round ligaments to stretch.[2,13] The round ligaments attach to the uterus at the top of the fundus, extend anteriorly and inferiorly to the oviducts, through the inguinal canal, and attach at the labia majora.

***Subjective Data.*** Usually in the second trimester, the client reports sharp or dull pain on either or both sides of the uterus. The pain often starts or worsens with twisting or quick movements. The client, however, does *not* report contractions, constipation, diarrhea, low-grade fever, anorexia, periumbilical pain, right lower abdominal flank pain, a tender lump in the groin that tends to worsen the longer she stands, or one-sided constant pain that increases (if the pregnancy is less than 14 to 16 weeks). These symptoms may indicate problems other than round ligament pain, and the possibility exists for medical referral.

***Objective Data.*** Diagnostic tests are not necessary. Physical examination and vital signs are within normal limits. Significant negatives include no contractions, cervical dilatation, effacement or softening, rupture of membranes, adnexal or abdominal masses, hernias, hyperactive or underactive bowel sounds, rebound tenderness, or tenderness on abdominal palpation other than along the round ligament.

***Differential Medical Diagnosis.*** Stretching of round ligaments ruling out preterm labor, ectopic pregnancy, rupture of an ovarian cyst, constipation, intestinal obstruction, gastroenteritis, appendicitis, and inguinal hernia.

***Plan***

Psychosocial Interventions. Explain to the client the underlying physiologic change causing the pain and inform her that the pain will resolve after pregnancy. Advise the client to notify the health care provider if any symptoms ruled out during history-taking occur in the future.

Lifestyle Changes. Advise the client to avoid sudden, twisting movements. Inform her that getting out of bed by turning onto her side and pushing up with her arm will reduce abdominal muscle and back strain.

Inform the client that she may apply heat to the painful area. Advise her to avoid excessive exercise, standing, or walking.

Follow-Up. Refer clients with symptoms of pathology to a physician.

### Excessive Salivation and Bad Taste in Mouth

***Etiology.*** The etiology of oral changes is not known. It is theorized that because swallowing saliva increases nausea, clients are reluctant to swallow, which results in their perception of more saliva.[19]

***Subjective Data.*** The client reports increased salivation or a bitter taste in her mouth. She does *not* report a sore throat, fever, flulike symptoms, heat, pain in the mouth, bad breath, upper abdominal pain, bloating, lethargy, dental problems, or pica. In addition, the client practices good dental hygiene and does not have symptoms of a psychiatric disorder.

***Objective Data.*** No diagnostic tests are necessary. Physical examination and vital signs, particularly the condition of the mouth and teeth, are within normal limits. Occasionally, perioral irritation, red-coated tongue, swollen glands, drooling, or speech difficulties may occur.

***Differential Medical Diagnosis.*** Excessive salivation related to pregnancy ruling out stomatitis, tonsillitis, gastric, hepatic or pancreatic disorders, dental problems, and pica.

***Plan***

Psychosocial Interventions. Reassure the client that the complaint is related to pregnancy and that the condition should resolve after the pregnancy. Also, inform the client that her breath does not smell unpleasant. Advise the client to notify the health care provider if any symptoms ruled out during the history-taking occur in the future.

Lifestyle Changes. Advise the client to maintain good oral hygiene.

Dietary Interventions. Advise the client to avoid excessive starch intake and to maintain a good diet and adequate hydration. Inform her that sucking hard candy or breath mints or chewing gum may improve the taste in her mouth.

Follow-Up. Refer a client with symptoms of pathology to a physician. Refer a client with symptoms of dental disease to a dentist.

### Pica and Changes in Taste and Smell

***Etiology.*** The physiologic change underlying pica (i.e., eating nonnutritive substances) is unknown. It occurs in all cultures but in some, for example, among Afro-American women in the southeastern United States, it is very common. Many clients notice a change in their senses of taste and smell but do not report pica.[1,2]

***Subjective Data.*** The client reports changes in her senses of taste and smell. Common changes include those in the taste of coffee, tobacco, alcohol, milk, eggs, and red meats. The client may report cravings for nonfood items or state that they are important for a healthy pregnancy, delivery, and baby and that not eating them may cause harm or birthmarks.

Pica may lead to constipation, bowel obstruction or perforation, parotid gland obstruction, anemia, lead intoxication, parasitic infection, or hypercalcemia (polyuria, kidney stones, anorexia, nausea and vomiting, constipation, weakness, and fatigue).[18]

Clients may also report financial problems affecting the food budget.

***Objective Data.*** Physical examination, particularly of the abdomen and mouth, and vital signs are within normal limits.

Diagnostic tests include the *urine dipstick,* which if negative for ketones rules out ketonuria, and a *complete blood count.*

***Differential Medical Diagnosis.*** Changes in taste and smell related to pregnancy ruling out pica. If pica is diagnosed, rule out anemia, ketonuria, obstruction, parasitic intestinal problems, hypercalcemia, and lead intoxication.

#### *Plan*

Psychosocial Interventions. Reassure the client that the changes in taste and smell should resolve after the pregnancy and may improve as pregnancy advances. While respecting cultural variations, explain that eating a particular nonfood item (e.g., starch) may hurt rather than protect the mother or fetus. Advise the client to notify the health care provider if any symptoms ruled out during the history-taking occur in the future.

Dietary Interventions. Evaluate the client's diet to determine its adequacy. If pica is diagnosed, explain the need to maintain a healthy diet and that problems could occur if the craved substance either is substituting for nutritious food or is harmful to the mother or fetus.

Follow-Up. Refer a client with symptoms of pathology to a physician or a client eating an inadequate diet to a dietitian. A client without adequate financial resources may be referred to a social worker.

## THIRD TRIMESTER

### Braxton–Hicks Contractions

***Etiology.*** During the sixth month of gestation, the uterus begins painless, irregular contractions known as Braxton–Hicks contractions. No cervical dilatation occurs. The contractions are thought to increase the tone of uterine muscles in preparation for labor.[2]

***Subjective Data.*** The client may report a sudden tightening or pressure in the uterus, without the sensation of building, that lasts from 30 seconds to 2 minutes. The contractions may decrease with position change or emptying of the bladder. The client does *not* report regular contractions, vaginal bleeding, bloody show, leaking or rupture of membranes, symptoms of urinary tract infection, constipation, diarrhea, fever, flulike symptoms, or cramping, as these symptoms/signs may indicate other conditions requiring medical follow-up.

***Objective Data.*** No diagnostic tests are necessary. Physical examination and vital signs are within normal limits. The pelvic exam, particularly cervical dilatation, effacement, and station, is within normal limits. No bleeding from the cervical os or pooling of amniotic fluid is evident. The abdominal exam does not reveal regular contractions or suprapubic tenderness. Bowel sounds are normal. The fetus should be normally active.

***Differential Medical Diagnosis.*** Braxton–Hicks contractions ruling out preterm labor, premature rupture of membranes, urinary tract infection, pyelonephritis, gastroenteritis, constipation, and normal fetal activity.

#### *Plan*

Psychosocial Interventions. Reassure the client that Braxton–Hicks contractions are normal and will resolve after delivery. Teach the client to differentiate between Braxton Hicks and labor contractions. Labor contractions grow longer, stronger, and closer together and occur at regular intervals. Often, activity strengthens labor contractions, but decreases Braxton–Hicks contractions. Labor is differentiated from Braxton–Hicks contractions by the presence of cervical changes.

Advise the client to notify the health care provider if any symptoms ruled out during the history-taking occur in the future.

Lifestyle Changes. Advise the client to empty her bladder frequently. Inform her that resting in a lateral recumbent position and walking or exercising lightly may relieve contractions.

As Lamaze breathing eases the discomfort of contractions, teach the client to breathe slowly and deeply at about half her normal rate. Make sure that she is inhaling and exhaling approximately equal amounts of air. Advise the client to contact the health care provider if contractions become strong or different in character from previous contractions.

Follow-Up. Refer a client with possible preterm labor, premature rupture of membranes, or symptoms of pathology to a physician.

### Dyspnea

***Etiology.*** The physiologic change underlying dyspnea is the enlarging uterus, which presses up against the abdominal organs and diaphragm, preventing full expansion of the lungs. The woman has an increased awareness of the need to breathe. Dyspnea can be aggravated by the pressure of the gravid uterus against the vena cava, reducing venous return to the heart.[1,2]

***Subjective Data.*** The client reports shortness of breath, which may or may not be associated with exercise, dizziness, or lightheadedness. There should be *no* history of headache, sore throat, coughing, flulike symptoms, chest pain, indigestion, or exercise intolerance with vomiting, sweating, or anxiety. Neither does the client smoke or have a history of respiratory or cardiac problems.

***Objective Data.*** Diagnostic tests are not necessary. Physical examination, particularly of the upper respiratory tract, heart, lungs, and vital signs are within normal limits.

***Differential Medical Diagnosis.*** Dyspnea related to pregnancy ruling out upper respiratory infection and pulmonary or cardiac problems.

#### *Plan*

Psychosocial Interventions. Reassure the client that her dyspnea is related to normal physiologic changes of pregnancy and that it will improve when the fetus drops into the pelvis. Inform her that it is not an indication that she or the fetus is receiving insufficient air. Advise the client to notify the health care provider if any symptoms ruled out during history-taking occur in the future.

Lifestyle Changes. Advise the client to avoid exercise that precipitates dyspnea, and to rest after exercise. Instruct her not to wear restrictive clothing. Inform the client that sitting up very straight or elevating her head with pillows may help relieve dyspnea, as may lying in the lateral recumbent position, which displaces the uterus off the vena cava.

Follow-Up. Refer a client with symptoms of pathology to a physician.

## Edema

***Etiology.*** The physiologic change underlying edema is increased capillary permeability caused by elevated hormone levels. Edema occurs most often in dependent areas. Moreover, the pressure of the gravid uterus slows down venous return to the heart. Consequently, more fluid passes into intracellular spaces.

***Subjective Data.*** The client reports mild edema in her hands and feet that worsens as the day progresses. Warm weather or prolonged sitting and standing may increase edema; it should improve by morning, however. Ask the client if she wears constrictive bands on her legs. Question her about her diet; a diet deficient in protein calories and fluids or high in sodium, fat, or sugar may increase edema.

The client does *not* report numbness or loss of sensation in the fingers of either or both hands. Edema is not generalized and improves after a night's sleep. There is *no* report or evidence of facial or upper extremity edema, confusion, headache, flashing lights, fatigue, nausea, vomiting, dyspnea, upper abdominal pain, decreased fetal movement, decreased urine output, or rapid weight gain (i.e., more than 2 pounds per week).[2]

***Objective Data.*** Physical examination, particularly of the heart, lungs, and abdomen, and vital signs are within normal limits. It is important to rule out pregnancy-induced hypertension,[1,2,13] By definition, pregnancy-induced hypertension occurs after 20 weeks of pregnancy except with a hydatidiform gestation. Hypertension before this time is considered preexisting, undiagnosed hypertension.[20] The client's systolic blood pressure has not risen 30 mm Hg, or her diastolic 15 mm Hg, above the baseline reading taken in the first trimester. The client's weight gain pattern is less than 2 pounds per week. Edema of the extremities is 0 (no swelling) to +1 (after pressing skin for 5 seconds, the indentation is slight and the contour normal). Deep tendon reflexes are also normal. Jaundice is not noted.

The *urine dipstick for protein* should be negative or show only a trace.

***Differential Medical Diagnosis.*** Physiologic edema of pregnancy ruling out pregnancy-induced hypertension, HELLP (i.e., hemolysis, elevated liver enzymes and low platelet count) syndrome, renal disease, varicosities, local trauma to extremities, carpal tunnel syndrome, and congestive heart failure.

### *Plan*

Psychosocial Interventions. Reassure the client that edema in pregnancy is normal and will resolve after pregnancy. Advise the client to notify the health care provider if any symptoms ruled out during the history-taking occur in the future.

Lifestyle Changes. Advise the client to lie in a lateral recumbent position for 1 to 2 hours twice a day and to sleep in that position at night. Also advise her to avoid long periods of sitting or standing. If a client must sit for extended periods, she should also stand—preferably walk—10 minutes every 1 to 2 hours, or vice versa.

Instruct the client not to wear constrictive bands on the legs and arms; however, she may wear support pantyhose if needed.

Inform the client that raising arms and legs above the level of the heart for short periods and pumping hands and feet may decrease edema. Advise her not to curl her hands under her head or pillow at night if they are swollen or numb. Use of wrists supports would decrease swelling and numbness.

Dietary Interventions. Advise the client to eat adequate protein and calories, drink 6 to 8 glasses of water a day, and avoid high intake of sugar and fats (they can cause water retention). Sodium intake should be moderate; a low intake may be detrimental to the pregnancy and a high intake may increase water retention.

Follow-Up. Refer a client with symptoms of pregnancy-induced hypertension or with symptoms of pathology to the physician. A dietitian may assist with special dietary needs.

## Dyspepsia

***Etiology.*** The physiologic changes underlying dyspepsia are the increase in levels of circulating progesterone that causes decreased gastrointestinal peristalsis and the relaxation of the hiatal sphincter. In addition, the pressure of the gravid uterus against the intestines and stomach increases the reflux of gastric contents into the esophagus.[2,13]

***Subjective Data.*** The client reports heartburn and bloating. The client may be under stress, depressed, swallowing air, or overweight. The client does *not* report chest pain; shortness of breath; exercise intolerance; palpitations; sweating; anxiety; upper abdominal pain, especially after heavy, fatty, or spicy meals; fatty, foul-smelling stools; nausea and vomiting; fever, or flulike symptoms, as these symptoms/signs may indicate other conditions requiring medical follow-up.

***Objective Data.*** No diagnostic tests are necessary. Physical examination, particularly of the heart and abdomen, and vital signs are within normal limits.

***Differential Medical Diagnosis.*** Dyspepsia related to pregnancy ruling out cardiac, gallbladder, epigastric, or pancreatic disease, gastroenteritis, and a hiatal hernia.

### Plan

Psychosocial Interventions. Reassure the client that the dyspepsia is related to pregnancy and should improve or disappear after pregnancy. Advise the client to notify the health care provider if any symptoms ruled out during history-taking occur in the future.

Medication. *Antacids* (Maalox, Mylanta) are indicated to relieve stomach hyperacidity and gas. Instruct the client to take antacids according to package instructions. Depending on the form of antacid, 2 to 4 tablets or 2 to 4 teaspoons are taken between meals and at bedtime. The medications are contraindicated for clients with renal disease or sensitivity to the medication. In addition, these medications are not taken if tetracycline has been prescribed. Teach the client to limit her daily dose of Mylanta to 24 tablets or teaspoons and of Maalox to 16 tablets per day. Antacids containing aluminum and magnesium hydroxides (Maalox, Mylanta) may impair iron absorption;[16] therefore, instruct the client to take iron and vitamin supplements at least 2 hours before or after taking these antacids. Advise the client not to take sodium bicarbonate.

*Calcium carbonate* is indicated for hyperacidity. One to two tablets are recommended every hour, as needed. Abdominal bloating may occur in some clients. Inform the client that calcium carbonate is an additional source of calcium.[16]

Lifestyle Changes. Advise the client not to lie down, bend, or stoop for 2 hours after eating. Inform her that for sleeping, the head of the bed may be elevated 6 inches. Instruct the client not to wear restrictive clothing around the abdomen or waist.

Teach the client to recognize her hyperventilation and swallowing of air, which may aggravate dyspepsia. Flying exercises may reduce discomfort: have the woman sit cross-legged, raise her arms above her head, and lower them quickly to waist level, several times.[3]

Advise the client to stop smoking.

Dietary Interventions. Advise the client to avoid hot, spicy, fatty, gas-forming foods; coffee; alcohol; and gum chewing. Instruct her to eat small, frequent meals and to chew slowly and thoroughly. Inform her that sipping water, milk, hot tea, or a tablespoonful of heavy cream, yogurt, or half-and-half may help dyspepsia.

Advise the client to avoid excessive weight gain.

Follow-Up. Refer any client with symptoms of pathology to a physician.

## Joint Pain/Ache

***Etiology.*** The physiologic changes underlying discomfort are hormonal. Hormone changes, primarily in relaxin, increase the mobility of the sacroiliac, sacrococcygeal, and pubic joints, which, in turn, slightly increases the size of the pelvis in preparation for delivery. The increased mobility of the joint is often painful.[2]

***Subjective Data.*** The client reports pain in the pelvis or hip joints. Pain often increases after fetal engagement. The client does *not* report contractions, symptoms of urinary tract infection, or transient pain, swelling, and redness in the joints with fever and other flu-like symptoms, as these symptoms/signs indicate other conditions requiring medical follow-up.

***Objective Data.*** Physical examination and vital signs are within normal limits; however, tenderness may be noted when palpating the symphysis pubis. There are no signs of labor.

***Differential Medical Diagnosis.*** Joint pain ruling out urinary tract infection, contractions, and rheumatic or joint diseases.

### *Plan*

Psychosocial Interventions. Reassure the client that the discomfort is limited to pregnancy. Advise her to notify the health care provider if any symptoms ruled out during the history-taking occur in the future.

Medication. Acetaminophen may be taken.

Lifestyle Changes. Advise the client to avoid excessive walking, high-heeled shoes, jarring movements, high-impact activities, or other movements that can cause pain. Inform her that she may apply a heating pad or warm moist heat to the painful area for 15 to 20 minutes and that good posture is helpful. Instruct the client that she may place pillows between the thighs and underneath her abdomen to support and align the back while sleeping.

## Emotional Lability

***Etiology.*** The physiologic change underlying lability is the constant rising and falling of hormonal levels during pregnancy. Progesterone has a depressant effect on the central nervous system. This, in addition to the psychosocial crisis pregnancy normally presents, results in frequent and unpredictable mood swings.[2,13]

***Subjective Data.*** The client may report emotional instability, mood swings, or frequent crying. She has adequate support systems and denies fatigue and physical or psychosocial problems.

***Objective Data.*** Physical examination and vital signs are within normal limits.

***Differential Medical Diagnosis.*** Emotional lability of pregnancy ruling out fatigue and physical or emotional disorders.

***Plan***

- *Psychosocial interventions* should be considered.
  - Reassure the client that mood swings are common and should improve after the postpartum period (see Chapter 16).
  - Explain the normal introversion that occurs in pregnancy and its role in mood swings.
  - Assess the adequacy of the client's support systems, including support and communication between partners. Encourage her to discuss her feelings with a trusted person.
  - Teach the client communication techniques. Use of "I" statements, which describe the feelings of the speaker without transferring blame to or labeling the feelings of the listener (i.e. "I am embarrassed by your behavior" rather than "You embarrassed me with that behavior.'). Encourage both the client and her significant other to observe the accompanying body language ("I'm OK" while crying indicates that the speaker may not be OK). Encourage clarification and guard against not fully listening to the speaker but instead formulating a response while listening. Instruct the client to use reflective responses for clarification (i.e. they reword and reflect what the listener has said). Advise her to use silence to encourage the speaker to continue or clarify his or her thoughts.
  - Encourage the client to participate in pleasurable activities and to take time for rest, sleep, exercise, and grooming.
- *Dietary Interventions.* Assess the adequacy of the client's diet and that caloric intake is spread throughout the day.
- *Refer a client* with symptoms of mental illness to a mental health care provider. Couples may also need specialized interventions.

## Altered Body Image

***Etiology.*** The physiologic changes underlying body image alterations result from hormonal fluctuations. Chloasma, uneven brown patches across the nose or cheeks and around the eyes, can appear lighter on black or brown skin. The areolae darken. The normally vertical, pale line that stretches from the umbilicus to the mons darkens (linea nigra). Some women experience acne as a result of increased levels of circulating progesterone, whereas others note improvement. Striae are stretch marks on the skin. Mild pruritus from dryness, as well as stretching, is frequent. Some clients develop spider nevi and palmar erythema. Breasts enlarge in preparation for lactation. The abdomen enlarges with the growing fetus.[2,13]

***Subjective Data.*** The client may report any of the previously described changes. Severe, generalized itching; jaundice; upper abdominal pain; bloating; malaise; constipation; diarrhea; change in stool color or shape; and severe psychosocial stress are *not* reported.

***Objective Data***

- Physical examination and vital signs are within normal limits.
- A *bile acid (cholylglycine) test* is done with severe abdominal pruritus to determine the level of bile acids in the serum. A venipuncture is performed and blood withdrawn for laboratory evaluation. The client must be instructed to fast for 8 hours before the test. The bile acid level is significantly elevated in pruritus gravidarum.

***Differential Medical Diagnosis.*** Changes in skin, breasts, and/or abdomen ruling out liver disease, pruritis gravidarum, scabies, and dermatologic or emotional problems.

### *Plan*

- *Psychosocial interventions* are predominantly to encourage verbalization of concerns.
  - Reassure the client that changes are due to pregnancy and will either fade (e.g., striae) or gradually disappear (e.g., nipple darkening, linea nigra) after delivery.
  - Encourage the client to verbalize her concerns, including her perception of her partner's reaction to the pregnancy and body changes. Encourage her to communicate with her partner. (See previous Plan section.)
- *Lifestyle changes* may improve disturbances in body image.
  - If acne is a problem, advise the client to wash her face carefully, to use a topical astringent, to avoid wearing makeup that clogs pores, and to apply a strong sunblock when in the sun (a strong sunblock may minimize chloasma).
  - Moisturizing lotions may reduce itching, but will not help striae.
  - Explain to the client to avoid irritating soaps (e.g., those with fragrance or deodorants), long, hot showers, and other drying agents.
  - Encourage the client to exercise regularly to control weight gain if no contraindications to exercise exist.
  - Encourage the client to consider breastfeeding, emphasizing that it will induce faster involution of the uterus and easier postpartum weight loss.
- *Dietary Interventions.* Advise the client to maintain a well-balanced diet (see Nutrition) with adequate fluids, which may help reduce acne breakouts and minimize unnecessary weight gain.
- *Refer a client* with symptoms of pathology to the physician. A client with severe relationship or psychosocial stress may be referred to a mental health care provider.

## ANTICIPATORY GUIDANCE DURING PREGNANCY

The issues of concern to pregnant women involve safety, comfort, and uncertainty about what to expect during pregnancy, labor, and delivery.

### CHEMICAL USE AND SAFETY

#### Tobacco

Smoking is related to bleeding, preterm rupture of membranes, premature birth, low birthweight, congenital anomalies, lags in developmental milestones, and low IQ in the child. The adverse effects of smoking increase with the number of cigarettes smoked each day and with the years that the client has smoked. Encourage the client to reduce or stop smoking during her pregnancy. Refer her to a smoking cessation clinic if needed.[21,22]

#### Alcohol

Alcohol use can cause low birthweight and fetal alcohol syndrome. Studies are not conclusive, but as little as 1 oz of alcohol per day (e.g., one beer or glass of wine or one shot of liquor) has been implicated.[21,22] Currently, the best advice for a pregnant woman is complete abstinence from alcohol.

- If the client is concerned about alcohol she consumed after her last menstrual period but before she knew she was pregnant, explain that all studies showing deleterious effects were done with women who consumed alcohol throughout pregnancy.[21,22] This information may be reassuring.

- Refer a client to a mental health care provider or Alcoholics Anonymous if needed.
- If the client is unwilling or unlikely to comply with abstinence, encourage her to reduce intake, as effects seem to be cumulative.[21]

## Caffeine

Caffeine has been implicated as a teratogen in some animal studies, but other research has not replicated this result.[21,22] It is important that the client be informed that the half-life of caffeine triples during the last trimester and it passes easily through the placenta to the fetus. Ideally, caffeine should not be consumed, but the risks are not as obvious as those of smoking and alcohol.[21,22]

Inform the client of caffeine sources: coffee, tea, chocolate, some sodas, and some over-the-counter pain and cold medications. Explain the physical effects of caffeine withdrawal (e.g., lethargy, irritability, headache) and their usual duration (3 to 4 days). Mixing decaffeinated and caffeinated products in increasing ratios to wean from caffeine use may reduce these effects.

## Illegal Drugs

The risks of using illegal drugs are fetal addiction, prematurity, low birthweight, placental abruption, stillbirth, and hepatitis B and HIV infection.[22] Advise clients to stop using drugs. Refer clients using illegal drugs to a drug detoxification center specializing in the needs of pregnant women or to a mental health care provider whose expertise is drug abuse.

## Over-the-Counter Medications

Health care providers do recommend some over-the-counter medications for minor complaints, such as colds and allergies. Some medications (e.g., pseudoephedrine) can restrict blood flow through the placenta to the fetus. Advise the client not to take any medication without first consulting a health care provider. Also advise her that megadoses of vitamins could harm both her and the fetus; she should take only a vitamin/mineral supplement prescribed by a health care provider.[23]

## Prescription Drugs

Many prescription drugs are harmful to the fetus. Advise the client to report all medications she is taking to her health care provider for evaluation.[22]

## Environmental Exposure

The client can be exposed to various chemicals in her work setting, home, or other environment. Ideally, the client should avoid exposure to chemicals, particularly during first trimester in which organogenesis occurs. To reduce exposure when using chemicals (e.g., household cleaning items), the client should ensure that area is well ventilated and wear protective gloves. Advise the client to avoid inhaling chemical fumes, particularly from paint or turpentine, and to wash off any chemicals on the skin immediately. Also advise her if she is in doubt about the toxicity of a chemical she should notify a health care provider or go to an emergency room.

Knowledge about teratogens is growing. To obtain the most current information, several hotlines are available.

- Reproductive Toxicology Center (1–202–293–5137), Columbia Women's Hospital, Washington DC. Information to professionals via on-line computer, FAX, or written request. A subscription service.
- National Institute for Occupational Safety and Health (1–800–356–4674). Research on occupational safety.

- National Pesticides Telecommunications Network (1–800–858–7378).

### Lead Poisoning

Lead poisoning can be a problem for clients who live in homes built before 1980. Lead-base paint on walls or lead pipes can be a source of lead contamination. Inhabitants of these homes should run the water several minutes before drinking. Advise clients who are planning home improvements during their pregnancy to check the house for lead first. Instruct clients to wash fruits and vegetables well to remove lead residue and to remove food from cans before storage, as the solder used to seam them may contain lead that could leach into food. (This effect could also be caused by drinking liquids stored in lead crystal or eating off lead-paint glazed dishes.) Hobbies of creating pottery with lead glaze or leaded glass work or occupations in lead smelting or printing could result in high blood lead levels.[24]

## THE WORKPLACE

In general, healthy women may work until delivery if they have an uncomplicated pregnancy and work at jobs where the potential hazard is no greater than that of normal community life.[25] Because of risk to the fetus in the first trimester, encourage clients to inform their employers of the pregnancy as early as possible.

### Modifications

Some modifications may be needed in employment.[25,26]

- The client should not work longer than 8 hours per day and 48 hours per week.
- The client should take two 10-minute breaks and one meal break each 8-hour shift.
- The client should have a place to rest on her side and should be able to elevate her legs and use the restroom.
- A client who must either sit or stand excessively should be allowed a short time every 1 to 2 hours to sit or walk, whichever is different from her work routine.
- The client should avoid exhaustion, discomfort, extreme temperatures, smoking areas, noxious odors, chemical fumes, activities that require good balance, and trauma to the abdomen.[26]
- Clients with strenuous jobs should avoid hard physical labor, stop or reduce work 2 to 4 weeks before the delivery date, and limit lifting to 10 to 15 pounds and use proper lifting technique.

### Variables

Several variables interact to determine the extent of a workplace hazard particularly in relationship to teratogen exposure: the type of hazard (see Table 13–4); the duration and level of exposure; the method of exposure, for example, inhalation, or ingestion; timing in relation to pregnancy, for example, first trimester; the health and genetic makeup of the client, for example, lead or benzene exposure induces or exacerbates anemia.

### Factors that Prohibit Work

Several physical conditions may make work impossible: incompetent cervix, history of fetal loss, cervical cerclage, heart disease classification greater than II (no symptoms at rest but minor limitations of physical activity due to fatigue, palpitations, or dyspnea),[2] uterine abnormalities, Marfan's syndrome, hemoglobinopathies, hypertension, retinopathy greater than stage 1, severe anemia, herpes gestationis if the pain is severe, diabetes, renal disease, severe disorders requiring medication, asthma, and disk or back problems.[26]

The Occupational Safety and Health Administration is a federal agency that determines and enforces standards regarding workplace safety.

## CONTACT WITH DISEASE

Ideally, clients should avoid persons with disease. In addition, immunizations should be up-to-date prior to pregnancy. The client should also be assessed for susceptibility to hepatitis B, rubella, toxoplasmosis, and varicella–zoster before pregnancy or early in the prenatal period (see Chapter 12).

### Toxoplasmosis

Advise clients to avoid *Toxoplasma* infection by not handling raw meat without gloves, outdoor sandboxes, or litter boxes. If the client must change a cat's litter, she should wear gloves. Afterward, hands are washed well. The route of transmission of *Toxoplasma* is hand to mouth.[27]

### Sexually Transmitted Diseases

Sexually transmitted diseases (STDs) pose a health threat to the fetus. Assess the client for a history of STDs; ask about the number of sexual partners she has and her use of condoms. Advise her to use condoms if she has multiple partners or a new partner, if she is unsure of her partner's sexual or drug use history, or if her partner has multiple sexual partners.

Advise clients who recognize symptoms of infection or are exposed to high-risk sexual partners to contact a health care provider as soon as possible (see Chapter 8).

## SEXUAL ACTIVITY

Many fluctuating factors—physical, hormonal, and psychosocial—influence sexual desire and sexual response throughout pregnancy.

### Normal Sexual Activity

Normal sexual activity is permissible, unless bleeding occurs, preterm labor is a risk, infection develops, intercourse is painful, or membranes rupture or are suspected of rupturing.

Assure the couple that the fetus will not be injured by intercourse nor is the fetus able to understand what is happening.

Encourage the couple to experiment with positions that may be more comfortable (e.g., woman on top, side lying).[2,23]

Inform couples that uterine contractions may occur with orgasm. This is safe if the client is not at risk for preterm labor.[22]

### Communication

A couple may require help adjusting to changes brought about by pregnancy. The woman often has an increased need for closeness during pregnancy but does not always desire intercourse; she should communicate this to her partner, stressing that she is not rejecting him. Emphasize to the couple that closeness and cuddling need not always culminate in intercourse. A mental health care provider may be consulted if necessary.

### Alternative Forms of Sexual Expression

If intercourse is prohibited, specify what is meant: orgasm, vaginal penetration, or unprotected penetration. Other forms of sexual expression (e.g., cuddling, kissing) may be advised.

## EXERCISE

Regular exercise during pregnancy increases a client's sense of well-being, improves sleep, helps her to control weight gain, tone muscles, and, after delivery, hastens her recovery.

**TABLE 13–4. SELECTED REPRODUCTIVE HAZARDS WITH EFFECTS AND PREVENTION BY OCCUPATION**

| Substance | Occupations | Effect | Prevention/ Treatment | Maximum Exposure Level |
|---|---|---|---|---|
| *Chemicals* | | | | |
| Lead | Autoworkers, ceramics workers, electronic workers, painters | Male: reduced sperm<br>Female: Stillbirths<br>CNS disorders in fetuses | Sample air, provide ventilation, clean work area | Inorganic: 0.1 mg/m³<br>Blood level: 60 μg/100 gm<br>Blood level in pregnancy: 40 μg/100 gm |
| Kepone (pesticide) | Agricultural workers, workers who manufacture kepone | Neurologic symptoms<br>Male: Reduced sperm counts | Avoid contact, use protective clothing, ventilation | 1 mg/m³ |
| Benzene (solvent) | Manufacturing of chemicals, artificial leather, dyes, varnishes | Chromosomal damage, CNS defects in fetuses | Avoid contact, good ventilation | 1 ppm |
| *Anesthetic Gases* | | | | |
| Nitrous oxide, halothane | Operating room personnel, dental workers | Spontaneous abortions, congenital defects: cardiovascular and musculoskeletal | Install scavenging devices, monitor levels in operating room air | Recommended limits: nitrous oxide—25 ppm; halothane—12 ppm |
| *Infections* | | | | |
| | Health care workers, teachers, parents, daycare workers | Effects of infection depend on gestational age at time of exposure | | |
| Rubella | | Deafness, microcephaly, CNS disease | Avoid contact if not immunized, vaccine when not pregnant | |
| Hepatitis B | | Prematurity, psychomotor retardation | Avoid contact (blood products), vaccination program: HBIG and vaccine to neonate of HBsAg-positive mother | |
| Cytomegalovirus | | Hearing loss, CNS disease, microcephaly | Handwashing, gloving when handling blood and body fluids | |
| Varicella-zoster (chickenpox) | | First trimester: Spontaneous abortion, muscle atrophy, clubbed foot, CNS disease, cataracts<br>Perinatally: Neonatal death | Avoid contact if not immune<br>VZIG (immune globulin) to exposed neonate at birth; delay delivery for five days after maternal rash in third trimester | |

**TABLE 13–4. CONTINUED**

| Substance | Occupations | Effect | Prevention/ Treatment | Maximum Exposure Level |
|---|---|---|---|---|
| *Infections (cont.)* | | | | |
| Toxoplasmosis | Animal laboratory workers | CNS disease, hydrocephaly, mental retardation | Handwashing, avoid cat feces and raw meat<br>Serial IgG titers; PUBS (percutaneous blood samples); experimental<br>Treatment: Pyrimethamine and sulfa, spiramycin | |
| HIV—AIDS | | Fetal infection | Appropriate isolation, precautions (blood and body fluids) | |
| Herpes simplex II | | Spontaneous abortions, prematurity, microcephaly, fetal infection | Handwashing, gloving | |
| *Stress* | | | | |
| | Most workers, dual job holders | Spontaneous abortions, prematurity, toxemia | Decrease sources of stress, relaxation techniques, good diet, exercise | |
| *Radiation* | | | | |
| Ionizing | Health care workers | Mutogenic: Dependent on dose and type of radiation, sensitivity of particular organs | Avoid during pregnancy, use proper shielding | 1.25 rad/3 mo., 5 rad/year<br>Pregnancy (fetus) 0.5 rad/full pregnancy equivalent to 1.5 rad/pregnant woman |
| Nonionizing video display terminals, microwaves | Office workers, cooks | No significant adverse effects | | |

CNS = central nervous system, HBIG = hepatitis B immune globulin, HbsAg = hepatitis B surface antigen, VZIG = varicella zoster immune globulin, IgG = immunoglobulin G, PUBS = percutaneous umbilical blood sampling.

*Reprinted with permission by Keleher, K.C. (1991). Occupational health: How work environments can affect reproductive capacity and outcome.* The Nurse Practitioner, *16(1), 23–27.*

## General Guidelines

A client who was physically active before conception should be able to engage in the same activities throughout pregnancy. You may need to advise clients not to take up new activities or sports if this activity requires balance because their sense of balance is decreased and their joints are looser, which increase the risk of injury.

Many exercise programs for pregnant women exist but because exercise specialists are not regulated, advise clients to consult their health care provider and to check the credentials of the instructor.

- The client should exercise three to four times per week, not sporadically.
- The client should drink water before, during, and after exercise to replace what is lost during exercise.
- The client should not exercise in hot, humid conditions or when feeling ill.
- The client should make a 5- to 10-minute warmup of stretching exercises routine. Heart rate is kept under 140 beats per minute during the intense portion of exercise, which should last no longer than 15 to 20 minutes. After a 5- to 10-minute cooldown period of stretching, the heart rate should be under 100 beats per minute. The total program lasts 30 to 60 minutes; beginners start with a shorter program. The length and intensity of the program are built gradually.
- The client should exercise on a floor that absorbs impact (e.g., rug-covered or wooden floor). The client should wear clothes that are loose or stretch and a well-fitting support bra. Sneakers are supportive and absorb impact. Deep knee bends should be avoided as should pointing toes, full situps, double leg raises, and straight toe touches; these exercises may injure joints or cause cramps.
- To avoid dizziness, the client should rise slowly following exercise.
- The client should avoid high-impact exercises (jumping, jerking, rapid direction changes), exercises that may force air into the vagina (upside-down bicycles), exercises that stretch the adductor muscles of the legs (putting soles of feet together and pushing down or bouncing legs), exercises that require uncomfortable positions, and exercises that exaggerate the normal curvature of the spine.[23]
- After 20 weeks of pregnancy, the client should not lie on her back for more than a few minutes at a time.
- The client should modify the exercise program as the physical load of pregnancy increases.
- The client should stop exercising and contact a health care provider if any of the following occur: pain, bleeding, dizziness that does not resolve quickly after rising, shortness of breath (unable to talk comfortably), palpitations, faintness, tachycardia, back pain, pelvic pain or pressure, or difficulty walking.

### Prohibited Sports

Advise the client to not participate in snow or water skiing, surfing, diving, scuba diving, ice or roller skating, sprinting, or any sport performed at altitudes higher than 10,000 ft, because they pose a risk of serious injury to mother and fetus.[23]

### Pregnancy Complications

Several complications of pregnancy may prohibit exercise. These include premature labor, placental abruption or previa, threatened abortion, a history of three or more spontaneous abortions, history of stillbirth, incompetent cervix, and medical diseases. Clients at risk should speak with a physician. Toning and stretching exercises, however, reduce the complications of bedrest.[13,23,28]

## SAUNAS, HOT TUBS, AND WHIRLPOOLS

Advise clients not to use such equipment. The high water temperature (higher than 100°F) could raise body temperature 1.5 to 2°F above normal, which is not considered safe. In addition, because blood is shunted to the skin in the sauna or whirlpool, the heart has difficulty maintaining circulation. Syncope could result.[23]

## RADIATION EXPOSURE

### Ionizing Radiation (X-ray, Radiation Therapy)

Dosage of ionizing radiation greater than 0.5 rad over an entire pregnancy may harm the fetus.[25] Total exposure during a barium enema series is 0.407 rad.[25] Several guidelines are suggested that pertain to exposure to diagnostic x-rays.

- Avoid unnecessary x-rays; use another diagnostic method if possible.
- Advise the client to inform anyone ordering or taking an x-ray that she is pregnant and to insist on lead shielding of the abdomen.
- Advise the client to follow exactly the directions of the technician to avoid having to retake x-rays.
- Advise a regularly inspected facility staffed with certified technicians and supervised by a radiologist.
- Advise the client that if x-rays are necessary, fetal risk is low, particularly as the pregnancy advances.

### Nonionizing Radiation

Emissions from video display terminals, televisions, and microwave ovens are very low. Although studies are not conclusive, the fetus does not appear to be at risk.[29]

### Ultrasound

The use of ultrasound, high-frequency sound waves, poses no risk to the fetus, according to several studies.[30]

## DENTAL CARE

Regular dental care is important during pregnancy. The dentist must be told of the pregnancy and x-rays performed only if necessary, with an abdominal shield. Local anesthesia is usually safe.

## TRAVEL

Generally, travel is best undertaken during the second trimester when risk of complications is low and the client is feeling her best.[13,23]

### General Guidelines

- The client should check with her health care provider prior to traveling. Travel may be contraindicated with certain complications: risk for preterm labor, repeated spontaneous abortions, pregnancy-induced hypertension, bleeding, or a medical condition, e.g., cardiac disease.
- If planning to fly, the client should check with the airline about its regulations concerning pregnancy. Pregnant women should not fly in unpressurized planes flying above 7000 to 9000 ft.
- The client should walk for 5 to 10 minutes every 1 to 2 hours while traveling. If driving, she should plan to make stops; if flying or traveling by train or bus, she should arrange for an aisle seat.
- The client should drink adequate fluids and urinate every 2 hours to increase comfort. Light snacks may help reduce nausea.
- The client should not take medication for motion sickness or constipation without first consulting a health care provider.
- The client should be provided with names of obstetricians in the area to which she will be traveling and given a copy of her prenatal record in case of unexpected complications.

### Foreign Travel Guidelines

- Immunizations should be up-to-date before departure.

- Use of chloroquine during pregnancy (to prevent malaria) is safe. Advise the client to start the medication 2 weeks before traveling to the risk area.[13] In some areas (East Africa, Thailand), the strains of malaria are resistant to chloroquine; no other safe medications are available. Because malaria during pregnancy carries increased risk to the mother and fetus, travel to these destinations should be postponed until after delivery.[13,23]
- In areas where water has been known to be contaminated, clients should avoid drinking it, as well as eating raw fruits and vegetables and using ice made from contaminated water or glasses washed in it. Water purification tablets containing iodine are not safe for pregnant women. She should drink only bottled water, soft drinks, or bottled fruit juices. Advise the client which medications and antibiotics to use if she should develop nausea, vomiting, or diarrhea and prescribe them for her if necessary.
- The American College of Obstetricians and Gynecologists publishes a directory of board-certified obstetricians practicing in foreign countries.

### Seat Belts

Advise the client to use shoulder and lap belts when traveling in a car. Correct positioning of a seat belt requires that the lap portion be placed below the abdomen, across the upper thighs. The shoulder belt should rest between the breasts. Both belts should be worn snuggly. If only the lap belt is available, it is used alone. Studies show that in most accidents the fetus recovers quickly from any damage caused by a seat belt, but not from impact against the dash or steering wheel.[13,22,23]

## CHILDBIRTH PREPARATION

Although all pregnant women do not have the same goals for their labor and delivery experience, most clients in their first pregnancy benefit from prepared childbirth classes. A birthing partner assists the client during her labor and delivery. The partner may be her husband, the baby's father, a friend, her parent, a sibling, or a paid birthing attendant.

### Three Philosophies

- Grantly Dick-Read uses education and relaxation techniques to reduce the fear–tension–pain cycle.[23]
- Bradley teaches nutrition, exercise to prepare muscles, relaxation techniques, and inward focusing with deep abdominal breathing to achieve labor and delivery without medication.[23]
- Lamaze uses relaxation techniques, contrived breathing techniques, outward focusing, and conditioned response to reduce the need for medication.[23]

### Shared Concepts

Some classes adapt parts of the three philosophies. The best classes usually comprise five to six couples, employ varied media to present materials, permit discussion, and ultimately prepare the client and her partner for many different experiences during labor and delivery.[23]

## VIVID DREAMS AND FANTASIES

Vivid dreams and fantasies are common, healthy, and normal during pregnancy. Most commonly, pregnant women dream or imagine they are unprepared, are being attacked, are hurt or trapped, have forgotten something, or are becoming physically unattractive. In addition, fantasies and dreams may focus on sex, death and resurrection, delivery at home, and the physical appearance of baby.[23] Recurrent themes may indicate an area of concern for the client.

Assess the need for intervention. Reassure the client that she is not mentally ill, that she will not be a bad mother, and that the dreams do not predict the future.

## CONCERN FOR BABY

Reassure the client that her concern about whether the baby will be normal is not unusual. The many tests that are available to diagnose problems prenatally may be discussed, if appropriate. If her concern seems excessive, refer the client for counseling.

## ACCIDENTS OR BLOWS TO THE ABDOMEN

Reassure the client that the amniotic fluid and abdominal structure protect the fetus, although a very serious blow to the abdomen could cause injury (e.g., hitting the steering wheel during an auto accident). Recommend that she contact a health care provider should such an accident occur, particularly if there is vaginal bleeding or fluid, abdominal pain, uterine contractions, or fewer or no fetal movements. Abusive relationships may intensify during pregnancy. If a woman is in a potentially abusive relationship, abuse may begin once she is pregnant. Refer her to a mental health care provider if abuse is evident (see Chapter 18).

## FETAL HICCUPS

Hiccups are common and do not harm the fetus.

## BATHING

Advise the client that she may take tub baths if ruptured membranes are not suspected and if she takes safety precautions in case she experiences syncope. Late in pregnancy, a woman may need help rising out of a low tub.

## INFANT SAFETY SEATS

By state law in many cases, most hospitals do not discharge infants unless the parents' car is equipped with an infant safety seat. These seats can be rented or purchased, and sometimes are available from charitable organizations and government social service offices. Hospitals, car dealers, baby stores, and consumer safety councils have the information.

## FEEDING METHOD

Whether to breastfeed or bottle feed is a woman's personal choice, although breast milk is the ideal infant food. Infants with cleft lip or palate or other mouth deformity have been successfully nursed using special techniques.[31]

### Advantages of Breastfeeding

Breast milk is ideally suited for the newborn and changes as the infant grows, adjusting to fulfill his or her nutritional needs. The milk is digestible, economical, and always ready. Breastfeeding encourages bonding between mother and child, speeds up uterine involution, suppresses ovulation (although not a reliable method of birth control), and helps weight loss. The sucking motion of nursing helps to develop the infant's jaws, teeth, and palate. Antibodies in breast milk provide protection against disease. Any adverse reaction to breast milk is usually related to the mother's diet, and removing the offending food often solves the problem.

### Disadvantages of Breastfeeding

Breast discomfort, sore or leaking nipples, increased incidence of mastitis, engorgement, less personal time than if bottle feeding, and vaginal dryness are often cited as disadvantages.

### Breastfeeding Contraindications

Breastfeeding is prohibited in the face of serious illness, very low maternal weight, certain infections (e.g., active, untreated tuberculosis, HIV disease or AIDS, hepatitis B, herpes lesion on the aerola). Breastfeeding is also contraindicated if the mother is taking certain medications or if the infant has certain metabolic disorders (e.g., phenylketonuria).

### Preparation for Breastfeeding

Educating a mother about breastfeeding will increase the likelihood of a successful breastfeeding experience. Encourage the client to attend a class (e.g., those offered by La Leche League), to read a good reference book about lactation (see Additional References), and to find a support person (a woman who had a successful nursing experience).

Nipple preparation is unnecessary unless nipples are inverted and do not become erect when stimulated. In such instances, advise the client to wear breast shells during the last 2 months of pregnancy. They are worn inside the bra with the nipples centered in the hole and a plastic dome fitted over it. The client should begin wearing the breast shells 2 hours a day for 1 week, and increase wearing time 1 hour each day until she is wearing the shells 8 hours a day. The client should maintain this schedule until after delivery, and then wear the shells 24 hours a day until the baby latches on easily when they are not used.

The nipples should not be rubbed roughly with a towel or rolled. No drying agents (e.g., alcohol, witch hazel, or soap) should be applied.

### Advantages of Bottle Feeding

The client can return to work more easily, go on a strict reducing diet, and have others share in the baby's feeding.

### Preparation for Bottle Feeding

If the client has chosen bottle feeding, emphasize that infant formula is recommended for the entire first year. Many formulas are available, for example, modified cow's milk and soy-based formulas with varied levels of iron and calories. Formulas are also designed for infants with special dietary needs. The pediatrician will advise the mother about the best formula for her baby. Formulas can be purchased in various forms: concentrated (need to be diluted with equal amounts of water); powdered (to be mixed with water); ready to use (poured directly into bottles); and prepackaged (ready to use in disposable bottles). Advise the client to follow directions carefully and never over- or underdilute the formula.

If a clean water source is available, bottles and nipples need only be cleaned carefully with soap and water and stored away from sources of contamination.

Infants should always be held during feedings. The bonding that occurs while an infant is held is essential to her or his emotional growth. The bottle should not be propped up against the infant. Propping can cause a newborn to aspirate formula. An older baby who lies down with a propped bottle is more likely to develop otitis media. Falling asleep with a bottle contributes to early dental caries.[2]

## CIRCUMCISION

The decision to circumcise is up to the parents. The procedure is usually performed before discharge from the hospital.

### Pro

Proponents argue that circumcision prevents urinary tract infection (rare), infection around the penis, and cancer. Cleanliness and personal, religious, or cultural preference are the most common reasons for circumcision.

### Con

Opponents argue that circumcision may cause injury, infection, and pain (local anesthesia is available). It is not medically indicated in normal circumstances and routine circumcision is not advised by the American Academy of Pediatrics.

## SIBLING RIVALRY

Many parents need reassurance that sibling rivalry is normal.

### Techniques to Minimize Rivalry

Parents can use the following techniques to minimize rivalry.

- Enroll the older child(ren) in sibling classes.
- Encourage the older child(ren) to verbalize his or her emotions and acknowledge the emotions.
- Expect and tolerate some regression.
- If the older child(ren) is to be moved from a crib to a bed or into another room to accommodate the baby, do so before the baby is born, preferably 2 to 3 months before.
- If the older child(ren) desires, buy a gift that she or he can give to the new infant. Be sure that the gift is safe for an infant and request that it be placed in the bassinette (purchase an item that can be cleaned or sterilized). The older child(ren) can then identify the infant in the nursery.
- The first time the child(ren) comes to visit, have the infant in the bassinette. Give the older child(ren) individual attention until he or she expresses an interest in the infant.
- It may also help to have a gift from the infant to the older child(ren).
- Encourage grandparents and visitors to pay attention first to the older child(ren) and to have her or him introduce the baby.
- Find time every day to be alone with the older child(ren).

## FAMILY PLANNING

Encourage the client to begin thinking about family planning methods before delivery.

### Spacing Births

Ideally, women should space births approximately 2 years apart to allow their bodies to recover and replace reserves.

### Breastfeeding Considerations

Although breastfeeding suppresses ovulation, it is not a reliable method of birth control. It should be combined with another form of birth control. Oral contraception is most often prescribed during the postpartum visit and is compatible with breastfeeding. The client should have lactation well established before starting combination pills, as they may reduce the milk supply.[32]

Norplant, according to the manufacturer, is safe for use during lactation. It can be implanted as early as 6 weeks postpartum.[33]

DepoProvera, recently approved by the Food and Drug Administration, is an injection that prevents conception for 12 weeks. It, too, is safe for use during lactation.[34]

### Interim Methods

Foam, suppositories, and lubricated condoms are recommended if a client has intercourse before obtaining contraception at the postpartum visit. They also counteract the normal vaginal dryness that occurs postpartum and with breastfeeding.

### Diaphragm

If the client used a diaphragm prior to conception and wants to use it again, it must be refitted.

### Intrauterine Devices

Intrauterine devices (IUDs) are usually inserted 6 weeks postpartum or after a menstrual period. In some settings, an IUD is inserted immediately after delivery.[33]

### Natural Family Planning

If this method is desired, refer the client and her sexual partner to classes. Advise them that the first ovulation following pregnancy can occur at any time; they should wait until after the first menses to use this method.

### Sterilization

If a client desires sterilization, the procedure may be done on the first postpartum day, during a cesarean section, or after her postpartum visit.

### Vasectomy

If the woman's partner decides to have a vasectomy, the procedure can be done at any time. Both partners, however, must be aware that a man is not sterile until his sperm count is zero. This usually takes 15 ejaculations and must be checked by a urologist.[33]

## DANGER SIGNS

Potential problems in pregnancy may be indicated by the development of particular signs. Should she recognize such a sign, the client should contact the health care provider as soon as possible.

### FIRST TRIMESTER

Signs in the first trimester include bleeding; cramping; painful urination; severe vomiting and/or diarrhea; fever higher than 100° F; low abdominal pain located on either side or in the middle; lightheadedness; and dizziness, particularly if accompanied by shoulder pain.

### SECOND TRIMESTER

Signs in the second trimester include all those noted for the first trimester plus regular uterine contractions; pain in one leg or calf with redness, heat, and tenderness, or coldness, numbness, and whiteness; symptoms of vaginal infection or sexually transmitted disease; sudden gush of fluid that cannot be controlled by Kegel exercises; absence of fetal movement for more than 24 hours; a sudden weight gain; periorbital or facial swelling; or severe headache with visual changes and/or photophobia.

### THIRD TRIMESTER

Signs in the third trimester (after 26 weeks) include all those noted for the first and second trimesters plus a decrease in the daily fetal movement indexes. To perform the fetal movement index, the client chooses four times during the day when the fetus is active, often after each meal and in the evening. She measures the time it takes to feel 10 fetal movements. This will vary with each pregnancy but should always take less than 3 hours. If movement is insufficient, she should contact the health care provider immediately.[1,2]

## INITIAL ASSESSMENT IN LABOR

### PRELABOR

The prelabor stage can begin 1 month to 1 hour before labor begins. It is a period of cervical softening, effacement, and descent of the presenting part into the pelvis. Dilatation of the cervix can also occur during this time.

#### Subjective Data

Lightening, dropping, or engagement occurs when the presenting part descends into the pelvis. The client notes easier breathing but increased pelvic pressure, cramping, low back pain, and more frequent urination. Among primiparas, lightening can occur 2 to 4 weeks before labor and, among multiparas, during labor. Either increasing (nesting) or decreasing energy levels are noted. Vaginal discharge increases and thickens. The client may notice loss of the mucous plug and/or bloody show if some cervical dilatation has occurred. The client may or may not observe a gelatinous, possibly bright red or brown, blood-tinged plug. (Bloody show is a pink or blood-tinged mucous discharge.) Braxton–Hicks contractions may increase and become more intense. They are irregular, feel high and in front, occur suddenly without buildup, and decrease after urinating or changing position.

Labor contractions are felt in the back, legs, or lower abdomen, and frequently are accompanied by menstrual-like or gastrointestinal cramping sensations. With walking or over time, they grow longer, stronger, regular, and closer together.

Diarrhea sometimes occurs.

#### Objective Data

Physical examination reveals a weight loss of 1 to 2 pounds since the last visit. Softening of the cervix, effacement, and possibly some dilatation occur; dilatation is occasionally as much as 4 cm. The cervix moves more anterior. With descent of the presenting part into the pelvis, the fundal measurement may decrease.

### DECISION TO GO TO HOSPITAL OR BIRTHING CENTER

#### Subjective Data

Usually, when contractions are 3 to 5 or 5 to 8 minutes apart with the characteristics of true labor, the client should go to the hospital/birthing center. This decision may be modified by physician preference or the distance the client lives from the hospital. Also, if the client was scheduled for a cesarean section, has a history of precipitous labor, or is labeled as a high-risk pregnancy, she may need to go to the hospital/birthing center earlier.

Signs indicating a client should be in the hospital include a significant decrease in fetal movement; menstrual-like bleeding; constant, severe contractions without relief; and rupture or suspected rupture of membranes. If the umbilical cord is in the vagina (see Chapter 14), the client should call an ambulance and assume a knee–chest position.

#### Objective Data

If the cervix is dilated 4 cm or greater, if amniotic fluid is present in the vagina, if the presenting part is not vertex and the client is having contractions (see Chapter 14), and if the uterus is hard and tender without relaxation, the client should be in the hospital.

Palpation of the umbilical cord during a pelvic exam signals a life-threatening emergency. The health care provider should attempt to push the presenting part back into the uterus while the physician is contacted immediately (see Chapter 14).

## NURSING DIAGNOSES

The following nursing diagnoses identified by the author are representative of those used in a health care plan for pregnant women; however, these diagnoses by no means constitute an inclusive list.

- Activity intolerance related to syncope
- Anxiety related to dyspnea in pregnancy
- Body image disturbance related to changes in the skin and figure
- Bowel elimination altered related to flatulence, constipation
- Comfort and nutrition altered related to dyspepsia, potential for less nutrition than body requirements
- Comfort altered with sleep pattern disturbance related to backache or calf, buttocks, or thigh cramps
- Comfort altered and verbal communication impaired
- Comfort altered related to Braxton–Hicks contractions; increased vaginal discharge; breast tenderness, enlargement, and pigmentation change; menstrual-like sensations in pelvis; increased salivation/bitter taste and/or speech difficulties
- Coping ineffective, individual and/or family, related to emotional lability
- Mobility impaired related to joint discomfort in pregnancy
- Nutrition altered, potential for more or less than body requirements related to changes in taste and smell and/or pica
- Sleep pattern disturbance related to insomnia or increased sleep needs during pregnancy
- Tissue perfusion altered related to edema
- Tissue integrity, altered oral and nasal mucous membranes related to epistaxis and/or epulis
- Urinary elimination, altered patterns related to urinary frequency and/or incontinence

## REFERENCES


1. Star, W.L., Shannon, M.T., Sammons, L.N., Lommel, L.L., & Gutierrez, Y. (1990). *Ambulatory obstetrics: Protocols for the nurse practitioners/nurse mid-wives* (2nd ed.) San Francisco: School of Nursing, University of California.
2. May, K.A., & Mahlmeister, L.R. (1990). *Comprehensive maternity nursing: Nursing process and the childbearing family* (2nd ed.). Philadelphia: Lippincott.
3. National Academy of Science. (1990). *Nutrition during pregnancy.* Washington, DC: National Academy Press.
4. Napier, K. (1991, March). The pregnant vegetarian. *American Baby,* pp. A1–102.
5. National Academy of Sciences. (1992). *Nutrition during pregnancy and lactation.* Washington, DC: National Academy Press.
6. Virginia Department of Health, Bureau of Immunizations. (1991). *Shots for tots* (Booklet No. 11551). Richmond, VA: Author.
7. American College of Obstetricians and Gynecologists. (1992, August). Rubella and pregnancy. *ACOG Technical Bulletin, 171.*
8. American College of Obstetricians and Gynecologists. (1988, March). Perinatal viral and parasitic infections. *ACOG Technical Bulletin, 114.*
9. American College of Obstetricians and Gynecologists. (1990, January). Guidelines for hepatitis B virus screening and vaccination during pregnancy. *Committee Opinion, Committee on Obstetrics: Maternal and Fetal Medicine, 78.*
10. American College of Obstetricians and Gynecologists. (1991, October). Immunizations

during pregnancy. *ACOG Technical Bulletin, 160.*

11. Madinger, N., & McGregor, J. (1992, January). Varicella during pregnancy. *Contemporary Obstetrics & Gynecology,* 83–88.
12. Amstey, M.S. (1988). Treatment and prevention of viral infections (HSV, CMV, HPV, HBV). *Clinical Obstetrics and Gynecology, 31*(2), 501–509.
13. Visscher, H.C., & Rinehart, R.F. (Eds.). (1990). *Planning for pregnancy, childbirth and beyond.* Washington, DC: American College of Obstetricians and Gynecologists.
14. DiIorio, C. (1988). The management of nausea and vomiting in pregnancy. *Nurse Practitioner, 13*(5), 23–28.
15. Wasson, J., Walsh, B.T., Tompkins, R., Sox, H., & Pantell, R. (1992). *The common symptom guide* (3rd ed.). New York: McGraw-Hill.
16. *Physicians' desk reference for nonprescription drugs* (13th ed.). (1992). Montvale, NJ: Medical Economics Data.
17. Poole, C.J. (1986). Fatigue during the first trimester of pregnancy. *Journal of Obstetrical, Gynecologic and Neonatal Nursing, 15*(5), 375–379.
18. Woodly, M. (1992). *Manual of medical therapeutics* (27th ed.). Boston: Little, Brown.
19. Van Dinter, M.C. (1991). Ptyalism in pregnant women. *Journal of Obstetrical, Gynecological and Neonatal Nursing, 20*(3), 206–209.
20. Hughes, E.C. (Ed.). (1972). *Obstetric–gynecologic terminology with section on neonatology and glossary of congenital anomalies.* Philadelphia: Davis.
21. Aaronsen, L.S., & Macnee, C.L. (1989). Tobacco, alcohol and caffeine use during pregnancy. *Journal of Obstetrical, Gynecologic and Neonatal Nursing, 19*(4), 279–287.
22. Corwin, R. (1991). Warning; Some things may be dangerous. *Baby on the Way, 2*(1), American College of Obstetricians and Gynecologists and Parenting Unlimited, 44–49.
23. Eisenberg, A., Murkoff, H.E., & Hathaway, S.E. (1988). *What to expect when you are expecting.* New York: Workman.
24. Barker, P., & Lewis, D. (1990). The management of lead exposure in pediatric populations. *Nurse Practitioner 15*(12), 8–16.
25. American College of Obstetricians and Gynecologists. (1980, May). Pregnancy, work and disability. *ACOG Technical; Bulletin, 58.*
26. Keleher, K.C. (1991). Occupational health: How work environments can affect reproductive capacity and outcome. *Nurse Practitioner, 16*(1), 23–27.
27. Corwin, R. (1991). Safe at work. *Baby on the Way, 2*(1), American College of Obstetricians and Gynecologists and Parenting Unlimited, 50–51.
28. Shaw, R. (1991). Exercise, how much, how often? *Baby on the Way, 2*(1), American College of Obstetricians and Gynecologists and Parenting Unlimited, 14–17.
29. Schnorr, T.M., Grajewski, B.A., Hornung, R.W., Thun, M.J., Egeland, G.M., Murray, W.E., Conover, D.L., & Halperin, W.E. (1991). Video display terminals and the risk of spontaneous abortion. *New England Journal of Medicine, 324*(11), 727–733.
30. Cunningham, F.G., MacDonald, P.C., & Gant, N.F. (1993). *Williams' Obstetrics* (19th ed.). Norwalk, CT: Appleton & Lange.
31. Kitzinger, S. (1989). *Breastfeeding your baby.* New York: Knopf.
32. Frigolette, F.D., & Little, G.A. (Eds.). (1988). *Guidelines for perinatal care.* Washington, DC: American Academy of Pediatrics and American College of Obstetricians and Gynecologists.
33. Hatcher, R.A., Stewart, F., Trussell, J., Kowal, D., Guest, F., Stewart, G., & Cates, W. *Contraceptive technology, 90–92* (15th ed.). New York: Irvington.
34. Grimes, D.A. (Ed.). (1992). Overview of DMPA. *Contraception Report, 3*(5), 3–8.

## ADDITIONAL REFERENCES

Arevalo, J.A., & Washington, A.E. (1988). Cost-effectiveness of prenatal screening and immunization for hepatitis B virus. *Journal of the American Medical Association, 259*(3), 365–369.

Bernhardt, J.H. (1989). Potential workplace hazards to reproductive health: Information for primary prevention. *Journal of Obstetric, Gynecologic and Neonatal Nursing, 19*(1), 53–62.

Briggs, G.G., Freeman, R.K., & Yaffer, S.J. (1986). *Drugs in pregnancy and lactation* (2nd ed.). Baltimore: Williams & Wilkins.

Davidson, E., Jr. (1991). Your pregnant body: Head to toe. *Baby on the Way. 2*(1), American College of Obstetricians and Gynecologists and Parenting Unlimited, 8–13.

Lee, R.V., McComb, L.E., & Mezzardi, F.C. (1990). Pregnant patients, painful legs: The obstetrician's dilemma. *Obstetrical & Gynecological Survey, 45*(15), 290–298.

National Research Council (U.S.), Subcommittee on the 10th edition of the RDA's. (1989). *Recommended dietary allowances.* Washington, DC: National Academy Press.

Wiggins, P.K. (1992). *Why should I nurse my baby?* (rev.) Franklin, VA: L.A. Publishing.

CHAPTER 14

# COMPLICATIONS OF PREGNANCY

*Joan Corder-Mabe*

*Ectopic pregnancy should be considered in diagnosis when any woman of childbearing age reports mild or severe abdominal symptoms.*

## *Highlights*

- Infections
  - *Hepatitis*
  - *Rubella*
  - *Varicella–Zoster*
  - *Cytomegalovirus*
  - *Parvovirus B19*
  - *Toxoplasmosis*
  - *Intraamniotic and Amniotic Infections*
- Bleeding
  - *Spontaneous Abortion*
  - *Ectopic Pregnancy*
  - *Gestational Trophoblastic Disease*
  - *Placenta Previa*
  - *Abruptio Placenta*
- Anemias
  - *Iron and Folate Deficiency Anemias*
  - *Thalassemia*
  - *Sickle Cell Anemia*
- Pregnancy-Induced Hypertension
- Diabetes
- Preterm Labor and Birth
- Substance Abuse
- Multiple Gestation

## INTRODUCTION

A high-risk pregnancy is one in which a condition exists that jeopardizes the health of the mother, her fetus, or both. The condition may be preexisting or may have occurred solely because of the pregnancy. In the last 50 years, the maternal mortality rate has been drastically reduced. Yet, one statistic raises much concern and many questions: Maternal mortality rate among African-American women and women of other minorities is more than two times that of white women.

Prenatal care has long been known to influence perinatal outcome. Of the women who experience a neonatal death, 15 percent have had little or no prenatal care.[1] Lack of or late prenatal care is associated with low-birthweight infants, who are at increased risk of neonatal mortality.[2] The reasons that women frequently give for not seeking prenatal care are lack of money, no transportation, and not being aware of their pregnancy.[2] Moreover, increased stress levels and inadequate support systems have been associated with complications of pregnancy.[3,4] Is it the lack of prenatal care or the social and behavioral factors associated with inadequate care that contribute to the increased maternal and fetal morbidity and mortality?

Optimal perinatal health care involves effective systems to assess all obstetrical clients for risk factors and to identify those women who are at risk. Appropriate interventions and procedures must then be implemented to minimize perinatal mortality or morbidity. Many perinatal centers have established antenatal care units to provide this specialized medical and nursing care.[5,6] Home care programs have also been developed that provide cost-effective, personal care to high-risk pregnant women in surroundings that are familiar to them.[7] Much needs to be learned about the effectiveness and efficiency of these strategies.

The advanced practice role in high-risk care includes several functions: assessment, anticipating concerns, education, advocating for the client, and counseling. The practitioner assesses the physical and emotional health of the woman; assists the family to activate their own strengths and develop strategies to deal with stressors of high-risk pregnancy; anticipates the needs and concerns the family may have and assists them to make appropriate plans to meet their needs; educates the woman and her family about all aspects of the treatment and care so that they can actively participate in the management; advocates for the woman and assists her to communicate and interact with the health care system; and counsels the client throughout her pregnancy.

The goal of care at all times is the best possible outcome for the woman and her family; the ultimate goal is a healthy mother with a healthy infant.

## INFECTIONS

### HEPATITIS

Hepatitis is an acute, systemic, viral infection and the most frequent cause of jaundice during pregnancy.[8,9] The most common forms are hepatitis A; hepatitis B; non-A, non-B (posttransfusion) hepatitis; and delta hepatitis. Hepatitis A is an RNA virus formerly known as infectious hepatitis, because it causes an acute, mild, self-limiting hepatitis without major risk to health. Liver enzymes are temporarily affected and the woman does not become a carrier. Hepatitis B, formerly known as serum hepatitis, is a DNA virus that causes an acute, more severe infection. Among its sequelae are chronic hepatitis, cirrhosis, and hepatocellular cancer. Pregnancy does not affect the severity or outcome of the disease. Non-A, non-B hepatitis is a viral syndrome that behaves much like hepatitis B. It does not, however, have markers for hepatitis A or hepatitis B. Delta hepatitis is a hybrid particle with a delta core and a hepatitis B surface antigen coat. It can only conflict with hepatitis B. Transmission is similar to hepatitis B. Generally a coexisting infection is not more virulent except in homosexuals and parenteral drug abusers when fatality can approach 5 to 10 percent. Hepatitis B vaccination seems reasonable to prevent delta hepatitis in the mother and therefore neonatal infection.

#### Epidemiology

Hepatitis A occurs throughout the population. Traditionally, risk populations for hepatitis B were defined by ethnic origin and historical data. Asians, Pacific Island residents, Eskimos, and certain African peoples are at increased risk. Groups at risk for hepatitis A and B are identified by a history of acute or chronic liver disease; potential exposure to infected blood or blood products, for example, repeated blood transfusions or hemodialysis; or employment in a high-risk environment, such as a labor and delivery or dialysis unit. Recently, however, evidence suggests a poor correlation between historical factors and positive hepatitis blood screens.

Transmission of hepatitis A virus (HAV) is via the fecal–oral route. Contaminated food, particularly milk, shellfish, and polluted water, are common agents. Hepatitis B virus (HBV) is transmitted through contaminated blood and blood products and through sexual intercourse. Skin punctures with contaminated needles, syringes, or medical instruments can also transmit the virus. The fetus is not at risk for the disease until it comes in contact with contaminated blood at delivery.

Incidence reports reveal that the hepatitis B carrier state affects 5 percent of the world population, with a higher percentage in tropical areas and Southeast Asia.

## Subjective Data

Hepatitis A produces flulike symptoms with malaise, fatigue, anorexia, nausea, pruritus, fever, and upper right quadrant pain. Symptoms of hepatitis B are similar to those of hepatitis A[9,10] but with less fever and skin involvement. The older the woman is, the more severe her symptoms.

## Objective Data

Physical examination may reveal a normal general appearance. Jaundice of the skin, sclera, or nail beds may be present.

The immunoglobulin M antibody response occurs 3 to 4 weeks after exposure to the virus and before elevation of liver enzymes. When the IgM level is elevated in the absence of IgG elevation, then acute infection is suspected. The level of IgM usually returns to normal in 8 weeks.

To do the test, obtain a serum sample and send it for laboratory evaluation. Explain to the client that the test will differentiate acute infection from chronic disease.

The immunoglobulin G antibody response occurs about 2 weeks after the IgM response begins. The level of IgG increases rapidly and slowly returns to normal. The IgG level may remain elevated for years. When the IgG is elevated in the absence of IgM elevation, chronic disease is suspected.

To do the test, obtain a serum sample and send it for laboratory evaluation.

Hepatitis B virus antigens and antibodies are identified in a laboratory screening. HBV, also called the Dane particle, consists of an inner core and an outer surface capsule. Laboratory screening is used to identify the presence of hepatitis B surface antigen in the blood, as well as antibodies to the virus surface or core. The hepatitis B surface antigen (HBsAg) screening test is most commonly performed, as a rise in HBsAg appears at the onset of clinical symptoms and generally indicates active infection. If HBsAg persists in the blood, the client is identified as a carrier. The hepatitis B surface antibody (HBsAb) appears 4 weeks after the surface antigen and indicates immunity. Elevation of hepatitis B core antibody (HBcAb) occurs in the period between disappearance of HbsAg and appearance of HBsAb. HBcAb is the only marker in this period that indicates a recent hepatitis infection.

To do the test, obtain a serum sample and send it for laboratory evaluation. Prepare the client for repeat testing, as HBV screening tests may also be used to monitor the progression of infection.

Serum levels of glutamic–pyruvic transaminase (SGPT) and serum glutamic–

oxaloacetic transaminase (SGOT), cellular enzymes found in the liver, are evaluated to determine liver damage. When liver damage occurs, increased amounts of these enzymes are released into the bloodstream.

To do the test, obtain a serum sample and send it for laboratory evaluation. As these enzymes are evaluated as part of a complete panel of blood work, usually following a positive screening for HBV or clinical signs of illness, inform the client that enzyme levels will be retested to monitor the severity and progression of disease.

### Differential Medical Diagnosis

Fatty liver disease, pregnancy-induced hypertension with HELLP (hemolysis, elevated liver enzymes, and low platelets) syndrome.

### Plan

***Psychosocial Interventions.*** Reassure the client that the fetus is at minimal risk. Family members should be encouraged to assist with household and child care duties to allow the client to rest.

***Medication.*** Immune globulin (gamma globulin) or immune-specific globulin (ISG) is indicated for any pregnant woman exposed to HAV, to provide passive immunity through injected antibodies. All household contacts should also receive gamma globulin. Gamma globulin is given intramuscularly. Immune globulin intravenous (IGIV) is available to provide passive immunity.

Hepatitis B immune globulin (HBIG) contains a high titer of hepatitis B surface antigen (HBsAg), which provides passive immunity to hepatitis B. Pregnant women with definite exposure to HBV should receive HBIG as soon as possible after contact and again 30 days later. The newborn of a woman positive for hepatitis should be given HBIG within 12 hours of delivery. If a woman is suspected of having an acute infection during pregnancy, serial HBsAg tests are done. Disappearance of HBsAg indicates that the fetus is no longer at risk. Close contacts of women with HBV should also receive HBIG.

Hepatitis B vaccine is indicated for the newborn of a woman who has tested positive for HBsAg to stimulate the newborn's active immunity. It should be given as soon as possible after birth up to 7 days of life, and again at 30 and 60 days. In many areas of the country, routine vaccination of all newborns is being recommended. The vaccination is not contraindicated during pregnancy.

***Hygienic Measures.*** All caregivers, whether health care providers or family members, should use universal precautions. Instruct family and friends concerning good handwashing and hygiene. Include the mode of transmission in the instruction.

***Diet.*** Recommend a bland diet with additional fluids, depending on the extent of a client's nausea and vomiting. Intravenous fluid hydration may become necessary.

***Follow-Up.*** Frankly discuss and assess possible drug use, as hepatitis is frequently associated with substance abuse. In addition, as hepatitis is sexually transmitted, recommend the use of condoms throughout the remainder of the pregnancy, and arrange to repeat screening tests for sexually transmitted diseases, especially human immunodeficiency virus (HIV) infection.

## RUBELLA

Commonly called German measles or 3-day measles, rubella is an acute, mild, contagious disease caused by the rubella virus.[9,10]

### Epidemiology

The etiology and risk factors of rubella are important in relation to pregnancy because of the potential teratogenic effects of the virus on the first-trimester fetus. The disease occurs worldwide, more frequently among adolescents and young adults.

Transmission occurs by direct contact with urine, stool, or nasopharyngeal secretions. The disease is transmitted to the fetus through transplacental infestation.

The low incidence of rubella and related congenital anomalies is attributed to the availability of rubella vaccine since 1969. It is estimated that 5 to 15 percent of women of childbearing age are susceptible to rubella.

### Subjective Data

The client reports a rash, fever, and a feeling of general malaise. She has no history of the disease or vaccination.

### Objective Data

Postauricular and occipital lymphadenopathy is present early in process. Fever may range from 99.5 to 101.7°F, and conjunctival erythema may be noted. The characteristic maculopapular rash starts on the face, spreads to the trunk, and disappears by the third day.

The diagnostic test used is hemagglutination inhibition (HI). A serum sample is obtained and sent for laboratory evaluation. When confirmation of rubella infection is important, as it is in pregnancy, an HI antibody titer is drawn immediately after exposure to the virus and repeated in 2 to 3 weeks. An initial titer of 1:8 indicates absence of previous rubella infection. A fourfold rise in antibody titer in 2 to 3 weeks indicates infection.

Prepare the client for repeat testing. When rubella affects the fetus, it is termed *rubella syndrome;* defects of the eyes (cataracts, retinopathy, glaucoma), ears (degenerative changes in inner ear, hearing loss), and heart (patent ductus arteriosus, pulmonary artery stenosis) may result. Also associated with the syndrome are decreased head circumference, mental retardation, and poor childhood growth and language and motor development. Seizures related to encephalitis from central nervous system damage also may occur.

### Differential Medical Diagnosis

Rubeola, scarlet fever.

### Plan

Ideally, all women have been vaccinated and have adequate immunity; however, it is recommended that all women be screened during the initial prenatal visit. Counsel clients who do not have adequate immunity to avoid situations where they may come in contact with infected persons. Vaccination is recommended during the immediate postpartum period.

If active disease occurs during the first trimester, counsel the client concerning the risks to her fetus. Support her decision to continue or terminate the pregnancy.

## VARICELLA–ZOSTER (CHICKENPOX)

Varicella–zoster is a highly contagious infection caused by a virus of the same name (varicella–zoster virus or VZV).[9,11] Like herpes, varicella can lay dormant in the dorsal root ganglia and reactivate later. It is a common benign childhood disease that can be more serious in adulthood. In pregnant women, the severity of the disease may be further increased, particularly if there is pulmonary involvement. Varicella, however, is rare in pregnancy; 95 percent of pregnant women have antibodies to VZV.

### Epidemiology

Pregnant women are at risk for developing varicella when they come in close physical contact with children who have active infection. (Most adults have had chickenpox.) The virus is transmitted through direct contact with respiratory tract secretions.

### Subjective Data

The client reports fever, malaise, and a generalized pruritic rash predominantly on the trunk. Usually, her history reveals exposure during the previous 2 weeks.

### Objective Data

Physical examination of the client reveals a characteristic rash. Fluid from the vesicles may be examined for diagnosis and several antibody tests performed. Later, congenital anomalies associated with varicella infection may be detected in the newborn.

Physical examination shows a maculopapular rash on the trunk. The rash quickly progresses to vesicles that erupt and then crust over. New vesicles form daily for 2 to 3 days. Consequently, a mixture of red papules, vesicles, and scabs appears at one time. Fever of 101 to 103°F may be present. Prenatal infection can lead to varicella embryopathy or varicella in the newborn. Congenital anomalies associated with varicella are limb atrophy, microencephaly, cortical atrophy, motor and sensory manifestations, and eye problems such as cataracts, chorioretinitis, microphthalmia, and Horner's syndrome.

Diagnostic methods include clinical evaluation of the virus isolated from vesicular fluid. Several antibody tests are also used to detect infection: enzyme-linked immunosorbent assay (ELISA), fluorescent antibody against membrane antigen (FAMA), and immune adherence hemagglutination (IAHA). None of these tests are in widespread use for screening at this time.

### Medical Differential Diagnosis

Rubella, rubeola.

### Plan

***Psychosocial Interventions.*** Focus on identifying women who are at risk prior to or shortly after exposure to the virus. Counsel any woman who has been exposed and has not previously had the infection to be tested for VZV antibody.

The primary care provider must educate all pregnant women to avoid situations where they may come in contact with varicella. When infection does occur, women require instructions on how to avoid spread of infection and how to relieve the discomforts of skin eruptions.

***Medication.*** Medication is given for symptomatic relief of pruritis; acetaminophen is given to control fever. For severe varicella infection in pregnancy involving pneumonia and high fever, intravenous acyclovir may be recommended.

Varicella zoster immune globulin is administered as soon as possible after a woman who has not had varicella infection is exposed to the virus. A newborn whose mother had an onset of varicella 5 days before or 2 days after delivery should receive varicella–zoster immune globulin.

***Other Interventions.*** Institute measures to prevent the spread of infection. Isolate the client until the rash has disappeared, which is usually about 7 days. Take respiratory and skin precautions if the client is in labor and in the hospital. Following delivery, she should be isolated with her neonate in a private room.

## CYTOMEGALOVIRUS

Cytomegalovirus (CMV) is a DNA virus that is widely spread throughout the human population.[9,12] Congenital infection is different from perinatal infection. Congenital CMV infections, especially those that occur in the first 20 weeks, are associated with symptomatic disease at birth and possible long-term problems of mental retardation, microencephaly, intracranial calcification, and chorioretinitis. On the other hand, perinatal CMV infection is not associated with any adverse effect unless it occurs in a very low birthweight infant.

### Epidemiology

The etiology of congenital disease involves in utero infection. Transplacental infection occurs secondary to primary maternal CMV infection. In women, the likelihood of seropositivity has been correlated with low socioeconomic status, older age, multigravidity, large number of sexual partners, and a first pregnancy before age 15. Women who fit these criteria are at most risk for primary CMV infection.

The virus is transmitted through contact with saliva, tears, urine, cervical secretions, and breast milk. Perinatal CMV is acquired through intrapartum exposure to secretions or postpartum exposure to CMV infection in breast milk or blood transfusions. Pregnant women acquire active disease mostly from sexual contact, blood transfusions, and contact with children in daycare centers. Reactivation of previous infection can also occur and cause congenital CMV.

Incidence reports reveal that congenital CMV occurs among 0.5 to 2.9 percent of all infants.

### Subjective Data

Most women with primary infections are asymptomatic. Clients may, however, report flulike symptoms, including myalgia, chills, and malaise.

### Objective Data

Blood work demonstrates leukocytosis and lymphocytosis; liver function tests are elevated. Diagnosis is most often made by means of antibody tests, including hemagglutination inhibition, ELISA, and fluorescent antibody. A positive CMV-specific IgM test confirms that infection occurred during the previous 60 days. A fourfold rise in IgG antibody titer indicates recent infection.

### Differential Medical Diagnosis

Mononucleosis, HIV disease.

### Plan

No therapy prevents or treats CMV infection. Screening for CMV using cervical cultures is not recommended. Women with documented infection may elect termination of their pregnancy, depending on the gestational age. Discuss the risks and be sensitive to the client's concerns and anxiety.

Teaching all pregnant women about good hygiene and handwashing helps decrease the spread of disease. Advise pregnant women to avoid exposure to individuals with CMV infection (e.g., persons with AIDS).

## ERYTHEMA INFECTIOSUM (FIFTH DISEASE)

This type of virus (parvovirus B19) usually does not cause infection in humans.[13,14] When, however, acute infection does occur during pregnancy, particularly before 18 weeks of gestation, fetal infection and stillbirth are possible.

### Epidemiology

The prevalence of infection among pregnant women and fetuses is not known. Among adults, 30 percent are carriers of antibodies for parvovirus. Infection is spread transplacentally and by direct contact through respiratory secretions. Estimating risk is impossible because studies are limited.

### Subjective Data

A client may report a facial rash and sometimes arthritic pain of the hands, wrists, and knees.[11]

### Objective Data

The most characteristic sign of parvovirus B19 infection is the "slapped-face" rash, a macular rash that may also be found on the trunk.

Blood work reveals aplastic crisis; IgG shows a 30 percent rise with acute infection. The serum maternal α-fetoprotein is also elevated.

A level II sonogram is ordered between 20 and 22 weeks to evaluate fetal structures and to detect the presence of hydrops. With hydrops, fetal edema and ascites are observed. There have been reports of subsequent sonograms that revealed resolution of previously detected hydrops.[14]

### Medical Differential Diagnosis

Rubella, rubeola, roseola, scarlet fever.

### Plan

With the sonographic findings that have reported resolution of Fifth disease, prognosis may not be as grave as earlier thought. The health care provider should share what information is available and be sensitive to the client's concerns.

## TOXOPLASMOSIS

Toxoplasmosis is a common infectious disease caused by the intracellular protozoan parasite *Toxoplasma gondii.*[10,15] Primary infection during pregnancy is associated with stillbirth or congenital infection. Symptoms usually appear at birth. About 10 percent of infected infants manifest severe disease characterized by chorioretinitis, cyanosis, pneumonia, hepatosplenomegaly, jaundice, and thrombocytopenia purpura. Infants who survive sustain some permanent neurological damage.

### Epidemiology

Risk factors for maternal infection include eating raw or undercooked meats and living in rural areas.

Usual transmission is through ingestion of tissue cysts in contaminated meat or through contact with oocytes in feces of infected cats or farm animals. During acute primary maternal infection, the fetus is transplacentally infected about 40 percent of the time. Any infection affords permanent immunity. Abortion, stillbirth, or severe congenital infection occurs in 10 to 15 percent of pregnancies complicated with toxoplasmosis.

The overall incidence is 0.25 to 1.0 per 1000 live births.

### Subjective Data

Although most women are asymptomatic, the client may report fatigue, fever, rash, depression, malaise, headache, and sore throat. Infection occurs 1 to 2 weeks after exposure, and the client may remain symptomatic for as long as several months.

### Objective Data

Physical examination reveals lymph node enlargement, particularly in the posterior cervical chain.

Diagnosis is made by means of serial toxoplasma antibody tests (two or more) done 3 weeks apart. The second sample shows significantly higher levels of antibodies if active infection is present. An indirect fluorescent antibody test of 1:512 or greater correlates with active infection.

Some countries screen all pregnant women for toxoplasmosis during the initial prenatal visit. That is not currently an acceptable approach in this country.

## Differential Medical Diagnosis

Infectious mononucleosis.

## Plan

***Psychosocial Interventions.*** Educate prenatal clients about the risk of toxoplasmosis and discuss prevention. Advise pregnant women to avoid handling cat litter, to wear gloves when gardening, to always wash their hands well after handling cats, and to avoid eating undercooked or raw meats. Prevention of disease is the key to management.

If primary infection occurs in the first trimester, discuss the option of terminating the pregnancy with the client and her family.

***Medication.*** Medications include pyrimethamine and sulfonamides. Some success may occur in treating maternal toxoplasmosis if the drugs are administered throughout pregnancy. Although the treatment reduces the severity of maternal toxoplasmosis, it is not currently standard therapy.

A newborn whose mother was treated antenatally for toxoplasmosis should be treated prophylactically with a combination of pyrimethamine and sulfadiazine (antimalarial drug). An infant with symptoms or an asymptomatic infant with positive cerebrospinal fluid should also be treated.

# INTRAAMNIOTIC INFECTION (GROUP B STREPTOCOCCI)

Intraamniotic infection (IAI) is any infection within the intrauterine structures.[9,16–19] Although in the past, the terms *chorioamnionitis* and *amnionitis* were used interchangeably, each is a specific diagnosis dependent on the structures affected. The conditions are frequently not detected until after delivery.

The organisms most often isolated from the amniotic fluid of infected women are Group B streptococci, *Bacteroides* species, *Bacteroides bivius, Escherichia coli, Clostridium,* peptostreptococci, and *Fusobacterium. Mycoplasma hominis* and *Listeria monocytogenes* have also been isolated, but not necessarily from infected women. How these organisms may affect preterm labor and neonatal sepsis is not clear. Group B streptococci are currently the most common cause of sepsis and meningitis in neonates and young infants.[16] Group A streptococci are not usually associated with neonatal sepsis.

## Epidemiology

In 5 to 25 percent of all pregnant women, group B streptococci can be cultured from amniotic fluid specimens; this rate does not vary with race, age, socioeconomic status, or parity. The amniotic cavity protects the fetus from ascending pathogens; however, with rupture of the membranes and onset of labor, ascending infection from the lower genital tract occurs more often. Group B streptococci is found in about 50 percent of infants whose mothers' cultures were positive for the organisms.

The incidence of neonatal sepsis is only 2 percent; however, infection can be fatal or lead to permanent neurodevelopmental defects.[20] The origin of group B streptococci in the genital tract is unclear, but the gastrointestinal tract seems the likely source. Reinfection is common through either autoinfection or sexual intercourse.

## Subjective Data

Women with colonies of group B streptococci in the genital tract are asymptomatic. With intraamniotic infection, however, the client may report vague symptoms of fever and malaise, usually in the third trimester after membranes have ruptured.

### Objective Data

Early diagnosis is difficult because symptoms do not occur until infection has progressed substantially.

The earliest sign of infection is most likely fever. Uterine tenderness and foul-smelling amniotic fluid are detected later, as are maternal leukocytosis and tachycardia.

Cultures can be done to isolate group B streptococci, but a minimum of 24 hours is needed for test results.

Gram stains can provide immediate results, but are not specific or reliable for group B streptococci.[18] Other methods to detect group B streptococcal infection are being studied.[19]

Routine antenatal screening has not been effective in detecting women at risk for delivering an infected neonate. Maternal colonization is frequently transient and intermittent; therefore, a positive antenatal culture does not indicate that a culture will be positive at the time of labor.

### Differential Medical Diagnosis

Pyelonephritis, bacterial vaginosis, gonorrhea.

### Plan

***Psychosocial Interventions.*** Educate the woman concerning the infection when it is diagnosed. It is not clear whether a woman who has had a child with neonatal sepsis is truly at risk during a subsequent pregnancy, but emotionally she is clearly at risk. Any history of neonatal sepsis can cause apprehension. The provider must recognize this and be sensitive to the client's concerns and questions.

***Medication.*** Broad-spectrum antibiotics are administered to symptomatic clients. Penicillin is prescribed by most providers if group B streptococci are detected during the antenatal period.

Routine intrapartum prophylaxis is controversial. Much depends on successful screening for group B streptococci at the time of labor. The neonate of a symptomatic woman is prophylactically treated.

***Delivery.*** The timing of delivery is debatable. Some physicians may deliver the fetus to drain the infected amniotic cavity. Others are more conservative and wait for spontaneous labor, which has resulted in good maternal and fetal outcomes.

## BLEEDING

Bleeding any time during pregnancy is serious and potentially life-threatening, and it occurs in 10 to 20 percent of all pregnancies.[9,10] The amount of bleeding and the time it occurs determine the urgency and management plan.

### SPONTANEOUS ABORTION

Spontaneous abortion is the termination of pregnancy before the point of fetal viability. Gestation should not be more than 20 weeks and conceptus should not weigh more than 500 g or be longer than 16.5 cm, crown to rump. *Miscarriage* is the lay term for spontaneous abortion.

### Epidemiology

A precise etiology of spontaneous abortion does not exist, but varied maternal and fetal factors are attributed to its incidence. Genetic abnormalities are the most common. Frequently, the embryonic sac is empty or a degenerated fetus is found; both conditions are referred to as *blighted ovum.* Another cause of spontaneous abortion is maternal infections. Both viral and bacterial infections can cause local infection of the conceptus, endometritis, or more generalized pelvic disease, all of which can lead to fetal death and abortion.

In addition, anatomic abnormalities of the reproductive tract are associated with abortion, usually in the second trimester. Some chronic diseases, such as diabetes, nutritional deficiencies, renal diseases, and lupus erythematosus, also affect a woman's ability to maintain her pregnancy. Moreover, lifestyle practices, such as smoking, substance abuse, and exposure to environmental hazards, are related to early pregnancy loss.

Incidence reports reveal that about 20 percent of all pregnant women experience some signs and symptoms of spontaneous abortion. About one half of those women continue through an uneventful pregnancy; the other half suffer pregnancy loss. Maternal age does increase the incidence of pregnancy loss.[9]

### Subjective Data

Varying degrees of vaginal bleeding, low back pain, abdominal cramping, and passage of products of conceptus are reported. Usually the severity of cramping progresses, and a change is seen in the type of blood lost.

Many women in early pregnancy report "spotting," a brown-red vaginal discharge that stains underwear or toilet tissue. Vaginal bleeding that becomes bright red is usually significant.

The amount of bleeding is ascertained by the saturation of sanitary napkins and the frequency with which the napkins must be changed. Saturation of one sanitary napkin every hour is significant.

### Objective Data

Data are established using categorizations based on the client's signs and symptoms and diagnostic test results.

Types of abortion are categorized according to signs and symptoms.

- A *threatened abortion* is possible pregnancy loss; however, pregnancy may continue without further problems. Slight bleeding usually occurs, and some uterine contractions are felt as abdominal cramping. Uterine size is compatible with dates, the cervical os is closed, and no products of conception are passed. Prognosis is unpredictable.
- An *inevitable abortion* is a pregnancy that cannot be salvaged. Moderate bleeding and moderate to severe uterine cramping occur, and the cervical os is dilated. Uterine size is compatible with dates. The products of conception are not passed. Prognosis is poor.
- In an *incomplete abortion,* some products of conception are passed. Moderate to severe uterine cramping and heavy bleeding occur. Uterine size is compatible with dates; the cervical os is dilated. Prognosis is poor.
- In a *complete abortion,* all products of conception are expelled. Bleeding may be minimal and uterine contractions have subsided. The uterus is normal prepregnancy size; the cervical os may be opened or closed.
- A *missed abortion* occurs when the embryo is not viable but is retained in utero for at least 6 weeks. Uterine contractions are absent. Bleeding may initially be absent, but spotting begins and later becomes heavier.
- *Habitual abortion* is the experience of three or more consecutive spontaneous abortions.

In the physical examination, uterine size is compared with expected gestational size. Fetal heart tones are reassuring and dictate a conservative management plan; their absence beyond the tenth week of gestation may indicate a missed abortion.

Real-time sonography, by 8 weeks, will determine the presence of an embryonic sac and detect fetal cardiac motion, which is reassuring and dictates a "wait and see" management approach. Absence of the embryonic sac in the uterus may indicate ectopic pregnancy and must be investigated further. Before 8 weeks, sonographic evidence of the embryonic sac without fetal cardiac motion does not rule out a viable pregnancy; pregnancy may not be at the expected gestational age.

Serial β-subunit human chorionic gonadotropin (hCG) measurements scheduled at least 2 days apart indicate pregnancy viability. Blood is collected for each measurement and sent to the laboratory. β-hCG levels should double every 2 days in early pregnancy, peak at about 10 weeks, then gradually decrease during the remainder of pregnancy. Doubling of levels indicates viability and favorable prognosis. Failure of the β-hCG level to double is suspicious of ectopic pregnancy or abortion.

Although the client requires no specific instructions for this test, waiting the 2 days between specimens may be distressing to her.

### Differential Medical Diagnosis

Malignancy, cervicitis, ectopic pregnancy, gestational trophoblastic disease (hydatidiform mole).

### Plan

***Psychosocial Interventions.*** Provide information for the client and her partner throughout all phases of threatened or eventual abortion. Blood tests and sonograms should be openly discussed. Explain to the client that all precautions will continue until an asymptomatic period of at least 48 hours has elapsed.

The health care provider should be tolerant of the many different responses to pregnancy loss. A response may be influenced by the value of the pregnancy to the client or couple, the desire for pregnancy, the length of gestation, history of other pregnancy losses, the couple's relationship, their social network and support, and religious beliefs.

***Medication.*** In some cases, progesterone supplementation via vaginal suppositories has been used successfully for women with known luteal phase deficit associated with spontaneous abortion defect.

***Specific Interventions.*** Threatened abortion requires conservative "wait and see" management, unless symptoms threaten the life of the mother. The client is at home on bed rest and pelvic rest, with instructions for hydration and when to report signs or symptoms. The client should be evaluated weekly in the health office to determine complete blood count, serial β-hCG levels, any signs of infection, or a missed abortion.

- Bed rest requires that the woman be away from her job, have no child care responsibilities at home, and rest in a horizontal position, except when bathing or using the toilet.
- Pelvic rest means no sexual intercourse and no douching or inserting anything into the vagina.
- Instructions for hydration are to drink a minimum of 32 ounces of noncaffeinated fluid every 24 hours.
- Clients are taught the signs and symptoms of infection and how uterine contractions and vaginal bleeding may progress.

Inevitable, incomplete, or missed abortion should be treated more aggressively as soon as a definitive diagnosis is made. To prevent infection and uterine hemorrhage, the uterus should be emptied of all products of conception. Whether instrumental evacuation is necessary in cases of complete abortion is controversial. If some products of conception remain in the uterus, suction curettage is recommended. Removal of necrotic decidua decreases the incidence of postaborion bleeding and shortens the recovery period.[20]

Missed abortion usually progresses to inevitable abortion, but a "wait and see" approach can be emotionally intolerable for some women. In such cases, suction curettage is recommended during the first trimester. In the second trimester, dilatation and evacuation may be performed or labor may be induced with an intravaginal prostaglandin $E_2$ ($PGE_2$) suppository. Some primary care providers use a laminarin to dilate the cervix overnight prior to the procedure, thereby facilitating a less stressful dilatation procedure. For some women, delaying the definitive diagnosis and treatment plan is necessary to help her accept the situation emotionally. The Rh factor should be assessed and immunoglobulin administered to Rh-negative, unsensitized women.

***Follow-Up.*** Instruct the client about the danger signs of problems she might encounter: fever, foul-smelling lochia, excessive bleeding, back or abdominal pain.

Inform the client that she will need to use some kind of contraception for at least 4 to 6 months to allow for complete maternal healing and regeneration of endometrial lining. Advise her to have a gynecological exam within 2 to 3 weeks of the abortion.

If a woman has had repeated pregnancy losses, complete evaluation is recommended to determine possible causes; appropriate treatment may be instituted prior to future pregnancies.

## ECTOPIC PREGNANCY

Ectopic pregnancy is the implantation of a fertilized ovum outside the uterine cavity.[21–23] Most ectopic pregnancies occur in a fallopian tube, but may also occur in the cervix, on an ovary, or in the abdominal cavity. Following implantation, the embryo grows, but no decidua is present. The structure of the implantation can sustain some growth; however, rupture is usually inevitable. Early signs of pregnancy, including uterine changes and amenorrhea, are present, secondary to hormonal influence. Ectopic pregnancy is a potentially life-threatening condition and almost always involves pregnancy loss.

### Epidemiology

The etiology of extrauterine implantation originates with an interference in normal ovum transport. Women at risk are those who have used an intrauterine device or who have a history of infertility, pelvic inflammatory disease, tubal surgery (e.g., ligation or reconstruction), or ectopic pregnancy.[21]

Some risk, although low, is associated with abdominal or pelvic surgery, postacute appendicitis, intrauterine exposure to diethylstilbestrol (DES), or use of drugs that slow ovum transport (e.g., minipill).[18]

Incidence worldwide has increased, but varies significantly among populations. In the United States, ectopic pregnancy occurs in approximately 1 in 80 pregnancies and is a leading cause of maternal mortality. It is more prevalent in poor, less advantaged countries. Although maternal mortality has decreased in the United States, the actual number of ectopic pregnancies has increased. The increase appears to be related to factors associated with infertility, such as chronic salpingitis.[23]

### Subjective Data

Classical and atypical presentations are used in diagnosis.

The classical clinical presentation includes many of the early signs of pregnancy: 1 to 2 months of amenorrhea, morning sickness, breast tenderness. Abdominal pain is unilateral, and mild vaginal bleeding is possible. The client is motivated to seek emergency care when her pain becomes sharper and she experiences more generalized discomfort.

She may report gastrointestinal disturbances and feelings of malaise and syncope. She may faint. Classically, pain is referred to the shoulder as the hemorrhage becomes extensive and irritates the diaphragm.

Atypical clinical presentations are not so clearly evident. Many clients report vague or subacute symptoms. They may report menstrual irregularity. Amenorrhea may not be obvious, as intermittent spotting or mild vaginal bleeding may mimic normal menses. Ectopic pregnancy should be considered in diagnosis when any woman of childbearing age reports mild or severe abdominal symptoms. Symptoms do not necessarily correlate with the severity of the condition; mild signs and symptoms may occur with massive hemorrhage.

## Objective Data

Diagnosis of ectopic pregnancy is difficult because so many other problems present with similar complaints.

Physical examination may reveal symptoms of shock. General signs of shock include cool, clammy skin and poor skin color and turgor. Late signs are changes in blood pressure and pulse. Abdominal examination may reveal some unilateral tenderness. A pelvic exam reveals a normal-appearing cervix, but marked tenderness is noted. The vaginal vault may be bloody, usually brick red to brown in color. There will be vaginal tenderness. A tender adnexal mass may be palpated, and the uterus may be slightly enlarged.

Levels of β-hCG are used to diagnose ectopic pregnancy. A small amount of functioning trophoblastic tissue, as is found in ectopic pregnancy, will produce a small amount of β-hCG without the doubling increases associated with normal pregnancy. Low β-hCG levels are therefore suggestive of an ectopic pregnancy and should be followed by a quantitative radioimmunoassay.

A sonogram is used to determine if the pregnancy is intrauterine.

Culdocentesis may be done to detect intraperitoneal blood. This procedure is carried out during a pelvic exam. The health care provider inserts a needle through the vaginal wall into the cul-de-sac and withdraws whatever fluid is present. Nonclotted blood indicates hemorrhage. The source of bleeding is then identified by means of laparoscopy or laparotomy, and measures are taken to control bleeding.

## Differential Medical Diagnosis

Pelvic inflammatory disease, ovarian cyst, ovarian tumor, intrauterine pregnancy, recent spontaneous abortion, early hydatidiform degeneration, acute appendicitis and other bowel-related disorders.

## Plan

***Psychosocial Interventions.*** Inform the client about procedures and support her as early diagnosis and appropriate medical referral are pursued. Because laparoscopy is frequently necessary for a definitive diagnosis, prepare the woman for safe and timely transfer to a hospital. Information about the procedure and management plan should be clearly stated for the client and her partner, a family member, or friend.

***Medication.*** Methotrexate is used in the management of ectopic pregnancy. The therapy is new for this condition and has been administered successfully either via local infiltration or orally. It clears remaining trophoblastic tissue and avoids the need for surgical intervention.[21–23]

***Evacuation of Conceptus.*** Immediately after ectopic pregnancy is diagnosed, the conceptus is evacuated. The success of conservative surgery is influenced by the condition of the client and the affected organ (e.g., fallopian tube, ovary), location of the conceptus, and the client's desire for future fertility. Two problems associated with surgery are uncontrolled bleeding and residual trophoblastic tissue. Because of the bleeding, a salpingectomy is necessary for many tubal ectopic pregnancies.

***Follow-Up.*** Postoperatively, all Rh-negative clients should be given Rh immunoglobulin. Discuss the normal body changes the client will experience. Instruct her concerning contraception, danger signals (e.g., signs of postsurgical infection or hemorrhage), and any further follow-up testing. The emotional needs of clients will vary. Pregnancy may not have been realized prior to diagnosis, and learning about the pregnancy and pregnancy loss in such a short period can be overwhelming. Pregnancy should be acknowledged and its meaning discussed. Explain to a client that having one ectopic pregnancy increases her chances for future ectopic pregnancies; review the signs and symptoms of repeated problems with her. Advise her to practice contraception for at least 2 months to allow for adequate healing and tissue repair. Schedule a follow-up appointment within 2 weeks of surgery, at which time some of these issues are best addressed.

Prevention of ectopic pregnancies through screening and client education is essential. Preventing tubal damage from, for example, sexually transmitted disease, can decrease the incidence of the disorder. Encouraging the use of condoms can decrease the incidence of many infections responsible for tubal scarring. Early detection and prompt treatment of gonorrhea and chlamydia, when they do occur, can decrease morbidity.

Appropriate selection of an intrauterine device (IUD) is important. Because IUD use may be associated with infections and tubal pregnancy, women need to be informed of the risk and effect of an IUD on future pregnancy.

## GESTATIONAL TROPHOBLASTIC DISEASE

Gestational trophoblastic disease is a group of neoplastic disorders that originate in the human placenta.[9,10]

- *Hydatidiform mole.* The most common type of gestational trophoblastic disease, hydatidiform mole is a benign neoplasm of the chorion in which chorionic villi degenerate and become transparent vesicles containing clear, viscid fluid. Recently, two types of molar gestations have been distinguished: partial and complete. No fetus or amnion is found in the complete mole, but in the partial mole, a fetus or evidence of an amniotic sac is present.
- *Invasive mole* (chorioadenoma destruens). Invasive mole is a complete molar gestation that has invaded the myometrium, metastasized to other tissues, or both. Karyotyping reveals abnormal genetic material resulting from an empty egg or diploid sperm.
- *Choriocarcinoma.* This rare chorionic malignancy may follow any type of pregnancy, even years later. Half of choriocarcinomas occur following hydatidiform molar pregnancy.

### Epidemiology

Etiology may be influenced by nutritional factors, such as protein deficiency. Such deficiencies would explain some of the race and geographical differences associated with gestational trophoblastic disease.

The incidence of molar pregnancy varies markedly around the world. Incidence in the Far East and Southeast Asia is 5 to 15 times greater than that in Western industrialized nations. The true incidence of partial mole is unknown, because many are diagnosed as spontaneous abortions and tissue karyotyping is not done.

Moles do recur in subsequent pregnancies. Age is also a factor; older women have a greater incidence of molar pregnancy.

## Subjective Data

Presenting symptoms are similar to those of spontaneous abortion. The client usually reports signs of early pregnancy (amenorrhea, breast tenderness, morning sickness) and presents with vaginal bleeding around the 12th week of gestation. Bleeding may begin as spotting, usually brownish rather than bright red. Some women experience severe nausea and vomiting and are treated for hyperemesis gravidarum. Fluid retention and swelling, usually associated with pregnancy-induced hypertension (PIH) later in a pregnancy, occur with molar pregnancy in the second trimester. Uterine cramping may or may not be present.

## Objective Data

Physical examination may reveal what is sometimes a first sign of molar pregnancy: expulsion of grapelike vesicles with or without a history of vaginal bleeding. Vital signs are usually stable; no medical emergency exists. The abdomen is soft and nontender; in the vagina, bloody or clear vesicles may be present. The uterus is usually enlarged beyond the point of expected gestation and has a "doughy" consistency. Ovaries may be enlarged and tender secondary to theca lutein cysts, which develop from ovarian hyperstimulation of high human chorionic gonadotropin levels. No fetal heart tones or fetal activity is detected.

The sonogram shows the absence of the gestational sac and characteristic multiple echogenic regions within the uterus.

Human chorionic gonadotropin levels are extremely high in molar pregnancies and continue to rise 100 days after the last menstrual period. No single value is diagnostic; therefore, serial values must be evaluated and compared with the normal pregnancy curve for hCG.

## Differential Medical Diagnosis

Normal pregnancy, threatened abortion: error in dates, uterine myomas, polyhydramnios, multiple gestation.

## Plan

Prompt identification of gestational trophoblastic disease and appropriate referral are essential to management.

***Psychosocial Interventions.*** Explain the diagnostic procedures and follow-up blood work to the client. Explore the meaning of the client's pregnancy with her and her partner, a family member, or friend. Support them in their grieving. Accounting for religious beliefs and cultural practices is crucial in counseling women concerning the necessity of contraception. Reassurance about future pregnancies is appropriate, because prognosis is good even for women with invasive molar pregnancies.

***Medication.*** No medication is indicated.

***Other Interventions.*** Evacuation of the uterus is recommended when diagnosis is made. *Dilatation and curettage* (suction curettage) is the safest, most effective method of emptying the uterus. Labor induction with prostaglandins or oxytocin is not recommended because these agents are inefficient in emptying the uterus of all trophoblastic tissue. Hospital admission is necessary for adequate anesthesia and nursing surveillance.

A *chest x-ray* is ordered to establish a baseline if there is any question later of invasive disease.

*Serial monitoring of hCG levels* is done weekly for 3 weeks and then monthly for 6 months after the evacuation procedure.

Levels of hCG are used to detect trophoblastic tissue. If any remains, it will regress spontaneously.

No further intervention is necessary if hCG levels decrease to normal, that is, become nondetectable. Pregnancy may be allowed after hCG levels remain normal for a minimum of 1 year. *Reliable contraception* must be used during this time because a positive pregnancy test cannot differentiate normal early pregnancy from beginning invasive disease. Oral contraceptives are desirable because they are reliable and safe following molar pregnancy.

If hCG levels either rise or plateau, *chemotherapy* is indicated for potential metastatic disease. For women who wish to protect their fertility, single-agent therapy is used, usually methotrexate administered orally.[22]

## PLACENTA PREVIA

In placenta previa, the placenta becomes implanted in the lower segment of the uterus and obstructs the presenting part prior to or during labor. When the cervix begins to dilate, the placenta is pulled away from the endometrial wall and bleeding can occur. Any significant bleeding that leads to hemorrhage can endanger the mother and, if allowed to persist, can interfere with uteroplacental sufficiency.

The three types of previa (total, incomplete, and marginal) are classified by the amount of cervix involved.

- In total or complete previa, the entire internal os is covered with placenta.
- In incomplete previa, the internal os is only partially covered by the placenta.
- In marginal or low-lying previa, the edge of the placenta is at the cervical os but does not obstruct any part of it.

The amount of cervical dilation can affect the classification system. Other systems are based on the amount of placental encroachment over the os at the point of full dilation.

### Epidemiology

The etiology of placenta previa is unknown, but certain women are at greater risk than others. Parity is the most common risk factor; old fundal implantation sites are scarred and not suitable for implantation. Other uterine surgical scars, such as those from cesarean section or myomectomy, increase the chance of placental implantation.

Incidence seems to vary with gestation, although the condition is reported in 1 of every 200 pregnancies. Better diagnostic techniques have revealed gestational differences. For example, in the second-trimester placenta previa is a prevalent finding on sonogram, but as pregnancy progresses the incidence falls. In the third trimester, however, as the lower uterine segment stretches and develops, the placenta seems to migrate away from the internal os, and the condition appears to resolve.

### Subjective Data

The characteristic symptom of placenta previa is painless bleeding during the third trimester of pregnancy. Bleeding may occur as early as 20 weeks of gestation and without any precipitating event. Blood is usually bright red. A woman may experience symptoms of shock, such as syncope. The first bleed, however, is usually not a significant amount.

### Objective Data

Vital signs are stable; fetal heart tones are normal and fetal activity is present. The uterus is nontender with a normal resting tone. Bright red blood is evident on sanitary napkins.

Diagnosis is best made by sonogram. No pelvic exam is done to avoid dislodging any clot that may have formed at the cervix. Historically, a sterile vaginal exam was done in a surgical suite to determine the diagnosis; if catastrophic bleeding occurred during the procedure, an emergency cesarean was performed. Now, however, with noninvasive accurate sonograms, such examination is rarely necessary or recommended.[9]

### Differential Medical Diagnosis

Abruptio placentae, genital lacerations, excessive show, cervical lesions and/or severe cervicitis, nonvaginal bleeding (urinary or rectal).

### Plan

The role of the primary care provider lies primarily in the early detection of placenta previa. Referral for appropriate intervention is necessary.

Medication is not indicated.

The medical plan depends on the extent of hemorrhage and length of gestation. If gestation is less than 36 weeks, an attempt is made to stabilize the mother, administer transfusions, and maintain the pregnancy. Strict hospital bed rest is employed, and the mother and fetus are closely monitored. If bleeding stops and the hematocrit is greater than 30 percent, then gradual ambulation may be allowed. Some women may be allowed to return home with limited activity until further problems arise or labor begins.

Provide the client with clear instructions about what pelvic rest entails and what she should do if she notes signs of impending labor or bleeding begins again.

During the "wait and see" period, amniocentesis may be done weekly after 36 weeks to document fetal maturity. In addition, serial sonograms are done to determine placement of the placenta and to note any "migration" if it occurs. Later in the pregnancy, placental problems can lead to uteroplacental insufficiency and intrauterine growth retardation.

Serial sonograms are also used to monitor fetal growth. If bleeding continues or recurs, then operative delivery may be forced. Once fetal maturity is accomplished, delivery is planned. The extent to which the os is covered by the placenta determines if vaginal delivery is considered. Cesarean delivery is usually recommended.

Postpartum follow-up is the same as for other postpartum women. The amount of blood loss is associated with perinatal outcome even though the number of bleeding episodes does not increase perinatal mortality or morbidity. A mother usually recovers readily from anemia and fluid loss. During the first month of life, the infant is at increased risk for death, compared with infants of the same gestational age and birthweight. The increased risk is probably related to transient episodes of fetal hypoxia.[9,10]

## ABRUPTIO PLACENTAE

Abruptio placentae is the partial or complete detachment of a normally implanted placenta at any time prior to delivery.[9] Detachment occurs more frequently during the third trimester, but may occur anytime after 20 weeks of gestation. The proposed mechanism is that maternal arterioles become thrombosed and lead to degeneration of decidua and, subsequently, to rupture of one vessel. The resultant bleeding forms a retroplacental clot, which increases pressure behind the placenta and adds to the separation process.

The classification of abruptio placentae is based on the signs and symptoms of abruption.

- *Revealed abruption.* Vaginal bleeding is evident. Maternal symptoms are consistent with amount of blood lost. Uterine tetany and tenderness, if present, are minor.
- *Concealed abruption.* No bleeding occurs. Uterine tenderness and tetany are

present. Fetal heart tones are usually absent.

- *Mixed abruption.* Bleeding and uterine tetany and tenderness are present.

## Epidemiology

The etiology of abruptio placentae is unknown. Multiparas, women older than 35, women with pregnancy-induced hypertension, and women who use cocaine are more likely to have premature separation.[9] These conditions suggest that underlying vascular problems can predispose a woman to abruption. Severe trauma, such as an automobile accident, has also been associated with abruption.

The true incidence is unknown because abruption occurs in varying degrees. Incidence ranges from 1 in 250 to 1 in 55 deliveries.[9]

## Subjective Data

Symptoms of abruptio placentae can vary significantly depending on the extent and location of separation. The client may report labor pains with some continual cramping. With more severe abruption, severe, sudden, knifelike pain may be described. The client may experience no bleeding, a small amount of dark old blood, or profuse bleeding. Depending on the amount of blood lost from the systemic circulation, she may experience symptoms of shock, such as syncope.

## Objective Data

***Physical Examination.*** May reveal vaginal bleeding (dark old blood or bright red blood), uterine tenderness (local or generalized), increased uterine tone, occasional boardlike quality with little or no relaxation between contractions, lack of fetal heart tones, or signs of fetal distress (such as tachycardia, loss of beat-to-beat variability, or late decelerations). No vaginal or rectal exam is done until placenta previa is eliminated as a diagnosis.

***Sonogram.*** Is frequently used to locate a retroplacental clot. If a clot is not seen on the sonogram, time is critical and diagnosis must be made on presumptive signs.

## Differential Medical Diagnosis

Placenta previa, hematoma of rectus muscle, ovarian cysts, appendicitis, degeneration of fibroids.

## Plan

Immediate identification of possible abruptio placentae dictates prompt referral for appropriate stabilization and treatment.

***Psychosocial Interventions.*** Allay the anxiety of a woman and her family. They need to be informed about impending diagnostic tests and treatment. In addition, maintain respiratory and cardiovascular support (intravenous fluid, oxygen) until the client is transported to the hospital. Because of the potential for hemorrhage, development of a coagulopathy disorder is a risk. Hemorrhage may occur into the postpartum period.

***Delivery.*** Delivery is accomplished once diagnosis is made. Whether the fetus is to be delivered by cesarean section or vaginally depends on the condition of both the mother and the fetus. If the mother's condition is stable, but the fetus is not viable, cesarean section is not indicated. Cesarean section is indicated with signs of fetal distress, maternal hemorrhage, maternal coagulopathy, or poor progress of labor.

***Follow-Up.*** After delivery, care for women with abruptio placentae is the same as that for other postpartum women. It may be necessary to deal with pregnancy loss or in some cases, when the infant survives, maternal grieving may occur over loss of a "normal" pregnancy. Infants may need care in a newborn intensive care unit, which adds to family stress.

## ANEMIAS

Anemia is the reduction of hemoglobin to below normal quantity.[10,24] In a normal pregnancy, concentrations of erythrocytes and hemoglobin fall because of a disproportional increase in the ratio of plasma volume to erythrocyte volume (physiological anemia of pregnancy). During pregnancy, plasma volume increases as much as 45 to 50 percent, but erythrocyte volume increases only 25 percent. Many women have borderline hemoglobin levels before pregnancy; therefore, they do not have the reserve necessary to support physiological changes. Hemoglobin concentration decreases after 8 weeks, drops to its lowest level at midpregnancy, and rises slightly or stabilizes near term. Anemia is not a disease, but a symptom of an underlying condition.

### IRON DEFICIENCY ANEMIA

In iron deficiency anemia, the hematocrit is less than 32 percent or the hemoglobin concentration is less than 10 g/dL. Many providers initiate treatment with a hematocrit of 34 percent.

#### Epidemiology

The cause of iron deficiency anemia is an inadequate iron supply usually secondary to poor dietary intake. Teenagers and women of low socioeconomic status are at greatest risk because of the likelihood of inadequate or improperly balanced diets. Women with short intervals between pregnancies are also at risk.

The incidence of iron deficiency anemia is highest among pregnant women.[9] Approximately 50 percent of all women are anemic in pregnancy.

#### Subjective Data

A woman may experience some fatigue or lassitude that may affect her ability to perform activities of daily living. In the second and third trimesters of pregnancy, she may notice shortness of breath on exertion.

#### Objective Data

All prenatal clients should be screened in the first trimester for anemia. Physical examination of a pregnant woman may suggest iron deficiency anemia; blood tests confirm it.

Physical examination may reveal pale conjunctiva and mucous membranes. Grade II systolic heart murmur may also be detected. Fetal iron stores are protected at the expense of maternal stores. Consequently, fetal effects are not noted unless the maternal hemoglobulin level is below 7 g/dL.

Diagnostic tests show decreased serum iron levels; the number of reticulocytes is low. A complete blood count (CBC) with indices is done showing mature red cells as microcytic and hypochromic. Two very sensitive and reliable laboratory tests for diagnosis of iron deficiency are serum ferritin (concentration of less than 12 μg/L) and free erythrocyte protoporphyrin (FEP). In the FEP test look for a fivefold increase over the normal of 15 to 80 μg/dL.

#### Differential Medical Diagnosis

Folate deficiency, thalassemia, sickle cell disease.

#### Plan

***Psychosocial Interventions.*** Inform the client of her need to eat a well-balanced diet, emphasizing foods that are high in iron. Explain why iron-rich foods are important for her health during and after pregnancy.

***Medication.*** Supplemental iron is administered. Whether it should be given to all pregnant women is controversial. The recommended daily dose of elemental iron for U.S. women is 60 mg. Most prenatal vitamins contain that amount of iron. Women with a hematocrit level of less than 32 percent should be treated for iron deficiency anemia.

The recommended dosage when deficiency is diagnosed is 120 to 180 mg of elemental iron per day; this amount is equivalent to the iron contained in two or three 300-mg tablets of ferrous sulfate. For women who cannot tolerate oral iron therapy, parenteral administration may be necessary.

A side effect of iron supplementation is gastrointestinal disturbance. To enhance its absorption, iron should be taken 30 minutes prior to a meal, preferably with a source of vitamin C. This timing, however, may lead to gastrointestinal effects, disturbances that can be decreased by taking the iron after meals. For pregnant women, taking iron following meals is less problematic because iron absorption is much more efficient during pregnancy. Instruct the client to drink extra fluids (not tea) to offset problems with constipation. Some clients may not be able to tolerate the maximum daily dose. To maximize patient compliance, individualize administration and dosage.

***Follow-Up.*** Schedule a repeat reticulocyte count in about 2 weeks. The count should rise significantly. All anemic women should be closely monitored for infection and signs of intrauterine growth retardation. Following delivery these women should remain on iron therapy and be monitored for recovery. More than 2 years may be needed to replenish iron stores from dietary sources. Counseling women about this period is important if other pregnancies are planned.[10]

## FOLIC ACID DEFICIENCY

Folic acid is a B-complex vitamin essential for cell growth and division. It promotes the maturation of red blood cells. Folic acid is stored in the liver for 4 to 6 weeks. Consequently, overt deficiency does not manifest until late in pregnancy or during the postpartum. Folic acid deficiency rarely occurs in the fetus and is not a cause of significant perinatal morbidity or mortality.

### Epidemiology

Folic acid deficiency is due to an inadequate iron supply usually secondary to poor dietary intake of folic acid. It is the most common cause of megaloblastic anemia.[10]

Teenagers and women of low socioeconomic status are at greatest risk for folic acid deficiency because of the likelihood of inadequate or improperly balanced dietary intake. (Green vegetables, peanuts, and animal proteins, especially liver and red meats, are good sources of folic acid.) Also at risk are women with hemoglobinopathies or those with a multiple pregnancy or pregnancies with a short interval between. Women taking hydantoin or ingesting ethanol are also at risk.

Folic acid deficiency is rare in the United States and is usually diet related. It is not unusual for folic acid deficiency to coexist with iron deficiency anemia.

### Subjective Data

A client with folic acid deficiency may experience symptoms, including nausea, vomiting, and anorexia during pregnancy, and possibly experience symptoms of iron deficiency if it coexists.

### Objective Data

Physical examination may reveal pale conjunctiva and mucous membranes, as well as a grade II systolic heart murmur. Signs of folic acid deficiency cannot be distinguished from those of iron deficiency anemia, as the two conditions are usually concurrent.

Diagnostic tests include determination of serum folate levels. Levels normally fall during pregnancy; however, a fasting folate level of less than 3 ng/mL in an anemic woman is a presumptive sign for diagnosis. Hypersegmented neutrophilic leukocytes and macrocytic red cells on peripheral smear are diagnostic, but definitive diagnosis is made by bone marrow examination. This should seldom be necessary.

### Differential Medical Diagnosis

Iron-deficiency anemia, thalassemia, sickle cell anemia.

### Plan

***Psychosocial Interventions.*** Provide the client with information about foods that are high in folic acid. Explain to the client the importance of eating healthful foods every day to benefit herself and her fetus.

***Medication.*** Prophylactic medication, a prenatal vitamin that contains 0.5 to 1.0 mg of folate, is given to most pregnant women. A full 1.0 mg per day is needed, if there is a deficiency.

***Follow-Up.*** The measures used for clients with folic acid deficiency are the same as those for women with iron deficiency anemia. The appropriate screening for iron deficiency should be performed and iron supplementation initiated when indicated.

## THALASSEMIA

Thalassemia is an autosomal recessive genetic disorder that causes a reduction in or the absence of the alpha or beta globin chain in hemoglobin.

Women with α-thalassemia have signs and symptoms of hemolytic anemia, namely, hemosiderosis, a condition characterized by deposition in organs of the iron-containing pigment hemosiderin, which is derived from hemoglobin degeneration. Symptoms may include chills, fever, hypotension, tachycardia, anxiety, nausea, vomiting, renal failure, and shock. Further discussion is beyond the scope of this chapter; however, medical referral is necessary.

A normal outcome is expected for mother and infant. Women with the disorder are at risk for pregnancy-induced hypertension. Folic acid and iron supplementation is necessary throughout pregnancy, but parenteral iron is contraindicated because of the possibility of exogenous hemosiderosis.

β-Thalassemia major (Cooley's anemia), which is homozygous, is rare. β-Thalassemia minor, the heterozygous form of the disease, is sometimes first identified in pregnancy. A good outcome is expected for both mother and infant. Administration of iron orally is controversial because hemosiderosis is possible. Parenteral administration is contraindicated.

## SICKLE CELL ANEMIA

Sickle cell anemia is an autosomal recessive inherited disease that results from abnormal hemoglobin (hemoglobin S) synthesis. Persons with sickle cell trait, on the other hand, are heterozygous for hemoglobin S and may go undiagnosed because of the lack of symptoms. Sickle cell trait, however, may be identified with routine prenatal screening. All women in high-risk groups should be screened during the initial prenatal visit.

In sickle cell trait, anemia and crisis states do not usually occur except in extreme cases. There is no increased risk for the fetus.

### Epidemiology

Sickle cell disease (sickle cell anemia) involves periods of hypoxia that lead to destruction of red blood cells, hemolytic anemia, and occlusion of blood vessels by abnormally shaped cells. Pregnancy can predispose to periods of hypoxia and trigger a crisis state. Infections, such as pyelonephritis, pneumonia, and osteomyelitis, occur more frequently among pregnant women with sickle cell disease. Other adverse effects that the disease has on pregnancy include an increased incidence of abortion, preterm labor, intrauterine growth retardation, and stillbirth. Sickle cell disease is found almost exclusively in African-Americans, but also among Greeks, Italians, Middle Easterners, and Asian Indians.

Sickle cell anemia is inherited as an autosomal recessive disorder.

The disease occurs in 1 in 400 adult African-Americans. The sickle cell trait is carried by 1 in 10 African-Americans.

## Subjective Data

The client reports multifocal pain, dyspnea, malaise, neurological symptoms, and gastrointestinal upset.

The crisis state is characterized by pain, dyspnea, and malaise. Pain can be multifocal, occurring in the extremities, chest, abdomen, or back. It frequently occurs in bones and joints. Neurological symptoms include headache, visual changes, and seizures. Liver and spleen involvement results in gastrointestinal symptoms, including nausea and vomiting or severe abdominal cramping.

## Objective Data

Physical examination of the mother reveals symptoms in several systems.

- Skin is pale and possibly jaundiced.
- Visual acuity and peripheral vision may decrease.
- Signs of distress are apparent. The client experiences shortness of breath and possibly signs of pulmonary embolus or pneumonia.
- Abdomen may be distended with hepatomegaly and palpable spleen. Fundal height may be equal to or less than expected, depending on the client's general health prior to the episode.
- Kidneys are unable to concentrate urine and signs of kidney failure may be evident.
- Fetal heart tones, if present, may suggest fetal stress.

Blood hemoglobin electrophoresis confirms the diagnosis. During their initial prenatal visit, all African-American women should be screened or have documentation of sickle cell hemoglobin.

## Differential Medical Diagnosis

Malabsorption syndromes, alcoholic cirrhosis, hookworm infestation.

## Plan

***Psychosocial Interventions.*** Make the client aware of the need to recognize symptoms of crisis or complication as soon as possible. Immediate attention can defer the effect on the fetus and frequently decrease the intensity of symptoms. Instruct the client to seek care at the first sign of a crisis. Teach the client the danger signs of pregnancy-induced hypertension and signs and symptoms of infection. Early treatment of common infections, particularly vaginitis and cystitis, may decrease the incidence of more advanced infections, such as pylonephritis and osteomyelitis.

Involve the client's family in every aspect of care. Provide information and clarification about the disease and its implication for pregnancy, delivery, and the fetus.

***Medication.*** There is no specific medication for sickle cell disease or the crisis state. Antibiotics are used for infection. Analgesics are used for pain during a crisis. Iron therapy should be initiated only if anemia is present.

Some authorities are concerned about iron overload.[10]

***Other Interventions.*** *Prophylactic transfusions* have been used throughout pregnancy with some success, but the practice is controversial.

*Blood samples* are taken throughout pregnancy to closely monitor cardiac, renal, and liver function. This procedure is especially critical during and after crises.

*A urine culture and sensitivity* should be performed at least once each trimester for women with sickle cell trait. They have an increased risk for bacteriuria, which, if undiagnosed, can progress to pyelonephritis.

*An early sonogram* is recommended to confirm dates; serial sonograms to assess fetal growth. Starting at 30 weeks, sonograms should be done weekly or biweekly to assess fetal well-being and amniotic fluid volume.

Sickle cell crisis requires hospitalization, enabling administration of transfusions, oxygen, intravenous therapy for hydration, and sedation and analgesia.

Delivery depends on the condition of both mother and fetus in relation to gestation and the risks and benefits that are presented. After 36 weeks, delivery should be initiated as soon as fetal lung maturity is documented. Vaginal delivery is preferred, if possible, and general anesthesia should be avoided because of the risk of hypoxia.

***Follow-Up.*** After delivery, recommend genetic counseling to assist the client and her family to plan future pregnancies. The newborn is screened within the first few days of life. The woman is observed closely for postpartum hemorrhage.

## PREGNANCY-INDUCED HYPERTENSION

Pregnancy-induced hypertension (PIH)[9,10] is characterized by hypertension, proteinuria, edema, or all of these conditions, after 20 weeks of gestation. Previously, PIH was known as toxemia of pregnancy. Pregnancy-induced hypertension is the same physiological condition as preeclampsia. *Eclampsia* refers to a convulsive state.

Mild PIH is characterized by a blood pressure of 140/90 on two occasions 6 hours apart, or a sustained rise of 30 mm Hg or more above baseline systolic blood pressure, or a sustained increase of 15 mm Hg or more in baseline diastolic blood pressure. Proteinuria is present, but is less than 300 mg in 24 hours. There may be slight edema.

In severe PIH, the blood pressure is higher than 160/110 on two occasions at least 6 hours apart. Proteinuria is greater than 500 mg in 24-hour urine collection, and oliguria (less than 400 mL in 24 hours) is detected. Severe PIH is diagnosed if pulmonary edema or thrombocytopenia with or without liver damage is present.

Pregnancy-induced hypertension develops when there is an imbalance in placental prostacyclin and thromboxane production. Prostacyclin is a potent vasodilator and inhibitor of platelet aggregation. A deficiency during pregnancy contributes to the occurrence of preeclampsia. Thromboxane, on the other hand, is a potent vasoconstrictor and stimulates platelet aggregation.

In normal pregnancy, thromboxane is increased: maternal plasma levels are higher late in pregnancy than in midpregnancy.[25,26] In normal pregnancy, prostacyclin and thromboxane levels are equal, but in a preeclamptic woman, the placenta produces seven times more thromboxane than prostacyclin. Vasoconstriction, platelet aggregation, and reduced uteroplacental blood flow result.

The disease is characterized by generalized vasospasm and a constant degree of tension in the vascular system. As a result, blood pressure rises and blood flow to target organs is reduced, giving rise to the various signs and symptoms of pregnancy-induced hypertension. In addition to the vascular system, the organs most affected are the brain, liver, kidneys, placenta, and lungs. Decreased blood flow to the brain leads to fluid shift, cerebral edema, and changes in sensorium. Cerebral edema also leads to central nervous system irritability, which can predispose to convulsions.

Endothelial damage leads to subsequent platelet adherence, fibrin deposition, and the presence of schistocytes. The fluid shift from intravascular to intracellular spaces cause generalized edema. Hemoconcentration occurs because of the decreased blood volume in the intravascular space. Decreased blood flow to the liver leads to microembolization, ischemia, possible infarct, and tissue damage. Subcapsular hemorrhage may occur.

Decreased blood flow to the kidneys normally initiates production of renin and angiotensin I which is converted to angiotensin II, the pressor agent that causes vasoconstriction and stimulates production of increased aldosterone. Aldosterone stimulates the reabsorption of sodium. In normal pregnancy, plasma renin and angiotensin II are elevated, but vasoconstriction does not occur because of the increased aldosterone. The higher levels of aldosterone indirectly increase blood volume and offset vasoconstriction. In PIH, the kidney becomes compromised.

Decreased uteroplacental blood flow can decrease fetal oxygen and lead to fetal stress or distress. Prolonged vasoconstriction can contribute to intrauterine growth retardation and premature separation of the placenta.

Fluid shift in the lungs leads to pulmonary edema.

## Epidemiology

Although it is not known why pregnancy-induced hypertension occurs, acceptable explanations are affected by several important observations.

- PIH occurs more frequently in primigravidas.
- PIH occurs more frequently with excessive placental tissue, as is seen in women with diabetes, gestational trophoblastic disease, and multiple gestation.
- PIH seems to have a genetic component.[27]
- Symptoms usually do not become evident until the third trimester, but there is evidence the process begins as early as the second trimester.
- Symptoms progress; early identification of symptoms and subsequent intervention can decrease the severity of disease and improve perinatal outcome.

Some evidence has been found that the genetic composition of fetal tissue may predispose a woman to the development of eclampsia.[27] An increased incidence of eclampsia among female relatives has been noted, but no conclusions have been drawn so far.

Five to seven percent of all pregnant women experience pregnancy-induced hypertension. It is responsible for more than 25,000 deaths annually. Women at risk for developing PIH include those at extreme ends of the childbearing age range (teenagers and women older than 35), women with preexisting vascular or renal disease, obese women, and women with lupus erythematosus.

## Subjective Data

The two most significant signs of PIH (proteinuria and hypertension) occur without the woman's awareness. By the time symptoms occur, PIH is severe. A woman may report headache, visual disturbances, facial, ankle, and finger edema, or severe heartburn. Therefore, frequent prenatal visits for all pregnant women are recommended for blood pressure and proteinuria screening. All women should be informed of the danger signals and directed to seek evaluation immediately.

## Objective Data

Woman may exhibit a decreased attention span, disorientation, sleepiness, or decreased alertness. Brisk reflexes or clonus may herald an imminent convulsive state; however, many normal women have hyperactive reflexes. Assessment may thus be helpful in monitoring drug therapy, but it cannot be diagnostic for determining status of PIH.

Retinal changes may include edema and arteriolar spasm. Rales and rhonchi can be heard in affected lobes when pulmonary edema is present. Hepatomegaly or upper right quadrant tenderness, or both, may be present. Oliguria (less than 400 mL of urine in 24 hours) is associated with severe hypertension.

Fundal height is usually as expected by dates. A nonreactive nonstress test may indicate fetal compromise. Blood pressure must be carefully and consistently measured to be meaningful. Consistent measurements are those obtained in the same arm with the client in the same position, using appropriate size cuff, and taken at least 6 hours apart.

The convulsive state is an emergency situation and can occur at any time, although the client has usually exhibited signs of severe PIH. Convulsive facial twitching and tonic—clonic contractions of the body occur. Gradually, movements subside, but the client may remain in a coma for an indefinite period. Following seizure, the client is hypoxic and acidotic and requires stabilization before delivery.

Measurements are done to detect changes in blood pressure, urine, and fluid retention. The mean arterial pressure (MAP), or the average pressure in the arteries, is calculated from a blood pressure reading using the formula $MAP = D + \frac{1}{3}(S - D)$, where $D$ is diastolic pressure, and $S$ is systolic pressure.[28,29]

In normal pregnancy, cardiac output increases, but peripheral resistance decreases. Arterioles relax to compensate for increased blood volume. MAP should decrease, particularly in the second trimester. The MAP should be 82 mm Hg or lower in the first and second trimesters and 89 mm Hg or lower in the third trimester.[28,29]

Weight is determined every visit; the client should gain no more than 4 pounds per month, or less than 2 pounds per week.

A urine dipstick is done at every prenatal visit to screen for proteinuria. The hematocrit is monitored to detect hemoconcentration.

## Differential Medical Diagnosis

Diseases that mimic severe PIH or HELLP syndrome (see below), including cholecystitis, viral hepatitis, idiopathic thrombocytopenia, hemolytic uremic syndrome, microangiopathic syndrome, and peptic ulcer.

Other hypertensive disorders may occur and become evident during pregnancy.

***Chronic (Essential) Hypertension.*** In this disorder, a blood pressure of 140/90 or higher either develops before pregnancy, is recognized before 20 weeks of gestation, or continues indefinitely postpartum. Chronic hypertension is seen more frequently in multiparous older women who had hypertension in previous pregnancies. Clinical signs are different from those of pregnancy-induced hypertension.

- Edema is usually absent.
- Proteinuria is absent.
- Hyperflexia does not occur.
- Weight gain is within normal limits.
- Physical signs associated with hypertension, such as retinal changes (arteriosclerosis and hemorrhages), occur.
- Fundal height may lag behind normal expectations, indicating possible intrauterine growth retardation. Fetal survival is related

to clinical course, maternal renal function, and gestation at delivery.

***Chronic Hypertension With Superimposed PIH.*** Signs of pregnancy-induced hypertension can occur in a woman who already has underlying hypertension. Proteinuria may or may not occur. Perinatal mortality increases significantly.

***Late, Transient, Gestational Hypertension.*** Some women experience elevated blood pressure late in the third trimester, intrapartally, or within the first 24 hours postpartally. Other signs of preeclampsia or chronic hypertension are absent, and blood pressure usually returns to normal limits by 10 days postpartum. Whether the occurrence is a sign of underlying chronic hypertension is unclear.

***HELLP Syndrome.*** HELLP is an acronym for hemolysis, elevated liver enzymes, and low platelets. Controversy surrounds the terminology, incidence, cause, diagnosis, and management of this syndrome. It is, however, considered a variant of severe preeclampsia and can develop prenatally, intrapartally, or postpartum.[30]

Symptoms and signs of HELLP syndrome include nausea, with or without vomiting, epigastric pain, upper quadrant tenderness, demonstrable edema, and hyperbilirubinemia. Blood tests reveal elevated serum glutamate–oxaloacetate transaminase (SGOT); elevated serum glutamate–pyruvate transaminase (SGPT); normal serum electrolytes; elevated blood urea nitrogen (BUN) and creatinine; normal prothrombin time (PT), partial prothrombin time (PPT), and fibrinogen; a peripheral blood smear indicating burr cells, schistocytes, or both; and thrombocytopenia (platelet count below 100,000/mm$^3$). Proteinuria is 2+ or greater.

***Disseminated Intravascular Coagulopathy.*** Disseminated intravascular coagulopathy is associated with severe PIH and HELLP syndrome. Most authors, however, do not consider HELLP syndrome a variant of disseminated intravascular coagulopathy because coagulation parameters in HELLP (PT, PTT, and fibrinogen) are usually within normal limits. Opinions vary, but the true relationship between these two processes is unclear.[31]

## Plan

***Psychosocial Interventions.*** The major role of the primary care provider in working with a client with a hypertensive disorder in pregnancy is providing education and support. Teaching about a healthy, balanced diet is important. The client may need to be taught to take her blood pressure or perform a dipstick urine test. All clients need to know the danger signals of PIH.

The provider must also be sensitive to the client's anxieties and concerns about the expected outcome and health of her unborn child. Women with PIH should be assisted and encouraged, within safety limits, to continue normal preparation for birth and the newborn.

***Medication.*** Drugs are given to decrease seizure activity and reduce blood pressure.

Low-dose aspirin therapy may be instituted if mild PIH is diagnosed because it is believed to decrease thromboxane production and platelet aggregation and may decrease the incidence of preeclampsia and fetal growth retardation.[26,32–35] No increased maternal or fetal risks have been demonstrated after administration of 60 to 80 mg of aspirin daily late in the third trimester.[34] More research is needed to define the length of therapy, the effective dose, and the appropriate client for this therapy. Aspirin should be administered with physician consultation.

To prevent the development of pregnancy-induced hypertension, prophylactic low-dose aspirin administration has been recommended for women in high-risk groups.

Women at high risk are those with chronic hypertension, a history of placental abruption, PIH in a previous pregnancy, or lupus erythematosus.

Magnesium sulfate is the drug of choice to control or prevent seizure activity (see Table 14–1). It is usually given as a bolus and subsequently in continuous intravenous infusion. Because magnesium sulfate readily crosses the placenta, the newborn will be affected by the sedative properties of the drug. The newborn may exhibit hypotonia, suppressed respiratory effort at delivery, and poor sucking. These effects subside as the newborn excretes drug over the following 3 to 4 days.

Antihypertensive therapy is initiated to decrease blood pressure enough to protect maternal organs without causing hypotension and threatening fetal oxygen supply.

Hydralazine, the drug used most often, relaxes smooth muscle and causes vasodilation. Blood pressure drops quickly; therefore, the client must be closely watched every 2 to 5 minutes until stabilization occurs, which is within 1 hour. If not controlled or corrected, blood pressure can drop rapidly, lead to fetal hypoxia and subsequent distress.

Whether pregnant women with chronic hypertension should be treated with antihypertensive agents is controversial. Most specialists agree that therapy should be continued for women who are already on a treatment regimen. Therapy for women on reserpine or propranolol should, however, be changed because of their fetal side effects. For women not taking a drug, hydralazine (Apresoline) or methyldopa (Aldomet) is recommended. Treatment is generally initiated when the blood pressure is 150/110.[9] Management is planned after accurate dates of pregnancy are determined.

**TABLE 14–1. MONITORING NEEDED TO ADMINISTER MAGNESIUM SULFATE**

| Activity to Monitor | Sign of Toxicity |
|---|---|
| Deep tendon reflexes | Hypoactivity |
| Respirations | <12 rpm |
| Urinary output | <25 mL/h |
| Blood pressure | Significant drop (>15 mm Hg) |
| Pulse | Tachycardia—sign of shock |

***Conservative Treatment.*** Bed rest, an adequate diet, and close monitoring are recommended for women with mild pregnancy-induced hypertension. Home care is successful when family support is adequate to afford the client appropriate rest.[35] Bed rest, preferably in the left lateral position at least intermittently throughout the day, and limited physical activity induce diuresis and, usually, a drop in blood pressure. A client who is not hospitalized should visit the health office two to three times a week for evaluation. Antepartal self-monitoring needs to be taught to the client (see Table 14–2).

Antepartal monitoring of pregnant women with known chronic hypertension involves obtaining a baseline serum creatinine, uric acid, and creatinine clearance. In addition, a baseline sonogram is done to confirm dates; sonograms are repeated in the second and third trimesters, and fundal height is carefully determined at regular prenatal visits. Moreover, the client must be taught how to take her blood pressure twice a day.

***Delivery.*** The only cure for PIH is delivery of the fetus. Primary goal of management is to allow pregnancy to progress as far as possible without jeopardizing maternal or fetal well-being. Timing and mode of delivery depend on stability of the maternal–fetal unit, gestation, and the cervix. For the woman with eclampsia, delivery should occur as soon as possible after the woman and fetus are stabilized. If the cervix is favorable and other factors are controlled, labor is induced with in-

**TABLE 14–2. ANTEPARTAL MONITORING OF PREGNANT WOMAN WITH MILD PREGNANCY-INDUCED HYPERTENSION**

| Home | Office Visit |
|---|---|
| Check blood pressure once or twice a day | Check blood pressure |
| Check weight every day | Check weight |
| Perform urine dipstick twice daily | Perform urine dipstick (protein) |
| Observe symptoms: occipital headaches, blurred vision, irritability or emotional tension, scotoma, epigastric pain or any signs and symptoms of labor | Assess symptoms: occipital headaches, blurred vision, irritability or emotional tension, scotoma, epigastric pain or any signs and symptoms of labor |
| Record fetal movements daily | Obtain baseline serum creatinine, uric acid creatinine clearance, total protein—repeat twice every week |
| | Obtain baseline liver enzymes, hematocrit, platelet count—twice a week |
| | Auscultate fetal heart tones, baseline fundal height, and weekly measurements |
| | Perform baseline nonstress test (NST) twice weekly |
| | Perform contraction stress test if NST is nonreactive |
| | Obtain baseline and serial sonograms |
| | Arrange for amniocentesis near term, starting at 33 weeks |

travenous oxytocin. Concurrently, magnesium sulfate therapy is administered to control or prevent seizures. Cesarean section is initiated if immediate delivery is indicated.

Some controversy exists as to use of epidural anesthesia. With proper blood pressure control, it can provide satisfactory anesthesia and permit the mother to be awake for delivery.

***Hospitalization.*** Hospitalization is usually essential in the treatment of chronic hypertension with superimposed PIH. The intrauterine environment becomes increasingly hostile to the fetus, and each day is a delicate balance between the risks and benefits of intrauterine and extrauterine existence.

Severe PIH is treated aggressively, as hypertension poses an immediate threat to mother and fetus. Aggressive therapy includes maternal and fetal assessments, medications to prevent seizure activity and stabilize blood pressure, and preparation for delivery. Hospitalization is indicated.

***System Support.*** For the client with eclampsia, airway maintenance and oxygen are necessary. Hemodynamic monitoring is useful for appropriate fluid management.

***Follow-Up.*** The prognosis for pregnancy depends on the severity of symptoms. With aggressive screening, identification, and treatment, maternal and fetal morbidity and mortality have decreased. Following delivery, most women recover quickly without any sequelae. The presence of contributing factors dictates the type of follow-up necessary. If underlying chronic hypertension or lupus erythematosus is suspected, then postpartally refer the woman to an internist for assessment.

Many women do not have problems in subsequent pregnancies; however, all women should be informed of the possibility and the need for early prenatal care and evaluation.

## DIABETES

Diabetes is a chronic disease characterized by a relative lack of insulin or absence of the hormone, which is necessary for glucose metabolism.[9,24] In normal pregnancy profound metabolic alterations occur to support the growth and development of a fetus. Maternal basal metabolism increases as a response to fetal growth. The increase contributes to increased glucose utilization and the risk of maternal acidosis. Glucose rapidly moves from maternal circulation to the fetus by simple diffusion; insulin does not cross the placental membrane.

Insulin, however, is present as early as 12 weeks in the fetal pancreas; it is stimulated by glucose from the maternal circulation. The increase in glucose to the fetus results in accelerated growth of the fetus. Human placental lactogen (HPL) and growth hormone (somatotropin) increase in direct correlation with the growth of placental tissue; it rises throughout the last 20 weeks of pregnancy and causes an increase in insulin resistance. HPL stimulates the mobilization of free fatty acids for maternal use, which can lead to maternal ketoacidosis.

The hormonal changes of pregnancy have conflicting but carefully balanced effects on carbohydrate metabolism. The increased estrogen acts as an insulin antagonist. Progesterone, on the other hand, augments insulin secretion while diminishing its peripheral effectiveness. In most cases, the maternal pancreas is able to increase insulin production to maintain normal glucose levels.

The woman with diabetes that has not been diagnosed is not able to cope with changes in metabolism resulting from insufficient insulin. The woman with suboptimal function who is not diabetic may not experience difficulty early in the pregnancy, but when pregnancy-related hormones are produced by the enlarging placenta and reach certain levels, her pancreas will not be able to accommodate the increased insulin demand. The increased need for insulin and the tendency toward hyperglycemia occur most often between 20 and 30 weeks of gestation.

In an attempt to predict client outcome and to establish treatment guidelines for diabetic clients, several classification systems are used. White's classification is based on age at onset of disease and degree of vascular involvement[10] (see Table 14–3). A general classification developed from the National Diabetes Data Group Classification of Diabetes Group has been used recently[10] (see Table 14–4).

### Diabetic Woman's Response During Pregnancy

A woman with diabetes may have several problems during pregnancy as a result of her diabetes, such as hypoglycemia, urinary tract infection, hypertension, hydramnios, and retinopathy.

***Hypoglycemia.*** Hypoglycemia occurs primarily in the first trimester in insulin-dependent, controlled diabetics. Because of its accelerated growth, the fetus uses glucose available in the maternal circulation, thereby decreasing her need for insulin. Women accustomed to a consistent diet and insulin intake are not able to adjust to their reduced need for insulin. Consequently, they commonly develop hypoglycemia in the first trimester.

**TABLE 14–3. WHITE'S CLASSIFICATION OF DIABETES IN PREGNANT WOMEN**

| | |
|---|---|
| A | Chemical diabetes |
| B | Maturity onset (age > 20 years), duration < 10 years, no vascular change |
| C | Age 10–19 years, duration 10–19 years |
| D | <10 years at onset; >20 years' duration, benign retinopathy, calcified vessels of legs, hypertension |
| E | Overt diabetes at any age |
| F | Nephropathy |
| R, RF, H, T | Combined retinopathy, renal disease, arteriosclerotic heart disease |

***Urinary Tract Infection.*** Urinary tract infection is common in diabetics because more glucose is filtered due to their increased glomerular filtration rate. Glycosuria predisposes to bacterial infection.

***Hypertension.*** Hypertension is related to the same factors that cause pregnancy-induced hypertension. Diabetics have a predisposition to PIH.

**TABLE 14–4. CLASSIFICATION OF DIABETES**

A. Insulin-dependent type (type I)
B. Non-insulin-dependent type (type II)
   1. Nonobese
   2. Obese
C. Other types (secondary diabetes)
   1. Pancreatic disease
   2. Hormonally induced
   3. Chemically induced
   4. Insulin receptor abnormalities
   5. Certain genetic syndromes
   6. Others
D. Impaired glucose tolerance (subclinical diabetes)
E. Gestational diabetes (pregnancy-induced glucose intolerance)

Source: *Buckley and Kulb.*[10]

***Hydramnios.*** Ten to twenty percent of diabetics have hydramnios. The reason is poorly understood, but it is explained as caused by fetal glycosuria. The urine in amniotic fluid attracts water to balance the high osmolarity of the fluid.

***Retinopathy.*** Diabetes is associated with retinal changes that may exacerbate during pregnancy and become more symptomatic.

## Effects on Fetus and Neonate

The fetus that remains in an environment of maternal hyperglycemia may demonstrate macrosomia, teratogenesis, or death.

***Macrosomia.*** The accelerated fetal growth that occurs when a mother is diabetic leads to a macrosomic or large-for-gestational-age infant.

***Teratogenesis.*** If significant maternal hyperglycemia continues, it can lead to maternal ketoacidosis and to movement of ketones across the placental membrane. These ketones have been associated with teratogenesis. Although rare, agenesis has been linked with ketosis between 5 and 6 weeks of gestation. Cardiac anomalies also occur. Ideally, preconception and early pregnancy glycemic control will prevent excess rates of congenital anomalies.[36]

***Death.*** Among mothers who develop ketoacidosis, 50 percent of infants die. Early first-trimester ketosis may cause early pregnancy loss. Hyperinsulinemia in the fetus may lead to delayed surfactant production in the lung and contribute to the incidence of respiratory distress syndrome.

***Other Effects.*** Neonates of diabetic women have more problems with hypoglycemia, hypocalcemia, and hyperbilirubinemia in the first days of life.

## Epidemiology

Diabetes is thought to have more than one cause. Insulin deficiency may be associated with damage to the pancreatic cells that make insulin, inactivation of insulin by antibodies, or increased insulin needs, as in pregnancy and obesity.

A genetic component, possibly an autosomal recessive trait, may exist but is not clearly understood. Diabetes is more prevalent in some families than others.

It is estimated that 2 to 3 percent of all pregnant women have diabetes mellitus; 90 percent of them have gestational diabetes. Annually, more than 90,000 women experience diabetes in pregnancy. Today, maternal mortality is negligible, but fetal mortality is 10 to 20 percent. Excluding death due to major congenital malformations, the perinatal mortality rate among newborns of diabetic women who receive optimal care approaches that observed during normal gestation.[37,38] (In the early 1970s, 30 percent of all diabetic women died from complications related to diabetes in pregnancy; 65 percent of their infants died.)

## Subjective Data

***Insulin-Dependent Diabetes.*** A woman who is insulin dependent may experience more problems with eating and nausea during early pregnancy. Insulin management is more difficult if she is nauseous and vomiting because eating patterns and insulin dosage are disrupted. If care is not taken, she may experience shock, coma, or both.

***Gestational Diabetes.*** The client with gestational diabetes is usually asymptomatic.

## Objective Data

Examination includes the procedures that are carried out for any pregnant woman. Certain signs are common in diabetes.

Insulin-dependent women may have retinal changes that occurred during a previous pregnancy. Retinal changes are also seen in older women or women who have been diabetic since early childhood. Fundal height may be greater than, equal to, or less than expected by dates, depending on the utero-placental unit.

Gestational diabetes does not generally cause retinal changes. Beginning in the second trimester, fundal height will exceed expected height by dates. Evidence of excessive uterine fluid is a tympanic, tight abdomen. Excessive weight gain is common. Glycosuria is present.

Women with gestational diabetes may be asymptomatic throughout pregnancy or have only subtle signs. Therefore, early testing to identify these women will facilitate prompt intervention. Identification is a three-step process.

The first step is to identify the population at risk. The client's history may suggest gestational diabetes.

- Family history of diabetes
- Poor obstetrical history, such as unexplained stillbirths or spontaneous abortions
- Previous unexplained birth of preterm or low-birthweight infant
- Previous newborn weighing 4000 g or more
- Infant with major congenital anomaly

The second step is to identify risk factors in the current pregnancy.

- Maternal age more than 35 years
- Obesity (weight more than 200 pounds)
- Recurrent monilial vaginitis
- Glycosuria determined with urine dipstick on two consecutive occasions
- Hydramnios
- Excessive weight gain or fundal height greater than expected, or both

The third step is to screen all prenatal clients. A reliable, specific, and cost-effective screening for gestational diabetes is the 1-hour post-50-g glucola plasma screen.[38] Optimal time is between 26 and 28 weeks of gestation. Women with risk factors should be screened earlier.

If the 1-hour glucola is greater than 140 mg/dL, the client should undergo a 3-hour glucose tolerance test (GTT) to establish the diagnosis. Two elevated values on the 3-hour GTT are diagnostic of gestational diabetes. If one value is elevated, repeat the screening at 32 to 34 weeks.[38]

## Differential Medical Diagnosis

Pancreatitis, malabsorption syndrome, hyperemesis gravidarum, hyperthyroidism.

## Plan

***Psychosocial Interventions.*** The primary care provider can play a major role in educating a client with diabetes and managing the condition. Encourage the client to continue preparing for birth of the child. Do not discourage her from attending childbirth classes. Because of the frequent prenatal visits and additional testing, the client may require help in rearranging and adjusting work responsibilities. Much depends on the maturity and motivation of the client. Normal daily activity should be continued.

Educating the client about treatment is critical to the successful management of diabetes. With appropriate counseling and information, the client and her family will be able to deal with all changes in her body as well as in their lifestyle.[39]

***Medication.*** The main goal of treatment is control of blood glucose levels. Ideally, blood glucose should remain under 120 mg/dL; levels above 150 mg/dL have been associated with increased perinatal morbidity.[38] Glucose levels can be lowered through diet control and insulin administration if indicated.

Insulin requirements for the previously diagnosed diabetic woman frequently decline in the first trimester and then gradually increase during the remaining months of pregnancy.

For a woman who has gestational diabetes, insulin therapy is initiated if, on more than two episodes within a 2-week interval, glucose levels are above 120 mg/dL.[40] Women who receive insulin should monitor their glucose levels at home daily; this includes a fasting level and at least one 2-hour postprandial level. Currently, insulin therapy is not recommended for all gestational diabetics, but it may be in some centers.

A mixture of intermediate and regular insulin is given in one to two subcutaneous doses daily. Only purified nonbeef insulin preparations should be used. Amounts are adjusted on the basis of daily glucose levels. Insulin dosages frequently are split between the morning and evening to provide around-the-clock coverage. Pregnant diabetics require a larger dose of insulin and their needs increase throughout pregnancy. A decrease in insulin needs during the third trimester may signal placental dysfunction, not stabilization of the diabetic process.

Oral hypoglycemic agents have been associated with teratogenesis, and their use is controversial. At this time, they are not recommended. The woman who was diabetic before pregnancy and taking an oral agent should immediately change to insulin on becoming pregnant.

***Diet.*** To accommodate pregnancy, 300 calories should be added to the diet of any woman each day. Diet counseling is initiated immediately after diagnosis of gestational diabetes. Ideally, a nutritionist should be available for instruction initially and consultation throughout pregnancy. The diet should contain 35 calories per kilogram of maternal weight (plus 300 calories for pregnancy), with 35 to 40 percent derived from complex carbohydrates. Additional fiber may help control glucose.

Some clients maintain adequate control of their diabetes with dietary changes alone. Differences occur in how to monitor glucose accurately in these clients. Some systems use weekly office visits and fasting blood sugar and 2-hour postprandial levels to monitor glucose. Other centers teach clients home glucose monitoring, which may be ordered two to four times a day, daily, or intermittently throughout the week.

***Exercise.*** Exercise can be a healthy adjunct in controlling glucose levels if it is not prolonged, overstrenuous, or contraindicated for other reasons.[41] It must be tailored to the individual's glucose–insulin balance with proper timing, intensity, and duration. The client should not exercise during states of fasting or hyperinsulinemia.

***Monitoring Techniques.*** Several tests may be done throughout pregnancy to provide information about maternal and fetal health.

The *glycosylated hemoglobin* $A_{1C}$ *(*$HbA_{1C}$*) test* measures glucose saturation of red blood cells, that is, the amount of glucose that will last the cell's lifetime. The test reflects serum glucose levels over the previous 4 to 6 weeks. Prolonged periods of hyperglycemia are evident in an elevated $HbA_{1C}$. The test is useful in evaluating past glucose control and client compliance. Any value less than 7.5 percent indicates good diabetic control; 7.6 to 8.9 percent, fair control; and 9 percent or higher, poor control. $HbA_{1C}$ does not correlate well with fetal well-being.

*Routine urine screening* is necessary because diabetic clients are predisposed to urinary tract infections.

*An eye examination* is recommended for established diabetics because of the proliferative retinopathy that occurs. Exacerbation occurs in about 15 percent of diabetics during pregnancy; laser coagulation may be required to control the process and prevent the possibility of blindness.

An early *sonogram* is recommended to confirm dates so that care may be planned and carried out at appropriate intervals. For established diabetics, serial sonograms starting at 26 to 28 weeks are helpful in assessment for intrauterine growth retardation. All women with diabetes have several sonograms to assess fetal size, amniotic fluid volume, and status of the placenta.

*α-Fetoprotein (AFP)* should be determined at 16 to 18 weeks of gestation to screen for spinal cord defects and Down syndrome. There is an increased incidence of neural tube defects in pregnant diabetics.

*Serial fetal monitoring* should start at 32 weeks and continue until delivery. Although the oxytocin challenge test is a more sensitive means of detecting fetal problems, most centers rely on biweekly nonstress tests because the oxytocin challenge test carries the risk of preterm labor. Currently, the biophysical profile and doppler studies are not routinely used for decision making; more investigation is required.

The *glucose level in amniotic fluid* may be measured during amniocentesis. Normally, levels decrease as pregnancy progresses. An elevated amniotic fluid glucose level is associated with neonatal respiratory depression and low Apgar scores; this information may help in making decisions concerning delivery.

***Delivery.*** Decisions concerning delivery can be difficult. Historically, the incidence of fetal death in the third trimester was decreased by arbitrary delivery at 36 to 37 weeks of gestation. Although infants survived, the incidence of respiratory distress syndrome and the complications of premature birth increased.

Newer technologies are used to document fetal maturity prior to delivery. The lecithin/sphingomyelin (LS) ratio of the amniotic fluid of diabetic women is not a reliable determinant of fetal lung maturation; however, the presence of phosphatidylglycerol (PG) strongly correlates with maturity. Samples are obtained by amniocentesis.

Vaginal delivery is attempted unless the fetus is estimated by sonogram to weigh more than 5000 g. In that case, a cesarean section may be initiated. Today, with adequate assessment of fetal well-being, clients may progress to term and deliver as normally as possible.

The key to intrapartum management of diabetic women is control of blood sugar within strict parameters. Clients are monitored with fingerstick blood samples every 1 to 2 hours and intravenous insulin is administered if necessary. An epidural is acceptable analgesia and anesthesia.

***Follow-Up.*** After delivery, insulin needs drastically decrease. The established diabetic may not need to return to insulin therapy for a couple of days. She should, however, resume her usual prepregnant glucose monitoring routine. The gestational diabetic who has been taking insulin will not need to continue. Screen the gestational diabetic with a glucose tolerance test at the 6-week postpartum exam to assess for underlying diabetes. Encourage the diabetic women to breastfeed, as it helps use glucose.

The primary health care provider must discuss future childbearing plans and contraception with clients. The risks should be discussed candidly. The gestational diabetic can return to whatever contraceptive method she prefers. For the established diabetic, oral contraceptives may be contraindicated because of the increased risk of thromboembolic disease and vasculopathy. The low-dose combination pill, minipill, or progestin iplant may be used by well-controlled diabetics.[38] Historically, intrauterine devices have been contraindicated for diabetics because of their association with infection, but this has recently been challenged.

Suggest sterilization if the woman has completed her family or the risks of future pregnancies warrant the procedure.

## PRETERM LABOR AND BIRTH

A preterm birth is one that occurs prior to 37 completed weeks of gestation.[10,42–44] Premature/preterm labor has its onset prior to 37 completed weeks of gestation.[44] The onset of labor, which is poorly understood no matter when it occurs, involves complex interaction among fetal, hormonal/endocrine, structural, and maternal changes. Until preterm labor is better understood, prevention and treatment will be inadequate.

### Theories of Labor

Several theories to explain the onset and maintenance of labor have been proposed; however, none by itself adequately explains the process.

***Uterine Stretch.*** The uterine stretch theory suggests that once the uterus reaches a certain size, it begins to contract to empty itself. The fact that premature labor occurs in most multiple gestations supports this theory; however, the theory does not explain why some women have excessively large newborns without premature labor or why women with small-for-gestational-age newborns have preterm birth.

***Progesterone Withdrawal.*** Another theory is progesterone withdrawal. Historically, it was believed that progesterone decreased immediately prior to birth and triggered labor. Clinically, however, the decrease has not been demonstrated; administration of progesterone does not slow or stop labor.

***Oxytocin Sensitivity.*** Oxytocin stimulation has also been proposed. More oxytocin receptors are present in the myometrium later in gestation; thus, the uterus becomes more sensitive to oxytocin as pregnancy progresses. Oxytocin causes increased uterine activity, but not necessarily cervical changes. It plays a major role in the second stage of labor and postpartum but not in the initiation of labor.

***Prostaglandins.*** The release of prostaglandins from the endometrium stimulates uterine activity, and prostaglandins have a significant role in the initiation of labor. (Oxytocin acts on the endometrium to release prostaglandins.) Use of prostaglandins any time during gestation induces labor.

***Fetal Influence.*** Finally, fetal–maternal communication is considered. The fetus may play a role in initiating labor. A stressor on the fetus will stimulate production of fetal cortisols. Cortisol production is communicated to the placenta or amniotic fluid, or both, thereby stimulating the production of prostaglandin precursors.

## Epidemiology

The causes of preterm labor are unknown, although several complications and conditions of pregnancy are associated with preterm birth[43–45] (see Table 14–5).

Demographic risks for preterm labor include age less than 17 years or greater than 34 years, African-American ethnicity, and poor socioeconomic status. These risk factors are probably not causative but do contribute to preterm labor because of their association with inadequate prenatal care.

Medical risks, such as hypertension and genetic disorders, that were present before a pregnancy occurred are associated with preterm birth.

Medical risks initiated by the current pregnancy constitute a considerable list. Renovascular disorders, such as abruptio placentae, are linked with preterm labor. Conditions that enlarge the uterus excessively, such as multiple gestation and macrosomia, are also associated with preterm labor. Any infection is a risk factor. Pyelonephritis during pregnancy has long been recognized as a risk factor.

**TABLE 14–5. PRINCIPAL RISK FACTORS FOR PRETERM LABOR AND BIRTH**

| |
|---|
| *Demographic Risks* |
| Age: <17 years or >34 years |
| Low socioeconomic status |
| Unmarried |
| Race: African-American |
| Low educational level |
| *Medical Risks Predating Pregnancy* |
| Parity: 0 or >4 |
| Nonimmune status for selected infections (e.g., rubella) |
| Genitourinary anomalies/surgery |
| Low birthweight, preterm birth |
| Multiple spontaneous abortions |
| Low weight for height |
| Selected diseases (e.g., hypertension) |
| Poor obstetric history |
| Maternal genetic factors |
| *Medical Risks in Current Pregnancy* |
| Multiple gestation |
| Hypotension |
| Hypertension/preeclampsia |
| First- or second-trimester bleeding |
| Spontaneous premature rupture of membranes |
| Anemia or hemoglobinopathy |
| Fetal anomalies |
| Hyperemesis gravidarum |
| Poor weight gain |
| Short interpregnancy interval: <1 year |
| Selected infections |
| Placental problems |
| Oligohydramnios or polyhydramnios |
| Isoimmunization |
| Incompetent cervix |
| *Behavioral and Environmental Risks* |
| Smoking |
| Alcohol and other substance abuse |
| High altitude |
| Poor nutritional status |
| Exposure to diethylstilbestrol and other toxic compounds |

Bacterial infection of the lower genital tract and amnion may lead to rupture of membranes and preterm labor. It is unclear whether premature cervical dilatation and uterine activity lead to rupture of membranes or whether rupture of membranes from other factors leads to preterm labor. It has been proposed that infection promotes the release of prostaglandins, which stimulate uterine activity and cervical change. Data are not conclusive as to whether treating maternal infection will subsequently prevent preterm labor.[46]

Behavioral and environmental risks include smoking, alcohol consumption, and substance abuse. Such activities inject possible toxins into the maternal–fetal unit and possibly induce prostaglandin production.

Premature birth occurs in 9 to 10 percent of all pregnancies and accounts for 50 to 70 percent of all perinatal deaths.[44]

### Subjective Data

Some women fail to recognize the signs and symptoms of preterm labor,[47] and thus it advances without successful intervention. Uterine contractions occur with or without pain or discomfort. Clients may complain of low backache, a sense of lower abdominal pressure, or lower abdominal or thigh pain. Some women experience a change in vaginal discharge from creamy white to more mucoid, blood-tinged, or watery.

### Objective Data

Cervical changes that indicate ripening (effacement, dilatation, or anterior position) and that occur prior to 35 weeks of gestation are signs of preterm labor. Any uterine activity assessed by electronic monitor or by palpation should be timed and considered preterm labor. Early engagement and zero station of presenting part may also be observed.

The diagnostic tests depend on the physical findings. A sonogram may be ordered to confirm gestational dates and assist in decisions about timing delivery. Serial sonograms can help identify a growth-retarded infant who may not necessarily be preterm but, instead, small for gestational age. Sometimes, true preterm labor is diagnosed in retrospect.

Significant numbers of women experience painful regular contractions during pregnancy without having a preterm birth.

Criteria have been developed for diagnosing preterm labor.

- Gestational age of 20 to 37 weeks
- Documented regular contractions: at least four in 20 minutes or eight in 60 minutes
- At least one of following: rupture of membranes, documented cervical change, cervix at least 2 cm dilated or 80 percent effaced[45] compared to initial cervical length (centimeters)

### Differential Medical Diagnosis

False labor/Braxton–Hicks contractions, urinary tract infection.

### Plan

The primary care provider works with several team members in managing the care of a client in preterm labor. Because preterm labor is a multifaceted problem, it requires a multidisciplinary approach. All members of the team provide information and support to encourage the client to participate in her care. All work toward the term delivery of a normal infant.

***Psychosocial Interventions.*** The best treatment for preterm labor is prevention.[45,47] To meet that end, providing general health education about pregnancy, birth, and prenatal care is essential. Generally, to address the risk of having a low-birthweight infant it is necessary to improve family planning services and provide accessible prenatal care for any woman regardless of her financial status.

A client often needs assistance with lifestyle changes. Many of these risk factors, such as smoking, substance abuse, poor nutrition, and job-related activities, are amenable to change. Educating and counseling women about these issues prior to and during pregnancy could have beneficial effects on the incidence of preterm labor.[48] In addition, helping the client to deal with stress, whether it is related to physical exertion from specific physical activities or occupational requirements or to emotional and financial factors, may lower the incidence of preterm labor.[49] Currently, however, the correlation between stress and preterm labor is unclear. All of these areas are difficult to research and only minimal attention has been given to them.

***Medication.*** Several types of drugs have been tried to prevent preterm labor and birth.[50] At present, the role of any tocolysis is questionable. Studies are inconclusive and debatable; placebos have a high rate of effectiveness. Overtreatment is probably occurring in women in whom preterm labor has been misdiagnosed.

Many drug therapies involve some type of home monitoring system once the client stabilizes.[51] The question that arises is whether self-palpation (which she must be taught) is as effective in detecting uterine contractions as use of a uterine monitoring device. Most programs employing devices also include home visits or phone calls from nurses. It is difficult to determine which is more effective: the uterine monitor or nursing contact. More research is needed.

One of several drugs may be used.

*Intravenous ethanol* has been used with some success until recently. It acts directly on the myometrium to cause uterine relaxation. Some use ethanol in conjunction with other drug therapies to reduce its dosage and unpleasant side effects. Because ethanol intake is correlated with a fetus's neurological status, possibly resulting in fetal alcohol syndrome (see Substance Abuse), long-term use is questionable.

*Magnesium sulfate* competes with calcium in smooth muscle and reduces the force and frequency of uterine contraction. The client with premature contractions must be hospitalized and the magnesium sulfate administered parenterally, usually intravenously. The client must be closely monitored by specially trained personnel.

*Beta sympathomimetics,* including ritodrine and terbutaline, are the most promising drugs currently available. They suppress the contractile response of the uterus.

- Ritodrine (Yutopar), the only FDA drug approved by the Food and Drug Administration for use in preterm labor, relaxes the uterus. Side effects are related to stimulation of the sympathetic nervous system: bronchial relaxation leads to pulmonary edema, hypotension can lead to fetal stress, glycogenolysis can lead to hyperglycemia, and cardiac stimulation leads to tachycardia. Ritodrine administration is initiated by intravenous therapy and requires hospitalization.
- Terbutaline (Brethine), like ritodrine, is administered for uterine relaxation. Initially, it is given by subcutaneous injection. Oral maintenance doses are continued unless uterine contractions return. Some evidence suggests that clients can learn to use a subcutaneous infusion pump and therapy continue parenteral therapy at home; however, the advantage of the pump over oral dosing has not been substantiated.[52]

*Antiprostaglandins, or prostaglandin synthetase inhibitors* (e.g., indomethacin [Indocin]), have been tried for some clients resistant to beta-adrenergic drugs. They have limited use in short-term intervals because of their association with closure of the ductus arteriosus.

*Calcium channel blockers* have been used to a limited extent to inhibit myometrial contractions. Oral nifedipine (Procardia) is being used with success for some women who do not respond to other therapies.

***Risk Screening.*** Although not proven reliable or sensitive in predicting preterm labor, risk screening is used by most primary health care providers to try to identify at-risk women and intervene to prevent preterm birth. Risk screening should be done during the initial prenatal visit and again at 25 to 28 weeks of gestation. A uniform tool for risk screening is not currently available.

***Education.*** The major component of a program to prevent preterm labor is education of the client and staff.[48]

Client education includes instruction about a variety of preventive measures. Information is provided about the signs and symptoms of labor. All pregnant women should be instructed to notify the health care provider if leaking of fluid begins, vaginal spotting or bleeding develops, or uterine contractions occur every 10 minutes or more frequently. The client may need instruction on how to time contractions.

A client may need to learn self-care strategies to decrease uterine activity. When uterine activity occurs, she should first lie down, preferably on her left side, drink fluids (at least 8 oz), palpate the uterus, and time contractions. The client must be instructed that if contractions do not subside in 30 to 60 minutes, she must be evaluated by a health care provider.

The client must also be informed about the specific drug therapy being administered.

The staff must be educated to be sensitive to a client's complaints and not to dismiss low backache, cramps, or descriptions of "the baby balling up" as normal discomforts of pregnancy. Emergency room caregivers and answering services should be apprised of the special needs of a preterm labor client.

***Traditional Approach.*** The traditional plan of care comprises bed rest, hydration, and sedation. Bed rest assists the cardiovascular return of fluid from the extremities and increases blood flow to the heart and subsequently to the uterus, causing uterine relaxation. Hydration also increases blood flow to the uterus. Sedation reduces the client's anxiety and helps her to rest. If, however, delivery is imminent, sedation poses the risk of neonatal respiratory suppression.

***Identifying Infection.*** The incidence of preterm labor is linked with genital tract infection. Any client showing possible preterm labor should have cervical, vaginal, and urinary cultures done and be treated with appropriate antibiotics.[46,53]

***Delivery.*** If labor is not halted, delivery management is based on fetal size and presentation. Delivery mode should be as atraumatic as possible; cesarean section is frequently performed with breech presentations. Cesarean sections should only be performed for the usual fetal and maternal indications.

Some providers administer betamethasone to the mother prior to delivery to stimulate surfactant production in the fetus and decrease the incidence of respiratory disease syndrome. To be effective, betamethasone must be given prior to 32 weeks of gestation, and maternal infection must not be present. Other centers have had success using surfactant replacement in the newborn to prevent or decrease the problems of respiratory distress syndrome. Neither of these treatments replaces the natural lung maturity that occurs in utero.

Preterm labor is not stopped if severe uterine bleeding or maternal disease or infection is present. Premature rupture of membranes is associated with preterm labor and genital tract infection; therefore, once rupture is suspected, cervical cultures, including those for group A beta streptococci, mycoplasma, gonorrhea, and chlamydia, should be obtained. Decision making with respect to delivery must balance the risk of prematurity with that of maternal/neonatal sepsis. Currently, the conservative approach of delaying delivery is more common, unless infection cannot be controlled with antibiotic therapy.

The client is hospitalized. Her temperature is monitored throughout the day, and the leukocyte count is evaluated every 2 to 3 days. An amniocentesis is considered to rule out subclinical infection. Tocolysis is contraindicated when chorioamnionitis is present.

## SUBSTANCE ABUSE

Research has documented a causal relationship between a woman's health behaviors and the health of her unborn child.[10,54] Ingestion of certain chemicals, legal and illegal, can be teratogenic. Indeed, the use of illegal chemicals (those that have no medically sanctioned use) is rising at an alarming rate in the United States. Cocaine, an amphetamine, is one example. Unfortunately, improper use of tobacco, alcohol, and caffeine is common and tolerated in our society.[55] In addition, certain controlled substances, such as sedatives, amphetamines, and narcotics, are misused.

Pregnancy affects a woman's response to certain drugs. Consequently, an amount of drug taken during pregnancy may have different, more unpleasant effects than it would in the nonpregnant state. Drugs cross the placenta but may not be able to cross back. The fetus, who usually requires more time to detoxify and excrete drugs, becomes a reservoir.

The timing of drug ingestion may also determine the type and severity of damage. Because many women are polyusers, the problem is compounded. Mixed-drug abuse may increase the incidence of adverse effects. It certainly complicates the primary care provider's ability to predict outcome and the counseling needs of clients.

Research on drug abuse has been extensive, but inconsistent and, in many cases, inconclusive. However, to assess clients effectively and intervene appropriately so as to promote and maintain health, the provider must be knowledgeable about current, accurate information.

### Epidemiology

Trying to explain or predict human behavior is a complex, usually unsuccessful endeavor. Because so many variables interact, research becomes difficult; however, several theories have been put forth about why drug addiction occurs.

The agent–host–environment theory proposes that an individual is susceptible because of an inherited genetic trait, a milieu that participates in drug use, or both. It becomes repetitious, almost semireflexive behavior. A pleasurable drug reaction reinforces participation.

The psychic pain theory states that drug use is an attempt to relieve "psychic pain." Feelings of depression, loneliness, or anger may lead persons to self-medicate. Some describe the use of drugs as a way to control their lives, which otherwise seem out of control, or to combat feelings of powerlessness and helplessness.

The World Health Organization[54] has summarized the following motives for drug use.

- To satisfy curiosity about a drug
- To achieve a sense of belonging
- To express independence or hostility
- To have new pleasurable experiences
- To break through to a new level of creativity
- To foster a sense of relaxation or to relieve tension
- To escape from problems

Addiction may have a genetic basis.

In several studies of obstetrical populations, 15 to 25 percent of clients reported their drug use during pregnancy. In reality, however, the incidence of drug use is higher, as many women deny use.

### Subjective Data

A client with substance abuse problems does not seek health care expressing her abuse as a chief complaint. Her complaints are usually vague, frequently cloaked by other problems for which she desires some relief. Often, she seeks prenatal care late or not at all. The client may arrive at the emergency room in labor or experiencing a complication that involves pain or bleeding.

Symptoms of withdrawal that may motivate a woman to seek care include nausea and vomiting, nervousness, tremors, and abdominal cramps. A woman abusing drugs often has a history of sexually transmitted disease. Other clues that place a woman at risk for substance abuse include a history of a low-birthweight infant, prostitution, poor self-care, or family violence.

### Objective Data

Effects of selected drugs in pregnancy and signs of recent drug use are listed in Tables 14–6 and 14–7, respectively. See Chapter 18 for more details on drug use.

Drug use is an important part of a client's history. The primary care provider must remember that the client may be involved in illegal activities, such as drug selling and prostitution, and may fear repercussions of seeking care. She often denies substance abuse. A caring, concerned manner is therefore critical to help the client feel "safe" and respond honestly. Indeed, many clients feel relieved because they want to discuss their problem. Pregnancy is the motivator for some who want to try treatment.

It is essential in discussions with clients about substance abuse to clarify the type of drug taken, the time during gestation when the fetus was exposed, and the amount of drug taken and to assess the client's concerns, level of knowledge, and fears. Such assessment depends on the adeptness of the provider. Questionnaires are available through drug and alcohol abuse centers to help the provider assess the type(s) and severity of an abuse problem.

The provider must not be judgmental toward clients who are abusing drugs. Many women use drugs to fill a need in their lives; they already suffer from low self-esteem and guilt feelings. Showing disapproval may increase their guilt, and the only way they may be able to deal with guilt is by using more drugs. The goal of therapy is to help the client deal with pregnancy by developing a trusting relationship with a person instead of the drug(s). Providing a full spectrum of medical, social, and emotional care is mandatory.

The initial prenatal visit should ideally provide an opportunity for all women to complete a confidential questionnaire that will provide a baseline for discussion. The provider should review the findings with the client in a private setting.

The interview should be done in a matter-of-fact manner. Questions should be phrased in a fashion that assumes drug use to decrease the client's defensiveness, for example, How many times do you drink beer in one week? In addition, the provider should ask about drinking and drug use prior to pregnancy. Evasive answers may indicate a problem.

### Differential Medical Diagnosis

These are medical problems associated with substance abuse in pregnancy: pelvic infections; sexually transmitted diseases including HIV infection and AIDS; irregular menses, amenorrhea, and uncertain date of last menstrual period; hepatitis; skin abscesses and

**TABLE 14–6. INCIDENCE AND EFFECTS OF USE OF CERTAIN DRUGS IN PREGNANCY**

| Substance | Incidence | Possible Effect on Pregnancy |
|---|---|---|
| Nicotine | 20–30% of women of child-bearing age | Vasoconstriction: decreased uteroplacental blood flow, decreased birth weight, prematurity, abortion, abruptio placentae |
| Alcohol | 96% of population at some time | Decreased folic acid and thiamine, inadequate weight gain, second-trimester abortion, fetal alcohol syndrome, alcohol-related birth defects |
| Caffeine | Average intake, 3 cups coffee daily | Fetal risks nebulous, caffeine present in newborn |
| Sedatives (barbiturates) | Widespread, not known | Teratogenic effects not known, newborn withdrawal, maternal seizures in labor |
| Amphetamines (cocaine) | 1 in 10 newborns exposed to illegal drugs | Vasoconstriction: pregnancy-induced hypertension, abruptio placentae, abortion; maternal starvation: ketosis and dehydration, "snow-baby syndrome," neonatal cerebral hemorrhage, preterm birth, increased incidence of sudden infant death syndrome, neural tube defects, failure to thrive |
| Narcotics: heroin morphine codeine meperidine opium | <1% of pregnant women | Maternal and fetal withdrawal, abruptio placentae, abnormal presentation, preterm labor, premature rupture of membranes, intraamniotic infections, postpartum endometritis, urinary tract infection, septic thrombophlebitis, increased incidence of pregnancy-induced hypertension, intrauterine growth retardation, small-for-gestational-age infant, neonatal jaundice, congenital anomalies, including cardiac and genitourinary newborn infection |
| Marijuana (cannabis) | 10% of all 18- to 25-year-olds | "Amotivational syndrome," no documented adverse effects on fetus, altered neonatal behavioral patterns |

Sources: *References 55–62.*

cellulitis; anemia and malnutrition; tuberculosis; urinary tract infection.

## Plan

Substance abusers are not going to stop because of any one intervention or because someone tells them to stop. The success rates of treatment programs are dismal. Nevertheless, many woman can be helped, as can their children, and that is the focus of the primary care provider. Multifaceted programs are needed to more adequately promote the health of these women and their unborn children.

***Psychosocial Interventions.*** The dangers of drug use in pregnancy need to be conveyed. Preconceptional counseling should include information about alcohol, smoking, caffeine, medications, and all other drugs, legal and illegal. The primary care provider should be supportive, yet provide clear directions to pregnant clients about avoiding smoking, drinking, and the use of drugs. Substance abuse crosses all socioeconomic and cultural groups; screening is not limited to low socioeconomic groups.

***Medication.*** See Chapter 18.

**TABLE 14–7. SIGNS OF RECENT DRUG USE**

| | |
|---|---|
| Sedatives | Unsteady gait, odor of fresh or stale alcohol, nystagmus, slurred speech |
| Amphetamines | Anxiety, paranoia, tracks or needle marks, tattoos or self-scarring over arms (to disguise needle marks), nasal irritation, frequent purposeless movements, excessive fetal activity |
| Narcotics | Depressed mood, nodding, pinpoint pupils, tracks or needle marks, tattoos, skin abscesses/cellulitis, fingertip burns (diminished pain sensation) |
| Hallucinogens | Paranoia, anxiety, thought disorders, impaired judgment, fingertip burns |

***Psychological Therapy.*** Once abuse has been identified, therapy should begin with the primary caregiver. Although the client may resist referral to a specialist and her personal freedom must be protected, adequate treatment is important. Specialized programs for pregnant women are designed to deal with substance abuse as well as the high-risk nature of pregnancy and birth.

***Delivery.*** Preparation for delivery and the infant is a positive activity and should be encouraged. Special classes will help her to prepare. Historically, these women do not receive gratification from infant care, but the programs preparing them for childbirth include strategies to boost self-esteem by helping the woman successfully parent her child.

A client should not be separated from her children, but instead involved in child care in a supportive, healthy environment. Children also need referral for close pediatric care.

## MULTIPLE GESTATION

Several complications of pregnancy are associated with multiple gestation.[9,63] Spontaneous abortion, for example, is more than twice as common in multiple gestation. Visualization of twins on an early sonogram of a woman who later delivered a single newborn has occurred and is known as the vanishing twin syndrome. It is believed that one or more embryos can be reabsorbed without jeopardizing the remaining embryo.

Overdistention can interfere with sustained functional labor contractions and affect dilatation and effacement; ineffective uterine activity results. It may also lead to uteroplacental insufficiency and fetal stress. Varied factors related to gestational age, general maternal health, labor pattern, and the maternal–placental unit determine fetal compensation in labor. The incidence of postpartum hemorrhage from uterine atony is significantly increased secondary to overdistention of the uterus during pregnancy. Overdistention of the uterus leads to uterine atony, thus increasing the incidence of postpartum hemorrhage.

### Development

Monozygotic (MZ) twins, also called identical twins, arise from a single fertilized ovum that divides during the early development phase into two embryos with identical genetic material.[63,64] The time of division determines fetal and placental morphology. Division occurring late, between 13 and 15 days postfertilization, will result in incomplete separation and, thus, conjoined twins.

Dizygotic (DZ) twins, also called fraternal twins, arise from multiple ova that are fertilized by multiple sperm. Multiple ovulation results from excessive gonadotropin stimulation. Fraternal twins are not true twins but siblings who share the same intrauterine environment. High-order multiple gestations (more than three fetuses) can result from monozygotic, dizygotic, or mono- and dizygotic division.

With a multiple gestation, blood volume increases 500 mL more; the volume of amniotic fluid in twin gestation may reach 10 L.

## Epidemiology

The incidence of multiple gestation worldwide is 1 in every 80 pregnancies.[65] The incidence of triplets is 1 in 6400 pregnancies, and that of quadruplets, 1 in 512,000 pregnancies. Incidence of multiple gestation varies among countries and races. Africa has the highest reported incidence, 1 in 22 pregnancies; Japan has the lowest incidence, 1 in 254 pregnancies. Within the United States, incidence varies among races: African-Americans experience multiple gestation in 1 in 100 pregnancies; caucasian women, in 1 in 110 pregnancies.

With identification of the vanishing twin syndrome, the incidence may be higher than previously thought. Early diagnosis by sonography has documented multiple gestations that resulted in single births.

A woman taking an ovulation induction drug or using an in vitro fertilization technique is at increased risk for multiple gestation. Other factors increase the risk of multiple gestation: dizygotic twins are more likely to occur among female relatives, women of advanced maternal age, and multiparas.

## Subjective Data

During early pregnancy, a woman with multiple gestation may experience more severe nausea and vomiting, which may last well into the second trimester. Hyperemesis gravidarum, probably related to increased human chorionic gonadotropin levels, may be the only diagnostic clue in the first trimester. The client may later experience excessive fetal movements. Neither sign, however, is reliable or helpful in early diagnosis.

## Objective Data

The data used to diagnose the presence of a multiple gestation are collected by physical examination, maternal serum α-fetoprotein testing, and sonography.[63,65,66]

In the second trimester, examination may reveal signs suggestive of multiple gestation. The most common early sign is a fundal height greater than expected for dates. Recently, however, the percentage of maternal abdominal length (PMAL) has been proposed as a more sensitive measurement than fundal height alone.[67] More than one heartbeat may be heard. Palpation of more than one fetus is not usually possible until the third trimester.

Maternal serum α-fetoprotein is measured between 15 and 18 weeks of gestation. If the α-fetoprotein level is elevated, multifetal gestation is suspected. Sonography is used for definitive diagnosis and to identify the number of fetuses.

## Differential Medical Diagnosis

Anemia, hyperemesis gravidarum, hyperthyroidism, gestational trophoblastic disease, gestational diabetes.

## Plan

Clinical goals[9,63,64,68–72] are to prevent premature birth and to detect fetal growth retardation early. The incidence of preterm delivery in multiple gestation is 20 to 50 percent. Fetal growth is usually satisfactory until 30 to 32 weeks of pregnancy. From 32 weeks onward, the total weight gain of fetuses is similar to the total weight gain of a single fetus.

Head circumference is similar, but fetuses have a low weight.

***Psychosocial Interventions.*** Support the client during diagnostic testing. Clarify the critical nature of such testing. Explain to her that a late diagnosis of multiple gestation is associated with poor perinatal outcome.

***Maternal Assessment.*** Carefully evaluate the usual pregnancy changes with particular attention to signs and symptoms of pregnancy-induced hypertension and preterm labor. In late pregnancy the incidence of PIH increases threefold; it also occurs earlier in pregnancy and is more severe.

The larger increase in maternal blood volume associated with multiple gestation increases the incidence of anemia.

***Fetal Surveillance.*** Sonography and a nonstress test are among the tests that may be carried out.

Sonography is done early in the second trimester to assess fetal structures for anomalies, to determine placental placement, and to identify chorionicity and amnionicity.[73] Fetal anomalies occur more frequently in monozygotic twins.

After 28 weeks, sonograms are done every 2 to 3 weeks to assess fetal growth. Biparietal diameter alone is an inadequate predictor of growth; the percentage of weight difference among fetuses must be assessed. A 15 percent or less difference is acceptable. Anything higher is suggestive of discordant growth.

Intrauterine growth retardation must be differentiated from discordant growth. Growth-discordant twins have lower Apgar scores, longer hospitalization, and higher perinatal death rates.

Malpresentation, which is common, is detected by sonogram. The most likely presentation is vertex/vertex; however, interlocking fetal parts can affect delivery. Crowding provokes less desirable presentations, such as vertex/breech, breech/breech, vertex/transverse, or several other combinations. Cord prolapse and cord entanglement are usually associated with malpresentation.

Nonstress tests start at 28 weeks and are done weekly. Each fetus should be monitored separately if possible.

Other tests that may be done are chorionic villus sampling and amniocentesis. These tests are carried out for the same reasons they would be during a single-gestation pregnancy. Preterm labor, if present, is treated as usual.

The lecithin/sphingomyelin ratio is used to make a decision about the timing of delivery, for example, in the case of a woman with twins and pregnancy-induced hypertension. As no significant difference is found in the lecithin/sphingomyelin ratio among sacs of laboring women, only one sac needs to be tapped.

Twin transfusion syndrome is uncompensated, unidirectional blood flow from one fetus to another. The donor twin becomes hypovolemic with suboptimal growth; the recipient becomes hypervolemic and hydropic.

***Selective Termination.*** Selective termination, the voluntary reduction of the number of embryos in a high-order multiple gestation, is performed as early as possible.[74–76] The intent is to increase the chance for survival for the remaining embryos. Among the various methods used is injection of potassium chloride into the embryonic sac to allow natural reabsorption. The number of embryos to be terminated is controversial. Because the perinatal outcome is significantly less favorable for more than two fetuses, most recommend reduction to two embryos. Many ethicolegal questions arise. The client and her family must have a thorough knowledge and understanding of the procedure and its implications.

***Comfort Measures.*** To address the intense discomfort associated with the exaggerated physiological changes of multiple gestation, various measures may be implemented. Nausea and vomiting may require intravenous hydration. Constipation, heartburn, sleeping disturbances, and low back pain can be alleviated by the usual measures. The overdistended uterus mechanically blocks the lower extremities, causing dependent edema and varicosities in the legs and labia. Maternity support hose may be recommended early in pregnancy.

Although excessive fetal movement is reported, it does not warrant intervention.

The health care provider can assist women in controlling and coping with changes with anticipatory guidance and education.[65]

***Diet.*** In addition to foods that are rich in iron, recommend a supplement of 60 to 80 mg per day. Encourage daily intake of prenatal vitamins with 1.0 mg folic acid. Monitor the woman's weight gain at each office visit.

***Bed Rest.*** Bed rest for women with a multiple gestation has been studied extensively with inconclusive results. Although bed rest has not prevented preterm birth, some evidence suggests that bed rest initiated at 26 to 32 weeks may increase birth weight and thereby improve perinatal outcome. Most providers limit a woman's activity based on her lifestyle and general health.

***Preparation for Childbirth.*** Classes should be begun earlier than usual, as immobility can be a problem in the later weeks of gestation.[65]

***Preterm Labor.*** Preterm labor is treated if signs occur. The use of tocolytic drugs to prevent preterm labor has not proven successful. Prophylactic cerclage has also not been beneficial, unless the client is experiencing premature cervical dilatation.

***Delivery.*** Decisions concerning delivery are based on gestational age, estimated fetal weights, presentations in relation to each other, and availability of adequate intrapartum monitoring. Cesarean section is performed frequently because of malpresentations and because of concern for the ability of preterm and low-birthweight fetuses to tolerate a difficult vaginal birth. An intrapartal sonogram is necessary to identify fetal presentations and establish a management plan for delivery.

***Follow-Up.*** Because of the increased chance of uterine atony and early hemorrhage following a multiple birth, caution is exercised to identify and treat it as soon as possible.

Although breastfeeding decisions are based on the same reasoning as that used following the birth of a single infant, a woman with more than one newborn will probably need additional education and support. More patience and time are needed to establish adequate lactation and feasible routines. Lactation consultants, lay groups such as the LaLeche League, and informed nurses within the health care system are available for referral.

Attachment takes longer when more than one infant is involved. Neonatal illness and separation can also interfere in parent–child bonding. Other factors affecting attachment include the meaning of the pregnancy to the couple, maternal health, and the general living conditions. If one or more of the siblings die, parents experience ambivalence in trying to grieve and at the same time celebrating the survival of one or more infants.[77]

Most communities have lay groups of parents who have had multiple births, such as Mothers of Twins and Mothers of Multiples. These groups provide sympathetic counseling, practical suggestions on how to cope with more than one infant at a time, directions for obtaining equipment and supplies, and referral for financial assistance which is frequently needed.

## NURSING DIAGNOSES

The following nursing diagnoses identified by the author are representative of those used in the health care plan of women with complications in pregnancy; however, these diagnoses by no means constitute an inclusive list.

Acute pain related to

- stretching of uterus
- pressure on surrounding tissue from enlarging gestational sac or blood in peritoneum
- uterine contractions and cervical dilatation

Alteration in

- nutrition related to lack of knowledge of healthy diet pattern
- parenting related to negative experiences in pregnancy, highly stressful delivery, or both

Altered nutrition, less than body requirements, related to fever, anorexia, or nausea of disease process

Altered sexual patterns related to medically imposed restrictions, couple's fear of harming fetus, or both

Altered maternal tissue perfusion related to hemodynamic changes

Altered family processes related to hospitalization

Altered health maintenance related to

- lack of knowledge about drug therapy or instruction in self-care at home
- lack of knowledge of medical management plan
- denial of problem and delay or rejection of management plan
- high-risk lifestyle practices (shared needles, unprotected sexual intercourse)

Anxiety (mild, moderate, severe) related to knowledge deficit about

- the diagnosis, treatment, and meaning to pregnancy
- preterm labor, its treatment, and the meaning to pregnancy
- diabetes and its meaning to the pregnancy

Body image disturbance related to

- swelling and changes from disease process
- physiological and anatomical changes of pregnancy

Decreased appetite and inadequate fluid intake

Decreased cardiac output related to hypovolemia

Disturbance in self-esteem related to inability to conceive "normal" pregnancy

Dysfunctional grieving related to anticipated loss of pregnancy and fetus

Fear related to threat

- to own well-being
- of pregnancy loss or birth of defective child

Fluid volume deficit related to

- peritoneal or other abnormal blood loss
- fluid shift out of the intravascular space

Grieving related to actual pregnancy loss or threat to fetal safety

Impaired health maintenance related to

- inadequate support systems

- lack of knowledge concerning necessary contraception and follow-up care postevacuation

Impaired skin integrity related to skin eruptions from infection

Ineffective coping related to the exaggerated discomforts of pregnancy

Potential for

- injury related to eclamptic seizures
- inadequate parenting/attachment related to birth of more than one offspring
- inadequate nutrition related to increased nutrient needs of more than one fetus

## REFERENCES


1. Atrash, H., Koonin, L.M., Lawson, H.W., Franks, A.L., & Smith, J.C. (1990). Maternal mortality in the United States, 1979–1986. *Obstetrics & Gynecology, 76,* 1055–1060.
2. Block, B. (1990). Evaluating the quality of perinatal health care. *American Journal of Perinatology, 7,* 146–153.
3. Aaronson, L. (1989). Perceived and received support: Effects on health behavior during pregnancy, *Nursing Research, 38,* 49–59.
4. Albrecht, S., & Rankin, M. (1989). Anxiety levels, health behaviors, and support systems of pregnant women. *Maternal–Child Nursing Journal, 18,* 49–60.
5. Loos, C., & Julius, L. (1989). The client's view of hospitalization during pregnancy. *Journal of Obstetric, Gynecologic, & Neonatal Nursing,* Jan./Feb., 52–56.
6. Williams, M. Lynne (1986). Long-term hospitalization of women with high-risk pregnancies. *Journal of Obstetric, Gynecologic, & Neonatal Nursing,* Jan./Feb., 17–21.
7. Dineen, K., Rossi, M., Lia-Hoagberg, B., & Keller, L.O. (1992). Antepartum home-care services for high-risk women. *Journal of Obstetric, Gynecologic, & Neonatal Nursing, 21,* 121–125.
8. Butterfield, C., Shockley, M., San Miguel, G., & Rosa, C. (1990). Routine screening for hepatitis B in an obstetric population. *Obstetrics & Gynecology, 76,* 25–27.
9. Scott, J., et al. (Eds.) (1990). *Danforth's obstetrics and gynecology* (6th ed.). Philadelphia: J. B. Lippincott.
10. Buckley, K., & Kulb, N. (Eds.) (1990). *High risk maternity nursing manual.* Baltimore: Williams & Wilkins.
11. Brunell, P. (1990). Varicella in the womb and beyond. *The Pediatric Infectious Disease Journal, 9,* 770–772.
12. Stagno, S. (1990). Significance of cytomegaloviral infections in pregnancy and early childhood. *The Pediatric Infectious Disease Journal, 9,* 763–764.
13. Shmoys, S., & Kaplan, C. (1990). Parvovirus and pregnancy. *Clinical Obstetrics and Gynecology, 33,* 268–275.
14. Torok, T. (1990). Human parvovirus B19 infections in pregnancy. *The Pediatric Infectious Disease Journal, 9,* 772–775.
15. Remington, J. (1990). The tragedy of toxoplasmosis. *The Pediatric Infectious Disease Journal, 9,* 762–763.
16. Klein, J. (1990). Bacteriology of neonatal sepsis. *The Pediatric Infectious Disease Journal, 9,* 778.
17. Edwards, M. (1990). Group B streptococcal infections. *The Pediatric Infectious Disease Journal, 9,* 778–781.
18. Carey, J.C., Klebanoff, M.A., & Regan, J.A. (1990). Evaluation of the gram stain as a screening tool for maternal carriage of group B beta-hemolytic streptococci. *Obstetrics & Gynecology, 76,* 693–697.
19. Wang, E., & Richardson, H. (1990). A rapid method for detection of group B streptococcal colonization: Testing at the bedside. *Obstetrics & Gynecology, 76,* 882–885.
20. Fletcher, J., and Gordon, R. (1990). Perinatal transmission of bacterial sexually transmitted diseases. *The Journal of Family Practice, 30,* 689–696.
21. Catlin, A., & Wetzel, W. (1991). Ectopic pregnancy: Clinical evaluation, diagnostic measures and prevention. *Nurse Practitioner, 16,* 38–46.
22. Rose, P., & Cohen, S. (1990). Methotrexate

for persistent ectopic pregnancy after conservative laparoscopic management. *Obstetrics & Gynecology, 76,* 947–949.

23. Stabile, I., & Grudzinskas, J.G. (1990). Ectopic pregnancy: A review of incidence, etiology and diagnostic aspects. *Obstetrical and Gynecological Survey, 45,* 335–347.
24. Hoffman, D.J., Knapp, C., & Giles, R. (1986). Anemias. In *Perinatal/neonatal nursing.* Boston: Blackwell Scientific.
25. Schiff, E., et al. (1990). The use of aspirin to prevent pregnancy-induced hypertension and lower the ratio of thromboxane $A_2$ to prostacyclin in relatively high risk pregnancies. *Obstetric Gynecology Survey, 45* (3), 179–180.
26. Walsh, S. (1990). Physiology of low-dose aspirin therapy for the prevention of preeclampsia. *Seminars in Perinatology, 14,* 152–170.
27. Cooper, D., et al. (1988). Genetic control of susceptibility to eclampsia and miscarriage. *British Journal of Obstetrics and Gynaecology, 95,* 644–653.
28. Easterling, T., Benedetti, T.J., Schmucker, B.C., & Millard, S. P. (1990). Maternal hemodynamics in normal and preeclamptic pregnancies: A longitudinal study. *Obstetrics & Gynecology, 76,* 1061–1069.
29. Youngkin, E.Q. (1991). Assessment and management of hypertensive disease in pregnancy for the primary care practitioner. *Nurse Practitioner Forum, 2* (1), 33–41.
30. O'Brien, W. (1992). The prediction of preeclampsia. *Clinical Obstetrics & Gynecology, 35,* 351–362.
31. Sibai, B. (1990). The HELLP syndrome (hemolysis, elevated liver enzymes, and low platelets): Much ado about nothing? *American Journal of Obstetrics and Gynecology, 162,* 311–316.
32. Sibai, B. (1990). A protocol for managing severe preeclampsia in the second trimester. *American Journal of Obstetrics and Gynecology, 163* (3), 733–738.
33. Nelson, M., & Walsh, S. (1989). Aspirin differentially affects thromboxane and prostacyclin production by trophoblast and villous core compartments of human placental villi. *American Journal of Obstetrics and Gynecology, 161,* 1593–1598.
34. Sibai, B. (1989). Low-dose aspirin in pregnancy. *Obstetrics & Gynecology, 74,* 551–556.
35. Sibai, B. (1992). Hypertension in pregnancy. *Obstetrics and Gynecology Clinics of North America, 19* (4), 615–632.
36. Kitzmiller, J., Gavin, L.A., Gin, G.D., Jovanovic-Peterson, L., Main, E.K., & Zigkang, W. D. (1991). Preconception care of diabetes. *Journal of the American Medical Association, 265,* 731–736.
37. Lorber, D. (1992). Complications of diabetes: Adverse outcomes of pregnancy. *Practical Diabetology, 11* (3), 12–17.
38. Ratner, R. (1993). Clinical review 47. Gestational diabetes mellitus: After three international workshops do we know how to diagnose and manage it yet? *Journal of Clinical Endocrinology and Metabolism, 77* (1), 1–4.
39. Leff, E., Gagne, M., & Jefferis, S. (1991). Type I diabetes and pregnancy. *American Journal of Maternal Child Nursing, 16,* 83–87.
40. Plovie, B. (1991). *Diabetes in Pregnancy.* White Plains, NY: March of Dimes Foundation.
41. Winn, H., & Reece, A. (1989). Interrelationship between insulin, dietary fiber, and exercise in the management of pregnant diabetics. *Obstetrical and Gynecology Survey, 44,* 703–710.
42. Bennet, N. (1989). New strategies for preterm labor. *Nurse Practitioner, 14,* 27–38.
43. Graf, R., & Perez-Woods, R. (1992). Trends in preterm labor. *Journal of Perinatology, 12* (1), 51–58.
44. Gjerdingen, D. (1992). Premature labor, part I: Risk assessment, etiologic factors, and diagnosis. *Journal of American Board Family Practice, 5,* 495–509.
45. Gjerdingen, D. (1992). Premature labor, part II: management. *Journal of American Board Family Practice, 5,* 601–615.
46. Reynolds, H.D. (1991). Bacterial vaginosis and its implication in preterm labor and premature rupture of membranes. *Journal of Nurse-Midwifery. 36* (5), 289–296.
47. Eganhouse, D., & Burnside, S. (1992). Nursing assessment and responsibilities in moni-

toring the preterm pregnancy. *Journal of Obstetric, Gynecologic, & Neonatal Nursing,* Sept./Oct., 355–363.

48. Freda, M.C., Damus, K., & Merkatz, I. (1991). What do pregnant women know about preventing preterm birth? *Journal of Obstetric, Gynecologic, & Neonatal Nursing,* Mar./Apr., 140–145.
49. Lynam, L., & Miller, M.A. (1992). Mothers' and nurses' perceptions of the needs of women experiencing preterm labor. *Journal of Obstetric, Gynecologic, & Neonatal Nursing,* Mar./Apr., 126–136.
50. Caritis, S., Darby, M., & Chan, L. (1988). Pharmacologic treatment of preterm labor. *Clinical Obstetrics and Gynecology, 31,* 635–651.
51. Koehl, L., & Wheeler, D. (1989). Monitoring uterine activity at home. *American Journal of Nursing, 89,* 200–203.
52. Sala, J. (1990). The treatment of preterm labor using a portable subcutaneous terbutaline pump. *Journal of Obstetric, Gynecologic, & Neonatal Nursing,* Mar./Apr., 108–115.
53. Gibbs, R. (1990). Subclinical infection as a cause of preterm delivery. *The Pediatric Infectious Disease Journal, 9,* 777.
54. Gillogley, K., Evans, A.T., Hansen, R.L., Samuels, S.J., & Batra, K.K. (1990). The perinatal impact of cocaine, amphetamine, and opiate use detected by universal intrapartum screening. *American Journal of Obstetrics and Gynecology,* Nov., 1535–1542.
55. Aaronson, L., & Macnee, C. (1989). Tobacco, alcohol, and caffeine use during pregnancy. *Journal of Obstetric, Gynecologic, & Neonatal Nursing,* July/Aug., 279–287.
56. Barbour, B. (1990). Alcohol and pregnancy. *Journal of Nurse-Midwifery, 35,* 78–85.
57. Chasnoff, I. (1989). Cocaine, pregnancy, and the neonate. *Women & Health, 15,* 23–35.
58. Janke, J.R. (1990). Prenatal cocaine use: Effects on perinatal outcome. *Journal of Nurse-Midwifery, 35,* 74–77.
59. Mastrogiannis, D., et al. (1990). Perinatal outcome after recent cocaine usage. *Obstetrics & Gynecology, 76,* 8–11.
60. Rosnak, D., Diamant, Y.Z., Yaffee, H., & Hornstein, E. (1990). Cocaine: Maternal use during pregnancy and its effect on the mother, the fetus, and the infant. *Obstetrical & Gynecological Survey, 45,* 348–359.
61. Little, B. (1990). Maternal and fetal effects of heroin addiction during pregnancy. *The Journal of Reproductive Medicine, 35,* 159–162.
62. Wolman, I., Niv, D., Yovel, I., Pausnek, D., Geller, E., & David, M.P. (1989). Opioid-addicted parturient, labor, and outcome: A reappraisal. *Obstetrical & Gynecological Survey, 44,* 592–597.
63. Creasy, R., & Resnik, R. (Eds.) (1989). *Maternal–Fetal Medicine* (2nd ed.). Philadelphia: W. B. Saunders.
64. Gabbe, S., Niebyl, J., & Simpson, J.L. (Eds.) (1991). *Obstetrics Normal and Problem Pregnancies* (2nd ed.). New York: Churchill Livingstone.
65. Spillman, J. (1987). The emotional impact of multiple pregnancy—The midwife's role in support of the family. *Midwives Chronicle & Nursing Notes,* Mar., 58–62.
66. O'Grady, J.P. (1987). Clinical management of twins. *Contemporary Obstetrics & Gynecology,* Apr., 126–142.
67. Faustin, D. (1991). Percentage of maternal abdominal length for detecting accelerated uterine growth from a twin gestation. *The Journal of Reproductive Medicine, 36,* 141–142.
68. Petrikovsky, B., & Vintzileos, A. (1989). Management and outcome of multiple pregnancy of high fetal order: Literature review. *Obstetrics & Gynecological Survey, 44,* 578–584.
69. Collins, M., & Bleyl, J. (1990). Seventy-one quadruplet pregnancies: Management and outcome. *American Journal of Obstetrics & Gynecology, 162,* 1384–1392.
70. Sassoon, D., Castro, L., Davis, J., & Hobel, C. (1990). Perinatal outcome in triplet versus twin gestations. *Obstetrics & Gynecology, 75,* 817–820.
71. Gonen, R., Heyman, E., Asztalos, E.V., Ohlsson, A, Pitson, L.E., Shennan, A.T., & Milligan, J.E. (1990). The outcome of triplet, quadruplet, and quintuplet pregnancies managed in a perinatal unit: Obstetric, neonatal, and follow-up data. *American Journal of Obstetrics & Gynecology, 162,* 454–459.

72. Brown, J., & Schloesser, P. (1990). Prepregnancy weight status, prenatal weight gain, and the outcome of term twin gestations. *American Journal of Obstetrics & Gynecology, 162,* 182–186.
73. Winn, H., Gabrielli, S., Reece, E.A., Roberts, J. A., Salafia, C., & Hobbins, J. C. (1989). Ultrasonographic criteria for the prenatal diagnosis of placental chorionicity in twin gestations. *American Journal of Obstetrics & Gynecology, 161,* 1540–1542.
74. Dommergues, M., Nisand, I., Mandelbrot, L., Isfer, E., Radunovic, N., & Damez, Y. (1991). Embryo reduction in multifetal pregnancies after infertility therapy: Obstetrical risks and perinatal benefits are related to operative strategy. *Fertility & Sterility, 55,* 805–811.
75. Evans, M., Max, M., Drugan, A., Fletcher, J.C., Johnson, M.P., & Solkol R.J. (1990). Selective termination: Clinical experience and residual risks. *American Journal of Obstetrics & Gynecology, 162,* 1568–1575.
76. Zaner, R., Boehm, F., & Hill, G. (1990). Selective termination in multiple pregnancies: Ethical considerations. *Fertility & Sterility, 54,* 203–205.
77. Johannsen, L. (1989). As birth and death coincide. *American Journal of Maternal Child Nursing, 14,* 89–92.

CHAPTER 15

# ASSESSING FETAL WELL-BEING

*Marion Herndon Fuqua*

*It is often a dilemma for the client to make the choices presented by screening and assessment tests.*

### *Highlights*

- Nursing Diagnoses
- Pregnancy at Risk
- Sequencing Advanced Fetal Testing
- Fetal Movement Counts
- Fetal Heart Rate
- Nonstress Test and Contraction Stress Test
- Ultrasound
- Biophysical Profile
- Doppler Flow Studies
- Screening for Size
- $\alpha$-Fetoprotein
- Chorionic Villus Sampling and Amniocentesis
- Rh Isoimmunization
- Perinatal Addiction
- Development of Screening Technology

## INTRODUCTION

The assessment of fetal well-being is both a subjective and an objective task, the success of which depends on open communication between the health care provider and the client. Very simple, noninvasive assessments, such as perception of fetal movement and fundal height measurement, have been used for years. Technological advances in assessing the fetus and improving the chances of fertility not only for older women, but also for women with disease, have required that the health care provider gain increasing knowledge and skill.

## NURSING DIAGNOSES FOR FETAL ASSESSMENT

Diagnosis, interpretation, and management or referral often are foremost in providing quality fetal assessment. Counseling, support, and education for mother and family are critical care elements that reduce anxiety about the unknown developing fetus and enable the health care provider to achieve continuity of care. The following list of nursing diagnoses, though by no means complete, does give insight into the time and attention needed for "supportive" care. Because the nursing diagnoses listed here apply to most of the tests described in this chapter, they are not repeated with the descriptions of the tests. Although only one or a few specific applications of the diagnosis may be given in this list, there are many other applications.

## GENERAL DIAGNOSES WITH FETAL TESTING[1]

- *Potential for Injury.* An obvious risk of invasive assessment techniques, such as chorionic villus sampling and amniocentesis, is the potential for injury. Such potential also exists for client and fetus with substance abuse and possibly also with oligohydramnios (compressed cord).
- *Powerlessness.* Once advanced fetal assessments begin, particularly daily or biweekly, a client may feel as though her body cannot properly care for the fetus or provide an adequate environment. Powerlessness applies, for example, to an isoimmunized client who cannot control the hemolysis of fetal red blood cells or who may be bleeding herself due to abruptio placentae or placenta previa. The client's control may be limited or lost because of the medical condition of the fetus or client.
- *Alteration in Comfort.* Comfort is disrupted by invasive tests or complete bed rest. Comfort is perceived differently by each individual and therefore should be explored with the client.
- *Anxiety.* Almost every woman with a normal pregnancy has some anxiety. Anxiety is heightened with complications and can be reinforced by additional fetal assessment. Some clients welcome the opportunity to follow their fetus more closely; others see testing as a reminder that their pregnancy is not normal. There may be uncertainty about whether the client will carry the fetus to term or whether delivery will be vaginal or cesarean.
- *Fear.* A woman with a history of fetal loss or complications is understandably fearful when faced with the possibility of fetal loss or fetal anomaly. Cultural and religious teachings or beliefs may increase fear if testing is not discussed thoroughly with the client.
- *Ineffective Individual or Family Coping.* Coping skills may be increasingly stressed during pregnancy if testing or procedures are begun early in gestation or if roles within the family are disrupted (e.g., when a client is on strict bed rest or hospitalized). If assessments are daily or weekly, continued support and encouragement are needed, as well as inquiries about how testing may be affecting the client, the father, and other family members. Ineffective coping is encountered with fetal demise, termination of pregnancy, and fetal anomalies. Culture may influence coping mechanisms.
- *Noncompliance.* A knowledge deficit or cultural or religious beliefs may cause noncompliance in fetal testing. Noncompliance is also seen among substance abusers, particularly those who fear legal repercussions. Furthermore, noncompliance may occur if a client is unable or unwilling to give up her career or her mother and wife roles.
- *Spiritual Distress.* Spiritual distress is an obvious diagnosis for a client considering termination of pregnancy and may also be significant if blood products or fetal surgery is required. A client may interpret poor outcome or pregnancy problems as punishment for something she has done.
- *Grieving, Anticipatory and/or Dysfunctional.* For a client carrying a fetus with structural or chromosomal anomalies or in the event of fetal demise, grieving is particularly evident. Allow the client to grieve the loss of a "perfect infant." Be attuned to the client or family unable to grieve or voice feelings or for whom there are no support systems. If a client has experienced a prior pregnancy loss, assess whether she resolved her grief before the current preg-

nancy. Consider also whether the fetus has a chromosomal or structural anomaly that is incompatible with life.

- *Social Isolation.* A client who is on strict bed rest or hospitalized may be socially isolated. Terminating a pregnancy without family or social support also may be difficult for a client. Fetal demise or an infant with an anomaly also causes isolation, as friends and family have difficulty responding to grieving parents.
- *Alteration in Parenting.* Parenting is certainly altered among substance abusers and women with problematic pregnancies. Testing and management may disrupt family roles and, consequently, parenting. A client may associate the infant with the financial and psychological stresses of pregnancy and perceive the infant differently than she does her other children.

## EMOTIONAL SUPPORT

- *Counsel the client before and after each test.* Prior to any test, ensure that the nature of the test, the information that it will provide, and the possibility of further intervention or testing are explained to the client. Counseling occurs before optional screening (e.g., α-fetoprotein) or testing to investigate a perceived risk to the client or fetus. It is often a dilemma for the client to make choices presented by some screening and assessment tests. Any risks to the client or fetus also are reviewed. To reinforce discussions and reduce anxiety, provide written information and answer questions thoroughly. Tell the client when test results are expected.

  If maternal or fetal risk is involved, for example, in cases of diabetes mellitus, the client needs to understand the particular risk, how it affects her pregnancy, and why various tests are important to assess fetal well-being. Depending on the clinical situation, several testing modalities are used. Often a client may become frustrated when one test cannot provide the necessary information, and it may be difficult for her to appreciate why different tests are required. Tolerance may be heightened if the health care provider conveys the need for assessment and the benefits for both fetus and client.

  If the client is upset over the need for tests or the results of tests, she may not "hear" what is being said. Therefore, include the support person or significant other in the counseling when possible. A support person can later help the client to recall the plan of care when her anxiety eases.
- *Acknowledge the normalcy of feelings of guilt.* A client may feel guilty if she feels inconvenienced by testing but realizes its importance. Having to put the fetus first for 9 months can be stressful during a healthy pregnancy, much less a complicated one requiring invasive or time-consuming procedures. With isoimmunization, for example, a client may feel guilty about her body "rejecting" or "harming" the fetus. Allow her to express those feelings. Reinforce the fact that she cannot control the actual isoimmunization process but can work with the health care team to provide the best care possible for her fetus.
- *Provide support when an infant has a chromosomal or structural anomaly.* The parents of a fetus with an abnormality may resent the invasive, lengthy procedures and wonder why they are necessary. The health care provider must be prepared to respond in such situations. The client must be informed of diagnoses and, where appropriate, referred to support groups for additional information. Support groups can be extremely helpful in assisting the client with the transition from being pregnant to caring for an infant with an abnormality. In addition, the client needs to grieve the loss of a "perfect child."

- *Provide support if the client chooses termination.* A client who chooses to terminate her pregnancy for any reason also needs support. This may be particularly true if termination is performed during the second trimester when the client has started "showing," heard the fetal heartbeat, felt movement, seen the fetus with ultrasound, and perhaps confided to friends and family that she is pregnant. The decision to terminate pregnancy is likely be a very difficult one.
- *Be aware of spiritual distress.* Spiritual distress may be encountered when the client or fetus requires blood (as with isoimmunization) or blood products (Rhogam). Although it is difficult, the client and health-care provider may need to consult with legal sources concerning client and fetus rights. Spiritual distress may also be encountered with termination of a pregnancy, spontaneous abortion, fetal demise, or neonatal death.

There may be situations in which the health care provider may not be able to attend to the needs of the client. Further psychological, spiritual, or financial intervention may be necessary. The health care provider can be a valuable mediator in such instances, especially by ensuring that appropriate follow-up for abnormal test results is made available to the client *before* she undergoes various tests.

## INDICATIONS FOR FETAL ASSESSMENT

### ROUTINE ASSESSMENT

Routine fetal assessment begins at the first prenatal visit. Fundal height is measured or a bimanual examination is performed to assess uterine size. If applicable, the fetal heartbeat is auscultated and the client's perception of fetal movement is determined.

This routine standard of care continues for all pregnancies until delivery. Some women begin pregnancy with risk factors (e.g., diabetes) that warrant further fetal surveillance. Furthermore, complications of fetal or maternal origin may arise during pregnancy and require fetal testing. Surveillance or testing is done to monitor a fetus that may be at risk for poor outcome. Some tests, such as α-fetoprotein, should be offered to all women as a screening method; a risk factor need not be present.

### ADVANCED ASSESSMENT

In general, advanced assessment is indicated when there is the risk of uteroplacental insufficiency, but it also can be indicated because of fetal factors, such as decreased movement. Each clinical situation is individualized for client and fetus. Not all health care providers believe that each of the following conditions warrants testing. Moreover, protocols concerning the onset and frequency of indications that warrant particular tests vary among institutions. As technology progresses and the etiology of fetal compromise is further understood, the list may grow.

*Fetal Conditions*[2,3]

- Twin–twin transfusion
- Premature rupture of membranes
- Isoimmunization
- Polyhydramnios
- Decreased fetal movement
- Congenital infection
- Any irregularity of fetal heartrate heard with Doppler ultrasound.
- History or presence of congenital anomalies

*Maternal Conditions*[2–4]

- Maternal age greater than 40 (35 or older for some genetic screening)

- Intrauterine growth retardation
- Chromosomally aberrant placenta
- Abruptio placentae, stable
- Placenta previa
- Oligohydramnios
- Unexplained vaginal bleeding
- Postdate pregnancy
- Multiple gestation
- Unexplained high α-fetoprotein
- Poor obstetric history, history of fetal loss, history of intrauterine growth retardation
- Premature rupture of membranes
- Maternal drug use

*Significant Maternal Disease*[2,3]

- Chronic hypertension
- Diabetes mellitus
- Pregnancy-induced hypertension
- Anemia
- Hemoglobinopathies
- Cardiac, renal, pulmonary, or connective tissue disease
- Hyperthyroidism
- Systemic lupus erythematosus

### ADVANCED ASSESSMENT FOR PREGNANCIES AT RISK

Disagreement exists about when advanced fetal assessment should begin, but the following guidelines generally can be used.

- *Begin as complications arise.* For example, if intrauterine growth retardation or preeclampsia is diagnosed, testing should begin.[2]
- *Anticipate events.* Begin 2 weeks before the time the problem arose during the previous pregnancy. If, for example, the client has a history of fetal demise, begin testing 2 weeks before the fetal problem was detected in the previous pregnancy.[2]
- *Begin at 28 weeks of gestation in the presence of maternal disease.* General testing should begin at 28 weeks of gestation, particularly with the risk of decreased placental perfusion or sooner if intrauterine growth retardation is diagnosed.[5,6] Druzin advocates testing at 26 weeks, because extrauterine life is possible at that time if delivery is indicated,[7] or at 20 weeks in presence of severe maternal disease, such as systemic lupus erythematosus.[7] Once testing is initiated, various options are available if the fetus is compromised. Delivery may not be a feasible option, depending on gestational age or the adequacy of premature-infant-care facilities. With the advances in technology, however, intervention on behalf of the fetus does not necessarily indicate delivery.[7]
- *Assess the postdate fetus (gestational age greater than 40 weeks).* The frequency of assessment ranges from daily to weekly depending on diagnosis severity (if applicable) and fetal and maternal status.[2,6]

### SEQUENCING ADVANCED FETAL TESTING

Testing can begin for a variety of reasons at any gestational age. Some tests are more appropriate than others. Appendix A provides an algorithm of fetal testing that might be used once problems arise.[3] It is one of many available frameworks to be adjusted within institutional protocols.

## FETAL ASSESSMENT

### FETAL MOVEMENT

Maternal perception of fetal movement correlates with fetal well-being.[4] Fetal movement should be perceived by a primigravida at 20 weeks of gestation, and by a multigravida at 16 to 18 weeks.[4] By the use of ultrasound, fetal movement has been noted as early as 8 weeks.[8] Opinions vary about the constancy of fetal movement as well as when movements are maximum.[8,9] Generally, from 24 weeks until term, frequency of fetal movement is fairly consistent if the fetus is not compromised.[8,9] Maternal perception of movement may diminish, however, as a result of decreasing amniotic fluid volume, improved fetal coordination, fetal sleep cycles, and increased fetal size.[8,9]

Even with a reassuring fetal heart rate, decreased fetal movement is a sensitive indicator of fetal distress. Decreased fetal movement is associated with more complications during the intrapartum period or in the neonate after delivery.[8]

Instruct all clients to perform fetal movement counts (FMCs) after 24 to 26 weeks gestation.[3,8] Clients with underlying "silent" problems but no obvious risk factors may be identified only through decreased fetal movement. Thirty to fifty percent of stillbirths occur in the absence of any maternal or fetal risk factors.[10]

### Significance of Fetal Movement

A normal fetus has coordinated movement by 16 to 20 weeks of gestation. Perceived fetal movement is most often related to trunk and limb motion and rollovers, or flips.[8]

Decreased fetal movement may be indicative of hypoxia, malformations, and severe intrauterine growth retardation. Studies have shown that with hypoxia, the fetus may move less to conserve energy and reduce oxygen consumption.[9] Less movement may also be noted in an isoimmunized fetus if anemia is severe.[8]

Fetal malformations include hydrocephaly, nonimmune hydrops, gastroschisis, and musculoskeletal deformities.[9] Some malformed fetuses, however, may have patterns of movement similar to those of normal fetuses.[8] Fetal movement may be perceived by mothers of fetuses with open neural tube defects, including those with anencephaly, but movements tend to be jerking and sporadic.[8]

Severe intrauterine growth retardation is characterized by fetal weight below the fifth percentile for the given gestational age. The fetus may have diminished activity. An underlying genetic, medical, or inflammatory process should be considered. Mild growth retardation, on the other hand, does not appear to reduce the number of fetal movements.[8]

### Factors That Decrease Fetal Movement

Maternal use of barbiturates, alcohol, methadone, narcotics, or cigarettes will decrease fetal movement.[8] The drug's effect depends on the amount used, concurrent use of other drugs, and the route by which the drug is taken (i.e., intravenous injection, inhalation, or oral).[11]

Fetal and placental factors that influence movement include congenital anomalies, decreased placental perfusion due to maternal disease, and fetal demise.[8,9] Decreased movement, however, may be due to fetal sleep cycles or to inactivity during a particular time of day. Fetal movement tends to be greatest during the evening.[8,9]

### Fetal Movement Counts

***Procedure.*** To heighten client awareness of fetal movement, instruct her to do a fetal movement count (FMC) daily using a procedure such as the following. (Several other counting methods have been devised.[8])

- Record the start time; then lie in the left lateral position, preferably after a meal or when the fetus is most active.
- Place a hand over the abdomen to palpate movement. (You may also sit or stand if you are able to detect movement.)
- Remain in this position until you have counted 10 fetal movements.[10]
- Record the end time.

To ensure continuity, fetal movement counts should be done at approximately the same time each day. If *10* movements are not obtained within *2 hours,* then further testing is indicated (e.g., a nonstress test).[2,3,8] Using this method, most clients feel 10 movements within 30 minutes; compliance is heightened when less than 1 hour is spent each day counting fetal movements.[12]

***Advantages and Disadvantages.*** Performing fetal movement counts (FMCs) is simple and inexpensive and does not require machinery. The client may proceed at her own convenience and in privacy. FMCs can promote maternal–fetal bonding. Fetal risk often can be noted using FMCs alone. Presence of adequate fetal movement offers some assurance of lack of fetal compromise.

There are also several disadvantages to FMCs. A pregnant woman who is busy throughout the day and unable to lie quietly and focus on her fetus may feel less movement. An obese woman may feel less movement, although this has not been well documented. A client may become anxious if movement is difficult to palpate or perceive, particularly if the pregnancy is problematic, or there is a history of fetal demise.

***Client Teaching and Counseling.*** Provide the client with detailed information concerning FMCs, including the significance of decreased fetal movement and the need to inform the health care provider promptly of any irregularity. Inquire about the client's FMCs at each visit to enhance your relationship and to stress the importance of FMCs.

## FETAL HEARTRATE

Auscultate the fetal heartrate (FHR) at each prenatal care visit for one full minute to note rate and rhythm. Take care not to mistake placental flow or maternal heart rate for FHR. Placental flow or souffle is a swishing sound different from the actual fetal heartbeat, which is a very distinct, clear beat. To ensure that you do not confuse maternal heartrate with FHR, palpate the client's pulse at the wrist while simultaneously auscultating the fetal heart through the abdomen with the Doppler or the fetoscope. Fetal heartrate should be auscultated by 12 weeks of gestation with Doppler ultrasound or at 20 to 22 weeks with fetoscope.[13,14]

### Procedure

Place a small amount of gel (with a water-soluble base) on the abdomen or directly on the Doppler. A fetoscope, which also can be used, does not require gel. Early in gestation (12 to 14 weeks), FHR is best auscultated just above the symphysis with the Doppler. As pregnancy progresses, the heart is usually heard in the lower abdominal quadrants; however, toward the end of pregnancy the fetus is not in the vertex position, and the FHR is often auscultated near or above the umbilicus. It is easiest to locate FHR with the client on her back, if she is able to tolerate that position. Most women can tolerate being supine for a few minutes. If you do not immediately detect the FHR, it may help to locate the fetal back by performing modified Leopold's maneuvers.

Four Leopold maneuvers may be performed[4]:

- With warm hands, gently outline the uterus to locate the fundus. While facing the client, ascertain what part of the fetus is at the fundus: Fetal breech feels nodular and large, and the fetal head feels hard and generally more movable.
- Facing the client, gently but firmly palpate the sides of her abdomen using the palms of your hands. The fetal back will be a hard, resistant structure; the opposite palm should feel nodularity of the extremities, such as knees or elbows. If the fetus is not

completely on its side, an additional moment of palpation may be needed to determine fetal orientation.

- Facing the client, grasp the lower portion of the maternal abdomen just above the symphysis pubis. If the presenting part is not engaged, it will be mobile. With careful palpation, noting cephalic prominence, it may be possible to determine whether the fetal head is extended or flexed.
- Facing the client's feet and using the tips of the first three fingers of each hand, gently but firmly palpate toward the axis of the pelvic inlet. If the fetal head presents, then the cephalic prominence will be noted first with one hand while the other hand will be able to descend more deeply into the pelvis. In vertex presentation, the cephalic prominence will be on the same side as the arms and legs, thereby confirming flexion of the fetal head. Cephalic prominence on the same side as the back suggests extension of the fetal head, or face presentation. The ease with which the cephalic prominence is noted provides information regarding descent: If the cephalic prominence is palpable, then the vertex has not reached the level of the ischial spines.

### Interpretation

The FHR should be 120 to 160 beats per minute (bpm), with allowance for accelerations.[4] *Mild bradycardia* is a baseline heartrate of 100 to 119 bpm, and *marked bradycardia* is a baseline heartrate of less than 100 bpm.[4] *Mild tachycardia* is a baseline heartrate of 161 to 180 bpm, and *marked tachycardia* is a baseline heartrate of more than 180 bpm.[4] Decelerations or variables may be heard, but they are identified and validated only with external FHR monitoring.

If fetal heartrate or rhythm abnormalities are noted, then a nonstress test is warranted to ascertain the FHR baseline and any periodic patterns. If FHR is absent, a second Doppler or fetoscope (if applicable) may be helpful. Ultrasound is indicated to document fetal viability if the FHR is not heard by a specified point in pregnancy or if it is absent after previously being documented.

### Factors That Influence Fetal Heartrate Detection

The fetal heart may be heard earlier than 12 weeks with Doppler if the uterus is anteflexed, not retroflexed, and if the client has little adipose tissue.[14] Adipose tissue may make it more difficult to hear the fetal heart early in gestation or later using a fetoscope. The type and age of the Doppler used may also affect ability to hear the fetal heart early in gestation.

### Advantages and Disadvantages

The procedure is noninvasive, and most clients enjoy hearing the fetal heart. Listening promotes bonding for mother, father, and siblings and may enable the mother to conceptualize her pregnancy early in gestation, prior to fetal movement. Often fetal movement can be heard with the Doppler and aids the client in distinguishing fetal movement from heart sounds.

On the other hand, the client may be anxious if the fetal heart is not detected immediately or is not heard at all, or if the fetus moves and the FHR is temporarily lost.

### Client Teaching and Counseling

Inform the client of the normal range of heartrate to decrease her anxiety; many women are unaware that FHR should be 120 to 160 bpm and worry that the fetal heart is beating too fast. Reassurance usually suffices.

## NONSTRESS TEST AND CONTRACTION STRESS TEST

The nonstress and contraction stress tests both reflect the status of fetal cardiac physiology, as well as the status of the central, peripheral, and autonomic nervous systems. Heartrate is continuously monitored.[7,13] The tests were developed to assess any indication of uteroplacental insufficiency, thereby predicting fetal ability to endure the stress of labor or the need for premature delivery if the fetus is distressed and could be better cared for outside the uterus.[2]

### Nonstress Test

The nonstress test (NST) can be performed reliably after 28 weeks of gestation when the above-mentioned fetal systems, particularly the autonomic nervous system, usually reach acceptable maturity and can be assessed.[3,17]

Because it is a noninvasive, basic procedure, almost any clinical situation is appropriate for the test. In cases of serious fetal or maternal disease, additional tests may be performed. As a reactive tracing cannot be obtained until 26 to 28 weeks of gestation, another test may be indicated earlier in gestation.[3]

***Procedure.*** The procedure involves the use of a fetal heart monitor. Two belts are secured around the abdomen; one holds the tocodynamometer over the fundus and the other holds a transducer over the fetal heart. Preferably, the client lies on her left side to avoid supine hypotension.[3] Fetal heart rate, fetal movement, and uterine contractions (if they occur) are assessed over 20 minutes and recorded on a monitor strip. The client notes fetal movement by using a hand-held "event marker" or by pushing a button on the monitor that marks the strip. Perceived fetal movement is thereby correlated with FHR.[4,7]

***Interpretation.*** The NST may be interpreted as reactive or nonreactive.

A *reactive NST* is characterized by two accelerations that last 15 seconds and reach 15 beats above baseline FHR in 20 minutes (15-by-15 criteria).[4] If a reactive NST cannot be obtained after 20 minutes, then monitoring is continued another 20 minutes.[3,15] According to some sources, the NST can be continued for a maximum of 90 minutes to reduce the potential for a false-positive result.[2,16]

When the NST is reactive, or "negative," it can be repeated at weekly intervals; in most cases, fetal well-being can be assured for 1 week.[4] Some clinical situations involving the client or the fetus may dictate more frequent testing, such as insulin-dependent diabetes.[3]

A *nonreactive NST* is characterized by the absence of two accelerations using the 15-by-15 criteria in a 20-minute time frame.[3] Other questionable patterns, such as lack of variability and presence of decelerations may be noted, however.[4] Additional testing, for example, a contraction stress test (CST) or biophysical profile, should be considered.[4,16]

Factors that influence reactivity include maternal sedatives, smoking, and hypoglycemia; fetal sleep cycles; and maternal or fetal disease and fetal anomalies. Lengthening the NST may be reasonable in order to rule out these variables.[16]

Patterns that may be viewed during NSTs and CSTs and require evaluation include fetal bradycardia, tachycardia, decelerations, and lack of variability.[4,17] Assess periodic patterns with a 10- to 20-minute tracing. The following definitions (variability, acceleration, deceleration, sinusoidal pattern), although helpful in understanding the fundamentals of interpreting FHR tracings, will neither replace diagnostic manuals nor diminish the expertise gained through experience in reading FHR tracings.

Variability. *Short term variability (STV),* considered the most important indicator of fetal well-being,[4,17] is the fluctuation of FHR from beat to beat, giving rise to a "saw-toothed" tracing. Variability reflects the pathway between the autonomic nervous system and the heart. Short term variability, however, can be truly documented only by using internal, not external, monitoring.

*Long term variability* is the fluctuation of FHR over 1 minute. It is assessed by noting the difference between maximum and minimum FHR, excluding accelerations, decelerations, and patterns exhibited during contractions.[4,17]

*Classification of Variability*[17]

- *Absent.* FHR changes of 0–2 bpm.
- *Minimal.* FHR changes of 3–5 bpm.
- *Average.* FHR changes of 6–10 bpm.
- *Moderate.* FHR changes of 11–25 bpm.
- *Marked.* FHR changes of greater than 25 bpm.

Essentially, FHR changes of 6 to 25 bpm are reassuring; however, minimal or marked variability does not always imply fetal distress.[4,17] *Questionable tracings always require a second opinion concerning intervention or further diagnostic testing, such as CST or biophysical profile.*

***Acceleration.*** Accelerations are increases in FHR over baseline, specifically a 15-bpm increase for 15 seconds.[4,17]

***Deceleration.*** Decelerations are decreases of FHR below baseline; they can be early, late, or variable.[4,17]

*Early decelerations* usually occur as a vagal response to increased intracranial pressure, although they also can occur with cord compression. A deceleration is uniform in shape with a contraction; it begins and ends with contraction. The FHR usually does not fall below 90 bpm, but that depends on the baseline FHR.[4,17]

*Late decelerations* occur as FHR begins to fall when contraction intensity peaks; FHR does not recover until contraction ends. The FHR usually does not fall below 100 bpm, but that depends on baseline FHR. Uteroplacental insufficiency should be questioned.[4,17]

*Variable decelerations* (i.e., mild, moderate, severe) have variable shape, depth, and duration due to cord compression and may occur at any time. Mild decelerations last less than 30 seconds, with FHR no less than 70 to 80 bpm for less than 60 seconds. Moderate decelerations last 30 to 60 seconds, with FHR no less than 70 to 80 bpm for less than 60 seconds. Severe decelerations last more than 60 seconds with FHR less than 70 bpm.[17]

***Sinusoidal Pattern.*** A sinusoidal pattern is characterized by an undulating FHR pattern of oscillations of 2 to 8 cycles per minute, with a flat baseline. Reactivity is absent, and the pattern lasts beyond 10 minutes. The pattern may be seen with severe fetal anemia, maternal narcotic use, and possibly hypoxia.[4,17]

***Vibroacoustic Stimulation.*** An artificial larynx, or acoustic stimulator, can be used to achieve a reactive tracing and reduce the length of the NST. No deleterious effects have been assessed, although research continues in this area.[18,19] If accelerations or fetal movement are not noted within 10 minutes during the NST, vibroacoustic stimulation is applied to the woman's abdomen over the fetal head for 1 to 3 seconds.[2,18] Acceptable accelerations usually result. One or two additional stimuli may be applied at 1- to 2-minute intervals if necessary.[2,18]

***Advantages and Disadvantages.*** The advantages of the NST are that it is easily performed and noninvasive. Furthermore, hearing and seeing the FHR recorded on the tracing may promote maternal–fetal bonding.

A disadvantage of the NST is that it requires someone with expertise to read the results, particularly suspicious patterns. In addition, the procedure may take longer if acoustic stimulation is not used. Continuous FHR tracing may be difficult to obtain if the client is obese or if the fetus is younger than 28 weeks. The NST is seldom reactive before 28 weeks,[2,7] and it cannot recognize impaired fetal growth or fetal anomalies.[20]

***Client Teaching and Counseling.*** Explain to the client the measurements taken by the transducer and tocodynamometer. Initially, to avoid client confusion and undue concern, explain the tracings of uterine activity and FHR. The client should also be told what the average FHR is and that variability is normal. Many women are alarmed when the FHR fluctuates (particularly with accelerations), or frightened if the FHR is temporarily "lost" as a result of a fetal or maternal position change. Explaining the different aspects of FHR monitoring can alleviate many fears. If vibroacoustic stimulation is used, have the client hear and feel the stimulus before applying it to the abdomen.

## Contraction Stress Test

Performed to note fetal response to uterine contractions, the CST mimics labor. It is theorized that if the fetus is hypoxic or has utero-placental insufficiency, late decelerations will occur with uterine contractions.[3] In many institutions, it is the test of choice. A CST may be indicated if a reactive NST cannot be obtained. If the CST is contraindicated, then a biophysical profile (BPP) or NST should be considered.[6]

***Contraindications.*** Premature rupture of membranes, history of premature labor with current pregnancy, incompetent cervix or presence of cerclage, previous vertical uterine incision, third-trimester bleeding, polyhydramnios, placenta previa, and multiple gestation are contraindications to performing the CST.[3]

***Procedure.*** The test procedure is much the same as that for the NST. The client is placed on an FHR monitor, and the fetus is monitored for 15 to 20 minutes prior to oxytocin release. Contractions are achieved by means of intravenous oxytocin infusion or nipple stimulation; nipple stimulation causes the release of endogenous oxytocin. Spontaneous contractions are acceptable, provided criteria are met (i.e., three contractions, each lasting at least 40 seconds, within a 10-minute period). Protocols vary among institutions.

Oxytocin infusion is begun at 0.5 mU per minute. The rate is doubled every 15 minutes until uterine response is noted; thereafter, smaller increments are used until criteria are met to evaluate tracing. Usually 4 to 8 mU is sufficient.[6]

To perform nipple stimulation, the client manually rubs one nipple through her clothing for 2-minute intervals, with 2-minute rests inbetween. If after four cycles adequate contractions have not occurred, one nipple can be stimulated continuously. Bilateral continuous stimulation can be performed if continuous unilateral stimulation is unsuccessful. As a last resort, oxytocin infusion may be started.[6]

***Interpretation.*** Interpreting a CST requires three contractions lasting at least 40 seconds each within a 10-minute period.[3]

- *Positive CST.* Late decelerations in more than 50 percent of contractions, regardless of contraction frequency. Delivery should be considered or further tests pursued, as the CST has a 30 percent false-positive rate.[5]
- *Equivocal CST.* Late decelerations in less than 50 percent of contractions.[3] The CST is also equivocal with hyperstimulation

(more than five contractions in 10 minutes or contractions lasting longer than 90 seconds).[5] Retesting should be done in 24 hours, or other tests pursued, such as a BPP.[6]

- *Negative or Normal CST.* No late or variable decelerations.[4,6] Subsequent testing is based on fetal and maternal conditions and the protocol of the institution.
- *Unsatisfactory CST.* Failure of adequate contractions to occur with either nipple stimulation or oxytocin infusion.[6] Consider doing a BPP.[3]

***Advantages and Disadvantages of the Contraction Stress Test.*** The CST determines fetal ability to endure labor. If the fetus cannot tolerate the stress of contractions in a controlled testing environment, then it is unlikely the fetus could tolerate labor. Therefore, this screening helps to avoid fetal distress. Furthermore, hypoxia may be detected earlier than if a NST or a BPP were employed.[6]

Nipple stimulation is less costly than oxytocin infusion and does not carry the possible complications associated with venipuncture, such as phlebitis and bruising. Hence, the client may prefer nipple stimulation if she is comfortable touching her breasts. Providing the client with privacy may reduce feelings of self-consciousness.

Theoretically, the CST carries the potential to induce labor; therefore, it is contraindicated if contractions are to be avoided.[6] In the event that contractions induce fetal distress, immediate intervention should be initiated. Another disadvantage is that the CST may take longer than the NST. Also, some clients may become upset with the invasive procedure of oxytocin infusion.

***Client Teaching and Counseling.*** Review those points included in the discussion of the NST. In addition, inform the client about the possible use of intravenous oxytocin. Clients should be aware that in most cases "manufactured" contractions do not prompt actual labor, but they may cause slight discomfort. Often contractions are painless.

## ULTRASOUND

Ultrasonography uses high-frequency sound waves to produce an image. A transducer directs sound waves toward an object (e.g., the fetus). When the waves interface with solid structures, energy is reflected back to the transducer, which creates electrical voltage. That voltage produces an image on screen. Real-time ultrasound differs from conventional ultrasound; real-time ultrasound uses a multiple-pulse system of sound waves to note movement, such as fetal breathing; conventional ultrasound uses only a single pulse.[4] Specialized training is needed to perform and interpret ultrasound. Abdominal ultrasound or a transvaginal probe may be used in assessment.

Ultrasound has no confirmed biologic adverse effects on the fetus.[5,21,22] Currently, ultrasound should be used only to medically benefit a mother or fetus, although many health care providers use ultrasound routinely.[4] Some feel it should be offered to all women in their second trimester to detect anomalies and to confirm gestational age.[23]

Most health care providers are familiar with the level I and II ultrasound terminology (see the following); however, with advances in the use of the transvaginal probe and in diagnosis of anomalies, the classification of ultrasonography may change. It may become more reasonable to establish criteria for ultrasonography based on what information should be assessed according to gestational age, rather than meet minimal criteria for a particular level. Should routine scanning for anomalies be justified, a level I ultrasound will not suffice.[24]

Generally, ultrasonography should provide the information sought (i.e., possible source of bleeding), as well as various parameters depending on gestational age. Although the content of each level has not been consistent[25] and may change, fundamental criteria have been established.

- *Level I, Basic Ultrasound.* Level I establishes gestational age, location and grade of placenta, presentation, number of fetuses, stage of fetal growth, cardiac activity, and amniotic fluid volume, and it detects maternal pelvic masses and gross fetal anomalies.[25,26]
- *Level II, Targeted Ultrasound.* Level II establishes information obtained in the level I exam and surveys the fetal anatomy for malformations.

## Indications for Ultrasound

***Gestational Age Determination.*** Ultrasound is used to establish gestational age in the first, second, or third trimester.

In the first trimester, fetuses are essentially the same size, regardless of eventual birthweight.[14] Gestational age is most accurately estimated by measuring crown-to-rump length (CRL) between 5 and 12 weeks.[14,27]

In the second and third trimesters, good estimates of gestational age are obtained from 12 to 20 weeks using biparietal diameter (BPD) and femur length.[27] BPD is unreliable if the cephalic index is below 0.75 or greater than 0.85; other measurements, such as head circumference, are then used.[25,28] After 20 weeks, head circumference and femur length provide better estimates of gestational age.[27] Ultrasound is most accurate when done before 26 weeks.[29]

***Growth Assessment.*** Ultrasound is indicated when a discrepancy exists between estimated gestational age and uterine size. The ultrasound is done to rule out abnormalities or to correct errors in dating. It is used serially to diagnose intrauterine growth retardation in clients at risk for decreased uteroplacental perfusion, for example, those with hypertension or a history of fetuses with intrauterine growth retardation.[30] Serial ultrasounds may also be used for an obese client, because accurate assessment of uterine size by means of fundal height measurement is difficult in obese women.

Ratios of various measurements are often given to provide an index for growth. If not, they can be calculated and compared with standardized charts to determine appropriate growth for a particular gestational age. The measurements most commonly used are biparietal diameter, femur length, and abdominal and head circumferences.[25]

***Detection of Fetal Anomalies.*** Fetal anomalies can be detected with ultrasound. Assessing fetal structures for anomalies is *fetal scanning.* With a level II assessment, craniospinal, cardiothoracic, urinary tract, and skeletal anomalies and gastrointestinal lesions should be detected. The ultrasonographer should be experienced.[25,26] Fetal scans are indicated for women with a family history of disorder or anomaly of the abdominal wall or central nervous, renal, cardiac, or skeletal system. Exposure to any teratogen that produces structural anomalies is also an indication for ultrasound. Use and image interpretation will become more complex and diverse as technology advances.[29,31–33]

***Assessment of Amniotic Fluid Volume.*** Amniotic fluid volume can be assessed by ultrasound. A decrease in volume may indicate fetal compromise. Several studies, for example, have correlated decreased amniotic fluid volume with intrauterine growth retardation and fetal hypoxia.[3,5]

***Monitoring of a Postdate Pregnancy.*** Surveillance has been considered for pregnancies longer than 40 weeks, beginning at 41 to 42 weeks.[3,6,34,35] Combining amniotic fluid volume and Doppler flow studies may be adequate to monitor a postdate fetus.[35] Even in the presence of a reactive NST, fetuses with decreased amniotic fluid volume have increased perinatal morbidity.[2–4] There is debate over the best method to measure amniotic fluid volume.[3,4]

***Detection of Placental Abnormalities.*** For women with a history of vaginal bleeding, ultrasound is needed to establish fetal viability and, if possible, to locate the origin of bleeding. Placenta previa or abruptio placentae may be diagnosed.

Ultrasound is also used to grade the placenta.[36–38]

- *Grade 0.* The placenta is homogeneous and immature without calcifications. A grade 0 placenta usually is not seen after 28 weeks. In a diabetic or Rh isoimmunized client, it may be present after 32 weeks.
- *Grade I.* Echogenic densities are noted at approximately 31 weeks. The chorionic plate has an undulating appearance, which may remain unchanged until term. A grade I placenta is rarely seen after 42 weeks.
- *Grade II.* Calcifications and indentations of chorionic plate are usually present at approximately 36 weeks. Basal echogenic densities are noted. These characteristics may remain unchanged until term.
- *Grade III.* Multiple indentations of the placenta, resulting in the "swiss cheese" formation, are present at approximately 38 weeks. With intrauterine growth retardation, hypertension, or preeclampsia, a grade III placenta may be seen before 35 weeks. Almost half of placentas at 42 weeks are grade III.

The incidence of abruption during labor and abnormal patterns of intrapartum FHR increases with grade III placenta.[36] Some classify a pregnancy as high risk if a grade III placenta is present prior to 36 weeks because of the potential for fetal compromise.[37]

***Documentation of Fetal Viability.*** When fetal heart tones are inaudible by Doppler at 12 weeks or with the fetoscope at 21 to 22 weeks, or if they are absent after previous documentation, ultrasound is indicated to verify cardiac activity.[13,14]

***Detection of Ectopic Pregnancy.*** Ectopic pregnancy is always a possible diagnosis in the first trimester in a client with abdominal pain and a positive pregnancy test. Abdominal ultrasound may be attempted first, depending on the protocol of the institution. If abdominal assessment is unsatisfactory, a transvaginal probe is used.

***Compilation of Biophysical Profile.*** The biophysical profile is compiled using ultrasound (see next section).

### Advantages and Disadvantages

Abdominal ultrasound is not invasive, and may promote bonding, particularly before quickening.[39] The transvaginal probe does not require a full bladder (as does abdominal ultrasound).

On the other hand, ultrasound must be performed and interpreted by a qualified individual. Depending on the test, expertise is required to collect correct data and interpret findings. Abdominal ultrasound presents a problem for a client experiencing nausea and vomiting during pregnancy, because she must drink approximately 1 quart of water in the hour before examination.

One study noted increased anxiety among women who were not given information during ultrasound concerning structures seen and the well-being of the fetus. Clients' fears lessened with positive feedback from the ultrasonographer.[39]

Loss of fetus or termination may be more difficult if the client has already viewed the fetus. If ultrasound has promoted bonding, a client may grieve more with demise or termination.

### Client Teaching and Counseling

Explain to the client what ultrasound is. Inform her that no cases of harm to a fetus have been documented. The client needs to be aware that a technician may perform the ultrasound, and, if so, that person can identify structures but cannot interpret findings. Depending on protocol, the radiologist, physician, or practitioner is responsible for discussing the results with the client.

For abdominal ultrasound, the client must drink approximately 1 quart of water 1 hour prior to procedure and, therefore, needs to be aware that there will be pressure on her bladder during ultrasound. If an ectopic pregnancy or any other diagnosis in which surgery may be indicated is to be ruled out, the bladder should be filled by catheter (usually by a technician), and the client should be informed of the need for catheterization.

For the client undergoing transvaginal ultrasound, explain that a probe will be inserted into the vagina. She can expect some pressure, but should not be uncomfortable. Briefly describe the probe and reassure the client that the probe will not hurt the fetus or cause miscarriage. A full bladder is not necessary for transvaginal ultrasound.

## BIOPHYSICAL PROFILE

Real-time ultrasound allows assessment of various parameters of fetal well-being: fetal tone, breathing, and motion and amniotic fluid volume. These four parameters together with the NST constitute the biophysical profile; however, not all facilities perform NST unless other parameters of the profile are abnormal.[40] BPP may best be used as a secondary method of testing fetal well-being, or perhaps used as an adjunct to NST.[41] For some, the BPP is fundamental to fetal assessment, particularly in high-risk pregnancies.[40]

### Procedure

Usually the profile is compiled in an outpatient testing center within a hospital. Skilled personnel are required to perform the NST, as well as to conduct and evaluate the ultrasound.

### Scoring

Each component of the BPP is scored as 2 (variable normal) or 0 (variable abnormal). A total score of 10 is possible, if the NST is used. Thirty minutes is allotted for testing, although less than 8 minutes is usually needed.[20] If the fetus is less than 28 weeks, BPP may need to be extended to 60 minutes.[40] In another scoring system under investigation, each component receives a score of 0, 1, or 2 and the placenta is graded.[36] The following criteria must be met to obtain a score of 2; anything less is zero.[40]

- *Gross body movements.* Three or more discrete body or limb movements.
- *Fetal tone.* One or more full extensions and flexions of a limb or trunk, or opening or closing of a hand.
- *Fetal breathing.* One or more breathing movements of at least 30 seconds' duration.
- *Amniotic fluid volume (AFV).* One or more pockets of fluid measuring 2 cm in vertical axis.
- *Nonstress test.* Performed prior to the ultrasound or in the event the first four parameters are abnormal; graded as normal (2) or abnormal (0). A normal NST is characterized by two accelerations greater than 15 bpm over baseline, each lasting at least 15 seconds within a 20-minute period. An abnormal NST characterized by fewer than two episodes of accelerations or accelerations less than 15 bpm above baseline within 20 minutes.[40]

### Interpretation

The BPP should be considered in view of the clinical history and the facilities available to care for mother and fetus. The recommendations in the table are to be used as guidelines within an existing protocol.[40]

Further testing, such as Doppler flow studies, may be required to validate clinical decisions.[4,40]

### Advantages and Disadvantages

As with ultrasound, the BPP can enhance maternal bonding and help the client recognize fetal movement. The BPP has the sensitivity to predict poor fetal outcome in high-risk pregnancies, as well as to permit assessment of amniotic fluid volume, placental characteristics, and the function of various fetal systems.

Research continues regarding questions of the effectiveness of the BPP as a screening test and the frequency with which it needs to be performed. Expertise is needed to perform and assess BPP accurately.[13]

### Client Teaching and Counseling

Teach the client about ultrasound (see preceding section), as the BPP is usually compiled through the use of abdominal ultrasound. If possible, point out the fetal anatomic structures and indicate the clinical parameters being assessed.

## DOPPLER FLOW STUDIES

Doppler ultrasound velocimetry is used to obtain hemodynamic information.[42] Although previously used only for cardiac diagnosis and to assess peripheral vasculature,[42] recent research in obstetrics has employed Doppler velocimetry to evaluate maternal and fetal blood flow. By transmission of an ultrasound beam across a blood ves-

**GUIDELINES FOR INTERPRETING THE BIOPHYSICAL PROFILE**

| | |
|---|---|
| 8/8 (without NST), 10/10 (with NST), and 8/10 (with normal AFV) | Testing may be repeated. |
| 8/10 with abnormal AFV | Consider delivery if gestation is greater than 36 weeks. If less than 36 weeks, serial testing is advised; consider delivery if the BPP is less than 6. |
| 6/10 with normal AFV | If the gestation is longer than 34 weeks, consider delivery; if less than 34 weeks, repeat the BPP in 24 hours. Consider delivery if the BPP score is less than 6. |
| 6/10 with abnormal AFV | Consider delivery if the gestation is longer than 26 weeks. |
| 4/10 with normal AFV | Consider delivery if gestation is greater than 32 weeks. If less than 32 weeks, repeat the BPP on the same day; consider delivery if that score is less than 6. |
| 4/10 with abnormal AFV | Consider delivery if longer than 26 weeks. |
| 2/10 | Extend the BPP to 60 minutes. Consider delivery if the score remains less than 6 and gestation is longer than 26 weeks. |
| 0/10 | Consider delivery if >26 weeks. |

sel, the velocity of blood flow can be measured.[42]

Serial Doppler studies may need to be performed. Because diastolic flow normally increases in relation to systolic peak throughout pregnancy, monitoring a pregnancy at risk for compromise includes noting decreased diastolic flow. Decreased diastolic flow indicates increased placental bed resistance and potential compromise for the fetus due to decreased placental perfusion.[43] Low or absent diastolic flow indicates high resistance in the placenta and is often seen in pregnancies complicated by preeclampsia or intrauterine growth retardation.[43]

If the potential for decreased placental perfusion exists, for example, in women with hypertension, Doppler predicts a poor outcome. Studies, however, question the ability of Doppler flow studies to detect fetal acidosis.[35,41,43] It is not a sensitive screening tool to predict intrauterine growth retardation among unselected populations.[43,44] The precise role of Doppler flow studies regarding screening, diagnosis, and management will continue to evolve.[45,46]

## Indications

Decreased placental perfusion caused by maternal disease or placental abnormalities is a potential indication for Doppler flow studies. Doppler has been used in pregnancies complicated by hypertension, diabetes mellitus, intrauterine growth retardation, and Rh isoimmunization.[47] Research continues with its use in preterm labor refractory to tocolysis, multiple gestation, and lupus anticoagulant positivity.[42,47]

## Procedure

Umbilical arterial, aortic, cerebral, and uteroplacental circulations can be assessed.[42] Fetal Doppler echocardiography is also used.[48] Currently umbilical arteries seem to hold the greatest promise for clinical evaluation.[49] To evaluate the umbilical artery, the blood flow is assessed during systole and diastole with a Doppler probe, thereby creating a waveform that can be plotted and measured. The systolic/diastolic (S/D) ratio is derived by dividing systolic peak by the end-diastolic component.[49]

A pulsed wave Doppler probe is used for flow studies. The client lies supine with the uterus slightly tilted, using a wedge or cushion. After transducer gel is placed on the abdomen, the fetus is located with Doppler probe. Flow within the umbilical artery is identified, and the difference between systolic and diastolic flow is displayed. Several readings are taken, and the S/D ratio calculated.[49] Other indices are also used.[42,43]

## Interpretation

A S/D ratio greater than 3 is considered abnormal.[42,49] The normal S/D ratio at midpregnancy ranges from 2.8 to 3.0 and it decreases to 2.2 at term.[5,49] Higher values may indicate increased resistance of the placental bed, resulting in decreased diastolic flow.[49]

Absence of end-diastolic flow is correlated with adverse perinatal outcome.[42] It is also associated with intrauterine growth retardation, preeclampsia, and hypertension.[42,43,49]

Reverse diastolic flow, which is caused by increased flow resistance in the placental bed, is an indication for hospitalization and evaluation for delivery. Reverse diastolic flow has been associated with fetal death.[44]

All abnormal results warrant further evaluation, such as fetal heart rate monitoring, biophysical profile, ultrasonography to monitor growth, or amniotic fluid indices.[5,43,49]

## Advantages and Disadvantages

Doppler has the potential to detect fetal compromise in high-risk pregnancies, it is noninvasive, it has no contraindications. Fetal growth retardation may be detected sooner with Doppler assessment than with ultrasonography.[42] In some instances of fetal compromise, changes in Doppler flow studies occur prior to detection of abnormalities with FHR monitoring.[42] Doppler flow studies may become abnormal 3 weeks before irregularities can be assessed using external fetal monitoring.[34,47]

There are also several disadvantages. An experienced individual must perform the test; up to 1 hour is required for a premature fetus. To date, studies question the indications for Doppler use; therefore it should be done as an adjunct with other studies.[5,42]

### Client Teaching and Counseling

Provide the same information given for ultrasound testing. The client needs to know why the test is being done, its implications, and how it complements other tests the client may need.

## SCREENING FOR SIZE/DATE DISCREPANCIES

When gestational age does not correlate with the apparent size of the uterus or fetus, further evaluation is indicated. The discrepancy may be noted during a bimanual exam or fundal height measurement at a regular prenatal visit, or at delivery when the Dubowitz examination is performed to estimate gestational age of the newborn. If the infant appears smaller or larger than would be expected for the dates, it is very important to determine the actual gestational age of the infant to the best of one's ability. This can impact decisions for interventions if needed. Regardless of when during a pregnancy or after delivery the discrepancy is detected, its cause should be investigated.

### Procedures

It is helpful to have good estimates of gestational age by means of pelvic examination or ultrasound in the first or second trimester.[29] The last menstrual period is recorded and used as the basis for actual gestational age if the client is certain she remembers the first day of her last normal period and if her cycles are about 28 days long. Then, during monthly visits, fundal height is measured or uterine size is assessed to correlate size with gestational age. The general rule is to consider ultrasound if uterine size is more than 2 weeks above or below the calculated gestational age, or fundal height is more than 2 cm above or below the calculated gestational age.[4]

Gestational age can be determined and the fetus assessed for abnormalities using ultrasound. A discrepancy in size may simply be the result of incorrect menstrual dates. It is, however, important to rule out other etiologies.

### Differential Medical Diagnoses

***Small for Gestational Age.*** A fetus that is small for gestational age (SGA) can be growth retarded (i.e., weight less than 10th percentile) or be small for genetic reasons (e.g., mother or father is of small stature).[4] The perinatal mortality of SGA infants is twice that of infants of appropriate weight.[14]

***Intrauterine Growth Retardation.*** Intrauterine growth retardation (IUGR) manifests as a fetal weight below the 10th percentile for age.[4,27] Growth retardation can be asymmetric, symmetric, or both.

*Asymmetric* growth retardation occurs primarily during the middle of the second trimester or the third trimester and results in decreased cell size. Certain cells are, however, spared, particularly brain cells.[4] Maternal disease or fetal insult may be the cause.

Maternal disease may be severe anemia, chronic hypertension, renal disease, or vascular disease.[4] Fetal insult can result from abruption (abruption is also caused by maternal disease); placenta previa; placental, cord, or uterine abnormalities; multiple gestation; postdates; and extrauterine pregnancy.[4,14,50]

*Symmetric* growth retardation occurs with fetal insult during the first trimester, when fetal growth is related to increase in cell number. It tends to be more severe than asymmetric growth retardation.[4] It has several causes.[4,14]

- A first-trimester infection, such as TORCH (toxoplasmosis, other, rubella, cytomegalovirus, herpesvirus), syphilis, varicella, hepatitis A and B, listeriosis, and tuberculosis
- Fetal organ and chromosomal anomalies, such as cardiac anomalies, dwarf syndromes, trisomy-13, trisomy-18, and anencephaly
- Poor maternal weight gain
- First-trimester radiation exposure (Five rads is the smallest dose causing teratogenic effects in the first trimester.)

*Combined symmetric and asymmetric* growth retardation is seen with severe maternal malnutrition and teratogenic drug use (alcohol, tobacco, narcotics, and some anticonvulsants).[4]

***Large for Gestational Age.*** A fetus may be large for gestational age (LGA), or macrosomic, because of a pathological process, such as diabetes, or because of genetic reasons (e.g., parents of large stature). An LGA fetus weighs more than 4000 g at birth or above the 90th percentile for age.[14,27]

Risk factors include genetic syndromes, excessive maternal weight gain, gestational or insulin-dependent diabetes, preconceptional obesity, multiparity, prolonged gestation, and previous delivery of infant weighing more than 4000 g.[4,14] The incidence of stillbirth, birth trauma, and neonatal metabolic abnormalities is increased in LGA fetuses.

***Other Diagnoses.*** Increased fetal or uterine size may also indicate twins, inaccurate dating, polyhydramnios, uterine fibroids, or a fetal anomaly such as hydrocephaly.[51] Decreased size may indicate fetal demise or oligohydramnios.[4] Both polyhydramnios and oligohydramnios may signify serious fetal anomalies.[14]

## Interventions

***Intrauterine Growth Retardation.*** Three variables are involved with treatment of IUGR: fetal environment, fetal assessment, and timing of delivery.

Improving the fetal environment involves consideration of nutritional supplementation, bed rest (to increase uterine blood flow), and cessation of drug use (alcohol, street drugs, smoking) and aggressive treatment of maternal disease (cardiac and renal conditions, hypertension, malabsorption syndrome).[14]

Fetal assessment may require ultrasound or karyotyping. Ultrasound is indicated to assess fetal growth, and measurements may be repeated at 2-week intervals. Abdominal circumference measurements that are two standard deviations below the mean for age are indicative of IUGR.[27] A less than 1-cm increase in abdominal circumference during a 2-week period confirms IUGR.[27]

Karyotyping from a fetal blood sample may be considered if a chromosomal anomaly is suspected.[4]

Other tests are the BPP, Doppler flow studies, amniotic fluid volume, NST, or any combination of these tests.[27,42]

Delivery may be considered if no fetal growth occurs in a 2-week interval or if the fetus has a better chance of survival outside the uterus. Survival depends on the facilities available to care for the infant.[4,14]

***Large-for-Gestational-Age Fetus.*** The mother is screened for gestational diabetes if the fetus is diagnosed as LGA, has no apparent anomaly, and parental stature is not a cause.[4]

Nutritional counseling for the mother includes information about appropriate weight gain and dietary needs of pregnancy.

Ultrasound surveillance should be considered to provide a close follow-up of estimated fetal weight. An abdominal circumference two standard deviations above the mean is suggestive of macrosomia.[27]

Delivery before the fetus reaches 4000 g may need to be considered to decrease the incidence of trauma. Establishing lung maturity first is essential.[27] Each situation should, however, be individualized, as ultrasound-based estimates of fetal weight have an error range of plus or minus 10 percent.[14]

### Client Teaching and Counseling

Describe to the client the interventions that are to be carried out. Emphasize that these interventions are necessary for a healthy, term infant (if possible) to heighten her compliance. For a client whose fetal growth retardation is due to drug use, further discussion about drug use is necessary. (See Perinatal Addiction.)

Many clients believe that a large infant is a sign of good health and that the mother has adequately cared for herself and her infant. The opposite, however, can be true for the mother of a small infant. When counseling clients, it may be difficult to overcome the positive cultural values associated with a large infant and equally difficult to overcome the negative connotations associated with a small infant. Educating the client concerning the underlying processes of abnormal growth patterns may encourage her participation in care.

## α-FETOPROTEIN

α-Fetoprotein (AFP), a glycoprotein produced by the fetal liver, gastrointestinal tract, and embryonic yolk sac, increases in the amniotic fluid through urination, gastrointestinal secretions, and movement across fetal blood vessels.[52] AFP crosses the placenta and fetal membranes into the maternal bloodstream, resulting in a rise in maternal serum AFP (MSAFP).[52] The level can be measured by taking a sample of maternal blood between 16 and 18 weeks of gestation.[52,53] Some centers can accurately assess MSAFP up to 23 weeks.

Measurement of MSAFP is primarily used to screen for open neural tube and ventral wall defects, although other conditions have been associated with abnormal levels of MSAFP (see Interpretation). MSAFP can be used as a marker for Down syndrome, especially when combined with other maternal blood tests, such as those for unconjugated estriol and the β subunit of human chorionic gonadotropin.[54] MSAFP screening should be offered to all women, but clients with a personal or family history of neural tube defects or chromosomal anomalies should also be offered more appropriate methods for diagnosis of chromosomal or structural anomalies[54] (e.g., chorionic villus sampling, amniocentesis, or ultrasonographic evaluation of fetus), depending on the client's risk factors and history[52].

### Interpretation

The level of MSAFP is reported as a multiple of the median (MoM) and adjusted in the laboratory for maternal weight, presence of diabetes, gestational age, multiple gestation, and race. In a singleton pregnancy, *elevated values* are greater than 2.5 MoM.[13,52] *Low values, however, are assessed with respect to maternal age* (maternal age-dependent threshold); elevated values are not.[52] With respect to low values, normal ranges of

MSAFP are established by each laboratory based on maternal age.

### Etiology of an Abnormal Result

The list of causes of an elevated or low level of MSAFP is lengthy and will grow longer as technology advances.

Elevated MSAFP levels are associated with incorrect gestational age; oligohydramnios; anencephaly; fetal death; multiple gestation; open neural tube defect; open ventral wall defect; fetomaternal hemorrhage; renal, pulmonary, abdominal wall, and placental anomalies: maternal liver disease; and malignancy.[13,53]

Low MSAFP levels are associated with Down syndrome or trisomy-18, hydatidiform mole, choriocarcinoma and fetal aneuploidy, and incorrect gestational age.[13,53]

### Clinical Management

Abnormal MSAFP levels may necessitate repeated testing, ultrasound, or amniocentesis.

An elevated MSAFP requires that the serum be retested. If the second MSAFP test is also elevated or if the initial value was low, ultrasound is performed alone or with amniocentesis.[52] Ultrasound can be used either to correct gestational age or to note a structural anomaly. If gestational age is incorrect or if another nonpathological cause of an abnormal value is noted (such as twins), the MoM is recalculated and usually found to be within normal limits. If a structural anomaly is noted, the fetus should be thoroughly assessed for other anomalies and amniocentesis encouraged to note genetic aberrations. If no anomaly is apparent and no other cause of an abnormal MSAFP is found, amniocentesis is indicated.[52]

Amniocentesis is done to assess amniotic fluid AFP (AFAFP) and perform chromosomal analysis. A positive AFAFP is validated by measuring the amount of acetylcholinesterase (AChE) in the amniotic fluid sample.[52] An elevated AChE level usually indicates an open neural tube defect. If the elevated AFAFP level is due to contamination with fetal blood, AChE will be absent. A low level of AChE or its absence suggests something other than open neural tube defect. Once contamination of the sample is excluded, a detailed ultrasonographic exam should follow.[52]

Ninety to ninety-five percent of clients with abnormal MSAFP levels have a normal level of AFAFP. Even though the AFAFP is normal, the risk for IUGR, premature labor, neonatal death, preeclampsia, fetal demise, and abruption is greater; the causes are not well documented.[14,52,53] These clients should undergo high-resolution ultrasounds and fetoplacental surveillance during the remainder of pregnancy.[53]

### Advantages and Disadvantages

Testing for MSAFP can be done in an office. If subsequent testing due to an abnormal AFP value reveals a fetal problem, treatment (if possible) may be instituted or the pregnancy terminated. A client can thus be prepared to plan care for a child with a chromosomal or structural anomaly.

There are disadvantages. MSAFP testing screens for abnormalities; it is not diagnostic. Further intervention is required to pinpoint the cause. The high rate of false-positive results may increase further if certain factors, for example, race and multiple gestation, are not taken into account, and clients may proceed with amniocentesis unnecessarily (see next section). Also, closed neural tube defects such as those associated with hydrocephaly cannot be detected by MSAFP testing.[52]

### Client Teaching and Counseling

Inform the client of possible test outcomes and recommendations that may be made.

Many clients can cope with having blood drawn, but the decision to do a chromosomal analysis may pose a cultural or religious dilemma for some. The sequence of events leading to diagnosis after an abnormal test result is unexpected. Some clients want to know if the fetus has some abnormality; others prefer not to know until the birth. The health care provider may be caught in the middle. As the fetus is assumed at risk, the client needs to be informed of the consequences of abnormal test results.

## CHORIONIC VILLUS SAMPLING AND AMNIOCENTESIS

Both chorionic villus sampling and amniocentesis aid in the diagnosis of chromosomal abnormalities in a fetus. Generally, prenatal diagnosis is offered to clients who will be age 35 or older at delivery, because the risk of a chromosomal abnormality outweighs the risks associated with amniocentesis and chorionic villus sampling. Before these tests are done, normal growth and fetal viability must be established by means of ultrasound.

### Chorionic Villus Sampling

Usually, chorionic villus sampling (CVS) is performed between 9 and 13 weeks. Sampling may occur transcervically, transabdominally, or transvaginally. There are reports of trials of transabdominal CVS at 6 to 7 weeks of gestation.[55,56] (MSAFP should be assessed at 15 weeks because CVS cannot detect open neural tube defects.[55]) With ultrasound for guidance, the villi are aspirated from the placenta and examined. A direct cell culture can be available in hours. Further cell culture is available in 8 to 14 days.[55,57] The methodologies for transcervical, transvaginal, and transabdominal CVS are slightly different.[55]

After the procedure, fetal cardiac activity is verified with ultrasound, and the client monitored for about 30 minutes to note any adverse effects. In addition, *Rhogam should be administered to unsensitized Rh-negative clients after the procedure.*

***Indications.*** Indications for CVS are maternal age greater than 35, previous child with a chromosome abnormality, balanced structural chromosome rearrangement in a parent, sex determination of a fetus in which X-linked disorders are in question, family history of detectable Mendelian disorders, and history of three or more spontaneous abortions.[55,58] If amniotic fluid is required for diagnosis, such as for neural tube defects, the client should be offered amniocentesis instead.[58]

***Contraindications.*** Chorionic villus sampling is contraindicated in the presence of cervicitis or vaginitis (for transvaginal or transcervical sampling) and maternal blood group sensitization.[13,55] Relative contraindications include multiple gestation, bleeding from the vagina 1 week prior to CVS, fibroids that obstruct the cervical canal, and a severely retroflexed uterus.[55] In the last two instances (obstructive fibroids and retroflexed uterus), a transabdominal or transvaginal approach may be preferred.[58]

***Advantages and Disadvantages.*** Compared with amniocentesis, CVS permits quicker diagnosis (hours for direct preparation and 8 to 14 days for cell culture, depending on health care facility) and, thereby, earlier recognition of a fetal abnormality. Earlier recognition is helpful if the client must make a decision concerning termination of the pregnancy.[57] Termination during the first trimester presents fewer risks to the client[13] and enhances her privacy, as pregnancy is not yet obvious to others. Moreover, early diagnosis can be essential to recognize and treat various chromosomal anomalies.[55] Although there is a risk of pregnancy loss (see Complications), very few failures occur in actually retrieving villi and performing chromosomal analysis.[59]

One disadvantage of CVS is that currently it is only done in large facilities; not all facilities have the capability or staff with sufficient expertise. Another disadvantage is that CVS tests only for chromosomal anomalies and cannot detect anatomic aberrations, such as neural tube defects. Also note the complications listed next.

***Complications.*** Pregnancy loss varies from 2 to 7 percent depending on the center; CVS carries a slightly higher rate of procedure failure and fetal loss than amniocentesis.[13,55,58–61] A landmark study of CVS found that after pregnancy losses were adjusted for maternal and gestational ages, the loss rate for CVS was 0.8 percent higher than that for amniocentesis (not statistically significant).[60]

Fetal loss may also be coincidental.[59] Women who are at increased risk for pregnancy loss secondary to their age or having a chromosomally abnormal fetus will have an increased rate of spontaneous abortion despite the risk of CVS. Those who calculate pregnancy loss from CVS or amniocentesis usually take this into account, but may specifically state "loss due to CVS."[59] Spontaneous fetal loss occurs with 1 to 2 percent of pregnancies.[4,13,59] Therefore, a total loss rate of 2 to 4 percent reflects an approximate 1 to 3 percent loss due to CVS over baseline loss. A study is currently being conducted to assess differences between transcervical and transabdominal sampling.[55]

Clinical infection is reduced if transabdominal sampling is used for a client with cervicitis or vaginitis.[55]

Damage to the fetus, placenta, or cord may cause clients to experience light vaginal spotting after the procedure, which often only needs to be monitored for increased flow or associated cramping.[62] Approximately 4 percent develop a subchorionic hematoma which resolves over 6 to 10 weeks.[13] Although damage to the fetus or cord does occur, the incidence tends to decrease with the use of ultrasound guidance.[33]

Subsequent limb anomalies have been linked to CVS. Conflicting reports exist concerning the incidence and etiology of limb reduction.[62–65] Theories suggest that CVS may be related to decreased fetal perfusion or thrombosis at the sampling site, resulting in embolization and subsequent vascular impairment.[62] Anomalies may also be related to gestational age at the time of CVS, catheter or needle size, and the clinician's experience in performing CVS.[63]

***Client Teaching and Counseling.*** Advise the client to call if she experiences moderate vaginal bleeding, severe cramping, leaking fluid, temperature higher than 100°F, or chills. Cramping may continue for up to 48 hours after CVS. The client should avoid strenuous activity and sexual intercourse for 48 hours.[66] Discuss each step of the procedure with the client to help decrease her anxiety.

The client should be aware of the potential risks to herself and the fetus. The consequences of an abnormal result should be discussed prior to the procedure. If a client chooses termination, counsel her appropriately and be knowledgeable about the location of centers for pregnancy termination.

### Amniocentesis

Amniotic fluid is withdrawn from the uterus, and the cells obtained are cultured to identify chromosomal and biochemical abnormalities; amniocentesis is performed at 15 to 18 weeks of gestation.[4,13] First-trimester amniocentesis has been investigated.[56,59] In the third trimester, the procedure has been used to determine fetal lung maturity.[13] The majority of amniocenteses are performed for advanced maternal age or abnormal MSAFP.[13] As with

CVS, ultrasound must be performed prior to the procedure to confirm gestational age and fetal viability.

The procedure is done with ultrasound guidance and surgical asepsis to avoid infection. After the abdomen is cleansed and the puncture site locally anesthetized, a 20- or 22-gauge, 3- to 6-in. needle is inserted. Amniotic fluid is aspirated and analyzed. After the procedure, fetal cardiac activity is verified, and the client monitored for 30 minutes for adverse effects.[4] *Rhogam is administered to Rh-negative clients after the procedure.*

***Indications.*** A repeatedly elevated MSAFP or an initial low MSAFP, maternal age greater than 35 years, history of chromosomal anomaly in a child or close family member, maternal carrier of X-linked disorder, parental chromosomal rearrangement, and a family history of detectable Mendelian disorders are indications for amniocentesis.[66]

***Advantages and Disadvantages.*** Amniocentesis is used to measure AFAFP. It is associated with an overall lower risk of complications than CVS, although the risk varies among institutions.[13]

Amniocentesis cannot detect a closed neural tube defect and is associated with some complications. If a fetal anomaly does exist and is not detected until the second trimester with amniocentesis, the client who chooses to abort is at greater risk for uterine perforation, hemorrhage, infection, or anesthetic complications than if she had aborted in the first trimester.[13]

***Complications.*** Maternal risks include hemorrhage, uterine cramping, infection, injury to abdominal viscera, leakage of amniotic fluid, and blood group sensitization.[66]

Fetal risks include needle injury, abortion, infection, and induced malformations due to amniotic bands.[62] Fetal injury is rare.[33] Pregnancy loss associated with amniocentesis approaches 0.5 to 1 percent over the baseline rate of pregnancy loss; the total risk of major complications with amniocentesis is 2 to 3 percent.[4,13]

***Client Teaching and Counseling.*** Inform the client that she may experience uncomfortable pressure during the procedure, mild cramping up to 48 hours after the procedure, and slight bruising around the insertion site. Reassure the client that fetal heartbeat will be verified after the procedure. Instruct her to telephone if she notes bleeding, leaking fluid, severe cramping, temperature higher than 100°F, chills, or quickening, as well as lack of fetal movement. Advise the client to avoid strenuous activity or sexual intercourse for 48 hours after the procedure.[66]

Inform the client of the possible risks to herself and the fetus, the meaning of abnormal values, and the possible consequences prior to the procedure. Be prepared to counsel the client about termination if she chooses and be knowledgeable about the location of centers for pregnancy termination.

## SCREENING AND PREVENTION OF RH ISOIMMUNIZATION

Maternal sensitization, or isoimmunization, may occur with exposure to blood or blood products that contain an antigen not found in maternal blood cells. Exposure prompts production of antibodies to that antigen.[4,63,64] Sensitization can occur following transfusion or exposure to fetal blood containing factors inherited from the father. The incidence of Rh isoimmunization has decreased because of the administration of Rh immune globulin (Rhogam) to unsensitized women[67]; however, Rh isoimmunization does occur. For example, an Rh-negative woman may unknowingly abort an Rh-positive fetus. Fetal sensitization can also occur according to the "grandmother" theory: An Rh-negative fetus is exposed to enough maternal Rh-positive red blood cells during delivery to cause fetal sensitization.[4,68]

## Rh Status

Rh status refers to presence (Rh-positive) or absence (Rh-negative) of Rh antigen on the red blood cell. More than 400 antigens of the Rh factor have been identified. They can all cause hemolytic disease; however, the "D" antigen causes 90 percent of cases of Rh isoimmunization.[4,68] Individuals lacking antigenic determinant D usually become immunized after a single exposure to D antigen.[4] Other antigens have various effects on fetuses as a result of diversified antibody responses and should be managed individually.[4] Because the vast majority of cases of isoimmunization are due to the D antigen, in the remainder of this section we use the D antigen as an example.

***Initial Screening.*** For all clients, determine blood type, Rh status, and antibody titer (indirect Coombs test) early in pregnancy.[67]

***Interpretation of Results and Management.*** If the client is D-negative or has a positive antibody screen, also determine the father's blood type and Rh and antigen status. If the father is D-negative and has no antigens to the corresponding antibodies that the mother has, then no further consideration is needed.[69] If, however, the father is Rh-positive and has a negative antigen screen, draw a maternal antibody titer at 28 weeks. If D antibody is absent, then give Rhogam. Rhogam is given specifically to prevent isoimmunization to D antigen. Rhogam is comprised of anti-D IgG antibodies and acts by binding with Rh-positive fetal cells if they are present in the maternal circulation. Through various means, it blocks maternal antigen processing.[70] Rhogam is of no value when isoimmunization has occurred.[67] Rhogam is also given within 72 hours of delivery if the fetus is Rh-positive.[69] In addition, Rhogam is given to Rh negative clients who undergo bilateral tubal ligation after delivery, because in the future they may decide to have the ligation reversed. Breastfeeding is not a contraindication to administration of Rhogam.

If the client has a positive antibody screen and the father is positive for antigen, maternal antibody should be characterized and the titer determined.[65] Titers must be followed through gestation if it is determined that antibodies are IgG; IgG can cross the placenta and cause hemolytic disease in the fetus.[69] A rising or elevated titer, greater than or equal to 1:16, indicates the need for further clinical assessment (see Management of an Isoimmunized Pregnancy later in this section).[69]

Of clinical importance is the need to notify the blood bank of the client's irregular antibody in the event a transfusion is needed at delivery.

***Other Indications for Administration of Rhogam During Pregnancy.*** Rhogam should be given anytime there exists a potential for mixing Rh-positive fetal and Rh-negative maternal blood.[4,67,70]

- Chorionic villus sampling
- Therapeutic or spontaneous abortion
- Ectopic pregnancy
- Hydatidiform mole
- Amniocentesis
- Antepartum hemorrhage
- Fetal blood sampling
- External version
- Fetal death
- Fetal surgery
- Transfusion of D-positive blood to D-negative mother

***Hemorrhage.*** If a large fetal-to-maternal hemorrhage is suspected to have occurred during pregnancy, or copious bleeding occurs at delivery, as with manual removal of the placenta, the Kleihauer–Betke test is performed on a sample of maternal blood to measure fetal blood in the maternal system. If fetal blood is present in maternal blood, then 10 µg of Rhogam is given per milliliter of fetal blood in the maternal system. The standard dose is 300 µg, which is effective for 30 mL of fetal blood. If more than 30 mL of blood is present in the maternal system, then the volume of fetal red cells can be estimated by analysis of maternal blood; the dose of Rhogam is adjusted accordingly.[4,67,68]

### Process of Isoimmunization

If the client does not receive Rhogam and is exposed to D antigen on fetal cells, she will produce anti-D IgM antibodies. This initial response usually is not problematic (unless the exposure is massive), as IgM antibodies do not cross placenta.[68] A second exposure to fetal cells with the D antigen will cause the development of IgG antibodies. No amount of prophylaxis at this point will prevent a hemolytic response.[70]

Anti-D IgG antibodies cross the placenta readily, coat fetal cells if they have D antigen, and cause hemolysis. If hemolysis is mild, fetus may compensate by increasing its production of red blood cells. If hemolysis is severe, the fetus maximizes red blood cell production in the liver and spleen. The increased demands on the fetal liver result in enlargement, altered function, and decreased albumin production, which lead to leakage of fluid from the fetal vasculature. Ascites and effusions thereby develop. As hemolysis continues, anemia worsens; liver failure and circulatory compromise result. Ultimately cardiovascular collapse and fetal death occur. These events describe the process of fetal hemolytic disease, or hydrops fetalis.[70]

***Management of an Isoimmunized Pregnancy.*** Management begins with assessment of maternal antibody titers and subsequently employs methods for fetal monitoring.

Maternal antibody titers are assessed early in pregnancy. If the titer is less than or equal to 1:8, it is assessed again at 16 to 18 weeks and every 2 to 4 weeks thereafter until it rises to 1:16.[69] If the initial titer is 1:16 or greater, ultrasound and amniocentesis should be considered to assess the possibility of severe hemolytic disease.[71] These titer values apply to anti-D sensitization only; other antibody responses may cause hydropic disease at a titer of 1:8.[70]

Ultrasound should be used when the maternal titer rises and abnormalities, such as ascites, are noted. The ultrasound may be done alone or with amniocentesis or percutaneous umbilical blood sampling.[69]

Amniotic fluid assays and percutaneous umbilical blood sampling (PUBS) may begin early in the second trimester, depending on the extent of disease. Bilirubin, the byproduct of red blood cell destruction, can be measured spectrophotometrically in amniotic fluid or fetal blood. PUBS may also be used to monitor the fetal hematocrit.[4,72] Through monitoring of the bilirubin level and fetal hematocrit, the necessity and frequency of fetal transfusion can be assessed. The frequency of monitoring depends on the severity of disease.[70]

Nonstress tests are recommended because hydrops-affected fetus may exhibit sinusoidal or other ominous patterns during heartrate monitoring.[16] Diminished fetal activity, however, may precede changes detected by external monitoring.[8] Therefore, fetal movement counts between ultrasound exams are advised to monitor an affected fetus.

***Treatment of Isoimmunization.*** Transfusions may be administered using the intraperitoneal, intracardiac, or intravascular route or via the intrahepatic portion of the umbilical vein. Although controversy remains as to which route is safest, transfusion is at present the only method that will save a hydropic fetus if delivery is remote.[73] A combination of intraperitoneal and intravascular routes is advocated.[69,71,73] Other methods have been investigated to minimize fetal hemolysis, but none has been successful.[4]

***Client Teaching and Counseling.*** Reinforce the need for Rhogam at 28 weeks and after delivery and encourage compliance with prenatal care visits. Because of her cultural or socioeconomic background, a client may consider home delivery even after receiving prenatal care, and postpartum administration of Rhogam may be bypassed.

Some clients feel that if they miscarry early in gestation and all tissue is passed and bleeding stops, they do not need to be evaluated in the health care setting. Stress the importance of evaluation and, at the same time, the necessity of receiving Rhogam when miscarriage occurs.

In the event of isoimmunization, carefully discuss all procedures with the client to encourage her compliance and fully explain the plan of care.

### ABO Incompatibility

ABO isoimmunization is not as severe because most antibodies to A and B antigens are IgM antibodies, which do not cross the placenta. Usually, the mother is blood type O, with anti-A and anti-B in her serum, and the infant is blood type A, B, or AB. Titers and amniocentesis are not required during pregnancy; however, treatment begins after delivery for the infant.

Jaundice becomes clinically apparent as the infant's red blood cells are hemolyzed as a result of ABO incompatibility. The infant's bilirubin levels are monitored and phototherapy is used to treat jaundice. Occasionally, a transfusion is required for the infant.[4]

***Client Teaching and Counseling.*** Most teaching centers on information concerning the infant's condition. The mother also needs reassurance.

Emphasize to the client that her infant's condition is not her fault and that she should not feel guilty about the infant undergoing treatment. Providing her with written material that explains ABO incompatibility and treatment will help.

The client needs to be prepared should the infant become frankly jaundiced. Tell her that the pediatrician may change the infant's feeding schedule or type of feeding to enhance the breakdown of bilirubin. Because the infant will be undergoing phototherapy a vast majority of the time, the mother will have less time to hold, feed, and bond with her infant. Assess this potential inability to bond and arrange to have the client provide as much care as possible. Also explain that the infant's eyes will be covered while undergoing phototherapy.

Discuss the possibility of transfusion. Discussion may assist the client in making decisions about problematic religious or cultural issues. Because transfusions can become a legal issue, every effort should be made to educate the client concerning the need for treatment. In this way, conflict may be avoided.

## PERINATAL ADDICTION

"A teratogen is any substance that alters the structure or function of the developing fetus, placing it in a compromised state. . . . A simple rule of thumb is that any drug that crosses the blood–brain barrier and has an effect on the central nervous system of the mother will also cross the placenta" (Hogerman et al., p. 559).[62] See also Substance Abuse in Chapter 14.

### Drug Effects

The effects of certain drugs are difficult to assign because often multiple drugs are used and nutritional status is also poor. Multiple drug use is associated with more severe intrauterine growth retardation and increased anomalies. Drug effects may also be enhanced by the duration of drug use and the amount and the timing in gestation.[63,64]

### Counseling

Ideally, counseling a client concerning substance abuse should begin prior to conception. Open discussions concerning substance use may make the client aware of the need to prevent pregnancy and to seek counseling if she is dependent. Clients who use substances occasionally need to be aware of the potential teratogenic effect of one exposure.

### Identifying Maternal Substance Abuse

Addicts often begin with "socially" acceptable drugs, such as alcohol and cigarettes, and then move on to common street drugs and hard drugs. Identifying maternal drug use as soon as possible is essential so that the client can enter a drug abuse program and thus decrease the potential for harmful effects on her and her fetus. The key to successful intervention is maintaining a nonjudgmental manner; a client who does not sense dismay or disgust is more apt to trust the health care provider and reveal abuse.

# POTENTIAL SCREENING METHODS FOR THE FUTURE

## FETOSCOPY

Direct visualization of the fetus has been attempted by fetoscopy, a procedure in which a scope is inserted *into* the amniotic cavity.[59] In addition to visualizing the fetus, it may also be used to sample fetal blood and obtain a fetal skin biopsy.[74] Its use is diminishing and development may be curtailed because of the fetal loss rate, the difficulty of the procedure, and advances in ultrasound.[4,33,59]

## EMBRYOSCOPY

Embryoscopy, which is currently under investigation,[29,59] is visualization of the embryo *through* the chorionic membrane using an endoscope. Advances in ultrasound and umbilical cord blood sampling have slowed the development of embryoscopy.[4]

Potential applications are in the diagnosis of fetal anomalies and the sampling of fetal blood and tissue. Serial views of the developing fetus may provide information concerning teratogenesis.[59]

The risks associated with embryoscopy include rupture of the amnion (less risk if embryoscopy is performed from 8 to 11 weeks), bleeding, pregnancy loss, infection, placental separation, and theoretic potential damage to the developing fetal eye from the halogen light source.[59]

## TROPHOBLAST ISOLATION

It is possible to assess fetal karyotype in fetal villous trophoblasts isolated from a maternal blood sample.[59] Fetal sex may be determined through use of polymerase chain reaction amplification with Y-chromosome DNA primers.[59]

A potential application of the technique, when it is perfected, is screening for conditions caused by single-gene disorders in which the DNA sequence is known, such as cystic fibrosis.[59]

There are no risks although bruising may occur during blood sampling.

Again, embryoscopy and trophoblast isolation are still under investigation and are not available as screening methods for fetal assessment in general practice.[59]

## ACKNOWLEDGMENT

The author expresses her thanks to Dr. Peter F. Boehling for his consultation.

## REFERENCES

1. Carpenito, L. (1991). *Handbook of nursing diagnosis.* Philadelphia: J.B. Lippincott.
2. McCaul, J., & Morrison, J. (1990). Antenatal fetal assessment: An overview. *Obstetrics and Gynecology Clinics of North America, 17,* 1–15.
3. Druzin, M. (1989). Antepartum fetal heart rate monitoring. *Clinics in Perinatology, 16,* 627–642.
4. Cunningham, G., MacDonald, P., & Gant, N. (1989). *Williams obstetrics* (18th ed.). Norwalk, CT: Appleton & Lange.
5. Gegor, C., Paine, L., & Johnson, T. (1991). Antepartum fetal assessment: A nurse-midwifery perspective. *Journal of Nurse Midwifery, 36,* 153–167.
6. Pircon, R., & Freeman, R. (1990). The contraction stress test. *Obstetrics and Gynecology Clinics of North America, 17,* 129–146.
7. Druzin, M. (1990). Fetal surveillance—Update. *Bulletin of the New York Academy of Medicine, 66,* 246–254.
8. Rayburn, W. (1990). Fetal body movement monitoring. *Obstetrics and Gynecology Clinics of North America, 17,* 95–110.
9. Baskett, T., & Liston, R. (1989). Fetal movement monitoring: Clinical application. *Clinics in Perinatology, 16,* 613–625.
10. Moore, T., & Piacquadio, K. (1989). A prospective evaluation of fetal movement screening to reduce the incidence of antepartum fetal death. *American Journal of Obstetrics and Gynecology, 160,* 1075–1080.
11. Chasnoff, I. (1991). Cocaine and pregnancy: Clinical and methodologic issues. *Clinics in Perinatology, 18,* 113–123.
12. Smith, C., Davis, C., & Rayburn, W. (1992). Patient's acceptance of monitoring fetal movement: A randomized comparison of charting techniques. *Journal of Reproductive Medicine, 37,* 144–146.
13. Newton, E. (1989). The fetus as a patient. *Medical Clinics of North America, 73,* 517–540.
14. Varner, M., & Hurst, B. (1989). Clinical assessment of fetal well-being. *Seminars in Ultrasound, CT, and MR, 10,* 367–382.
15. Hurst, B., & Varner, M. (1989). Nonimaging methods for assessment of fetal well-being. *Seminars in Ultrasound, CT, and MR, 10,* 396–404.
16. Devoe, L. (1990). The nonstress test. *Obstetrics and Gynecology Clinics of North America, 17,* 111–128.
17. Murray, M. (1988). *Antepartal and intrapartal fetal monitoring.* Washington, DC: NAACOG.
18. Auyeung, R., & Goldkrand, J. (1991). Vibroacoustic stimulation and nursing intervention in the nonstress test. *Journal of Obstetric, Gynecologic, and Neonatal Nursing, 20,* 232–238.
19. Arulkumaran, S., Skurr, B., Tong, H., Kek, L., Yeoh, K., & Ratnam, S. (1991). No evidence of hearing loss due to fetal acoustic stimulation test. *Obstetrics and Gynecology, 78,* 283–285.
20. Manning, F. (1990). The fetal biophysical profile. *Obstetrics and Gynecology Clinics of North America, 17,* 147–162.
21. Maulik, D. (1989). Biologic effects of ultrasound. *Clinical Obstetrics and Gynecology, 32,* 645–659.
22. Reece, A., Assimakopoulos, E., Zheng, X., Hagay, Z., & Hobbins, J. (1990). The safety of obstetric ultrasonography: Concern for the fetus. *Obstetrics and Gynecology, 76,* 139–146.
23. Rottem, S., & Chervenak, F. (1990). Ultrasound diagnosis of fetal anomalies. *Obstetrics and Gynecology Clinics of North America, 17,* 17–40.
24. Romero, R., Oyarzun, E., Sirtori, M., & Hobbins, J. (1991). Prenatal detection of anatomic congenital anomalies. In A. Flasher, R. Romero, F. Manning, P. Jeanty, & E. James (Eds.), *The principles and practices of ultrasonography in obstetrics and gynecology* (pp. 193–211). Norwalk, CT: Appleton & Lange.
25. Committee on Technical Bulletins of the American College of Obstetricians and Gyne-

cologists. (1988). Ultrasound in pregnancy. *ACOG Technical Bulletin, 116,* 1–4.

26. Murphy, P. (1990). Assessment of fetal status. In K. Buckley & N. Kulb (Eds.), *High risk maternity nursing* (pp. 44–58). Baltimore: Williams & Wilkins.
27. Hadlock, F. (1989). Computer-assisted, multiple-parameter assessment of fetal age and growth. *Seminars in Ultrasound, CT, and MR, 10,* 383–395.
28. Jeanty, P. (1991). Fetal biometry. In A. Flasher, R. Romero, F. Manning, P. Jeanty, & E. James (Eds.), *The principles and practice of ultrasonography in obstetrics and gynecology* (pp. 93–108). Norwalk, CT: Appleton & Lange.
29. Nelson, L. (1989). Fetal imaging in prenatal diagnosis. *Pediatric Annals, 18,* 726–735.
30. Hamilton, L. (1986). Intrauterine growth retardation, intrauterine fetal demise, and postterm pregnancy. In N. Hacker & G. Moore (Eds.), *Essentials of obstetrics and gynecology* (pp. 214–220). Philadelphia: W.B. Saunders.
31. Rodis, J., & Vintzileos, A. (1991). A sound way to diagnose congenital anomalies. *Contemporary Obstetrics and Gynecology, 36(7),* 65–76.
32. Rodis, J., & Vintzileos, A. (1991). Scanning to diagnose congenital anomalies. *Contemporary Obstetrics and Gynecology, 36(8),* 45–54.
33. Committee on Technical Bulletins of the American College of Obstetricians and Gynecologists. (1987). *Antenatal Diagnosis of Genetic Disorders, 108,* 1–8.
34. De Vore, G., & Hebertson, R. (1990). The temporal association of the implementation of a fetal diagnostic and surveillance program and decreased fetal mortality in a private hospital. *Obstetrics and Gynecology, 75,* 212–213.
35. Pearce, J., & MacPharland, P. (1991). A comparison of Doppler flow velocity waveforms, amniotic fluid columns, and the nonstress test as a means of monitoring the post-dates pregnancy. *Obstetrics and Gynecology, 77,* 204–208.
36. Vintzileos, A., Campbell, W., & Rodis, J. (1989). Fetal biophysical profile scoring: Current status. *Clinics in Perinatology, 16,* 661–669.
37. Bezjian, A. (1988). Sonographic evaluation of the placenta. *Contemporary Issues in Obstetrics and Gynecology, 3,* 41–60.
38. Hobbins, J., Winsberg, F., & Berkowitz, R. (1983). *Ultrasonography in Obstetrics and Gynecology.* Baltimore: Williams & Wilkins.
39. Lumley, J. (1990). Through a glass darkly: Ultrasound and prenatal bonding. *Birth, 17,* 214–217.
40. Manning, F., Harman, C., Menticoglou, S., & Morrison, I. (1991). Assessment of fetal well-being with ultrasound. *Obstetrics and Gynecology Clinics of North America, 18,* 891–905.
41. Vintzileos, A., Winston, C., Rodis, J., Mclean, D., Fleming, A., & Scorza, W. (1991). The relationship between fetal physical assessment, umbilical artery velocimetry, and fetal acidosis. *Obstetrics and Gynecology, 77,* 622–626.
42. Maulik, D., Yarlagadda, P., & Downing, G. (1990). Doppler velocimetry in obstetrics. *Obstetrics and Gynecology Clinics of North America, 17,* 163–186.
43. Cook, C., Connelly, A., & Trudinger, B. (1989). Doppler assessment of the umbilical circulation. *Seminars in Ultrasound, CT, and MR, 10,* 417–427.
44. Morrow, R., & Ritchie, K. (1989). Doppler ultrasound fetal velocimetry and its role in obstetrics. *Clinics in Perinatology, 16,* 771–778.
45. Bruinse, H., Sijmons, E., & Reuwer, P. (1989). Clinical value of screening for fetal growth retardation by Doppler ultrasound. *Journal of Ultrasound in Medicine, 8,* 207–209.
46. Rotmensch, S., Copel, J., & Hobbins, J. (1991). Introduction to Doppler velocimetry in obstetrics. *Obstetrics and Gynecology Clinics in North America, 18,* 823–841.
47. Maulik, D. (1991). Doppler for clinical management: What is its place? *Obstetrics and Gynecology Clinics of North America, 18,* 853–873.
48. Reed, K. (1989). Fetal Doppler echocardiography. *Clinical Obstetrics and Gynecology, 32,* 728–736.

49. Cundiff, J., Haubrich, K., & Hinzman, N. (1990). Umbilical artery Doppler flow studies during pregnancy. *Journal of Obstetric, Gynecologic, and Neonatal Nursing, 19,* 475–481.
50. Otto, C., & Platt, L. (1991). Fetal growth and development. *Obstetrics and Gynecology Clinics of North America, 18,* 907–931.
51. Nichols, C. (1985). Clinical management of size/dates discrepancy. *Journal of Nurse-Midwifery, 30,* 15–24.
52. Committee on Technical Bulletins of the American College of Obstetricians and Gynecologists. (1991). Alpha-fetoprotein. *ACOG Technical Bulletin, 154,* 1–6.
53. Martin, J., & Cowan, B. 1990. Biochemical assessment and prediction of gestational well-being. *Obstetrics and Gynecology Clinics of North America, 17,* 81–93.
54. Canick, J., & Knight, G. (1992). Multiple-marker screening for fetal Down syndrome. *Contemporary Obstetrics and Gynecology, 36,* 25–42.
55. Elias, S., & Simpson, J. (1991). Sampling the chorionic villi. *Contemporary Obstetrics and Gynecology, 4,* 11–25.
56. Brambati, B., Tului, L., Simoni, G., & Travi, M. (1991). Genetic diagnosis before the eighth gestational week. *Obstetrics and Gynecology, 77,* 318–321.
57. Carlson, D. (1991). Prenatal diagnosis: Ultrasound advances. *Obstetrics and Gynecology Clinics of North America, 18,* 797–808.
58. Shulman, L., & Elias, S. (1989). Chorionic villus sampling. *Pediatric Annals, 18,* 714–725.
59. Viscarello, R., Gollin, Y., & Hobbins, J. (1991). Alternate methods of first-trimester diagnosis. *Obstetrics and Gynecology Clinics of North America, 18,* 875–889.
60. Rhoads, G., Jackson, L., Schlesselman, D., de la Cruz, F.F., Desnick, R.J., Colbus, M.S., Ledbetter, D.H., Lubs, H.A., Mahoney, M.J., & Pergament, E. (1989). The safety and efficacy of chorionic villus sampling for early prenatal diagnosis of cytogenetic abnormalities. *New England Journal of Medicine, 320,* 609–617.
61. Canadian Collaborative CVS–Amniocentesis Clinical Trial Group. (1989). Multicentre randomized clinical trial of chorionic villus sampling and amniocentesis. *Lancet, 1,* 1–6.
62. Burton, B., Schulz, C., & Burd, L. (1992). Limb anomalies associated with chorionic villus sampling. *Obstetrics and Gynecology, 79* (5, pt 1), 726–730.
63. NICHHD Workshop. (1993). Report of National Institute of Child Health and Human Development workshop on chorionic villus sampling and limb and other defects, October 20, 1992. *American Journal of Obstetrics and Gynecology, 169,* 1–6.
64. Brambati, B., Simoni, G., Travi, M., Danesinos, C., Tului, L., Privitera, O., Stioui, S., Tedeschi, S., Russo, S., & Primignani, P. (1992). Genetic diagnosis by chorionic villus sampling before 8 gestational weeks: Efficiency, reliability and risks on 317 completed pregnancies. *Prenatal Diagnosis, 12,* 789–799.
65. Lippman, A., Tomkins, D., Shime, J., & Hamerton, J. (1992). Canadian multicentre randomized clinical trial of chorionic villus sampling and amniocentesis: Final report. *Prenatal Diagnosis, 12,* 385–476.
66. Morgan, C., & Elias, S. (1989). Prenatal diagnosis of genetic disorders. *Journal of Perinatology and Neonatal Nursing, 2,* 1–12.
67. Committee on Technical Bulletins of the American College of Obstetricians and Gynecologists. (1990). Prevention of D isoimmunization. *ACOG Technical Bulletin, 147,* 1–4.
68. Tabsh, K., & Monoson, R. (1986). Rhesus isoimmunization. In N. Hacker & G. Moore (Eds.), *Essentials of obstetrics and gynecology* (pp. 230–236). Philadelphia: W.B. Saunders.
69. Committee on Technical Bulletins of the American College of Obstetricians and Gynecologists. (1990). Management of isoimmunization in pregnancy. *ACOG Technical Bulletin, 148,* 1–6.
70. Harmon, C. (1989). Fetal monitoring in the alloimmunized pregnancy. *Obstetrics and Gynecology Clinics of North America, 17,* 691–731.
71. Queenan, J. (1991). Rh and other blood group

immunizations. *Contemporary Obstetrics and Gynecology, 36,* 25–46.

72. Dunn, P., Weiner, S., & Ludomirski, A. (1988). Percutaneous umbilical blood sampling. *Journal of Obstetric, Gynecologic, and Neonatal Nursing, 17,* 308–313.
73. Copel, J., Cullen, M., Grannum, P., & Hobbins, J. (1990). Invasive fetal assessment in the antepartum period. Obstetrics and Gynecology Clinics of North America, 17, 201–220.
74. Tabsh, K., & Fox, M. (1986). Genetic counseling and prenatal diagnosis. In N. Hacker & G. Moore (Eds.), *Essentials of obstetrics and gynecology* (pp. 64–72). Philadelphia: W.B. Saunders.

# APPENDIX: AN ALGORITHM OF FETAL TESTING THAT MIGHT BE USED WHEN A PROBLEM ARISES

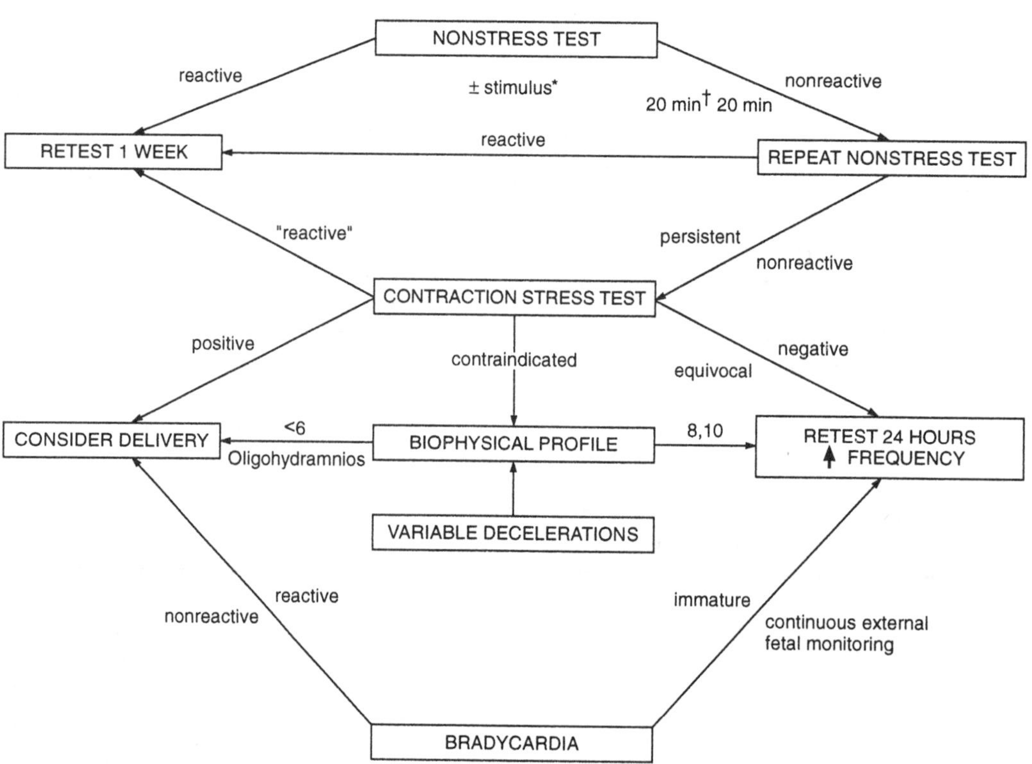


*Reprinted with permission from Druzin, M. (1990). Fetal surveillance—Update.* Bulletin of the New York Academy of Medicine, 66, *246–254.*

CHAPTER 16

# POSTPARTUM AND LACTATION

*Kathleen M. Akridge*

*The support and experience previously provided by the extended family are not easily accessible for families of today.*

## *Highlights*

- Two-Week and Four- to Six-Week Assessments
- Post-Cesarean Section Assessments
- Normal Postpartum Assessments
  - *Pelvic Musculature*
  - *Breasts*
  - *Contraception*
- Postpartum Complications
  - *Gestational Diabetes*
  - *Persistent Hypertension*
  - *Hemorrhage*
  - *Uterine Subinvolution*
  - *Mastitis*
  - *Metritis With Pelvic Cellulitis*
  - *Thyroiditis*
  - *Urinary Tract Infection*
  - *Acute Appendicitis*
- Early Discharge
- Adjusting to Parenting
  - *Barnard and Mercer Models*
  - *Factors Inhibiting Attachment*
  - *Family Relationships, Single Parent*
- Children With Malformations
- Postpartum Depression
- Perinatal Loss
- Breast- and Bottle-Feeding

## INTRODUCTION

Knowledge of the normal physiologic changes and complications of the postpartum period, parental roles, perinatal loss, and lactation is essential in managing the care of a client and her family postpartum. The health care provider must be familiar with assessment, diagnosis, management, and follow-up and know when referral is needed for further evaluation and management.

In the diagnosis and management of complications, it may be necessary to implement emergency measures until definitive care from a consulting medical professional arrives. The postpartum woman may be assessed in a hospital setting or alternative birthing site such as a birthing center.

The extended family of 40 or 50 years ago has been replaced by nuclear families and such nontraditional families as single-parent and blended (two partial families joined to become one) families. The support and experience previously provided by the extended family are not easily accessible for families of today. Early hospital discharge means that many of the nurturing and infant care skills previously taught by health professionals on the second postpartum day are now crammed into a short time frame just prior to hospital discharge, when the client's attention is often focused on what awaits her at home. To meet the health needs of today's new mother, many hospitals provide follow-up telephone calls or home visits.

Many women choosing to breastfeed may be deterred when faced with engorgement, tender nipples, and nonsupportive family and friends. Women who deliver twins may believe that breastfeeding is not possible. A unique opportunity exists to make this a successful experience for the breastfeeding family.

The postpartum experience is not always joyful. Many women or couples are left to deal with the loss of the fantasized infant as they struggle with the reality of a miscarriage, deformity, or perinatal death. Knowing how to help the woman and her family and suggest appropriate referral is imperative. There is a list of Support Groups at the end of this chapter.

Health care during the postpartum period focuses on evaluation of the physiological and psychological changes that normally occur. Any abnormal findings or dysfunctional behavior detected during the antepartum and postpartum periods should continue to be evaluated.

## THE PUERPERIUM

Postpartum, also referred to as the *puerperium,* is the period from delivery of the placenta and membranes to the return of the woman's reproductive organs to their nonpregnant state. It generally lasts about 6 weeks and is divided into three segments. The immediate puerperium is the first 24 hours after delivery; the early puerperium extends from the second day postpartum to the end of the first postpartum week; and the remote puerperium continues to the end of the sixth week.

### IMMEDIATE POSTPARTUM

- *Uterine Involution.* This process includes shedding of the decidua and endometrium. It is monitored by assessing the amount of lochia and uterine size and tone.
  - Immediately after delivery the uterus is approximately two thirds to three fourths of the way between the umbilicus and the symphysis pubis; after a few hours, the uterus rises to the level of the umbilicus and remains there or one fingerbreadth below for about 2 days before gradually descending into the pelvis. Any time the top of the fundus is above the umbilicus, bladder or uterine distention from blood or clots is possible.
  - Lochia is the uterine discharge during the puerperium that escapes vaginally. Lochia rubra is the earliest lochia and is red because it contains blood and decidual tissue. It begins immediately after delivery and continues the first 2 to 3 days postpartum.
- *The Vagina and Perineum.* These structures are quite stretched and edematous following a vaginal delivery. The vagina gapes at the introitus; it is also smooth-walled and generally lax. Hematoma should be suspected if the woman reports excruciating pain or is unable to void, or if a tense, fluctuant mass is noted. Inspect the episiotomy for hematoma. Vulvar and rec-

tal hemorrhoids are often present and must be observed for evidence of thrombosis. After delivery, ice bags may be applied to the perineum and hemorrhoids for 30 to 60 minutes; ice bags are removed then to prevent a secondary effect, vasodilation.

- *Vital Signs.* Blood pressure, pulse, and respirations should be stabilized to within normal limits. Fever is indicative of infection, probably in the genitourinary tract.
- *Bladder.* The bladder is edematous, hypotonic, and congested immediately postpartum. Consequently bladder distention, incomplete emptying, and excessive urine residual may develop unless the woman is encouraged to void periodically even when she does not feel the need.
- *Breasts.* Lactation naturally begins unless the woman is given a lactation suppressant. Lactation suppressants, however, may fail in their action. Colostrum is the first fluid the infant receives from the breast. Engorgement commonly occurs 48 to 72 hours after delivery. The nonlactating woman may receive some relief from engorgement if an ice bag is applied to the breasts for 30 to 60 minutes, then removed for 1 hour before being reapplied.
- *Abdominal Muscles.* The muscles are flabby and all have some degree of diastasis recti. If cesarean section was performed, a dressing usually covers the incision; the dressing should be dry.
- *Postpartum Blues and Grief.* Descriptions are provided in the sections on Psychiatric Disturbances and Perinatal Loss.

## EARLY PUERPERIUM

From the second postpartum day to the end of the first postpartum week additional changes evolve.

- *Uterus.* The uterus is approximately 12 weeks' size and is barely palpable just above the symphysis pubis.
- *Lochia Serosa.* The normal uterine discharge from the vagina that occurs during postpartum days 4 to 10 is lochia serosa. It contains primarily serous fluid, decidual tissue, leukocytes, and erythrocytes. Flow is decreasing. Encourage use of sanitary pads rather than tampons.
- *Vagina and Perineum.* The vagina remains smooth, and the perineum may be slightly uncomfortable. If an episiotomy was performed, the sutures will still be palpable. Attention should be given for signs of infection or hemorrhoids. Discourage douching as it may alter vaginal pH and wash out protective vaginal organisms. Bathing can soothe and cleanse the perineum. Oils and fragrances should not be used in bath water. If hemorrhoids are present, relief can be obtained with Tucks, Nupercaine ointment, dermaplast, increased fluid and fiber intake, stool softeners as needed, and warm or cool Sitz baths. Urinary incontinence may indicate cystocele (see Chapter 9).
- *Breasts.* By this time, breasts contain milk for those women who are breastfeeding. Breast milk usually appears on postpartum days 3 to 5, and is a bluish white. A mother may need reassurance that the color is normal and her milk has not become "weak" (see Breastfeeding section).
- *Abdominal Muscles.* These muscles are lax, and a woman needs reassurance that it is normal. Walking and swimming may help tone muscles without exerting undue stress.
- *Diuresis and Profuse Perspiration.* These conditions are normal as long as the woman is afebrile.

## LATE PUERPERIUM

From the end of the first postpartum week to the end of the sixth week maternal change continues.

- *Uterus.* The uterus returns to its nonpregnant size 4 to 6 weeks following birth.
- *Lochia Alba.* The last lochia, lochia alba, begins at about day 10 and continues until approximately day 35 postpartum. It is scant, composed primarily of leukocytes and decidual cells, and is creamy white.
- *Vagina and Perineum.* These structures begin to regain tone by 6 weeks postpartum. Rugae are normally present by that time. Atrophy, however, may still be evident in the lactating woman. Of concern are maintaining and strengthening vaginal tone, preventing pelvic relaxation, and promoting nonpainful resumption of intercourse.
- *Breasts.* The breasts begin to adapt to the nutritional needs of the baby, but engorgement and mastitis remain primary concerns. Assess the breastfeeding process and family support. The breasts of a nonlactating woman may contain milk for up to 3 months postpartum.
- *Renal System.* Urinary tract infection (UTI) may occur, and continuing assessment is of particular concern for clients with a history of UTI.
- *Abdominal Muscles.* Abdominal wall musculature becomes firmer by the end of the sixth postpartum week but may never regain its prepregnant appearance if the muscles remain weakened and stretched.

## THE FOUR- TO SIX-WEEK POSTPARTUM ASSESSMENT

### SUBJECTIVE DATA

Generally review the woman's systems. Specific determinations also need to be made:

- Number of weeks postpartum
- General adaptation to motherhood; assess client's rest and sleep habits, appetite, activity level, exercise program, and nutrition.
- Coping ability in caring for baby and making family adjustments
- Problems with baby (feeding, health, first exam)
- Family adjustments caring for baby
- Sexual intercourse (resumption, type of contraceptive used, dyspareunia and other problems)
- Family planning method desired; assess previous methods used, length of time used, satisfaction with methods, and reason for discontinuance.

Ask the client if she has called a health care provider or gone to an emergency room and whether she was admitted or readmitted. In addition, ask if she has had fever, chills, or flu.

- *Breasts.* Assess engorgement and breastfeeding.
  - Determine when engorgement occurred, how long it has lasted, if it has been treated, and whether it continues to be a problem or has resolved.
  - If breastfeeding is discontinued, determine the length of breastfeeding and the reason for stopping.
  - If the client is currently breastfeeding, ask her about problems, frequency, nipple soreness, breast care, and enjoyment of breastfeeding.
- *Lochia.* In the postpartum period, assess the duration of each lochia color in sequence, presence of odor, excessive bleeding, clots, and pain.
- *Return of Menses.* Several factors influence the return of menses. Nonlactating women menstruate 6 to 8 weeks following delivery, and lactating women 2 to 18 months following delivery. The first postpartum menstruation is heavier than normal menstruation and often anovulatory. Menses returns sooner in the multipara than the primipara.

## OBJECTIVE DATA

### Physical Examination

Generally assess the client.

- *General Appearance and Vital Signs.* Compare blood pressure with range during pregnancy. Compare weight with prepregnant weight and weight at delivery.
- *Neck.* Determine that the thyroid is nonpalpable. If thyromegaly or nodules are palpated, order thyroid function tests (TFTs) and refer client for medical evaluation (see Normal Postpartum Health Assessment).
- *Breasts.* Evaluation is influenced by whether the client is lactating.
  - Lactating breasts should be full, without erythema, masses, or lymphadenopathy. Milk should be easily expressed.
  - Nonlactating breasts are soft, without masses or lymphadenopathy. Bilateral galactorrhea may be present in nonlactating women for up to 3 months postpartum; these women should re-turn for evaluation of galactorrhea beyond 3 months postpartum. Mechanical stimulation of nonlactating breasts may lead to persistence of milky discharge, but more serious causes should be ruled out.
- *Extremities.* Assess for varicosities and phlebitis.
- *Cardiovascular and Respiratory Systems.* Rate and rhythm should be regular without murmurs or extra heart sounds. Clear, equal breath sounds should be evident bilaterally. Blood volume returns to normal by approximately 1 week postpartum.
- *Abdomen and Musculoskeleton.* Assess for costovertebral angle tenderness (CVAT) and tenderness along paraspinous muscles. In addition, inspect for striae, diastasis, hernias, masses, tenderness, and lymph nodes. If a cesarean section was done, assess healing. Abdominal musculature involution may require 6 to 8 weeks.
- *Genitalia and Reproductive Organs.* Several structures are involved.
  - External genitalia should be without edema or lesions and nontender.
  - Vagina should appear rugated, except in lactating women when rugae may be decreased secondary to hypoestrogenic state. Episiotomy should be intact, well healed, and nontender.
  - Cervical internal os should be closed. If it is open, determine whether placental products have been retained. After childbirth, the cervix appears as a transverse slit. It appears stellate if severe lacerations were sustained during childbirth.
  - Uterine corpus at 4 to 6 weeks postpartum is nonpregnant size. If uterine tenderness is detected, consider infection and prepare appropriate cultures (e.g., chlamydia, gonorrhea).
  - Involution of ovaries and fallopian tubes is complete by 6 to 7 weeks postpartum.
  - Inspect rectum for hemorrhoids. Assess sphincter control, especially if third- or fourth-degree laceration was sustained during childbirth.
- *Psychological Factors.* Assess affect, mood of mother, and her interaction with infant.

### Diagnostic Tests

Various tests need to be performed.

- Compare antenatal and postnatal hemoglobin levels and hematocrits.
- Check immunity status for rubella and, if not immune (titer $\leq$ 1:10), confirm that rubella vaccine was given prior to hospital discharge. Nursing mothers may be vaccinated.
- If client is Rh-negative, check Rh status of infant and, if clinically indicated, determine whether Rho(D) immune globulin was given to mother postpartum.

- Check when last Pap smear was done and results.

### PLAN

- *Psychosocial Intervention.* Counseling may be helpful about available social services, public health nursing, and child protective services (see Postpartum Depression Support Groups at the end of this chapter).
- *Medication.* Ask the client whether she was satisfied with previously used methods of contraception. Ask about her concerns regarding the method she wishes to use now. Base your instructions about a method of contraception on the client's level of comprehension.
- *Preventive Measures.* Encourage health maintenance/health promotion activities, such as breast self-examination, Kegel exercises, annual Pap examination, not smoking, weight reduction, and exercise.

### FOLLOW-UP

- *Pap Smear.* Perform if due or if previously abnormal.
- *Colposcopy.* Perform or refer if clinically indicated.
- *Culture.* Culture for chlamydia or gonorrhea if indicated.
- *Urine Testing.* Culture urine if bacteriuria occurred during pregnancy or if physical exam warrants.
- *Blood Tests.* Obtain hemoglobin level, hematocrit, or complete blood count if indicated.
- *Immunization.* Request rubella immunization if indicated.
- *Intravenous Pyelogram and Urology.* Refer client for intravenous pyelogram and urology consultation if she has a history of pyelonephritis or hematuria of unknown etiology.
- *Glucose Testing.* Request 75-g glucola (i.e., 2-hr oral glucose tolerance test) if the client was gestational diabetic. Protocols vary depending on the setting. A 3-hour test may be used. However, since glucose tolerance testing in the immediate postpartum period is unreliable, there must be a wait of at least 6 weeks postpartum for a reliable testing of carbohydrate intolerance.

## NORMAL POSTPARTUM HEALTH ASSESSMENT

Essential aspects of normal postpartum health assessment are pelvic musculature and breast evaluations and contraception counseling. See Chapter 10 for information on breast self-examination. Evaluation of pelvic musculature and contraception counseling are discussed here.

### PELVIC MUSCULATURE

Pelvic musculature is assessed following pregnancy to evaluate involution and resumption of nonpregnant function (see Chapter 9). The general function of pelvic musculature is to support pelvic organs and assist urinary continence.

#### Etiology of Relaxed Pelvic Musculature

Relaxed musculature may be related to childbearing, age, obesity, or lack of exercise.

- Closely spaced pregnancies or large fetuses can stretch and traumatize pelvic musculature and contribute to relaxation.
- Aging, because of decreased estrogen production, contributes to loss of elasticity.
- Obesity increases intraabdominal pressure and contributes to relaxation of vaginal muscles.
- Failure to perform Kegel exercises permits continued relaxation.

### Subjective Data

A woman may report sensations of pelvic pressure, urinary incontinence, and lack of perineal support during defecation.[1] Specific information needs to be pursued.

- Involuntary loss of urine during an activity that increases intraabdominal pressure
- Age of onset and circumstances of incontinence
- Increase in severity or number of pelvic symptoms, or both
- Day and night voiding patterns
- Frequency and severity of wetting
- Amount of urine lost (drops, teaspoon, tablespoon, quarter of cup, layer of clothing soaked)
- History of and reasons for previous vaginal or urinary tract surgery
- History of lower back surgery (The pudendal nerve innervates pelvic floor muscles and could have been damaged in surgery.)
- Past history of stress urinary incontinence and method of treatment

Stress urinary incontinence (SUI) and detrusor instability should be differentiated. SUI results from an incompetent urethra. Urine is lost immediately with an event that increases intraabdominal pressure.[1] With detrusor instability (involuntary contraction) the bladder itself is the cause of incontinence. A delay occurs between the precipitating event and urine loss; urine loss may also be sudden and without warning.[1]

### Objective Data

Data are determined by preliminary diagnostic tests followed by measurement of pelvic muscle strength.

***Preliminary Assessment.*** The first test requires that the client not urinate for 2 hours prior to the exam. She should stand with legs apart, hold a folded paper towel against her perineum, and cough vigorously. The amount of urine lost can be seen on the towel.[1]

The urine stop test shows significant negative correlations with pelvic muscle strength: the greater the time needed to stop urine flow, the weaker the musculature. The client sits on a standard commode with the knees about 16 inches apart to discourage use of gluteal or abdominal muscles. The examiner must be able to hear the onset of urination, and the client must be able to hear the "stop" command. Five seconds after onset of urination, the client is told to stop. Women with adequate muscle control should stop urination completely within 2 seconds.[1]

***Digital Examination.*** Digital measurement of pelvic muscle strength scale assesses vaginal muscles. The examiner inserts index and middle fingers 6 to 8 cm into the introitus on an anteroposterior plane and ask the client to contract her vaginal muscles around the fingers for as long as possible and as forcefully as possible. The scoring criteria are pressure, duration of pressure, and alteration in plane of examiner's fingers.[1] Scores range from 1 to 4, with 4 denoting the greatest muscle strength (Table 16–1).

The next step is to assess for cystocele, urethrocele, rectocele, and enterocele. Firmly exert pressure with fingers posterior to the vaginal wall and ask the client to bear down or cough. Observe the vaginal wall to detect an anterior bulge (cystocele or urethrocele). Continue pressing posteriorly with fingers while simultaneously separating them; ask the client to cough or bear down and observe the posterior wall for a bulge (rectocele or enterocele).

### Plan

Pelvic muscle exercise benefits women with cystocele, urethrocele, rectocele, or enterocele that bulges into the vaginal vault but not

**TABLE 16–1. PELVIC MUSCLE STRENGTH RATING SCALE**

| Characteristic | 1 | 2 | 3 | 4 |
|---|---|---|---|---|
| Pressure | None | Weak, feel pressure on fingers, but not all way around | Moderate, feel pressure all around | Strong, fingers compress override |
| Duration | None | <1 s | >1 <3 s | >3 s |
| Displacement in plane | None | Slight incline, base of fingers move up | Greater incline of fingers along total length | Fingers move up and are drawn in |

*From C. Sampselle and C. Brink (1990). Pelvic muscle relaxation.* Journal of Nurse Midwifery, 35*(3), 130. Copyright American College of Nurse Midwives. Reprinted with permission.*

outside the introitus. It may be done in any position as long as knees are 16 to 18 inches apart. Instruct the client to contract vaginal muscles as tightly as possible for as long as possible; the goal is to hold each contraction for 5 to 10 seconds. Initially, the client should contract her pelvic muscles while slowly counting to 5, hold, and gradually release to the count of 5. The aim is 80 contractions per day (groups of 5 to 20 per session).[1]

Refer the client to a urologist or gynecologist if she has a "cele" that descends beyond the introitus.

## CONTRACEPTION COUNSELING

### Assessment

Assess a woman's knowledge of and preference for available contraceptive methods (see Chapter 6). She should be instructed in her choice of a temporary or permanent method. Temporary methods include barrier, hormonal, and spermicidal devices and periodic abstinence. Permanent methods are female sterilization and male sterilization.

### Oral Combination Contraception

A breastfeeding woman may begin a low dose (35 μg or less) of estrogen 4 to 6 weeks postpartum; at the time of discharge, a progestin-only may be started.[2] Estrogen may decrease the amount of milk produced.

### Breastfeeding

Breastfeeding can be used to delay subsequent pregnancies; however, a principal problem is to determine when ovulation occurs. Ovulation can be predicted using basal body temperature determination and observation of cervical mucus changes and cervical position in conjunction with breastfeeding. Ovulation is much more difficult to assess for a woman who is breastfeeding.

An upward thermal shift in basal body temperature (BBT) occurs after ovulation; intercourse should be avoided until the third day after the temperature rise. Temperature is monophasic during the preovulatory period of lactation; sexual abstinence is indicated when using BBT until ovulatory cycles have resumed.[3]

Cervical mucus changes may be misleading during anovulatory postpartum, as dry mucus is similar to that of preovulatory days during an ovulatory cycle; profuse, thick mucus makes identification of mucous patterns for prediction of ovulation difficult.

- Take basal body temperature if cervical mucus appears or the cervix opens or becomes elevated.

- Infertility of breastfeeding can be reasonably assumed if cervical mucus remains tacky for 3 weeks and does not become clear and stretchy.[3]
- With intermittent signs of cervical mucus discharge, begin BBT. When mucus lasts 3 or more days and its cessation is accompanied by continued low temperature, breastfeeding infertility can be assumed 2 days after mucus disappears.[3]

If weaning occurs slowly after 3 to 4 months, daily BBT should be continued and cervical mucus checked for onset of ovulation. Coitus is allowed throughout a 10-day weaning period. The couple should consider themselves fertile on the eleventh day until cervical and thermal signs show ovulation has occurred.[3] If weaning occurs naturally, the client should monitor for signs of ovulation after the ninth postpartum month.[3]

The importance of complete breastfeeding, as well as the importance of continuing breastfeeding to maintain postpartum infertility, should be taught to clients and their partners. Infants are not introduced to solid foods until approximately 6 months old and they may be slowly introduced to taking liquids by cup. Refer clients to breastfeeding support groups and local lactation consultants. It should be stressed that breastfeeding is not an effective method of birth control but, if used solely to supply the infant with food, it is used to space pregnancies in many cultures.

# ASSESSMENT OF POSTOPERATIVE CESAREAN SECTION AND STERILIZATION

Following a cesarean section, women are encouraged to ambulate to decrease the risk of thrombosis and embolism. Analgesics are given shortly before ambulation. Intake and output are monitored, and the wound observed for infection and hematoma. In addition, contact should be encouraged between mother and infant.

Following a sterilization procedure, mild analgesia is provided for pain. The site is observed for infection and hematoma. Prior to and after surgery, the mother's contact with her infant should be encouraged.

## TWO-WEEK POST-CESAREAN SECTION ASSESSMENT

### Subjective Data

Several points of information may be gained from the mother or from hospital records at the 2-week postcesarean assessment.

- Reason for cesarean section, type of section and anesthesia
- Length of labor, how long membranes were ruptured
- Support system during labor and delivery
- Weight and sex of baby
- Number of days in hospital, general well-being
- Medications, allergies
- Incision
- Pain, fever
- Lochia
- Bladder and bowel function
- Diet/appetite, sleep patterns/fatigue
- Family adjustments/support since discharge home
- Infant feeding, emotional state

Review the mother's feelings about delivery and her understanding of the medical reasons for her cesarean section.

### Objective Data

***Physical Examination.*** Evaluate the woman's general appearance. Check her vital signs and weight. Compare her blood pressure with the range during pregnancy; compare her weight with prepregnant weight and weight at last antepartum visit.

- *Neck.* Examination should reveal a nonpalpable thyroid. If, however, thyromegaly or nodules are palpated, order thyroid function tests and refer the client for medical evaluation (see Postpartum Thyroiditis in next section on complications).
- *Cardiovascular and Respiratory Systems.* Rates and rhythms should be regular without murmurs or extra sounds. Clear, equal breath sounds should be heard bilaterally.
- *Breasts.* Examination depends on whether the client is breastfeeding. A lactating woman will have full breasts without erythema, masses, or lymphadenopathy. Milk should be easily expressed. A nonlactating woman will have soft breasts without masses or lymphadenopathy. Bilateral galactorrhea may be present in nonlactating women for up to 3 months postpartum.
- *Abdomen and Musculoskeleton.* Assess to detect costovertebral angle tenderness and tenderness along the paraspinous muscles. Fundus is usually several fingerbreadths below the umbilicus and is not tender when palpated gently. The incision is healed, without exudate, and not tender.
- *Genitalia and Reproductive System.* Evaluation is generally deferred until the 6-week postpartum assessment.

***Psychological Assessment.*** Assess the mother's feelings and her understanding of the labor or cesarean birth, or both. Assess her support system. Review the type of uterine incision with the client and the issue of vaginal birth after cesarean section.

***Laboratory Tests.*** Determine rubella immunity. Obtain documentation that rubella vaccine was given during the postpartum. For Rh-negative mothers, determine whether $Rh_o(D)$ immune globulin was given if the infant was Rh-positive.

### Health Teaching

Use the same material focused on during the 6-week postpartum assessment.

### SIX-WEEK POST-CESAREAN SECTION ASSESSMENT

The 6-week postpartum evaluation of a woman who had a cesarean section is the same as that of a woman who delivered vaginally, except that the abdominal incision is assessed following a cesarean section as well as the perineum and vulva.

## COMMON POSTPARTUM COMPLICATIONS

Table 16–2 summarizes the postpartum complications.

### GESTATIONAL DIABETES

Gestational diabetes is carbohydrate intolerance that is induced by pregnancy (see Chapter 14).

***Epidemiology.*** Among women with gestational diabetes, 40 percent may persist with diabetes in the postpartum; 60 percent of obese women with gestational diabetes develop diabetes later in life.[4]

***Subjective Data.*** The client states she had diabetes during her pregnancy.

***Objective Data.*** The 2- or 3-hour oral glucose tolerance test detects diabetes in nonpregnant women. In women previously diagnosed with gestational diabetes, it is administered 6 weeks postpartum. The test measures the rate at which a concentrated amount of glucose is removed from the bloodstream (see Chapter 17). The healthy person almost immediately produces a surge of insulin that removes a large amount of the

**TABLE 16–2. SUMMARY OF POSTPARTUM COMPLICATIONS**

| Complication | Signs and Symptoms | Management |
|---|---|---|
| Postpartum hemorrhage (early) | Soft, boggy uterus; cool, clammy skin; fever; tachycardia; vertigo; tachypnea | Maintain patent IV line and begin second line; call physician; type and cross for blood; bimanual uterine massage if boggy uterus; oxytocic agents; elevate right hip; CBC and coagulation studies<br>Breastfeeding if possible |
| Postpartum hemorrhage (late) | Heavy lochia; foul lochia; fever; opened cervical os; pelvic or back pain; uterine tenderness; prolonged bleeding | Bed rest and oral oxytocic agents; physician consultation<br>Breastfeeding if possible |
| Subinvolution | Painless, heavy vaginal bleeding; uterine size larger than expected; uterine tenderness; fever | CBC; endocervical cultures; quantitative β-hCG<br>Meds: Methergine 0.2 mg q3–4h × 2 d<br>Augmentin or amoxicillin 500 mg tid × 7–10 d<br>Tetracycline 500 mg qid × 10 d<br>Breastfeeding |
| Mastitis | Flulike symptoms; malaise; fever and chills; erythema and swelling of affected breast with possible pitting edema | Milk culture; bed rest; continue breastfeeding; ice packs/warm packs; increased fluid intake;<br>Meds: Dicloxacillin sodium 250–500 mg qid × 10 d |
| Metritis with pelvic cellulitis | Unilateral/bilateral abdominal pain; foul lochia; fever; parametrial tenderness; leukocytosis | Endocervical cultures (gonorrhea and chlamydia); endometrial cultures (aerobic and anaerobic); medical consultation; hospitalization; rest<br>Meds: Erythromycin 500 mg qid × 10 d<br>Tetracycline 500 mg qid × 10 d<br>Augmentin or amoxicillin 500 mg tid × 10 d<br>Cephalosporin 500 mg qid × 10 d |
| Postpartum thyroiditis (thyrotoxicosis) | Weight loss; increased fatigue; palpitations; heat intolerance; sinus tachycardia | Radioactive iodine uptake; physician referral |
| Postpartum thyroiditis (transient hypothyroidism) | Pronounced fatigue; continued weight gain; coarse hair; dry skin; delayed reflexes; psychological reactions mimicking depression | Elevated TSH; thyroxine therapy; physician consultation |
| Urinary tract infection | Spiking fever; costovertebral angle tenderness; dysuria; urgency; oliguria | Urinalysis with culture and sensitivity<br>Meds: Amoxicillin 500 mg tid × 10 d<br>Macrodantin 100 mg qid × 10 d |
| Appendicitis | Right upper quadrant or entire right abdominal tenderness; positive Bryan's sign (pain elicited when enlarged uterus moved to right); positive Alder's test (pain elicited when provider maintains constant pressure at area of maximal tenderness and woman rolls from supine to left position) | Endocervical and lochial cultures; CBC; urinalysis; medical referral; hospitalization |

glucose, with insulin peaking in 30 to 60 minutes. Serum glucose levels return to normal within 3 hours.

The test procedure requires that for the 3 days preceding the test, the client consumes a diet containing at least 150 g of carbohydrate (300 g preferred) per day. After overnight fasting (12 hours), a sample of blood is taken. The client then drinks a preparation containing 75 g of glucose. She must drink all of the solution. Blood samples are then taken at 30 minutes, 1 hour, 1½ hours, and 2 hours.

Counsel the client regarding the purpose of the test and the need for a high-carbohydrate diet during the 3 days prior to the test. Remind the client that overnight fasting is required. In addition, advise her not to drink alcohol and caffeine the evening prior to the test and not to smoke during the 2-hour blood testing.

#### Differential Medical Diagnosis

- *Normal Values.* Fasting, <115 mg/dL; 1/2-hour, 1-hour, 1½-hour, and 2-hour blood sugars, <140 mg/dL.[4]
- *Impaired Glucose Tolerance.* Fasting, <140 mg/dL and 2-hour plasma glucose ≥140 and <200 mg/dL with one intervening value ≥200 mg/dL after 75-g glucose load.[5]
- *Diabetic Values.* Unequivocal elevation of plasma glucose ≥200 mg/dL and classic symptoms of diabetes, including polydipsia, polyuria, polyphagia, and weight loss; fasting, ≥140 mg/dL on two occasions; fasting, <140 mg/dL and two oral glucose tolerance tests with the 2-hour plasma glucose ≥200 mg/dL and one intervening value ≥200 mg/dL after 75-g oral glucose tolerance test.[5]

#### Plan

- *Psychosocial Intervention.* Assess client's lifestyle and knowledge of diabetes and its management. If lifestyle changes are indicated, counsel the client about the specific change (e.g., diet or exercise). Provide clear, accurate information regarding nongestational diabetes and its usual signs and symptoms and management. Refer the client to support groups if indicated. Frank diabetes may develop as she ages.
- *Medication.* Medication is not usually needed after 1 to 2 days postpartum.
- *Follow-Up.* Refer client to a diabetologist if frank diabetes is revealed.

## PERSISTENT HYPERTENSION

Persistent hypertension is blood pressure that remains significantly elevated in the postpartum period. It is usually indicative of chronic vascular disease. (See Chapter 17 for information about hypertension in nonpregnant women.)

***Subjective Data.*** The client may report a family history of hypertension or a diagnosis of pregnancy-induced hypertension. She may have no specific symptoms.

***Objective Data.*** Physical examination reveals a systolic blood pressure equal to or greater than 140, a diastolic blood pressure equal to or greater than 90, or both. No edema is evident. Reflexes are within normal limits. Other findings are normal.

Diagnostic tests include a urine dipstick for protein, baseline electrolyte, blood urea nitrogen (BUN), and creatinine levels, urinalysis for protein urea, and baseline albumin, calcium, and phosphorus levels. More extensive testing (e.g., electrocardiogram) is indicated by extent of findings.

***Differential Medical Diagnosis.*** Essential hypertension, hyperaldosteronism, hyperthyroidism, pheochromocytoma, renovascular disease.

#### Plan

- *Psychosocial Intervention.* Determine stress levels and sources of stress and counsel client regarding ways to reduce stress. Referral for support and counseling may be appropriate.

- *Medication.* The safety of medications must be considered if the client is breastfeeding.
- *Lifestyle Changes.* Provide dietary counseling to help client reduce fat, sodium, and refined sugar intake. She should maintain adequate complex carbohydrate, protein, and polyunsaturated fats. Counsel regarding exercise for aerobic health. Lactating mothers require information about specific dietary modifications and exercise. Advise mothers to stop smoking; explain cardiovascular changes that occur with smoking. In addition, advise client not to consume alcohol.
- *Follow-Up.* Postpartum follow-up should occur 1 week after hospital discharge; if hypertension persists, consult with a physician or refer the client for management.

## POSTPARTUM HEMORRHAGE

Hemorrhage during the postpartum period is blood loss in excess of 500 mL in 24 hours. Blood is measured by weighing pads and linens. The best method of estimation is use of laboratory data: There is a decrease in hemoglobin of 1 to 1.5 g/dL for every unit (450–500 mL) of blood loss.[6] Factors contributing to hemorrhage are uterine atony, coagulopathy, birth canal trauma, and poor general health.

### Early Postpartum Hemorrhage

Early hemorrhage refers to that which occurs during the first 24 hours postpartum. Several risk factors have been identified.

- Uterine overdistention (macrosomic infant, multiple fetuses, hydramnios)
- Midforceps delivery, forceps rotation
- Delivery through incompletely dilated cervix
- Intrauterine manipulation
- High parity
- Use of drugs to induce or augment labor or of halogenated anesthetics
- History of previous postpartum hemorrhage
- Chorioamnionitis
- Retained placental tissue
- Coagulation defects
- Fibroids
- Placenta previa or abruptio placentae

***Subjective Data.*** The client may report vertigo, extreme fatigue, chills, or a history of anemia.

***Objective Data.*** Physical examination reveals cool, clammy skin; fever; rapid, thready pulse; tachypnea; pallor of nail beds and mucous membranes. Bleeding may not be massive; however, a steady seepage may continue until significant hypovolemia has occurred. If uterine atony is the cause of blood loss, uterine assessment will show that the uterus feels boggy and that clots are easily expressed with massage.

The complete blood cell count (CBC) provides a reliable measurement of blood loss. Blood studies will show a decrease in the hemoglobin level of 1 to 1.5 g/dL for every unit (450–500 mL) of blood lost; the hematocrit will decrease by about 2 to 4 percent for same amount of blood loss.[6]

Coagulation studies are done to determine the nature and extent of coagulation disorders contributing to the abnormal bleeding.

***Differential Medical Diagnosis.*** Early postpartum hemorrhage secondary to uterine atony, early postpartum hemorrhage secondary to lacerations, hemorrhage secondary to blood coagulopathies.

### Plan

***Psychosocial Intervention.*** Provide emotional support. Inform the client in a calm tone of the procedures that are being instituted. Make instructions specific, for example, "I'm going to give you some oxygen through this mask. I want you to try to breathe normally so that the oxygen will help you." Encouraging the woman to breastfeed will help in the release of oxytocin and therefore help facilitate natural uterine contractions.

### *Medication*

*Oxytocin*

- *Indication.* Uterine stimulation.
- *Administration.* Diluted in intravenous fluids per hospital or agency protocol; usually 10 to 40 units in 1000 mL of intravenous solution given at 20 to 40 mU/min.
- *Side Effects.* Hypertension, uterine tetany, nausea, vomiting, bradycardia, tachycardia, premature ventricular contractions, water intoxication.
- *Contraindication.* Hypersensitivity to oxytocin.
- *Anticipated Outcomes on Evaluation.* Decreased uterine bleeding and increased uterine tone.
- *Client Teaching.* Inform the client that she will experience increased uterine contractions, which may be quite uncomfortable.

*Methylergonovine Maleate (Methergine)*

- *Indications.* Uterine and vascular smooth muscle constriction.
- *Administration.* Intramuscularly, orally, and, in an emergency, intravenously.

| | |
|---|---|
| Intramuscular | 0.2 mg, repeated in 2 to 4 hours |
| Oral | 0.2 to 0.4 mg every 6 to 12 hours, usually for 2 days |
| Intravenous | Hazardous; should be reserved for emergency control of postpartum hemorrhage. If methylergonovine maleate is given intravenously, 0.2 mg is infused over 60 seconds or longer. |

- *Side Effects.* Headache, dizziness, nausea, vomiting, chest pain, palpitation, hypertension (especially when given intravenously).
- *Contraindications.* Hypertension, hypersensitivity to ergot alkaloids, respiratory disease, cardiac disease, peripheral vascular disease.
- *Anticipated Outcome on Evaluation.* Decreased uterine bleeding.
- *Client Teaching.* Inform the client about possible side effects and increased uterine cramping.

*Prostaglandins*

- *Indication.* Uterine contraction.
- *Administration.* Intramuscularly—prostin 15/M (Carboprost) 250 μg, repeated as necessary every 15 to 90 minutes—and intravaginally—prostin E2 (PGE2, Dinoprostone) 20-mg vaginal suppository.
- *Side Effects.* Mild fever, diarrhea, abdominal cramping, vomiting.
- *Contraindications.* Hypersensitivity, respiratory disease.
- *Anticipated Outcome on Evaluation.* Decreased uterine bleeding.
- *Client Teaching.* Counsel the client regarding possible side effects, including abdominal cramps, low-grade fever, and diarrhea. The following steps must be taken.
  - Maintain patent intravenous line in client, and begin second intravenous line.
  - Elevate right hip to prevent vena cava syndrome.
  - Begin oxygen therapy with face mask at 6 to 8 liters per minute; provide positive-pressure ventilation if needed.
  - Inform physician about client's status and corrective measures already done.
  - Assess client's response by determining vital signs; insert Foley catheter to measure urinary output.
  - Anticipate blood transfusion and request cross-matching of blood.

***Follow-Up.*** Advise client to eat foods high in protein and iron. Iron supplements will be needed for an additional 2 to 3 months postpartum.

### Late Postpartum Hemorrhage

Late hemorrhage occurs after the first 24 hours and up to 1 month postpartum. Its usual onset is 6 to 10 days after delivery. Several risk factors have been identified:

- Retained placental tissue
- Uterine subinvolution
- Infection

***Subjective Data.*** The client may report pelvic or back pain, uterine tenderness, or bleeding for more than 2 weeks.

***Objective Data.*** Physical examination may reveal heavy lochia with a foul odor, fever, an open cervical os after the first week postpartum, and hematoma.

A complete blood count is ordered (see Early Postpartum Hemorrhage).

***Differential Medical Diagnosis.*** Trauma, blood coagulopathy.

***Plan***

- *Psychosocial Intervention.* Provide emotional support by assisting to calm the client and her family—speaking calmly and giving information about procedures (see Early Postpartum Hemorrhage). She may need help obtaining child or infant care.
- *Medication.* Methylergonovine maleate was discussed under Early Postpartum Hemorrhage.
- *Ultrasound.* Ultrasound examination is done to detect retained placental fragments.

***Follow-Up.*** Consult with a physician to determine need for hospital admission or other management.

## SUBINVOLUTION OF THE UTERUS

Subinvolution of the uterus is the arrest or prolongation of the normal involution process that occurs following pregnancy.[7] Complications of subinvolution include hemorrhage, pelvic peritonitis, salpingitis, and abscess formation.

***Epidemiology.*** Several risk factors are identified in the etiology of subinvolution:

- Distended bladder
- Retained placental fragments
- Endometritis
- Cesarean section
- Uterine myoma
- Multiparity

***Subjective Data.*** The client may report painless, excessive vaginal bleeding; chills and fever; pelvic or back pain; or leukorrhea.

***Objective Data.*** Physical examination of the genitalia and reproductive tract reveal whether the uterus is larger than expected for the period of puerperium and whether fundal height is normal—midway between the umbilicus and symphysis following the third stage of labor and at the level of the bony pelvis 2 weeks postpartum. The uterus should return to nonpregnant size at 4 to 6 weeks postpartum.[8] With subinvolution the uterus feels boggy and soft and may be tender. Uterine bleeding, excessive lochia, and leukorrhea are possible. Fever may also be present.

Diagnostic tests include serum blood tests, culture of cervical discharge, and ultrasound. Clients must be prepared for venipuncture.

- A complete blood count is performed to detect anemia and infection.
- An erythrocyte sedimentation rate (ESR) is a diagnostic evaluation for occult disease.
- Cervical discharge is cultured to identify a specific infective agent. Before a cervical specimen is obtained, the client should be informed about the use of the speculum,

the testing to be done, and the reason for the test.

- Quantitative determination of the β subunit of human chorionic gonadotropin (hCG) assists the health care provider in detecting pregnancy, trophoblastic tumors, and tumors that ectopically secrete hCG. Explain the rationale for requesting the test to the client.
- Pelvic ultrasound is done to evaluate whether placental fragments were retained. Instruct the client to drink four glasses of water 1 hour prior to the ultrasound exam. While she is supine on examining table, the transducer is placed in contact with her skin and swept over the area being studied.

***Differential Medical Diagnosis.*** Distended bladder, ovarian cyst, pelvic adhesions, malignant uterine tumors, cystitis, gestational trophoblastic disease, anemia, uterine leiomyoma, retained placental fragments.

## Plan

***Psychosocial Intervention.*** Inform the client about the diagnosis, suspected etiology, and plan of treatment. Explain that methylergonovine may cause painful uterine contractions. Advise her of the need to rest and avoid overexertion.

***Medication.*** For information on methylergonovine maleate, see Early Postpartum Hemorrhage.

*Amoxicillin or Augmentin*

- *Indication.* Infection. Because augmentin contains a β-lactamase inhibitor, it is effective against bacteria that produce β-lactamase.
- *Administration.* One 500-mg tablet orally every 8 hours for 10 days.
- *Side Effects.* Nausea, vomiting, diarrhea, vaginitis, eosinophilia, leukopenia.
- *Contraindication.* History of penicillin allergy.
- *Anticipated Outcome on Evaluation.* Clinically decreased evidence of infection. Check culture and sensitivity report from earlier cultures to confirm effectiveness of chosen antibiotic.
- *Client teaching.* Instruct the client to complete the 10-day medication regimen. Tell the client to telephone if side effects make compliance difficult.

*Tetracycline*

- *Indication.* Infection.
- *Administration.* One 500-mg tablet orally every 6 hours for 10 days.
- *Side Effects.* Nausea, vomiting, diarrhea, increased BUN, rash, urticaria, photosensitivity, increased pigmentation, hepatotoxicity, pseudomembranous colitis.
- *Contraindications.* Hypersensitivity to tetracyclines, kidney dysfunction, pregnancy, lactation.
- *Anticipated Outcome on Evaluation.* Decreased clinical evidence of infection. Check culture and sensitivity report to confirm organism's responsiveness to tetracycline.
- *Client Teaching.* Explain to the client that effects of tetracycline decrease when antacids, dairy products, or kaolin/pectin are also consumed. Advise the client to avoid sun exposure (sunscreen does not seem to decrease photosensitivity), to contact the health care provider if significant diarrhea develops, and to complete the 10-day medication regimen.

*Doxycycline*

- *Indication.* Infection.
- *Administration.* One 100-mg tablet orally every 12 hours for 10 days.
- *Side effects.* Same as for tetracycline.
- *Contraindications.* Hypersensitivity to tetracyclines, pregnancy, lactation. Because elimination is primarily nonrenal, doxycycline, unlike tetracycline, may be used for patients with renal failure.

- *Anticipated Outcome on Evaluation.* Decreased clinical evidence of infection.
- *Client Teaching.* Emphasize the need to complete the 10-day medication regimen. Instruct the client to avoid sun exposure (sunscreen does not seem to decrease photosensitivity) and to take doxycycline with a full glass of water. Do not lay down sooner than one hour after administration to avoid epigastric discomfort. In addition, let the client know that the drug may be taken with meals, as its absorption is not affected by food.

***Hospitalization.*** Hospitalization may be necessary if infection is severe, if pelvic structures in addition to the uterus are involved, or if uterine bleeding is excessive.

***Follow-Up.*** Reassess the uterus in 1 to 2 weeks. Report signs and symptoms of hemorrhage, pelvic peritonitis, salpingitis, or abscess to physician for further evaluation and management.

## MASTITIS

Mastitis, an inflammation of the breast, may be caused by tight clothing, missed infant feedings, poor drainage of duct and alveolus, or an infecting organism (*Staphylococcus aureus, Escherichia coli, Streptococcus*).[7,9]

Infection may be transmitted from lactiferous ducts to a secreting lobule, from a nipple fissure to periductal lymphatics, or by hematogenic means. Five percent of lactating women develop mastitis.[10]

***Subjective Data.*** A woman may report flu-like symptoms, including malaise, fever, and chills. She may also describe a tender, painful area or lump in the breast.

***Objective Data.*** Physical examination is usually sufficient to diagnose mastitis. Assess vital signs. Fever is often high; tachycardia is common. Examination of the breast reveals increased warmth, redness, tenderness, and swelling. The affected lobule is often in the outer quadrant and wedge-shaped; the nipple is cracked or abraded; and the breast distended with milk. If an abscess has formed, pitting edema is possible and fluctuation may be felt over the affected area. The remainder of the exam is usually normal.

Diagnostic testing may include a culture and sensitivity, although it is seldom used; diagnosis is generally made without culture. Culture and sensitivity identifies the causative infectious agent using an expressed sample of breast milk. Test results may not be available for 72 hours, but antibiotic therapy needs to be started immediately.

***Differential Medical Diagnosis.*** Clogged duct, simple breast engorgement, breast abscess, viral syndrome.

### Plan

***Psychosocial Intervention.*** Counsel the client regarding the etiology of mastitis. Unless she has been prescribed a sulfa drug (see below), encourage her to continue breastfeeding emphasizing that her medication is safe to use during lactation. Inform the client of the signs and symptoms of worsening mastitis and the need to call the health care provider should they develop.

***Medication.*** Sulfa drugs should not be prescribed if the nursing infant is less than 1 month old.

*Dicloxacillin Sodium (Dynapen, Dycill, Pathocil)*

- *Indication.* Treatment of penicillinase-resistant organisms.
- *Administration.* 250 to 500 mg orally every 6 hours for 10 days.
- *Side Effects.* Nausea, vomiting, diarrhea, vaginitis.
- *Contraindication.* Hypersensitivity to penicillins.

- *Anticipated Outcome on Evaluation.* Resolution of mastitis.
- *Client Teaching.* Instruct the client to complete the 10-day medication regimen even if she feels better before medication is finished; if medication is not taken for all 10 days, the risk for relapse increases.[7,9,10] The medication is category B for pregnancy.

*Acetaminophen (Tylenol)*

- *Indications.* Antipyretic and analgesic.
- *Administration.* 325–650 mg orally every 4 hours as needed, not to exceed 4 g per day.
- *Side Effects.* Few if taken in therapeutic doses. Acetaminophen does not cause gastric bleeding or inhibit platelet aggregation. No relationship to Reye's syndrome has been found. Overdosage can cause hepatic necrosis.
- *Contraindication.* None are known.
- *Anticipated Outcome on Evaluation.* Decreased pain and fever.
- *Client Teaching.* Inform the client about the effects of overdosage; instruct her to take no more than 4 g per day. She should know the early symptoms of hepatic necrosis: nausea, vomiting, diarrhea, sweating, abdominal discomfort. Tell the client to telephone the health care provider if she experiences symptoms of overdosage.

***Breast Care.*** Ice or warm packs may be applied to the breast, whichever is more comfortable. The client should continue to nurse her infant on both breasts, but begin on the unaffected breast and thus allow the affected breast to "let down." Review breastfeeding techniques with the client.

Complications of mastitis require special breast care measures.

- Candidal invasion, described as incredible pain like "hot cords," is a fungal infection of milk ducts. Nystatin cream (Mycostatin or Mycolog) should be massaged into the nipple and areola after each feeding. The infant must simultaneously be given oral nystatin or the mother will be reinfected.
- Abscess formation requires incision and drainage, antibiotics, rest, warm soaks, and complete emptying of breast at least every few hours. If feeding is discontinued, milk is expressed manually until sufficient healing occurs.[9]

***Fluid Intake.*** The client should increase fluid intake.

***Lifestyle Changes.*** Bed rest, with bathroom privileges, is necessary in the treatment of mastitis to prevent the client from becoming exhausted and thereby worsening the mastitis.9

***Follow-Up.*** Referral to a breastfeeding support group or lactation consultant may be necessary (see Support Groups).

## METRITIS WITH PELVIC CELLULITIS (ENDOMETRITIS)

This form of endometritis is inflammation of the decidua, myometrium, and parametrial tissues following childbirth.[11] Bacteria from an infected surgical incision and from a colonized cervix and vagina enter amniotic fluid during labor. Once in amniotic fluid, bacteria invade uterine tissue postpartum. Bacteria invade the remaining uterine decidua up to a few days postpartum.

Endometritis may have an early onset, generally following cesarean section, or late onset, usually after vaginal delivery and tends to be mild.[11]

***Epidemiology.*** Risk factors include cesarean section, membranes ruptured for longer than 3 hours, prolonged labor, numerous cervical examinations, internal fetal monitoring, and cervical lacerations.[11,12]

Transmission occurs via several routes.

- Lymphatic transmission may be from an infected cervical laceration, uterine incision for cesarean section, or uterine laceration.

- Direct invasion occurs when cervical laceration extends into connective tissue at the base of broad ligaments, providing direct access to infective organisms.
- Transmission may be secondary to pelvic thrombophlebitis. A thrombus may become purulent, resulting in necrosis of venous walls and pathogenic access to surrounding connective tissue.[11]

Metritis with pelvic cellulitis occurs among 3 to 6 percent of vaginal deliveries and 90 percent of operative deliveries done for cephalopelvic disproportion without perioperative prophylaxis.[11,12]

***Subjective Data.*** A client may report unilateral or bilateral abdominal pain; foul-smelling lochia; fever, which is minimal if confined to decidua, but more commonly 39°C (102.2°F) or higher; malaise; and anorexia.[11]

***Objective Data.*** The client appears wan and lethargic. She also appears to have pain.

- Vital signs show a fever of about 38°C (100.4°F); tachycardia may or may not be present.
- Abdominal and musculoskeletal examinations reveal significant lower abdominal pain with tenderness and rebound. Paralytic ileus may cause distention and vomiting.[13]
- Genitalia and reproductive organs have parametrial tenderness on bimanual exam. The pelvic exam may be normal even with severe endometritis. Uterine subinvolution is possible. Discharge is increased, dark red/brown, and foul smelling. Cervical motion tenderness is also possible.

A complete blood count is ordered to detect infection or anemia. Leukocytosis (15,000 to 30,000 cells per microliter) may be noted on testing of the serum sample. The client should be counseled regarding the purpose of the test and the method used to obtain the serum sample.

Chest radiography is used to diagnose pulmonary diseases, to detect mediastinal abnormalities, and to assist in assessment of pulmonary status. Request upright anterior, posterior, and lateral views of chest. Inform the client about the test's purpose. She should be told that the radiology technician will ask her to remove her clothing to the waist, take a deep breath and exhale, and take a second deep breath and hold it while the x-ray is taken. Assure the client that the procedure takes only a few minutes, is painless, and may be safely performed during lactation.

Cervical cultures are done to identify *Neisseria gonorrhoeae, Chlamydia,* or other pathogens, such as group B streptococci and *Staphylococcus aureus.*

- A sterile speculum exam is conducted with the client in the lithotomy position. *No* lubricant is used on the speculum. Excess cervical mucus is gently removed with a large cotton-tipped applicator. Next, a sterile swab, specific for the test desired, is inserted into the endocervical canal. The swab is not removed from the endocervical canal for several seconds to allow absorption of organisms. Swabs are placed into the appropriate culture container for transport to laboratory.
- Inform the client about the test, including its rationale. The health care provider obtaining the cultures should wear disposable gloves according to the facility's protocol and Centers for Disease Control guidelines.

A urine culture and sensitivity is done to diagnose urinary tract infection. Urine is collected in a sterile container. Ask the woman to remove her lower undergarments and thoroughly wash her hands with soap and water and dry her hands with a disposable towel. To prepare for urine collection, instruct the woman to remove the cap from the sterile container and place its outer surface down on a clean surface. Then she should cleanse the area around the urinary meatus from front to back with an antiseptic sponge. She should separate the labia with one hand before collecting the specimen. A small amount of urine is passed into the toilet bowl before the remaining urine is collected in a sterile container.

***Differential Medical Diagnosis.*** Metritis with pelvic cellulitis, cystitis, pyelonephritis, mastitis, appendicitis, viral disease, septic pelvic thrombophlebitis, toxic shock syndrome, paralytic ileus.

## Plan

***Psychosocial Intervention.*** Inform the client of her diagnosis and treatment plan and inquire about her support systems.

Medication. One of the following drugs is selected, as clinically indicated. Hospitalization is required for intravenous administration of antibiotic to clients with moderate to severe infections.

*Erythromycin*

- *Indication.* Infection.
- *Administration.* 500 mg orally every 6 hours for 10 days.
- *Side Effects.* Gastrointestinal disturbances, vaginitis. Cholestatic hepatitis is caused by erythromycin estolate but not by other forms of erythromycin. Symptoms of cholestatic hepatitis include nausea, vomiting, abdominal pain, jaundice, and elevated levels of serum bilirubin and liver transaminases. Erythromycin can increase plasma levels and half-lives of theophylline, carbamazepine, and warfarin.
- *Contraindication.* Hypersensitivity to the drug.
- *Anticipated Outcome on Evaluation.* Resolution of infection.
- *Client Teaching.* Instruct the client to complete the medication regimen, even if she feels better sooner. Advise her to take the medication with a full glass of water; she should not take erythromycin with fruit juice.

Tetracycline and amoxicillin are broad-spectrum antibiotics (previously discussed) used to treat metritis with pelvic cellulitis.

The cephalosporins include cephradine (Velosef), cephalexin (Keflex, Keftab, Ceporex), cefaclor (Ceclor), and cefadroxil (Duricef, Ultracef) and are broad-spectrum antibiotics with β-lactamase activity.

- *Administration.* Cefaclor: 500 mg orally every 8 hours for 10 days, not to exceed 4 g per day. Cephradine and cephalexin: 500 mg orally every 6 hours for 10 days. Cefadroxil: initial loading dose of 1 g, then 1 to 2 g every day or every 12 hours for 10 days.
- *Side Effects.* Maculopapular rash, urticaria, and gastrointestinal upset. Discontinue medication if allergy symptoms appear (urticaria, rash, hypotension, difficulty breathing).
- *Contraindication.* Hypersensitivity to cephalosporins and penicillins.
- *Anticipated Outcome on Evaluation.* Resolution of symptoms and clinical improvement.
- *Client Teaching.* Stress the importance of completing the medication regimen. Instruct the client to report signs of allergy.

Conservative management with antibiotics usually produces a response in 48 hours. A poor response indicates abscess, retention of placental parts, or incorrect diagnosis.[13]

***Fluid Intake.*** Women with metritis with pelvic cellulitis should increase fluid intake.

Lifestyle Changes. Explain to the client and her partner the client's general need for rest, as well as her need for pelvic rest (including no sexual intercourse).

***Follow-Up.*** Medical consultation is required. In addition, telephone the client daily and schedule a return appointment 48 to 72 hours after treatment begins. Complications of endometritis can be severe.

- With septic pelvic thrombophlebitis pain typically develops after the second or third postpartum day. Fever spikes continue despite antimicrobial treatment. Diagnosis is established using computerized tomography or magnetic resonance imaging (MRI).[11] Refer the client for immediate medical treatment.
- Pelvic abscess is usually unilateral. Clinical presentation is 1 to 2 weeks postpartum and surgical drainage is most likely necessary, as rupture can cause peritonitis.[11]

## POSTPARTUM THYROIDITIS

Postpartum thyroiditis is an autoimmune thyroid disease that results from transient rebound of the autoimmune process following delivery or abortion.[14] It is differentiated from other forms of thyrotoxicosis by the lack of thyroid pain, its transient symptoms with spontaneous remission, and elevated serum antibodies and thyroid hormones (hyperthyroid phase) with concomitant suppression of radioactive thyroid uptake.[15]

***Epidemiology.*** The risk factors involved include a personal history of known or suspected thyroid disease (a genetic or family history is not a predictor); small, soft, diffuse goiter; any pituitary gland dysfunction; psychological distress that intensifies over time and requires intervention; and symptoms that persist despite the absence of external stressors or that persist after stressors abate.[15]

Postpartum women account for 10 percent of all individuals with thyroiditis.[15]

***Subjective Data.*** A client may report symptoms of thyrotoxicosis during the first postpartum month and transient hypothyroidism with symptoms that peak after 3 to 5 months.

Thyrotoxicosis has a rapid onset in the latter half of the first postpartum month and persists for 2 to 4 months, usually resolving by the fourth postpartum month. The client reports weight loss, fatigue that occurs easily, heat intolerance, palpitations, hand tremors, nervousness, or other psychoneurotic reactions.[15]

In transient hypothyroidism, clinical signs peak between 3 and 5 months postpartum. The client shows progressive and pronounced fatigue, continued weight gain in the latter months of first postpartum year, coarse hair, dry skin, and psychological reactions that mimic depression.

***Objective Data.*** Physical examination reveals signs unique to both phases of postpartum thyroiditis. In the thyrotoxicosis phase, the client exhibits sinus tachycardia, stare or lid lag, brisk reflexes, and a firm, nontender thyroid. Only 50 percent of women have thyroid enlargement.[15] The transient hypothyroidism phase involves delayed reflexes, psychomotor retardation, and psychological reactions that mimic depression.

The thyroid-stimulating hormone (TSH) test is done to diagnose primary hypothyroidism, differentiating primary from secondary hypothyroidism. In addition, an elevated level of serum thyroid-stimulating hormone is noted in the hypothyroid phase. The test procedure requires a blood sample. Inform the client of the venipuncture procedure and the rationale for the test, and explain test results to her.

The antithyroglobulin antibody test differentiates thyroid diseases such as Hashimoto's thyroiditis and thyroid carcinoma. A blood sample is also used in this test. Inform the client of the venipuncture procedure and the purpose of the antithyroglobulin antibody test.

Antimicrosomal antibody test (MsAb) is a diagnostic evaluation for the presence of thyroid microsomal antibodies. As a blood sample is required, advise the client about the venipuncture procedure. Tell the client that positive antimicrosomal antibody titers are found in 50 to 80 percent of affected postpartum women. Antimicrosomal antibody titers equal to or more than 1:1000 require follow-up to detect signs of subclinical, transient hypothyroidism. The facilities to assess clients for antimicrosomal antibodies are not readily available in all community settings.[15]

The radioactive iodine uptake test (contraindicated for pregnant or lactating women) reveals increased uptake in hyperthyroidism of Graves' disease, but decreased uptake in hyperthyroidism of thyroiditis.[15] This diagnostic test evaluates the thyroid's ability to concentrate and retain iodine and is indicated in the diagnosis of thyroid disease.

The test procedure is done in conjunction with a thyroid scan and assessment of thyroid hormone levels. A liquid form or capsule of radioiodine is administered orally. The radioactivity of the thyroid gland is measured by scanning the gland 2, 6, and 24 hours later.

Provide the client with information about factors that interfere with, or lower, radioactive iodine uptake: iodized foods and iodine-containing medications (1 to 3 weeks' duration), vitamin preparations that contain minerals (1 to 3 weeks' duration), antithyroid medications (2 to 10 days' duration), thyroid medications (1 to 2 weeks' duration), antihistamines, corticosteroids, isoniazid, thiocyanate, perchlorate, sulfonamides, orinase, Butazolidin, adrenocorticotropin, aminosalicylic acid, coumadin anticoagulants.

Medications and conditions that increase uptake include thyroid stimulating hormone, pregnancy, cirrhosis, barbiturates, lithium, phenothiazine, iodine-deficient diets, and renal failure. Tell the client that the test is painless, but requires 24 hours to perform. Restrict iodine intake (e.g., iodized salt, seafood) for at least 1 week prior to the test.

***Differential Medical Diagnosis.*** Graves' disease, postpartum depression, Sheehan's syndrome.

## Plan

***Psychosocial Intervention.*** Reassure the client regarding the validity of her symptoms. Explain to her the etiology and management of postpartum thyroiditis. Counsel the client regarding spontaneous resolution as well as possible recurrence of the condition with future births.

***Medication.*** Levothyroxine (T4) is administered to treat hypothyroidism. Initial doses should be low, increasing gradually every 2 weeks until full replacement doses have been achieved (0.025–0.4 mg orally every day). Replacement doses have been achieved when repeat thyroid function tests are within normal limits.

- *Side Effects.* Rare when given in therapeutic doses. Excessive doses of levothyroxine may cause thyrotoxicosis; symptoms are anxiety, insomnia, tremors, tachycardia, angina, palpitations, hyperthermia, and sweating.
- *Contraindications.* None are known.
- *Anticipated Outcomes on Evaluation.* Reversal of signs and symptoms of hypothyroidism and a decline in serum TSH levels.
- *Client Teaching.* Instruct the client to take the medication on an empty stomach to enhance absorption; morning administration decreases sleeplessness. Medication should be kept in a light-resistant container. Advise the client to report excitability, irritability, or anxiety. Also advise her

not to switch brands of levothyroxine unless approved by the health care provider.

***Follow-Up.*** Referral to a physician is required. Regular checkups are scheduled for laboratory assessment of thyroid function. Assessment should continue for 2 years postpartum.

## URINARY TRACT INFECTION

***Epidemiology.*** Risk factors for infection, caused by bacteria in the urinary tract (see Chapter 17), include trauma to the bladder or urethra, such as that resulting from catheterization; history of urinary tract infection; sickle cell trait; and diabetes mellitus. Infection is transmitted in vaginal secretions via sexual intercourse and perineal pads.

***Subjective Data.*** A client may report dysuria, oliguria, urinary frequency or urgency, nausea and vomiting, chills, and abdominal pain or cramping.

***Objective Data.*** Physical examination usually reveals that general appearance and vital signs are within normal limits. Fever, however, may be present and is indicative of upper urinary tract infection (pyelonephritis). The abdomen and musculoskeletal system exam is done to detect costovertebral angle tenderness and suprapubic tenderness.

A urinalysis determines the properties of urine and abnormal products. Pyuria (white blood cells in urine), hematuria (red blood cells in urine), and positive nitrite indicate a urinary tract infection and warrant a urinary culture. The test procedure for urinalysis requires a routine urine sample obtained by voiding. Instruct the client about the purpose of the test and the method of collection.

A urine culture and sensitivity is done to diagnose bacterial infection and identify offending organisms (see Metritis With Pelvic Cellulitis for a description of the test procedure and client teaching).

***Differential Medical Diagnosis.*** Urinary tract infection (lower or upper tracts).

### Plan

***Psychosocial Interventions.*** Provide the client with information and counsel her regarding the suspected diagnosis and pathophysiology of urinary tract infection.

***Medication.*** One of the following drugs is administered.

*Amoxicillin*

- *Administration.* One 250-mg to 500-mg tablet orally every 8 hours for 7 days.
- *Side Effects.* See Subinvolution of Uterus.
- *Contraindication.* Sensitivity to penicillins.
- *Anticipated Outcomes on Evaluation.* Reduction in client's symptoms and negative urine culture following treatment.
- *Client teaching.* See Subinvolution of Uterus.

*Nitrofurantoin (Macrobid)*

- *Administration.* One 100-mg tablet orally every 12 hours for 7 days.
- *Side Effects.* Gastrointestinal reactions (nausea, vomiting), headache, vertigo, drowsiness.
- *Contraindications.* Hypersensitivity to the drug, glucose-6-phosphate dehydrogenase (G6PD) deficiency, renal disease.
- *Anticipated Outcomes on Evaluation.* Resolution of client's symptoms and negative urine culture following treatment.
- *Client Teaching.* Advise the client to complete the 7-day medication regimen even if symptoms disappear before that time. Medication is taken with food or milk. The client should be told to return for a follow-up visit if indicated.

*Trimethoprim–Sulfamethoxazole (Bactrim-DS, Septra-DS, Cotrim-DS)*

- *Administration.* One tablet orally every 12 hours for 10 days.

- *Side Effects.* Gastrointestinal reactions (nausea and vomiting), rash, blood dyscrasias (hemolytic anemia, leukopenia, thrombocytopenia).
- *Contraindications.* Hypersensitivity to trimethoprim or sulfonamides, G6PD deficiency, first 12 weeks or last trimester (28 to 42 weeks) of pregnancy, megaloblastic anemia.
- *Anticipated Outcomes on Evaluation.* Resolution of client's symptoms and negative urine culture following treatment.
- *Client Teaching.* Instruct the client to complete the 10-day medication regimen even if symptoms improve or disappear before that time. Medication should be taken with a full glass of water; water intake is increased to decrease crystallization in kidneys. Advise the client to avoid sunlight to prevent burns and to contact the care provider if side effects occur.

For information on cephalosporins, see Endometritis.

***Follow-Up.*** Review proper perineal hygiene with the client. In addition, reemphasize her need to increase fluid intake. (Additional follow-up is outlined in Chapter 17.)

## ACUTE APPENDICITIS

The appendix may become inflamed as a result of obstruction of the appendiceal lumen by hardened stool, hypertrophy of lymph follicles in the wall of the appendix, or strictures.

***Epidemiology.*** In a pregnant woman, the appendix is atypically positioned, as it is in obese individuals. Chronic constipation is another risk factor. Adolescents and young adults, however, are at greatest risk; the incidence of acute appendicitis is rare among pregnant women.

***Subjective Data.*** The client may report loss of appetite, abdominal distention, and abdominal pain.

***Objective Data.*** Physical examination may reveal the client to be distressed, obviously in pain. Her vital signs are likely to be within normal limits; temperature may be elevated.

Abdominal muscles do not show the classic signs of appendicitis (abdominal guarding and rigidity) in early puerperium, as the appendix does not return to its usual location until involution is completed (6–8 weeks).[13]

- Tenderness is common in the right upper quadrant or entire right abdomen when uterine size is 12 weeks or greater.
- Psoas, obturator, and Rovsing's signs are not predictive of appendicitis in pregnant or postpartum women.
- Bryan's sign is positive if moving the enlarged uterus to the right elicits pain,[13] and may be a more reliable indicator of appendiceal pathology.
- Alder's test requires the health care provider to maintain constant pressure at an area of maximum tenderness while the client rolls from the supine position onto her left side. Alder's test assists in differentiating pain of uterine etiology from that of extrauterine origin;[13] pain of uterine origin may be relieved by change in position, whereas pain of extrauterine origin will not be relieved regardless of position.

Examination of the genitalia and reproductive tract reveals that the lochia is not excessive and has no foul odor, the cervix is closed, and the uterus is nontender.

Diagnostic tests assess blood, urine, and endocervical tissue.

A complete blood count identifies anemia and specific infections. Leukocytosis is nonspecific and does not differentiate appendicitis from other inflammatory causes of abdominal pain. White blood cell (WBC) counts of

20,000 to 25,000/mm$^3$ and increased neutrophils are not uncommon in appendicitis during the first 10 to 14 days postpartum. A blood sample must be obtained, and the client counseled regarding the purpose of the test and the method used to obtain the sample.

The erythrocyte sedimentation rate (ESR) is used to monitor an inflammatory or malignant disease. The test also helps to detect and diagnose occult disease. A blood sample must be obtained, and the client counseled regarding the purpose of the test and method of collection.

Urinalysis determines the properties of urine, including abnormal products. Pyuria (white blood cells in urine), hematuria (red blood cells in urine), and positive nitrite are indicative of urinary tract infection and warrant urine culture. Sterile pyuria (>5 WBCs per high-power field) and hematuria are seen in 15 to 30 percent of pregnant and puerperal women, in whom the appendix lies proximal to the ureter.[13] (See Urinary Tract Infection for details of the test procedure and nursing implications.)

The urine culture and sensitivity is discussed under Urinary Tract Infection.

Endocervical cultures are discussed under Endometritis.

***Differential Medical Diagnosis.*** Appendicitis; endometritis; pyelonephritis; tubo-ovarian abscess.

***Plan.*** Counsel the client and her family about the diagnosis and assist the family to arrange for child care. Immediate referral to a surgeon is mandatory, as complications include death and appendiceal perforation.

## EARLY DISCHARGE

Early discharge follows a hospital stay of 48 hours or less. It subjects a woman to certain risk factors. For example, physical complications may occur: discomfort at an episiotomy or cesarean incision site, endometritis, mastitis. Physiologic changes may be affected: uterine involution, increased edema and hyperemia of the bladder with possible atony, and diuresis. The client will confront other changes, such as fatigue, meeting the needs of her infant, role conflict, and adjustment within parental and family relationships.[16]

Follow-up care in the home or by telephone should be pursued to assess the health needs (physical, psychosocial, and educational) of the mother, the family, and the infant in the early puerperium and to implement nursing plans to meet assessed needs. Criteria for prospective payment and a shorter hospital stay will need to be complied with as various insurance policies mandate shorter hospital stays. Referral to support groups may be helpful (see Support Groups at the end of this chapter).

### HOME VISITS

Home visits are made within the first week of discharge, and should be available to any childbearing family. The family should live within a reasonable radius of the health agency. If they do not, referral to a closer agency is indicated.

### FOLLOW-UP TELEPHONE CALLS

Telephone calls are made within the first week after hospital discharge to all families who elect not to have home visits.

### MATERNAL ASSESSMENT

Physical inspection, psychological evaluation, and assessment of feeding technique are parts of the maternal exam.

***Physical Examination.*** Focus on answering several questions.

*General Appearance and Vital Signs*

- Does the client appear rested or exhausted?
- Are her blood pressure and pulse within her normal limits, based on her baseline vital signs as an inpatient (assuming no pregnancy-induced hypertension)?
- Does the client complain of chills or fever? If so, determine her temperature.
- In a client with a history of pregnancy-induced hypertension, how does current blood pressure compare with in-hospital blood pressure?

*Breast Health and Care*

- Is the client lactating?
- Are the breasts soft or hard and painful (engorged)?
- Is the client wearing a supportive bra?
- If the client is breastfeeding, how often is the infant nursing?
- Is the client experiencing pain or nipple tenderness when she breastfeeds?
- Does the client feel comfortable with breastfeeding or insecure or worried?

*Abdomen and Musculoskeletal System*

- Does the client have discomfort or difficulty urinating?
- Is she constipated or does she have hemorrhoids?
- If the client had cesarean section, how does the incision appear? Are staples present? What is the color of the skin and skin integrity? Is the incision draining? If so, what color is the drainage?

*Genitalia and Reproductive Organs*

- What is the fundal height?
- Is there uterine tenderness?
- How much lochia is evident and what color is it? Has there been any change in these qualities?
- If an episiotomy was done, is the incision erythematous? draining? intact?

***Psychological Evaluation.*** Assess the client's ability to cope: What is her financial status? Did she recently relocate? Are her family and significant other supportive? What is her housing situation? Is she homeless, or living in overcrowded conditions?

Provide anticipatory guidance for a client concerning her neonate's behavior. Assess her and her family's knowledge of neonatal and infant development and infant cues. Assess their adjustment to the infant.

***Feeding Technique.*** Assess feeding technique—breast or bottle—during follow-up visits or phone calls. Who is the primary provider of care for the infant? Does another person in the client's family influence infant feeding, for example, the type of milk given, the frequency of feedings, the introduction of solids?

Breastfeeding technique may be assessed by asking specific questions. How often does the infant nurse? Do her breasts feel soft after feeding? Ask the client to describe the infant's suck: Is it strong and vigorous, or does the infant frequently stop sucking and cry? Are supplemental feedings given? If so, ask the client the reason for supplementation.

Consider observing the mother and infant during a feeding session to assess the effectiveness of breastfeeding technique. Bottle feeding technique may also be assessed by questioning. How often is the infant fed and by whom? What type of milk is given—commercially prepared formula or table milk? How is the infant held during feeding? Is the bottle propped? Is the nipple properly positioned? Are solids given? If so, why and how is infant fed the solid food?

***Infant Care.*** Assess the client's or caregiver's knowledge of infant cues, infant sleep and awake states, and child developmental stages (see Neonatal Assessment below.)

***Health Teaching.*** Provide the client with information about exercise, nutritional needs, postpartum sexuality and fertility, health care, and the nurturing needs of the infant.

## NEONATAL ASSESSMENT

Physical inspection, home safety assessment, and identification of engagement and disengagement cues are parts of the neonatal evaluation.

***Physical Examination.*** The physical examination is directed to answering several questions.

*General Appearance and Vital Signs*

- Has the infant gained weight since hospital discharge? Weigh the infant if a portable scale is available.
- Does the infant appear healthy?
- When awake, does the infant appear alert, wan, irritable?
- What color is the infant's sclera? If yellow, was bilirubin tested prior to discharge?
- When is the infant's follow-up appointment?
- Is the infant's skin clean, without lesions, bruises, or unexplained markings?

Cardiovascular and respiratory assessments include the infant's apical pulse and respiratory rate. If either is elevated, inquire regarding infant's sucking strength, frequency of feedings, and type of cry (absent, weak, vigorous). If assessment indicates possible infection, refer the client and infant for follow-up.

Abdominal assessment determines the amount and frequency of the infant's voidings and the amount and consistency of stool. Assess the abdomen for softness and tenderness.

In a male infant the circumcision site, if present, is assessed for type of discharge and evidence of healing. If circumcision was not done, instruction should be given regarding proper care: Wash external penile skin only, as foreskin of infants and young children cannot be retracted.

Genitalia of a female infant may show a small amount of vaginal blood, which is the result of maternal estrogen in utero.

***Home Safety.*** A hazard-free environment is important. Anticipatory guidance is useful for potential safety problems at different developmental stages of the infant and child. Suggest to the client, for example, that she tie knots in plastic bags before throwing them away, use child-safety gates, and select toys with no sharp edges or separable, hazardous parts.

***Child Development.*** Observe nonverbal and verbal cues used by the infant to initiate or stop interaction with the caregiver. An infant's demonstration of disengagement behaviors warrants cessation of caretaking activity and then reassessment of the infant. Evaluate the infant's sleep states (deep or light sleep) and awake states (drowsy, quiet alert, active alert, crying). An infant is most conducive to learning and taking in environmental stimuli when in an active alert state.

*Engagement Cues*

- Verbal cues are feeding sounds (sucking) and crying.
- Nonverbal cues are rooting; alerting signs; facial brightening; smooth cyclic movements of the extremities; mutual gaze; feeding posture; brow raising; and facing gaze (infant looks at parent's or caregiver's face).[17]

*Disengagement Cues*

- Verbal cues are spitting; vomiting; hiccoughs; whimpering; crying during caregiving activity; and fussing.
- Nonverbal cues are lip compression; clenching eyes; gaze aversion; yawning;

tongue show; increased foot movement; and hand-to-ear movement.[17]

## ADJUSTING TO PARENTING

Parenting is a skill that is often learned, to varying degrees of success, by trial and error. Attachment is a process whereby affection develops between infant and parent or caregiver. The process of attachment has been defined as an emotional or affectional commitment to an individual, facilitated by positive interaction between the two and mutually satisfying experiences.[18] Maternal attachment begins during pregnancy as the result of fetal movement and maternal fantasies about an infant.[19–21]

A mother's attitudes about pregnancy may influence her feelings about the infant. Maternal grief over the loss of a fantasized perfect child may result in delayed bonding or attachment if, for example, the infant is born prematurely or with obvious birth defects. The infant's behavior can also affect maternal bonding. The infant's crying, avoidance of eye contact, refusal of breast, or withdrawal of a hand when touched is negative reinforcement for a mother.

Nursing Child Assessment Satellite Training tools have been developed to enable the health care provider to identify families that need intervention.[17]

### BARNARD MODEL FOR ATTACHMENT AND PARENTING

Adaptation is a result of caregiver–environment–infant interaction. Kathryn Barnard noted that the infant has the tasks to produce clear clues and to respond to the caregiver. If the infant is unable (due to immaturity, illness, or other physical/neurological problems), the adaptive process is interrupted. The mother/caregiver, in turn, cannot respond to the infant's needs, resulting in feelings of maternal inadequacy. Tasks for the mother/caregiver include being able to respond to the infant's cues, to allay distress, and to provide a growth-stimulating environment. Failure interferes with the infant's ability to adapt. The infant, in turn, becomes frustrated, and learns inappropriate interaction behaviors.[17] The environment is also influential. For example, the family is impacted by the actual birth of the child, or social deprivation, or an alternate family style, such as single parenting.

Stress or interference may cause parental insensitivity to an infant's cues, failure of the infant to give reliable cues, and failure of the infant to respond to the parent.

### MERCER MODEL FOR ATTACHMENT AND PARENTING

Mercer's definition of attachment—a process affected by positive feedback through mutually enjoyable experiences—stresses "process" (progressive nature, occurring over time), "positive feedback" (social, verbal, nonverbal, real or perceived responses of one partner to another), and "mutually satisfying experience" (environment can have positive or negative impact on the mother–infant interaction).[18]

Four stages of attachment are identified:

- *Anticipatory:* Mother seeks out role model.
- *Formal:* This stage begins with the birth of the child and continues for 6 to 8 weeks; the mother's behaviors are affected primarily by the expectations of others.
- *Informal:* Mother begins to develop her own unique role behavior.
- *Personal:* Mother feels comfortable with role and others accept her role performance.[22,23]

## INHIBITORS OF ATTACHMENT

***Maternal Factors.*** Among high-risk and low-risk women and partners, parental competence is a major predictor of parent–infant attachment.[24] Facilitating parental competence thereby increases parent–infant attachment.[24] Parental competence may be defined as the real or perceived ability to care for the physical and psychosocial needs of the infant.

Several factors inhibit attachment and decrease competence.

- Medication, such as narcotics, sedatives, and some forms of anesthesia
- Physical problems from pregnancy, such as long labor, difficult delivery, or chronic illness
- Lack of experience in caring for newborns/older infants
- Learned maternal behaviors that have a negative influence
- A negative self-concept
- Lack of a positive support system
- Grieving a significant loss
- Anticipatory grieving over an imagined loss of infant, resulting from, for example, complicated pregnancy or postnatal problems
- Psychological unpreparedness due to premature birth
- Escape mechanisms, such as alcoholism and drugs[20]

***Infant Factors.*** Several factors may inhibit attachment.

- Neonatal complications in full-term infants
- Infant abnormalities
- Immaturity resulting from premature birth
- Multiple births
- Feeding difficulties[20]

***Paternal Factors.*** A father may exhibit behaviors that inhibit his attachment with the infant.

- Difficulty adjusting to new dependent
- Failure to relate to newborn
- Escape mechanisms, such as alcohol and drugs
- Separation from mother and child because of business or military responsibilities[21]

***Hospital Factors.*** Hospital procedure may inhibit attachment.

- Separation of infant and mother immediately after birth, at night, and for long periods during day
- Policies that discourage or inhibit unwrapping and exploring the infant, limiting mother's caretaking
- Restrictive visiting policies
- Hospital/intensive care environment
- Staff behavior not supportive of mother's caretaking attempts and abilities[20]

## PARENTS OF INFANTS WITH MALFORMATIONS

***Stages of Adjustment.*** A wide range of change occurs during adjustment.

- Shock, irrational behavior
- Denial
- Grief/anger/anxiety
- Equilibrium; lessening of anxiety and intense emotional reactions
- Reorganization[25]

***Long-Range Impact.*** Caring for a child with malformation affects all aspects of the parents' lives.

- Financial cost for surgery, medical care for chronic problems, or early stimulation, for example, physical therapy sessions
- Guilt over time spent with affected infant compared with that spent with other child(ren)
- Social support from family and friends having adverse effect on family relationship

***Therapeutic Approach.*** The health care provider should realize that the infant is a complete distortion of the parents' fantasized infant and that a therapeutic approach is necessary to address their feelings.

- Parents must mourn the loss of the fantasized child before they can fully attach to the living "defective" infant.
- Guilt accompanies their mourning.
- Resentment and anger are often directed at health care personnel. Allow parents to express their feelings and take the time necessary to experience the full extent of their grief.
- The demands of the "imperfect" newborn retard mother's attempt to mourn the fantasized child.
- Mourning is asynchronous; that is, progress through the stages of mourning varies for each parent.[25]
- Parents should not be given conflicting information concerning their infant.
- The health care provider may be a role model for parents by responding to the infant with smiles; the infant's positive features should be pointed out to parents.
- Social services may provide financial assistance, and a support group social, interpersonal, or medical support.

## FAMILY RELATIONSHIPS

***The Secundigravida.*** The concerns of a woman experiencing her second pregnancy are primarily for her other child and the expectation of caring for two children.

- Concern for first child may cause grieving over the dyadic relationship with the first child and her anticipation of the first child's pain.
- Managing the care of two children may cause a mother to feel overwhelmed. She may have increased expectations of the first child and may doubt her own ability to love two children equally.
- The second pregnancy may not be as exciting or as desired as the first. The mother may not be totally engrossed in mothering her second baby as she was with the first. She may feel sad or guilty.
- Maternal self-perception changes[26,27] and she sees herself as experienced. She recognizes her needs as separate from those of her role as mother.

***Readjustment with the Infant's Father.*** A negative effect of childbirth may be the breakup of the marriage or relationship. The mother may lack support in child care and household tasks. Spouse abuse or child abuse may increase. In assessing the couple, focus on their sharing of tasks, sexual relationship, leisure activity, and financial management.

- Sharing of family tasks and responsibilities often occurs following agreement before childbirth on the division of tasks. Equal sharing of child and infant care may be agreed on, or the parents may prefer that the father be primary caregiver for the older child or children. Other parents may prefer that the father assume more household tasks and the mother have the responsibility for infant and children.
- Assess the parenting roles of the mother and father. Assess their self-expectations and their expectations of each other. Parenting behavior can be adaptive (constructive) or maladaptive (nonconstructive, harmful).
- The sexual relationship may be safely resumed 2 weeks postpartum.[28] Physiological responses in the puerperium may cause a decrease in the intensity of the sexual experience. The decrease is due to thin vaginal walls in the hypoestrogenic state, especially during lactation; delayed congestion of the labia majora and minora until the plateau phase, and decreased strength of orgasmic contractions. Sexual activity is decreased because of fatigue, weakness, vaginal discharge or spotting, perineal

pain, tight or lax vaginal muscles, breast discomfort, and decreased vaginal lubrication. Client teaching may include suggestions to enhance sexual comfort.

- Saliva (after postpartum exam) or water-soluble gel may be used for lubrication.
- The female-superior or side-to-side positions may help control the depth of thrusting.
- Gentle rotation of two fingers around the vagina may aid vaginal relaxation.
- Other displays of affection (holding, cuddling) are pleasurable if intercourse is not desired.
- The woman may assist partner to orgasm with masturbation or fellatio. Her partner may help her also achieve orgasm without intercourse.
- The client should perform Kegel exercises to regain vaginal tone.
- A nutritious diet will promote healing and a sense of well-being.

- Leisure time for the couple should include time alone. They may enlist the help of family and friends to watch the infant and children. Encourage communication between the couple ("I love you," "You are special to me," "Thanks for your help"). Simple gestures of affection (romantic card or flowers for him or her) provoke loving feelings.
- Management of finances may require referral to a community food bank, social services, or the Women, Infants, and Children Program (WIC).

***Single Parent/Working Mother.*** Address the parent's child-rearing difficulties, financial insecurity, role conflict, or social isolation.

- Encourage the parent to verbalize feelings on how absence of one parent may affect parent–infant relationship or child development.
- Identify for the working mother the positive aspects of separation (daily break from infant and child care while at work).
- Stress the importance of quality rather than quantity of time spent with the infant and children.
- Assess the parent in developing confidence in parenting skills through parenting classes that include information about infant behavior, home visits, and telephone calls.
- Encourage inexpensive activities that are relaxing and enjoyable for parent and infant.
- Financial insecurity may benefit from referral to community food bank, social or legal services, or WIC. In addition, referral for housing or job training may be necessary.

A parent experiencing role conflict and uncertainty concerning responsibilities may benefit from assistance in establishing priorities and assigning appropriate tasks to older children. Referral to appropriate resources may also be necessary to develop essential skills in caretaking and home management.

Social isolation and loneliness may be eased by client's involvement in parental and social groups (apartment complex, church, extended family) and support groups (see list of Support Groups at the end of this chapter).

***Lesbian Families.*** Such families may include legal guardian relationships, working collectives, roommates, ex-lovers now considered family members, and couples with or without children.[29]

The health care provider should be knowledgeable regarding lesbian issues and health care concerns, comfortable providing health care to the gay population, and supportive of the lesbian family.[30]

Lesbian concerns range from unique to common.

- Fear of custody battles require referral for legal advice on custody, because a nonbiological lesbian parent may not have a legal right to parent a child if the biological parent, her partner, dies.[29,31]

- Fear of HIV infection is possible. An alternative insemination/unscreened donor may have been used for conception. One partner may use intravenous drugs or may have intercourse with men. The mother may receive fluid (vaginal fluid, menstrual blood) from an HIV-infected partner. One means of exchanging fluid is sharing a dildo without using a condom.[31] If HIV infection is a concern, counsel women regarding safer sex (see Chapter 8).
- Battering—physical, emotional, or verbal—is possible. Refer the woman for counseling, to a shelter, or to a support group.
- Alcoholism affects lesbian relationships and families as it does heterosexual relationships and families.
- Support may be lost from family and friends and her job.[23,31]

A role model should be available to assist with maternal tasks.

- Determine the coparent's involvement in infant care and with partner.
- Encourage the partner's role in parenting.
- Encourage the partner's presence during health care visits.
- Referral to appropriate support groups may be helpful.

***Families With Human Immunodeficiency Virus Infection.*** HIV-infected families are those families in which one or more persons are infected with the virus. Persons may be asymptomatic carriers or exhibit AIDS, having been diagnosed with opportunistic infections and malignancies. The epidemiology of AIDS is described in Chapter 8.

The health care provider must maintain a nonjudgmental attitude and should not assume heterosexuality. Do not record the client's sexual preference in her records without her permission. Offer nonheterosexual educational materials and, if necessary, educate yourself about lesbian lifestyles. Suggest HIV testing if the client expresses concern. Identify what the family sees as its needs; many HIV-infected families are living in unsanitary, crowded, and physically hazardous environments and may not be enrolled in basic public assistance programs. Establish a trusting relationship; be aware of family-member attempts to manipulate.

Teach clients about infection control, such as hand washing, avoiding exchange of body fluids or sharing of razors and toothbrushes, wrapping soiled peripads in sturdy plastic containers, and cleaning soiled surfaces with a dilute bleach solution of 1 part bleach to 10 parts water. Review safer sex practices with clients.

Advise clients to contact the health care provider should they note signs of infection: fever, foul smell of lochia, excessive amount of bleeding, return of bright red bleeding. Clients should also contact the health care provider if there are signs of worsening HIV infection: fatigue, anorexia, weight loss, sore throat, cough, dermatologic disorders, or unusual vaginal discharge. The infant's health care provider should be contacted if the infant exhibits fever, poor feeding, oral thrush, diarrhea, cough, or flulike symptoms.

Instruct the client on how to avoid other infection, for example, not ingesting raw meat or eggs to avoid *Salmonella* infection, not emptying cat litter to avoid the risk of toxoplasmosis, not sharing needles, and discontinuing substance abuse, including tobacco and alcohol.[32,33]

***Homeless Families.*** More than two thirds of homeless families are headed by single women.[23] Approximately one third of homeless people are women.[34] Their education most likely does not exceed high school.

Health issues for homeless families are staggering.

- Social isolation
- Lack of access to health care
- Physical violence on the streets and in shelters
- Spouse abuse, child abuse, or both
- Substance abuse
- Chronic health problems
- Obesity
- Inadequate diet: insufficient iron, folic acid, calcium; excessive intake of saturated fats[35–37]

Arrange for nursery services so that the client may attend classes in parenting skills and learn about infant behavioral cues. Evaluation and care are provided at times and locations convenient to the population to be served. Assist in providing nutritional information to volunteers at "soup kitchens." Refer families to community resources for lodging and job training. WIC, substance abuse programs, and domestic violence programs may also be suggested.

### PLAN

The plan to assist families in their adjustment to parenting should offer many alternatives to address the multitude of needs.

- *Practical Guidance.* This can include the simple suggestion to lay out clothes at night for the next day to decrease tension in the morning while dressing the infant and older child (children) for day care or school.
- *Child Development and Behavior.* Teaching a client about child development enables her to better understand older children and the new infant; counseling should address infant's cues and states.
- *Referral.* Individual counseling may be necessary for a client who feels excessively guilty or angry about her first child's reactions to the infant. After counseling the client regarding daily nutritional needs of adults, infants, and children, referral for specific dietary needs may be helpful. Refer the client for legal assistance and domestic violence counseling and assistance if appropriate (see Parenting/Family Support Groups at end of chapter).

## PSYCHIATRIC DISTURBANCES

Psychiatric disturbances occur during the puerperium. The disturbances are classified on the basis of their severity:

- *Maternity Blues or "Baby Blues."* Transient, emotional disturbances commonly occurring around the second or fourth postpartum day, lasting from a few hours to 2 weeks.
- *Postpartum Depression.** Characterized by lowered mood, irritability, fatigue, feelings of worthlessness, sleeping and eating changes, and subtle changes of personality.
- *Postpartum Psychosis.** Severely impaired ability to perform daily living tasks.[38]

### Epidemiology

***Etiology and Risk Factors.*** Risk factors for postpartum depression are listed in Table 16–3.

Maternity Blues. Maternity blues are the mildest form of depression and are usually self-limiting. They begin on the second or third postpartum day and last up to 14 days.

Physiological factors are rapid hormonal changes (decreased estrogen, human placental lactogen, progesterone, human chorionic gonadotropin, plasma renin, aldosterone);[38,39]

*Conditions are prolonged beyond usual period expected for "blues."

**TABLE 16–3. RISK FACTORS FOR POSTPARTUM DEPRESSION**

1. Woman feels increased anxiety/worry during this pregnancy.
2. Woman has history of perimenstrual mood swings.
3. Woman has history of depression following previous pregnancy.
4. Woman does not feel in control of life.
5. Woman perceives self as nervous person or a worrier.
6. Woman believes she has lack of family or friends she can call for support.
7. Woman expresses feelings of depression or sadness with this pregnancy.
8. Woman regrets she is pregnant and feels child unwanted.
9. Woman had unhappy childhood.
10. Woman has financial/housing/personal problems.
11. Woman has history of emotional problems.
12. Woman was previously treated for mental illness.
13. Woman feels anger at life situation or at family or acquaintances.
14. Woman blames self when things go wrong.
15. Woman feels unloved by infant's father.

*Note:* Preliminary research done by D. Boyer suggests that women with three to six risk factors are at risk for postpartum depression, and women with more than six risk factors are at high risk.
*From D. Boyer (1990). Prediction of postpartum depression. In 1990,* NAACOG's Clinical Issues in Perinatal and Women's Health Nursing, 1*(3), 364. Copyright 1990 by NAACOG. Adapted by permission.*

lack of sleep and less effective sleep; and increased energy expenditure. Psychological factors include the conflict caused by cultural expectations to bear children and pursue personal goals and the economic cost of childbearing and childrearing.

Postpartum Depression. Postpartum depression has a slow, insidious onset over several weeks postpartum. It usually begins within 2 or 3 weeks postpartum and may last up to a year. There is no definite etiology.

Physiological factors are hormonal, neurotransmitter, and genetic.[40] Psychological factors include isolation from the extended family, a dearth of cultural role models for pregnant and postpartum women, and lack of cultural support in a career-oriented society.

Postpartum Psychosis. Postpartum psychosis has its onset within a few weeks or, at most, 3 months postpartum; the affected woman is 16 to 20 times more likely to require hospital admission in the 3 months postpartum than in an equivalent period preconceptually. Primiparas are at greatest risk. The symptomatology may resemble that of maternity blues.[40,41]

Physiological factors are theorized; there is no definite etiology. Theories involve hormonal, neurotransmitter, and genetic factors. Psychological factors reflect no definite etiology; the primary risk factor seems to be a history of manic–depressive psychosis.[40]

***Incidence.*** Incidence varies among the three classifications. Maternity blues affect 50 to 70 percent of postpartum women. Postpartum depression affects 10 to 15 percent of women during the first 3 months postpartum; 25 percent of these women are likely to develop chronic, severe depression.[42] Postpartum psychosis affects 1 to 2 per 1000 new mothers.[43]

## Subjective Data

***Current Symptoms.*** Symptoms may be similar among the three classifications; however, distinct differences are reported by clients. It is important to identify the major problems causing the client to seek help: severe mood swings, hyperactivity, irritability, depression, obsessional thoughts, insomnia, lack of appetite, difficulty with concentration, hallucinations, delusion, inability to care for herself or child, suicidal or homicidal thoughts.

Maternity Blues. Women with maternity blues report weeping, often alternating with periods of elation; irritability; anxiety; headaches; confusion; forgetfulness; depersonalization; disturbances in sleep pattern; and fatigue.[40]

Postpartum Depression. Women with postpartum depression report symptoms similar to those of maternity blues but without periods of elation. In addition, these symptoms are more intense and last longer. The client considers herself a failure as a mother; she looks for reasons for the perceived failure and associates it with real or imagined character weaknesses and questions self-worth. She experiences excessive fatigue and excessive weight gain or weight loss. Thinking and speaking may be slow. Suicide is a serious hazard and the method is often well planned.[39,42]

Postpartum Psychosis. Women with postpartum psychosis report variable symptoms. Three expressions, or phases, of psychosis are possible: manic phase, delirious state, and psychotic depression.

- Manic phase, with symptoms similar to those of the manic phase of manic–depressive illness, is characterized by racing thoughts, hyperactivity, and mood swings.
- Delirious state symptoms include confusion, dissociative episodes with confusion, dissociative episodes with hostility, and anxiety.
- Psychotic depression symptoms include suicidal tendencies, desire to harm the infant or others, psychomotor retardation, and prominent delusions that are often related to the infant.[38,43]

***History of Present Illness.*** Ask the client to describe the onset of symptoms. What symptoms were present during pregnancy or after the infant's birth? When were symptoms more severe or less severe, and how long did they last? Have symptoms caused her to make unexpected changes in lifestyle?

***Past Psychiatric Condition.*** Ask the client if she has a history of depression, manic–depressive illness, or other psychiatric illness. Were any of the illnesses related to childbearing? Did she receive any psychotropic medication? Did the medication help?

***Medical–Surgical–Obstetrical History.*** Was the pregnancy planned or unplanned? Were there complications with this pregnancy? Have the client describe her labor and delivery. Does she have a history of medical illness (thyroid disease, other endocrinological problems)? Did the newborn have any serious health problem?

***Family History.*** Does any family member have psychiatric problems (depression, manic–depressive illness, schizophrenia, alcoholism or other substance abuse, anorexia nervosa, bulimia)? What type of help was received? Was medication received and what was the response? What was the client's childhood like? Ask her to describe her relationship with parents and her perceptions of their effectiveness as role models. Is there a history of physical or sexual abuse?

***Social History.*** With whom does the client live? Is there someone with whom she can share the responsibility of caring for the child and house? Are there financial problems? Is she planning to work full- or part-time outside the home or full-time in the home? Is her partner emotionally supportive?

## Objective Data

***Physical Examination.*** Excessive weight loss or gain is possible. Affect may be flat; speech and thinking processes may be slow; the woman may be weepy, agitated, or irritable. She may exhibit confusion, hostility, or anxiety. The remainder of the physical examination is most likely within normal limits.

***Edinburgh Postnatal Depression Scale.*** The Edinburgh Postnatal Depression Scale (EDPS) is employed in determining objective data (see Table 16–4). The scale has a higher sensitivity (95 percent) than the Beck Depression Inventory (68 percent)[44] and is used to detect major postpartum depression and changes in the severity of depression. It can also be used to monitor the effectiveness of treatment. The scale has been administered 6 weeks postpartum, but recent study showed significant positive correlation between EPDS scores at 5 days and 6 weeks.[45]

Ask the client to complete the scale alone, without other family members present. She should underline those responses that come closest to how she felt during the previous 7 days; she should answer all 10 items. A score of 12/13 indicates the likelihood of depression, but not its severity. Have the client verbalize her feelings by responding to open-ended questions.

## Differential Medical Diagnosis

Maternity blues, postpartum depression, postpartum psychosis.

## Plan

***Psychosocial Intervention.*** During the antepartum period, provide the client with information related to maternal changes that could occur after birth: mood swings and lifestyle changes. Suggestions should include coping strategies related to the birth:

- Get plenty of rest.
- Allow family and friends to help with household tasks and the care for older children.
- Eat a well-balanced diet that is low in salt and sugar and high in complex carbohydrates, protein, and green leafy vegetables.
- Drink plenty of fluids, especially water, and limit caffeine intake.
- Continue prenatal vitamins.
- Perform light exercise daily.
- Ensure some personal time and adult relationships.
- Avail oneself of support groups and other community resources (see Breastfeeding/Information Support Groups at the end of this chapter.)

***Medication.*** Antidepressants are most useful for women with pronounced vegetative signs of depression: fatigue, poor concentration, feelings of hopelessness and helplessness, irritability, suicidal thoughts, no appetite. Lithium, an antimanic, or carbamazepine, an anticonvulsant, are used to manage manic episodes. Antipsychotic drugs may be prescribed for women with postpartum psychoses who are experiencing hallucinations or other distortions of reality.

Tricyclic Antidepressants. Tricyclic antidepressant administration is begun after physician consultation and referral. More sedating tricyclic antidepressants, such as doxepine (Sinequan), trazodone (Desyril), and imipramine (Tofranil) are useful for women with insomnia, agitation, and anxiety attacks.[38] Less sedating tricyclic antidepressants, such as desipramine (Norpramine) and protriptyline (Vivactyl) are more useful for clients with severe fatigue, difficulty waking up in the morning, or concern they may not hear their infant cry if they are too sedated.[38]

- *Administration.* Initially, 25 mg per day, increasing by 25 mg in divided doses every other day as tolerated until a therapeutic range is reached. Blood levels must be drawn to determine the therapeutic range. The dosage range for doxepin, imipramine, and desipramine is 150 to 200 mg per day.
- *Side Effects.* Oversedation, dry mouth, constipation.

**TABLE 16–4. EDINBURGH POSTNATAL DEPRESSION SCALE (EPDS)**

Name:

Address:

Baby's age:

As you have recently had a baby, we would like to know how you are feeling. Please **underline** the answer which comes closest to how you have felt **in the past 7 days**, not just how you feel today. In the past 7 days:

*1. I have been able to laugh and see the funny side of things.
  As much as I always could
  Not quite so much now
  Definitely not so much now
  Not at all

2. I have looked foward with enjoyment to things.
  As much as I ever did
  Rather less than I used to
  Definitely less than I used to
  Hardly at all

*3. I have blamed myself unnecessarily when things went wrong.
  Yes, most of the time
  Yes, some of the time
  Not very often
  No, never

4. I have been anxious or worried for no good reason.
  No, not at all
  Hardly ever
  Yes, sometimes
  Yes, very often

*5. I have felt scared or panicky for no very good reason.
  Yes, quite a lot
  Yes, sometimes
  No, not much
  No, not at all

*6. Things have been getting on top of me.
  Yes, most of the time I haven't been able to cope at all
  Yes, sometimes I haven't been coping as well as usual
  No, most of the time I have coped quite well
  No, I have been coping as well as ever

*7. I have been so unhappy that I have had difficulty sleeping.
  Yes, most of the time
  Yes, sometimes
  Not very often
  No, not at all

*8. I have felt sad or miserable.
  Yes, most of the time
  Yes, quite often
  Not very often
  No, not at all

*9. I have been so unhappy that I have been crying.
  Yes, most of the time
  Yes, quite often
  Only occasionally
  No, never

*10. The thought of harming myself has occurred to me.
  Yes, quite often
  Sometimes
  Hardly ever
  Never

Response categories are scored 0, 1, 2, and 3 according to increased severity of the symptom. Items marked with an asterisk are reverse scored (i.e., 3, 2, 1 and 0). The total score is calculated by adding together the scores for each of the ten items. Users may reproduce the scale without further permission providing they respect copyright (which remains with the *British Journal of Psychiatry*) by quoting the names of the authors, the title and the source of the paper in all reproduced copies.

*From J.L. Cox, J.M. Holden, R. Sagovsky (1987), Detection of Postnatal Depression: development of the 10-item Edinburgh Postnatal Depression Scale.* British Journal of Psychiatry, 150, *786. Copyright 1987 by the British Journal of Psychiatry. Reprinted by permission.*

- *Contraindications.* Hypersensitivity to tricyclic antidepressants, urinary retention, narrow-angle glaucoma. Concomitant use of a tricyclic antidepressant and a monoamine oxidase (MAO) inhibitor can lead to severe hypertension from excessive adrenergic stimulation of the heart and blood vessels. Tricyclics potentiate activity of direct-acting sympathomimetic and anticholinergic drugs and decrease response to indirect-acting sympathomimetic drugs.
- *Anticipated Outcome on Evaluation.* Remission of symptoms of depression.
- *Client Teaching.* Include information on relieving side effects. If the client feels oversedated, the dosage can be increased more slowly and the majority of dose taken at night. Dry mouth can be moistened by chewing gum or sucking lemon drops. Constipation can be relieved by drinking more fluids and eating more fiber. Psyllium laxatives, such as Metamucil, are also helpful. Advise clients that there is a 2- to 3-week lag time before depression clinically improves.

Serotonin Uptake Inhibitors. Selective serotonin uptake inhibitors are also indicated to treat depression. Fluoxetine (Prozac) is administered initially, 20 mg in the morning with dosage increased according to response; it may be given in divided doses in the morning and at noon. The dosage should not exceed 80 mg per day.

Sertraline (Zoloft) administration begins at 50 mg orally daily. Dosage adjustments should be made at no less than weekly intervals. The dosage range is 50 to 200 mg daily.

Paroxetine (Paxil) administration begins at 20 mg orally daily. Dosage may be increased in 10-mg increments up to a maximum of 50 mg daily.

- *Side Effects.* Nervousness, anxiety, insomnia, headache, somnolence, tremor, nausea, vomiting, dry mouth, arrhythmias, dyspepsia, weight loss, rash, pruritus, urticaria. Selective serotonin uptake inhibi-tors may prolong the half-life of diazepam. Use with tryptophan can cause agitation, gastrointestinal distress, and restlessness. Avoid use with tricyclic antidepressants because of the increased adverse effects on the central nervous system. Interaction with warfarin or other highly protein-bound drugs can increase serum level. Advise the client of the 4-week lag before clinical improvement of depression.
- *Contraindications.* Hypersensitivity to any of the selective serotonin re-uptake inhibitors. In addition, the drug should not be used within 14 days of cessation of MAO inhibitors. Cimetidine may increase the plasma concentration of paroxetine.
- *Anticipated Outcome on Evaluation.* Remission of symptoms of depression.
- *Client Teaching.* Include information about side effects.

Lithium. Lithium is indicated if antidepressant treatment precipitates a manic episode, with symptoms of racing thoughts, hyperactivity, pressured speech, increased energy, and impulsive behavior.[38] Discontinue the antidepressant if manic episodes occur, and begin lithium. Long-term use of lithium can induce goiter and has been associated with degenerative renal changes. Therefore, baseline thyroid function tests ($T_3$, $T_4$, thyroid-stimulating hormone) and renal function tests (BUN, creatinine) should be obtained as a baseline. Thyroid stimulating hormone and renal function tests should then be done every 6 months.

- *Administration.* Therapeutic range: 0.5 to 1.0 mEq/L; higher levels can produce toxicity (nausea, vomiting, diarrhea, shakiness) and extremely high levels can produce death. Subtherapeutic levels do not provide an adequate clinical response.[38] Serum values should be drawn weekly, then every 2 to 3 months. Lithium is the drug of choice for clients with postpartum psychosis with manic features.

- *Side Effects.* Nausea, vomiting, diarrhea, thirst, polyuria, lethargy, slurred speech, muscle weakness, fine hand tremor. When administered above the therapeutic range, lithium may cause headache, persistent gastrointestinal upset, confusion, hyperirritability, drowsiness, dizziness, tremors, ataxia, dry mouth, hypotension, rash, and pruritus.
- *Contraindications.* Hepatic disease, renal disease, pregnancy, lactation, severe cardiac disease.
- *Anticipated Outcome on Evaluation. The* abatement of manic symptoms.
- *Client teaching.* Include information related to side effects.

Carbamazepine. Carbamezepine (Tegretol) can be used by clients who cannot tolerate or who do not respond well to lithium. Because carbamazepine has been associated with the development of potentially fatal blood cell abnormalities (leukopenia, thrombocytopenia, agranulocytosis, aplastic anemia), a baseline complete blood cell count should be obtained followed by repeated complete blood counts.

- *Indications.* Seizure disorders, trigeminal and glossopharyngeal neuralgias, manic–depressive disorder.
- *Administration.* Initially 200 mg orally per day, gradually increasing by 200 mg per day in divided doses. Optimal dosage is 600 to 1800 mg per day. The serum therapeutic level is 4 to 12 μg/mL.[38]
- *Side Effects.* Sedation, ataxia, nausea, and vomiting. Carbamazepine accelerates the metabolism of oral contraceptives and coumadin-type anticoagulants.
- *Contraindications.* Hypersensitivity to carbamazepine or tricyclic antidepressants, bone marrow depression, and concomitant use of MAO inhibitors.
- *Anticipated Outcome on Evaluation.* Abatement of manic behaviors.
- *Client teaching.* Include information concerning side effects and contraindications.

Antipsychotic Drugs. Antipsychotic drugs such as trifluoperazine (Stelazine), haloperidol (Haldol), and thioridazine (Mellaril) are also prescribed. See the current *Physicians' Desk Reference* (PDR) or a pharmacotherapeutic resource for detailed information.

***Follow-Up.*** Home visits, telephone calls, and psychiatric referral may be part of follow-up care.

Consider telephone calls 3 days after hospital discharge and a home visit 7 days after discharge to assess the client's adaptation to motherhood and family responsibilities. If she is adapting well, repeat contact after another 7 to 10 days. On the other hand, if she is experiencing difficulty, refer her to appropriate agencies or support groups (see Breastfeeding Information/Support Groups at the end of this chapter).

- Cognitive and supportive therapies help identify and correct distorted perceptions of reality and encourage the partner or other family member(s) to assist with household and child care tasks.
- Concurrent marital therapy, in conjoint sessions, is especially helpful if the partner exhibits narcissistic behavior or is a substance abuser.[38]
- Support groups (group therapy) complement individual therapy. They help decrease the sense of isolation.
- Hospitalization should include admission of both mother and infant.[42]

## PERINATAL LOSS

Perinatal loss involves perinatal mortality, both stillbirth and neonatal death.[46] A perinatal loss may also involve a perceived loss, including loss of expectation or giving one's infant up for adoption.

Stillbirth or neonatal death (death within the first 30 days of life) is obviously a loss for the mother and the family. Less obvious may be the loss felt by a woman who miscarries or elects to terminate a pregnancy. All of these losses are irrevocable.

Loss of expectation is also a real loss for some women and their families. It may be experienced in the birth of a viable infant who is premature or has congenital anomalies or deformities. Loss of expectation may also be experienced when the birthing act causes losses that precipitate maternity blues even though the infant is healthy. For example, postpartum fatigue may make daily tasks difficult to perform and contribute to postpartum blues or depression.

The woman or couple who gives up an infant for adoption experience loss, especially if they bonded with the infant before birth; giving up the infant does not eliminate these bonds.[47]

## Epidemiology

In 1990 the United States ranked 17th among other nations in infant mortality, with a rate of 10.4 per 1000 live births.[48] Sixty percent of the infants that die within the first year of birth are of low birthweight.[49] African-American mothers are twice as likely as white mothers to have low-birthweight babies; 12.4 percent of African-American infants weigh 5.5 pounds or less compared with 5.6 percent of white infants. The infant mortality rate for African-Americans (17.6 percent per 1000 live births) is twice that of white infants (8.5 percent per 1000 live births).[49,50]

Out of 3.3 million babies born alive in the United States, 30,000 die during the first 28 days of life from genetic disease and congenital malformations; they constitute 10 percent of total neonatal deaths.[51,52] Approximately 33 percent of stillbirths have a congenital defect.[52] Miscarriages occur in approximately 43 percent of pregnancies; approximately 50 percent are caused by chromosomal anomalies.[53]

## Subjective Data

A client may report sadness, loss of appetite, inability to sleep, increased irritability or hostility toward others, preoccupation with the lost infant, inability to return to normal activities, and somatic distress.[54] The client may also have feelings of guilt and preoccupation with her negligence or minor omissions.[47,54]

## Objective Data

Data are determined concerning the client and her family's grieving by means of observation and counseling. The primary health care provider can then help them cope with their loss.

***Phases of Mourning.*** Progression through the five stages of mourning varies among individuals and regression may occur. Perinatal grieving involves acute grief, which is most intense during the 4- to 6-week period following loss and less intense in the subsequent 4 weeks. The normal grief reaction may last from 6 months to 2 years or may never resolve. The anniversary of the loss may reactivate grief reactions.[55]

- The shock and numbness stage (denial) is expressed as impaired normal functioning. The individual has difficulty making decisions and may be aloof.
- Searching and yearning (anger) constitute the second stage of mourning. Anger and bitterness can be transferred to other people, especially health care professionals. Restlessness and guilt feelings may also be experienced.
- Bargaining, which is usually a brief phase, attempts to delay loss.
- Disorganization (depression) is the phase when the reality of the loss occurs. Depres-

sion may occur as the full impact of loss is felt. Guilt feelings remain.

- Resolution may be seen as the individual begins to function better at home and at work. Self-confidence increases. The individual is able to place the loss in perspective with life.[55,56]

***Parental Tasks.*** Following perinatal loss, parents must work through the loss and make it real. The parents must allow the normal grief reaction to progress. During this time, parents should meet their own needs as well as those of their other children and communicate their feelings to the children.

***Multiple Gestation.*** Parents who experienced a multiple gestation may have an additional or more acute sense of loss from conflicting emotions. Parents need to grieve their deceased infant(s) before relating to the survivor(s). Parents may experience grief from loss of prestige as parents of twins. In addition, they may have a sense of inadequacy, as the death of one child may be perceived as the inability to raise more than one child.

## Plan

***Psychosocial Interventions.*** Measures are directed toward helping parents work through loss and make it real. Their coping abilities are assessed and, if indicated, the parents are referred to support groups for counseling.

- Telephone parents (especially important on what had been due date or on the anniversary of death) to reevaluate coping and readjustment. Call during the evening to involve the partner. Provide parents with the phone number of the hospital's maternity floor.
- Advise parents to join support groups (see Parental/Family Support Groups and Perinatal Loss Support Groups at the end of this chapter).
- Provide anticipatory guidance, counseling parents about the normalcy of grief, its stages, and the varying duration. In addition, prepare parents to deal with the reactions of others. The most difficult time is the 2 to 4 months after death (acute grief).
- Recommend postponing pregnancy until both parents have worked through their grief.
- Provide suggestions for dealing with grief.
  - Communicate with partner, family, and friends.
  - Eat a well-balanced diet and drink adequate fluids; avoid caffeine and alcoholic beverages.
  - Exercise daily.
  - Avoid tobacco as it depletes the body of vitamins, increases stomach acidity, decreases circulation, and can cause palpitations.
  - Rest daily; rest at night even if unable to sleep.
  - Read books, poems, and articles that comfort; avoid "scare" literature and technical medical bulletins.
  - Keep a diary or journal of thoughts, memories, and mementos.
  - Write poems or letters to the infant.
  - Avoid making big decisions or changes for 24 months, and do not let others make decisions for you; put away baby clothes and articles when you are ready.
  - Accept help from others; request help from clergy if desired.[52]

***Medication.*** Medication is not indicated.

***Follow-Up.*** Follow-up involves continuing observation for resolution of grief. Grief is completed when an individual is able to turn outward and think of others and to formulate plans for the future. If grief remains unresolved, refer parents to a skilled professional counselor. Unresolved grief may be observed in several behaviors:

- Persistent yearning for recovery of lost objects
- Overidentification with the deceased

- Inability to cry or rage despite desire to do so
- Misdirected anger or ambivalence toward infant
- Lack of support group
- Presence of secondary gain, e.g., increased attention to mother

## BREASTFEEDING

In 1984, 25 percent of American women breastfed for 6 months[9]; in 1987, the number of women breastfeeding infants at 6 months dropped to 21 percent.[9] In Third World countries and in acute poverty-stricken areas in the United States, an infant who is bottle fed has a greater morbidity and mortality risk within the first year than an infant who is breastfed.[57,58] Despite the increased safety of commercial infant formulas, breastfeeding has distinct advantages for both mother and infant, and almost no contraindications. Human milk is physiologically compatible with the human infant's digestive tract, and provides the exact balance of nutrients, electrolytes, and immunological factors necessary for optimal growth and development. Even the act of suckling employs the use of different muscles and feeding mechanism than bottle feeding.[9,59] Breastfeeding is easier, nothing to heat or spoil, no extra bottles to transport. And an emotional bond develops between mother and nursing infant that does not occur when an infant is bottle fed.[9,31]

A mother who is breastfeeding for the first time may not have the support of family and friends, and needs encouragement, support, and accurate information to become self-assured about breastfeeding. The health care provider should help the first-time breastfeeding mother and her infant to successfully breastfeed.

### TYPES OF BREASTFEEDING

#### Unrestricted Breastfeeding

The infant is put to breast immediately after delivery and then on demand. Breast milk is the major source of nourishment for the first year of life.

The advantages of this type of breastfeeding are that less illness occurs during first year of life,[9] infant has mouth–nipple contact and body contact, and the breast is associated with comfort as well as food. The disadvantage is that breastfeeding requires the mother's dedication.

#### Token Breastfeeding

Restrictions are placed on the duration of breastfeeding and the length of each time at the breast; feedings are scheduled. The infant is offered water or glucose water between feedings. Weaning occurs by the third month or earlier.

The advantage is that other family members can participate in feeding the infant. The disadvantages are that the milk supply may decrease, the infant is more susceptible to illnesses, and the infant learns bottle-sucking techniques, which may lead to nipple confusion.

### BREAST ANATOMY

Breast tissue comprises glands, supporting connective tissue, and fatty tissue. The primary structures are skin, subcutaneous tissue, and the corpus mammae.

The skin includes the nipple, areola, and general skin. Each nipple contains 15 to 25 milk ducts; each of the tubuloalveolar glands opens separately onto the nipple. The nipple also contains smooth muscle fibers, sensory nerve endings, and sebaceous and apocrine glands. Nipple erection is caused by tactile, sensory, or autonomic sympathetic stimuli. Montgomery's tubercles contain the ductular openings of sebaceous and lactiferous glands. They secrete a substance that protects and lubricates the nipple and areola during pregnancy and lactation.

Subcutaneous tissue lies just below the dermis.

The corpus mammae is divided into the parenchyma and stroma. Parenchyma includes the ductular–lobular–alveolar structures. The lactiferous ductal system connects the alveoli to the nipple. Fifteen to twenty tubuloalveolar glands are embedded in fat.[9] They open into lactiferous ducts, which open into lactiferous sinuses, which, in turn, open onto the nipple. The stroma comprises connective tissue, fat, blood vessels, nerves, and lymphatics.

## PHYSIOLOGY OF LACTATION

Lactation is hormonally controlled. The physiological changes that occur are directed toward mammogenesis, lactogenesis (milk secretion), and galactopoiesis (milk maintenance). Most milk is synthesized in the acini and smaller milk ducts during suckling.[9]

### Mammogenesis

Mammogenesis is the development of the mammary glands to their functional state.

Estrogen stimulates parenchymal proliferation and ductal growth. Luteal and placental hormones increase ductular and lobular formation; placental lactogen, prolactin, and chorionic gonadotropin accelerate mammary growth.[9] Prolactin (from the anterior pituitary gland) stimulates glandular production of colostrum; human placental lactogen stimulates secretion of colostrum by the second trimester[9]; and progesterone stimulates lobular growth.

### Lactogenesis

Milk production by the mammary glands proceeds in two stages.

Stage I of lactogenesis begins 12 weeks before parturition and is preceded by significant increases in lactose, total proteins, and immunoglobulins and decreases in sodium and chloride.[9] Stage II clinically begins on days 2 and 3 postpartum with copious milk secretion; mature milk is established in approximately 10 days.[9]

### Galactopoiesis

Prolactin stimulates and sustains lactation (milk secretion); oxytocin stimulates milk ejection. An intact hypothalamic–pituitary axis regulates prolactin and oxytocin levels and is essential for the maintenance of milk secretion. Ejection reflex is dependent on receptors in the canalicular system of the breast. Dilation or stretching of the canalicules causes a reflex release of oxytocin. Tactile receptors for both oxytocin and reflex prolactin release are located in the nipple.[9]

Prolactin secretion is controlled by prolactin inhibitory factor (PIF) produced by the hypothalamus.[60] Suppression of PIF allows the anterior pituitary gland to secrete uninhibited amounts of prolactin. Catecholamine levels in the hypothalamus control PIF. Drugs and events that decrease catecholamines also decrease PIF, thereby causing an increase in prolactin.[9] Among nonnursing mothers, prolactin levels drop to normal in 2 to 3 weeks, independent of lactation suppression therapy.

Release of oxytocin into the circulation is stimulated by sucking. Two minutes of sucking may be required for a full oxytocin response.[61] Release of oxytocin peaks 6 to 10 minutes after sucking begins.[61] The hormone causes the ejection of milk (milk ejection reflex) from alveoli and smaller milk ducts into larger lactiferous sinuses and ducts. It also stimulates myometrial contraction and uterine involution.

## Composition of Human Milk

Milk varies with the stage of lactation, time of day, sampling time during a given feeding, maternal nutrition, and the individual. Initially, colostrum is produced. A transitional phase in production leads to secretion of mature milk.

***Colostrum.*** A yellowish, thick fluid produced during the first postpartum week. It contains higher concentrations of sodium, potassium, and chloride than mature milk. Protein, fat-soluble vitamins, and minerals are also in larger concentration than in transitional or mature milk. This high-protein, low-fat milk meets the needs and reserves of the newborn.9 The mean energy value is 67 kcal/100 mL of mature milk. Colostrum facilitates the establishment of bifidus flora in the digestive tract and the passage of meconium. It contains abundant antibodies.

***Transitional Milk.*** Secreted beginning 7 to 10 days postpartum and continuing until 2 weeks postpartum. The concentration of immunoglobulins decreases, although lactose, fat, and total caloric content increase. Water-soluble vitamins increase and fat-soluble vitamins decrease to approach the level found in mature milk.[9]

***Mature Milk.*** The only necessary source of nutrition for an infant's first 4 to 6 months of life and should be the primary source for the first year.[9,62]

- Water is the major constituent. A lactating woman requires an increased water intake. If water intake is decreased, sensible and insensible water loss are decreased before water for lactation is decreased.
- Lipids, the second most plentiful constituent, and the most variable, provides the major portion of kilocalories. It is almost completely digestible.
- Proteins constitute 0.9 percent of human milk content.[9]
- The predominant carbohydrate is lactose. Synthesized by the mammary gland, it is specific for newborn growth and enhances calcium absorption. Lactose appears to be critical for the prevention of rickets, as human milk is relatively low in calcium.
- Minerals essential to the newborn are potassium and iron.
  - Potassium levels are higher than sodium in breast milk (similar to intracellular fluids). Sodium levels in cow's milk are 3.6 times greater than those in human milk.[9]
  - The concentration of exogenous elemental iron in human milk is 100 μg/1100 mL.[9] Normal infants need 8 to 10 mg per day in the first year of life. Prepared formulas provide 10 to 12 mg per day; infants breastfed for the first 6 months are not at increased risk for iron-deficiency anemia or depletion of iron stores.[9,63] Although its concentration in human milk is low, iron is absorbed more readily than iron from other sources. Thus, infants are not at risk for iron deficiency anemia or deple-tion of iron stores if they are breast-fed totally during the first 6 months of life.
- An adequate supply of vitamins A, E, and C is present in breast milk.
  - The amount of vitamin A in mature human milk is 280 IU and in cow's milk, 180 IU; an infant consuming 200 mL of breast milk every day obtains an adequate amount of vitamin A.
  - Serum levels of vitamin E in breastfed babies rise quickly at birth and are maintained by approximately 4 weeks postpartum with only breast milk intake.[9]

• Vitamin C and other water-soluble vitamins in human milk reflect maternal dietary intake.[9] Human milk is an excellent source of these water-soluble vitamins.[9]

### Resistance Factors and Immunological Significance

Breastfeeding significantly decreases infant morbidity and mortality by protecting against enteropathogens that may contaminate other food or formula. The protective factors contained in breast milk are both cellular and humoral.[9]

Cellular factors include macrophages, polymorphonuclear leukocytes, and lymphocytes. These cells are phagocytes and they stimulate antibody formation. The humoral factors are immunoglobulins.

- Immunoglobulin A (IgA) is the most important immunoglobulin in terms of biological activity, and it is the most concentrated. IgA also has antitoxin activity against *Escherichia coli* and *Vibrio cholerae* and thereby prevents diarrhea.[9]
- Bifidus factor is responsible for the growth of *Bifidobacterium bifidum,* the predominant bacteria in the gut of breastfed infants. The flora of bifid bacteria inhibits pathogenic *Staphylococcus aureus, Shigella,* and *Protozoa* and encourages growth of *Lactobacillus bifidus,* which crowds out other bacteria. Lysozyme and lactoferrin act directly to inhibit pathogen growth. The resistance factor protects against *Staphylococcus* infection.[9]
- Breast milk contains antibodies against poliovirus, coxsackievirus, echovirus, influenza virus, and rhinovirus and, thus, helps to prevent viral infections.
- Breast milk protects against the development of allergies. An infant begins to produce antibodies to cow's milk within 18 days of ingestion. Syndromes associated with cow's milk allergy include gastric enteropathy, atopic dermatitis, rhinitis, chronic pulmonary disease, eosinophilia, and failure to thrive.[9]

## CONTRAINDICATIONS TO BREASTFEEDING

***Breast Cancer.*** Controversy regarding the role of prolactin in the progression of mammary cancer may be a reason to contraindicate breastfeeding for pregnant women.[9] The risk of developing breast cancer is the same for women who breastfeed and those who do not.[9,64]

***Hepatitis B Virus.*** Breastfeeding is permitted for immunized infants in all countries.[65] Many hospitals immunize all newborns so that breastfeeding can occur even with cracked nipples.

***Cytomegalovirus.*** Breast milk also contains appropriate antibodies that protect the infant against cytomegalovirus. There does exist a risk for the infant who is exposed to virus but not a daily dose of antibodies.[9,62]

***Human Immunodeficiency Virus.*** For women in the United States who test positive for HIV, breastfeeding is contraindicated.[9,66,67] Breastfeeding, however, remains the feeding method of choice in countries where the death rate in the first year of life is 50 percent, compared with the 18 percent risk of dying from AIDS when born to an infected mother.[9]

***Augmentation or Reduction Mammoplasty.*** If milk ducts were cut during mammoplasty, breastfeeding may not be possible.[9] Incisions around the areola usually indicate that some milk ducts were cut and possible nerve damage occurred.[62,68]

***Active Tuberculosis.*** Breastfeeding is permitted if the mother's skin test is positive, and if at the same time there is no radiologic indication of disease and the client has started antituberculin medication. If the mother has a positive tuberculin skin test and positive chest film, she may breastfeed if she is taking antituberculous medication and the sputum culture is negative.[9,68] If the sputum culture is positive, breastfeeding may be possible after the mother has taken medication for at least 1 week. Limited isolation from the mother with active disease may be required. The breastfeeding infant may be treated prophylactically by the pediatrician.

## ELEMENTS OF BREASTFEEDING

***Compression of Lactiferous Sinuses.*** Externally, the infant's mouth should cover the lactiferous sinuses, whereas internally, the correct movement of the infant's tongue provides areolar compression between the infant's tongue and palate. The lactiferous sinuses lie underneath the areola; compression of the lactiferous sinuses removes milk from the breast. Sucking may need to continue for 2 minutes for the full response to oxytocin release.

***Number of Feedings per Day.*** A minimum of eight feedings are necessary in 24 hours, with each feeding providing a minimum of 5 to 10 minutes of swallowing at each breast. The milk ejection reflex takes 2 to 3 minutes before it is effective[9]; limiting nursing to 2 to 3 minutes does not permit the infant to obtain milk. Suck efficiency is critical to breastfeeding success.

***Systematic Assessment of Infant at Breast.***[61] Assessment of a breastfeeding session requires direct observation. Observe positioning and alignment, areolar grasp, and sucking.

Positioning and Alignment. The infant should be relaxed, in a responsive state, and displaying early hunger cues—rooting and hand-to-mouth activity. Crying is a late hunger cue.

The infant's body should be flexed with the head and trunk aligned so that the head is straight on the breast, not turned laterally or hyperextended (head and body are at breast level). The infant should be brought to the breast, not the breast to the infant. Proper alignment decreases traction on the mother's nipples; the areola and nipple are more easily kept in the infant's mouth; swallowing is facilitated.

The mother's hand should cup her breast, with her fingers supporting the lower portion of the breast and her thumb resting on the upper portion. The infant should be permitted to grasp at least one-half inch of areolar tissue. This position is the "C-hold," and permits the mother to support her breast without distorting the nipple.

The traditional "scissors" or "cigarette" hold in which the breast is held between the mother's middle and index fingers has two disadvantages: (2) the mother's fingers cannot spread apart as far as in the C-hold and may interfere with the infant's latching on, and (2) breast tissue can be restricted by the scissors hold to such a degree that ducts become plugged.[62]

Areolar Grasp. The infant must have a correct mouth opening, correct lip flanging, and correct tongue placement. To elicit the grasp gently, tickle the infant's lips with the nipple to stimulate the mouth to open. When the mouth is opened wide, quickly pull the infant close to the breast and center the nipple in infant's mouth. Move the infant's head and trunk as a unit to avoid hyperflexion, hyperextension, or lateral turning of the head. Avoid holding the back of the infant's head to maneuver it onto the breast, because it does not allow the mother to feel rapid arm motion and erodes her confidence if the infant latches on. Placing a hand on the mother's arm and moving it quickly toward her breast allows the mother to feel the quick arm movement.

Breastfeeding Problems. May be determined during systematic assessment of the infant at the breast.

- Problems with grasping the areola may be caused by "prissily pursed" lips. The infant appears to be drinking through a straw. Only the nipple is grasped, and the mother often experiences nipple pain. The infant receives little milk because the lactiferous sinuses are not compressed. Break the suction by inserting a finger into the corner of infant's mouth and stimulate the mouth to open wide. Alternate sucking of the nipple and the areola through pursed lips will traumatize the nipple and the suck will become inefficient.[61] Friction may abrade the mother's areolar tissue and result in ineffective sucking.
- Another grasping problem is negative pressure in an infant's intraoral cavity, which results in retention of the nipple and areolar tissue in the infant's mouth. This counteracts the naturally retractile nature of nipple tissue, helps to refill the lactiferous sinuses with milk from the lactiferous ducts, and conveys milk to the oropharynx. Negative pressure is achieved when an infant forms an effective seal with the border of his or her mouth.
- Sore nipples cause discomfort, and breastfeeding should not hurt. If the mother has sore, cracked nipples, the cause must be found: Review positioning and latch-on of the infant. A variety of measures may be tried to relieve sore nipples.
  - Some milk may be expressed before feeding to stimulate the milk ejection reflex, thus allowing for softening of the areola before the infant latches on.
  - Some milk may be expressed onto the nipples after feedings and allowed to air dry.
  - The flaps of the nursing bra may be left open after feedings.
  - Nursing pads with plastic liners should be avoided. Nipple shields also compound the problem by increasing nipple irritation and confusing the baby so that the baby sucks improperly and further irritates the nipple.[9,62]

Sucking. Correct sucking requires that the infant's tongue cover the mandibular–alveolar ridge on the lower gum line and curve beneath the areolar tissue.

Evaluate tongue placement by gently pulling infant's lower lip downward. Incorrect tongue placement is indicated by clicking or smacking sounds and drawing in of cheek pads with each suck, or by the loss of large amounts of milk over the infant's chin.[61,62] A short tongue or one with a short lingual frenulum may not extend over the lower alveolar ridge.

Evaluate areolar compression by carefully noting the type of sucking and swallowing. A sustained slower mandibular motion indicates nutritive sucking; rapid mandibular motion indicates nonnutritive sucking. Audible swallowing is the most reliable indicator of milk intake. Documentation of an infant's breastfeeding should state: "Breastfed with audible swallowing at each breast."[61]

***Breastfeeding Positions.*** Whichever position (four are listed below) the mother uses to nurse her infant, she should be comfortable. Pillows should be used to help support her arm and help her hold the baby close to her breast, relaxed and without muscle strain.

- *Cradle Hold.* The mother sits up, the infant faces her, and the infant's head or arm rests on the mother's forearm or in the crook of her arm. The cradle hold is a good choice for a mother whose infant has low muscle tone, for example, an infant with Down syndrome.
- *Football Hold.* The mother sits up, the infant's head faces her breast, and the body is tucked under her arm at her side. The baby's bottom should be resting on a pillow near the mother's elbow to provide additional support for the mother and avoid muscle strain. The football hold is a good choice for a mother who recently had ab-

dominal surgery, as the position does not put pressure on the incision.

- *Side-Lying Position.* Both the mother and infant lie on their sides, facing each other, with the infant's feet pulled in close to his or her body. Pillows under the mother's head, behind her back, and under the knee or her upper leg may provide comfort.
- *Slide-Over Position.* This position is especially useful with infants who refuse one breast. The mother can begin nursing the infant on the preferred side, then slide the infant over to the less preferred side once the milk ejection reflex has occurred. The infant's body position is not changed; he or she merely "slides over."

***Breast Preparation.*** To prepare breasts for feeding, first assess them by palpating the tissue and inspecting the nipples and areolae; then teach the mother proper care of the breasts.

Palpate to detect inelastic breast tissue. Skin that is taut and firm and difficult to pick up is more prone to engorgement. Tissue can be improved by prepartum massage (see Chapter 13) and measures to prevent engorgement.[9]

Assess the nipples and areolae by gently compressing each areola between the thumb and forefinger. The normal nipple everts with gentle pressure; the inverted or tied nipple inverts more with gentle pressure.[9] Inverted nipples may be treated with a nipple shell worn during last trimester (see the list at the end of this chapter). Exercises to evert the nipple are rarely successful and can lead to premature labor.[9]

Stress the importance of avoiding soap and other drying agents on the nipples. Teach the mother to wash breasts with water only.[62,66] Routine use of ointments and creams is discouraged, as some have irritants, such as lanolin;[9,10,62] Vitamin E or hormone creams or ointments are unsafe on the nipples unless prescribed for a specific problem, and they then should be used only in minute amounts.[9,62] Sebaceous glands and tubercles of Montgomery are easily plugged by repeated application of oily substances.

***Extrinsic Factors Contributing to Breastfeeding Problems.*** Separation, delayed feedings, and introduction of bottle feedings interfere with breastfeeding.

Separation of mother and infant interferes with milk ejection reflex; the infant is not able to nurse on demand, causing a delay that contributes to milk stasis and engorgement. If in the mother's absence, the infant learns to suck on a bottle, then sucking at the breast becomes incorrect, causing pain and trauma.

Delaying first feedings to a healthy infant—an infant is most receptive to nursing in the first 90 minutes after birth—can erode the mother's self-confidence when a sleepy infant is later brought to her to feed. Delay can also decrease the milk ejection reflex.

Limiting the frequency and duration of feedings contributes to breastfeeding problems. The milk ejection reflex occurs 2 to 3 minutes after sucking is initiated.[9] Limiting nursing interferes with the reflex and the infant's milk supply. The limited feedings contribute to milk stasis and engorgement and sore nipples.

Introducing bottles to an infant interferes with the milk ejection reflex by suggesting to the mother that her milk is insufficient. Bottles cause the infant to become confused as sucking at the breast differs from sucking on a commercial nipple or pacifier. An infant may reject the breast or, on the other hand, suckle frequently and for prolonged periods to be satisfied.

***Breastfeeding Infants in Multiple Births.*** The advantages of breastfeeding infants in a multiple birth are similar to those of breastfeeding a single child: breastfeeding provides a perfect food that is easily digested and provides immunities; the milk is easily accessible; financial savings are substantial; and a special relationship is promoted between mother and infants. The mother may find a support group helpful (see Appendix IA).

The amount of milk produced is influenced by the size of the infants and the number of breastfeeding sessions. The mother should begin breastfeeding at the earliest possible time. An electric piston-type pump (Medela or Ameda/Egnel) may be needed if infants are unable to suckle.[69] Optimal milk production with minimum pumping will most likely involve five pumping sessions per day, at least 10 to 15 minutes per breast. A minimum total of 100 minutes pumping over 24 hours is recommended[69]; short, frequent sessions to express milk are more effective and stimulate more milk production than longer sessions with longer intervals.[69] It is not necessary for the mother to waken at night and pump.[69]

If only one infant can feed and the other is hospitalized the mother has two options: (1) Nurse twin A while simultaneously pumping for twin B; breast milk obtained can be taken to twin B. This schedule is rigorous and may be exhausting for the mother. (2) Begin pumping for twin B a few days prior to the infant's discharge.

Feedings may be simultaneous or individual. Simultaneous feedings are advantageous because both feedings are completed in one session. Simultaneous feedings save time and may take advantage of simultaneous letdowns. A disadvantage is that the mother loses individual time with each infant.

Individual feedings are advantageous because modified scheduling may be employed. For example, the hungrier infant sets the pace, and the second infant is awakened for feedings. A disadvantage of this type of feeding is that it is time consuming.

***Simultaneous Feedings.*** Proper positioning is particularly important for breastfeeding two infants so that the mother does not bear the weight of the infants. Pillows should support the infants' weight.

- The double football hold is used for simultaneous feedings. The head and neck of each infant are supported by the mother's hands, with each infant's body tucked under one of the mother's arms and their feet toward her back. The infants' abdomens face up or are rotated in toward the mother's chest or side. An advantage of the double football hold is that the mother can assist with head control; the more difficult to manage infant should be placed on the side easiest for the mother to manage.[69] The mother should not bend over to nurse but, instead, bring the infants close to her.
- In the combination cradle/football position, twin A is held like football and approaches the breast at 12 and 6 o'clock. Twin B is cradled across the mother's chest with her or his abdomen tucked in tightly toward the mother's abdomen and approaches the breast at 9 and 3 o'clock.[69] Two advantages of this position are that it is the most inconspicuous for nursing outside the home, and it is easily mastered if one or both infants have difficulty latching onto the breast.
- In the parallel hold both infants are angled in the same direction. Twin A is cradled, held with legs behind twin B; the legs simultaneously support Twin B's head. The advantage of the parallel hold is that the weight of one twin keeps the second infant attached to the breast. In addition, the mother's arms can rest comfortably on pillows.[69]
- In the crisscross hold both infants are in cradle position, with the legs of one crossing over those of the other. The infants are in the crook of the mother's arms and are rotated toward her abdomen. The mother supports the infants by holding their but-

tocks. A disadvantage is that this position is difficult for infants to maintain; it requires head control.[69]

- "V" position is similar to crisscross. The mother is lying nearly flat on her back with pillows under her head. The infants' heads are at their mother's breasts, forming a "V," with their knees touching her upper abdomen.[62] This position allows the mother to rest more comfortably; it can be used for night feedings. The disadvantage is that it requires infants to have more head control and assistance in grasping the nipple.[69]

## DRUG TRANSMISSION IN BREAST MILK

Transmission of a drug in breast milk from mother to infant depends on several factors:

- Absorption of drug by mother's body: half-life or peak serum time, absorption rate, route of administration
- Lipid solubility and plasma protein binding properties of drug
- Movement of drug from maternal plasma to milk: cell diffusion or active transport
- Amount of drug ingested by infant
- Concentration of drug in milk
- Size and relative metabolic maturity of infant
- pH of substrate[70]

The effect of the drug can be minimized in several ways:

- Do not use a long-acting form of the drug. Infants have difficulty with excretion and detoxification usually occurs in liver; however, the infant liver is immature.
- Schedule the doses so that the least amount of the drug enters the milk: Have the mother take medication immediately after breastfeeding.
- Choose drug that passes least into milk.
- Advise the mother to take medication as directed and to watch the infant for unusual signs and symptoms or a change in feeding pattern or activity. She should contact her health care provider if she has any concerns or questions.

***Contraindications.*** Certain drugs are contraindications to breastfeeding:

- Alcoholic beverages (interfere with ejection reflex)
- Chronic aspirin use may cause metabolic acidosis in infant and affect platelet function (aspirin or acetaminophen in single dose is not significantly transferred)
- Cocaine
- Chloramphenicol (potential for bone marrow toxicity)
- Cimetidine (unknown effect in nursing infant)
- Cyclosporine
- Doxorubicin
- Gold salts (rash, kidney and liver inflammation)
- Iodine (preferentially concentrated in milk with concentrations 20 to 30 times those of maternal serum)
- Lithium (infant hypotonia, lethargy)
- Methotrexate
- Minor tranquilizers (barbiturates, benzodiazepines)
- Narcotics (methadone for maintenance therapy reported safe)
- Phencyclidine (PCP)
- Thiouracil (not, however, propylthiouracil)
- Tobacco (smoking more than 20 cigarettes per day decreases milk supply; passive, inhaled smoke increases risks for allergies, sudden infant death syndrome, pneumonia, and bronchitis)[62,71,72]

Drugs requiring temporary interruption are radiopharmaceuticals including indium-111 and gallium-67.[69]

The effects of metoclopramide on nursing infants are unknown. No adverse effects have been reported; however, there is the potential for central nervous system effects.[71]

Drugs that have caused significant effects in some nursing infants and should be used with caution include clemastine, phenobarbital, primidone, and sulfasalazine.[71]

A mother who uses recreational drugs should not breastfeed.

Amphetamines (crack, speed, ups, uppers) are excreted in breast milk; levels in milk exceed those in maternal serum. Abstinence from amphetamines is recommended until more information is available.[62,73]

Cocaine (snow, coke, crack, champagne, tool, pearl flake, blow, gold dust, dama blanca) appears to be excreted in breast milk[73]; cocaine intoxication has been reported in 2-week-old infants. Mothers should not apply cocaine to sore nipples[73]; seizures, apnea, and cyanosis were reported in an 11-day-old infant whose mother applied cocaine to sore nipples.[73]

Heroin ("H," junk, smack, China white, black tar) crosses into breast milk to cause addiction in breastfed infants.[73]

Hallucinogens have not been reported in breast milk. Hallucinogens include LSD (acid, lysergic diethylamide), mescaline (peyote), psilocybin (found in certain mushrooms) and Ts and blues (combination of pentazocine and tripelennamine).[73]

Marijuana (dope, weed, herb, grass, pat, hashish, hash) has unknown long-term effects on infants; the concentration transferred into breast milk is eight times that in maternal blood.[73]

***Compatible Drugs.*** Certain drugs are usually compatible with breastfeeding:

- Amoxicillin
- Azithromycin
- Cefoxitin
- Cisplatin
- Diltiazem
- Erythromycin
- Hormones (oral contraceptives, including those with estrogen which may decrease milk production)
- Labetalol
- Methimazole
- Mexilitine
- Minoxidil
- Piroxicam
- Procainamide
- Suprafen
- Terbutaline
- Ticarcillin
- Tolmetin
- Verapamil.[9,62,71]

## BREAST PUMPS

Mothers of preterm infants or of newborns hospitalized for other reasons and mothers who work may use breast pumps. An infant's suckling, however, remains the most efficient pump. Infants suck at approximately 55 to 220 mm Hg.[74] Pumps that match suckling stimulate the milk ejection reflex and promote milk production most effectively. The vacuum produced by a pump should not exceed the vacuum created by an infant.

Infants nurse in a burst-pause pattern. Suckling has three phases: suction, release, and relaxation. The actions are carried out approximately 60 times per minute.[74] Infants apply suction for less than 1 second each time.[75]

A correctly fitting flange surrounds the areola and allows the nipple to move back and forth during pumping.[73] The flange should engulf and firmly support the breast and allow maximum nipple stretch, yet be small enough to provide gentle nipple friction.

There are different types of pumps. An electric pump obtains more milk and is easier to use than a hand-operated pump or manual expression.[76] The double pump expresses milk most quickly and can be rented for about one dollar per day. An intermittent draw pump is less likely to cause trauma and provides better stimulation of the milk ejection reflex.[76]

Manual expression of milk might be necessary in the event a part of the mechanical pump is lost or the pump is left at home. To manually express (pump) milk, the mother first washes her hands. She positions her thumb and first two fingers about 1 to 1½ in. behind her nipple, forming a "C" with her hand. She should then push straight into the chest wall and roll her thumb and fingers forward. The movement is repeated rhythmically; the thumb and fingers are rotated to milk other sinuses. She should express each breast until milk flow decreases, then gently massage the breasts to stimulate milk ejection.[62]

*Not recommended* for pumping breasts is the bicycle horn pump. It cannot be sterilized, milk can be easily contaminated, and it has no collection mechanism for milk, it is difficult to clean, it can damage breast tissue, and it expresses milk ineffectively.

***Using a Pump.*** Practicing with pump before actual need for milk will facilitate successful use. A woman should become knowledgeable about the pump several weeks before milk is actually needed; she should practice putting the pump together and using it. Hands should be washed before beginning breast pumping, and manufacturer's instructions followed for cleaning the pump.

The mother moistens the breast with water (to form a seal), centers the nipple in the proper size nipple adapter, and begins pumping at the lowest setting. To stimulate the milk ejection reflex she should interrupt milk expression several times to gently massage the breast. She should switch breasts when milk flow begins to decrease.

***Storing Milk.*** If milk is to be used within 48 to 72 hours refrigeration is sufficient for storage. Milk should be frozen if storage will be longer than 24 hours. Do not freeze in glass containers. Frozen milk can be stored for 1 month in the freezer compartment of a refrigerator or 6 months in a deep freeze. Frozen milk should be thawed quickly; the most effective way is to prop stored milk in drinking glass into which warm water is poured. Then the bag or glass of milk is shaken to bring separated particles back into suspension.[62,76] Milk should not be heated in a microwave oven, as it can become too warm and have isolated hot spots which may burn the infant.

## RETURNING TO WORK AND BREASTFEEDING

***Pumping/Expressing Milk.*** Advise the client to begin freezing milk for later use approximately 14 days before returning to work. She should pump at least three times per day, after breastfeeding the infant. A formula is used to estimate the amount of milk needed per feeding:

$$\frac{\text{infant weight} \times 2.5}{\text{number of feedings}} = \text{ounces per feeding}$$

For example, for a 10-pound infant,

$$\frac{10 \times 2.5}{8} = \frac{25}{8} = \text{approximately 3 oz of milk needed per feeding}$$

A Nuk-type nipple should be used when bottle feeding, as it most closely resembles breast.

***Baby's Refusal of Bottle.*** Refusing to drink from a bottle occurs most often among infants approximately 3 months old. Using a bottle along with breastfeeding in the first month of life increases the likelihood of nipple confusion; poor suckling at breast results and establishment of a milk supply that meets the infant's needs is delayed.[76] Someone other than mother should use a second feeding skill with the infant, for example, offering milk in a cup or spoon rather than the bottle.[74]

***Preparing for Absence.*** Some guidelines might help the client adapt to the challenges of breastfeeding and spending time away from the infant.

- Suggest to the client that she pack an extra bra and wear a two-piece outfit to facilitate pumping and to camouflage leakage of milk.
- Advise the client to ensure that the infant's caregiver is comfortable with the mother's desire to breastfeed and knows how to handle breast milk.
- Suggest to the client that she pack several diaper bags to obviate the need to return home for forgotten articles.
- Refer the client to a breastfeeding support group (see Breastfeeding Information/Support Groups at the end of this chapter).

## BOTTLE FEEDING

Although breast milk is the perfect food for infants, not all mothers choose or are able to breastfeed their infants. Formula feedings should be given to an infant for the first year of life. If the infant is allergic to cow's milk, soy-based formulas may be used.

An amendment was passed in 1980 by Congress to the Food, Drug and Cosmetic Act specifying new regulations for commercially prepared infant formulas. This act, the Infant Formula Act of 1980, gave the Food and Drug Administration (FDA) the authority to establish quality-control procedures for infant formula, to establish recall procedures, to establish and revise nutrient levels, and to regulate labeling. Manufacturers were also required to analyze each batch of formula to ensure all nutrients were present in the correct amounts, to ensure that the formula was stable over the period of recommended shelf life, and to make all records available to the FDA. The year 1986 saw the requirement for standard labeling of nutrition information and directions for preparation become mandatory.[70]

*Teaching Bottle Feeding*

- Point the nipple directly into the mouth and on top of the tongue, rather than toward the palate. The nipple should be full of milk at all times to avoid ingestion of air. The nipple hole should be large enough so that milk flows in drips when inverted; if it is too large, the infant can eat too fast and regurgitate or overeat.
- Stroke, cuddle, and talk to the infant during feedings.
- Never prop bottles or feed infant in totally recumbent (flat) position which can result in positional otitis media.
- Avoid warming bottles in a microwave oven, as milk can become too hot and burn the infant. Formula should be at room temperature.
- Avoid reusing milk from a previous feeding.

## NURSING DIAGNOSES

The following nursing diagnoses identified by the author are representative of those used in the health care plan of women during postpartum and lactation; however, they by no means constitute a complete list.

- Alteration in parenting related to: conflict of roles; fatigue; poor nutrition; work overload; lack of support of significant others; unrealistic expectations for self, partner, child
- Disturbance in self-concept, maternal role performance, related to: discrepancy between perceived and actual role behaviors; fatigue; inability to achieve self-ideal mothering roles
- Altered family processes: poverty; economic crisis; loss of home

- Ineffective family coping, disabling: rejection; abandonment; abuse
- Altered nutrition, more than body requirements: knowledge deficit regarding components of daily nutritional requirements; lack of storage/cooking facilities
- Compromised family coping related to: lack of support or positive reinforcement for primary caregiver; psychological illness of family member; conflict of roles (mother, career, and wife); fatigue/poor nutrition/work overload; minimal reserves (financial, housing, child care)
- Impaired parenting related to lack of effective role-model
- Impaired home maintenance related to: morbidity of parent (depression); knowledge deficit of management problems and solutions
- Impaired social interaction with infant related to: fatigue, illness; role conflicts; work overload; negative infant behaviors; minimal support of significant others; unwanted pregnancy
- Disturbance in self-concept, maternal role performance, related to: discrepancy between perceived and actual role behaviors; fatigue; inability to achieve self-ideal mothering roles.

## SUPPORT GROUPS

### Breastfeeding Information/ Support Groups

- Ameda/Egnell
  765 Industrial Drive
  Cary, IL 60013 (800) 323–8750
  Breast pumps and breastfeeding accessories
- Gentle Expressions
  Graham–Field
  400 Rabro Drive East
  Hauppauge, NY 11788
  In New York: (800)632–8390
  Outside New York: (800)645–8176
- International Childbirth Educators' Association
  P.O. Box 20852
  Milwaukee, WI 53220
  (414)476–0130
- International Lactation Consultant Organization
  P.O. Box 4031
  University of Virginia Station
  Charlottesville, VA 22903
- La Leche League International
  9616 Minneapolis Avenue Box 1209
  Franklin Park, IL 60131–8209
  (708)455–7730
- Medela, Inc.
  P.O. Box 660
  McHenry, IL 60051–0660
  (800)435–8316
  Breast pumps, breast pump rentals (including double-pumping system), breastfeeding products
- Women, Infants, and Children (WIC) and Food Stamp Programs (administered by local health departments)

### Cesarean Birth Support Groups

- Cesarean Prevention Movement
  P.O. Box 152
  Syracuse, NY 13210
- Cesarean Support Education and Concern
  22 Forest Road
  Framington, MA 01701

### Parenting/Family Support Groups

- Al-Anon Family Group Headquarters
  One Park Ave.
  New York, NY 10016

- Alcoholics Anonymous
  Park Avenue South
  New York, NY 10017
  Resource material and referral service
- Alcoholics Anonymous
  (Gay AA groups)
  P.O. Box 459
  Grand Central Station
  New York, NY 10017
- Alcoholism for Women
  1147 South Alvarado Street
  Los Angeles, CA 90006
  Recovery center with services available to all women who have primary problem with alcohol misuse
- Alliance of Genetic Support Groups
  35 Wisconsin Circle, Suite 440
  Chevy Chase, MD 20815
  (800)336–GENE
- American Council of Blind Parents
  6209 Lycoming Road
  Montgomery, AL 26117
  (205)277–2798
- Association of Birth Defect Children
  3201 East Crystal Lake Avenue
  Orlando, FL 32806
- Association for Maternal and Child Health and Crippled Children's Programs
  P.O. Box 95007
  301 Centennial Mall, South
  Lincoln, NE 68502
- Center for Sickle Cell Disease
  2121 Georgia Avenue, NW
  Washington, DC 20059
- Custody Action for Lesbian Mothers
  P.O. Box 281
  Narbeth, PA 19072
- Down's Syndrome International
  11 North 73rd Terrace, Room K
  Kansas City, KS 66111
  Parent-to-parent counseling and referral
- Fragile X Foundation
  P.O. Box 300233
  Denver, CO 80233
  (800)835–2246 ext. 58
- Fragile X Program
  Duke University
  P.O. Box 3364
  Durham, NC 27710
  (919)684–5513
- Institutes for the Achievement of Human Potential
  8801 Stenton Avenue
  Philadelphia, PA 19118
- International Center for the Disabled
  340 East 24th Street
  New York, NY 10010
- Klinefelter Syndrome & Associates
  P.O. Box 119
  Roseville, CA 95661–0119
  (Enclose stamped, self-addressed envelope)
- Lesbian Mothers' National Defense Fund
  P.O. Box 21567
  Seattle, WA 98112
- Little People of America, Inc.
  P.O. Box 9897
  Washington, DC 20016
- National Association for Gay and Lesbian Alcoholism Professionals
  204 West 20th Street
  New York, NY 10011
  (212)713–5074
- National Center for Lesbian Rights
  1663 Mission Street
  San Francisco, CA 94103
  (415)621–0674
  Nonprofit, public interest law firm dedicated to preserving and increasing the legal rights of lesbians and gay men

- National Center on Child Abuse and Neglect
  Department of Health & Human Services
  U.S. Children's Bureau/NCCAN
  P.O. Box 1182
  Washington, DC 20013
  Information on programs in individual states, publications, and training materials
- National Domestic Violence Hotline
  (800)333–7233
  Makes referrals to lesbian or lesbian-friendly support and shelter services
- National Gay and Lesbian Task Force (NGLTF)
  1734 14th Street NW
  Washington, DC 20009
  (202)332–6483
- National Information Center for Handicapped Children and Youth
  Box 1492
  Washington, DC 20013
- Neurofibromatosis, Inc.
  3401 Woodridge Court
  Mitchellville, MD 20721–2817
  (301)577–8984
- Parents Anonymous
  22330 Hawthorne Boulevard, Suite 208
  Torrance, CA 90505
- Parents of Down Syndrome Children
  11600 Nebel Street
  Rockville, MD 20852
- Parents of Prematures
  13613 Northeast 26th Place
  Bellevue, WA 98005
- Parents of Premature & High-Risk Infants International
  33 West 42nd Street, Room 1127
  New York, NY 10036
  Provides education and directory of support groups
- Spina Bifida Association
  4590 MacArthur Boulevard, Suite 250
  Washington, DC 20007
  (800)621–3141
- Support Organization for Trisomy
  478 Terrace Lane
  Tooele, UT 84074
- Twin Line
  P.O. Box 10066
  Berkeley, CA 94709
  (415)644–0861
- Your Twins/NOMOT (National Organization of Mothers of Twins Clubs, Inc)
  5402 Amberwood Lane
  Rockville, MD 20853
  (301)460–9108

### Postpartum Depression Support Groups

- Depression after Delivery (D.A.D.)
  P.O. Box 1282
  Morrisville, PA 19067
  (212)295–3394
- Postpartum Support International
  927 North Kellogg Avenue
  Santa Barbara, CA 93111
  (206)881–6580 or (805)682–7529

### Perinatal Loss Support Groups

- National Sudden Infant Death Syndrome Foundation
  Two Metro Plaza, Suite 205
  8240 Professional Place
  Landover, MD 20785
- The Compassionate Friends
  P.O. Box 3696
  Oak Brook, IL 60522–3696
  (708)990–0010
- International Council for Infant Survival
  P.O. Box 3841
  Davenport, IA 52808

Offers consolation and information to members of families who have lost a child to sudden infant death syndrome and who may blame themselves for the death

- Resolve Through Sharing
  La Crosse Lutheran Hospital
  1910 South Avenue
  La Crosse, WI 54601
  (608)785–0530 ext. 3693

## REFERENCES


1. Sampselle, C., & Brink, C. (1990, May/June). Pelvic muscle relaxation: Assessment and management. *Journal of Nurse Midwifery, 35*(3), 127–132.
2. Hatcher, R., Stewart, F., Trussell, J., & Kowal, D. (1990). Combined oral contraceptives. In *Contraceptive technology* (15th ed., pp. 227–299). New York: Irvington.
3. Lethbridge, D. (1989, Jan./Feb.). Use of breast feeding as a contraceptive. *Journal of Obstetric, Gynecologic, and Neonatal Nursing 18*(1), 31–37.
4. Chez, R.A., Coustan, D.R., Gabbe, S.G., & Langer, O. (1989, September). Meeting the challenge of gestational diabetes. *Contemporary Obstetrics and Gynecology, 34*(3), 120–122, 125–126, 128, 131, 135–136, 138, 140.
5. American Diabetes Association. (1991, March). Office guide to diagnosis and classification of diabetes mellitus and other categories of glucose intolerance. *Diabetes Care, 14*(Suppl. 2), 3–4.
6. Luegenbiehl, D.L. (1991). Postpartum bleeding. In D. Wooley Perlis (ed.), *Bleeding in women,* Vol. 2(3): *NAACOG's clinical issues in perinatal and women's health nursing* (pp. 402–409). Philadelphia: Lippincott.
7. Cunningham, F.G., MacDonald, P., & Gant, N. (1992). Other disorders of the puerperium. In *Williams obstetrics* (19th ed., pp. 643–659). Norwalk, CT: Appleton & Lange.
8. Star, W.L., Shannon, M.T., Sammons, L.N., Lommel, L.L., & Gutierrez, Y. (1990). *Ambulatory obstetrics: protocols for nurse practitioners/nurse midwives* (2nd ed.). San Francisco: University of California.
9. Lawrence, R. (1989). *Breastfeeding: A guide for the medical profession* (3rd ed.). St. Louis: C. V. Mosby.
10. NAACOG. (1991, Nov.). Facilitating breastfeeding. *OGN nursing practice resource.* Washington, DC: NAACOG.
11. Cunningham, F.G., MacDonald, P., & Gant, N. (1993). Puerperal infections. In *Williams Obstetrics* (19th ed., pp. 627–642). Norwalk, CT: Appleton & Lange.
12. Soper, D. (1988, Jan.). Postpartum endometritis: Pathophysiology and prevention. *Journal of Reproductive Medicine, 33* (1, Suppl.), 97–100.
13. Brennan, D.F. (1989, Jan.). Postpartum abdominal pain. *Annals of Emergency Medicine, 18*(1), 83–89.
14. Heath, G.C. (1988, Nov.). Postpartum thyroiditis. *Journal of the National Medical Association, 80*(11), 1231–1232, 1235.
15. Affonso, D., Andreyko, J., & Mills, K. (1987, September/October). Postpartum thyroiditis: A new challenge in nurse midwifery. *Journal of Nurse Midwifery, 32*(5), 308–316.
16. Evans, C. (1991, March/April). Description of a home follow-up program for childbearing families. *Journal of Obstetric, Gynecologic, and Neonatal Nursing, 20*(2), 113–118.
17. Barnard, K. (1978). *Learning resource manual.* Seattle: University of Washington, Nursing Child Assessment Satellite Training.
18. Mercer, R.T. (1983). Parent–infant attachment. In L. Sonstegard, K. Kowalski, & B. Jennings (eds.), *Women's health,* Vol. II: *Childbearing.* (pp. 17–42). New York: Grune & Stratton.
19. Cranley, M.S. (1981). Roots of attachment: The relationship of parents with their unborn. In *Birth defects: Original article series* (Vol. 17(6), pp. 59–82). White Plains, NY: March of Dimes Birth Defects Foundation.
20. Cropley, C. (1986). Assessment of mothering behaviors. In S. H. Johnson (ed.), *Nursing assessment and strategies for the family at risk* (2nd ed., pp. 15–40). Philadelphia: Lippincott.

21. Davis, M., & Akridge, K. (1987, Nov./Dec.). The effect of promoting intrauterine attachment in primiparas on postpartum attachment. *Journal of Obstetric, Gynecologic, and Neonatal Nursing, 16*(6), 430–437.
22. Mercer, R.T. (1985, July/Aug.). Process of maternal role attainment over the first year. *Nursing Research, 34*(4), 198–204.
23. Mercer, R. (1990). *Parents at risk.* New York: Springer.
24. Mercer, R.T. & Ferketich, S. (1990, March). Predictors of parental attachment during early parenthood. *Journal of Advanced Nursing, 15*(3), 268–280.
25. Klaus, M., & Kennell, J. (1983). Adjusting to malformation. In *Bonding: The beginnings of parent–infant attachment* (pp. 140–161). St. Louis: C. V. Mosby.
26. Merilo, K. (1988, May–June). Is it better the second time around? *MCN, 13*(3), 200–204.
27. Sammons, L.N. (1990). Psychological aspects of second pregnancy. In S. Flagler (ed.), *Psychological aspects of pregnancy,* Vol. 1(3): *NAACOG's clinical issues in perinatal and women's health care* (pp. 317–324). Philadelphia: Lippincott.
28. Cunningham, F.G., MacDonald, P., & Gant, N. (1993). The puerperium. In *Williams Obstetrics* (19th ed., pp. 459–473). Norwalk, CT: Appleton & Lange.
29. Zeidenstein, L. (1990, Jan./Feb.). Gynecological and childbearing needs of lesbians. *Journal of Nurse Midwifery, 35*(1), 10–18.
30. Harvey, S.M., Carr, C., & Bernheine, S. (1989, May/June). Lesbian mothers: health care experiences. *Journal of Nurse Midwifery, 34*(3), 115–119.
31. Boston Women's Health Book Collective. (1992). *The new our bodies, ourselves: A book by and for women.* New York: Touchstone.
32. Bastin, N., Tamayo, O.W., Tinkle, M., Amaya, M.A., Trejo, L.R., & Herrera, C. (1992, March/April). HIV disease in pregnancy: Part 3. Postpartum Care of the HIV-positive woman and her newborn. *Journal of Obstetric, Gynecologic, and Neonatal Nursing, 21*(2), 105–111.
33. Efantis, J. (1990). In-patient maternity care for the HIV-positive woman and her newborn. In B.P. Sinclair & A.M. McCormick (eds.), *AIDS in women,* Vol. 1(1): *NAACOG's clinical issues in perinatal and women's health care* (pp. 47–52). Philadelphia: Lippincott.
34. Robert Wood Johnson Foundation. (1991). *Challenges in health care: A chartbook perspective 1991* (pp. 80–81). Princeton, NJ: Author.
35. Bachrach, L.L. (1987). Homeless women: A context for health care. *The Milbank Quarterly, 65*(3), 371–396.
36. Drake, M.A. (1992, May–June). The nutritional status and dietary adequacy of single homeless women and their children in shelters. *Public Health Reports, 107*(3), 312–319.
37. Wiecha, J.L., Dwyer, J.T., & Dunn-Strohecker, M. (1991, July–August). Nutrition and health services needs among the homeless. *Public Health Reports, 106*(4), 364–374.
38. Casiano, M.E. (1990). Outpatient management of postpartum psychiatric disorders. In D.M. Semprevivo (ed.), *Postpartum depression,* Vol. 1(3): *NAACOG's clinical issues in perinatal and women's health* (pp. 395–401). Philadelphia: Lippincott.
39. Hansen, C. (1990). Baby blues: Identification and intervention. In D.M. Semprevivo (ed.), *Postpartum depression,* Vol. 1 (3): *NAACOG's clinical issues in perinatal and women's health nursing* (pp. 369–374). Philadelphia: Lippincott.
40. Boyer, D. (1990). Prediction of postpartum depression. In D.M. Semprevivo (ed.), *Postpartum depression,* Vol. 1(3): *NAACOG's clinical issues in perinatal and women's health nursing* (pp. 359–368). Philadelphia: Lippincott.
41. Hamilton, J. A. (1989, March). Postpartum psychiatric syndromes. *Psychiatric Clinics of North America, 12*(1), 89–103.
42. Kumar, R. (1990). An overview of postpartum psychiatric disorders. In D.M. Semprevivo (ed.), *Postpartum depression:* Vol. 1(3): *NAACOG's clinical issues in perinatal and women's health nursing* (pp. 351–358). Philadelphia: Lippincott.
43. Theesen, K., Alderson, M., & Hill, W. (1989, Feb.). Caring for the depressed obstetric pa-

tient. *Contemporary Obstetrics and Gynecology, 33*(2), 123–126, 129.

44. Harris, B., Huckle, P., Thomas, R., Johns, S., & Fung, H. (1989). The use of rating scales to identify postnatal depression. *British Journal of Psychiatry, 154,* 813–817.
45. Hannah, P., Adams, D., Lee, A., Glover, V., & Sandler, M. (1992, June). Links between early postpartum mood and postnatal depression. *British Journal of Psychiatry, 160,* 777–780.
46. Cunningham, F.G., MacDonald, N.G., & Gant, N. (1993). Obstetrics in broad perspective. In *Williams Obstetrics* (19th ed., pp. 1–9). Norwalk, CT: Appleton & Lange.
47. Rubin, R. (1984). *Maternal identity and the maternal experience.* New York: Springer.
48. U.S. Bureau of the Census. (1991). *Statistical Abstract of the United States* (111th ed., p. 77). Washington, DC.
49. Robert Wood Johnson Foundation. (1991). *Challenges in health care: a chartbook perspective 1991* (pp. 27–38). Princeton, NJ: Author.
50. Arnold, L., Brecht, M., Hackett, A., Amspacher, K., & Grad, R. (1989, March /April). Lessons from the past. *MCN, 14*(2), 75, 78, 80, 82.
51. Lynch, M. (1989, March/April). Congenital defects: Parental issues and nursing supports. *Journal of Perinatal and Neonatal Nursing, 2*(4), 53–59.
52. Limbo, R., & Wheeler, S.R. (1986). *When a baby dies: A handbook for healing and helping.* LaCrosse: Gunderson Clinic, Ltd.
53. Cunningham, F.G., MacDonald, P., & Gant, N. (1993). Abortion. In *Williams Obstetrics* (19th ed., pp. 661–690). Norwalk, CT: Appleton & Lange.
54. Kennell, J., Slyter, H., & Klaus, M. (1970). The mourning responses of parents to the death of a newborn infant. *New England Journal of Medicine, 283*(7), 344–349.
55. Limbo, R., & Wheeler, S.R. (1986). Coping with unexpected outcomes. In *NAACOG Update Series,* (Vol. 5, Lesson 3). Princeton, NJ: Continuing Professional Education Center.
56. Szgalsky, J. (1989, Oct.). Perinatal death, the family, and the role of the health professional. *Neonatal Network, 8*(2), 15–19.
57. Kovar, M.G., Serdula, M.K., Marks, J.S., Fraser, D.W. (1984). Review of the epidemiologic evidence for an association between infant feeding and infant health. *Pediatrics, 74,* 615–638.
58. Kramer, M.S. (1988, Jan.). Infant feeding, infection, and public health. *Pediatrics, 81*(1), 164–166.
59. Newman, J. (1990, Feb.). Breastfeeding problems associated with the early introduction of bottles and pacifiers. *Journal of Human Lactation, 6*(2), 59–63.
60. Guyton, A. (1982). Pregnancy, lactation, and fetal and neonatal physiology. In *Human physiology and mechanisms of disease* (3rd ed., pp. 648–664). Philadelphia: W. B. Saunders.
61. Shrago, L. (1990, May/June). The infant's contribution to breastfeeding. *Journal of Obstetric, Gynecologic, and Neonatal Nursing, 19*(3), 209–215.
62. Mohrbacher, N., & Stock, J. (1991, Aug.). *The breastfeeding answer book.* Franklin Park, IL: La Leche League International.
63. Schulz-Lell, G., Buss, R., Oldigs, H-D, Dörner, K. & Schaub, J. (1987, July). Iron balances in infant nutrition. *ACTA Paediatrica Scandinavica, 76*(4), 585–591.
64. Speroff, L., Glass, R.H., & Kase, N.G. (1989). The breast. In *Clinical gynecologic endocrinology and infertility,* (4th ed., pp. 283–315). Baltimore: Williams & Wilkins.
65. Cohen, M., & Cohen, H. (1990, Nov.). Current recommendations for viral hepatitis. *Contemporary Obstetrics and Gynecology, 35*(11), 56–58, 61, 65–70, 72, 74–75, 79.
66. Fekety, S. (1989, Sept./Oct.). Managing the HIV-positive patient and her newborn in a CNM service. *Journal of Nurse Midwifery, 34*(5), 253–358.
67. American College of Obstetricians and Gynecologists. (1992, June). *Human immunodeficiency virus infections* (Technical Bulletin No. 169). Washington, DC: Author.
68. Niebyl, S. (1986, Sept.). Making the breastfeeding decision. *Contemporary Obstetrics and Gynecology, 28*(3), 43–44, 46, 51–52, 54.
69. Sollid, D., Evans, B., McClowry, S., & Gar-

rett, A. (1989, July). Breastfeeding multiples. *Journal of Perinatal and Neonatal Nursing, 3*(1), 46–65.

70. Beal, M. (1987, Feb.). Breastfeeding: Some drug admonitions. *Contemporary Obstetrics and Gynecology, 29*(2), 49–52, 54.
71. Toll, L. (1990, June). A review of the new AAP guidelines of drugs and human milk. *Journal of Human Lactation, 6*(2), 73–74.
72. Bronner, Y.L., & Paige, D.M. (1992, March/April). Current concepts in infant nutrition. *Journal of Nurse-Midwifery, 37*(2, Suppl.), 43S–58S.
73. Hansen, B., & Moore, L. (1989, Dec.). Recreational drug use by the breastfeeding woman. *Journal of Human Lactation, 5*(4), 178–180.
74. Zinamon, M.J. (1987, October). Breast pumps: Ensuring mothers' success. *Contemporary Obstetrics and Gynecology, 30*(Special Issue), 55–57, 60–62.
75. Walker, M. (1987, July–Aug.). How to evaluate breast pumps. *MCN, 12*(4), 270–276.
76. Auerbach, K. (1990, Jan./Feb.). Assisting the employed breast-feeding mother. *Journal of Nurse Midwifery, 35*(1), 26–34.

# PRIMARY CARE PROBLEMS AFFECTING WOMEN'S HEALTH

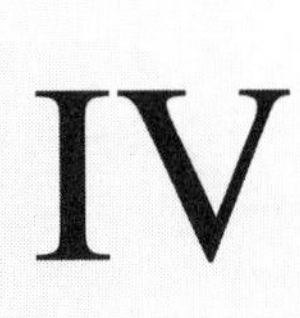

CHAPTER 17

# MEDICAL PROBLEMS IN PRIMARY CARE

*Linda C. Hancock • Patricia M. Selig*

*Among women with a urinary tract infection, 80 percent will have another within the year.*

### *Highlights*

- Anemia
- Cardiac Disease
- Gastrointestinal Disease
- Headache
- Respiratory Infections
- Skin Cancer
- Thyroid Dysfunction
- Urinary Tract Infections

## INTRODUCTION

It is beyond the scope of this book to address all medical problems seen in clinical practice. Those that are included were chosen for their clinical significance to women or because of their frequency in the general population. The provider is encouraged to consult chapter references for guidance in finding more in-depth information.

The provider's level of comfort and competence in managing medical problems is dependent on her or his experience, medical resources, location of practice, access to diagnostic testing, practice protocols, and scope of practice.

## ANEMIA

Anemia is a *sign* of an *underlying* problem; it is not a diagnosis. Identifying anemia is the beginning of a workup, much as identifying a fever is the start of a diagnostic workup. Correcting the anemia may be of little importance compared with finding its cause.[1]

In general, anemia is defined either as a reduction in red blood cell (RBC) volume measured by hematocrit (Hct) or a decrease in the percent concentration of hemoglobin (Hgb) in the peripheral blood. The World Health Organization defines anemia in women as a hemoglobin less than 12 g/dL and in pregnant women as a hemoglobin less than 11 g/dL.[1,2] Clinical practice sites and laboratories may vary in their parameters.[3]

Laboratory values may be affected by age, sex, altitude, smoking, and hydration state. Beware of "spurious anemia" caused by hemodilution during pregnancy and congestive heart failure. Look at the individual's clinical picture.[2] All blood cell types (RBCs, white blood cells [WBCs], and platelets) are derived from the pluripotent stem cells in the marrow. Pancytopenia, or a decrease in all cell types—WBCs (leukopenia), RBCs (anemia), and platelets (thrombocytopenia)—requires referral to a hematologist.[2,4]

Three mechanisms cause anemia: blood loss; decreased red cell production, usually as a result of insufficient building supplies such as iron, vitamin $B_{12}$, and folate; and increased red cell destruction (hemolysis). To determine the mechanism, ask the following three questions.[2]

*What Is the Mean Corpuscular Volume?* Mean corpuscular volume (MCV) is one of three RBC indices and indicates blood cell size. Normal MCV is approximately 80 to 100 fL. According to the MCV, anemias are categorized as microcytic, normocytic, or macrocytic (see Table 17–1).

*What Is the Reticulocyte Count?* Reticulocytes are immature RBCs that retain nuclear particles for 24 hours after leaving the marrow. Normally, reticulocytes constitute about 1 to 1.5% of circulating RBCs.[5] Increased reticulocyte count (>3%) may be an indication of rapid bleeding or hemolysis as the body attempts to replenish lost RBCs. Reticulocyte counts less than 1 percent may indicate nutritional deficiencies or marrow dysfunction.[5,6]

*What Is the Clinical Picture?* Based on the client's demographic characteristics and problem list, certain types of anemia would be suspected (see Table 17–2).

Among the many types of anemia (most of them rare), three account for approximately 90 percent of the anemias in the United States. They are iron-deficiency anemia (IDA), thalassemia, and the anemia of chronic diseases (ACD).[7]

## IRON-DEFICIENCY ANEMIA

Iron-deficiency anemia can be caused by inadequate dietary intake of iron or by loss of iron through bleeding. Because the body aggressively recycles iron, adults with reasonable nutrition do not experience deficits. Nutritional inadequacies occur primarily in infants, children, and pregnant women. In a woman who is not pregnant, blood loss is assumed to be the cause of iron-deficiency anemia.[5,7] In premenopausal women, menstruation is the primary cause of blood loss. In postmenopausal women and in men, IDA is

**TABLE 17–1. DIFFERENTIAL DIAGNOSES OF ANEMIA BY ERYTHROCYTE MORPHOLOGY**

| Microcytic Anemia (MCV[a] <80) | Macrocytic Anemia (MCV >100) | Normocytic Anemia (MCV 80–100) |
|---|---|---|
| Iron deficiency | $B_{12}$ deficiency | Anemia of chronic disease[b] |
| Thalassemias | Folate deficiency | Endocrinopathy |
| Anemia of chronic disease[a] | Liver disease | Hemolysis |
| Sideroblastic | Alcoholism | Myeloma |
| Aluminum toxicity | Myelodysplastic syndromes | Renal disease |
| | Marked reticulocytosis | Sideroblastic[a] anemia |
| | Spurious anemia | Bleeding |
| | | Aplastic anemia |

[a] Mean corpuscular volume.
[b] Some overlap can occur depending on stage of disease.
Sources: *References 2, 5, 6.*

**TABLE 17–2. DIFFERENTIAL DIAGNOSIS SUGGESTED BY CLINICAL PICTURE**

| | |
|---|---|
| Female | Iron deficiency |
| Race | |
| Blacks | G6PD[a], thalassemia, hemoglobinopathies |
| Mediterranean origin | G6PD, thalassemia |
| Southeast Asians | Hemoglobinopathies (e.g., –HgB E) |
| Infections | G6PD, immune hemolysis |
| Thyroid disease | IDA, pernicious anemia |
| Alcoholism | Bleeding, folate deficiency, IDA, sideroblastic anemia, hemolysis, hypersplenism |
| Renal failure | Decreased production, hemolysis, bleeding |
| Connective tissue disorders | Anemia of chronic diseases, IDA, hemolysis |
| Cancer | Anemia of chronic diseases, hemolysis |
| Lead exposure | Sideroblastic anemias, IDA |
| Drugs | |
| Sulfa | G6PD |
| Dilantin | Megaloblastic anemia (folate), pure red cell aplasia |
| Antitubercular drugs | Sideroblastic anemia |
| Gold | Aplastic anemia |

[a]G6PD, glucose-6-phosphate dehydrogenase deficiency; IDA, iron-deficiency anemia.
Sources: *References 2, 5.*

presumed to result from occult gastrointestinal blood loss (rule out colon cancer) until proven otherwise.[1,2,5,7]

## Epidemiology

Studies reveal that IDA among pregnant women is caused by nutritional deficits, and among nonpregnant women, primarily by blood loss. Risk factors for bleeding include frequent heavy menses, miscarriages, abortions, deliveries, and surgeries. On average, women lose about 50 mL of blood per month as a result of menses; women with heavy menses may lose five times this amount. Oral contraceptive use decreases menstrual blood flow 30 to 60 percent and thus protects against IDA. Progestin-containing contraceptive devices may also decrease blood loss.[3] Risk factors for occult bleeding include a family history of colon cancer or hemolytic anemias.[2]

Incidence reports show that IDA is the most common nutritional disorder in the world. It is seen primarily in children; however, it is estimated to occur in 20 percent of adult women, 50 percent of pregnant women, and 3 percent of adult men.[5]

## Subjective Data

Subjective data vary for premenopausal and postmenopausal women. Premenopausal women report heavy or frequent menses. Acute loss of large volumes of blood may cause the sudden onset of shortness of breath, faintness, thirst, weakness, and rapid pulse. More commonly, however, blood loss is slow and subtle, especially in postmenopausal women. In that manner, the body is able to adjust to the gradual decrease in RBCs; no symptoms develop until the hemoglobin is 6 to 8 g/dL. In severe chronic cases, symptoms may include fatigue, dysphagia, sore tongue or mouth, and pica.

History-taking should focus on sources of blood loss or hemolysis. Ask about blood donations, recent surgeries, melena (rectal bleeding), family history of colon cancer, medications, diet, smoking, alcohol use, previous anemia, and splenectomy.[1,5]

## Objective Data

***Physical Examination.*** May reveal nothing abnormal. Occasionally, however, signs of anemia may be detected.

- *General appearance.* Fatigue, tachypnea.
- *Vital signs.* Increased pulse and respirations; may be orthostatic, with decreased blood pressure on standing.
- *Skin.* Pallor, tenting, pale palpebral conjunctiva, nails with spooning, separation, and ridges.
- *Mouth.* Angular stomatitis (sores at corners of mouth), cheilosis (red, sore lips), glossitis (beefy red tongue consistent with vitamin $B_{12}$ deficiency).
- *Chest.* Rapid respiratory rate, rales.
- *Heart.* Flow murmurs, tachycardia.
- *Abdomen.* Splenomegaly (hemolysis), hepatomegaly (liver disease, alcoholism), masses (colon cancer).
- *Pelvic exam.* Rule out mass.
- *Rectal exam.* Rule out mass, guaiac stool.
- *Central nervous system.* Altered mental status (rule out lead poisoning and vitamin $B_{12}$ dementia), paresthesia (pernicious anemia).[1,2,5]

***Diagnostic Tests.*** Performed in stages; avoid the expensive shotgun approach to ordering tests. Initial tests help support diagnosis; later tests, after treatment has begun, confirm the diagnosis.2,6

Initial laboratory tests include a baseline complete blood cell count (CBC) with indices (MCV, mean corpuscular hemoglobin [MCH], mean corpuscular hemoglobin concentration [MCHC]) and reticulocyte count. A fecal test for occult blood is done on the basis of the clinical picture.[2,5,6]

Initial findings are evaluated. If data reveal microcytic (MCV < 80), hypochromic anemia with a low reticulocyte count, the diagnosis is most likely IDA. Confirm the diagnosis prior to treatment by ordering an iron panel, which usually comprises a serum iron, total iron binding capacity (TIBC), and percent saturation. Also order a serum ferritin test. (*Note:* Iron-deficiency anemia usually occurs gradually. Consequently, laboratory values change slowly over time. The continuum of change begins with decreased serum ferritin and progresses to decreased serum iron, increased TIBC with decreased percent saturation, and finally to decreased MCV and hemoglobin [indices usually are normal until hemoglobin is 10 g/dL].[2,5])

Consult the physician if laboratory data are not consistent with the clinical picture or the hematocrit is less than 25%/dL. Also plan consultation if the client has a positive stool guaiac, history of bleeding, or family history of anemia, or if you suspect underlying chronic disease.[1]

Follow-up tests are crucial to ensure that the diagnosis is correct and that anemia is resolving with treatment. At 1 week, the reticulocyte count should increase 5 to 10 percent; at 1 month, the hemoglobin should increase 2 points; at 2 to 3 months, all normal levels should be reached. Iron is continued another 3 months or more.[1,2,5]

## Differential Medical Diagnosis

See Tables 17–1 and 17–2.

## Plan

***Psychosocial Interventions.*** Reassure the client with iron-deficiency anemia secondary to menses or pregnancy that her condition is common. Advise her that it takes at least 6 months to completely refill iron stores. Stress the importance of follow-up laboratory tests to confirm the diagnosis. Encourage compliance with oral iron and dietary measures. If the client is postmenopausal, explain the need for further testing to locate the source of blood loss.[2,5]

***Medication.*** Ferrous sulfate is given once iron-deficiency anemia has been documented and confirmed by laboratory tests.

- *Administration.* A 325-mg tablet is taken three times a day, with orange juice, for a minimum of 6 months.[1,2]

- *Side Effects.* The most frequent are gastrointestinal: nausea, constipation, and black stools. The difficulty tolerating iron may be minimized if the client consumes the dose with food, starting slowly with one tablet per day and increasing as tolerated.
- *Contraindications.* Do not administer iron if a deficiency has not been documented by laboratory tests. Iron overload can be fatal and hard to reverse. Mistakenly treating other types of anemia, such as sideroblastic anemia and anemia of chronic diseases, with iron can lead to overload and death.[2,5]
- *Client Teaching.* After diagnosis, explain to the client that follow-up and treatment will continue for about 6 months. Stress the importance of obtaining follow-up laboratory tests at 1 and 3 months and continuing medications as ordered. Advise the client to keep iron out of the reach of children.

***Dietary Interventions.*** The diet should include foods high in iron: lean meats, egg yolk, shellfish, leafy greens, raisins, and dried apricots and peaches. Advise the client to avoid taking iron with tea and antacids.[1,3]

The iron supplement contained in multivitamins (18 mg iron) will not correct iron-deficiency anemia but will help prevent recurrences of the problem in menstruating women. The average American diet contains 10 to 15 mg of iron per day; only about 1 to 2 mg per day is absorbed. Dietary measures alone are usually insufficient to correct the iron losses from heavy menstruation. Generic one-a-day multivitamins with iron are a reasonable approach to avoiding IDA in otherwise healthy women, but will not correct an anemia.[3]

***Follow-Up.*** All clients should be retested to confirm the IDA diagnosis and to determine if the anemia is improving. (As stated earlier, after 1 month with adequate treatment the hemoglobin should increase 2 points; at 2 to 3 months the ultimate goal of the hemoglobin within normal range should be reached. Iron supplementation is continued for 3 months thereafter.) If the client is compliant, yet no improvement occurs, reconsider the diagnosis and refer her to a physician for further evaluation.[1,2,5]

## THALASSEMIA

Thalassemia encompasses a group of hereditary anemias in which synthesis of one or both chains of the hemoglobin molecule (α and β) is defective. A low hemoglobin level and a microcytic, hypochromic anemia result. Individuals who are heterozygous for α- or β-thalassemia have *thalassemia minor;* those who are homozygous have *thalassemia major.* β-Thalassemia major (Cooley's anemia) is a fatal condition that results in the deaths of more than 100,000 children worldwide each year.[7] The most severe form of α-thalassemia major results in hydrops fetalis syndrome.

### Epidemiology

In the United States, β-thalassemia minor occurs primarily among African-Americans and persons of Mediterranean descent. α-Thalassemia occurs primarily among Southeast Asians. Its transmission is genetic. β-Thalassemia minor is a silent "carrier" state in which the individual fails to produce a β hemoglobin chain. The body compensates by selectively producing hemoglobin $A_2$, which does not require a β chain.[2,8] α-Thalassemia minor is a more benign state and more difficult to diagnose, as hemoglobin $A_2$ does not increase and other confirmatory tests are not readily available for adults.[2,10]

### Subjective Data

Thalassemia minor is an asymptomatic condition, diagnosed inadvertently primarily by abnormal laboratory findings.

### Objective Data

Physical examination reveals nothing abnormal.

A routine CBC will indicate a combined extremely low MCV (usually less than 65 fL) and only a slightly decreased hemoglobin (usually between 10 and 12 g/dL).[2,10]

Hemoglobin electrophoresis can confirm a diagnosis of β-thalassemia because of the increased level of hemoglobin $A_2$; the test cannot confirm α-thalassemia. The clinical picture and other laboratory results must be evaluated.

The test for α-thalassemia is not easily available. If, however, a client has a clinical picture consistent with β-thalassemia trait (very low MCV and mild anemia) yet hemoglobin electrophoresis does not show an increase in hemoglobin $A_2$, suspect the α-thalassemia trait. Refer the client for genetic counseling.

### Differential Medical Diagnosis

See Table 17–1.

### Plan

***Psychosocial Interventions.*** Make the appropriate genetic counseling referral and support the client as she makes decisions regarding childbearing. Reassure her that she is not "sick" and does not need lifelong treatment for anemia.

***Medication.*** None is required. Caution the client that blindly and constantly supplementing her diet with iron tablets is dangerous and a needless expense.[2,8]

## ANEMIA OF CHRONIC DISEASES

Anemia of chronic diseases (ACD) is a common but poorly understood condition. It is seen in clients with cancer or chronic inflammatory disorders, such as lupus and rheumatoid arthritis. Despite adequate iron supplies, the body cannot use its stored iron. Red blood cells may be normocytic or microcytic; no uniform hematologic picture can be outlined.[7]

### Epidemiology

The cause of anemia of chronic diseases is unknown, although it is associated with chronic inflammatory conditions.

### Subjective Data

The condition is usually asymptomatic. When anemia becomes severe, symptoms relative to the coexisting chronic disease may exacerbate. In addition, symptoms of anemia, such as fatigue and shortness of breath, may be present.

### Objective Data

For information on the physical examination, see Iron Deficiency Anemia.

No specific diagnostic tests are conclusive; the anemia is primarily a diagnosis of exclusion. A CBC may reveal normocytic or microcytic anemia; however, no consistent pattern is found in other tests. The serum ferritin is usually adequate. For diagnosis, refer to a physician.

### Differential Medical Diagnosis

See Table 17–1.

### Plan

***Psychosocial Interventions.*** Support the client in dealing with chronic illness.

***Medication.*** None is required. Caution the client to avoid taking iron unless prescribed: excess intake may cause iron overload.[8] Ask the client if she is taking a nonsteroidal anti-inflammatory drug. Gastrointestinal bleeding and subsequent iron deficiency may confuse the clinical picture.

***Follow-Up.*** Consultation with a physician is necessary for all clients with ACD. If anemia is severe, refer the client to a hematologist.

## LESS COMMON ANEMIAS

Less common types of anemia may need to be identified. They may be caused by dietary deficiencies or genetic defects.

*Glucose-6-phosphate dehydrogenase deficiency* (G6PD deficiency), which is inherited, causes a hemolytic anemia. The enzyme protects RBCs against breakdown by free oxygen. Until an acute hemolytic episode is triggered, the client remains asymptomatic. Hemolysis can be precipitated by viral or bacterial infections or by certain oxidizing drugs.

Glucose-6-phosphate dehydrogenase deficiency is usually discovered accidentally; for example, a pregnant woman who is followed with serial hematocrits may be diagnosed when a marked anemia develops after treatment with an antibiotic, such as sulfa. If hemolysis is severe, she is referred to a hematologist. The woman is instructed to avoid aspirin, sulfa, nitrofurantoin, primaquine, phenacetin, and some vitamin K derivatives.[2,8]

Glucose-6-phosphate dehydrogenase deficiency is seen primarily in African-Americans and persons of Mediterranean descent.[2,9]

*Sickle cell anemia* and *sickle trait* are caused by various genetic defects in hemoglobin chains. Sickle cell disease (Hgb SS) occurs in 0.25 percent of African-Americans, and sickle cell trait (Hgb AS), among 8 percent of African-Americans. Occasionally, sickle cell trait occurs in persons of Mediterranean, Arabian, or East Indian descent.

Most often persons with sickle trait are asymptomatic; occasionally, however, episodes of hematuria, increased bacteriuria, and pyelonephritis during pregnancy are associated with sickle trait. Hemoglobin electrophoresis is used in diagnosis. Test results indicating sickle trait show 25 to 40 percent hemoglobin S and the remainder hemoglobin A with small amounts of hemoglobins F and $A_2$.[2] Management consists primarily of documenting the condition, encouraging genetic counseling, and reassuring the woman that sickle trait is benign.[2]

A discussion of sickle cell disease is beyond the scope of this chapter.

*Anemia caused by vitamin $B_{12}$ deficiency* is megaloblastic, most often caused by pernicious anemia and occasionally by gastrointestinal disorders that result in gastrectomy. Lack of dietary vitamin $B_{12}$ is rarely a problem, as body stores last 3 to 5 years. Vitamin $B_{12}$ absorption, however, may be affected. It requires the intrinsic factor produced by the stomach lining and an intact ileum, where absorption actually occurs. Pernicious anemia is an autoimmune disorder that usually becomes symptomatic around age 60 when the stomach is unable to produce intrinsic factor; as a result, the small intestine is unable to absorb vitamin $B_{12}$. The "classic triad" of vitamin $B_{12}$ deficiency includes weakness, sore tongue, and paresthesias (particularly loss of vibratory sense). The Schilling test is used for diagnosis. Treatment involves monthly vitamin $B_{12}$ injections.[2,10]

*Folate deficiency,* related primarily to inadequate nutrition, may cause a megaloblastic anemia. Folate does not accumulate in the body; therefore, the anemia is more common than that caused by vitamin $B_{12}$ deficiency. Folate deficiency most commonly occurs during pregnancy and among alcoholics. Lab work reveals a megaloblastic anemia (MCV $> 100$) and a decreased folate level. Diagnosis is confirmed by an appropriate clinical response to administration of folic acid, usually 1 mg per day. Management should also address the underlying condition, such as alcoholism. Sources of folic acid (leafy vegetables, fruits, nuts, and liver) should be increased in the diet. Certain drugs, for example, dilantin and trimethoprim, inhibit folate absorption.[11] It is interesting to note that the macrocytic anemias caused by vitamin $B_{12}$ and folate deficiency can cause false-positive Pap smears. Abnormal Pap smears should be repeated after adequate treatment with vitamin $B_{12}$ or folic acid.[2,5]

# CARDIAC DISEASE

The four cardiac diseases considered in this chapter are coronary artery disease, hyperlipidemia, hypertension, and mitral valve prolapse.

## CORONARY ARTERY DISEASE

Coronary artery disease (CAD) is caused by altered blood flow in the coronary arteries and, consequently, reduced oxygenation of the myocardium. Myocardial ischemia occurs when oxygen demand exceeds oxygen supply. The supply–demand balance may be disturbed by coronary atherosclerosis, vasospasm, thrombus formation, or cardiomyopathy.

### Epidemiology

Coronary artery disease was once considered a male affliction, although women are now recognized to be at equal and, in some circumstances, greater risk.[12] Men and women, however, may differ in the onset, distribution, and presentation of disease.

***Modifiable Risk Factors.*** Factors that may influence the development of CAD include cigarette smoking, obesity, physical inactivity, hypertension, and hyperlipidemia.

Cigarette smoking is largely responsible for cardiovascular events in premenopausal women.[13] It increases the risk of CAD two to three times that of a nonsmoker, but the risk is reversible within a year of cessation of smoking. Smoking low-tar and low-nicotine cigarettes does not reduce the risk of cardiovascular events. With the substantial increase in the number of women smoking, the incidence of CAD is expected to rise. Moreover, women who smoke *and* use oral contraceptives are more likely to have a heart attack.[14] In addition, the use of estrogens by smokers may exacerbate the chance of thrombus formation.

Obesity also presents a formidable risk. Clients who are more than 30 percent overweight are more likely to develop heart disease even if it is their only risk factor.[14]

Physical inactivity—a sedentary lifestyle—contributes to CAD by unfavorably altering serum lipid ratios.

Hypertension and hyperlipidemia and their specific contributions to risk are discussed later under Cardiac Disease.

***Nonmodifiable Risk Factors.*** Nonmodifiable risk factors for CAD are family history, age, gender, and diabetes.

A strong family history of CAD is significant. Early sudden cardiac death of a first-degree relative warrants a more aggressive approach in controlling modifiable risk factors, even if the client is asymptomatic.[15]

Age and gender differences are difficult to distinguish because research studies on women and cardiovascular disease are inadequate. Current research shows that the average age of onset of CAD among men is between 40 and 44 years. Women tend not to develop heart problems until after menopause, most likely because of the cardioprotective effects of estrogen. After menopause the risk of CAD increases steadily. If menopause is iatrogenic (the uterus and ovaries are surgically removed), the risk of a heart attack rises more sharply than if menopause occurs naturally. Exogenous estrogen replacement after menopause may reduce the risk of cardiovascular events by as much as 50 percent.[15]

Morbidity and mortality associated with myocardial infarction are higher among women,[12] because of the failure to identify CAD earlier in women. Anginal symptoms more likely are attributed to noncardiac causes. In addition, noninvasive testing for CAD is less accurate in women.[16,17] Invasive correction of vascular disease in women is more challenging because the condition is usually more advanced when the procedure is done and the diameter of their coronary arteries is smaller.[14]

Diabetes mellitus not only increases the risk of CAD, but is a major predictor of mortality following a myocardial infarction.

The incidence of coronary artery disease is distributed throughout the population. It is the leading cause of death in women older than 50. More than 500,000 Americans die each year of heart attacks. Almost half of these are women.[18] CAD is the most common cause of heart attacks. It is more prevalent among minorities, particularly African Americans.

## Subjective Data

Women are likely to report chest pain (angina) as their first symptom. Men typically present with a myocardial infarction or sudden cardiac death. A thorough history includes the onset, character, location, radiation, frequency, duration, precipitating factors, relieving factors, and associated symptoms. If the client reports a clear relationship between her symptoms and physical exertion, a cardiac origin is highly suspected.

Intensity of pain does not always correlate with severity of disease. Angina may be described as a minor ache or crushing chest pain. Clients may relate only associated symptoms such as dyspnea and diaphoresis with exertion. Treatment of silent ischemia is based more on objective than on subjective findings.[19]

## Objective Data

***Physical Examination.*** May reveal nothing abnormal; however, signs of CAD may include:

- *General Appearance.* Obese, anxious, dyspneic.
- *Vital Signs.* High or low blood pressure, tachycardia or bradycardia, fever.
- *Skin.* Cyanosis, diaphoresis.
- *Eyes.* Arcus senilis, xanthomas, hypertensive retinopathy.
- *Neck.* Jugular venous distention, carotid bruits.
- *Chest.* Adventitious or diminished breath sounds.
- *Heart.* Murmurs, gallops, rubs, clicks, irregular rhythms, displaced point of maximal impulse (PMI), heaves, and thrills.
- *Vascular System.* Absent or diminished peripheral pulses, edema, mottling.
- *Abdomen.* Hepatomegaly, bruits.

***Diagnostic Tests.*** Involve lab work, x-ray, electrocardiogram, exercise tolerance testing, radionuclide studies, coronary arteriography, and echocardiography.

Laboratory testing includes a *CBC* and *kidney and liver function tests* to determine underlying disease and identify risk factors.

A *roentgenogram* (chest x-ray) is used to evaluate CAD, congestive heart failure, valvular disease, and pulmonary abnormalities. The chest x-ray assists in differential diagnosis and in evaluating the progress of disease. It may reveal increased pulmonary markings or cardiomegaly. The client lies supine for the roentgenogram; radiation exposure is minimal. It is contraindicated for pregnant women.

*Electrocardiography* (ECG) permits myocardial ischemic changes to be seen in ST segment elevation or, more commonly, depression. Dysrhythmias, such as ventricular premature beats (VPBs), or premature ventricular contractions (PVCs), may be detected. This noninvasive test is essential to detection of myocardial ischemia; however, a normal ECG does not exclude the diagnosis of CAD. The procedure lacks specificity and sensitivity in women, particularly younger women and those with atypical chest pain.

*Exercise tolerance testing* (ETT), a stress test, identifies the location of ischemic vessels by recording the changes that occur during exercise on an ECG. When evidence of ischemia is presented early in testing, the likelihood of multivessel involvement is increased. The client walks on a treadmill while ECG activity is monitored. As a precautionary measure, an intravenous catheter is inserted for venous access. Approximately 40 percent of women have a false-positive reading. The test helps determine the need for further evaluation or medical treatment.

*Radionuclide studies* include dipyridamole/thallium/dobutamine imaging, with or without active exercise. Coronary blood flow is visualized using the radioactive dye. The studies are recommended when exercise tolerance testing does not yield conclusive information or the client is deconditioned or disabled, prohibiting her from sustaining a level of exertion necessary to complete the testing. An intravenous catheter must be placed. The procedure is invasive and the client may develop allergic reactions to the dye. A day is usually required to complete the test; an overnight stay is usually not necessary.

*Coronary arteriography*, or cardiac catheterization, is the most definitive test to determine the location and extent of CAD. It is performed in a catheterization laboratory by a cardiologist. A catheter is threaded through the coronary vessels retrograde from the femoral arteries or a brachial artery.

The client should anticipate an overnight stay and that a standard preoperative workup is done. Specific preoperative and postoperative teaching should be done by the cardiologist or designated staff member.

*Echocardiography* is the most sensitive, noninvasive diagnostic test used to measure cardiac size and function. It determines abnormalities in the motion of the myocardium, abnormalities in structure and ventricular function, and hypertrophy. The procedure is noninvasive. In the future, exercise echocardiograms may be more sensitive in detecting CAD than stationary echocardiograms or electrocardiograms.[19]

## Differential Medical Diagnosis

Thoracic outlet syndrome, mitral valve prolapse, anemia, substance abuse, costochondritis, reflux esophagitis, esophageal spasm, panic disorder.

## Plan

As interventions are employed, continued surveillance of symptoms, medications, and risk factors is required.

***Psychosocial Interventions.*** Provide anticipatory guidance about diagnostic testing and the nature of the disease. Assist clients in gaining a sense of control over the disease through risk reduction. Clients need to know the risks and benefits of all treatment options to make informed decisions about their lives and health.

***Medication.*** Coupled with a reduction in modifiable risk factors, medication is a viable option for up to two thirds of clients with CAD. In weighing medical against surgical intervention, the key factors are the extent and location of damage.[15]

- *Nitrates.* Nitrates may be used independently or with other medications, such as angiotensin-converting enzyme inhibitors and calcium channel blockers.[15,20] Although nitrates have been the drug of choice, they are being replaced by calcium channel blockers. Nitrates are used as an antianginal agent because of their vasodilating effect.

- *Administration.* Sublingual, topical, transdermal, and oral (long-acting or chewable tablet) forms are available. The sublingual form acts within 15 seconds and has a 15- to 30-minute duration of action. Ointments and transdermal patches may last 12 hours or longer.
- *Side Effects.* Headaches are common. They may be relieved by changing the dosage or route of administration. Other reactions to nitrates are hypotension, dizziness, and palpitations.
- *Contraindications.* Do not administer to clients with severe hypotension.
- *Anticipated Outcome on evaluation.* Anginal episodes decrease or are eliminated.
- *Client Teaching.* Include information about all possible side effects and indications for intermittent use of nitrates as needed.

■ *Aspirin.* Aspirin lowers the risk of myocardial infarctions in persons at increased risk for atherosclerosis and thrombogenesis, including persons who have had a myocardial infarction, unstable angina, or postcoronary artery bypass grafting.[21] Aspirin inhibits platelet aggregation and prevents formation of arterial thrombi on atherosclerotic plaques. It is recommended for men at risk for CAD or for men older than 40 with known cardiac disease; aspirin appears to have the same therapeutic benefits for women. It is considered prudent therapy for women with known cardiac disease.[21]

- *Administration.* One enteric coated 325-mg aspirin is taken daily.
- *Side Effects.* Gastrointestinal upset and bleeding.
- *Contraindications.* Do not administer to clients with ulcerative disease and coagulopathies.
- *Anticipated Outcomes on Evaluation.* Progression of atherosclerotic disease slows, and the likelihood of thrombolic events decreases.
- *Client Teaching.* Include information about the side effects of aspirin. Medication needs to be used consistently to be an effective preventive measure.

■ *β-Adrenergic Receptor Antagonists.* Beta blockers (as they are more commonly called) may be indicated for hypertension and ischemic heart disease. These drugs attenuate increased blood pressure and heart rate during activity, thereby decreasing the workload of the heart.

- *Administration.* Lipids are administered twice a day because their action is of shorter duration; most are metabolized by the liver. Water-soluble agents are given once daily and are eliminated primarily by the kidneys; they may be $\beta_1$ or $\beta_2$ selective.
- *Side Effects.* Depression, impotence, peripheral vascular ischemia, and palpitations are known to occur.
- *Contraindications.* Do not administer to clients with heart failure, sick sinus syndrome with atrioventricular block, bradycardia (fewer than 50 beats per minute), and asthma.
- *Anticipated Outcomes on Evaluation.* Symptoms of angina, as well as blood pressure, decrease.
- *Client Teaching.* Prepare the client for gradual discontinuance of the beta-blocker. The beta blocker may decrease the effectiveness of other medications such as oral hyperglycemic agents.

- *Calcium Channel Blockers.* Calcium channel blockers decrease vascular resistance, thereby increasing blood flow. Generally the drugs are longer acting than beta blockers and nitrates with a better side effect profile. They are also used for hypertension and cardiac arrhythmias, particularly supraventricular rhythms. Eighty percent of the dose is orally absorbed, but because of extensive hepatic metabolism, a much smaller dose reaches the systemic circulation.
  - *Side Effects.* Side effects are specific to the agent and include hypotension, dizziness, constipation, headache, and peripheral edema.
  - *Contraindications.* Do not administer to clients with hypotension, heart failure, and slow or altered cardiac conduction.
  - *Anticipated Outcomes on Evaluation.* Episodes of angina and blood pressure decrease.
  - *Client teaching.* Make clear to the client that calcium channel blockers are more expensive than other antihypertensive medications, but may not require as frequent monitoring of side effects.

***Surgical and Other Interventions.*** In percutaneous transluminal coronary angioplasty (PTCA), a balloon is introduced into an artery and inflated at the site of an atherosclerotic plaque. In dilating the vessel, the balloon flattens the plaque against the arterial wall, reducing its thickness. About one third of arteries restenose. Complications include acute restenosis or vessel dissection, with the possibility of open heart surgery or death.[15]

Coronary artery bypass grafting (CABG) is performed for select groups of clients with multivessel disease, left main coronary artery disease, or ventricular aneurysm. Generally, anginal symptoms markedly improve and improvement persists at least 10 years. Surgical risks may be increased or decreased, depending on the extent of disease and the presence of other underlying medical problems at the time of surgery.[15]

***Lifestyle/Dietary Changes.*** Such changes can dramatically reduce morbidity and mortality. Primary prevention focuses on modifying risk factors: hypertension, hyperlipidemia, cigarette smoking, obesity, and physical inactivity.[22] Advise the client to follow a low-cholesterol and low-fat diet (see Hyperlipidemia).

Physical activity is tailored to the individual client, considering her overall physical condition and cardiac history. Advise the client to avoid exertional activities during extreme weather conditions or after a heavy meal. The client should always carry nitroglycerin and alert the health care provider of any change in symptoms.

Cigarette smoking is a significant risk factor and should be discontinued. Involve the client in a smoking cessation program.

Intravascular stents, atherectomy, and laser therapy are viable options for a subset of clients.[15] A discussion of these invasive procedures is deferred to the cardiologist.

## HYPERLIPIDEMIA

Hyperlipidemia is an increased plasma lipid concentration of cholesterol, triglycerides, or both. Water-insoluble lipids are carried in the bloodstream by lipoproteins, which are complex molecules made up partly of cholesterol and triglycerides. Lipoproteins transport both dietary and endogenous lipids from sites of absorption or synthesis to sites of storage or metabolism.

High levels of low-density lipoprotein are injurious to the vascular intima and lead to the deposition of cholesterol (see Table 17-3). This and other thrombolic events combine to form atherosclerotic plaques within the vessel, narrowing the lumen and eventually reducing blood flow to many tissues.[23]

**TABLE 17–3. CLASSIFICATION OF LIPIDS**

| | Level (mg/dL) | | |
|---|---|---|---|
| | *Desirable* | *Borderline* | *High Risk* |
| Total cholesterol | <200 | 200–239 | >240 |
| High density lipoprotein cholesterol | >40 | 35–55 | <35 |
| Low density lipoprotein cholesterol | <130 | 130–159 | >160 |
| Triglycerides | <250 | 250–500 | >500 |

## Classification of Lipoproteins

Four principal classes of lipoproteins have been determined.[24]

- Chylomicrons are the major transporters of dietary triglycerides.
- Very low density lipoproteins (VLDLs) are responsible for the transport of endogenous triglycerides.
- Low density lipoproteins (LDLs) are the major transporter of cholesterol.
- High density lipoproteins (HDLs) collect cholesterol from the tissues to return it to the liver, thereby acquiring the pseudonym "good cholesterol."

## Epidemiology

Genetic factors and lifestyle are major forces in the development of hyperlipidemia.

Risk factors are a high-fat diet, genetic predisposition, sedentary lifestyle, cigarette smoking, and underlying diseases (diabetes mellitus, hypothyroidism, chronic renal disease, liver or gastrointestinal disorders). These may all contribute to an alteration in lipid values.

Levels of LDLs and HDLs are predictors of risk. Although LDL level is a powerful predictor of CAD in men, HDL level appears to be a better predictor of risk for CAD in women. Even with a higher average total cholesterol and higher LDL levels, women have fewer cardiovascular events than men possibly due to their higher HDL levels. Recently, more weight has been given to the ratio of LDLs to HDLs in both sexes than any one single measurement in predicting risk. A ratio of 4 or less is considered acceptable; a ratio of 6 or above warrants an aggressive approach.[25] Research is almost exclusively based on men; until further studies of women are completed, it is considered clinically prudent to apply to women the same recommendations used in the care of men.

Hyperlipidemia occurs in 50 percent of the U.S. adult population.[26]

## Subjective Data

The client reports a first-degree relative with known hyperlipidemia, a family history of premature CAD, or a medical condition associated with hyperlipidemia.

## Objective Data

Although the physical examination may be entirely normal (see Coronary Artery Disease), physical findings that are consistent with hyperlipidemia are obesity, xanthomas, lipemia retinalis, corneal arcus, and hepatosplenomegaly.

***Hyperlipidemia Screening.*** Diagnostic laboratory testing includes screening asymptomatic clients for hyperlipidemia every 5 years (see Table 17–3). It is done more often if there are additional risk factors.

The test procedure, a fasting serum lipid profile study, involves venipuncture, which is more accurate than a fingerstick. The blood sample is drawn after a minimum of 8 hours of fasting. Values that classify clients as moderate to high risk are based on at least two separate studies by venipuncture, drawn 2 months apart. If the difference is less than 30 mg/dL, the two values are averaged. If the difference is more than 30 mg/dL, another sample is obtained and the three values are averaged.[27]

Inform the client that she may drink water when fasting. Fasting is most important in the assessment of hypertriglyceridemia. A random (nonfasting) total cholesterol can be done as a screening measure in low-risk individuals.

The client should understand that every 1 percent decrease in a high serum cholesterol reduces her risk for coronary artery disease by 2 percent.[28,29] Triglyceride levels above 1000 mg/dL should be treated to prevent pancreatitis.

## Differential Medical Diagnosis

Diabetes mellitus; liver disease (obstructive, hepatocellular, or hepatic storage disorder); hypothyroidism; renal disease (nephrosis and renal failure); hormonal imbalance (estrogens, progestins, and androgens); hyperuricemia; acute intermittent porphyria; alcoholism.

## Plan

A majority of clients with hyperlipidemia are managed by their primary care provider. Treatment must be individualized with respect to age, risk factors, clinical status, and the presence or extent of CAD (see Table 17–4).

***Psychosocial Interventions.*** Support and encourage clients who are changing their diet and level of physical activity to reduce lipid blood levels. Clients should have realistic expectations and be given objective evidence of their efforts. If medications are indicated, reinforce the information that nonpharmacological interventions are also essential to lowering lipids. Some individuals may have a genetic predisposition to elevated serum cholesterol and, consequently, have less response to nonpharmacologic interventions. Avoid attributing high levels to noncompliance without adequate evaluation.

***Medication.*** Discontinue medications that may adversely influence lipid levels.[29,30] Medication chosen to lower lipid levels is specific to the client and the desired effect on lipid profile. Adherence to any drug regimen necessitates that the client be informed of the benefits of the drug, its potential side effects, cost, and convenience. A motivational feedback mechanism is provided by repeated serum cholesterol evaluation, which reflects the progress made.

- *Fish Oil.* Fish is recommended in the diet; however, the benefits of fish oil (long-chain, highly unsaturated omega-3 fatty acids in coldwater fish) in capsules have not been proven.
- *Psyllium.* Psyllium hydrophilic mucilloid is the active ingredient in many bulk-forming laxatives (e.g., Metamucil). It binds with cholesterol for removal via the gut. Psyllium hydrophilic mucilloid is an option for clients with mild to moderately elevated lipid levels and for whom a bulk laxative is indicated. Dosage varies with the individual: Begin with the smallest recommended dose and increase as needed. Drink sufficient fluids to avoid constipation and gas pains.
- *Bile Acid Sequestrants (Cholestyramine and Colestipol).* These agents reduce cholesterol by binding bile acids in the gut.
  - *Administration.* A powder, which is mixed with a liquid, or chewable bars are taken in two to four divided doses. Usual dosage for cholestyramine is 12–24 g p.o.; for colestipol is 15–30 g.
  - *Side Effects.* Gastrointestinal complaints are common. Bile acid sequestrants may interact with fat-soluble vitamins. Triglycerides tend to increase.

**TABLE 17–4. RECOMMENDED INTERVENTIONS FOR GROUPS AT RISK FOR CORONARY ARTERY DISEASE**

| Client Group | Recommendations |
|---|---|
| 1. All adults > 20 years of age | Measure TC[a] every 5 years |
| 2. TC < 200 mg/dL | Desirable range<br>General dietary and risk reduction counseling<br>Repeat in 5 years |
| 3. TC 200–239 mg/dL | Borderline high risk; confirm with fractionated lipid profile |
| 4. If no CAD and fewer than two risk factors | Phase I diet<br>Reevaluate in 1 year; goal is to lower LDLs < 160 |
| 5. If definite CAD or two risk factors and LDLs > 160 | Lower LDLs < 130 by diet |
| 6. If definite CAD or two risk factors and LDLs > 190 | Give medication; goal is to lower LDLs < 160 if no CAD or fewer than two risk factors; otherwise lower < 130 |
| 7. TC > 240 mg/dL | High risk; same as for groups 3–6 |

[a]TC, total cholesterol; CAD, coronary artery disease; LDL, low density lipoprotein.
Source: *Adapted from NIH Adult Treatment Panel's Recommendations for Measuring and Classifying CAD risk.*[26]

- *Contraindications.* Do not administer to pregnant women.
- *Anticipated Outcome on Evaluation.* Both LDL and total cholesterol levels decrease.
- *Client Teaching.* Include information about the expense of the medication. Also advise the client that the preparations have a gritty quality and should be taken several hours apart from other medications.

■ *Nicotinic Acid (Niacin).* Nicotinic acid reduces cholesterol by inhibiting its synthesis in the liver.

- *Administration.* Usual drug dosage is 2–3 g t.i.d. in three divided doses. Start with the smallest dose and gradually increase as tolerated until the desired effect is achieved.
- *Side Effects.* Pruritus, gastrointestinal distress, and severe flushing are known side effects.
- *Contraindication.* Do not administer to clients with liver abnormalities.
- *Anticipated Outcome on Evaluation.* All lipoprotein levels are normal.
- *Client Teaching.* Advise the client that nicotinic acid is the least expensive of the medications. Flushing, a side effect, may be controlled by not drink-ing alcohol or warm fluids and taking one 325-mg aspirin tablet 30 minutes before the nicotinic acid, if there is no contraindication to the use of aspirin.

■ *Gemfibrozil (Lopid).* Gemfibrozil is a fibric acid derivative that is indicated primarily to lower plasma triglycerides. It also lowers cholesterol, but to a lesser extent, and may raise high density lipoprotein.

- *Administration.* Give 600 mg orally twice daily, 30 minutes prior to a meal.
- *Side effect.* Gastrointestinal distress is known to occur.
- *Contraindications.* Do not administer to clients with impaired renal or hepatic function or to pregnant or breastfeeding women.
- *Anticipated Outcome on Evaluation.* Total cholesterol decreases, with a greater effect on triglycerides.

- *Client Teaching.* Counsel the client to be alert for drug interactions.

- *Probucol (Lorelco).* Probucol lowers serum cholesterol levels by reducing low density lipoprotein concentrations.
  - *Administration.* A 500-mg tablet is taken twice daily with meals.
  - *Side Effects.* Probucol is generally well tolerated. Side effects are infrequent; however, diarrhea may occur. Ventricular arrhythmias may be a serious side effect.
  - *Contraindications.* Do not administer to pregnant or breastfeeding clients. Safe use has not been established.
  - *Anticipated Outcomes on Evaluation.* All cholesterol levels, including that of HDL, decrease.
  - *Client Teaching.* Inform the client that a favorable decline in cholesterol levels should be seen in about 2 months. It is generally thought that if probucol is not effective after 4 months, it should be discontinued. Probucol accumulates slowly in adipose tissue and may persist 6 months or longer after the last dose. Advise clients to discontinue use at least 6 months prior to conception.
- *Hydroxymethylglutaryl Coenzyme A (HMG-CoA) Reductase Inhibitors.* These agents reduce cholesterol by inhibiting the enzyme that catalyzes the rate-limiting step in cholesterol synthesis. Slowing down the rate of cholesterol synthesis decreases the release of cholesterol into the bloodstream.
  - *Administration.* This drug is taken once a day with the evening meal or twice daily with meals. Lovastin is usually given as 20–80 mg p.o. in one or two doses; Simvastatin as 40–80 mg p.o. in one or two doses; Pravastatin as 40 mg p.o. in one to two doses. Both Simvastatin and Pravastatin are pending approval by the FDA.
  - *Side Effects.* Myalgias and elevated liver enzymes are known side effects; however, the inhibitors are generally well tolerated.
  - *Contraindication.* Do not administer to clients with liver disease.
  - *Anticipated Outcome on Evaluation.* Cholesterol levels decrease.

**Surgical Intervention.** Surgery may be an option. Refer the client to a cardiac surgeon for atherectomy.

**Lifestyle Changes.** Focus on diet (primary intervention), physical activity, and not smoking.

Physical activity might include 30 minutes of aerobic exercise daily to increase HDL levels and facilitate weight loss.[28,29]

Cigarette smoking increases LDL levels. All nicotine use should be discontinued.

**Dietary Interventions.** Refer to the American Heart Association's progressive dietary plan for hyperlipidemia. Clients may benefit from consultation with a dietitian, especially if the diet becomes more complex with additional restrictions imposed because of other illnesses.[26] Dietary measures are safe and cost effective and may eliminate the need for drugs to lower cholesterol.

Phase I of American Heart Association diet calls for considerable restriction of fats and carbohydrates. All family members should be involved. Meet with them collectively or at least with the primary meal provider. Emphasize the foods that can be eaten rather than those that cannot.

- *Fat* intake is reduced to 30 percent or less of the diet. A high-fat diet without cholesterol raises serum cholesterol levels by increasing bile reabsorption from the gut, which, in turn, limits the amount of cholesterol that can be excreted. Decrease saturated fats to 10 percent of caloric intake.
- *Cholesterol* is limited to no more than 300 mg per day.

- *Complex carbohydrates* include water-soluble fiber and are increased in small amounts as tolerated.
- *Weight* is maintained at ideal body weight.
- A *food diary* is recorded to target problem areas and provide feedback for the client and provider.
- A specific *food plan is* described during dietary counseling. For example, recommend mozzarella cheese made with skim milk or any dairy product with less than 1 percent fat. Recommend chicken or fish instead of beef. Offer suggestions on how to cook meat (broil, boil) to reduce fat content.

Phase II of the American Heart Association diet further restricts fat intake to 20 to 25 percent of total calories. Saturated fats are reduced to 6 to 8 percent of total fat intake and cholesterol to 150 to 200 mg per day.

***Follow-Up.*** Ascertain whether the expectation of a 10 to 20 percent decrease in total cholesterol was reached after approximately 6 weeks of dietary modification. Before considering any change in the treatment plan, individuals who have no additional risk factors should continue dietary interventions for at least 6 months. Most medications reduce total cholesterol an average of 20 to 25 percent, and triglycerides 40 to 50 percent, within 6 weeks. Much remains to be learned concerning the management of hyperlipidemia as it relates to age and risk of CAD.

## HYPERTENSION

Hypertension (HTN) is a systolic blood pressure (SBP) of 140 mm Hg or greater, a diastolic blood pressure (DBP) of 90 mm Hg or greater, or both (see Table 17–5).

### Epidemiology

Essential hypertension is idiopathic and most common. Risk factors are a genetic predisposition, age older than 40, minority status, and alcoholism. Although nicotine transiently increases blood pressure, prolonged use is not associated with an increased prevalence of hypertension.

**TABLE 17–5. CLASSIFICATION OF BLOOD PRESSURE IN ADULTS AGED 18 YEARS OR OLDER**

| Blood Pressure Range (mm Hg) | Category |
|---|---|
| Diastolic blood pressure | |
| < 85 | Normal blood pressure |
| 85–89 | High to normal blood pressure |
| 90–104 | Mild hypertension |
| 105–114 | Moderate hypertension |
| > 115 | Severe hypertension |
| Systolic blood pressure when diastolic < 90 mm Hg | |
| < 140 | Normal blood pressure |
| 140–159 | Borderline isolated systolic hypertension |
| > 160 | Isolated systolic hypertension |

Source: *Reference 31.*

Secondary hypertension, which is uncommon, may be caused by polycystic kidneys, renovascular disease, aortic coarctation, Cushing's syndrome, and pheochromocytoma. Reversible risk factors include medication, alcohol abuse, and excessive dietary sodium.

Incidence reports show hypertension among 58 million people in the United States. Its prevalence increases with age and is higher among African-Americans than caucasians.[31]

### Subjective Data

A client with hypertension is most often asymptomatic. She may report a family or personal medical history of hypertension, diabetes, kidney disease, hypothyroidism, or cardiovascular disease. Be alert for deviations from usual blood pressure readings or a history of elevated blood pressure. Note results and side effects of previous treatments. Identify risk factors including recent weight gain or loss, changes in exercise or diet, or increased sodium or alcohol intake. Obtain a complete psychosocial history including socioeconomic status, emotional stress, coping mechanisms, and cultural habits. List all prescription and nonprescription medications that may contribute to hypertension.[31]

## Objective Data

Hypertension is not diagnosed by a single measurement. Three elevated readings on three separate visits are required to diagnose mild hypertension. Moderate or severe hypertension warrants a more immediate and aggressive approach.

***Physical Examination.*** Begins by assessing the client's general appearance. Determine if she is uniformly obese or, as in Cushing's syndrome, has truncal obesity and pigmented striae.

Blood pressure findings that are abnormal are episodic elevations, discrepancies between blood pressures in contralateral arms, and decreased pressures in the lower extremities. Specific measures may be taken to ensure accurate blood pressure readings.

- Seat the client with her arm supported and positioned at the level of her heart.
- Cigarettes should not be smoked or caffeine ingested within 30 minutes of the measurement.
- Have the client rest for about 5 minutes before measuring blood pressure.
- Use appropriate cuff size. The rubber bladder should be two-thirds the size of the arm.
- If not contraindicated, check readings in both arms. If there is a discrepancy, as in peripheral atherosclerosis, use the higher value.

Examine the eyes for arteriolar narrowing, arteriovenous compression, arteriovenous nicking, hemorrhages, exudates, and papilledema. Use a fundoscope.

Examine the neck for an enlarged thyroid gland and carotid bruits.

Check the heart for murmurs, gallops, rubs, and the displaced point of maximal impulse (PMI). Perform a vascular exam to detect diminished or absent extremity pulses, bruits, and edema.

Evaluate the abdomen for the presence of abdominal bruits, enlarged kidneys, or masses or dilation of the aorta.

***Diagnostic Tests.*** Include blood and urine analyses, echocardiogram, and electrocardiogram. Laboratory tests include a CBC, chemistries to evaluate kidney and liver function, lipid profiles, and urinalysis. The evaluations are done to rule out secondary causes, identify the risk for heart disease, provide baseline values for the selection and surveillance of medications, and monitor for sequelae from hypertension. The test procedure requires that a serum sample be obtained. Nursing implications are for continued surveillance.

The echocardiogram (ECHO) and electrocardiogram (ECG) are used to detect left ventricular hypertrophy (LVH), the result of cardiac adaptation to increased pressure and increased afterload imposed by an elevated blood pressure.[31] Left ventricular hypertrophy is a significant independent risk factor of cardiac dysrhythmias and sudden death.

## Differential Medical Diagnosis

Pheochromocytoma, thyroid disease, renal disease, Cushing's syndrome, primary aldosteronism, alcoholism, iatrogenic.

## Plan

The goal of intervention is to prevent the morbidity and mortality associated with high blood pressure. The severity of hypertension, complications, and other risk factors for cardiovascular and cerebrovascular disease guides intervention.

***Psychosocial Interventions.*** Involve the client in decisions concerning treatment. Acknowledge hypertension as a chronic disease that can be controlled but not cured. Contract with the client for follow-up at predetermined intervals.

***Medication.*** Medication for moderate or severe hypertension decreases cardiovascular mortality and morbidity. Clients with mild hypertension benefit from medication in that it arrests the progression to a more severe condition and reduces the risk of cerebrovascular accidents. In individuals with a blood pressure persistently higher than 94 mm Hg, the benefits of drug therapy outweigh the risks.[31]

Single-dose therapies are usually a first choice to improve compliance and reduce side effects and expense. Combinations of medications often achieve better blood pressure control with smaller doses, thereby minimizing dose-dependent side effects.

- *Diuretics.* Diuretics reduce blood pressure by decreasing volume and thereby decreasing preload. They are classified by mechanism and site of action.

  Thiazides and sulfonamides are relatively contraindicated in persons with sulfa allergies. These agents may raise lithium blood levels and serum cholesterol. Concomitant administration of nonsteroidal anti-inflammatory drugs may antagonize thiazide or sulfonamide effectiveness or cause electrolyte disturbances and sexual dysfunction.

  Potassium-sparing agents are dangerous for clients with renal compromise and/or using angiotensin-converting enzyme inhibitors.

  Loop diuretics cause electrolyte disturbances. Potassium supplementation is often required.

- *Angiotensin-Converting Enzyme Inhibitors.* Angiotensin-converting enzyme (ACE) inhibitors are indicated to suppress the renin–angiotensin–aldosterone system. Structure, absorption, and duration of action differ slightly among these drugs. They are particularly effective for congestive heart failure.

  Administer ACE inhibitors once or twice daily. Although they are generally well tolerated, adverse effects may include cough (persistent and nonproductive), angioedema, hypotension, rash (most common with captopril), and hyperkalemia. Monitor renal function.

- *Other Medication.* Beta blockers and calcium channel blockers (see Coronary Artery Disease) are also used for hypertension.

***Lifestyle/Dietary Changes.*** Encourage the client to make changes in diet and lifestyle if the diastolic blood pressure falls between 90 and 94 mm Hg. Recommend a nonpharmacological approach, as the risk of developing cardiovascular disease is low. Involve the client and target one area at a time. Build on changes as they occur.

Dietary modification may be an essential lifestyle change. Weight should be kept within 15 percent of desirable weight.

Advise the client to limit alcohol intake to one 8-oz glass of wine, three 8-oz glasses of beer, or 2 oz of liquor daily.

Sodium should be limited to a moderate intake between 70 and 100 mEq per day. Usually this amount is achieved by not adding salt to foods.

Fats should be limited to 30 percent of caloric intake for weight control and hyperlipidemia.

Physical activity may include a 30-minute aerobic exercise program at least three times a week. The program should be initiated gradually. An overall increase in physical activity is encouraged; the benefits are numerous. Exercise increases fibrinolytic activity, prevents the deformation of red blood cells, and expands plasma volume, which reduces blood viscosity.

- High-density lipoprotein levels increase.
- Arterial blood pressure decreases.
- Glucose intolerance improves.
- Stress decreases.

Advise the client to stop smoking. Cessation reduces the risk of coronary artery disease. The most successful strategies are those that involve both pharmacological (nicotine replacement) and behavioral methods.[18,19]

Biofeedback and relaxation have been demonstrated to have modest results in reducing blood pressure in selected groups and may be the most useful treatment for mild hypertension.

***Follow-Up.*** Arrange for periodic evaluation for hypertension and left ventricular hypertrophy. It is not known whether the reversal of hypertension-induced cardiac hypertrophy decreases its associated risks, but evidence of its presence, even mild hypertension, requires aggressive therapy.[31] Intervals between office visits vary and depend on the degree and lability of hypertension. Adjust medication after 1 to 3 months if the client's response is inadequate.

Address reasons for unresponsiveness to therapies (see Table 17–6). For clients who are following nonpharmacological therapeutic recommendations in addition to medications, a trial of step-down therapy and drug withdrawal may be considered after blood pressure has been at goal level for 1 year.

**TABLE 17–6. POSSIBLE CAUSES OF HYPERTENSION TREATMENT FAILURE**

1. Nonadherence
   A. Side effects
   B. Cost
   C. Frequency of dosage
2. Drug Related
   A. Inappropriate choice or combination
      Blacks and older clients tend to do better with diuretics and calcium channel blockers.
      Combinations of similar classes/drugs are ineffective.
   B. Rapid inactivation
   C. Drug interactions
      Sympathomimetics
      Antidepressants
      Adrenal steroids
      Nonsteroidal anti-inflammatory drugs
      Nasal decongestants
      Oral contraceptives
3. Associated conditions
      Increasing obesity
      Excessive alcohol intake
      Renal insufficiency
      Renovascular hypertension
      Malignant/accelerated hypertension
4. Volume overload
      Inadequate diuretic therapy
      Excess sodium intake
      Fluid retention from reduction of blood pressure
      Progressive renal failure

Source: *Adapted from the 1988 National Committee Report on Hypertension.[31] The Committee is part of the National Heart, Lung, and Blood Institute, Bethesda.*

## MITRAL VALVE PROLAPSE

Mitral valve prolapse (MVP) is a relatively benign and common disorder. Its distinguishing pathology is ventriculovalvular disproportion. The chordae tendinae, which suspend the mitral valve, are too large for the left ventricular cavity. Valve leaflets are also enlarged and thickened. The primary causative factor seems to be characteristic dysgenesis of collagenous valvular tissue.[32]

### Epidemiology

Mitral valve prolapse is a genetic disorder of autosomal dominance; offspring have a 50 percent chance of being affected if one parent has the disorder. MVP occurs in several connective tissue diseases, other cardiovascular processes, and miscellaneous muscular and thyroid abnormalities.[33]

Studies show that MVP is the most common valvular abnormality in the United States, with about 5 percent of the general population affected. Mitral valve prolapse is most commonly found among females 14 to 30 years of age but may be discovered at any age.[34] Prevalence varies from 2 to 40 percent, depending on the method of diagnosis (auscultation or echocardiography).[32] The prevalence of "clinically significant" MVP is estimated to be 2 to 4 percent.

Complications are mitral regurgitation, infective endocarditis, thromboembolism, and cardiac arrhythmias. They may occur but usually are not serious and can either be prevented or treated. Sudden death is rare. The role of MVP in thromboembolic disease is less clear. It is often considered a factor in unexplained cerebral ischemic events; however, the incidence of transient ischemic attacks is quite low, at 0.02 percent. With no complications, activities and exercise are not limited.

Mitral regurgitation is caused most often by MVP, although only a very small percentage of clients with MVP progress to mitral regurgitation. Moreover, a small number within that group become hemodynamically impaired.[35]

Anxiety is not a causative factor in the development of MVP but it can be a manifestation. Heart, hormone, and chemical disturbances may account for the symptomatology of panic disorder; however, they are not yet understood.[35]

## Subjective Data

A client with mitral valve prolapse is usually asymptomatic; however, she may report chest pain. The exact etiology of pain is unknown. The chest pain is atypical for angina and usually nonexertional. It may result from mechanical stress on the papillary muscle, from coronary artery spasm or embolism, left ventricular dysfunction, rate-related supply/demand imbalance, independent coronary artery disease, or extracardiac conditions.[32] Heart palpitations are also common. Other symptoms include complaints of fast heart rate, skipped beats, lightheadedness, fatigue, weakness, dyspnea, anxiety, and postural phenomena.

## Objective Data

Mitral valve prolapse is identified by means of physical examination, electrocardiogram, and echocardiogram. Laboratory tests are done to rule out other suspected medical problems.

***Physical Examination.*** Usually normal unless MVP is associated with other conditions. The client's general appearance is slender. Cardiac symptoms include an isolated, high-pitched, mid- to late systolic click. The client may have a late systolic murmur (late or pansystolic murmurs indicate mitral regurgitation). Chest auscultation is best done with the diaphragm over the cardiac apex. Examine the client in the supine and left lateral recumbent positions. The click is heard earlier and occupies much of systole when sitting or standing. Postural auscultation is the key to diagnosis. If the client is squatting, the click may be closer to S2, and murmur may be delayed but more intense.36 Murmur often disappears during pregnancy because of expanding blood volume and the subsequent increase in left ventricular cavity size.

***Diagnostic Tools.*** See Coronary Artery Disease and Hypertension sections for tests done to rule out medical problems that may be associated with MVP.

Electrocardiogram abnormalities are present in up to 50 percent of clients, but do not usually account for subjective complaints.[32,36]

The echocardiogram confirms the diagnosis and extent of disease. It is recommended to determine whether mitral valve leaflets have hypertrophied, which increases the risk of infective endocarditis and progression to mitral regurgitation. The policy of obtaining an echocardiogram to confirm MVP is not universally indicated.[32]

## Differential Medical Diagnosis

Marfan's syndrome, rheumatic fever, trauma, hypertrophic cardiomyopathy, atrial septal defect, anorexia nervosa, pectus excavatum, connective tissue disorders.

## Plan

***Psychosocial Interventions.*** Educate the client about her common, benign condition. The valve functions properly, and usually no treatment is needed. Mitral valve prolapse does not appear to alter the course of pregnancy. Periodic auscultatory examinations are necessary to note any changes.

***Medication.*** Although not usually required, medications may be prescribed.

*β-Adrenergic or calcium channel blockers* are usually effective in controlling symptoms (palpitations).[32] Their use is described under Coronary Artery Disease.

*Anxiolytic drugs* are recommended ***only*** if there is an underlying anxiety disorder.

*Anticoagulants and antiplatelet medications* are a possible therapeutic intervention for those at high risk for thromboembolic disease. Their effectiveness in terms of primary prevention remains unknown.

*Antimicrobial prophylaxis* is recommended for clients with mitral valve prolapse ***and*** mitral regurgitation or those who have MVP associated with thickening and redundancy of the valve leaflets. Prophylaxis is ***not*** recommended for prolapse without valvular regurgitation[37] (see Table 17–7). Prophylaxis may prevent risk of endocarditis in clients with valvular disease who must undergo procedures that may cause transient bacteremia, although bacterial endocarditis may occur despite preventive measures. Guidelines for administration have been established and are considered standard practice; however, controlled clinical trials are inadequate. Bacteremia should be considered if a client experiences unexplained malaise or fever following a surgical or dental procedure. Poor dental hygiene or periodontal infections may produce bacteremia in the absence of dental procedures.

**TABLE 17–7. RECOMMENDED PROPHYLAXIS FOR DENTAL, ORAL, OR UPPER RESPIRATORY TRACT PROCEDURES IN PATIENTS WHO HAVE MITRAL VALVE REGURGITATION[a]**

| Drug | Dosing Regimen |
|---|---|
| Amoxicillin[b] | 3.0 g orally 1 hour before procedure; then half the dose 6 hours after initial dose |
| *In Amoxicillin/Penicillin-Allergic Patients* | |
| Erythromycin[c] | Erythromycin ethylsuccinate (E.E.S.) 800 mg or erythromycin stearate (Erythromycin Stearate Filmtab) 1.0 g orally 2 hours before procedure; then half the dose 6 hours after initial dose |
| or | |
| Clindamycin (Cleocin) | 300 mg orally 1 hour before procedure; then half the dose 6 hours after initial dose |

[a]Prolapse alone does not warrant medication.
[b]The antibiotics amoxicillin, ampicillin, and penicillin V are equally effective in vitro against beta hemolytic streptococci (the most common cause of endocarditis following dental procedures); however, amoxicillin is now recommended because it is better absorbed from the gastrointestinal tract and provides higher and more sustained serum levels.
[c]These forms of erythromycin are recommended because of more rapid and reliable absorption.
Source: *Reference 37.*

***Surgical Interventions.*** Valve repair or replacement is indicated for symptomatic and hemodynamically significant mitral regurgitation. The procedure depends on the extent and etiology of disease.

***Follow-Up.*** Recommend follow-up in 2 to 5 years for asymptomatic clients without murmurs.

## GASTROINTESTINAL DISEASE

### GASTROESOPHAGEAL REFLUX DISEASE

Gastroesophageal reflux disease (GERD) is a clinical syndrome characterized by heartburn, a burning sensation resulting from the backward flow of gastric contents into the esophagus. The most common form is idiopathic lower esophageal sphincter incompetence. Contributing factors include gastric hyperacidity, impaired esophageal clearance, increased volume of gastric contents, and altered mucosal resistance.[38]

#### Epidemiology

Etiology reveals that hiatal hernias predispose to GERD, but are not pathognomonic. Other conditions may exacerbate symptoms: scleroderma, pregnancy, and obesity. Cigarette smoking and some medications (tetracycline, doxycycline, quinidine, slow-release potassium supplements, iron, calcium channel blockers, and nonsteroidal anti-inflammatory drugs) also aggravate GERD. The higher incidence of GERD among asthmatics may be related to medications. Delayed gastric or esophageal emptying and prolonged exposure to gastric acid increase the frequency and severity of symptoms, complications, and recurrence of gastroesophageal reflux.[39]

Reports reveal that the condition is common at all ages, but more prevalent among persons 60 to 70 years old. Incidence is reported to be as high as 30 to 40 percent in the general population and accounts for almost half of all noncardiac chest pain.[40] GERD is reported in 46 percent of all asthmatics.

#### Subjective Data

The client describes a burning sensation or pain underneath the sternum followed by a bitter taste. It may be related to certain foods. Intensity varies, but the sensation usually increases after eating, with forward bending, when supine, or with vigorous exercise. Less common symptoms that may be reported are odynophagia, dysphagia, and pulmonary manifestations, such as nocturnal coughing, wheezing, and hoarseness.

#### Objective Data

Physical examination is usually benign.

Diagnostic tests are done most often for clients older than 50 whose histories indicate the need. Early diagnosis and appropriate treatment can prevent secondary complications, such as esophageal strictures, ulcers, Barrett's esophagus, bleeding, pulmonary disease, and hoarseness.

Diagnostic testing for clients older than 50 is done if heartburn is a new complaint, if the symptom cannot be explained by a recent change in lifestyle (starting to smoke or snacking before bedtime), if the client has a history of ulcerative disease, or if symptoms persist despite conservative therapy.[38,41]

***Endoscopy.*** The most definitive approach to diagnosis. It allows direct visualization and biopsy and is 100 percent sensitive. Endoscopy is performed under anesthesia.

Advise the client of the disadvantages of the procedure. It is expensive and is associated with increased risks for clients who have cardiopulmonary disease, are elderly, or otherwise debilitated.

***Upper Gastrointestinal X-ray.*** Determines the extent of damage to esophageal mucosa. It detects ulcers, strictures, hiatal hernias, and masses. Double-contrast studies are more sensitive and specific than single-contrast studies. They have a sensitivity of 80 to 90 percent, which decreases with ulcers less than 5 mm in diameter. Barium is used as contrast in x-rays of the upper gastrointestinal tract.

Inform the client that spontaneous reflux is uncommon. In addition, describe the disadvantages of the test: it is associated with high false-positive and false-negative results and cannot evaluate the gastric mucosa. If an esophageal lesion is detected, a biopsy cannot be done to exclude malignant disease.

***A 24-Hour pH Monitor (a portable unit).*** Useful in determining the total acid exposure and identifying episodes of nocturnal reflux. The pH probe is manually placed in the esophagus; reflux is defined by a distal esophageal pH less than 4.

***The Bernstein Test.*** Used to demonstrate the relationship of symptoms to pain. Symptoms are simulated: hydrochloric acid and normal saline are alternately infused into the esophagus, while the patient's response is recorded. The test is provocative and potentially uncomfortable for clients.

***Esophageal Manometry.*** Indicated for clients who are not responding to conventional medical therapy or for whom surgery is being considered. Lower esophageal pressure is measured, and esophageal peristalsis and the competence of the lower esophageal sphincter are assessed. Normal lower esophageal sphincter pressure ranges between 10 and 25 mm Hg. A pressure of 6 mm Hg or less or inappropriate sphincter relaxation is also highly diagnostic.

## Differential Medical Diagnosis

Peptic ulcer disease, esophageal strictures, Barrett's esophagus, angina, pancreatic disease, esophageal candidiasis, Zollinger–Ellison syndrome, respiratory disease.

## Plan

In determining the management of symptoms, consider their severity, as well as the cost of procedures, the risk–benefit of diagnostic testing, and the age and health status of the client.

***Psychosocial Interventions.*** Involve the client as an active partner in management. She should know that the condition is chronic but manageable.

***Medication.*** Medications are not corrective but protect the mucosa from chronic insult. They suppress and neutralize acid and are cytoprotective.[42]

*Antacids* neutralize gastric acid.

*Alginic acid* (Gaviscon) forms a foamy coating over gastric contents, protecting the esophageal mucosa during regurgitation.

*H2 receptor agonists* block parietal cell actions and thereby decrease gastric acid formation. Few side effects are noted; however, close observation for drug interactions is important.

*The dopamine antagonist/protokinetic agent metoclopramide hydrochloride* (Reglan) increases esophageal sphincter pressure and enhances gastric emptying. It may be given in conjunction with an H2 blocker.

*The "acid proton pump" inhibitor omeprazole* (Prilosec) inactivates the hydrogen–potassium ATPase enzyme that drives the proton pump of the parietal cell. It is indicated for intractable reflux esophagitis, Zollinger–Ellison syndrome, and hyperhistaminic states.

*Cholinergic drugs* (e.g., bethanecol hydrochloride) increase lower esophageal sphincter pressure.

*Anticholinergic agents* reduce acid secretion but are rarely used because of their adverse effects.

*Sucralfate* (Carafate tablets) binds bile salts and pepsin, aids mucosal regeneration, and enhances prostaglandin synthesis, making it cytoprotective.

*Misoprostol* (Cytotec), a synthetic prostaglandin analog, reduces mucosal injury related to use of nonsteroidal anti-inflammatory drugs. Diarrhea may preclude prolonged use.

***Surgical Interventions.*** Surgery may be indicated for clients who have evidence of reflux and failed a 6-month trial of medical management.[40] Surgery is reserved for those who have not responded to simple therapeutic maneuvers or medications, or have advanced disease or complications, such as esophageal stricture, severe bleeding, and pulmonary aspiration. A hiatal hernia is not an indication for surgery. Surgery is effective in 90 percent of cases; the Nissen fundoplication procedure restores sphincter competence.

***Lifestyle/Dietary Changes.*** Lifestyle and dietary changes may be effective initial and adjunctive therapies.[38] Controlled studies, however, show their benefits are limited.

The diet should not include offending foods (spicy foods, high-fat foods, citrus juices, chocolate, peppermint, onions, and coffee). Ideal body weight should be maintained and alcohol eliminated. Advise the client to take the following measures:

- Avoid recumbent positions within 3 hours of a meal.
- Elevate the head of the bed on 4- to 6-in. blocks or on a bed wedge.
- Avoid bending forward.
- Discontinue cigarette smoking and use of all nicotine products.

***Follow-Up.*** Refer client with respiratory symptoms to a specialist, as such symptoms may indicate other underlying disease.[37]

## PEPTIC ULCER DISEASE

Peptic ulcers are small sores, or lesions, in the lower end of the esophagus or the lining of the stomach, duodenum, or jejunal side of the gastrojejunostomy. The two main types of peptic ulcer disease (PUD) are duodenal and gastric.

Pepsin, the chief enzyme of gastric juices, combines with hydrochloric acid to digest food in the stomach. Normally the lining of the stomach resists corrosion, but for unclear reasons, resistance can break down and an ulcer develops. Because most clients with these ulcers demonstrate normal acid production, research is directed toward mucosal defense mechanisms.[43,44]

### Epidemiology

Risk factors include cigarette smoking, medical or family history, and medication. Nonsteroidal anti-inflammatory drugs (NSAIDs)/aspirin or steroids in high doses or used long term can contribute to the development of PUD, particularly among women older than 65 years.[44] The risk is the same for plain or buffered aspirin but less if it is enteric coated, because with the coating the tablet dissolves in the small intestine.

Medical conditions predisposing individuals to PUD are hyperparathyroidism (secondary to increased calcium, which increases gastric secretion), cirrhosis, chronic pulmonary disease, and renal failure. The evidence that increased stress causes or activates ulcer formation is not conclusive.

In clients older than 50, it is necessary to rule out gastric cancer as an etiology, especially if symptoms have a recent onset or are persistent despite treatment.

Transmission may involve *Helicobacter pylori (Campylobacter pyloris),* although its role in the pathogenesis of ulcers is unclear. Investigators believe that gastroduodenal mucosa infected with the organism is more likely to undergo ulceration.[45] It is agreed that it is the causative organism in type B antral gastritis.[45]

Incidence reports estimate that 4 million Americans suffer from PUD at any given time. It rarely occurs as a new condition before puberty or after age 65 and peaks between ages 55 and 65.[43] Between 4 and 8 percent of females develop an ulcer at some time in their life. Duodenal ulcers are more common than gastric ulcers.[44] The incidence of gastric ulcers is similar among men and women.

## Subjective Data

Less than half of clients with PUD present typically. Clinical features in the elderly are often vague or may be absent until a complication occurs.

Gnawing, burning, epigastric or upper abdominal pain radiating to the back may awaken clients in the night or early morning. Typically, symptoms of a peptic ulcer are brought on by an empty stomach and may be relieved by eating.

On the other hand, gastric ulcers are usually aggravated by eating. Pain begins almost immediately after eating. It is not uncommon for months or years to pass without pain. Associated symptoms include dyspepsia, heartburn, and nausea or may be more severe with vomiting and weight loss. Bowel habits generally remain unaltered.[43]

## Objective Data

Diagnostic tests and other procedures are the sources of objective data. Physical examination rarely helps in diagnosis. Epigastric tenderness is neither specific nor sensitive.

Diagnostic laboratory tests are used to evaluate a client for complications, such as bleeding, or indications of malabsorption.[42] Blood is drawn by venipuncture for CBC and chemistries; a test for fecal occult blood is also done. The sensitivity of fecal occult blood testing varies from 20 to 70 percent. False-positive results may be due to the use of laxatives or NSAIDs, peroxidase-containing foods, or hemorrhoids. False-negative results are related to the technique by which the sample was collected or tested.

The upper gastrointestinal x-ray and endoscopy are explained under Gastroesophageal Reflux Disease.

## Differential Medical Diagnosis

Esophageal stricture, Barrett's esophagus, angina, respiratory disease, gallbladder disease.

## Plan

***Psychosocial Interventions.*** Provide information and support concerning diet and possibly long-term medications.

***Medication.*** See Gastroesophageal Reflux. Treatment of *H. pylori* infection with medication as a routine course of action is not recommended, especially if the client is asymptomatic.[46] If upper GI symptoms are present, treatment by a GI specialist is indicated only if duodenal ulcer disease is present and "is a significant management problem." If PUD is documented by endoscopy and is unresponsive to H2 blockers, treatment by a specialist is advised.

Ulcer recurrence may be prevented with chronic H2 blockers at half the initial therapeutic dose among persons at high risk for recurrence (asthmatics, cigarette smokers, and diabetics) or clients at high risk for complications (renal transplant recipients and clients with systemic disease)[38,41] (see Table 17–8).

**'TABLE 17–8. MANAGEMENT OF PEPTIC ULCER DISEASE**

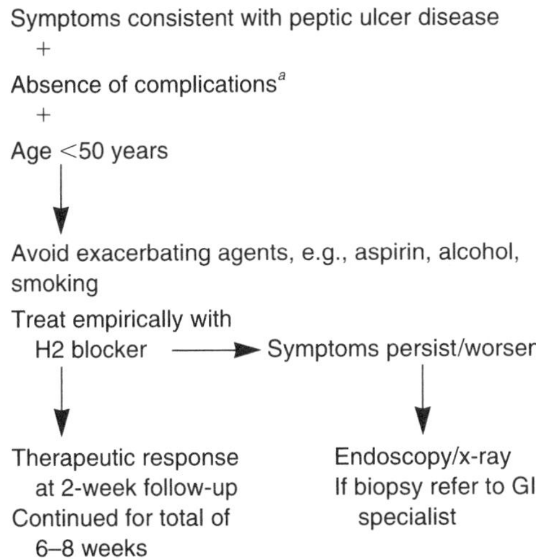


[a]History of GI/peptic ulcer disease, bleeding, weight loss, persistent pain, vomiting.
Sources: *References 42, 43.*

***Dietary Interventions.*** Have the client eliminate from her diet any offending foods, aspirin/NSAIDs, and alcohol. Ask her to keep a food diary.[43] Frequent, small bland meals with milk were encouraged for years; however, that diet is now known to increase acid production.

***Follow-Up.*** Follow-up differs for gastric and duodenal ulcers. Gastric ulcers take longer to heal and require a full 8 weeks of treatment. Duodenal ulcers may heal more quickly but recur in about 80 percent of clients within 1 year and are more likely to be a chronic condition. Refer clients with ulcers that are unresponsive (persistent symptoms) to a GI specialist.

## GALLBLADDER DISEASE

The two gallbladder diseases discussed in this chapter are cholecystitis and cholelithiasis.

*Cholecystitis* is acute inflammation of the gallbladder, usually caused by a gallstone blocking the outlet of the gallbladder or cystic duct. Edema, infection, and ulceration result. If this process continues, necrosis, perforation, and peritonitis may result.

*Cholelithiasis* is the presence or formation of gallstones. Generally, gallstones form whenever cholesterol is oversaturated. Gallstones are classified by composition.[47]

Cholesterol stones constitute 80 percent of all gallstones in the United States and contain, in addition to cholesterol, bile acids, calcium salts, proteins, and phospholipids.

Pigment stones are black or brown. Black pigment is more common in the United States, brown among native Asians. The brown stones sometime form in the bile duct following cholecystectomy.[48]

### Epidemiology

Risk factors are multiparity, use of estrogens (including oral contraceptives), obesity, rapid weight loss, high-fat diet, Crohn's disease (involving the ileum or ileal resection), regional enteritis, cirrhosis, diabetes, a family history of gallbladder disease, and any condition in which there is an excess of cholesterol. There is a 50 percent chance of recurrence with a previous history of gallbladder disease.[45]

Gallbladder disease occurs primarily among overweight women 55 to 65 years of age. The incidence among women is almost three times that among men and increases with age.[45,47]

### Subjective Data

Initially, a client reports diffuse, intermittent right upper quadrant pain, an ache or pressure that occurs at night or early in the morning. It progresses to a continuous, more severe pain and may radiate to the epigastrium or right shoulder. Onset of pain may be sudden and last from 20 minutes to 5 or 6 hours; it may continue as a dull ache for 24 hours or longer. Intervals between episodes vary considerably, from weeks to years. Pain may be accompanied by nausea, vomiting, constipation, or fever.[45]

## Objective Data

Physical examination during the acute phase of disease may be helpful along with blood tests and visualization methods.

***Physical Examination.*** Not helpful in the nonacute phase. During the acute symptom phase, specific changes may be observed:

- The client appears restless and jaundice may be apparent. No position is comfortable.
- The client may have a fever.
- The eyes are icteric.
- The client may splint the chest during respiration.
- The abdomen is tender above the right upper quadrant. A palpable globular mass lies behind the lower border of the liver. Murphy's sign is positive. (To determine Murphy's sign, place your fingertips along the right costal margin and ask the client to inhale. The client will report a sharp pain on deep inspiration with respiratory splinting.)

***Diagnostic Laboratory Tests.*** May reveal elevations of serum transaminases, alkaline phosphatase (due to obstructed biliary tract), or serum lipase or amylase (gallstone pancreatitis). An increase in white blood cells with a left shift denotes cholecystitis or cholangitis. A venipuncture is required for blood tests.

*Ultrasonography* is used to diagnose about 75 percent of gallstones in affected clients. The method is noninvasive and requires no preparation. Explain to the client that gallstones measuring 4 mm or larger can potentially obstruct the bile duct. "Silent stones" (radiologic evidence of stones less than 4 mm in asymptomatic clients) do not, however, necessitate treatment.

*The hepato-iminodiacetic acid (HIDA) scan* is the diagnostic test (radioisotope test) of choice when a problem is acute. It provides additional information on gallbladder function and cystic duct patency. Before the procedure, the client fasts for a minimum of 8 hours. Technetium-labeled iminodiacetic acid is injected and the scan done 60 minutes later.

If the gallbladder can be visualized, the cystic duct is not obstructed. The scan also provides information about hepatocellular disease.

An *oral cholecystogram* is a diagnostic evaluation for cholelithiasis. The client takes iopanic or tyropanoic acid tablets the night before the exam. The dye concentrates in the gallbladder and permits its visualization the following day. The method is well tolerated. It is 90 to 95 percent accurate in detecting stones.

## Differential Medical Diagnosis

Angina, peptic ulcer disease, esophageal spasm, appendicitis, intestinal obstruction, pancreatitis, myocardial ischemia, pyelonephritis.

## Plan

***Psychosocial Interventions.*** Discuss with the client that surveillance of recurrence alone may be suitable management for infrequent symptoms and little disability.

***Medication.*** Use of oral bile salts is limited to clients with small radiolucent stones (indicating cholesterol composition) and a functioning gallbladder and to clients with mild or infrequent symptoms. Oral salts are also given to clients who refuse surgery or who are poor surgical candidates. The medication is taken daily for 6 months to 2 years. Treatment requires follow-up visits and ultrasound examination. Medication is expensive.[45]

Bile salts alter the ratio of bile acids to cholesterol and lecithin as well as reduce HMG-COA reductase activity, thereby reducing hepatic cholesterol synthesis.

***Surgical Interventions.*** A cholecystectomy is the best choice for frequent, severe biliary pain, acute cholecystitis, or suspected gallbladder cancer. It is essentially a cure. Stones may be retained or recur in the biliary ductal system after cholecystectomy.[44]

The laparoscopic approach to cholecystectomy is becoming the surgical method of choice for select clients in many medical centers. Not every client is a candidate for this method, as many require an incisional approach secondary to disruption of the ducts.

Lithotripsy, extracorporeal shock-wave therapy of gallstones, is gaining popularity but its use is limited. Its distinct advantage is that it is noninvasive. More research is needed to determine the rate of recurrence, adverse sequelae, and cost effectiveness.

***Follow-Up.*** Refer clients with acute cholecystitis to a collaborating physician, gastrointestinal specialist, or surgeon for evaluation and treatment. Acute cholecystitis can be a life-threatening emergency. Major complications are perforation of the gallbladder with resultant peritonitis and internal biliary fistula. Fever, severe pain, and elevated white blood cell counts are indications for prompt surgical referral. The size, number, and location of gallstones influence the decision to treat aggressively versus conservatively. A more aggressive approach will likely be based on greater pain and disability from biliary attacks.

## IRRITABLE BOWEL SYNDROME

The etiology of irritable bowel syndrome (IBS) is probably multifactorial. Contraction of colonic smooth muscle is controlled by cyclic alterations of smooth muscle membrane potential. In IBS, the normally orderly movement of colonic contents is altered. The entire gut, particularly the colon, is affected.[48]

### Epidemiology

Etiology reveals a threefold increase in psychiatric illnesses (anxiety, hysteria, and depression) among persons with irritable bowel syndrome. When psychiatric illness is a cofactor, clients are more often middle-aged.[49]

Irritable bowel syndrome occurs most often among women between the ages of 20 and 50 years, but it may develop at any age. It is one of the most common reasons for referral to gastrointestinal specialists. About 30 percent of the general population may have symptoms, but only 14 percent seek medical attention.

### Subjective Data

A careful history is the key to diagnosis. Acute stressful events, such as acute illness, job demands or loss of job, financial pressures, and illness or death of a close friend or relative, seem to precipitate attacks. Poor dietary habits may also be influential. About 50 percent of clients report nausea, heartburn, and dyspeptic symptoms. Colic abdominal pain varies in intensity. It may be precipitated by eating, but is typically relieved by a bowel movement. A client may experience diarrhea, constipation, or both. In addition, she may report abdominal distention, increased amounts of rectal mucus, and a feeling of incomplete evacuation. The condition does *not,* however, awaken clients from sleep, does *not* usually result in any appreciable weight loss (if any, it is less than 10 percent of body weight), and does *not* cause rectal bleeding.[49,50]

### Objective Data

Diagnosis is often made only after other gastrointestinal disorders have been excluded.

Consequently, expensive and unnecessary testing may occur. A detailed history guides the workup.

***Physical Examination.*** May reveal diffuse abdominal tenderness. A rectal exam is essential. Hemorrhoids and anal fissures are evaluated.

***Diagnostic Laboratory Tests.*** CBC, chemistries, urinalysis, and examination of stools for ova and parasites (particularly Giardia). Stools for culture, white blood cells, red blood cells, and an elevated erythrocyte sedimentation rate are done to rule out inflammatory bowel disease. A lactose tolerance/hydrogen breath test may be done.

*Flexible sigmoidoscopy* is used to rule out polyps, malignancy, and inflammatory bowel disease. The procedure is usually well tolerated. In the absence of organic lesions, irritable bowel syndrome is strongly suspect.

*A colonoscopy or double-contrast barium enema* is indicated for clients older than 40 years or with a strong family history of colon cancer. The tests rule out polyps and malignancy. The client is given a cathartic 24 hours prior to procedure to evaluate bowel debris. Usually, preprocedure medication is given via an intravenous catheter. Advise the client that she will need to be accompanied to and from the test.

## Differential Medical Diagnosis

Laxative abuse, lactose intolerance, Crohn's disease, ulcerative colitis, colon cancer, parasitic infestation.[50]

## Plan

***Psychosocial Interventions.*** Explain to the client that she should avoid stressful situations. Although symptoms are stress related, overemphasizing the role of stress can induce confusion and guilt in the client. She should know that irritable bowel syndrome is a chronic condition that can be managed. Reassure her that her condition is not cancer and will not progress to inflammatory bowel disease. Symptoms are controllable, although it may take time and a trial-and-error approach to find the right therapeutic management for an individual. A plan should focus on diet and lifestyle.

***Medication.*** Medications that may be used address a variety of symptoms.[48,49]

*Psyllium* is a bulk laxative that improves regularity and is the main pharmacotherapeutic intervention.

*Calcium channel blockers* decrease smooth muscle response to neurohumoral stimulation.

*Nitrates* stimulate production of cyclic guanosine monophosphate within the cell, inhibiting smooth muscle contractions.

*Anxiolytics* are nonspecific in their action and reserved for underlying anxiety disorders.

*Cholestyramine* is used if increased fecal bile salts are suspected of contributing to diarrhea.

*Antispasmodic* agents such as dicyclomine hydrochloride (Bentyl) are used for abdominal pain and cramping.

*A tricyclic antidepressant* is used only if depression is evident. Amitriptyline hydrochloride (Elavil) given at night is a good choice because it has anticholinergic properties.

***Lifestyle/Dietary Changes.*** These changes include modifications in diet, exercise, and elimination.

A low-residue diet is recommended for diarrhea and a high-fiber diet for constipation. Advise the client to avoid gas-producing foods (eg, cabbage and beans) and to eat at regular hours; to chew food thoroughly; and to increase intake of fluids, especially fruit juices and water.

Daily exercise is helpful. Also advise the client to avoid straining at bowel movements; the urge to defecate should be promptly followed by elimination.

***Follow-Up.*** A diagnosis of irritable bowel syndrome does not require frequent x-rays or colonoscopic examinations. The frequency of follow-up visits depends on the severity of the client's symptoms. Systems are reviewed, the effectiveness of intervention assessed, and a physical examination done. Encourage the client to return should her symptoms exacerbate or change. Irritable bowel syndrome is a chronic illness that requires support and reinforcement of the prescribed therapeutic regimen.

## ANAL FISSURES

An anal fissure is a linear ulcer on the margin of the anus.

### Epidemiology

Anal fissures are a secondary irritation from diarrhea or straining related to constipation, laxative overuse, or trauma. Their exact incidence is unknown.

### Subjective Data

A client may report bleeding and pain with and often after defecation. Pain may be severe and last 30 minutes or more following a bowel movement. Pruritus ani may occur.[50]

### Objective Data

Internal hemorrhoids may be found. Lateral traction on buttocks should expose the fissure. If not, referral is made for inspection using an anoscope. In the acute stage, tissues are erythematous and inflamed. Chronic fissures may erode the anoderm and expose the base of the internal sphincter.

### Differential Medical Diagnosis

Primary lesion of syphilis, tuberculosis ulcerations, herpes, malignant epithelioma, abscesses, anorectal fistulas, cancer, Crohn's disease.

### Plan[50]

***Psychosocial Interventions.*** Address the client's acute fear of cancer that may be aroused by her pain or bleeding. Reassure her that symptoms will resolve and can be prevented.

***Medication.*** Stool softeners and lubricating anesthetic ointments (short-term) are used for severe pain. Avoid laxatives and suppositories.

***Surgical Interventions.*** An internal sphincterotomy is usually performed to decrease the pressure of chronic fissures in the anal canal. A short 2- to 3-day hospital stay is required, the wound heals quickly, and the procedure is curative in 90 to 95 percent of cases.

***Lifestyle/Dietary Changes.*** Advise the client to follow a high-fiber diet. Sitz baths are of no proven value.

***Follow-Up.*** Most symptoms resolve within 2 to 4 weeks. If, however, no improvement occurs, refer the client to a surgeon.

# HEADACHE

In 1988, the Headache Classification Committee of the International Headache Society adopted 13 categories to help clarify the confusing differential diagnosis of headache.[51,52] This chapter focuses on the two most common types: tension and migraine.[53] Most experts agree that tension and migraine headaches are on a continuum, with some overlap and shared characteristics and etiologies.

Prior to discussing the common and more benign headaches, it is best to understand rare headache variants and potentially more dangerous headaches. Only 2 percent of headaches fall into a category that has been labeled traction or inflammation.

Traction and inflammation headaches are precipitated by organic conditions, for example, brain tumors, bleeding, and meningitis. Often, no characteristic history indicates the cause, but red flag signs may be detected[54,55] (see Table 17–9).

## UNCOMMON HEADACHE VARIANTS

Several uncommon headache variants must be considered in diagnosis: cluster headaches, complex migraines, and headaches caused by pseudotumor cerebri, temporal (giant cell) arteritis, and subarachnoid hemorrhage.

Keep in mind that systemic illnesses can affect headaches. Look at the total picture including the possibility of referred pain from sinus infections or dental infections.

### Cluster Headaches

Cluster headaches are a rare variant type of migraine, seen in 0.07 percent of the population. Reports show that 90 percent occur among men. Attacks usually begin between ages 20 and 40 and occur in "clusters," usually nightly in 6-week cycles. Excruciating pain lasts about 1 hour and is described as "boring" around one eye. Tearing and nasal congestion often occur on the affected side. Cluster headaches are frequently triggered by alcohol or histamine. Refer the client to a neurologist.[56]

**TABLE 17–9. RED FLAG SYMPTOMS FOR DANGEROUS HEADACHES**

| |
|---|
| No recognizable benign pattern for headaches |
| Client description: "Worst headache ever" |
| Onset of headache with exertion (cough, strain, Valsalva maneuver) |
| Vomiting without nausea |
| Personality changes (decreased alertness or cognition) |
| Any abnormality on physical exam |
| Neck not supple, pain with flexion |
| Fever |
| Focal neurological signs |
| Seizure(s) |
| Sudden change in headache pattern |
| Progression of symptoms |

### Complex Migraine Headaches

Complex migraines are associated with focal neurological signs, which may continue after the prodrome and into or past the headache phase. They may be confused with stroke. Always refer the client to a neurologist.

### Pseudotumor Cerebri

Headaches may be caused by pseudotumor cerebri (benign cranial hypertension). The hypertension, of unknown etiology, is most often seen among children or obese young pregnant women. It has been associated with use of tetracycline, vitamin A, or a steroid. A client is in no apparent distress. She may report "mild headache"; papilledema is noted on the physical exam. Partial or complete visual loss occurs in 5 to 10 percent of cases not treated. Refer the client to a neurologist immediately.

### Temporal Arteritis

Headaches may also result from temporal (giant cell) arteritis. The arteritis is of unknown etiology and occurs primarily after age 40. Incidence is estimated at 24 per 100,000. Clients may have associated fever, malaise, and muscle aches. Clients usually, although not always, have a headache. Visual symptoms occur among 50 percent. Temporal arteritis is also associated with proximal muscle weakness (polymyalgia rheumatica). Tenderness over temporal arteries can be elicited. The erythrocyte sedimentation rate is dramatically elevated, often greater than 100 mm per hour. Refer the client to a neurologist immediately. Treatment with steroids is initiated to prevent blindness.

### Subarachnoid Hemorrhage

Subarachnoid hemorrhage may be reported as the "worst headache in my life." The hemorrhage is usually secondary to trauma or a congenital aneurysm and is most common between ages 25 and 50. The individual may collapse and lose consciousness. Neck stiffness and neurological signs almost always occur. Refer the client to a neurologist immediately or an emergency room if a neurologist is not immediately available.

## TENSION HEADACHES

The pathophysiology of tension headaches is poorly understood. Although once referred to as muscle contraction headaches, current research indicates that muscle contraction is not always present with this type of headache. Stress or tension is almost always involved, but the exact pathophysiology is unknown. Tension headaches can be episodic or chronic daily headaches.

### Epidemiology

Studies reveal that 90 percent of headaches are tension headaches. Episodic tension headaches are the classic stress-related headaches. Chronic daily headaches, on the other hand, are often associated with depression that requires treatment. (see Table 17–10).

### Subjective Data

A headache history, taken with interest and concern, is the key to the diagnosis. Patterns should be established (see Table 17–11). Rule out a history of trauma, neurological signs, and concurrent disorders.

Have the client keep a headache diary. She should record the day and time of the headache and surrounding events, such as diet, physical activity, and menstrual cycle. She should note aggravating and relieving factors.

When taking a history, it is important to have a client identify different types of headaches, as she may easily have more than one. Ask her to describe specific symptoms (see Table 17–11). General symptoms apply to all headaches and must be evaluated (see Table 17–12).

### Objective Data

Data are based on a complete physical examination and, in some instances, diagnostic tests. Physical examination includes examination of the nervous system and eyes, nose, and throat (see Table 17–13).

**TABLE 17–10. EPIDEMIOLOGY OF TENSION AND MIGRAINE HEADACHES**

| | Tension Headache | Migraine Headache |
|---|---|---|
| Prevalence | Almost universal | 15% of population |
| Family history | 40% with family history | 70% with family history |
| Age of onset | Any age; however, rare in childhood and common in adulthood | 5–40 years, rare after 40 |
| Sex distribution | 75% female | Male:female the same until puberty, then female:male 3:2 |

Source: *Reference 57.*

**TABLE 17–11. HEADACHE SYMPTOM PATTERNS IN HISTORY**

| Symptom | Migraine Headache | Tension Headache | Traction and Inflammation |
|---|---|---|---|
| Onset | 10% have aura; may awake with headache | Gradual; often begin during times of stress | Varied (tumors may have periods of pain remission, but pain returns with increased severity) |
| Duration | Usually 8–12 hours; range 3 hours to rarely 3 days | Usually 8–12 hours; may last days, weeks, months | Varied, but tumor symptoms progressive |
| Frequency | Usually one or two per month or less, rarely one per week | Wide range (daily to rarely) | Varied |
| Pain location | Approximately 60% unilateral; may switch side or become bilateral | Approximately 90% bilateral; frontal area, "hat band" area, or back of neck | Often unilateral |
| Pain quality | Throbbing; moderate to severe | Constant; nagging to severe | Varied |
| Associated symptoms | Nausea, vomiting photophobia, phonophobia | None | Varied (vomiting without nausea) |
| Triggers | Stress; menses; alcohol; food; "letdown" after stress | Stress | None known (mass lesion headache worse after cough or Valsalva maneuver) |
| Relieving factors | Rest in dark room; sleep | Relaxation exercise; Tylenol/NSAID[a] | Varied |

[a]Nonsteroidal anti-inflammatory drug.

Usually no diagnostic tests are indicated for tension headaches. For any patient older than 40 with a new type of headache, order a CBC and erythrocyte sedimentation rate to rule out temporal arteritis.

## Differential Medical Diagnosis

See Table 17–14.

## Plan

***Psychosocial Interventions.*** It is crucial to reassure the client that tension-type headaches are usually not associated with any severely negative consequences. A thorough physical exam can greatly decrease the woman's anxiety level. Once reassured, she can better focus on lifestyle changes and stress management techniques that might help to decrease the frequency of headaches.

***Medication.*** Nonsteroidal anti-inflammatory drugs are very helpful for tension headaches as well as migraine and perimenstrual headaches. Ibuprofen (Advil, Motrin) is the first choice; naproxen sodium (Naprosyn) is helpful for perimenopausal headaches. Refer to a pharmacotherapeutics textbook for further information.

- *Side Effects.* Gastrointestinal distress and bleeding may occur.
- *Contraindications.* Do not administer to those clients with a history of peptic ulcer disease, bleeding disorders, pregnancy, kidney problems, or allergic reactions to NSAIDs.

**TABLE 17–12. GENERAL SYMPTOMS AND MENSTRUAL PATTERN PERTINENT TO ANY HEADACHE HISTORY IN WOMEN**

*General Symptoms*[a]

*Sleep pattern:* Depression is associated with early-morning wakening. Trouble falling asleep is associated with anxiety.

*Past Medical History:* Allergies, medications (especially "withdrawal" from substances such as caffeine, alcohol, and over-the-counter medications), habits, family history, history of head trauma, previous tests, or coexisting illnesses.

*Diet:* Often related to migraine; unrelated to tension-type.

*Emotional status:* Ask open-ended questions, such as "Tell me about yourself." "How are things at home? At work?"

*Menstrual History and Headache*

*Migraine:* Strong association between migraines and the menstrual cycle. Up to 60 to 70 percent of female migraine sufferers may have exacerbations of migraines around menses. About 50 percent of women experience migraine remission during pregnancy. Have client keep menstrual and headache diary.

*Perimenstrual headaches:* Many women not identified with classic migraines suffer from perimenstrual headaches. Perimenstrual headaches usually occur the week before or the week of menses. Women often do not complain to health care providers despite severe, sometimes incapacitating symptoms. Because perimenstrual headaches are predictable, they may be less threatening; therefore women do not seek help. Perimenstrual headaches are thought to be vascular. Falling estrogen levels may prime cerebral vessels, allowing migraine inducers, such as serotonin, to induce headache.

[a]General well-being and overall lifestyle.
Source: *Reference 58.*

- *Anticipated Outcome on Evaluation.* Headache is relieved.
- *Client Teaching.* Advise the client that NSAIDs are most effective when taken at onset of pain. Encourage her to break the pain cycle and give adequate amounts of medication. Narcotics should not be given for this diagnosis, as clients may become physically dependent and experience withdrawal and rebound headaches.

***Lifestyle/Dietary Changes.*** The client may require support in evaluating current life situation and stressors. Help her to prioritize activities and to let go of unnecessary tasks and difficulties. Teach general stress management principles. Refer the client for counseling if indicated.

Dietary changes are not applicable unless over- or undereating is a source of tension or stress.

Exercise or other physical activity is an effective stress reducer. Encourage and support lifestyle changes that incorporate 30 minutes of aerobic exercise 3 to 5 days a week.

***Follow-Up.*** Plan a follow-up visit 2 weeks after the initial visit to support and reassess the client. If headaches have not significantly improved or if the client has experienced any new symptoms, such as those listed in Table 17–11, refer her to a neurologist. Depression may also be a cause of the headaches.

## MIGRAINE HEADACHES

Migraine headaches are recurrent headaches that may or may not be accompanied by visual and gastrointestinal disturbances. The prodromal symptoms (aura) may result from an intracerebral vasoconstriction.[57,58] Vasodilation follows, resulting in a sterile inflammation (causing the head pain) and edema. Secondary muscle contraction headache may also develop.

In migraines with an aura, previously called "classic migraines," focal neurological symptoms usually precede the headache and may last up to about 20 minutes. Auras are often visual; they may include visual field deficits, a scintillating scotoma (a luminous

**TABLE 17–13. PHYSICAL EXAM FOR HEADACHE**

*General appearance:* Note affect, photophobia.

*Vital signs:* Blood pressure and temperature must be charted.

Blood pressure—Hypertension (HTN) rarely causes headaches; pain with diastolic > 120–140. HTN may aggravate migraine.

Temperature—Fever, rule out meningitis, arteritis, sinusitis, abscess.

*Mental status:* Usually assessed within framework of interview.

| | Cranial Nerves[a] | Head, Eyes, Ears, and Throat |
|---|---|---|
| (If normal, efficient charting states "cranial nerves II–XII intact.") | | |
| I. | Olfactory: usually not done | |
| II. | Optic: visual acuity, visual fields by confrontation | Disc flat (rule out papilledema) |
| III, IV, VI. | Oculomotor, trochlear, abducens<br>PERRLA,[b] EOMs, note ptosis of upper lids | |
| V. | Trigeminal<br>Motor—palpate masseter, open and close jaw<br>Sensory—touch forehead, cheek, jaw | Palpate "click" from temporo-mandibular joint<br>Palpate temporal area (rule out arteritis) |
| VII. | Facial<br>Observe facial symmetry<br>Raise eyebrows, frown<br>Close eyes, resist opening<br>Smile, puff out cheeks | Check tenderness over sinuses (rule out sinusitis) |
| VIII. | Acoustic: hearing watch tick | Look at tympanic membrane |
| IX, X. | Glossopharyngeal, vagus<br>Symmetrical movement soft palate | Check teeth |
| XI. | Spinal accessory<br>Atrophy, shrug upward against hands<br>Turn head against your hands | Check nodes<br>Check neck stiffness<br>Bruits<br>Tender neck muscles |
| XII. | Hypoglossal<br>Tongue movement, fasciculations | |

*Screening motor*

Walk note gait, heel/toe walk

Hop on one foot, Romberg

Deep knee bend, check arms pronator drift

*Screening sensory*

Pain and vibration (tuning fork), hands and feet

Stereognosis

*Reflexes*

Check deep tendon reflexes, Babinski, and other systems if indicated by history

[a]For efficiency, examine cranial nerves and head, eyes, ears, nose, and throat system simultaneously.

[b]PERRLA, pupils equal, round, reactive to light and accommodation; EOM, extraocular movement.

**TABLE 17–14. DIFFERENTIAL DIAGNOSES OF HEADACHES**

| Tension Headache (90% of headaches) | Vascular Headache (8% of headaches) | Traction and Inflammation Headache (2% of headaches) |
|---|---|---|
| Episodic/chronic | Migraine | Mass lesions (tumors, hematomas, edema) |
| Temporomandibular joint (TMJ) syndrome | With aura | Head, eye, ear, nose, and throat diseases, such as sinusitis, tooth abscess |
| Chronic myositis | Without aura | Temporal arteritis |
| Cervical osteoarthritis | Complicated | Cranial neuralgias |
| | Cluster | Occlusive vascular disease |
| | Hypertension | Pseudotumor cerebri |
| | Fever (toxic vascular) | |

patch with irregular outline in the visual field), or a fortification spectrum (a dark patch with zig-zag outline). Other neurological auras, such as aphasia and hemiplegia, occur occasionally. When the aura fades, the headache usually begins.

Migraines without an aura, previously called "common migraines," have the features of classic migraines, such as throbbing pain, nausea, vomiting, photophobia, and phonophobia, but no aura.[59]

## Epidemiology

The cause of migraine headaches is unknown. The use of oral contraceptives may be a risk factor for more frequent, more intense migraines; on the other hand, oral contraceptives may make migraines better. Any increase in frequency or intensity of migraines among women taking an oral contraceptive is a contraindication to that contraceptive drug (see Table 17–10).

Incidence reports show that 8 percent of headaches are migraine or vascular headaches.

## Subjective Data

Obtaining a compete history is essential (see Tables 17–11 and 17–12). The history is used to differentiate between migraines and tension headaches because their treatments differ. The criteria for migraine without an aura include a recurring idiopathic headache with at least two of the following: nausea (with or without vomiting), unilateral pain, throbbing, photophobia or phonophobia, association with menstrual cycle, positive family history.

## Objective Data

A physical examination is done (see Table 17–13). For recurrent migraines no diagnostic workup is necessary. For an initial diagnosis, a CBC and chemistries may be helpful. Anemia, electrolyte imbalance, and increased calcium can aggravate migraines.

## Differential Medical Diagnosis

See Table 17–14.

## Plan

***Psychosocial Interventions.*** Psychosocial intervention is critical, especially for a client who has migraines with an aura, as these can be very frightening. Reassure the client that she is not having a stroke and involve her as an active participant in measures to prevent and abort attacks.

**TABLE 17–15. OVERVIEW OF MEDICATIONS FOR MIGRAINES[a]**

**Abortive Measures:** Appropriate for clients experiencing occasional headaches, not more than one a month.

*NSAIDs*[b]*:* Very effective, especially if taken early because they block the sterile inflammation of migraines. Any NSAID may be tried. Naproxen sodium (Naprosyn, 550 mg p.o. b.i.d.) helpful for women suffering with perimenstrual vascular headaches.

*Antiemetics:* Oral or per rectum. Prochlorperazine (Compazine) suppositories are an example. Help nausea and aid client in "sleeping off" the headache.

*Ergots:* Potent vasoconstrictors. May be given intramuscularly, orally, sublingually, by inhalation, or rectally. Most helpful if client has "aura" and can take immediately. Example: Ergotamine tartrate SL (Ergostat) 2 mg at onset and 1 mg every 30 minutes until headache is relieved or to a maximum of 6 mg per day, 12 mg per week.

A widely recognized, effective treatment for acute migraine is dihydroergotamine mesylate (D.H.E. 45 injection) given 1 mg IM. Give antiemetic first or concurrently.[61]

**Caution.** Be familiar with doses of medications used. Overuse can lead to "ergotism" (prolonged vasoconstriction that can cause tissue ischemia and gangrene). Beta blockers increase the risk for ergotism; simultaneous use is contraindicated.

**Preventive Measures:** Indicated for three or more attacks per month or one prolonged attack per month. Give adequate trial of 3–6 months of therapy.

*Beta-blockers:* Numerous types (propranolol, long-acting preparation increases compliance). Effective in 50 percent of cases.

**Caution**. Contraindicated with such conditions as asthma and congestive heart failure.

*Tricyclics:* Numerous types (amitriptyline [Elavil] often used, starting with a 25-mg dose at bedtime, increasing as necessary).

*NSAIDs:* Ibuprofen, naproxen sodium. Observe for gastrointestinal side effects.

*Calcium channel blockers:* Numerous types (verapamil [Calan, Isoptin] p.o. 240–360 mg per day). Usually ordered by neurologist.

*Methylsergide (Sansert):* **Last choice**. Ordered only by a neurologist. Can cause fibrosis of heart valves and peritoneum if given longer than 6 months.

[a]Please consult a current pharmacotherapeutics text for details.
[b]Nonsteroidal anti-inflammatory drugs.
Source: *Reference 60.*

**TABLE 17–16. DIETARY FACTORS AND MIGRAINE HEADACHES**

| Direct Vasoactive Substances | Indirect Triggers |
|---|---|
| Tyramine | Caffeine |
| Aged cheeses | Nicotine |
| Pickled foods | Ergotamine |
| Fresh baked bread | Hypoglycemia |
| Marinated foods | Ice cream |
| Nitrates (cured meats) | Monamine oxidase inhibitors |
| Chocolate | |
| Monosodium glutamate (MSG) | |
| Alcohol | |

***Medication.*** See Table 17–15.[60]

***Lifestyle/Dietary Changes.*** Focus primarily on what triggers the migraine. Often there is a "letdown" trigger; for example, the headache starts Saturday morning following a stressful week. Counsel the client to readjust her lifestyle and help her with stress management.[61]

Diet may be a factor in the occurrence of migraines. The most common triggers are chocolate, alcohol, and aged cheeses (see Table 17–16). Ask the client to keep a diary of foods eaten and to avoid foods associated with the onset of migraine.

Advise the client that physical activity, including aerobic exercise for 30 minutes three to five times a week, helps to reduce stress.

***Follow-Up.*** Teach the client the warning signs of headaches with serious underlying causes (see Table 17–9). If such a warning sign occurs, refer her to a neurologist immediately. Otherwise, arrange to see the client about every 4 to 6 weeks until the migraines improve. If no improvement is seen in 8 weeks or the migraines worsen, refer her to a neurologist.

# RESPIRATORY INFECTIONS

## COMMON COLD

The common cold is a mild, self-limited condition caused by a viral infection of the upper respiratory mucosa. The nasal mucosa is prominently involved.[62]

### Epidemiology

Studies of the common cold demonstrate that age and environmental contacts are the two major factors influencing the extent of illness.[62] Numerous groups and hundreds of viral strains cause "cold" symptoms. Rhinoviruses are the most common group. Others include coronaviruses, respiratory syncytial virus, adenovirus, echovirus, coxsackievirus, and parainfluenza virus.[62,63]

Transmission is primarily via direct contact with infected secretions, usually hand-to-hand and subsequent hand-to-face contact. It is evident that good handwashing is crucial in breaking the chain of transmission. Less often, transmission occurs via respiratory droplets from coughs or sneezes. Crowds and poor ventilation promote transmission.[62,63] The incubation period is usually 48 to 72 hours.[62,63]

Incidence of the common cold among average adults is 2 to 4 colds per year; the average child has 6 to 12 colds per year; parents of small children have about 6 colds per year.[62,63] People seek primary care most often for viral upper respiratory conditions. The vast majority of these illnesses are benign and self-limited; however, they have a major social and financial impact. They are responsible for more absences from work and school than any other type of illness.[63]

### Subjective Data

The client's chief complaints are malaise, rhinorrhea, and a "scratchy" throat. Nasal secretions are usually clear and copious at onset, changing to mucoid appearance later in the illness. Mucopurulent secretions *do not* necessarily indicate a secondary bacterial infection. Fever is rare in adults. Symptoms peak in 2 to 4 days, then gradually resolve. The total course of the illness is usually 5 to 10 days. When nasal symptoms last longer than 10 to 14 days, the client needs to be evaluated for sinusitis or allergies.[62,63]

### Objective Data

Physical examination reveals a benign general appearance. Fever is either low grade or absent. Nasal mucosa is often edematous with clear discharge.

The pharynx appears to have mild erythema. Lymphoid hyperplasia of the posterior pharynx is more common than tonsillar enlargement. Lymph nodes are usually nonpalpable, but small anterior cervical nodes may be palpable. Lungs are clear.

### Differential Medical Diagnosis

Bacterial infections (*Mycoplasma pneumoniae, Chlamydia psittaci,* group A beta hemolytic streptococcus); viral syndromes (Epstein–Barr or mononucleosis, cytomegalovirus); allergic rhinitis (seasonal, associated itching and copious clear nasal discharge).[62,63] Colds resolve in a few days; other syndromes are more severe and/or long lasting.

### Plan

A large part of intervention is helping the client care for herself.

***Psychosocial Interventions.*** Educate the client on the expected course of her illness and the need for self-care. Empower her to pursue self-care when appropriate. Provide information about the difference between viral and bacterial infections; tell her that antibiotics do not treat viral infections.

***Medication.*** See Table 17–17.

**TABLE 17–17. OVERVIEW OF ORAL MEDICATION TYPES USED FOR THE COMMON COLD[a]**

| Class | Indications | Side Effects | Contraindications |
|---|---|---|---|
| Decongestants | Shrink swollen nasal mucosa | Neurologic agitation, increased blood pressure | Avoid with hypertension. |
| Antihistamines | Dry up mucous membrane secretions | Drowsiness (no effect on blood pressure) | Avoid with asthma and history of asthma "flair" with use of antihistamines. Avoid giving with sedating medications or alcohol. |
| Antipyretics/ analgesic | Relieve discomfort or fever | Gastrointestinal irritation with nonsteroidal anti-inflammatory drugs | Aspirin is associated with Reye's syndrome; use acetaminophen, especially in clients under age 18. |

[a]Numerous drugs are included in each class. See specific pharmacotherapeutics texts for details.
Sources: *References 62, 63.*

***Lifestyle Changes.*** Lifestyle changes may help prevent the spread of colds. Advise clients to practice good handwashing and to avoid hand-to-face contact. Increasing fluid intake helps keep secretions loose and moving. Physical activity may be carried out as tolerated.

Strongly encourage cessation of smoking, as it increases the risk for secondary bacterial infections affecting ears, sinuses, and the lungs.

***Follow-Up.*** Teach clients to look for pain (in ear, face, or chest), fever (fever higher than 102°F or fever that recurs after initial few days), and distressing cough that is associated with dyspnea, fever, or localized chest pain, or that is persistent and progressive.[62,63]

## OTITIS MEDIA

Otitis media (OM) is an acute infection of the middle ear. The majority of infections are caused by eustachian tube dysfunction, which in adults is caused primarily by edema from viral upper respiratory infections and allergies. Barotrauma (flying/scuba diving) and cancer can also impair eustachian tube function. Chronic negative pressure in the middle ear leads to serous effusion and overgrowth of respiratory tract bacteria, with subsequent purulent discharge and inflammation.[64,65]

### Epidemiology

Studies indicate that otitis media is a bacterial disease of the respiratory tract mucosa. The three primary pathogens are *Streptococcus pneumoniae, Hemophilus influenzae,* and *Moraxella catarrhalis* (previously *Branhamella catarrhalis*).[66] Resistant strains of *M. catarrhalis* and *H. influenzae* can produce β-lactamase, which inactivates penicillin and amoxicillin.[64,66]

Transmission of otitis media as a primary viral upper respiratory infection occurs in the usual way; however, it is most often a secondary bacterial infection following a viral upper respiratory tract infection or problems with allergies.

Incidence reports show otitis media most common among children; however, at least 4.4 percent of the adult population has one episode per year.[67]

### Subjective Data

Usually the client reports a history of viral respiratory infections, allergies, or barotrauma. She describes unilateral or bilateral ear pain associated with decreased hearing. Systemic symptoms are uncommon in adults. New onset of recurrent otitis media with no preceding history of upper respiratory infections or allergies may be indicative of cancer, especially in women who smoke and drink alcohol.[63]

### Objective Data

Data are gathered primarily from physical examination of the ears.

Physical examination reveals a general benign appearance. Vital signs are usually normal, fever rare. The external canal of the ear should appear normal, with no tragus or mastoid tenderness. Otoscopy is used to evaluate five parameters of tympanic membrane appearance:

- *Color.* Erythema is consistent with acute infection.
- *Contour.* The membrane may be bulging in acute suppurative otitis media, and retracted in serous otitis.
- *Translucence.* The membrane may be thick and opaque in chronic otitis.
- *Structural Changes.* An irregular light reflex or blisters indicate infection.
- *Mobility.* A light reflex should move with insufflation; immobility is consistent with infection.[63,67]

If the canal is obscured by copious purulent drainage and the possibility of rupture exists, do not instill anything into the ear or attempt to clean it out.

The throat appears benign, although it may have changes associated with allergies or other causes of pharyngitis. The neck usually shows no change, although small anterior nodes may be present. The mastoid should not be tender.

Diagnostic tests are not usually indicated. An audiogram may be helpful in assessing hearing, and tympanometry may help assess mobility.

### Differential Medical Diagnosis

Several conditions of a serious nature should be considered.

External otitis is also called "swimmer's ear." The canal is usually swollen with exudate and tender with external manipulation of the ear. *Treatment with otic drops, usually Cortisporin otic suspension, is required.*

Serous otitis media is characterized by a retracted tympanic membrane, possibly an air–fluid level, and often decreased hearing. There is no erythema, and the condition is common with allergies and upper respiratory infections.

Mastoiditis is a life-threatening condition caused by the spread of infection from the middle ear to the air cells of the mastoid process. Any tenderness over the mastoid should lead to suspicion of mastoiditis. Refer the client immediately for hospitalization.

Meningitis usually causes the client to appear toxic; severe neck pain occurs with flexion.

Malignant otitis externa is associated with a 50 percent fatality rate and is seen in diabetics and in those immunocompromised with external otitis. Refer the client to a physician immediately.[63,65,66]

### Plan

***Medication.*** Use of antibiotics and other medication is debatable. In European countries, such as The Netherlands, antibiotics are not prescribed because improvement is seen in 10 days regardless of treatment. In this country, however, it is felt that the risk of suppurative complications is too great, supporting aggressive treatment with antibiotics.[65,66]

In general, the first choice is amoxicillin (Polymox) 250 or 500 mg orally three times daily for 10 days; the second choice is trimethoprim–sulfamethoxazole double-strength tablets (Bactrim DS) twice daily for 10 days. Third-choice antibiotics include cefaclor (Ceclor) and amoxicillin/clavulanate potassium (Augmentin). (Augmentin is made of amoxicillin and clavulanic acid and works against the β-lactamase-producing resistant bacteria.[64,66]) For analgesia, acetaminophen and NSAIDs usually suffice. Decongestants have never been proven to shorten the course of otitis media[68] and are used only symptomatically for nasal congestion. Refer to a pharmacotherapeutics text for details.

Tympanostomy (myringotomy) is not usually required for adults. Refer the client to an ear, nose, and throat specialist if she does not improve after two or three 10-day treatment regimens.

***Lifestyle Changes.*** Advise the client to avoid vigorous nose blowing and to increase fluid intake. Encourage the client to stop smoking, as smoking increases the risk of otitis media.

For fluid behind the ear, teach the client to carry out gentle autoinsufflation: She manipulates the posterior pharynx (swallowing, chewing gum, yawning) to speed drainage of fluid from the middle ear.

***Follow-Up.*** Ask the the client to return to the clinic if acute symptoms, such as pain, are not improved in 48 hours or if she is not asymptomatic in 10 days.[66,67]

## ACUTE SINUSITIS

Acute sinusitis is infection of one of the four sinuses: maxillary, frontal, ethmoid, and sphenoid. The mucosal lining becomes swollen and occludes air exchange and mucous drainage, resulting in inflammation, bacterial replication, and purulent discharge.[69]

### Epidemiology

Studies reveal that numerous conditions can predispose an individual to acute sinusitis. The most common risk factors are viral upper respiratory infections, allergic rhinitis, and dental extraction and abscesses. Barotrauma (flying or diving), foreign bodies, tumors, and polyps are less common but they can block the ostia (or openings) to the sinuses.[69]

The primary organisms causing acute sinusitis are *Streptococcus pneumoniae, Haemophilus influenzae, Moraxella catarrhalis,* group A streptococci, and staphylococci.[69] Organisms involved in chronic infections include those already listed as well as mixed anaerobes, which are often difficult to treat.

Incidence reports show acute sinusitis as a common condition; it complicates about 0.5 percent of all upper respiratory infections.

### Subjective Data

Taking a detailed history is imperative, as a physical exam is of limited use in making the diagnosis. The classic history is a preceding upper respiratory infection lasting 5 days or longer, with subsequent development of copious yellow-green nasal discharge and intense, localized facial pain, worse on forward bending. Discomfort is often intense and constant. Depending on which sinus is infected, the pain may be referred to the teeth or palate (maxillary), the eyebrow area (frontal), or behind the eyes or at the top of the head (ethmoid and sphenoid). Note whether symptoms are unilateral or bilateral. Some infections present with only a history of purulent nasal discharge and fatigue, with no associated face pain.[63,69,70]

Infection can be acute (1 day to 3 weeks), subacute (3 weeks to 3 months), or chronic (more than 3 months). The time frame is important to ascertain, and then treat the infection aggressively, as chronic infection is more difficult to treat and at times can require surgical intervention.[71]

## Objective Data

***Physical Examination.*** Reveals a benign general appearance. Vital signs are usually normal; fever is rare. If fever is high, consider referral. (Caution: Clients are in pain and may be taking analgesics that mask fever; ask if they have taken any acetaminophen, aspirin, or NSAIDs in the previous 4 hours.)

Abnormal eye movements, facial edema, and erythema around the eyes suggest spreading cellulitis; Immediate referral is necessary.[71]

A purulent nasal discharge and edematous turbinates may be noted, as may a purulent postnasal drip.

Sinuses are difficult to assess; percussion for tenderness and transillumination are often unreliable.[69,71]

***Diagnostic Tests.*** Although not usually indicated, tests may include special x-rays. The x-rays, however, are difficult to interpret and are best ordered by a specialist.

## Differential Medical Diagnosis

Viral upper respiratory infections, allergic rhinitis, rebound medicamentosa from topical decongestants, dental extractions and abscesses, nasal polyps and tumors.[69]

## Plan

***Psychosocial Interventions.*** Encourage the client to comply with the 10- to 14-day antibiotic regimen. Educate her about the warning signs and symptoms of complications: facial swelling, eye problems, high fever, increased pain.[63]

***Medication.*** Antibiotics, decongestants, and analgesics may be helpful. Refer to a current pharmacotherapeutics text for details.

The *antibiotic* of first choice is amoxicillin, 500 mg orally three times daily for 10 to 14 days. An alternative is trimethoprim–sulfamethoxazole double strength (Bactrim DS) twice daily for 10 to 14 days.

*Decongestants* may help to shrink tissue and drain infection. Note the contraindications, especially for hypertensive clients.

*Analgesics* include NSAIDs, which help to ease the pain and edema.

*Antihistamines* are usually avoided, as they may dry mucous membranes and impair ciliary movement to clear sinuses.[63,69]

***Surgical Interventions.*** Surgical management may be recommended by an ear, nose, and throat specialist if the client's symptoms do not improve.

***Lifestyle Changes.*** Use of a room humidifier, hot showers, and nasal saline nose drops may keep mucous membranes moist and draining. Application of warm packs to the affected area may provide comfort.[71] Increasing fluid intake also helps to keep secretions loose. Advise physical activity as tolerated, and discourage smoking.

***Follow-Up.*** Consider the potentially lethal complications of acute sinusitis, including periorbital cellulitis and abscess leading to meningitis, osteomyelitis, or cavernous sinus thrombosis.[71] Refer clients to a physician if they appear toxic, have a high fever, or exhibit redness or swelling around the eyes, difficulty moving the eyes, or double vision. Consult a physician with any concern.

Symptoms should improve greatly 48 hours after starting antibiotics. If not, refer the client to a physician. All symptoms should resolve before completion of medications. If not, or if they recur, refer the client to a physician. Rule out nasal allergies, tumors, and polyps if acute episodes recur or if symptoms persist with treatment.[63,71]

## PHARYNGITIS

Pharyngitis, an inflammatory condition of the pharynx, has numerous causes. Three causes discussed here in depth are group A beta hemolytic streptococci (GABHS), infectious mononucleosis, and *Neisseria gonorrhoeae* (see Table 17–18).

### Epidemiology

Identification of GABHS necessitates immediate treatment, because these organisms can cause rheumatic fever if untreated and if associated with local suppurative complications such as tonsillar abscess.[72,73] Infectious mononucleosis is acute infection with the Epstein–Barr virus. Although pharyngitis caused by mononucleosis cannot be treated, it should be identified so that the client can be monitored for potentially lethal complications, such as airway compromise and splenic rupture. Pharyngitis caused by *N. gonorrhoeae* may be confused with pharyngitis caused by GABHS or mononucleosis, but it must be identified so that sexual partners can be treated.[72,73]

Transmission of GABHS (scarlet fever) occurs primarily among children of school age or people living under crowded living conditions, such as college dormitories and military barracks. Mononucleosis is primarily a disease of the young passed though mucous membrane secretions. Gonorrheal pharyngitis is most commonly seen among homosexual males, but should be considered in any sexually active adult with a sore throat who fails to respond to treatment.[72,73]

Incidence reports show that GABHS are responsible for about one third of the sore throats seen in primary care. GABHS commonly occur among children between 3 and 15 years of age; however, these organisms cause 5 to 20 percent of sore throats among persons older than 15.[63] Ninety percent of the population has had mononucleosis by age 40. Most adults are not aware that they had it in childhood. The infection tends to be more severe if contracted as an adult.[63,74]

Gonorrhea is responsible for about 1 percent of pharyngitis infections among adults treated in primary care.[74]

### Subjective Data

Histories reported by women vary, depending on the etiology of pharyngitis. Pharyngitis caused by GABHS is associated with a classic history of sudden onset of malaise, fever (usually higher than 101°F), tender anterior cervical nodes, headache, and a severe sore (not "scratchy") throat. Nasal symptoms are infrequent and cough is rare. Often a woman has been exposed to small children. If an abscess is present, the client may experience excruciating unilateral pain and may report drooling or spitting saliva, rather than swallowing it. Ask the client about a history of abscesses, as recurrence is common.[63,72]

Infectious mononucleosis in adults usually presents with a history of gradual onset of fatigue that becomes severe (sleeping 12 to 14 hours per day). Appetite decreases. Sore throat begins, and the client complains of "aches" around the neck caused by prominent neck adenopathy. Fever is variable; temperature may be normal to greater than 103°F. Side tenderness and jaundice may be caused by hepatosplenomegaly. Symptoms are most prominent in the first 2 weeks, and gradual full recovery usually occurs in 6 weeks.[63,74]

Gonorrheal pharyngitis may be mild or severe. The diagnosis is suspected if a client reports a new sexual partner and oral sex. The diagnosis is primarily suspected if persistent sore throat is not cured by usual management.[62]

## Objective Data

Because physical examination cannot differentiate between viral and bacterial causes of pharyngitis, specific laboratory tests are required for diagnosis.

***Physical Examination.*** Findings depend on the etiology (see Table 17–19). The client may be flushed, appear sick and have fever. A fine, red, sandpaper-like rash is consistent with GABHS (scarlet fever). A maculopapular rash is consistent with mononucleosis and hemorrhagic pustules with gonorrhea. Jaundice can occur in mononucleosis.[63]

Nasal congestion and a hoarse voice are primarily of viral origin and are rare in pharyngitis caused by GABHS, mononucleosis, or gonorrhea. "Hot potato" voice and drooling are red flags and may indicate an abscess. In pharyngitis caused by GABHS, tonsils are often large and beefy red with a thick white exudate. Suspect an abscess or peritonsillar cellulitis if the soft palate shows unilateral bulging, the uvula is deviated or edematous, or if the client will not open her mouth because of pain.[63,74] Never force a client's mouth open; if epiglottitis is present it may cause spasm and occlusion of the airway.

Neck adenopathy is nonspecific. As a rule, however, large, very tender anterior nodes are consistent with pharyngitis caused by GABHS or gonorrhea; posterior cervical nodes and generalized adenopathy are more consistent with pharyngitis caused by mononucleosis.

The lungs should be clear. Abdominal examination may reveal side tenderness, indicating hepatosplenomegaly from mononucleosis or the mononucleosis-like cytomegalovirus.

Genitalia are examined only if gonorrhea is suspected.

***Diagnostic Tests.*** Specific for bacterial and viral infections. For pharyngitis caused by GABHS, in-office rapid strep tests or cultures are helpful. The white blood cell count may be slightly elevated in streptococcal pharyngitis, but may be greater than 15,000 if an abscess exists.[73]

For infectious mononucleosis, the mononucleus spot test (or heterophile antibody test) often does not turn positive for 5 to 12 days or longer after onset of illness. The CBC is usually normal or shows a slightly decreased white blood cell count with a predominance of lymphocytes and monocytes. The diagnosis may be made with a blood smear showing 20 percent atypical lymphocytes. If the client exhibits the classic clinical picture of mononucleosis but the monospot remains negative, consider ordering a battery of tests to rule out cytomegalovirus, toxoplasmosis, and histoplasmosis.[63,74]

For gonorrheal pharyngitis, order a throat culture; use calcium alginate swabs, plate on Thayer Martin medium, and incubate.[62,74]

## Differential Medical Diagnosis

See Tables 17–18 and 17–19.

## Plan

***Psychosocial Interventions.*** Explain to the client her condition or the differential diagnoses being considered if tests were inconclusive. Inform her about the course of treatment to expect and the red flag symptoms that should prompt her to call the health care provider.

***Medication.*** Refer to a current pharmacotherapeutics text for details.

For pharyngitis caused by GABHS, penicillin V (Betapen-VK) 250 to 500 mg orally four times daily for 10 days (administer erythromycin if the client is allergic to penicillin V.)

**TABLE 17–18. DIFFERENTIAL DIAGNOSIS OF PHARYNGITIS**

| Bacterial Diseases | Viral Diseases | Other Diseases |
|---|---|---|
| **GABHS**[a]<br>Large tonsils beefy red ± exudate<br>Fever (>101°F)<br>Nodes anterior and very tender<br>Rash, scarlatina sandpaper-like<br>Often headache<br>Often vomit once<br>No cough | **Mononucleosis**<br>Large tonsils, palatine petechiae ± exudate<br>Fever may or may not occur<br>Nodes posterior or generalized<br>Rash, faint, maculopapular<br>Headache may or may not occur<br>Persistent anorexia/fatigue<br>Rare cough<br>30% splenomegaly<br>10% hepatomegaly | **Mycoplasma**<br>Rarely diagnosed in absence of bronchitis/pneumonia |
| **Gonorrhea**<br>1% of sore throats in adults ± exudate<br>History of oral sex | **Common cold**<br>URI caused by rhinovirus etc usually nasal symptoms may be hoarse | **Candida**<br>"Thrush," rule out AIDS, cancer, and diabetes |
| **Diphtheria**<br>Pseudomembrane<br>Unimmunized population | **Herpes simplex**<br>Ulcers on gums, hard palate tissue and lips | **Allergies**<br>Consider if "cold lasts > 3 weeks," worse in morning and nighttime, postnasal drip |
| ***Haemophilus influenzae***<br>Rare in adults<br>Epiglottitis in children | **Coxsackievirus**<br>Ulcers on soft palate and tonsillar pillars | **Spirochetes**<br>Syphilis<br>Acute necrotizing ulcerative gingivitis<br>Ulcers on gums<br>"Trench mouth" |
| **Group D and C streptococci**<br>Rarely cause suppurative complications, therefore not treated | **Cytomegalovirus**<br>Mononucleosis-like syndrome may be asymptomatic or quite ill, will shed virus, dangerous to pregnant women with no immunity | **Dehydration** |
| **Tuberculosis** | **Measleas, mumps, rubella, varicella** | **Irritant gases** |
| | | **Trauma** |
| | | **Foreign body** |
| | | **Neoplasm** |

[a]GABHS, group A beta hemolytic streptococci; URI, upper respiratory infection.
Sources: *References 63, 72, 74.*

*Note:* Although amoxicillin is effective against GABHS, do not give it when the strep test is negative and mononucleosis cannot be ruled out as cause of exudative pharyngitis. Clients with mononucleosis develop a total body maculopapular rash if given amoxicillin.[63,72]

For pharyngitis caused by infectious mononucleosis, analgesics such as ibuprofen may be given. Steroids may be used if tonsillar enlargement threatens the airway.[63,74]

For gonorrheal pharyngitis, if uncomplicated, inject ceftriaxone sodium (Rocephin) 125 to 250 mg (by weight) intramuscularly (see Chapter 8 for recommendations). Also administer oral doxycycline (Vibramycin) or tetracycline (Achromycin) to treat the possibility of concurrent chlamydial infection.[63]

***Surgical Interventions.*** Surgery may be needed if abscess is present. Refer the client for needle aspiration and possible incision and drainage.

**TABLE 17–19. DIFFERENTIAL DIAGNOSIS OF INFECTIOUS PHARYNGITIS: EXUDATIVE VERSUS NONEXUDATIVE**

| Exudative | Nonexudative |
|---|---|
| Group A beta hemolytic streptococci | Rhinovirus |
| Mononucleosis | Coronavirus |
| Adenovirus | Respiratory syncytial virus |
| *Neisseria gonorrhoeae* | Influenza virus |
| Mixed anaerobic bacteria | Parainfluenza virus |
| Herpes simplex virus | |

Sources: *References 62, 63.*

***Lifestyle Changes.*** If pharyngitis caused mononucleosis is diagnosed, encourage the client to listen to her body and to rest when she feels tired. She should avoid vigorous activity for about 6 weeks and protect her sides because of the risk of rupturing the spleen.[74] Otherwise, activity is as tolerated. Warn the client to avoid hepatotoxins, such as alcohol. The client may use warm saline gargles and lozenges if she feels they help.

If gonorrheal pharyngitis is diagnosed, education about safer sex practices should be discussed and all sex partners should be tested and treated.

If pharyngitis caused by GABHS is diagnosed, decreased activity and alcohol intake are recommended. In general, encourage clients to increase fluids and nutrition. Discourage smoking.

***Follow-Up.*** Follow-up is specific to the condition.

Pharyngitis caused by GABHS should improve greatly in 48 hours; otherwise have the client return to rule out abscess or other infection.

Clients with pharyngitis caused by mononucleosis are sickest on about days 4 to 8 of illness and should be followed on the basis of the clinical picture. Observe for airway obstruction, hepatitis, and splenic enlargement.

Clients with gonorrheal pharyngitis are at risk for numerous complications, such as disseminated gonococcal infection with bacteremia and purulent arthritis.[63] Ensure that all sexual contacts are treated.

## INFLUENZA

Influenza, an acute, usually self-limiting upper respiratory infection, may be caused by influenza A, B, or C virus. Strains of the A virus are the most common and most virulent. B virus infection has some increased association with Reye's syndrome. C virus infection is a mild illness, usually not significant or identified clinically.[63,74]

### Epidemiology

Etiology of the influenza virus reveals the unique ability to vary antigenically from year to year, hence the terms *antigenic drift* (minor variations) and *antigenic shift* (major variations). Prior exposure provides limited immunity. Epidemics occur every 2 to 3 years; about every 10 years the strains vary dramatically and produce a "pandemic."[75]

Transmission is primarily through aerosolized particles from a cough or sneeze, although the virus can be spread by close or hand contact. The incubation period is about 18 to 72 hours. Infectious viral shedding occurs for 10 days but is most prominent in the first 48 hours of illness.[62,63]

In an epidemic year 20 to 30 percent of the population may contract influenza. Deaths are usually due to pneumonia (influenza pneumonia is the sixth leading cause of death in the United States) or to cardiovascular decompensation related to the influenza.[63,75]

### Subjective Data

History reveals the four hallmarks of influenza: headache; myalgias, especially in the legs and back; fever, often 102 to 104°F for 3 to 4 days or longer; and nonproductive cough, which usually is not prominent at the beginning of illness but increases over time. Watery eyes and dry throat may be present, but nasal symptoms are usually absent.[62,63]

## Objective Data

On physical examination, the client may be flushed and sweating. She appears ill. High fever is common, usually greater than 102°F, but rarely 106°F or higher. Heart and respiratory rates are increased.

The eyes, ears, nose, and throat usually appear normal. The lungs are clear. If crackles or rhonchi are heard, obtain a chest x-ray to rule out influenza pneumonia.

Monitor the heart to assess cardiovascular status. Influenza may precipitate cardiovascular failure in cardiac clients.[62,63]

Diagnostic tests are usually not required unless the fever lasts longer than 4 days, in which case a white blood cell count should be ordered. If the white blood cell count is greater than 12,000, suspect pneumonia and order a chest x-ray.[62,63]

## Differential Medical Diagnosis

Parainfluenza virus, respiratory syncytial virus, adenovirus, other viral syndromes. In the absence of an epidemic, it is difficult to identify influenza from many other viral syndromes. Note that influenza is always associated with cough.[62,63]

## Plan

***Psychosocial Interventions.*** Inform the client about the expected course of disease, and teach the warning signs of influenza pneumonia and cardiac complications. Reassure her that taking acetaminophen is permitted. Aspirin, however, should be avoided because of its association with Reye's syndrome. Comfort will be increased and myalgias decreased if fever is controlled by acetaminophen.[62,76]

***Medication.*** Medication is administered for prophylaxis and treatment.

- *Amantadine.* Amantadine (Symmetrel) is the only drug approved for both prophylaxis and treatment in influenza A; it is not effective against influenza B.[76,77]
  - *Administration.* For prophylaxis, administer for 2 weeks with a late vaccine in the midst of an outbreak. For treatment, amantadine must be given within 24 to 28 hours of the onset of symptoms.

    The usual adult dose for adults 65 years or younger is 200 mg twice daily for 10 to 14 days.
  - *Side Effects.* Side effects are infrequent and cease when medication is stopped. The client may experience central nervous system symptoms, including nervousness, dizziness, and insomnia.[63]
  - *Contraindications.* Do not administer to any client with renal compromise or clients older than 65 years. Refer to a pharmacotherapeutics text for doses for clients older than 65 for those with decreased creatinine clearance.
  - *Anticipated Outcome on Evaluation.* When used for treatment, amantadine should decrease the severity and duration of illness.
  - *Client Teaching.* When amantadine is given for prophylaxis, inform the client that the drug is 70 to 90 percent effective in preventing influenza A but does not replace the vaccine, as it fails to work against influenza B and is only protective for the duration of therapy.[75–77]
- *Influenza Trivalent Vaccine.* Influenza trivalent vaccine (two strains of A and one of B) is administered annually beginning in September. Vaccinations begin protection in 2 weeks; protection peaks in 1 to 2

months and gradually declines over time. Vaccines may be given anytime after an outbreak begins, but should be supplemented with 2 weeks of amantadine treatment until the vaccine can induce an immune response.[77]

The high-risk groups for whom annual administration of vaccine is currently recommended are persons with heart disease (congenital or acquired), chronic lung disease, chronic renal disease, chronic severe anemia, and immunocompromising illness (diabetes, cancer). Others for whom the vaccine is indicated are persons between the ages of 60 and 65, those living in chronic care/nursing homes, and those at risk of exposure and subsequent transmission to high-risk groups, which includes health care providers as well as family members who take care of high-risk clients.

- *Side Effects.* Side effects are rare with modern inactivated vaccines. Less than 5 percent of recipients develop a febrile reaction; some local soreness may be noted.
- *Contraindications.* Do not administer to individuals with egg allergy or febrile illness.
- *Anticipated Outcome on Evaluation.* The vaccine will be 80 percent effective in preventing disease. If, however, disease is contracted, the course of illness will be less severe.
- *Client Teaching.* Encourage the client to comply each year and receive the vaccine instead of waiting for symptoms to develop.[75–77]

***Lifestyle Changes.*** Encourage the client to increase intake of fluids, as high fevers lead to diaphoresis and dehydration. Bed rest is advised. Also, advise the client to avoid unnecessary contact with others to decrease spread of illness. In addition, discourage smoking.

***Follow-Up.*** Educate the client about symptoms of influenza pneumonia, which has its onset about 1 week after onset of influenza symptoms. Pneumonia accounts for one half of the deaths associated with influenza. It is characterized by severe dyspnea, cyanosis, and often scanty blood-tinged sputum. There are few physical signs, for example, change in respiratory rate and vital signs (lungs may sound clear); therefore, focus on the client's history. Influenza can lead to a rapidly progressing pneumonia with a high fatality rate in the very young, the very old, and those with preexisting disease. Refer the client to a physician if you suspect pneumonia.[75,76]

Preventing influenza is crucial. Only 20 percent of the high-risk population are vaccinated against this deadly disease and amantadine is underused in epidemics.[77] To facilitate implementation of vaccination guidelines in an office setting, one staff member may be designated each fall to head the effort. During that season, charts of high-risk patients should be flagged and posters placed in waiting and examination rooms.[75–77]

## LOWER RESPIRATORY TRACT INFECTIONS: PNEUMONIA AND BRONCHITIS

Pneumonia, an acute infection of the alveolar spaces or interstitial tissues (or both) of the lung, is broadly defined as an inflammation of the tracheobronchial tree. There are four classifications of pneumonia: "typical," or classic bacterial pneumonia; atypical pneumonia; aspiration pneumonia, which occurs mainly in alcoholics or hospitalized, debilitated patients; and hematogenous pneumonia.[63,78] This chapter focuses on the two types seen most often in primary care, typical and atypical (see Table 17–20).

Bronchitis is clinically defined as "an acute cough with sputum in the absence of pneumonia."[79] Bronchitis is most often caused by

**TABLE 17–20. PNEUMONIA PATHOGENS OBSERVED IN PRIMARY CARE**

| Classic | Atypical |
|---|---|
| ***Common*** | |
| *Streptococcus pneumoniae* (also called pneumococcal) | *Mycoplasma pneumoniae*<br>Viral |
| ***Uncommon*** | |
| *Haemophilus influenzae*<br>*Staphylococcus aureus*<br>*Klebsiella pneumoniae* | *Legionella pneumophila*<br>*Chlamydia psittaci*<br>*Francisella tularensis* |

Sources: *References 62, 63, 78.*

viruses (influenza, rhinovirus, adenovirus) or mycoplasma. Secondary bacterial bronchitis is often a complication of viral respiratory infection. Invaders include the usual respiratory pathogens, such as *Streptococcus pneumoniae* and *Haemophilus influenzae.*[79,80] Acute bronchitis is not to be confused with the chronic inflammatory condition associated with continual irritation of the airways, usually induced by smoking.[79]

## Epidemiology

Studies show that lower respiratory tract infection affects the normal function of the tract, resulting in intermittent production of small amounts of aspirate. All individuals aspirate small amounts of gastric contaminants most of the time. The lung has defense mechanisms to clear the aspirate. Pneumonia is more common among those who aspirate larger amounts, that is, those who have had a stroke or are in a coma, those who have poor dentition, alcoholics, and those who take drugs for sedation. Also at risk are those who are immunocompromised, have impaired cough, or had a preceding viral infection.[78]

More than 3 million cases of pneumonia are diagnosed annually. It is the most common cause of infectious death in the United States. The very young and the very old are at greatest risk for death. Bronchitis is common.[63,78]

## Subjective Data

The symptoms reported by clients with pneumonia and bronchitis are compared in Table 17–21.

Pneumococcal pneumonia has a classic history of sudden onset of "teeth-rattling" chill (rigor) and fever of 101° to 106°F. Clients often report a rusty-colored or purulent sputum, chest pain, and shortness of breath.[81]

Mycoplasma pneumonia, on the other hand, has a less dramatic clinical picture and history. The cough is paroxysmal and may be nonproductive. Fatigue and shortness of breath are common.[82]

## Objective Data

A physical examination is done (see Table 17–21). Lab work is ordered only if pneumonia is suspected.

The serum white blood cell count is often higher than 12,000 in pneumonia and normal in bronchitis.

Chest x-ray is indicated if pneumonia is suspected. It may help to guide treatment and follow-up. Lobar or segmental consolidation is strongly suggestive of pneumococcal pneumonia. The x-ray may be false negative if the client is dehydrated.

A Gram stain of sputum may be helpful if an adequate sample is obtained. Good smears have fewer than 10 squamous epithelial cells and more than 25 neutrophils per high-power field. These results can guide empirical therapy if one organism predominates. Gram-positive diplococci suggest *Streptococcus pneumoniae;* Gram-negative coccobacilli suggest *Haemophilus influenzae;* absence of a predominant bacterium with neutrophils suggests mycoplasma.

**TABLE 17–21. HISTORY AND EXAMINATION TO DIFFERENTIATE BRONCHITIS AND PNEUMONIA**

| Symptoms/Signs | Bronchitis | Pneumonia |
|---|---|---|
| *History* | | |
| Onset | Gradual, over 5–10 days, usually preceded by URI[a] | Acute onset, ± preceding URI |
| Fever | Mild or absent | Usually 101–106°F |
| Chills | Mild, recurring, or intermittent | True "rigor," teeth-rattling chill |
| Chest pain | Vague "tightness" or chest congestion | Intense, pleuritic, localized |
| Sputum | Scant to copious | "Rusty"-colored in pneumococcal or mucopurulent |
| Dyspnea | Rare | Common |
| *Examination* | | |
| General appearance | Not toxic, no apparent distress | Often toxic, weak, may use accessory muscles |
| Vital signs | Often normal | Often tachycardia, tachypnea, fever |
| HEENT[a] | May be consistent with URI | Normal or findings consistent with URI |
| Lungs | Usually clear, may have rhonchi or wheeze that clears with cough | Crackles, won't clear with cough; signs of consolidation (E to A changes, dull to percussion) ± rub |
| Heart | At normal baseline | Tachycardia |

[a]URI, upper respiratory infection; HEENT, head, eyes, ears, nose and throat.
Sources: *References 62, 63, 78.*

A sputum culture (send specimen prior to beginning medication) confirms diagnosis and is critical for immunocompromised clients.

## Differential Medical Diagnosis

Infectious causes (see Table 17–20) and noninfectious causes, including asthma, inhalation of chemicals, pulmonary infarct, tumor, pulmonary edema, and foreign body.

## Plan

***Psychosocial Interventions.*** Reassure the client and teach her the warning signs of potential complications. In addition, advise her to notify the health care provider if symptoms of complications develop (see Table 17–22).

***Medication.*** Antibiotics and vaccine are used in treatment.

- *Antibiotics.* See Table 17–23.
- *Pneumococcal Polysaccharide Vaccine.* Pneumococcal polysaccharide vaccine (Pneumorax 23), a 23-valent vaccine is in-

**TABLE 17–22. CRITERIA FOR OUTPATIENT MANAGEMENT OF PNEUMONIA[a]**

1. Able to take fluids and oral medications
2. Not toxic, no respiratory distress, only single lobe involvement
3. No underlying chronic disease, such as chronic obstructive pulmonary disease or diabetes
4. Pneumonia not related to aspiration (alcoholism or sedation, for example)
5. Adequate support system at home to provide care, observation, and immediate transportation to hospital if condition worsens

[a]Client must meet the following criteria.
Sources: *References 78, 79.*

**TABLE 17–23. ANTIBIOTICS FOR LOWER RESPIRATORY INFECTIONS[a]**

| | |
|---|---|
| Pneumococcal pneumonia: | Penicillin V (Betapen) 250–500 mg p.o. q.i.d. × 14 days |
| Mycoplasma pneumonia | Erythromycin 250–500 mg p.o. q.i.d. × 14 days |
| Pneumonia, etiology unknown | Erythromycin 250 mg p.o. q.i.d. × 14 days |
| Bronchitis: | Usually of viral origin; no antibiotics indicated. If mycoplasma bronchitis or secondary bacterial bronchitis is suspected, erythromycin 250 mg p.o. q.i.d. × 10 days is treatment of choice. Smokers are highly likely to develop a secondary bacterial bronchitis. Trimethoprim–sulfamethoxazole or amoxicillin may be administered to treat mixed organisms or *Haemophilus influenzae*. |

[a]For details, see a current pharmacotherapeutics text.
Sources: *References 62, 78, 79, 81, 82, 84.*

dicated for protection against pneumococcal pneumonia. It is recommended for healthy adults older than 65; anyone with heart, lung, liver, or renal disease; diabetics; alcoholics; immunocompromised adults (including those with HIV and splenectomized clients); and children older than 2 years who have risk factors for pneumococcal infection, such as sickle cell disease, HIV, and nephrotic syndrome.

Recent recommendations are to revaccinate after 6 years individuals at highest risk and to revaccinate without waiting those individuals who are at highest risk who have received the 14-valent vaccine.[83,84] Refer to a current pharmacotherapeutics text.

- *Administration.* The vaccine is given in a single intramuscular dose.
- *Side Effects.* Side effects are minor and local. Fifty percent of clients experience pain or redness at the site of injection; 1 percent have a fever or rash.
- *Contraindication.* Do not administer to any client who has had a reaction to the vaccine.
- *Anticipated Outcome on Evaluation.* Overall, the vaccine has a protective effect in 64 percent of recipients.[83]
- *Client Teaching.* Encourage the client to receive vaccine as recommended. Emphasize that more than 500,000 cases of pneumonia occur every year with a 5 percent mortality rate. Prevention is the most effective intervention.

***Lifestyle Changes.*** Advise the client to humidify the environment if possible; to increase intake of fluids and nutrition, to rest. Cough suppressants are used only if cough is excessive and disrupts rest. Discourage smoking.

***Follow-Up.*** Assess the client for outpatient management (see Table 17–22). Any client with pneumonia should be reevaluated every 24 hours. Most clients with pneumococcal pneumonia are afebrile in 3 days. Refer for hospitalization any client who does not rapidly improve. Possible complications of pneumonia include pleural effusion, empyema (suspect lung abscess if fever persists), disseminated intravascular coagulation, and nephritis.[84]

Clients with bronchitis should gradually improve and the cough resolve while on medications. Any client with a cough lasting 6 weeks requires a chest x-ray and in-depth evaluation to rule out such conditions as lymphoma, tuberculosis, and asthma.[62,79]

## SKIN CANCER

The three most common types of skin cancer in the United States are basal cell cancer, squamous cell cancer, and malignant melanoma. Basal and squamous cell cancers are the most common; however, malignant melanoma accounts for almost all the deaths. Women, because of their sun bathing, are particularly at risk.

## BASAL CELL SKIN CANCER

Basal cell cancer (BCC) arises from epidermal keratinocytes. It grows by direct extension and destruction of surrounding tissue. Metastasis is uncommon.[85,86]

### Epidemiology

Risk factors are similar for all types of skin cancer:

- Fair skin that burns easily (see Table 17–24)
- Substantial time spent outdoors, particularly occupational, for example, farmers and sailors
- Family history of skin cancer
- X-ray or radiation burn sites
- Arsenic ingestion

Fair skin and sun exposure are the key risk factors. More than 90 percent of basal cell cancer occurs on sun-exposed areas of the head and neck but are rare on the back of the hand. The cancer may occur at sites of previous trauma, such as in thermal burns and scars. Basal cell cancer has many clinical forms which vary in appearance and malignant potential.

It is estimated that one in seven Americans will develop basal cell cancer. It is the most common type of skin cancer in the United States. Basal cell cancer is common among caucasians and rare among African-Americans. It may occur at any age but the incidence markedly increases after age 40.

### Subjective Data

Basal cell cancer is primarily asymptomatic; its course is unpredictable. The lesion may remain small with almost no perceptible growth for years or it may grow rapidly. Symptoms such as enlargement, change in color, pain, itching, and bleeding should be investigated. If a client is uncertain about how long a crust lesion has been present, have her return for follow-up in 2 weeks. If the suspicious lesion remains unchanged, refer her for biopsy.[87]

### Objective Data

Because the early stages of skin cancer are primarily asymptomatic, screening is crucial. A complete physical exam reveals more than six times the pathology revealed by exams limited to normally exposed sites.

Physical examination should employ a magnifying lens and good lighting to observe suspicious lesions. It is helpful to wet the lesion with oil or an alcohol swab and stretch the lesion between two fingers to check for color patterns. Look for signs of dysplastic nevus syndrome (see Table 17–27). In addition to good visualization, careful palpation for lymphadenopathy is necessary.

Basal cell cancer usually begins as a small shiny papule that enlarges over months and develops telangiectasias and a pearly border. After time, it develops a central ulcer that recurrently crusts and bleeds. Less common forms of basal cell cancer appear as flat plaques.

Diagnostic tests may be performed by a dermatologist following referral. A suspicious lesion is evaluated and skin biopsy may be necessary.

### Differential Medical Diagnosis

See Table 17–25.

### Plan

***Psychosocial Interventions.*** Help the client to understand the importance of compliance with referrals and treatment regimens.

**TABLE 17–24. SKIN CANCER PREVENTION GUIDELINES**

*1. Avoid sun exposure*

- Skin types I–IV are especially susceptible.
- Protect infants and children. Children cannot protect themselves and significant increased risk may be associated with exposure in first decade.
- Use caution with sun-sensitizing medications: tetracycline, tricyclics, antihistamines, antipsychotics, hypoglycemics, diuretics, antineoplastics, retin A.

*2. When you must be in the sun, protect yourself*

- Avoid peak times for ultraviolet B: 10 AM to 2 PM.
- Wear protective clothing: hats, light-colored clothing.
- Beware of reflective surfaces: snow and cement.
- **Use sunscreen or sun block whenever going outdoors:** Choose strong enough sun protective factor (SPF). See guidelines below. Apply adequate amounts of sunscreen; manufacturer's directions are more than most people use. Apply lotion 30–60 minutes before expected sun exposure, as it takes time for *para*-aminobenzoic acid (PABA) to bind in the stratum corneum. Reapply at least every 40–80 minutes and more frequently if swimming or perspiring.

*3. Types of sunscreens/sunblocks*

- Chemical sunscreens
  - PABA and PABA esters: they are the first choice because they effectively block ultraviolet B (UVB), which is associated with skin cancers.
  - Non-PABA sunscreens include benzophenones and cinnamates, which weakly block UVB; use if allergic to PABA.
- Physical sunblocks: zinc oxide and titanium dioxide; opaque and often cosmetically unacceptable.

*4. Skin type and choice of sun protection factor (SPF)*

| Skin Type | Skin Color and Sunburn History | SPF |
|---|---|---|
| I | Very fair: always burns, never tans | ≥15 |
| II | Fair: burns easily, tans minimally | ≥15 or more |
| III | Light brown: burns moderately, tans gradually and uniformly | 10–15 |
| IV | Moderate brown: burns minimally, always tans well | 6–15 |
| V | Dark brown: rarely burns, tans profusely | 6–15 |
| VI | Deeply pigmented: never burns | None |

Sources: *References 90–92.*

***Medication.*** None is administered.

***Surgical Interventions.*** Surgical excision may be recommended following skin biopsy.

***Lifestyle Changes.*** There is no safe tan.[88] Sun exposure accelerates photoaging.[89] Convincing young women to avoid sun tanning is *very* difficult because of cultural norms and feelings of invulnerability. In prevention education, an emphasis on photoaging may be more effective. All people wrinkle; the question is how much and how soon. Have the woman look at how smooth and soft the skin of her upper inner arm is and compare it with that on the back of her hand. This demonstrates photoaging. Encourage all women to follow the skin cancer prevention guidelines in Table 17–24.[90–92]

Also encourage the client to stop smoking.

***Follow-Up.*** Referral to a dermatologist is necessary after identification of a suspicious lesion.

**TABLE 17–25. DIFFERENTIAL DIAGNOSIS OF SKIN CANCER**

| | |
|---|---|
| Benign skin lesions: | Nevi, seborrheic keratosis, cysts, skin tags, dermatofibromas, keloids |
| Dermatoses: | Seborrhea, eczema, psoriasis, human papillomavirus, fungi |
| Lesions with premalignant potential | Actinic keratosis, leukoplakia, dysplastic nevus syndrome |
| Skin cancers | Basal cell cancer, squamous cell cancer (Bowen's, Paget's), malignant melanoma, mycosis fungoides (rare T-cell lymphoma that originates in skin) |
| Cutaneous metastasis | 3–5% of those with metastatic disease develop secondary skin cancers |

[a]See Table 17–19.

## SQUAMOUS CELL CANCER

Squamous cell cancer (SCC) arises in the epithelium. Like basal cell cancer, squamous cell cancer is most common on areas exposed to the sun; however, distribution is somewhat different. SCC is commonly found on the scalp, the back of the hand, and the ear. It often arises from a precursor lesion called *actinic keratosis.* Actinic keratosis, a premalignant skin condition of the elderly, may appear as flat tan or brown spots with adherent scales and mild surrounding erythema. These often feel rough. Induration, inflammation, and oozing suggest degeneration into malignancy. Squamous cell cancer arising from actinic keratoses is not aggressive but can eventually metastasize.

Squamous cell cancers that arise at thermal burn sites or sites of chronic inflammation have a higher metastatic potential than squamous cell cancers evolving from actinic keratoses.

### Epidemiology

The etiology of squamous cell cancer differs somewhat depending on the type; however, all of these cancers usually appear on sun-exposed areas of fair-skinned persons. These types (simplified here) and their locations include Bowen's disease, on the trunk and extremities; erythroplasia of Queyrat, on the glans penis; Paget's disease, on the areola, nipple, and vulva; and extramammary Paget's disease, on the anogenital region, axilla, external ear canal, and eyelids.

Paget's disease of the areola manifests as a sharply demarcated area of erythema and scaling, often with oozing and crusting. It is associated with breast cancer, but easily confused with eczema. By contrast, eczema is bilateral and resolves with treatment; Paget's lesions are mostly unilateral and progressive.

Squamous cell cancer is common in the oral cavity of women who smoke and drink, often on the posterior lateral borders of the tongue. Leukoplakia, a white opaque patch found on the lips, oral mucosa, and vulva, is a precursor lesion that may degenerate into squamous cell cancer.

Hairy leukoplakia is different from leukoplakia; it is unique to AIDS and associated with the Epstein–Barr virus and human papillomavirus. White and hairy papillary projections are found primarily on the lateral border of the tongue.

Incidence reports show that squamous cell cancer is the second most common skin cancer among the general population. It is the most common among African-Americans.[93]

### Subjective Data

Squamous cell cancer is primarily asymptomatic, but a client may report itching, irritation, bleeding, or a change in skin appearance.

## Objective Data

See Objective Data under Basal Cell Cancer.

Physical examination reveals a variable appearance among clients, but the lesion usually begins as a reddish papule or plaque with a scaly or crusted surface. It may mimic dermatitis. Later, the lesion may appear nodular or warty. Eventually, it ulcerates and invades underlying tissue.

Diagnostic evaluation and management are carried out by a dermatologist.

## Differential Medical Diagnosis

See Table 17–25.

## Plan

***Psychosocial Interventions.*** Emphasize the importance of skin cancer prevention (see Table 17–24). Some actinic keratoses may regress if the client avoids sun exposure. Stress the importance of the treatment regimen outlined by the specialist.

***Medication.*** Topical tretinoin (Retin-A) or 5-fluorouracil (Efudex) may be used.

***Surgical Interventions.*** Excision, cryosurgery, or electrodesiccation and curettage may be performed depending on the extent of the lesion.

***Lifestyle Changes.*** See those recommended for clients with basal cell cancer.

***Follow-Up.*** Continue to monitor the client for new lesions and teach her how to perform monthly self-examinations of the skin.

## MALIGNANT MELANOMA

Malignant melanoma (MM) arises from melanocytes.[94] It is associated primarily with sun exposure. Because 40 to 50 percent of malignant melanomas arise from pigmented moles, any change in a mole is always of concern. Removal of benign moles does not decrease the risk for malignant melanoma. It may also develop anywhere there are melanocytes or pigmented skin, such as mucous membranes, eyes, and the central nervous system. Malignant melanoma may arise de novo, that is, from sites where no mole is visible.

Malignant melanoma is deadly. Early identification and prompt surgical excision offer the only chance for cure. The radial growth phase is a "window of opportunity" during the first several months to years of a malignant melanoma. A mole removed while it is less than 0.76 mm deep is associated with a 98 percent cure rate. Excision of vertical growths greater than 3 mm results in only 50 percent survival at 10 years.[95]

Dysplastic nevus syndrome (DNS) is a familial syndrome found in 2 to 5 percent of the population. Individuals with dysplastic nevus syndrome have at least a 6 percent lifetime risk for malignant melanoma. Clients exhibit large asymmetric and irregularly pigmented nevi. If they have a family member with malignant melanoma, their lifetime risk for developing malignant melanoma is 100 percent.

## Epidemiology

An epidemic of skin cancers has occurred since the 1920s when tans became "fashionable." More than 300,000 new skin cancers are diagnosed each year in the United States. Malignant melanoma accounts for only 3 percent of these cancers, yet it is responsible for two thirds of the deaths from skin cancer.[96]

Risk factors for malignant melanoma include a history of six or more serious sunburns; excessive sun exposure during the first decade of life; an indoor occupation with intermittent, intense sun exposure; large congenital hairy nevus; and family history of malignant melanoma and dysplastic nevus syndrome. Immune dysfunction may also be a risk factor. Recent research indicates that immunocompromise may allow transformation of dysplastic nevi into malignant melanoma.

The incidence of malignant melanoma has increased from 1 in 1500 persons in 1930 to 1 in 250 persons in 1980. Projections are that by the year 2000, 1 in every 90 persons will develop malignant melanoma. It is now the leading cause of cancer deaths in women younger than 35.[88]

### Subjective Data

Four major symptoms are enlargement, color change, pain (sometimes "itch"), and bleeding. Most clients present with only one symptom, and any symptom warrants referral for evaluation. Refer to a dermatologist all women with a family history of dysplastic nevus syndrome, especially if they also have a family history of melanoma.

### Objective Data

A physical examination will help identify suspicious changes. The ABCDs (asymmetry, border, color, diameter, surface/sensation) can assist practitioners, as well as clients, in performing skin exams (see Table 17–26).

Physical examination focuses on sun-exposed areas (back, head, and neck) where most malignant melanomas occur. Acrolentiginous melanoma is a rare, but rapidly fatal lesion, occurring most often among African-Americans on their palmar, plantar, or nail bed surfaces. Each of the several types of melanoma has its own particular idiosyncrasies and growth patterns. Be suspicious of variegated color, irregular borders, and an increase in size (see Table 17–26).

**TABLE 17–26. ABCDs OF SKIN CANCER**

| | | |
|---|---|---|
| A | *Asymmetry* | One half shaped unlike the other |
| B | *Border* | Irregular, notched, or scalloped |
| C | *Color* | Haphazard shades of brown, red, blue, gray |
| D | *Diameter* | Greater than 6 mm (size of the tip of a pencil eraser) |
| s | *Surface or sensation* | Surface distortion may be subtle or obvious, assess by focusing light at side of lesion; sensation refers to itch, burn, or pain |

Small dysplastic nevi may be difficult to differentiate from common moles on physical exam. If the client has a family history of dysplastic nevus syndrome and any questionable lesion, refer her to a dermatologist.

Diagnostic tests are conducted by a dermatologist. Refer any suspicious lesion for evaluation and probable biopsy.

### Differential Medical Diagnosis

See Table 17–27.

### Plan

***Psychosocial Interventions.*** Educate the client about moles and reassure her that not all moles are harmful. In general, people are born without moles. Small, flat, "common" moles develop in childhood and increase in size and number after puberty. They may become smooth domes. By early adulthood, individuals average 12 to 25 moles. In individuals who live long lives, the moles recede and disappear before death.

***Medication.*** Refer to dermatologist.

***Surgical Interventions.*** Surgical excision may be performed.

***Lifestyle Changes.*** Encourage the client to follow skin cancer prevention guidelines (see Table 17–24). She should also perform monthly self-exams of the skin and stop smoking.

***Follow-Up.*** Refer a client with any suspicious lesion to a dermatologist. If dysplastic nevus syndrome is suspected, refer the client. With numerous dysplastic nevi, baseline pho-

**TABLE 17–27. DIFFERENTIAL DIAGNOSES OF DYSPLASTIC NEVI**

| Sign | Common Mole | Dysplastic Mole |
|---|---|---|
| Shape | Round or oval | Irregular |
| Margins | Sharp, well circumscribed | Hazy, indistinct |
| Color | Light brown to black, uniform pigmentation | Variegated tan, dark brown on pink background |
| Topography | Flat or smooth dome shape | "Fried egg" shape, papular center with macular periphery or pebble contour |
| Size | Usually <6 mm | Usually >6 mm, up to 12 mm |
| Number | Usually 12–25 | One or many, often >100 |
| Location | Usually face and upper extremities | Mostly on covered areas: buttocks, scalp, and female breasts |
| Age of onset | Few appear after early adulthood | Continue to appear after age 35 |

tographs and perhaps serial photodocumentation are needed.

Immunocompromised clients may be seen every 3 to 4 months by the dermatologist. Family members of clients with dysplastic nevus syndrome must be screened; often an early operable melanoma is found in a distant relative. All women should be taught the ABCDs of melanoma (see Table 17–26). A complete skin exam should be conducted at the time of the client's annual physical. Encourage women to examine their skin monthly at home.

# THYROID DYSFUNCTION

## HYPOTHYROIDISM

Hypothyroidism is a clinical syndrome associated with subnormal levels of circulating thyroid hormones. A client may be asymptomatic; the condition may be mild or severe. Myxedema is the advanced form of hypothyroidism characterized by proteinaceous infiltration of the skin and subcutaneous tissues with multiple organ–system involvement.[97]

### Epidemiology

The cause differs among the four types of hypothyroidism: primary, secondary, goitrous, and transient.

Primary hypothyroidism is characterized by atrophy or destruction of thyroid tissue due to an autoimmune response. Primary hypothyroidism accounts for more than 90 percent of hypothyroid disease. Primary hypothyroidism may also be iatrogenic (following radioiodine therapy or thyroid-ectomy for hyperthyroidism), idiopathic, or the result of a congenital disorder (cretinism).[98]

Secondary hypothyroidism results from insufficient stimulation of an intrinsically normal gland. It may occur in primary disorders of the pituitary or hypothalamus, which result in deficiencies of thyroid-stimulating hormone (TSH) or thyrotropin-releasing hormone (TRH).

Goitrous hypothyroidism is due to defective thyroid hormone synthesis and is characterized by development of a goiter. Goitrous disorders include Hashimoto's thyroiditis; iodine deficiency; acquired hypothyroidism, caused by the use of goitrogens (propylthiouracil, methimazole, lithium, or iodine);

peripheral resistance to thyroid hormone; and infiltrative disorders (amyloidosis, sarcoidosis, lymphoma; or malignancy).[99]

Transient hypothyroidism sometimes occurs after pregnancy.

Hypothyroidism is an autoimmune disease; the exact etiology remains unknown.

Hypothyroidism onset is most common among women between 30 and 60 years of age. It develops in both men and women. It is a common disorder of the elderly. One to two percent of individuals older than 65 have hypothyroidism; almost 85 percent of them are women.[99]

Routine screening of asymptomatic adults is not recommended. It may be clinically prudent, however, to screen those at increased risk, namely, elderly women.

## Subjective Data

Hypothyroidism is easily misdiagnosed because its presentation is nonspecific and it involves multiple organ systems. Less than one third of older persons manifest typical symptoms: cold intolerance; weight gain; dry skin; weakness; fatigue; hoarseness; inattention or difficulty concentrating; dizziness; constipation; arthralgias; muscle cramps; menstrual irregularities, particularly menorrhagia; galactorrhea.[99]

## Objective Data

***Physical Presentation.*** Depends on the progression of disease from a subclinical one to a medical emergency, such as that which often precedes myxedema coma.

Physical examination is complete.

- *General Appearance.* Skin possibly dry, cool, and coarse with a diffuse waxy pallor; depressed affect; low-pitched, slow speech.
- *Vital Signs.* Bradycardia, hypertension.
- *Skin.* Thin, brittle nails with transverse grooves; dry, scaly skin.
- *Head.* Coarse, dry, brittle hair with alopecia; facial edema; enlarged tongue; thinning or absence of the lateral eyebrows.
- *Neck.* Normal, enlarged, small, or absent thyroid; thyroid nodules; tracheal deviation.
- *Chest.* Exertional dyspnea, pleural effusions.
- *Heart.* Cardiomegaly, arrhythmias.
- *Abdomen.* Gastrointestinal hypomotility, ascites.
- *Neurologic Exam.* Cerebellar dysfunction, delayed deep tendon reflexes, parasthesias, peripheral neuropathies.
- *Endocrine System.* Galactorrhea.

***Diagnostic Laboratory Tests.*** Reveal levels of circulating thyroid hormones. The active thyroid hormones are tetraiodothyronine (thyroxine or T4) and triiodothyronine (T3). Both T3 and T4 circulate in the serum, bound to three proteins: thyroxine-binding globulin (TBG), thyroxine-binding prealbumin (TBPA), and albumin. The small fractions of T3 and T4 that circulate free (not bound to protein) are the active forms. Alterations in TBG (e.g., with pregnancy, estrogen replacement, or the use of oral contraceptives) may change total circulating T3 and T4 levels but do not affect free unbound forms.100

Primary hypothyroidism is confirmed by a high level of thyroid-stimulating hormone (TSH) and a low level of $T_4$/free thyroxine. A serum TSH is the most sensitive test; it is elevated in more than 95 percent of clients with primary hypothyroidism.[101]

Secondary hypothyroidism is differentiated from primary hypothyroidism by the thyrotropin-releasing hormone (TRH) test of pituitary–thyroid regulation. This test should be ordered by an endocrinologist.

## Differential Medical Diagnosis

Virtually every possible diagnosis may be considered. Cardiac disease, renal disease, and neuromuscular disorders are common diagnostic considerations.

## Plan[98,99]

***Psychosocial Interventions.*** It may be necessary to address acute anxiety reactions, which are often among the manifestations of this multisystem disorder. Reassure the client that her symptoms will gradually abate with treatment.

***Medication.*** Levothyroxine (Levothroid, Synthroid), a synthetic $T_4$ hormonal replacement, is used.

- *Administration.* Begin with levothyroxine 25 to 50 μg daily and increase by 25 μg every 4 to 6 weeks. Dosages need to be initiated and adjusted with caution in the elderly and in clients with cardiac disease.
- *Side Effects.* Palpitations and dysrhythmias are known to occur.
- *Contraindications.* Contraindications are outweighed by the risk of not treating the hyperthyroidism. Use caution, however, in clients with cardiac disease.
- *Evaluation of Drug Action.* Measure serum TSH values no sooner than 4 to 6 weeks after initiating therapy and again 3 to 4 months after a maintenance dose is reached, to ensure equilibrium. Annual exams are then done to monitor therapy, as needs may change with time.
- *Client Teaching.* Alert the client to the possibility of hypo/hyper reactions, which may indicate the need for medication change.

Subclinical disease, in which individuals are asymptomatic, does *not* benefit from treatment. Treatment may be advisable if other medical problems are exacerbated.

Early treatment is clearly beneficial and indicated in congenital hypothyroidism.[98]

***Surgical Interventions.*** Surgery is an option for a small percentage of clients (those with goitrous disease or suspected cancer). Part or all of the thyroid gland may be removed. Defer discussion to an endocrinologist.

***Lifestyle Changes.*** The daily medication regimen and chronic condition may cause the client to alter her self-perception. Encourage positive, affirming activities. Diet and exercise are not restricted.

***Follow-Up.*** Once the client is stable, teach her the symptoms of her condition. Reinforce the need for annual visits.

# HYPERTHYROIDISM (THYROTOXICOSIS)

Thyrotoxicosis is a hypermetabolic state that results from an excess of circulating thyroid hormone. Excessive thyroid hormone does not always result from thyroid gland hyperactivity; thus thyrotoxicosis, not hyperthyroidism, is the preferred term.

The most common condition is Graves' disease, an autoimmune disorder.[102,103] Thyroid-stimulating immunoglobulins (TSIs) bind to thyroid cell receptors and stimulate overproduction of thyroid hormones $T_4$ and $T_3$. The cause of TSI production is unknown. Graves' disease is characterized by diffuse thyroid enlargement (goiter), hyperthyroidism, ophthalmopathy, and occasionally pretibial myxedema.

Other causes of thyrotoxicosis include toxic multinodular goiter, toxic adenoma, subacute thyroiditis, autoimmune thyroiditis, and excessive exogenous thyroid hormone.

## Epidemiology

Graves' disease, which accounts for up to 90 percent of all cases of thyrotoxicosis, appears to be familial. Family history also shows an increased incidence of other autoimmune disorders. Toxic multinodular goiter is usually seen after age 50 in individuals with preexisting nontoxic nodular goiter. Silent thyroiditis occurs fairly frequently in postpartal women.[98,104]

Graves' disease occurs predominantly among women 20 to 40 years old. Up to 2 percent of women are affected. Either sex at any age may be affected, however.[98,102,105]

### Subjective Data

Clients may report tremulousness; palpitations; heat intolerance; increased perspiration; eye irritation, excessive lacrimation, photophobia, and diplopia; dyspnea; unexplained weight loss, despite increased appetite; frequent bowel movements; fatigue; weakness, especially of the proximal muscles; and decreased menstrual flow or amenorrhea.[103]

### Objective Data

Symptoms are related to excessive sympathomimetic activity and increased catabolic activity. The elderly do not usually present with classic symptoms. Cardiac symptoms, including atrial fibrillation, are more common among the elderly, whereas goiter and eye symptoms may be absent.[99,105]

***Physical Examination.*** It is comprehensive.

- *General Appearance.* Rapid, rambling, anxious speech.
- *Vital Signs.* Tachycardia, systolic hypertension, widened pulse pressure.
- *Skin.* Warm, smooth, moist skin and onycholysis.
- *Eyes.* Exophthalmus, proptosis, upper lid retraction, periorbital swelling.
- *Neck.* Enlarged, soft thyroid gland, nodules, thyroid bruits.
- *Chest.* Tachypnea.
- *Heart.* Atrial fibrillation, hyperdynamic apical impulse, systolic flow murmur.
- *Vascular System.* Bounding peripheral pulses.
- *Abdomen.* Hyperactive bowel sounds.
- *Musculoskeletal System.* Myopathy, especially in lower extremities.
- *Central Nervous System.* Fine tremor, hyperreflexia.

***Diagnostic Laboratory Tests.*** Show an elevated serum free T4 and a low TSH. If results are normal yet suspicion remains high, refer the client to an endocrinologist for further evaluation. Additional studies might include a serum T3 or thyrotropin-releasing hormone test.

### Differential Medical Diagnosis

Amphetamine or cocaine abuse, anxiety states/panic disorder, chronic obstructive pulmonary disease, pheochromocytoma, myeloproliferative disease, diabetes.

### Plan

Treatment must be individualized with consideration to the etiology and severity of disease, client's age, concomitant disease, and risks and benefits of therapeutic modalities.[103,105]

***Psychosocial Interventions.*** Reassure the client that her condition is not a malignant process.

***Medication.*** Antithyroid drugs, beta blockers, and radioactive iodine are used.

- *Antithyroid Drugs.* Antithyroid drugs are recommended for pregnant women.
  - *Administration.* Medication is taken daily.
  - *Side Effects.* The most frequent side effects are rash, malaise, fever, urticaria, arthralgias, gastrointestinal disturbances, and loss of taste. Transient leukopenia occurs in about 12 percent of adults.
  - *Contraindication.* Do not administer antithyroid drug to clients with cardiac disease.

- *Anticipated Outcome on Evaluation.* Level of circulating thyroid hormone decreases.
- *Client Teaching.* Inform the client that although the duration of therapy is controversial, it is rarely longer than 2 years.

- *Beta Blockers.* Beta blockers are indicated to alleviate symptoms of thyrotoxicosis: tachycardia, palpitations, hypertension, tremor, heat intolerance, and anxiety. Beta blockers are used as an adjunct to radioactive iodine until its therapeutic effect is achieved. See Coronary Artery Disease.
- *Radioactive Iodine.* Radioactive iodine is the treatment of choice for clients older than 40 years.
    - *Administration.* The tracer dose of radioactive iodine in tablet form is administered and followed by irradiation.
    - *Side Effect.* Within the first year, hypothyroidism occurs in 10 percent of those treated. The likelihood of hypothyroidism developing increases by 5 percent each subsequent year over the next 20 years.
    - *Contraindication.* Radioactive iodine is never administered to pregnant women.
    - *Anticipated Outcome on Evaluation.* If an adequate dose of RAI is given, it will be 100 percent effective. Approximately 20 percent require a second dose. Complete resolution of symptoms occurs within 6 months of treatment.
    - *Client Teaching.* Inform the client that RAI is inexpensive and effective. Many clients then exhibit hypothyroidism and require $T_4$ replacement. Periodic testing for hypothyroidism should be done indefinitely. The amount of radiation received is comparable to the amount necessary to perform a barium enema. Clients should not become pregnant for 6 months following treatment.

***Surgical Interventions.*** Surgical intervention is limited and controversial. It may be an option for pregnant women or for those who do not respond to antithyroid medications.[105]

***Follow-Up.*** Treatment dictates follow-up. Educate clients about the symptoms of hyper- and hypothyroidism.

## THYROID NODULES

A thyroid nodule is a mass that presents as a single palpable nodule or as part of a multinodular gland.[105] The diagnostic challenge is to distinguish a benign nodule from a malignancy.[106]

### Epidemiology

Studies often reveal a history of radiation exposure. The period of latency ranges from 5 to 35 years, with an average of 20 years. A family history of thyroid malignancies or endocrine tumors is common. About 20 to 30 percent of persons exposed to ionizing radiation develop palpable thyroid abnormalities; 50 percent have nodules. Of those nodules, 30 to 50 percent are malignant. Single nodules are more likely to be malignant than a multinodular gland.[106]

Incidence reports reveal that about 4 percent of the adult population has thyroid nodules; incidence increases to 5 percent among individuals older than 60 years. Nodules are four times more common in women than men; however, malignant nodules are more common in men. At least 95 percent of all palpable nodules are benign.[107]

Thyroid cancer is rare and deaths from thyroid cancer are even rarer.

### Subjective Data

A client may report a medical history of thyroid disorders, endocrine tumors, and/or head or neck irradiation. Although most women are asymptomatic, a client may have hoarseness, vocal cord paralysis, and dysphagia.[107]

## Objective Data

***Physical Examination.*** May be unremarkable or reveal symptoms of hypo- or hyperthyroidism. Nodules range from barely palpable to visible; their physical characteristics do not secure a diagnosis of benign or malignant. Although nodules may be tender, most are nontender. Thyroid malignancy is suggested by a solitary firm nodule with associated nontender cervical lymphadenopathy.105

***Diagnostic Methods.*** These include laboratory tests, biopsy, and imaging. Laboratory tests usually show normal thyroid function.

*A fine-needle aspiration biopsy* is the most reliable diagnostic method. If the aspirate shows malignancy, the probability is that it is 95 percent correct. If suspicious, a 45 percent chance of malignancy is probable. Biopsy determines which nodules will be surgically excised; biopsy is the only truly definitive evaluation and surgery the definitive treatment.

The test procedure requires an experienced cytologist. It is safe, inexpensive, and accurate. Fine-needle aspiration biopsy followed by a thyroid scan for suspicious lesions seems to be the most cost-effective approach.

*Ultrasonography* determines consistency but does not define benign versus malignant disease. It is used as a guide for fine-needle aspiration.

*Radionuclide imaging* classifies nodules as "hot" or "cold." A malignant lesion incorporates less iodine than normal thyroid tissue; therefore, it should appear "cold." This technique is not sensitive; although a "hot" nodule reduces the likelihood of malignancy, it does not exclude the possibility.

*Thyroid suppression* is controversial and logistically difficult to interpret because of clinical limitations in sizing nodules.

## Differential Medical Diagnosis

Hemorrhagic cysts, Hashimoto's thyroiditis.

## Plan

***Psychosocial Interventions.*** Inform the client that although it is rare for a nodule to be malignant, the risk is real.

***Surgical Interventions.*** Surgical management of thyroid cancer is controversial. It is generally agreed that the nodule be removed and suppressive therapy used. The amount of thyroid to be removed (one lobe or total thyroidectomy) and the method of follow-up may vary.

***Follow-Up.*** Refer all clients with thyroid nodules to an endocrinologist who will manage treatment.

# URINARY TRACT INFECTIONS

Urinary tract infection (UTI) denotes the presence of microorganisms anywhere from the kidney (acute pyelonephritis), to the bladder (cystitis), to the distal urethra (urethritis).[108] Urine is sterile, with the possible exception that the normal urethra may be colonized by diphtheroids, lactobacillus, and alpha hemolytic streptococci.[109] Ascent of pathogenic bacteria typically begins with the rectal flora moving upward to the vaginal introitus, distal urethra, bladder, and finally, occasionally, the kidney. The population of bacteria established in the bladder may double every 40 minutes.

With repeated infections, it is important to differentiate between reinfection and relapse. Reinfection denotes infection by a different organism, and its source is usually vaginal or fecal flora. Relapse refers to recurrence of the same organism, usually from an incompletely treated focus in the kidneys.[110]

## Epidemiology

***Etiology.*** In a bladder infection, a combination of specific host and pathogen factors are involved. Bacteria with little or no pathogenic mechanisms can cause infection in immunocompromised hosts.[111] In healthy women, however, a few serotypes of *Escherichia coli* are responsible for more than 85 percent of bladder infections, yet these serotypes constitute only 1 percent of rectal flora. A specific interrelationship between bacterial adhesion and epithelial cell receptors in women predisposes them to infection.[112]

Periurethral cells in infection-prone women more readily bind *E. coli* cells than do periurethral cells in women who are not prone to infection. In women with recurrent UTIs, periurethral tissue is laden with pathogenic bacteria. Any additional factor, such as the motion of sexual intercourse, may cause these women to develop infection.[113] Surface mucin that coats the bladder helps prevent bacterial attachment. That lining may decrease with age, however.[114]

Risk factors for infection vary depending on the location of infection (see Table 17–28).[115]

Sexual activity places women at risk for all types of UTIs. The risk for cystitis is highest with vaginal intercourse. Any manipulation of the urethra, however, such as oral sex and masturbation, has some associated risk. Voiding prior to intercourse has not been shown to decrease risk of infection; however, voiding after intercourse decreases infection rates.[116] Diaphragm use greatly increases risk. Recent studies suggest that diaphragm spermicides may predispose women to UTIs by altering vaginal flora.[117]

***Transmission.*** Most often women serve as their own reservoir for pathogenic bacteria. Bacterial growth in the urinary tract of women is primarily related to urethral manipulation, most often as a result of intercourse. Residual urine, blockage of urine flow, or decreased voiding due to dehydration can also promote bacterial growth. Common pathogenic organisms in the urinary tract of women are listed in Table 17–29.

Urethritis may be caused by sexually transmitted diseases; primarily gonorrhea, chlamydia, and herpes. Urethritis and dysuria in males are usually secondary to sexually transmitted diseases; therefore, male partners with suspected urinary tract infections should be carefully assessed and treated for sexually transmitted diseases as appropriate. Some men develop dysuria in the presence of *Urea-*

**TABLE 17–28. RISK FACTORS FOR URINARY TRACT INFECTIONS**

| Cystitis | Acute Pyelonephritis | Urethritis |
|---|---|---|
| Childhood UTI[a] | Childhood UTI | New sex partner |
| Sexual activity ("honeymoon cystitis") | Prior history of pyelonephritis | Male partner with recent dysuria (rule out sexually transmitted diseases) |
| Diaphragm use | Three UTIs in past year | |
| | Known structural abnormality or stone | |
| | Urban indigent | |
| | Immunocompromised status | |
| | Pregnancy | |

[a]Urinary tract infection.
Source: *Reference 115.*

**TABLE 17–29. COMMON PATHOGENIC ORGANISMS IN WOMEN**

| Gram-Negative Pathogens | Gram-Positive Pathogens |
|---|---|
| *Escherichia coli* (responsible for >85% of UTIs)[a] | *Staphylococcus saprophyticus* (previously thought not to be a pathogen; now second most common cause of UTI in women) |
| *Proteus mirabilis* (a urea-splitting organism, associated with stone formation) | *Staphylococcus aureus* |
| *Klebsiella* species | Group A beta hemolytic streptococci |
| | Enterococci |

[a]Urinary tract infections.

*plasma urealyticum,* which is not currently considered a cause of sexually transmitted disease.

***Incidence.*** Approximately 10 to 25 percent of women will experience a lower urinary tract infection.[118] Among women with a UTI, 80 percent will have another within the year.[119,120] UTIs may occur at any time in the life span, but are more common with increasing age. The high prevalence rate with increased age is associated with an increase in chronic systemic problems, concurrent diseases, bowel incontinence, overuse of catheters, and poor nutrition.

## Subjective Data Interpretation

After data are collected, the primary care provider must discern whether symptoms are vaginal or urinary (see Table 17–30) and whether the upper urinary tract is involved (see Table 17–31). It is important to review a woman's history of UTIs or urinary problems and any recent medications; antibiotics will yield negative urine findings, and medications such as pyridium can make urine orange or green. Cystitis that occurs for no obvious reason in children, men, or a previously well woman older than 50 requires that the individual be referred to a urologist to rule out structural pathology.

An accurate sexual history is crucial. Women do not always volunteer important information such as having vaginal discharge or a new sex partner and, consequently, need to be questioned carefully. Women can usually discern whether dysuria is internal or an external burning as the urine passes over the labia. Vaginal infections, such as *Trichomonas, Candida,* bacterial vaginosis, and herpes simplex, may cause external dysuria.

Most often, urethritis in women is caused by *Chlamydia trachomatis,* the most prevalent bacterial sexually transmitted disease in the United States. Infrequent infections of the urethra may include *Neiserria gonorrhoeae, Trichomonas,* herpes simplex, and *Candida.*

Dysuria occurring gradually over 5 to 7 days is more characteristic of urethritis and acute pyelonephritis than cystitis, which usually has an abrupt onset. Urethritis symptoms, such as dysuria, with no recognized pathogens and no pyuria may be secondary to trauma or postmenopausal estrogen deficiency.[117]

Accurate discrimination between upper and lower UTIs by means of a history or physical exam is difficult. Of women diagnosed with lower UTI (cystitis), 30 percent actually have occult pyelonephritis.[121] Because pyelonephritis can cause permanent renal damage or death, it is crucial to try to make the correct diagnosis using a history

**TABLE 17–30. HISTORICAL CLUES TO DYSURIA**

| Cystitis | Vaginitis | Urethritis |
|---|---|---|
| Abrupt onset | Gradual onset | Gradual onset |
| Internal dysuria | External dysuria | Internal dysuria |
| Change in voiding: frequency, urgency, small volumes, possibly nocturia and/or incontinence | No change in voiding pattern | May have some change in voiding pattern, no nocturia |
| Symptoms aggravated by voiding | Symptoms more continuous | Symptoms primarily associated with voiding |
| May have grossly bloody or odorous urine | No change in urine appearance | No change in urine appearance |
| No vaginal discharge | Vaginal discharge odor, itch, or irritation | May or may not have vaginal discharge |
| 10% complain of suprapubic tenderness | No abdominal symptoms | Abdominal pain if associated with pelvic inflammatory disease |

(see Table 17–31). Differences may distinguish lower UTI (cystitis) from upper UTI (acute pyelonephritis). The typical presentation of acute pyelonephritis is abrupt onset of fever and flank pain; it may also be associated with generalized symptoms, such as nausea, vomiting, and chills. Pain may be perceived as low back or abdominal. Women with acute pyelonephritis may have no symptoms of dysuria or other common bladder symptoms.

History must confirm the presence or absence of any systemic symptoms: fever, chills, nausea, vomiting, diarrhea, headache, or malaise. Cystitis is rarely associated with fever or systemic symptoms; therefore, the presence of fever or systemic symptoms is strongly suspicious of pyelonephritis. Risk factors for upper UTIs also need to be assessed (see Table 17–28).

## Objective Data

***Physical Examination.*** The client is generally assessed; occasionally a pelvic exam is necessary.

- *General Appearance.* A client with acute pyelonephritis may appear toxic.
- *Vital Signs.* Blood pressure and temperature are elevated.
- *Costovertebral Angle Tenderness.* Determine whether it is present.
- *Abdomen.* Check for suprapubic tenderness; a more extensive exam is done if the abdomen is very tender or if the bladder is palpable from distention.
- *Pelvic Exam.* A pelvic exam may or may not be indicated based on the history and results of lab tests. When it is done, examine Skene's and periurethral glands. A pelvic exam may be necessary if the client has a history of external dysuria or gradual-onset dysuria especially with vaginal discharge or other vaginal symptoms; new or multiple sex partners; or internal dysuria (but the urinalysis appears benign with no pyuria).

***Diagnostic Tests.*** Methods of testing include urinalysis, urine culture and sensitivity, vaginal wet mounts, and various cultures.

*Urinalysis* is the cornerstone of diagnosis. It is important to teach women how to collect

**TABLE 17–31. DIFFERENTIATION OF UPPER AND LOWER URINARY TRACT INFECTIONS BY MEANS OF HISTORY AND PHYSICAL EXAMINATION**

| Lower UTI[a] (Cystitis) | Upper UTI (Acute Pyelonephritis) |
|---|---|
| Usually sudden onset | Often gradual onset over >5 days |
| Dysuria and voiding symptoms | ±Voiding symptoms |
| No systemic symptoms | Fever, chills, nausea, vomiting |
| No costovertebral angle tenderness | Often costovertebral angle tenderness |
| Serum WBC count normal | Serum WBC count often elevated |
| No WBC casts | May have WBC casts |

[a]UTI, urinary tract infection; WBC, white blood cell.

a urine specimen* and to examine urine within 1 hour of collection, because bacteria multiply[122] (see Table 17–32).

*A urine culture and sensitivity test* is beneficial in determining the type of bacteria and its sensitivity to antibiotics. It was previously believed that a true infection was represented by a colony count of $10^5$ microorganisms. Current research, however, shows that by using a colony count of $10^5$, health care providers miss the diagnosis of acute bacterial cystitis in about half the women presenting with clinical symptoms. A colony count of $10^2$ (100 colonies) in a symptomatic female is considered sufficient to cause a true, treatment-worthy infection.

Traditionally urine cultures were done prior to and following treatment of any urinary tract infection. As a result of cost–benefit analysis, a more rational approach is recommended, based on the individual's clinical profile.[123]

With uncomplicated cystitis, urine pretreatment cultures are not recommended unless the diagnosis is in question. The purpose of posttreatment cultures is to rule out relapses or untreated foci of infection.

Pretreatment urine cultures are recommended in specific circumstances.

- All complicated urinary tract infections, including suspected pyelonephritis, history of structural abnormalities, and history of frequent urinary problems/infections
- Uncertain diagnosis
- Symptoms present longer than 7 days
- History of UTI within preceding 3 weeks (possible relapse)
- History of recent catheterization or urologic surgery
- Pregnancy or suspected pregnancy
- Diabetes or other immunocompromising disorders

Posttreatment cultures are recommended in the following circumstances.

- Failure to improve with treatment
- Diagnosis of acute pyelonephritis
- Presence of complications

*Vaginal wet (KOH and saline) mounts* are used to rule out *Trichomonas, Candida,* and bacterial vaginosis (see Chapter 8).

*STD cultures* are done to rule out gonorrhea and chlamydia.

## Differential Medical Diagnosis

Primary differential diagnoses are urethritis, cystitis, and pyelonephritis (see Tables 17–30

*Studies reported in the *Journal of Pediatrics, American Journal of Medicine*, and *New England Journal of Medicine* have shown that the procedure to obtain a clean catch urine specimen does not reduce bacterial contamination of urine cultures. A study of 100 women was reported in 1993 by the University of Virginia Health Sciences Center. It confirmed that to obtain a good urine sample for culture, it is not necessary to first clean the urinary meatus or to hold the labia apart while voiding. From, *American Journal of Nursing,* August 1993, p. 2.

**TABLE 17–32. URINALYSIS FINDINGS ALTERED BY URINARY TRACT INFECTIONS[a]**

| | |
|---|---|
| *Color/appearance* | Often dark, turbid with foul smell; may be grossly bloody (hemorrhagic cystitis) |
| *Dipstick* | |
| Specific gravity | If too dilute, may be false-negative reading (i.e., low count of WBCs, RBCs, bacteria). |
| pH | If very high pH, may be associated with urea stone-forming *Klebsiella*; low pH retards bacterial growth |
| Nitrites | Confirms presence of bacteria that convert nitrates to nitrites (does not always mean infection if asymptomatic; see asymptomatic bacteriuria section) |
| Protein | May have 1+ or 2+ protein with lower UTI; however, 3+ or 4+ urine deserves special attention and follow up to rule out kidney damage.<br>Vaginal secretions may contaminate urine and give false positive for some protein; deserves follow-up |
| Leukocyte esterases | Quick way to determine pyuria, not as accurate as microscopic. |
| *Microscopic Exam* | Usually performed on spun urine; in women, normal urinary sediment may contain one or two RBCs and up to 4 WBCs per high-power field |
| RBCs | 40–60% of women with cystitis have some microscopic hematuria; most common cause of hematuria is infection; also seen with stones, glomerulonephritis, neoplasm, tuberculosis |
| WBCs | May come from any part of urinary tract; "clumping" may be seen in infection; presence of 5–10 WBCs per high-power field is suspicious for UTI, although false positives are common in women |
| Bacteria | Usually visible in true infection |
| Casts | RBC and/or WBC casts indicate kidney involvement |
| Epithelial cells and mucous | Large amounts of either suspicious for vaginal contamination |

[a]WBC, white blood cell; RBC, red blood cell; UTI, urinary tract infection.

and 17–31). Differential diagnoses also include asymptomatic bacteriuria, interstitial cystitis, and renal calculi.

***Asymptomatic Bacteriuria.*** Asymptomatic bacteriuria is defined as bacteria in the urine with no symptoms of urinary tract infection. Whether to treat is debatable. Current recommendations are to treat pregnant women as if the condition were a urinary tract infection. Elderly women, who have a high incidence of bacteriuria, have not been harmed by asymptomatic bacteriuria nor do they benefit from treatment.[124]

***Interstitial Cystitis.*** Interstitial cystitis is a syndrome of painful bladder without infection, characterized by urinary frequency, urgency, nocturia, and bladder pressure sensations that are often relieved by voiding. The urologist diagnoses interstitial cystitis by excluding other causes of painful bladder (cancer, tuberculosis, cystitis, herpes). Diagnosis is supported when cystoscopy reveals mucosal bleeding after distention of the bladder. Etiology is uncertain.[125]

***Renal Calculi.*** Renal calculi, called kidney stones, may cause intermittent flank pain or pain that radiates around to the abdomen. They are associated with hematuria. Clients may develop superimposed urinary tract infections. Most calculi are composed of calcium oxalate and phosphate and can be visualized on x-ray of the kidney, ureter, and bladder. Uric acid stones, on the other hand, do not show up on x-rays and are associated with urea-splitting bacteria, such as *Proteus mirabilis*. UTIs with *Proteus* must be evaluated to rule out calculi.[126]

## Plan

***Psychosocial Interventions.*** Discuss pain/discomfort management with the client and explain the mechanisms of urinary tract infections. Reassure her that a UTI is not a sexually transmitted disease, although intercourse may be mechanically related to the condition. Inform the woman so that she can identify her own precipitating factors and use appropriate preventive measures.

***Medication.*** Table 17–33 lists the management options for cystitis[127–129] and Table 17–34 describes outpatient management of acute pyelonephritis.

***Surgical Interventions.*** Women with recurrent cystitis rarely have anatomic abnormalities that require surgical intervention. Referral, however, is suggested for women with recurrent problems who have a history of childhood infections, more than one episode of acute pyelonephritis, possible nephrolithiasis, relapsing infections, infections caused by *Proteus mirabilis,* or painless hematuria.[130]

***Lifestyle Changes.*** Teach the client healthy voiding practices: void at first urge, void after intercourse. Encourage the client to make these practices routine. Advise her to maintain adequate hydration and to avoid use of contraceptive methods associated with increased UTI risk, such as a diaphragm.

***Follow-Up.*** Women should feel much improved within 24 to 48 hours of starting medication; if not, they should be instructed to telephone or return to the clinic. Teach clients the warning signs and symptoms of pyelonephritis and instruct them to telephone immediately if any of the symptoms develop.

For management of urethritis and vaginitis, see Chapter 8. For pregnant women, aggressive screening for urinary tract infection and treatment is recommended. UTIs and asymptomatic bacteriuria in pregnancy are associated with increased fetal and maternal morbidity.

**TABLE 17–33. TREATMENT OPTIONS FOR UNCOMPLICATED AND RECURRENT CYSTITIS**

| | |
|---|---|
| *Uncomplicated Cystitis:* rare or infrequent episodes of cystitis | |
| ***First-Line Medications*** | |
| 1. Single-dose therapy | |
| Advantages | Low cost, infrequent side effects, high compliance |
| Disadvantages | High failure rate (often >20%), does not treat unsuspected pyelonephritis |
| Medication of choice | TMP/SMX,[a] two double-strength tablets, stat; ampicillin and cephalosporins avoided due to high failure rate/resistance |
| Client teaching | Even if organism is eradicated with single-dose therapy, it may take 2 or 3 days for symptoms to resolve; client should immediately report any increase in symptoms or symptoms of pyelonephritis (e.g., fever, flank pain, nausea, etc.) |

*(continued)*

**TABLE 17–33. CONTINUED**

| | |
|---|---|
| 2. Three-day treatment | |
| Advantages | New area of study that combines decreased cost and decreased side effects |
| Disadvantages | Twice the side effect rates as single dose; more research on effectiveness needed |
| Medications of choice | TMP/SMX double-strength tablets b.i.d. × 3 days OR nitrofurantoin (Macrodantin) 50–100 mg q.i.d. × 3 days |
| Client teaching | Call or return to clinic stat if not improved or symptoms reappear |
| 3. Traditional 7- to 10-day treatment | |
| Advantages | Only a 5% failure rate; most research done with this approach |
| Disadvantage | Twice the side effect rate of single dose, increased cost, decreased compliance |
| Medication of choice | TMP/SMX DS b.i.d. × 7 days OR nitrofurantoin 50 mg q.i.d. × 7 days; |
| Client teaching | encourage finishing medication as ordered; if side effects occur, stop medications and telephone primary health care provider |
| ***Second-Line Medications*** | |
| Several new, expensive medications are now available for urinary tract infections. They should be reserved for clients with allergies or with resistant organisms, e.g., ciprofloxacin (Cipro) 250 or 500 mg b.i.d. × 7 days OR norfloxacin (Noroxin) 400 mg b.i.d. × 7 days | |
| *Recurrent Cystitis:* arbitrarily defined as three or more episodes of cystitis per year | |
| 1. Postcoital prophylaxis | |
| Indications | Highly effective for the 85% of women who have onset of symptoms 24 to 48 hours after intercourse; intercourse does not occur as frequently as daily |
| Medications | Oral antibiotic is taken just prior to or just after intercourse |
| Options | 50 mg nitrofurantion, 250 mg cephalosporin, half single-strength TMX/SMX |
| 2. Intermittent self-start therapy | |
| Indications | Client must be motivated and reliable about following directions<br>Home dipslide cultures are prepared by client at onset of symptoms and the client self-starts traditional first-line antibiotics as prescribed; dip slides are inexpensive and save cost of two office visits; client must demonstrate a clear knowledge of the procedures and the signs of relapse and pyelonephritis |
| Medications | 7-day course of traditional antibiotics<br>TMP/SMX double strength b.i.d. × 7 days OR nitrofurantoin 50 mg q.i.d. × 7 days p.o. |
| 3. Low-dose continuous prophylaxis | |
| Indications | Method of choice with high or daily sexual frequency; absence of any infection must be documented by urine culture prior to start |
| Medications | Cephalexin (Keflex) 250 mg, trimethoprim 100 mg, Cinoxacin 250–500 mg<br>Given daily at bedtime or three times weekly; nitrofurantoin avoided, as long-term exposure may cause hypersensitivity reactions in the lung and kidney; breakthrough infections treated with the full traditional 7-day therapy as indicated |

[a]See a current pharmacotherapeutics text for details.
[b]TMP/SMX, trimethoprim–sulfamethoxazole (Bactrim).
Sources: *References 127–129.*

**TABLE 17–34. ACUTE PYELONEPHRITIS: OUTPATIENT MANAGEMENT[a]**

*Criteria for Outpatient Management[b]*

1. Diagnosis is secure (consult with physician)
2. No underlying, complicating disease, such as diabetes
3. Not pregnant
4. No history of recent urinary tract instrumentation
5. Not toxic, must be able to tolerate oral therapy and fluids
6. Follow-up must be easily accessible in 24 hours
7. Culture and sensitivity must be sent the day treatment is initiated

*Medications*

1. Must be broad spectrum (ampicillin and first-generation cephalosporins should not be used; trimethoprim–sulfamethoxazole (Bactrim) double strength b.i.d. or ciprofloxacin hydrochloride (Cipro) 500 mg b.i.d. for 14 days
2. Addition of a stat dose of intramuscular gentamicin (dose based on weight) used by some clinicians
3. Client should improve substantially in the first 24 hours; consult/refer if not improved.

[a]Consult a pharmacotherapeutics text for details.
[b]Woman must meet these criteria to attempt outpatient management.

## NURSING DIAGNOSES

The following nursing diagnoses identified by the author are representative of those used in the health care plan of women with medical problems; however, these diagnoses by no means constitute an inclusive list.

- Activity/rest deficit related to poor self-worth or time management
- Airway clearance ineffective related to infection or cough suppressants; potential for aspiration, at risk for pneumonia
- Alteration in comfort related to biliary pain
- Alteration in patterns of urination related to discomfort/dysuria
- Alteration in sleep pattern related to nocturnal nonulcerative dyspepsia
- Alteration in tissue perfusion related to coronary artery disease
- Body image disturbance related to malformation of cardiac structure
- Constipation related to fear of painful defecation
- Excess fluid volumes related to intake of more than daily sodium requirements
- Exogenous obesity related to excessive caloric intake
- Fear related to possibility of malignancy
- Impaired swallowing related to mechanical obstruction by tonsils, at risk for choking
- Impaired tissue integrity related to prolonged exposure to corrosive gastric contents
- Inability to identify health risks related to lack of knowledge
- Ineffective individual coping related to a physiologic hyperkinetic state
- Ineffective thermoregulation related to low metabolic state
- Knowledge deficit related to
  —dietary sources of iron, inappropriate treatment with iron
  —diagnostic testing
  —prescribed dietary regimen
- Mucous membrane alterations, at risk for bacterial secondary infections
- Noncompliance in avoiding ultraviolet light, related to client's value system and cultural norms
- Noncompliance to pharmacotherapeutic regimens related to a lack of subjective physical evidence of disease

- Nutrition less than body requirements
- Pain related to psychological factors and underdeveloped stress management skills
- Potential for cellulitis and spread of septicemia related to knowledge deficit of early warning signs
- Potential for pulmonary aspiration related to esophageal reflux
- Sensory/auditory alteration related to fluid behind tympanic membrane
- Sexuality alterations required related to risk of urinary tract infection

## REFERENCES


1. Lubkin, I. (1982). Evaluating iron deficiency anemia. *Nurse Practitioner, 7,* 34–38.
2. Waterbury, L. *Hematology for the house officer.* Baltimore: Williams & Wilkins.
3. Kitay, D. (1991). The pregnant patient with anemia. Part 1. *The Female Patient, 16,* 23–34.
4. Brown, R. (1991). Determining the cause of anemia. *Postgraduate Medicine, 89,* 161–170.
5. Branch, W. (1987). *Office practice of medicine* (2nd ed.). Philadelphia: W.B. Saunders.
6. Welborn, J., & Meyers, F. (1991). A three point approach to anemia. *Postgraduate Medicine, 89,* 179–186.
7. Beutler, E. (1988). The common anemias. *Journal of the American Medical Association, 259*(16), 2433–2437.
8. Froberg, J. (1989). The anemias: Causes and courses of action. *R.N., 52*(1,3,5), 24–29, 52–56, 42–50.
9. Goodman, K., & Salt, W. (1990). Vitamin $B_{12}$ deficiency. *Postgraduate Medicine, 88,* 147–155.
10. Esposito, N. (1992). Thalassemias: Simple screening for hereditary anemias. *Nurse Practitioner, 17,* 50–61.
11. Stander, P. (1989). Anemia in the elderly. *Postgraduate Medicine. 85,* 85–92.
12. Steingart, R.M., Packer, M., Hamm, P., Coglianese, M.E., Gersh, B., & Geltman, E.M. (1991). Sex differences in the management of coronary artery disease. *New England Journal of Medicine, 325*(4), 226–230.
13. Langer, R.D., & Connor, E.B. (1991). Epidemiology and prevention of cardiovascular disease in women. *Contemporary Internal Medicine,* 50–63.
14. Eaker, E. (1991, May). Coronary heart disease in women. In *Women and heart disease.* Annual Conference of the American Heart Association, Virginia Affiliate.
15. Chapman, D.W. (1991). Angina pectoris. *Consultant, 31*(3), 21–35.
16. Wexler, A., et al. (1991). Differences in use of procedures between women and men hospitalized for CAD. *New England Journal of Medicine, 325* (4), 221–230.
17. Bush, T.L., Fried, L.P., & Barrett-Connor, E. (1988). Cholesterol, lipoproteins and coronary heart disease in women. *Clinical Chemistry, 34,* B60.
18. Eaker, E.D., Packard, B., & Thom, T.J. (1989). Epidemiology and risk factors for coronary artery disease in women. *Cardiovascular Clinics, 19,* 129–145.
19. Smith, M.A., & Johnson, D.G. (1991). Evaluation and management of coronary artery disease: Guidelines for the primary care nurse practitioner. *Nurse Practitioner Forum, 2*(1), 19–26.
20. McMahon, J.K., & Briggs, G.C. (1991). Ace inhibitors and calcium channel antagonists: A practical approach. *Nurse Practitioner Forum, 2*(1), 61–69.
21. Manson, J.E., Stampfer, M.F., Colditz, G.A., Willett, W.C., Rosner, B., Speizer, F.E., & Hennekens, C.H. (1991). A prospective study of aspirin use and primary prevention of cardiovascular disease in women. *Journal of the American Medical Association, 266* (4), 521–527.
22. Report of the U.S. Preventive Services Task Force. (1989). *Guide to clinical preventive services.* Baltimore: Williams & Wilkins.
23. Jones, P.H., & Gotto, A.M. (1987). Hyperlipoproteinemia. *Consultant, 27*(11), 126–47.

24. National Cholesterol Education Program. (1991). *Archives of Internal Medicine, 151,* 1071–1084.
25. Forster, C.J. (1992). LDL should be shelved as a guide to making cholesterol-lowering treatment decisions. *Modern Medicine, 60*(2), 12–23.
26. Panel on Detection, Evaluation, and Treatment of High Blood Cholesterol in Adults. (1988). *Archives of Internal Medicine, 148*(2), 36–69.
27. Dujovne, C.A., & Harris, W.S. (1990). Variabilities in serum lipid measurements. *Archives of Internal Medicine, 150,* 1583–1585.
28. Lipid Research Clinics Program. (1984). Research clinics coronary primary prevention trial results. *Journal of the American Medical Association, 251*(3), 351–364.
29. Naito, H.K. (1987). Reducing cardiac deaths with hypolipemic drugs. *Postgraduate Medicine, 82*(6), 102–112.
30. Long, K., & Long, R. (1991). Lowering cholesterol pharmacologically. *Nurse Practitioner Forum, 2*(1), 11–12.
31. The 1988 Report of the Joint National Committee on Detection, Evaluation and Treatment of High Blood Pressure. (1988). *Archives of Internal Medicine, 148,* 1023–1036.
32. Cheng, T.O. (1990). Mitral valve prolapse. *Postgraduate Medicine, 88*(7), 93–100.
33. Cornell, L.V. (April 1985). Mitral valve prolapse syndrome: Etiology and symptomatology. *Nurse Practitioner, 10*(4), 25, 26, 29, 34.
34. Wooley, C.F. (1983). Mitral valve prolapse syndrome. *Hospital Practice, 18*(6), 163–174.
35. Clinical Experience Column (1987). Mitral valve prolapse. *Hospital Practice,* March, 40–57.
36. Hunt, A.H. (April 1985). Mitral valve prolapse: physical assessment, complications and management. *Nurse Practitioner, 10*(4), 15, 17, 20, 21.
37. Dajani, A.S., Bisno, A.L., Chung, K.J., Durack, D.T., Freed, M., & Gerber, M.A. (1990). Prevention of bacterial endocarditis. *Journal of the American Medical Association, 264*(22), 85–89.
38. Kitchin, L.I., & Castell, D.O. (1991). Rationale and efficacy of conservative therapy for gastroesophageal reflux disease. *Archives of Internal Medicine, 151,* 448–453.
39. Heading, R.C. (1989). Epidemiology of esophageal disease. *Scandinavian Journal of Gastroenterology, 24*(Suppl. 168), 33–37.
40. Sutherland, J. E. (1991). Gastroesophageal reflux disease. *Postgraduate Medicine, 89* (7), 45–53.
41. Rogers, A. I. (1990). Medical treatment and prevention of peptic ulcer disease. *Postgraduate Medicine, 88*(5), 57–60.
42. Rosen, S.D., & Rogers, A.I. (1990). Clinical recognition and evaluation of peptic ulcer disease. *Postgraduate Medicine, 88*(5), 42–55.
43. Fenner, L. (1984). *When digestive juices corrode, you've got an ulcer.* Department of Health and Human Services Consumer Report, HHS Publication No 84-1113 (FDA).
44. Katz, K.D., & Hollander, D. (1988). Outpatient management of duodenal ulcer disease. *Hospital Medicine,* Jan., 95–114.
45. Dudley, S.L., & Starin R.B. (1991). Cholelithiasis: Diagnosis and current therapeutic options. *Nurse Practitioner, 16*(3), 12–24.
46. DeCross, A.J. and Marshall, B.J. (1993). Eradication of *Helicobacter pylori:* Which patients, which drugs? *Physician Assistant,* 65–78.
47. Schoenfield, L. (1988). Gallstones. *Clinical Symposium, 40*(2), 2–4.
48. Snape, W.J. (1987). Irritable bowel syndrome. *Postgraduate Medicine, 88*(5), 57–60.
49. Danilewitz, M. (1991). Irritable bowel syndrome. *Consultant, 31*(6), 50–2.
50. Guthrie, J.F., Hines, C., Muldoon, J.P., Pennington, E.E., Weakley, F.L., & Ganz, S.B. (1986). Detecting and treating anal fissures. *Patient Care,* 111–116.
51. Olsen, J. (1988). Classification and diagnostic criteria for headache disorders, cranial neuralgias and facial pain. *Cephalalgia, 8* (Suppl. 7), 9–96.

52. Kunkel, R. (1991). Diagnosis and treatment of muscle contraction (tension-type) headaches. *Medical Clinics of North America, 75,* 595–603.
53. Diamond, S., & Medina, J. (1989). Headaches. *Clinical Symposia, 41,* 2–32.
54. Smith, L. (1988). Evaluation and Management of Muscle Contraction Headache. *Nurse Practitioner, 13,* 20–27.
55. Edmeads, J. (1989). The worst headache ever. *Postgraduate Medicine, 86,* 93–110.
56. Gabai, I., & Spierings, E. (1990). Diagnosis and management of cluster headaches. *Nurse Practitioner, 15,* 32–36.
57. Diamond, S. (1991). Migraine headaches. *Medical Clinics of North America, 75,* 545–566.
58. *Perimenstrual headache pain.* (1990). A NAACOG Continuing Education Program for Nurse Practitioners, Syntex.
59. Solomon, S. (1988). Common migraine: Criteria for diagnosis. *Headache, 28,* 124–129.
60. Walling, A. (1990). Drug prophylaxis for migraine headaches. *American Family Physician, 42,* 425–432.
61. Kudrow, L. (Oct. 1993). Migraine in women: Recognizing hormonal influences. *The Female Patient, 18,* 33–38.
62. Pearlman, P., & Ginn, D. (1990). Respiratory infections in ambulatory adults. *Postgraduate Medicine, 87*(1), 175–184.
63. Wilson, D. (Ed.) (1990). *Harrison's textbook of internal medicine.* New York: McGraw-Hill.
64. Bernstein, J. (1990). Applying today's concepts on pathogenesis of otitis media. *Journal of Respiratory Diseases, 11,* 402–418.
65. Facione, N. (1990). Otitis media: An overview of acute and chronic disease. *Nurse Practitioner, 15,* 11–20.
66. Klingman, E. (1991). Treatment of otitis media. *American Family Physician, 45*(1), 242–250.
67. Stool, S. (1989). Otitis media: Update on a common and frustrating problem. *Postgraduate Medicine, 85*(1), 40–53.
68. Woolbert, L. (1990). Do antihistamines and decongestants prevent otitis media? *Pediatric Nursing, 16,* 265–267.
69. Herr, R. (1991). Acute sinusitis: Diagnosis and treatment update. *American Family Physician, 44*(6), 2055–2062.
70. Sande, M. (1989). Managing sinus infection: Efficient diagnosis, effective therapy. *Modern Medicine, 57,* 103–106.
71. Gray, W., & Blanchan, C. (1987). Sinusitis and its complications. *American Family Physician, 53*(3), 232–243.
72. Huovinen, D. (1990). Causes, diagnosis and treatment of pharyngitis. *Comprehensive Therapy, 16,* 59–65.
73. Hedges, J., & Lowe, R. (1987). Approach to acute pharyngitis. *Emergency Clinics of North America, 5,* 335–349.
74. Komaroff, A. (1987). Pharyngitis and related infections in adults. In *Branch's office textbook of medicine* (2nd ed.). Philadelphia: W.B. Saunders.
75. Douglas, G. (1988). Influenza prevention and treatment. *Postgraduate Medicine, 83* (5), 207–212.
76. Dowling, C. (1989). Preventing pneumonia and influenza deaths in 1989–90. *Consultants, 11,* 25–31.
77. Dolin, R. (1990). Influenza: Current practices in prevention and treatment. *Journal of Respiratory Diseases, Supplement,* s14–s19.
78. Amin, N. (1989). Evaluation and treatment of pneumonia in adult patients. *Modern Medicine, 57,* 58–73.
79. Biller, P. (1987). Diagnosis and management of acute bronchitis and pneumonia in the ambulatory setting. *Nurse Practitioner, 12,* 13–27.
80. Brown, R. (1989). Acute and chronic bronchitis. *Postgraduate Medicine, 85,* 249–254.
81. Markowitz, S. (1990). Pneumococcal pneumonia. *Postgraduate Medicine, 88*(7), 33–47.
82. Stinger, S., & Anderson, W. (1990). Mycoplasma pneumonia. *Postgraduate Medicine, 88*(7), 61–70.
83. Marion, G. (1992). Preventing tetanus, influenza, and pneumococcal infection in adults. *Physician Assistant,* Oct., 27–50.
84. Rytel, M. (1990). Pneumococcal pneumonia: Still a serious problem. *Journal of Respiratory Diseases, 11,* 83–95.

85. Habif, T. (1990). *Clinical dermatology.* St. Louis: C.V. Mosby.
86. Tubinick, E. (1987). Basal cell cancer. *American Family Physician, 36*(3), 219–224.
87. Elwood, J. (Ed.). (1988). *Melanoma and naevi.* Basel: Karger.
88. Greeley, A. (1991). No safe tan. *FDA Consumer. 25*(4), 17–21.
89. Burke, K. (1990). Facial wrinkles: Prevention and non-surgical management. *Postgraduate Medicine, 88,* 207–227.
90. Pathak, M. (1986). Sunscreens: Topical and systemic approaches for the prevention of acute and chronic sun-induced reactions. *Dermatologic Clinics, 4,* 321–333.
91. Potts, J. (1990). Sunlight, sunburn and sunscreens. *Postgraduate Medicine, 87,* 52–63.
92. Lawler, P., & Schreiber, S. (1989). Cutaneous malignant melanoma: Nursing's role in prevention and early detection. *Oncology Nursing Forum, 16*(3), 345–352.
93. Hadler, R., & Bang, K. (1988). Skin cancer in blacks in the United States. *Medical Clinics of North America, 6*(3), 379–405.
94. Finley, C. (1986). Malignant melanoma: A primary care perspective. *Nurse Practitioner, 11,* 22–38.
95. Crutcher, W., & Cohen, P. (1990). Dysplastic nevi and malignant melanoma. *American Family Physician, 42,* 327–382.
96. Becker, J., Goldberg, L., & Tschen J. (1989). Differential diagnosis of malignant melanoma. *American Family Physician, 39,* 203–214.
97. Sakiyama, R. (1988). Common thyroid disorders. *American Family Physician, 38*(1), 227–38.
98. Whiteside-Yim, C., & Mac Adams, M.R. (1987). Thyroid disorders. *Postgraduate Medicine, 81*(5), 231–240.
99. Mazzaferri, E.L. (1986). Adult hypothyroidism. *Postgraduate Medicine, 79*(7), 75–86.
100. Schultz, A.L. (1986). Thyroid function tests. Selective use for cost containment. *Postgraduate Medicine, 80*(2), 219–228.
101. Wilbur, J.F. (1988). Hypothyroidism. In *Medicine for the Practicing Physician* (2nd ed.). Boston: Butterworth.
102. McFarland, K.F., & Saleeby, G. (1988). Graves' disease. *Postgraduate Medicine, 83* (4), 275–281.
103. Safrit, H.F. (1979). Diagnosis and management of Graves' disease. *Hospital Medicine,* Oct., 74–87.
104. Gardner, D.F. (1988). Thyroid disease. In *Medicine for the practicing physician* (pp. 479–484). Boston: Butterworths.
105. Geelhoed, G.W., & Proye, C.A. (1991). Partial and total thyroidectomy. *Hospital Medicine,* May. 91–98.
106. Burch, W.M. (1984). *Endocrinology for the house officer.* Baltimore: Williams & Wilkins.
107. Hamburger, J.I., & Hamburger, S.W. (1986). A practical guide to thyroid nodules. *Contemporary Obstetrics and Gynecology, Special Issue: General Medicine Update,* 97–100.
108. Thompson, F. (1987). *Disorders of the kidneys and urinary tract.* London: Edward Arnold.
109. Kamoroff, A. (1989). Acute dysuria in women. *New England Journal of Medicine, 310*(6), 368–375.
110. Johnson, C. (1991). Definition, classification and clinical presentation of UTIs. *Medical Clinics of North America, 75,* 241–253.
111. Sobel, J. (1991). Bacterial etiologic agents in the pathogenesis of UTI. *Medical Clinics of North America, 75,* 253–273.
112. Measley, R., & Levinson, M. (1991). Host defense mechanisms in the pathogenesis of urinary tract infections. *Medical Clinics of North America, 75,* 275–286.
113. Schaeffer, A. (1987). Recurrent urinary tract infections in women: pathogenesis and management. *Postgraduate Medicine, 81,*51–58.
114. Millette-Petit, E. (1988). Urinary tract infections in older adults. *Nurse Practitioner, 13,* 21–29.
115. Stamm, W. (1988). Dysuria: Establishing a diagnostic protocol. *Contemporary Obstetrics and Gynecology, 10,* 81–89.
116. Strom, B., et al. (1987). Sexual activity, contraceptive use and other risk factors for symptomatic and asymptomatic bacteriuria. *Annals of Internal Medicine, 107,* 816–823.
117. Hooten, T., & Stamm, W. (1991). Manage-

ment of acute uncomplicated UTI in adults. *Medical Clinics of North America, 75,* 339–357.

118. Rakel, R. (1990). *Textbook of family medicine.* Philadelphia: W.B. Saunders.

119. Johnson, M. (1990). Urinary tract infections in women. *American Family Physician, 41,* 565–571.

120. Thomas, S., & Bhatia, N. (1989). New approaches in the treatment of UTIs. *Obstetrics and Gynecology Clinics of North America, 16,* 897–909.

121. Johnson, J., & Stamm, W. (1989). Urinary tract infections in women: Diagnosis and treatment. *Annals of Internal Medicine, 111* (11), 906–917.

122. Pappas, P. (1991). Laboratory in the diagnosis and management of UTIs. *Medical Clinics of North America, 75,* 313–327.

123. Patton, J., Nash, D., & Abrutyn, E. (1991). UTI: Economic considerations. *Medical Clinics of North America, 75,* 495–511.

124. U.S. Task Force. (1990). Screening for asymptomatic bacteriuria, hematuria and proteinuria. *American Family Physician, 8,* 54–59.

125. Fletcher, S. (1988). Interstitial cystitis: Painful bladder syndrome. *Nurse Practitioner, 13,* 7–12.

126. LaPorte, J., & Blaum, N. (1990). Kidney Stones. *Postgraduate Medicine, 87,* 219–223.

127. Bump, R. (1990). Urinary tract infections in women: Current role of single dose therapy. *Journal of Reproductive Medicine, 35,* 785–791.

128. Fihn, S. (1988). Trimethoprim–sulfamethoxazole in acute dysuria in women: A single dose or a 10 day course. *Annals of Internal Medicine, 108,* 350–357.

129. Stapelton, A. (1990). Postcoital antimicrobial prophylaxis for recurrent urinary tract infections. *Journal of the American Medical Association, 204*(6), 703–706.

130. Shalom, R. (1987). Problem areas in the management of urinary tract infections. *Journal of the American College Health Association, 36,* 165–169.

# CHAPTER 18

# PSYCHOSOCIAL HEALTH CONCERNS

*Nancy L. Harris and Belinda Seimer*

*For a woman to achieve changes for herself and her family, she must acknowledge her own self-worth. The health care provider can play a vital supporting role.*

*Highlights*

- Women as Victims
  - *Sexual Harassment*
  - *Violence*
  - *Sexual Abuse*
- Substance Abuse
- Depression
- Anxiety
- Stress, Post-traumatic Stress Disorder
- Anorexia Nervosa
- Bulimia
- Compulsive Overeating
- Alternative Lifestyle

## INTRODUCTION

To thoroughly address women's health, the health care provider must consider the potential psychosocial problems that women face. Some specific problems are sexual harassment, physical and verbal abuse, and sexual assault; depression, stress, and anxiety; substance abuse; and eating disorders. Identifying women at risk for these health problems and managing their care is the role of a primary care provider. A common thread throughout this chapter is the influence of low self-esteem, feelings of inadequacy, and the socialization of "learned helplessness" on the psychosocial health of women.

Prevention of these complex psychosocial problems requires that women, and society as a whole, acknowledge their existence. Community education, referrals, support systems, and counseling should be used extensively in recovery. If encouraged, women can develop coping mechanisms that promote wellness and a positive self-concept through assertiveness training and learning to take responsibility for self. It is essential for them to learn what is appropriate behavior for themselves and people close to them rather than what may be accepted as the norm, for example, physical or verbal abuse. For a woman to achieve changes for herself and her family, she must acknowledge her own self-worth.

The health care provider can play a vital supporting role.

## WOMEN AS VICTIMS

### SEXUAL HARASSMENT

Sexual harassment encompasses unwelcome sexual advances, requests for sexual favors, and other verbal or physical conduct or written communications of an intimidating, hostile, or offensive nature or action taken in retaliation for reporting such behavior, regardless of where such conduct might occur.[1] Sexual harassment is most common among women working in a male-dominated profession, but may occur in any work environment.

Overt discrimination in the workplace has decreased since passage of the Civil Rights Act in 1964; however, subtle discrimination continues to persist, as does sexual harassment against women.[2] A random survey of 10,000 women employed by the federal government in 1981 found that 62 percent had experienced sexual touching and 20 percent, actual or attempted sexual assault on the job.[3]

#### Subjective Data

A woman may express an inability to concentrate, reduction in confidence, decreased motivation that affects her job, tension, nervousness, anger, fear, or helplessness. These feelings may or may not carry over into her home. Physical complaints may include nausea, headaches, and chronic fatigue, which may lead to use or abuse of alcohol, prescriptive drugs, or nonprescriptive drugs to reduce stress-related symptoms.

The history includes several specific points of information.

- Chief complaint, with brief description in chronological order of present problem
- Medical history noting childhood illnesses; injuries (be observant for injuries that are not consistent with explanation); hospitalizations and surgeries; previous major illnesses; allergies; habits (start with less offensive), including caffeine, tobacco, alcohol, and illicit drugs; and medications, prescriptive and nonprescriptive
- Family medical history noting substance abuse and any mental health problems
- Social history noting family relationships (married/divorced/single); support system; occupational history (time at present job, recent loss of job or job change); and economic status
- Psychological system, with cognitive abilities (orientation to present, memory, history of psychiatric illness) and cultural implications
- Nutrition and rest and exercise patterns

#### Objective Data

A complete physical examination and wide range of diagnostic tests are carried out.

***Physical Examination***

- *General Appearance.* The client may or may not be well groomed, may be over- or underweight, and may appear anxious or nervous.
- *Eyes.* Circles may be visible under eyes. Eyes may be red and puffy from lack or sleep or crying.
- *Neck.* Neck muscles may be tense and tender from stress or tension.
- *Skin.* Skin may be bruised, lacerated, burned, dry, or cold and clammy.
- *Nails and Hair.* The nails and hair may be dull and brittle.
- *Chest.* Respiratory rate may be increased.
- *Vascular System.* Blood pressure and heart rate may be increased.
- *Abdomen.* Bowel sounds may be hypoactive or hyperactive. Abdomen may be tender on palpation.

- *Musculoskeletal System.* Examination may reveal bruising, redness, edema, joint pain or swelling, poor posture, tense muscles, or limited range of motion.
- *Nervous System.* Poor coordination, unsteady gait, abnormal cranial nerve evaluation, sluggish speech, flight of ideas, inability to concentrate, and poor memory are possible findings.
- *Genitalia.* If indicated. See Sexual Abuse.

***Diagnostic Tests***

- Electrocardiogram
- Electroencephalogram, if indicated
- Complete blood count to rule out anemia and infection
- Thyroid panel to rule out thyroid disease
- Stool guaiac if diarrhea is present
- Upper and lower GI series, if indicated
- Urinalysis to rule out urinary tract infection and diabetes

### Nursing Implications

Throughout the physical examination, validate all normal findings and reassure the client. In a positive way, explain any abnormal findings. Prior to laboratory tests, explain the test, review what is involved and why the test is being done.

### Differential Medical Diagnosis

Depression, chronic fatigue syndrome, gastroenteritis, dyspepsia/ulcers, migraine or cluster headaches, panic/anxiety attacks, stress.

### Plan

***Psychosocial Intervention.*** Be active and supportive, and provide information about the emotional, physical, economic, and family effects of harassment. Identify the source of physical and emotional symptoms and explore the impact of harassment on marital and family life.[2] Validate the client's experience and help her resist devaluing herself. Discuss options and their ramifications. Encourage assertiveness training and stress management, and review existing coping skills. Help refine coping skills as needed.

***Follow-Up.*** Refer the client to a psychotherapist or other mental health practitioner for individual or group counseling. Referral for legal counsel may also be appropriate.

## VIOLENCE

Abuse is seen in many forms, from forceful physical abuse to less obviously damaging verbal abuse. Intent to hurt the victim ranges from slapping, beating, pushing, biting, and threats to attack with a weapon. Psychological aggression and abuse not only refer to verbal abuse, such as insults, constant negative feedback, screaming, and swearing, but may include depriving a woman of sleep and food. This violence often involves a combination of abusive acts.[4]

### Epidemiology

***Etiology.*** Violence and abuse are often the result of inefficient coping and stress-reducing skills. Frequently the abuser's behavior is learned; the abuser may have witnessed abuse or been abused.[5,6]

The battering cycle, or cycle of violence, is characterized by tension-building incidents.[5,7]

- Tension builds with acts of intimidation and initial, though lesser, physical abuse (shoving, pushing, name calling). As it does, the woman first tries to placate her partner. When this does not work, she withdraws to prevent a confrontation. During this time, the woman's repressed anger can contribute to her sense of guilt and low self-esteem. He may become more aggressive as she withdraws.

- Explosion occurs following mounting tension with physical and verbal attack and subsequent injury. The woman often feels she was at fault and the outburst is justified. The explosive phase usually lasts 24 hours or less which allows the abuser to release tension.
- During the honeymoon that follows the explosion, the abuser repents and promises never to abuse again.[5,7] The abused woman wants to believe that the abuse will stop and stays in the relationship.

In the repetitive cycle, abuse does not stop with one incident, but increases in frequency and severity. Learned helplessness, low self-esteem, feelings of guilt, lack of resources, and anticipatory fear eventually immobilize a woman to the point where she feels there is no way to escape.[7,8] The abused woman usually has a small social network with whom she can confide, but probably will not because of her shame and guilt. She is usually dependent on her abuser, both emotionally and financially, and makes excuses for the abuser's behavior.[5,9] Abused women are caught between maintaining the relationship, economic survival, and the well-being of her partner and children on the one side, and her own physical and emotional well-being on the other.[10]

***Risk Factors.*** History of abuse as a child, poor self-esteem, limited resources, and absence of support persons are risk factors.

***Incidence.*** Violence against women occurs in at least 1 of every 8 to 10 families; it is as common as hypertension and more common than breast cancer or gestational diabetes.[10] The Federal Bureau of Investigation (FBI) estimates that in the United States the following statistics reflect violence against women.

- A woman is beaten every 18 minutes.
- Of all women who use emergency rooms 21 percent are battered women, yet only 1 of 25 women is recognized as such by health care providers and offered appropriate treatment.
- Of all women who are murdered, 30 percent are murdered by their husbands, boyfriends, or ex-partners.
- Battering is a cause in one of two suicide attempts by African-American women and one of four suicide attempts by all women.[10]

## Subjective Data

Few women who seek medical care will state the cause of their injuries. Health care providers seeing nonacutely ill women in an office setting will not be confronted with any specific sign or symptom pathognomonic for battering.[4,10]

Vague symptoms may present during the tension building phase secondary to increased stress. Symptoms may include backaches, headaches, fatigue, anxiety, stress, insomnia, anorexia, indigestion, hypertension, allergic skin reactions, palpitations, hyperventilation, chest pain, choking sensation, claustrophobic feelings, and pelvic pain.[9,11,12]

In relating her history, a client may be hesitant, embarrassed, or evasive. She may be depressed, abuse alcohol and medications, and have a history of suicide attempts.[4,9,10] A complete social history should be obtained, including substance use and abuse, family situation, and support systems. The interview should focus on present injuries, and if the client admits to abuse, then the provider should question her about past abusive incidents.[12]

Indicators of possible battering include change in appointment pattern (increased or frequently missed appointments), complaints of problems at home or with partner (partner jealous, possessive), making excuses for partner's behavior, and ambivalent statements about battering or signs of fear when discussing it.[12,13] The client should be interviewed in a nonjudgmental manner and in private. If the abuser is with her, try to speak to her alone without raising the abuser's suspicion.

## Objective Data

A complete physical is carried out and carefully documented. Throughout the examination assure the client that the assault was not her fault. Explicitly document all findings and note if the client's explanation is not consistent with her injuries. Encourage the client to respond to questions; however, if she becomes upset, explain concern and describe the cycle of violence, emphasizing its repetitive and escalating nature.[12,13]

In the physical examination, a body map should be used to document current injuries, healing injuries, and scars.

- *General appearance.* The client may appear well groomed or chaotic with torn clothes. She may be nervous and emotional or calm and collected. There may be injuries that require immediate attention or no visible signs of injury.
- *Head, face, and throat.* These are the most typical locations of injury.[4,10]
- *Skin.* Lacerations, burns, and bruises of the skin, both old and new, may be noted. Be sure to examine all areas covered by clothing.[10,11] Clothes should be inspected for evidence of violence, although such evidence will probably not be seen in an office setting.
- *Chest.* Chest exam may reveal difficulty breathing because of pain from fractured ribs.
- *Vascular system.* Blood pressure and heart rate are increased.
- *Abdomen.* Abdominal pain may be evident with palpation. In pregnant women, the breast and abdomen are targets of assault.[10,11]
- *Genitalia.* See the section on Sexual Abuse.
- *Musculoskeletal system.* Fractures of the extremities, ribs, and skull may be found; pain with palpation, redness and swelling.

Photographs may be taken if signed consent is obtained. Color photographs of injuries with her face or hand for identification are recommended.[10,11] All signed and dated evidence should be placed in a sealed envelope marked confidential and filed in a secure place.[11]

## Differential Medical Diagnosis

Trauma not related to abuse, suicide attempt, self-mutilation.

## Plan

***Psychosocial Intervention.*** Ideally, intervention should begin during the tension-building phase or immediately after an abusive incident, because intervention is usually unsuccessful during the reconciliation phase.[8] The health care provider's role, however, is that of giving permission and information. In that role, the provider carries out many functions.

- Identifies the problem
- Supports the client in acknowledging a problem
- Affirms that abusive behavior is unacceptable
- Assists the woman to gain access to available community resources, such as housing, counseling, and legal services (The provider does not, however, initiate contact.)[8,10,12,13]
- Helps the client to identify options, as she may believe she has none
- Assists the client to develop an escape plan if she plans to stay in the abusive situation. (This includes placing clothes, money, and copies of necessary documents in an easily accessible, secret, and secure place.)

***Follow-Up.*** Counseling is essential and should be encouraged. Often, however, the client is not ready to seek assistance, and the decision must be respected.[8,12,13] Treatment of all injuries is pursued and x-rays ordered as needed.

## SEXUAL ABUSE OR RAPE

Sexual abuse or rape is forced sexual intercourse perpetrated against the will of a victim.[14] Force may be employed by physical violence, coercion, or threat of harm. Acquaintance rape usually occurs in a dating situation and is perpetrated by someone the woman knows and trusts.[15] Sexual assault involves actions other than rape: sodomy, forced anal intercourse; oral copulation, forced copulation of mouth of one person with sexual organ or anus of another; rape with a foreign object, forced penetration of genital or anal openings with a foreign object; and sexual battery, unwanted touching of an intimate part for the purpose of sexual arousal.

### Epidemiology

***Etiology.*** Rape challenges a woman's ability to maintain her defenses and arouses feelings of guilt, anxiety, and inadequacy.[16] The overwhelming experience heightens her sense of helplessness and intensifies her conflict about dependence and independence.[16] The survivor's response is determined by her stage in life, her defensive structures, and her coping ability.[16]

Rape trauma syndrome comprises the sequential reactions of the survivor in dealing with her experience. The syndrome is described as a two- or three-stage process.

The immediate response, or acute phase, occurs immediately after the assault or the disclosure of assault.[14,17] The survivor's lifestyle is completely disrupted and reactions are tearfulness and agitation or a relaxed calm.[14,16,17] This stage can last as long as 3 to 6 months, with typical symptoms being anxiety, fears and phobias, suspiciousness, major depressive symptoms, feelings of inferiority, inability to think clearly, and difficulty functioning at home, work, or school.[14,17] In addition, feelings of guilt, shame, embarrassment, and self-blame are common. Psychophysiological disturbances affect eating, sleeping, gastrointestinal function, and sexual intimacy.[4] Ensuring safety and regaining control over her life are the survivor's main emotional needs during this time.[14,17]

Medical attention is important as 66 percent of women will show trauma of a mild to moderate degree, and 4.5 percent will have serious physical injuries.[16]

The middle phase, or readjustment stage, is a period of transition when the survivor rationalizes that she could have prevented the assault and develops unrealistic plans to avoid another.[14,17]

The final stage, or reorganization phase, may last 2 years or longer and is difficult and painful.[14,17] During this stage, the survivor begins to deal with the reality of her victimization and may make changes in lifestyle, relationship, and work.[14,16,17]

***Risk Factors.*** Any woman is at risk; however, dating situations, unfamiliar partners, alcohol and drug use, and miscommunication create additional risk.

***Incidence.*** Rape is one of the most frequently committed and underreported violent crimes in the United States. Taking unreported rapes into consideration, one of every three women will be raped during her lifetime.[6] Sexual assault occurs every 1 to 10 minutes, and it is believed that only 1 in 10 of these women will seek professional help.[17]

### Subjective Data

A client may report various physical and psychological problems. Careful recording of the details of the assault, in addition to the client's gynecological, sexual, and social histories, is essential.

Symptoms may include headaches, sleep disturbance, loss of appetite with weight loss or gain, nausea, vomiting, constipation, diarrhea, sexual dysfunction, menstrual irregularities, abnormal vaginal discharge, and urinary dysfunction. The client may report difficulty in relationships with others and in functioning at home, work, or school.

The history of assault will include date, time, location, description, use of a weapon, and type of weapon; the part of the body penetrated, the object used to penetrate (body part or foreign object); occurrence of ejaculation; and involvement of alcohol or other drugs. Record any information about the assailant. Question the client about her activities after the assault: Did she shower, change clothes, urinate, or defecate?

The obstetric and gynecological history includes the date of the client's previous menstrual period, pregnancies, abortions, and miscarriages; contraceptive methods used; and history of sexually transmitted infections.

The sexual history includes information about the client's sexual activity: Was she sexually active within 1 week before or after assault? Has she been the victim of past sexual assaults (give dates)? Does she have any HIV high-risk sexual contact.

The social history includes information about whether the survivor lives alone, has a support system, wants someone notified, needs social service assistance, or wants police notified if they are not aware of assault.

## Objective Data

Data are recorded from a physical examination and a variety of forensic tests. Most jurisdictions do not accept evidence collected more than 72 hours following an assault.[17]

Physical examination and sexually transmitted disease (STD) testing are indicated after major injuries have been treated, no matter how much time has elapsed since the assault. If the woman has not showered or changed clothes since the assault, have her disrobe while standing on a sheet to collect any evidence. Then, give her a gown. Place any clothes that may contain evidence in a labeled paper bag.

### *Physical Examination*

- *General Appearance.* The survivor may be calm and relaxed or tearful and emotional. Her clothes may be torn and stained; injuries may be visible.
- *Head, Face, and Throat.* There may be lacerations, abrasions, and bruising. Dried secretions may be present on the face, mouth, or ears.
- *Chest.* There may be bruising, lacerations, and abrasions and tenderness on palpation. Increased respirations, difficulty breathing, or hyperventilation may be observed.
- *Abdomen.* Bruising, lacerations, abrasions, and tenderness may be evident, indicating potential internal injuries.
- *Musculoskeletal System.* Potential fractures are indicated by lacerations, abrasions, bruising, and tenderness of the back and extremities.
- *Genitalia and Reproductive Tract.* The perineum, rectal area, and vagina may have bruises, lacerations, and abrasions. Bartholin's and Skene's glands and the urethral meatus may be tender. Uterine size, shape, and consistency may be abnormal. Tenderness with cervical motion and uterine and adnexal palpation may be noted. Tears or pain may also be noted on rectovaginal examination.

A body map is used to document all injuries, including their size, location, and coloration. Photographs of abrasions may be helpful if the survivor plans legal action.

***Diagnostic Tests.*** Done within 24 to 72 hours of the assault. Forensic specimen collection should ideally be done by an experienced practitioner, but someone with less experience can do the tests using a forensic kit. Instructions for using the kit may change; therefore, its use is not discussed here. The health care provider must read the instructions for the forensic kit, step by step, prior to the exam. Use a Wood's lamp to detect semen stains, especially on the perineum and inner thighs.[18] If the mouth, ears, or other area was penetrated, swab it for specimens.

- Gonorrhea and chlamydia cultures are obtained from the endocervix, vaginal vault, rectum, and oropharynx, as indicated by history or evidence of penetration.
- Urine is collected for microscopic examination and pregnancy test.
- Wet mount specimens can show trichomonas, clue cells, and motile sperm for up to 72 hours. Include the pH of vaginal discharge and presence of positive whiff test.
- Vaginal smear is taken to detect sperm and p30 prostate specific antigen; considered more reliable than phosphatase determination.
- Bloodwork includes blood type/Rh, hepatitis antigen, rapid plasma reagin (RPR), and HIV antibody titer serum can be frozen.
- Fingernail scrapings should be collected from each hand and saved in separately labeled bag.
- Hair samples are collected by combing both head and pubic hair; specimens are placed in labeled bags.
- Blood and dried fluids found on the survivor's body and clothing are collected and labeled.

## Nursing Implications

In caring for a victim of sexual abuse or rape, it is important to understand that evaluation and treatment of the survivor require a multidisciplinary approach.

If a woman calls and reports rape, instruct her to avoid showering or changing her clothes. Encourage her to go to the emergency room nearest her or to the health care provider's office.

Prior to taking a complete history, explain that the information is needed for her medical management as well as for forensic use. Determination of rape is made in a court of law; therefore, the wording in the history should reflect only the client's report of the incident.[18] It is important to record, sign, and date all information. A consent form and release of information form must also be signed. Reassure the woman that questions, especially those covering her sexual history, are asked to ensure proper medical treatment. Throughout her visit, explain each procedure and why it is being done, and restore her sense of control. Give her options and seek consent with each procedure. Reinforce that rape was not her fault. Provide information about available social services, including a crisis hotline. Assist her to decide whether to report the crime, and encourage her to seek follow-up care.

## Differential Medical Diagnosis

Trauma not related to sexual assault.

## Plan

***Psychosocial Intervention.*** Refer the client for counseling. Women who do not deal realistically with rape and resolutions of issues may develop severe, long-term sequelae, such as depression, substance abuse, anxiety disorder, and suicide.[17] If legal action is desired, assist the woman in contacting the proper authorities.

***Medication.*** Medication may be needed for sexually transmitted diseases or possible pregnancy.

Treatment for STDs (antibiotic prophylaxis) should be offered because of the 5 percent risk that infection was transmitted.[16,17] Review the risks and benefits of both treatment and observation. If the client refuses prophylactic antibiotics, then follow-up cultures are done at the 6-week visit. If the client consents to prophylactic antibiotics, then treat her according to current Centers for Disease Control (CDC) guidelines for chlamydia, gonorrhea, syphilis, and trichomoniasis.

Postcoital contraceptive (PCC) medication may be offered to the client. A 5 percent risk of pregnancy exists if she was not using a contraceptive. Postcoital medication has a 1 percent failure rate.[17] Postcoital contraception is a safe, effective tool in avoiding unintended pregnancy.

The most common regimen is taking two Ovral tablets (ethinyl estradiol 50 μg and 0.5 mg norgestrel progestin) within 72 hours of coitus and two more 12 hours after the first dose. A pregnancy test is performed before any administration of medication. A history of thrombosis or perhaps of hypertension would be potential contraindications. Review with the client the side effects, including nausea and vomiting; and danger signs, including abdominal pain, chest pain, headache, blurred vision, and leg pain. Other alternatives that have been suggested are Lo-Ovral, Nordette, Triphasil yellow pills, or Tri-Levlen yellow pills given in appropriate doses (4 pills each time).

Hepatitis B vaccination may be indicated.

***Follow-Up.*** Telephone or personal contact with the client is recommended within 24 to 48 hours of initial treatment to allow for ongoing evaluation of problems and concerns.[17] An appointment is scheduled for 1 week after initial treatment to evaluate physical and emotional status. If the client has no complaints, a physical exam is not needed. Inquire about counseling. If the client is not involved in counseling encourage her to begin and provide a referral. The last required visit is scheduled at 6 weeks. At that time, a physical exam is done, specimens are taken for repeat cultures for STDs, rapid plasma reagin, and HIV antibody. A pregnancy test is done as needed.

## SUBSTANCE ABUSE

### ALCOHOL, COCAINE, SEDATIVES, AND CANNABIS

A maladaptive pattern of psychoactive substance use is indicated by at least one of the following: The client continues to use a psychoactive substance despite her awareness of persistent or recurrent social, occupational, psychological, or physical problems that are caused or exacerbated by its use; the client continues to use the substance in situations where use is physically hazardous; some symptoms of disturbance persist for at least 1 month or occur repeatedly over a longer period; the client does not fulfill criteria for psychoactive substance dependence.[19] Substance abuse is multidimensional with interacting factors that predispose the client to addictive use. Gender, age, race, physiology, and genetics all contribute to development of addictive disease.[20]

#### Epidemiology

***Etiology.*** Substance abuse and the risk factors for addiction are in many instances predictable.

Genetic research indicates that addiction in a family places a person at risk for addiction to drugs and compulsive behaviors.[20]

Female physiology may be influential. Research concerning the role that hormones play in the development of alcoholism is unclear.[20] Clinical research has been done on the role of hormones in the development of long-term effects on various organs of chronic alcohol consumption. There appears to be a relationship between the menstrual cycle and consumption and the effects of alcohol. Female physiology is believed to influence the metabolism of alcohol and the dose-related effects of other drugs, resulting in different patterns of morbidity and mortality. Given the lower body fluid ratios and lower body weight, the effects of drugs on the central nervous system are evident sooner.[20]

Psychological factors are influential. Psychopathology and psychological conflicts place women at risk for substance abuse. Traditional patterns of women's socialization include the belief that the needs of spouse, children, and others come before their own and that the expression of such feelings as anger and competition is unfeminine. Women may attempt to deal with their negative feelings through pharmacological suppression or drinking.[20]

***Risk Factors.*** Specific risk factors have been recognized.

- An addictive parent
- Divorce or separation
- Living alone with children
- Lesbian lifestyle
- Reliance on pharmacological agents or alcohol to relax, sleep, feel more comfortable in social settings, or control unpleasant feelings

***Incidence.*** The incidence of substance abuse is gender related.

- Women represent a growing percentage of drinkers.
- Among younger women in the general population, the proportion of drinkers is beginning to approximate that of men.[21]
- Women are more likely than men to become addicted to prescription drugs and use them with alcohol, as they outnumber men in their reported abuse of over-the-counter medications in combination with alcohol.[21]

## Subjective Data

Careful observation and listening may reveal symptoms of abuse of a specific substance. Histories are also essential.

Symptoms of abuse are often specific to a particular substance.

- Alcohol abusers often report gastritis, vomiting, and diarrhea. They may lose or gain weight. In addition, a client may report nervousness, anxiety, depression, sleep disturbances, pelvic pain, abnormal vaginal discharge, infertility, or sexual dysfunction.
- Cocaine abuse may lead to sinusitis and upper respiratory infection, allergic rhinitis, nasal congestion, and epistaxis. Weight loss may be experienced. Abstinence from cocaine may produce anxiety, fatigue, depression, irritability, and sleep disturbances.
- Abuse of sedatives (benzodiazepines) may cause headaches, nausea, paranoia, and sleep disturbances. Withdrawal may cause insomnia and irritability. When used with alcohol, sedatives increase central nervous system depressant effects.
- Cannabis (marijuana) abuse may provoke fatigue, decreased motivation, panic attacks, anxiety, and paranoia.[22,23]

Histories are the best indicators of early substance abuse. An alcohol history may use a screening questionnaire such as the CAGE questionnaire, which looks at patterns and consequences, or the Short Michigan Alcoholism Screening Test (SMAST), which deals with consequences. Diagnosis should not rest solely on the questionnaire; rather, the questionnaire is used to determine the index of suspicion for abuse.[24]

The health care provider should always approach the client in a nonjudgmental manner.

When questioning about abuse *always* begin with questions about less sensitive substances: How many cups of coffee do you drink per day? How much tobacco do you use per day? How many drinks per day? Then ask about tolerance (How many drinks does it take for you to feel high?) and the occurrence of blackouts. Inability to remember what happened when drinking is a probable sign of alcoholism.[19,25]

- *The drug history* includes information about prescription medication, over-the-counter medication, and illicit drugs (substance abuse may progress from alcohol, to cannabis, to cocaine, and so on). Inquire if one drug is taken in conjunction with another or with alcohol.
- *The social history* includes information about marital or family problems, job or promotion loss due to poor performance or absenteeism, and multiple arrests for disorderly conduct or driving under influence of a drug. Inquire about behavior changes, such as termination of old friendships and loss of interest in favorite pastimes. Whether financial difficulties have occurred should also be queried.[22,23,25]
- *Past medical history* includes questions about accidental injuries and illnesses related to abuse. For example, individuals who abuse cocaine have frequent urinary tract infections, sinusitis, nosebleeds, and burns if the drug is smoked; alcohol abuse may cause gastroenteritis, ulcers, hepatitis, and pneumonia; and cannabis frequently causes urinary tract infections.[22,23,25]
- *The sexual history* includes questions about pregnancies, abortions, sexually transmitted infections, pelvic inflammatory disease, abnormal Pap smears, menstrual irregularities, sexual dysfunction, and HIV risk factors. Substance use and abuse decrease inhibitions. Consequently, a woman is more likely to engage in sexual intercourse, which may increase the risk of sexual abuse. Substance abuse may lead to frequent partners if sex is exchanged for substance; intravenous drug use increases the risk of hepatitis B and HIV infection.[22,23,25]
- *Family medical history* includes information about mental illness, dysfunctional family, and substance abuse.[22,23,25]

## Objective Data

Although histories and observation are important investigative tools, diagnosis is rarely made without laboratory tests and physical examination.

***Alcohol.*** Alcoholism may be diagnosed with the use of physical examination and a variety of diagnostic tests: blood, liver, electrolyte, thyroid, glucose, and stool.

*Physical Examination*[22,23,25]

- *Skin.* Cigarette burns, seborrheic dermatitis, palmar erythema, and spider veins (particularly on the chest) may be evident.
- *Head and Eyes:* Poor dentition is likely, with possible lesions on the posterior lateral tongue (increase risk for oropharyngeal cancer with alcohol and tobacco abuse) and alcohol odor to the breath. The face may be red and puffy; the nose enlarged with prominent veins; the eyes puffy with erythematous conjunctiva; the voice hoarse with or without cough; and the parotid gland enlarged.
- *Chest.* Auscultation of rates "E" to "A" changes indicate possible pneumonia. Point tenderness may be caused by ribs fractured during falls.
- *Vascular System.* Examination may reveal cardiac arrhythmias, tachycardia, and hypertension.
- *Abdomen.* The liver is palpable and tender in hepatitis. The spleen may be enlarged. Ascites may be present. Abdominal pain suggests gastritis, ulcers, duodenitis,

esophagitis, ileitis, irritable bowel syndrome, or pancreatitis.

- *Musculoskeletal System.* Bruises or fractures indicate trauma. An abnormal gait and decreased muscle strength are related to myopathy. Gout causes red, tender, and edematous joints.
- *Genitalia and Reproductive Tract.* Menstrual irregularities, unplanned pregnancy, abnormal vaginal discharge, and pelvic pain with adnexal and cervical motion tenderness are possible findings.
- *Nervous System.* Examination may reveal abnormal cranial nerve findings, peripheral neuropathy, cerebral degeneration, optic neuropathy, and presence of tremors or seizures.

*Diagnostic Tests*

- *Blood Tests.* Hemoglobin and hematocrit decreased (anemia); mean corpuscular volume decreased (common finding in alcohol abuse); prothrombin time prolonged; platelets decreased (clotting disorder).
- *Liver Function Tests.* Serum $\gamma$-glutamyltransferase (SGGT) (most sensitive), alanine aminotransferase (ALT), aspartate aminotransferase (AST), lactate dehydrogenase (LDH), amylase, alkaline phosphatase, total bilirubin, cholesterol, and triglycerides all increased (indicative of alcoholic liver disease).
- *Electrolytes.* Serum magnesium, calcium, phosphorus, and potassium usually decreased.
- *Thyroid Function.* Abnormal (especially in stimulant users).
- *Glucose.* May be increased or decreased.
- *Stool.* Occult blood present.

***Sedatives.*** Sedatives (benzodiazepines) produce no significant findings except in an overdose. Clients who overdose are seen in the emergency room.

***Cannabis.*** Cannabis abuse may be detected by means of physical examination, with close attention to the eyes, and an electrocardiogram.

*Physical Examination*

- *General Appearance.* Dreamlike state.
- *Skin.* Burns on fingers or around mouth if cannabis is smoked.
- *Eyes.* Conjunctival injection often the only objective sign.
- *Vascular System.* Tachycardia and hypertension (especially if multiple drugs are used).

A diagnostic electrocardiogram may show nonspecific ST-T wave changes related to rate.

***Cocaine.*** Cocaine abuse may be detected by examining the nose, chest, and cardiovascular system and by carrying out various diagnostic tests.

*Physical Examination*

- *Nose.* Nasal bleeding, erythematous nostrils, nasal septal atrophy with perforation.
- *Chest.* Increased respiratory rate, abnormal breath sounds.
- *Vascular System.* Increased heart rate, palpitations, cardiac arrhythmias, hypertension (possibly), elevated body temperature.

*Diagnostic Tests*

- Hepatitis panel
- Rapid plasma reagin (RPR)
- HIV infection
- Urine toxicology (for cocaine, cannabis, sedatives)

## Nursing Implications

The primary health care provider's role is to help the client recognize and accept the negative relationship between her substance abuse and the consequences of abuse.[25] If substance use causes problems (physical, mental, legal, or financial), then use is abuse. The client needs to be told that a problem exists and given evidence to support this conclusion. Subsequently, the client should be directed to the proper resources.

If, on the other hand, substance use is detected, the woman should be educated about the potential problem of abuse in an effort to prevent it.

### Differential Medical Diagnosis

Depression, anxiety, hyperthyroidism, viral or bacterial gastroenteritis, upper respiratory infection, chronic sinusitis.

### Plan

***Psychosocial Interventions.*** Involve others close to the client in the treatment plan and inform them about the disease process. Use a positive approach and emphasize that the disease is treatable. Dealing with denial is critical. The first priority is to stop substance use, not to determine the cause of abuse. Total abstinence is the ideal; however, ability to abstain does not mean elimination of the problem. The inability of a woman to use a substance in moderation indicates that a problem may exist. Contracts with self may be useful if the client is motivated to change her behavior. A contract should have realistic goals within a definite time frame. One way to help a woman realize that she has a problem is to have her contract to use a limited amount of substance (within reason) for a set time (3 months) in her usual pattern. If she finds she is using more than she contracted to use, then a potential problem exists.

***Medication.*** Disulfiram is recommended for alcohol abuse; the use of sedatives is not desirable. Disulfiram 500 mg, administered orally daily (after abstention for 12 hours) and reduced to 250 mg after 1 week, may be a deterrent. Disulfiram blocks metabolism of alcohol with acetaldehyde buildup, resulting in headaches, flushing, and nausea. Extreme side effects include hypertension, shock, and coma. The client must be taught about the medication and its potential danger. Side effects, without concomitant alcohol use, include impotence, liver damage, drowsiness, and fetal anomalies if taken by pregnant women. Contraindications are pregnancy, cardiac disease, and psychoses.[26]

***Follow-Up.*** Refer the client for psychiatric consultation or other mental health services. In addition to mental health resources, a client often needs help accessing financial aid, job training, and insurance benefits.[21] Women in all socioeconomic groups may face legal problems in relation to child custody, drug theft, and driving infractions; therefore, they may need information about the legal system.[21] Encourage the client to become involved in Alcoholics Anonymous or a similar group. Significant others should become involved in a support group that deals with enabling behaviors. Biofeedback and relaxation training may also be helpful.

At first, the client should be followed closely. A minimum of one weekly visit is recommended, with additional phone contact if necessary.

## MENTAL HEALTH PROBLEMS

### DEPRESSION

The DSM-III-R (*Diagnostic and Statistical Manual of Mental Disorders,* 3rd ed., revised) classification of depression is descriptive, based on clinical features of the depressive disorder.[19] (Publication of DSM-IV is planned for late 1994.) Depression, classified as an affective disorder, includes major depression, other specific affective disorders, and atypical affective disorders. In this chapter, three types of depression are defined: major depression, dysthymia, and depression reactive to psychosocial factors.

Major depression occurs as a single episode or recurrent condition independent of life events. The client loses interest or pleasure in all or almost all her usual activities and experiences four of the following conditions: significant weight loss or gain or changes in appetite; sleep disturbances; psychomotor agitation or retardation; fatigue or loss of energy; feelings of worthlessness or inappropriate guilt; diminished ability to concentrate; recurrent thoughts of death.[19]

Dysthymia is a chronic, less acute affective disorder. The client must experience depressed mood for more than 2 years without being symptom free for more than 2 months and two of the following conditions: poor appetite or overeating; sleep disturbance; low self-esteem; fatigue; poor concentration or difficulty making decisions; feelings of hopelessness.[19] Dysthymia is frequently a consequence of a preexisting, chronic nonmood disorder, such as anorexia nervosa, psychoactive substance dependence, or anxiety disorder.[19]

Depression reactive to psychosocial factors occurs following some life event. The event is usually associated with loss and accompanied by anger and guilt.[26] This depression is often self-limiting, and no therapy is necessary.[26]

## Epidemiology

***Etiology.*** Depression can be a normal reaction to everyday life. If it is appropriate to the life event and not severe, treatment may not be necessary. Current theories focus on different factors, but the cause of depression is believed to be multifactorial.

Psychological models include psychosocial stresses and developmental problems (personality defects, childhood events).[26] Sense of loss, failure to live up to one's ego ideal, and a sense of hopelessness and helplessness are all important concepts in the etiology of depression.[27] Often, loss or perceived loss precedes the onset of depression. Loss may involve a person, expectation, or job. Common ideals are to be loved, to be good and kind, to be recognized for achievements, and to attain goals.[27] With disappointments and failures comes the feeling of not living up to one's ego ideals. Guilt felt because of failure can lead to anger and self-hatred with feelings of hopelessness and helplessness. These feelings are related to one's negative self-concept, negative interpretation of one's experiences, and negative view of the future.[27]

Biological models include genetic and biochemical factors. Depression appears to have some familial pattern or predisposition; however, the exact familial role is not known.[27] The biochemical model postulates a decrease in available biogenic amines at the postsynaptic membrane.[27] Many studies have used this model with inconsistent results.

***Risk Factors.*** Risk factors include a family history of depression, poor self-concept or self-esteem, female gender, chronic nonmood disorders, substance abuse, loss or death, and stressful life event. Suicidal risk factors include previous attempted suicide, depression, dysfunctional family, battering, alcoholism, and chronic illness.

***Incidence.*** Reports reveal that 20 percent of women and 10 percent of men will have a major depressive episode in their lifetime; 4.5 to 9.3 percent of females and 2.3 and 3.2 percent of males suffer from depression in the United States and Europe.[26]

### Subjective Data

Women frequently report somatic symptoms rather than depression, and several conditions are typically revealed in history taking, including chronic illness and substance abuse.

Symptoms that the depressed woman frequently reports include headaches, constipation, sleep disturbance, loss of energy, change in appetite with weight loss or increase, decreased libido, and chronic pain. These symptoms are somatic complaints, and a woman will more often present with them than complaints of depression. Unidentifiable somatic complaints frequently indicate depression and fatigue, but often women with these symptoms are labeled hypochondriacal.[26,27] When asked about her feelings, a woman may admit to sadness; decreased mood; feelings of guilt, worthlessness, or hopelessness; loss of interest in daily events; or withdrawal from work and recreation. She may complain of difficulty concentrating and thinking or an inability to make decisions.

History incorporates five areas: medical, family medical, gynecological obstetric, social, and psychological.

- *Medical history* is taken with the realization that any illness may cause depression, but chronic illness is the most likely cause. Questions regarding hospitalizations and injuries may provide important clues, especially if injuries are related to events such as violence or numerous accidents. Substance use should be included in the history, as it is often related to depression. In addition, include prescription and over-the-counter medications that are being taken, because some are associated with symptoms of depression. Stimulants can cause depression during withdrawal; certain antihypertensive agents, oral contraceptives, and corticosteroids may also cause depression.
- *Family medical history* includes questions about the family's history of depression, mental illness, suicide, and substance abuse.
- *Gynecological obstetric history* includes the date of the previous menstrual period and cycle length to determine the possibility of premenstrual syndrome (PMS); PMS is associated with depression.
- *Social history* includes marital status, home or work problems, job changes, economic status, and support systems.
- *Psychological history* includes information about previous psychiatric illness, suicide attempts, and cognitive abilities (memory and thought process). Always ask about suicidal ideation, what means would be used, if a plan has been established, and when the plan is to be carried out.[28]

### Objective Data

A physical examination is done, as are several diagnostic tests, including those ruling out substance abuse.

***Physical Examination.*** Begins with evaluation of the client's general appearance. She may be over- or underweight, be unkempt, have poor affect, or move sluggishly.

- *Skin, nails, and hair.* Hair may be dirty and uncombed, and nails brittle and dry. Scars may be visible on the wrist or other parts of body.
- *Eyes.* The eyes may appear dull with fixed gaze, poor eye contact, circles under eyes from lack of sleep, and pale conjunctiva and mucosa.
- *Mouth.* Oral hygiene may be poor.
- *Neck.* Thyroid may be palpable or with nodules.
- *Nervous system.* See Substance Abuse and Violence sections. Mental status may require qualitative scales to determine degree of depression.

Diagnostic tests are varied. Hematocrit and hemoglobin tests rule out anemia. The thyroid panel rules out thyroid disease. See Substance Abuse section for specific tests.

### Nursing Implications

The health care provider must give full attention to the client in the privacy of an office. If the client does not feel comfortable, she will probably not be honest about her problem. A nurse practitioner may provide care for a mildly depressed woman usually in collaboration with a physician, but referral should be made to a psychiatric specialist for a seriously depressed woman. It is critical to know when to refer. *Always refer a client if suicidal ideation is expressed.*

### Differential Medical Diagnosis

Chronic illness, hypothyroidism, depressive side effects from medication, premenstrual syndrome, substance abuse.

### Plan

***Psychosocial Intervention.*** The type of intervention depends on the type of depression. Individuals with major depression may benefit from antidepressant medication, education, supportive counseling, psychotherapy, and family therapy.[29] Individuals with dysthymia are often given antidepressant medication for symptom relief, but are not as responsive as clients with major depression.[29] The client with dysthymia should also receive psychotherapy or supportive counseling.[29] The client with reactive depression usually requires no antidepressant medication, but responds well to education, supportive counseling, and family therapy. When precipitated by an illness, depression often resolves as the illness improves.

- Client education should include information about depression and the relationship of its symptoms to medical illness, stressors, and situational crisis. It should be stressed that depression is a medical illness, not a character defect or weakness. Treatments are effective, and there are many treatment options. An effective treatment can be found for nearly every client. Recovery is the rule, not the exception. The goal is complete symptom remission. Recurrence is a risk; therefore, the client should be encouraged to return with any recurrent signs and symptoms.[28] Teaching stress reduction, coping styles, and assertiveness may be beneficial. Help the client identify and express her feelings of anger, hostility, sadness, and anxiety.
- Supportive counseling focuses on encouraging the client to develop a social network and increase her activity. Participation in support groups may be beneficial for the client and her family. When appropriate, always involve persons who are important in the client's life.
- Family counseling may be beneficial because episodes of depression have been associated with family dysfunction.[29]
- Psychotherapy's goal is to correct specific aspects of depression, including thoughts, behavior, and affect.[28,29] Its purpose is not to change the client's personality.

***Treatment of Depression.*** Consists of three phases.[28]

- Acute treatment (6 to 12 weeks) aims at remission of symptoms. If medication is used, it should be individualized to the client to optimize treatment benefits and lower risk. Considerations in choosing a medication include short- and long-term side effects, past experience with medications, possible drug interactions, presence of other conditions, and age. Acute treatment should be monitored every 1 to 2 weeks. Evaluation at 6 weeks determines if the client is responding. If the desired response occurs, continue treatment for another 6 weeks. If the client experiences some improvement, but not the desired response, consider adjusting the dosage. If there is no response, the treatment may need to be changed. Continue to monitor every 1 to 2 weeks. Consult if the desired response does not occur.

- Continuation treatment (4 to 9 months) aims at preventing relapse. Medication should be continued at full dosage.
- Maintenance treatment aims at preventing recurrences in clients with prior episodes.

The objective throughout each treatment phase is attainment of a sustained asymptomatic state. The essential features of the plan should include education; regular monitoring of side effects and depressive symptoms; and adjustment or changes in the plan if response is not timely or complete.[28]

***Medication.*** Medication includes antidepressant drugs, which work to elevate mood. Three major types are tricyclic antidepressants, monoamine oxidase inhibitors, and heterocyclic antidepressants. Most antidepressants may take several weeks before clinical improvement. Consequently, tell the client not to expect sudden improvement. Stress compliance. Instruct the client to avoid alcohol and other mood-altering substances. Tables 18–1 and 18–2 provide overviews of the side effect profiles and pharmacology of antidepressant medications.[28]

Caution clients to notify the provider if they have thoughts of suicide. Consultation with a physician is indicated.

***Follow-Up.*** Initially, follow-up should be weekly, with telephone backup. The health care provider may counsel the reactive depressed client without referral for therapy. The client with major depression or dysthymia, however, should be referred for family counseling and psychotherapy. If a client exhibits a personality disorder or suicidal tendencies or the cause of depression is unidentifiable, a referral should also be made.[28,29] After medication is determined, collaboration with a physician and follow-up may be indicated.

The suicidal client should always be referred. If a client telephones and states she is suicidal, find out her location, keep her on the line, and telephone emergency medical services if another line is available. If she has not yet attempted suicide, try to persuade her to postpone suicide for a set period; if she has attempted suicide, try to find out what method was used.

## ANXIETY

Anxiety may be defined as a normal emotional experience (part of normal stress reduction), a pathological cognitive/physiological symptom, or an abstract theoretical construct.[19] DSM-III-R classifies anxiety disorders as panic disorder, agoraphobia, social phobia, simple phobia, obsessive–compulsive disorder, post-traumatic stress disorder, and generalized anxiety disorder. The disorders may overlap. With striking regularity, concomitant medical illness occurs in psychiatric patients.[30] Indeed, medical illness may cause psychiatric symptoms or exacerbate underlying psychiatric symptomatology.[31]

### Types of Anxiety

Four types of anxiety are described below.

- Panic disorders are short-lived, recurrent, unpredictable episodes of intense anxiety accompanied by physiological symptomatology.[26,31] Episodes of apprehension, fear, and a sense of doom may be precipitated by a stimulus or may arise spontaneously.[32]
- Generalized anxiety is the most common anxiety disorder.[19] Unrealistic or excessive anxiety and worry about two or more life circumstances occurs for 2 months or longer.[19]
- Phobic disorders use the mechanism of displacement. Clients transfer their feelings of

anxiety from the true object to one that can be avoided.[26]

- Obsessive–compulsive disorder involves an irrational idea or impulse that persistently intrudes into awareness.[26] The client recognizes its absurdity, but anxiety is relieved only with ritualistic perfor-mance, impulse, or entertainment of an idea.[26]

## Epidemiology

***Risk Factors.*** Physical and mental illness, life situations or crises, and family history of anxiety disorders are risk factors for anxiety.

***Incidence.*** Incidence varies among the four types of anxiety.

- *Panic disorder.* 2:1 prevalence among women; onset younger than 25; affects 3 to 5 percent of population.[26,29]
- *Generalized anxiety.* Questionable slight predominance among women; onset 20 to 35 years of age.[19,26,32]
- *Phobic disorder.* Depends on type of pho-

**TABLE 18–1. SIDE EFFECT PROFILES OF ANTIDEPRESSANT MEDICATIONS**

| | Side Effect[a] | | | | | | |
|---|---|---|---|---|---|---|---|
| | | Central Nervous System | | Cardiovascular | | | Other |
| Drug | *Anticholinergic*[b] | *Drowsiness* | *Insomnia/ Agitation* | *Orthostatic Hypotension* | *Cardiac Arrhythmia* | *Gastrointestinal Distress* | *Weight Gain (>6 kg)* |
| Amitriptyline | 4+ | 4+ | 0 | 4+ | 3+ | 0 | 4+ |
| Desipramine | 1+ | 1+ | 1+ | 2+ | 2+ | 0 | 1+ |
| Doxepin | 3+ | 4+ | 0 | 2+ | 2+ | 0 | 3+ |
| Imipramine | 3+ | 3+ | 1+ | 4+ | 3+ | 1+ | 3+ |
| Nortriptyline | 1+ | 1+ | 0 | 2+ | 2+ | 0 | 1+ |
| Protriptyline | 2+ | 1+ | 1+ | 2+ | 2+ | 0 | 0 |
| Trimipramine | 1+ | 4+ | 0 | 2+ | 2+ | 0 | 3+ |
| Amoxapine | 2+ | 2+ | 2+ | 2+ | 3+ | 0 | 1+ |
| Maprotiline | 2+ | 4+ | 0 | 0 | 1+ | 0 | 2+ |
| Trazodone | 0 | 4+ | 0 | 1+ | 1+ | 1+ | 1+ |
| Bupropion | 0 | 0 | 2+ | 0 | 1+ | 1+ | 0 |
| Fluoxetine | 0 | 0 | 2+ | 0 | 0 | 3+ | 0 |
| Paroxetine | 0 | 0 | 2+ | 0 | 0 | 3+ | 0 |
| Sertraline | 0 | 0 | 2+ | 0 | 0 | 3+ | 0 |
| Monoamine oxidase inhibitors (MAOIs) | 1 | 1+ | 2+ | 2+ | 0 | 1+ | 2+ |

[a]0 = absent or rare, 1+, 2+ = inbetween, 3+, 4+ = relatively common.
[b]Dry mouth, blurred vision, urinary hesitancy, constipation.
*From U.S. Department of Health and Human Services, Public Health Service, Agency for Health Care Policy and Research. (1993).* Clinical practice guideline No. 5: Depression in primary care: Detection, diagnosis, and treatment *(Publication No. 93-09553). Rockville, MD: AMPCR.*

bia (animal phobias and agoraphobia are more common among women).[19]

- *Obsessive–compulsive disorder.* Occurs equally in women and men; 2 to 3 percent incidence in the United States; highest rates among young, divorced, separated, and unemployed.[19,26]

## Subjective Data

The client may report dyspnea, shortness of breath or smothering sensation, palpitations, tachycardia, chest pain, flushing, sweating or cold clammy hands, abdominal discomfort, diarrhea, nausea, dry mouth, difficult swallowing, urinary frequency, headache, muscle tension, aches, soreness, trembling, twitching, or shakiness.

Psychological complaints may include restlessness, fatigue, sleep disturbances, irritability or edginess, exaggerated startle response, and difficulty concentrating.

Anxiety produces symptoms that involve multiple organ systems and causes confusion and frequent medical consultation and testing. Moreover, certain medical conditions and medications produce symptoms of anxiety disorders.[31] In taking a history, explore the client's chief complaint, including precipitating factors, duration of symptoms, and use and effectiveness of self-treatment.

- *Past medical history* includes chronic disease, illness, hospitalizations, and surgeries.
- *Medication* use includes present and past prescription medications and over-the-counter medicines.
- *Habits* include caffeine intake and use of tobacco, alcohol, and illicit substances.
- *Family medical history* includes chronic diseases, substance abuse, and mental illness.
- *Gynecological/obstetric history* includes date of last (previous) menstrual period, cycle, and premenstrual symptoms.
- *Social history* includes support systems, lifestyle, abusive home life, and job.

## Objective Data

An extensive physical examination is done and a variety of diagnostic tests are performed.

### *Physical Examination*

- *General appearance.* The client may appear restless, trembling, or emotional.
- *Eyes.* Circles under the eyes indicate a lack of sleep. Nystagmus may be elicited with different maneuvers.
- *Ears.* Rule out otitis externa or media.
- *Mouth.* Rule out large tonsils, lesions, and polyps in throat causing difficult swallowing.
- *Neck.* Enlarged, tender, or nodular thyroid indicates thyroid disorder.
- *Skin.* Skin may be cold, clammy, sweaty, flushed, or pale.
- *Chest.* Respiratory rate may be increased. The client may hyperventilate. Wheezing may indicate asthma.
- *Vascular system.* Blood pressure and heart rate may be increased. A murmur, gallop, or click may indicate mitral valve prolapse or arrhythmias. Rule out heart disease with chest pain.
- *Abdomen.* The client may experience pain with palpation. Bowel sounds may be absent or hyperactive.
- *Musculoskeletal system.* Gait may be unsteady. Joints may be red and edematous and a source of pain. Muscle strength may be abnormal. Signs of trauma may be evident.
- *Nervous system.* Examination may reveal hyperreflexia, positional vertigo, and abnormal cranial nerve findings.

**TABLE 18–2. PHARMACOLOGY OF ANTIDEPRESSANT MEDICATIONS**

| Drug | Therapeutic Dosage Range (mg/d) | Average (Range) Elimination Half-Life[a] | Potentially Fatal Drug Interactions |
|---|---|---|---|
| *Tricyclic Antidepressants* | | | |
| Amitriptyline (Elavil, Endep) | 75–300 | 24 (16–46) | Antiarrhythmics, MAOIs |
| Clomipramine (Anafranil) | 75–300 | 24 (20–40) | Antiarrhythmics, MAOIs |
| Desipramine (Norpramin, Pertofrane) | 75–300 | 18 (12–50) | Antiarrhythmics, MAOIs |
| Doxepin (Adapin, Sinequan) | 75–300 | 17 (10–47) | Antiarrhythmics, MAOIs |
| Imipramine (Janimine, Tofranil) | 75–300 | 22 (12–34) | Antiarrhythmics, MAOIs |
| Nortriptyline (Aventyl, Pamelor) | 40–200 | 26 (18–88) | Antiarrhythmics, MAOIs |
| Protriptyline (Vivactil) | 20–60 | 76 (54–124) | Antiarrhythmics, MAOIs |
| Trimipramine (Surmontil) | 75–300 | 12 (8–30) | Antiarrhythmics, MAOIs |
| *Heterocyclic Antidepressants* | | | |
| Amoxapine (Asendin) | 100–600 | 10 (8–14) | MAOIs |
| Bupropion (Wellbutrin) | 225–450 | 14 (8–24) | MAOIs (possibly) |
| Maprotiline (Ludiomil) | 100–225 | 43 (27–58) | MAOIs |
| Trazodone (Desyrel) | 150–600 | 8 (4–14) | — |
| *Selective Serotonin Re-uptake Inhibitors (SSRIs)* | | | |
| Fluoxetine (Prozac) | 10–40 | 168 (72–360)[b] | MAOIs |
| Paroxetine (Paxil) | 20–50 | 24 (3–65) | MAOIs[c] |
| Sertraline (Zoloft) | 50–150 | 24 (10–30) | MAOIs[c] |
| *Monoamine Oxidase Inhibitors (MAOIs)*[d] | | | |
| Isocarboxazid (Marplan) | 30–50 | Unknown | For all three MAOIs: Vasoconstrictors,[e] decongestants,[e] meperidine, and possibly other narcotics |
| Phenelzine (Nardil) | 45–90 | 2 (1.5–4.0) | |
| Tranylcypromine (Parnate) | 20–60 | 2 (1.5–3.0) | |

[a]Half-life is affected by age, sex, race, concurrent medications, and length of drug exposure.
[b]Includes both fluoxetine and norfluoxetine.
[c]By extrapolation from fluoxetine data.
[d]MAO inhibition lasts longer (7 days) than drug half-life.
[e]Including pseudoephedrine, phenylephrine, phenylpropanolamine, epinephrine, norepinephrine, and other drugs.
*From U.S. Department of Health and Human Services, Public Health Service, Agency for Health Care Policy and Research. (1993).* Clinical practice guideline No. 5: Depression in primary care: Detection, diagnosis, and treatment *(Publication No. 93-09553). Rockville, MD: AMPCR.*

***Diagnostic Tests***

- Electrocardiogram
- Electroencephalogram
- Urinalysis to rule out urinary tract infection and diabetes
- Thyroid panel as indicated
- Complete blood count to rule out anemia and infection
- Electrolytes as indicated
- Glucose tolerance test to rule out diabetes and hypoglycemia
- Upper and lower GI series if indicated

### Nursing Implications

Showing genuine concern and empathy decreases the chance that the client will perceive the health care provider as unsympathetic to her problem. Use open-ended questions when interviewing to allow the client to disclose information she may not otherwise have revealed. Permit the client to ventilate her concerns and, at the same time, to prioritize them. Reassuring her may also be helpful.[32]

### Differential Medical Diagnosis

Hyperthyroidism, hypoglycemia, cancer, organic brain syndrome, depression, substance abuse, hypertension, side effects of prescription or over-the-counter medication, physical or sexual abuse.

### Plan

***Psychosocial Intervention.*** During an acute anxiety episode, stay with the client, decrease environmental stimuli, and, above all, remain calm. Counseling that focuses on the present, using reflection and clarification, is most effective.[32] Deal with issues of fears, self-concept, self-esteem, problem solving, and coping mechanisms. Acknowledge and express acceptance of anxiety. Relaxation techniques and imagery may help decrease anxiety. Assist the client to identify sources of anxiety, to develop plans to deal with them, and to modify her lifestyle.

***Medication.*** Benzodiazepines (Dalmane, Librium, Valium) are the drugs of choice. They should be considered only for clients with disabling or severe symptoms and for clients who are unlikely to abuse them.[32] Duration of therapy should be short and dosage tailored to the individual. Progress must be monitored.[32] Addiction and withdrawal are possible.

β-Adrenergic blockers (propranolol) can be used to reduce peripheral somatic symptoms.[26,32] Antidepressants may also be used (see Depression).

- Common side effects of benzodiazepines are dizziness, drowsiness, fatigue, confusion, disorientation, and, above all, psychological addiction.
- Contraindications are pregnancy, known hypersensitivity to benzodiazepines, and use with alcohol and other central nervous system depressants.
- Weekly follow-up visits are encouraged. Discontinue medication as soon as possible.
- Provide information about side effects and contraindications and when to contact provider. Emphasize the need to use an effective contraceptive and avoid alcohol and other central nervous system depressants. Caution clients not to drive or use potentially dangerous equipment because of the sedative effects of anxiolytic agents.

***Follow-Up.*** Follow-up is weekly; however, during an acute episode, daily clinic visits may be necessary. Referral depends on the health care provider's expertise, the severity of the client's symptoms and functional impairment, her response to intervention, and her receptiveness and motivation.[32] Consultation with a physician, referral, or both are indicated when medication is used or if signs of underlying physical or emotional problems are present. Immediately refer a client with any suicidal ideation.

## STRESS

Stress is a unique and individual expression in response to any number of events. It occurs when the adaptive or coping mechanism is overwhelmed by events. An event is not always negative; but may be positive, such as marriage or a promotion. Stress is the result of an intertwine of forces: stressors, perceptions of those stressors, emotional and physiological responses to those perceptions, and efforts to cope.[33] The degree to which a certain stressor causes stress is determined by the perception of that stressor.[33] Stressors may include interpersonal problems, time demands, and internal conflicts.[33]

Risk factors are poor support systems, ineffective coping skills and psychopathological conditions. No precise data are available about the incidence of stress; however, all individuals experience it to some degree.

### Subjective Data

A woman may react to stress by becoming anxious or depressed, developing physical symptoms, or using substances. See Anxiety, Depression, and Substance Abuse sections.

### Objective Data

See Anxiety, Depression, and Substance Abuse sections.

### Differential Medical Diagnosis

Coronary heart disease, chronic pain, headaches, hypertension, asthma, rheumatoid arthritis, irritable bowel syndrome, ulcers, eczema, anxiety, depression, muscular tension, insomnia, fatigue.

### Plan

***Psychosocial Intervention.*** Discuss with the client ways to avoid a stressful situation. If a stressful situation cannot be avoided, discuss ways to minimize stress by altering the stressor.[33] If a stressor cannot be avoided or altered, the client needs to develop coping skills to deal with it. Coping can be accomplished through a healthy lifestyle (sleep, balanced nutrition, exercise, relaxation).[33] Help the client to identify self-induced stress, which may be caused by unrealistic expectations, and to correct the stress-producing thoughts.[33] Encourage the client to try to develop a relaxation program; it might include progressive muscle relaxation, meditation, and breathing exercises. Time management and assertiveness training may also be helpful.

***Follow-Up.*** Refer the client when problem areas could be more appropriately addressed by a specialist.[33]

## POST-TRAUMATIC STRESS DISORDER

Symptoms of post-traumatic stress disorder (PTSD) develop following a psychologically distressing event that is outside the range of usual human experience.[19] The affected client reexperiences the traumatic event, avoids stimuli associated with the event, and exhibits a numbed general responsiveness and increased arousal.[19] The trauma that is experienced may be a serious threat to life or physical integrity, a serious threat or harm to someone close to the client, sudden destruction of one's home or community, or seeing someone recently injured or killed.[19]

### Subjective Data

According to DSM-III-R diagnostic criteria, the traumatic event is persistently reexperienced in at least one of several ways: recurrent and intrusive recollection of event; recurrent distressing dreams of the event; sudden acting or feeling as though traumatic event were recurring; and psychological distress at exposure to events.

Persistent avoidance of stimuli associated with the trauma and numbed responsiveness are indicated by at least three of following: efforts to avoid thoughts or feelings associated with trauma, efforts to avoid activities or situations that arouse recollections, inability to recall an important aspect of the trauma, diminished interest in significant activities, feelings of detachment from others, restricted range of affect, sense of shortened future.[19]

Persistent symptoms of increased arousal are indicated by at least two of following: sleep disturbances, irritability or anger outburst, physiological reactivity on exposure to events that symbolize or resemble an aspect of the traumatic event.[19]

### Objective Data and Differential Medical Diagnosis

See Anxiety, Depression, and Substance Abuse sections.

### Plan

***Psychosocial Intervention.*** Focus on counseling that emphasizes the here and now and strengthens existing defenses.[26] Helping clients to clarify the problem allows them to begin viewing it within its proper context and facilitates decision making.[26] Instructing clients about stress reduction techniques and encouraging them to develop relaxation and exercise programs may help them to reduce stress by providing other outlets for their feelings.

***Medication.*** Medication may include limited use of sedatives for acute anxiety symptoms. (See Anxiety section.)

***Follow-Up.*** Refer the client to a psychiatrist or mental health counselor for psychotherapy and medication. As with anxiety, referral for other manifestations of stress depends on the health care provider's expertise, the severity of symptoms and functional impairment, the client's response to intervention, and her receptiveness and motivation.[32]

## EATING DISORDERS

Eating disorders are complex psychological problems that affect the client's general health. That eating disorders have evolved is not surprising; this nation spends an estimated $150 million to $500 million annually on diet products and weight loss programs.

The largest percentage of clients with eating disorders are female. Motivation to control weight differs in males and females. Males wish to increase physical effectiveness, females to decrease body weight and increase "attractiveness."[34]

A client may exhibit behaviors seen in different types of eating disorders, or her behavior may change over time from that which is more typical of anorexia to that which is typical of bulimia. Health care providers must be aware that various terms exist for the same condition, for example, anorexia nervosa and restrictive anorexia. Similarly, there are anorexics who purge (bulimarexia or bulimia nervosa) and bulimics who do not purge (compulsive overeaters).

Several characteristics, however, are frequently reported by women with an eating disorder. For example, one or both parents or a sibling is preoccupied with weight and food. Or, a crisis, such as loss, may precipitate an eating disorder; loss may be real (death) or psychological (breakup of a relationship or a move from familiar surroundings).

Another characteristic is family chaos, such as alcoholism, drug addiction, violence, sexual abuse, compulsive gambling, affective disorder, and depression. The client's behavior is a symptom of the family's ineffective coping style, not the cause of it. She has learned that unpleasant emotions, such as anger, disappointment, sorrow, and loss, are to be avoided. Consequently, she becomes accomplished at denial and may be unable to recognize the normal range and expression of human emotions.

In addition, a client's independence or autonomy from her family may have been stifled, allowing little control over her life. Control of her body is control of something.

Finally, the common denominators of any eating disorder are low self-esteem and a distorted body image.

Eating disorders include a wide spectrum of gross disturbances in eating behaviors. Generally, however, anorexics control weight by restricting food intake and excessive exercise; bulimics alternate strict dieting with episodes of binging and purging; compulsive overeaters also alternate strict dieting with binges but do not purge. It is important to differentiate compulsive overeating from obesity: although the two have similar long-term health risks, *obesity* is a term based on weight that does not address psychological issues.

Unfortunately, predictors of outcome and prognosis for clients with anorexia and bulimia vary considerably because of diverse methodology, inconsistent utilization of diagnostic criteria, and lack of specifically defined criteria for recovery, relapse, and recurrence. DSM-III-R also includes the category Eating Disorders Not Otherwise Specified. An example of such a disorder is evident in a person of average weight who does not have binge eating episodes, but frequently engages in self-induced vomiting for fear of gaining weight.[19] One consistent finding of studies is that the prevalence of eating disorders is increasing.[35,36]

## ANOREXIA NERVOSA

Essential features of anorexia nervosa according to DSM-III-R criteria are refusal to maintain body weight above minimal normal weight for age and height; intense fear of gaining weight or becoming fat, even though underweight; distorted body image ("feel fat" when obviously underweight or even emaciated); and amenorrhea (absence of at least three consecutive menstrual cycles when otherwise expected to occur or menstruation that occurs only following hormone administration).[19]

The client is preoccupied with food, weight, and diet (e.g., she counts the calories in one Lifesaver candy when keeping a food diary) and weighs herself more than once a day. She exhibits compulsive behaviors and low self-esteem. The client hoards food, has bizarre eating behavior, and limits selections to a few low-calorie foods. She may over-exercise to the point of exhaustion or injury.

### Epidemiology

***Risk Factors.*** Among the risk factors are female gender (9:1 female:male ratio); age range of 15 to 50; career choice that stresses thinness, competition, perfection, or self-discipline (modeling, theater, ballet, competitive athletics); parent or sibling with eating disorder, affective disorder, or substance abuse problem; psychiatric illness or depression; or being achievement-oriented, compliant, "model" child, or perfectionist. Some studies suggest an increased incidence of eating disorders among young women with insulin-dependent diabetes; this association remains controversial.[37]

***Incidence.*** Incidence varies from 1 in 800 to 1 in 100 females between ages 12 and 18. Onset is usually in early to late adolescence. The mortality rate is between 5 and 18 percent. Anorexia nervosa usually occurs among females of upper-middle socioeconomic status.

### Subjective Data

The client may report feeling bloated, fatigue, constipation, diarrhea, decreased libido, cold intolerance, insomnia, sore tongue, frequent upper respiratory infections, muscle weakness and cramps, dizziness, social isolation, nausea, fainting spells. She may deny hunger or exhaustion. Amenorrhea or infertility is associated with anorexia and bulimia.[38,39] (An October 1990 study from

Canada found that 7 percent of women aged 21–39 at an infertility clinic were currently suffering from anorexia or bulimia, a rate two to four times that in the general population; this study also demonstrated that women had failed to discuss their eating disorder with their gynecologists.[38])

Subtle clues may be detected by a health care provider who is attuned to the client. For example, the client may be oversensitive when weighed or have excessive concerns about being overweight, even if she appears normal or under normal weight. She may request advice about fad diets and weight loss programs, may claim she "does not have enough time to eat," may dress in oversized clothes or layers of clothing to hide weight or health (yet she denies a problem), and may be compulsive about exercise. A wide discrepancy may exist in caloric intake and expenditure, leading to caloric deficit and subsequent weight loss.

Thorough medical and psychosocial histories are of utmost importance. Various screening tools are available and most often used in psychotherapy: Eating Attitudes Test (EAT), Diagnostic Survey for Eating Disorders (DSED), Eating Disorder Inventory (EDI), and bulimia test (BULIT). A pertinent history that is applicable to any eating disorder addresses five topics.

- *Attitude.* Weight attitudes and problems may be detected by asking several questions. Do you like yourself at current weight? What would you like to weigh? What was your weight in the past month? The past 6 months? What are your highest and lowest weights? Have you always been over/underweight? Are other family members over/underweight?
- *Diet History.* Ask the client to complete a 24-hour dietary intake record of the previous day including breakfast, lunch, dinner, snacks; caffeine (sodas, tea, coffee); alcohol, recreational drugs, and tobacco; and medications (prescription and over-the-counter). Ask the client what constitutes a binge? A reasonable meal? Note her reluctance or resistance to respond during the diet history. Assign the client the task of keeping a food/mood diary for several days: time of day eating occurred, food or beverage consumed, amount eaten, calories, food group supplied, how quickly meal was eaten, degree of hunger, feelings and circumstances that prompted eating, where eating took place, names of persons who ate with client, activities while eating (e.g., sitting, standing, walking, lying down).
- *Exercise.* Describe frequency (per day or week) and type of exercise. Differentiate compulsive exercise and athletic exercise. The athlete participates in purposeful training with an athletic goal and has high exercise tolerance, good muscle development, body fat within normal limits, and, most importantly, an accurate body image. The pressure to excel, especially among elite athletes, has brought attention to the "female athlete triad": disordered eating, amenorrhea, and osteoporosis. This is especially common among athletes competing in appearance or endurance sports. Parents, coaches, athletic trainers, team physicians, and athletic association administrators must also recognize their roles in the development of this pattern and consider the lifelong consequences for the athlete.[38,40] If the client is a competitive athlete, she must learn at what point exercise loses its beneficial quality and becomes harmful. Reasons for excessive exercise should be evaluated: Is it the demand of a coach or sport or is it compulsive behavior to manage anxiety or purge the effects of eating? Also, can the athlete with an eating disorder stop dieting, binging, or purging when the season is over? Does the

athlete realize that the behavior may compromise, rather than enhance, performance?

- *Menstrual History.* At what age did menarche occur and at what age did regular menses begin? Is the client currently menstruating? Has the client experienced a recent change in menstrual pattern (in 20 percent of anorexics, this may be the first sign before low body weight)? What contraceptive method does she use? How many pregnancies? Abortions?
- *Social History.* Does the client live alone? Does she cook or eat alone? Have friends and family complained of a change in her behavior? Ask the client to describe the number and character of her relationships. How many hours per week does she devote to school, work, or both? Has she undergone a recent crisis? Has she ever had psychological counseling? Is she now undergoing counseling? Does she vomit frequently or use laxatives, diuretics, or appetite suppressants? Does she use syrup of ipecac? Ipecac is an inexpensive, over-the-counter drug that can be lethal. Repeated use results in chronic absorption causing myopathy, which is reversible on discontinuation of the drug. However, potentially fatal cardiomyopathy may also be a consequence of chronic use.[41] If a client reports taking laxatives, inform her that they are ineffective for weight loss: If 2100 calories are consumed followed by 50 laxative tablets, the net calorie savings is only 252.[42]

## Objective Data

Data are determined by means of specific calculations to measure body fat and mass, physical examination, and several diagnostic tests to identify anemia and rule out imbalances in body chemistry and other metabolic reasons for weight loss.

### *Measurements*

- Measure frame size and compare height and weight with Metropolitan Insurance Height/Weight tables.[43]
- Measure percentage of body fat using skin fold calipers (healthy for men is 15 percent, for women 22 percent).[43,44]
- Plot body mass index [weight (kg)/height $cm^2$]; indexes greater than 27.2 and 26.9 indicate obesity in men and women, respectively.[45]
- Calculate ideal body weight. For women, this is 100 pounds plus 5 pounds for every inch over 5 ft; for men, 110 pounds plus 5 pounds for every inch over 5 ft.[45]

### *Physical Examination*

- *General Appearance.* The client appears pale and emaciated, and manifests delayed sexual maturation.
- *Skin.* The client may have lanugo (fine, downy hair that covers extremities and face), brittle nails, dry skin, hair loss or thinning, and carotenemia evidenced by yellowing palms and soles.
- *Throat.* Buccal mucosa may be erythematous.
- *Breasts.* Breasts may be atrophied or poorly developed.
- *Vascular System.* Arrhythmias (secondary to electrolyte abnormalities) and peripheral edema may be detected.
- *Abdomen.* The abdomen may appear scaphoid. Bowel sounds may be hypoactive.
- *Genitalia and Reproductive Tract.* The client may have primary or secondary amenorrhea, irregular menses (may not be identified if she takes oral contraceptives), and decreased fertility.
- *Rectal Area.* Hemorrhoids (secondary to constipation) may be present.
- *Musculoskeletal System.* The client may exhibit overuse injuries (stress fractures,

joint or tendon problems). A client with severe anorexia is at risk for osteoporosis.

- *Nervous System.* Determine if the client is suicidal.
- *Endocrine System.* Thyroid abnormalities may be detected.

#### Diagnostic Tests

- *Urinalysis.* A urinalysis is done to evaluate carbohydrate metabolism and specific gravity. Elevated ketones and protein indicates low carbohydrate metabolism (due to poor intake). Specific gravity is increased if the client is dehydrated and decreased if she is drinking excessive water (common before being weighed). A urine pregnancy test is done if amenorrhea is a symptom and the client is sexually active.
- *Blood Chemistry.* A complete blood count is done to determine anemia and neutropenia. Electrolytes are evaluated. Decreased potassium may cause arrhythmia, then death. In addition, decreased calcium, magnesium, chloride, sodium, albumin, and globulin and increased BUN are typical with anorexia nervosa.
- *Liver Function Tests.* To help rule out other causes of weight loss, some values may be affected by malnutrition.
- *Endocrine Tests.* Levels of follicle-stimulating hormone and luteinizing hormone may be decreased. Prolactin, thyroid-stimulating hormone, and thyroxine levels may be normal. Thyroid function tests may be borderline low.[46]
- *Electrocardiogram.* An electrocardiogram is indicated to determine the presence of arrhythmias, especially if the health care provider suspects poor follow-up or severe disease.

### Differential Medical Diagnosis

Weight loss: rule out anorexia nervosa, hyperthyroidism, malabsorption syndrome, mesenteric artery syndrome, Addison's disease, Alzheimer's disease, Crohn's disease, depression, ischemic heart disease, carcinoma, other chronic diseases.[47]

Amenorrhea, primary: rule out pituitary adenoma, ovarian failure, genital tract obstruction. (See Chapter 5.)

Amenorrhea, secondary: rule out pregnancy, pituitary failure, weight loss or decreased body fat due to body building or sports. (See Chapter 5.)

### Plan

***Psychosocial Interventions.*** It is vital that a trusting relationship be established between the primary health care provider and the client; this process takes time. Support the client, and remain nonjudgmental if she reveals bizarre food habits. Help the client to find appropriate alternative coping behaviors and reestablish a healthy attitude regarding food and weight. In addition, act as role model by accepting your own body size and weight and by maintaining healthy eating and exercise habits.

Other resources are essential, for example, individual and/or group therapy (group therapy reduces secrecy and allows sharing of concerns), assertiveness training, self-esteem and body image groups, family therapy.

***Medication.*** Tricyclic antidepressants may be prescribed and monitored by a psychiatrist. A small volume is prescribed to avoid lethal dose if the client is suicidal. (See Depression section.)

***Diet.*** Diet modification includes psychological measures, as well as careful nutritional planning, preferably by a nutritionist.

- A computer nutritional analysis is helpful in comparing the client's intake with healthy percentages of fat, carbohydrates, and protein. Estimate her basal metabolic rate.[45] This method provides reality-based information to help dispel the client's nutritional myths.

- Contract negotiation between client and health care provider focuses on an acceptable weight range and plan for exercise, food intake, and follow-up. Self-contract enhances the client's control in that she is responsible both for changing her behavior and identifying the reward to reinforce health-promoting behavior. The ultimate responsibility for recovery lies with the client. If, however, the provider feels the client is endangering herself (low weight, excessive purging, refusing to eat, suicidal gestures), the provider must recommend inpatient therapy, which requires breaking confidentiality.
- The American Diabetes Association's guidelines are used in nutritional planning. The client chooses foods in all food groups. Urge her to use servings, *not* calories, as a basis for planning: no less than 2 or 3 servings of meat or other protein, 6 to 11 of grains, 2 to 4 of fruits, 3 to 5 of vegetables, and 2 to 3 of milk. Smaller, more frequent meals may be more acceptable to a client who "feels full" quickly. Incorporate previously "forbidden" foods, that is, carbohydrates, into plan. Increase calories enough to elicit a 1- to 2-pound per week increase in weight.

***Exercise.*** Exercise should be modified. Encourage the client to decrease the amount and intensity, for example, change from high-impact aerobics to strengthening/stretching, low-impact aerobics, or walking several times a week. If the client refuses to decrease exercise, she must substantially increase her food intake.

***Follow-Up.*** Monitor the client's well-being. Assess weight weekly; the client should wear similar clothes each time. Assuming that the client weighs herself several times daily, encourage her to limit weighing to once a day or less.

Hospitalization criteria are made clear to client at her initial visit. This places the responsibility for control on the client.

- *Medical Indications for Hospitalization.* Severe emaciation, laboratory tests showing decreased sodium and potassium, abnormal electrocardiogram, minimal or no food intake, persistent weight loss, and need to facilitate differential diagnosis.
- *Psychiatric Indications for Hospitalization.* Moderate to severe depression (suicide risk); inability to function at home, work, or school; inability of family or current living arrangement to provide adequate psychological environment for improvement to occur;[40,52,53] and lack of improvement in outpatient treatment.[35,47,48]

## BULIMIA

Specific criteria characterize bulimia.[19] Most characteristic, perhaps, are the recurrent episodes of binge eating. A binge is described as the rapid consumption of a large amount of food in a discrete period. To be diagnosed with bulimia, a client must have had, on average, a minimum of two binge eating episodes per week for at least 3 months. During binges, clients often consume high-calorie, sweet, salty, or starchy food (junk food) that is easily and rapidly eaten. The binge is terminated by abdominal discomfort, sleep, social interruption, or induced vomiting. The client feels a lack of control over eating behavior during binges. Moreover, the client is often self-critical and depressed following a binge.

In addition, self-induced vomiting, use of laxatives or diuretics, strict dieting or fasting, or vigorous exercise is used to prevent weight gain. The client is persistently overconcerned with body shape and weight.

Frequent weight fluctuations (10 pounds per month) due to alternating binges and fasts are common; most bulimics are within the normal weight range. Bulimics also exhibit poor impulse control (promiscuity, shop-lifting, self-mutilation) and may be multiple substance abusers (most frequently sedatives, amphetamines, cocaine or alcohol).

## Epidemiology

Bulimia occurs most often among females aged 13 to 50. Males are also diagnosed, but to a lesser degree.

***Risk Factors.*** Obesity during adolescence (may have started restrictive diet, now out of control), substance abuse, depression, and family history of alcoholism or affective disorder are risk factors.

***Incidence.*** The condition is estimated to occur among 4.5 percent of female college freshmen and 0.4 percent of male college freshmen. Bulimia is also reported among middle- and upper-class women.[19]

Onset occurs in adolescence and early adulthood or during developmental transitions (college, marriage, breakup of relationship). Mortality is rare. It is usually related to unintended aspiration of vomitus or electrolyte abnormalities that cause cardiac arrhythmias or sudden death.

## Subjective Data

The client usually acknowledges and is disturbed by her abnormal eating behavior. She may report abdominal distention, cramping, and constipation secondary to chronic laxative abuse. She may seek advice or prescriptions for laxatives, diuretics, or diets. The client may also describe muscle weakness and fatigue, depression, chronic pharyngitis, difficulty swallowing, esophageal irritations, frequent dental problems, shortness of breath, palpitations, and chest pain. She may spontaneously regurgitate food, may skip heartbeats, and may be able to consume large amounts of food that are inconsistent with her weight.

She may be secretive and plan binges. Family or roommates report that the client is frequently in the bathroom after meals with the shower or water running. She may steal money to buy food or steal food or laxatives. Binges may cost up to $60 or $70 per day; consequently the woman is always without money.

Weight fluctuations occur as a result of binges, which vary from 1000 to 5000 calories. Binging and purging may be carried out from a few times per month to 20 times per day. Injuries result from excessive exercise (3 to 5 hours per day); the client may be an aerobics instructor at more than one fitness center. She may be a high achiever, but passive and nonassertive.

## Objective Data

A complete physical examination is done as are several diagnostic tests.

### *Physical Examination*

- *General appearance.* The client appears to be of normal weight for her height, although she may be slightly overweight.
- *Skin.* There may be scars on the dorsum of the hand from induced vomiting.
- *Head.* Examination may reveal bilateral parotid gland enlargement and "chipmunk" appearance.
- *Eyes.* Conjunctival hemorrhages may result from forceful vomiting.
- *Throat.* The dental enamel on inner aspects of the teeth may be eroded.
- *Chest.* Aspiration pneumonia from vomitus is most likely to occur with concomitant alcohol or drug ingestion.
- *Breasts.* Striae may be the result of weight fluctuations.
- *Vascular system.* Examination may reveal

arrhythmias and peripheral edema secondary to laxative withdrawal (related to electrolyte disturbances). Sudden death may result from the cumulative ingestion of syrup of ipecac.

- *Abdomen.* There may be esophageal tears or rupture. Abdominal striae and poor musculature are due to rapid weight changes.
- *Genitalia and reproductive tract.* Pregnancy is a risk if the client vomits after taking oral contraceptives.
- *Rectum.* Tearing and fissures may be caused by frequent enemas or hemorrhoids.
- *Musculoskeletal system.* Overuse injuries may be evident.
- *Nervous system.* Convulsions may be due to electrolyte imbalances.
- *Endocrine system.* Menstrual irregularities may be experienced. The client who is an insulin-dependent diabetic is at risk for hyper- or hypoglycemia and ketoacidosis.

#### Diagnostic Tests

- Urinalysis
- Complete blood count (anemia, neutropenia)
- Electrolytes (decreased chloride, increased phosphorus, decreased total protein)
- Liver function tests (especially with alcohol or substance abuse)
- Electrocardiogram (indicated especially with Ipecac use)
- Amylase test (differing reports use it as an indication of bulimia)
- Chest x-ray (may be indicated to rule out aspiration pneumonia)

### Differential Medical Diagnosis

Digitalis or pilocarpine toxicity, gastrointestinal carcinoma, malignant hypertension, pyloric obstruction, mesenteric artery syndrome, metabolic alkalosis, migraine, pinealoma, postconcussive syndrome, posterior fossa tumor.[47]

### Plan

***Psychosocial Intervention.*** See Anorexia section.

***Medication.*** See Depression section.

***Diet.*** Dietary intervention includes identifying "triggers." In addition, the client should be instructed in several steps toward recovery: to keep binge foods out of sight (or not purchase them); to be with other people at times known to be vulnerable (weekends, evenings) or to change her environment; to learn to nurture self in ways other than eating (taking bubble baths, reading, pursuing hobbies, telephoning a friend).[43]

The client should plan three to four regularly scheduled meals per day and eat them regardless of binges and purges. Nonemaciated bulimics should be encouraged to maintain weight or to gain gradually by consuming no fewer than 1800 to 2400 calories per day.

***Lifestyle Changes.*** See Anorexia.

***Follow-Up.*** Follow-up is weekly or every 2 weeks to assess the client's weight. More crucial than weight evaluation, however, is monitoring the frequency of binge/purge behavior, exercise, and abuse of laxatives, appetite suppressants, and diuretics.

Hospitalization criteria are described under Anorexia. Other indications for hospitalization are vomiting of all food eaten; two purges per day; refusal to stop using laxatives, ipecac, diet pills, and other substances; electrolyte imbalances, abnormal electrocardiogram; and problems related to self-induced vomiting, such as esophageal tears or rupture. In these circumstances, hospitalization is needed to interrupt the binge/purge cycle.[35]

## COMPULSIVE OVEREATING

Compulsive overeating is uncontrolled overeating not related to hunger, followed by guilt and shame about the behavior and consequent weight gain; fear of not being able to stop eating voluntarily; and awareness that the eating pattern is abnormal. A cyclical pattern emerges: binging, rigid dieting, feelings of deprivation and increasing anxiety, followed by binging again in response to anxiety or feelings of failure and despair due to inability to maintain diet.

Food is used to cope with stress, emotional conflicts, daily problems, boredom, depression, anxiety, loneliness, and anger.[49–51] A compulsive overeater may or may not be obese (body weight 20 percent over ideal body weight for height, age, and gender). In contrast, a body builder may be overweight for height due to muscle mass, but not have excessive body fat.

## Epidemiology

Compulsive overeating begins during early childhood when eating patterns are developed. The condition continues through life. A parent may comfort an infant by feeding; a family may use eating as an escape from feelings or as an activity when bored. The client as a consequence responds to external cues (sight or smell of food) rather than internal cues (hunger or satiation following eating). Weight gain may be unremarkable until metabolic needs decrease as a young adult.

Incidence studies show no specific statistics on compulsive overeating.

## Subjective Data

From the client's history, it becomes evident that she overeats compulsively; she eats little in public, yet high weight is maintained due to private binges. One study found that obese subjects who failed to lose weight underreported their actual calorie intake and overestimated their physical activity.[52] The client binges on any available food, most likely at night or on weekends. She has a long history of unsuccessful diets and restricts social activities because she is embarrassed about her weight (inability to fit in normal-size seats). The client may attribute social and career failures to weight (false belief that she would be a better person if thin) and may fear medical complications such as diabetes, hypertension, and heart disease.

## Objective Data

A physical examination and several diagnostic tests are done.

### *Physical Examination*

- *General Appearance.* The client appears healthy, but has excessive body fat on the extremities as well as the trunk.
- *Vital Signs.* Tachycardia and hypertension (use appropriately sized blood pressure cuff) are possible.
- *Skin.* Skin breakdown is observed at intertriginous areas (beneath abdomen, vulva, groin, breasts, axillae); wound healing is poor. If obesity is accompanied by androgen excess, acne and hirsutism of the face, lower abdomen, thighs, and chest may be observed.
- *Chest.* Respirations are increased. There is dyspnea on exertion.
- *Breasts.* Hair surrounds the areolae in women with androgen excess.
- *Vascular System.* Varicosities and thrombophlebitis may be present.
- *Abdomen.* Abdomen is protuberant.
- *Genitalia and Reproductive Tract.* There may be a history of pregnancy or delivery complications, newborn complications, or male hair pattern in females (if androgen excess).
- *Musculoskeletal System.* Examination may reveal osteoarthritis (especially of the hips and knees), sciatica, and lower extremity injuries.
- *Nervous System.* Depression may be revealed.

- *Endocrine System.* Hyperglycemia and amenorrhea are possible findings.

### *Diagnostic Tests*

- Complete blood count
- Glucose and lipid profiles (cholesterol, high density and low density lipoproteins, fasting triglycerides)
- Electrolyte analysis (especially if using fad diets)
- Urinalysis
- Electrocardiogram
- Endocrine studies when indicated (follicle-stimulating hormone, thyroid-stimulating hormone, prolactin, luteinizing hormone, free testosterone, dehydroepiandrosterone sulfate)

## Differential Medical Diagnosis

Obesity with amenorrhea—rule out polycystic ovary syndrome/anovulation; obesity due to compulsive eating disorder; complications of obesity, such as hypertension, gallbladder disease, hyperlipidemia, and non-insulin-dependent diabetes.

## Plan

***Psychosocial Interventions.*** See Anorexia section. Suggest to the client that she join a support group, such as Overeaters Anonymous.

***Medication.*** Antidepressants may be indicated (see Depression). Appetite suppressants are not recommended.

***Diet.*** Dietary interventions are numerous (also see Anorexia). No fewer than 1200 calories should be consumed per day; otherwise essential nutrients are restricted and metabolism decreased, possibly prompting a binge.

Suggest to the client that she replace problem behaviors with alternative behaviors.[43] Provide accurate information regarding weight loss programs, including the risks involved with fad diets or "powdered formula" diets. The following questions are helpful in evaluation of weight loss programs.[53]

- Is this a diet the client could live with indefinitely?
- What is the recommended rate of weight loss?
- Does the program take individual differences into account to determine caloric needs?
- To what extent does the plan educate the client about nutrition, behavior modification, and the importance of exercise?
- Does the program put the client in contact with professionals such as physicians, registered dietitians, and psychotherapists?
- What percentage of clients reach goal weight and maintain their losses?
- Does the program offer a maintenance plan once weight is lost?
- What is the nature of the advertisements and endorsements?
- How much does the program cost?

***Exercise.*** Exercise needs to be incorporated into lifestyle. Inform the client about the health benefits of regular exercise. Exercise increases basal metabolic rate, which increases calorie use and promotes weight loss. Exercising at least four times per week for 20 to 30 minutes is recommended.

Devise a mutually agreeable plan for aerobic exercise; calculate the target heart rate.[54] Weight loss cannot occur and be maintained if the client is unwilling to continue exercise and reasonable caloric restriction.

Explain to the client that weight may not change drastically; rather, she should use as a guide how she feels physically and how her clothes fit. Encourage the client to wear flattering clothing to boost self-esteem.

***Follow-Up.*** Follow-up visits are scheduled for every 2 weeks or monthly to evaluate weight and blood pressure and review exercise, dietary goals, and compliance problems.

## HEALTH CONCERNS OF LESBIAN CLIENTS

*Lesbian* describes sexual preference and is not a clinical entity.[55] Lesbians are reported to constitute 2 to 12 percent of the general population; however, the percentage may be underestimated.[56,57] The concerns and needs of lesbian women are similar to those of heterosexual women, yet unique. Lesbian clients experience menstrual problems, sexually transmitted infections, and many other problems seen in the heterosexual woman. Special health concerns include substance abuse, depression, cervical cancer, sexually transmitted infections, and pregnancy.

### TROIDEN'S FOUR-STAGE MODEL

The Troiden model addresses gay/lesbian identity development and may provide insight into the increased risk of depression and substance abuse among the homosexual population. The health care provider must understand that no individual fits the model perfectly or always progresses in the projected linear pattern.[58]

#### Stage 1

Sensitization usually occurs before puberty. Children do not see themselves as homosexual, but begin to see themselves as different from their peers. Homosexual/heterosexual issues have no meaning to children before puberty and should not be the focus. Health care providers can help children integrate these concerns about feeling different.

#### Stage 2

Identity confusion in a lesbian adolescent is the beginning of the realization that she may be homosexual. Anxiety and inner trauma may result. Most lesbians realize their homosexuality, on average, at age 18. The stigma, inner turmoil, and fear create difficulty for lesbian youths in discussing their homosexuality. Typically, they respond to identity confusion by denying their feelings, striving to repair themselves, and avoiding all situations that might increase their homosexual feelings. They also may respond by rationalizing their behavior as only a phase and escape through drugs and alcohol, and even pregnancy. Denial of their homosexuality, for whatever reason, may last months, years, or a lifetime. Adolescents who accept it seek information and resources. The health care provider can help them to validate their sexual feelings.

#### Stage 3

Identity assumption is the stage when homosexual identity is assumed and shared with others. Typically, it occurs for lesbians between 21 and 23 years of age. Realization usually occurs through an intense love relationship with another woman. The outcome of her experiences affects how she perceives and accepts herself. The woman may deal with societal stigma by avoiding homosexual activity, behaving in a stereotyped gender-inappropriate way, becoming involved in the lesbian community, or concealing sexual preference and leading a double life.

The health care provider can provide factual information on homosexuality and resources such as support groups.

#### Stage 4

The stage of commitment is characterized by involvement in intimate relationships. Internally, it validates identity as a lesbian and develops satisfaction with that identity. Externally, it discloses homosexual identity to others who are not homosexual. The client now manages societal stigma by acting in gender-appropriate ways, without expressing or denying homosexuality.

The health care provider must realize that the client may lack the trust to reveal her concerns and needs and that disclosure may be very difficult. She may fear that if she discloses her homosexuality to the health care provider, she will be denied care or rejected, or her confidentiality may be violated. Many lesbian clients may not offer their sexual orientation but, if asked directly in an unbiased manner, will disclose such.[55–58]

## HEALTH CONCERNS

In a study of physical health problems and concerns of lesbians, it was found that clients sought health care primarily for menstrual problems (painful and irregular periods), sexually transmitted diseases and vaginitis (vaginal infections were predominant), other reproductive system problems (pelvic pain, uterine infections, and painful sexual relations), bladder and kidney infections, musculoskeletal problems, and breast problems.[59]

The lesbian population is at increased risk for substance abuse, depression and suicide, sexually transmitted diseases, cervical cancer, and vaginitis.

### Substance Abuse

A high incidence of alcoholism is reported among lesbians.[57] Suggested reasons include socialization in gay bars (not well substantiated), difficulty accepting gay identity, and isolation and rejection by society and family.

### Depression and Suicide

The lack of lesbian role models for the adolescent population makes it difficult for a lesbian to feel positive about herself.[60] The isolation experienced by many lesbian women may lead to depression and suicide, a major health issue. Attempted suicides are significantly higher among lesbians than among their heterosexual counterparts. In the general adolescent population, suicide is also a major problem; however, the research related to homosexual youth reveals that feelings of self-hatred and self-destructiveness are very strong.[60]

### Sexually Transmitted Diseases, Cervical Cancer, and Vaginitis

Often, a lesbian client is reluctant to seek care for gynecological problems.[56,57] Exclusive lesbians with no history (or partner history) of bisexual contact or no intravenous drug use within the last 10 years have the lowest risk of contracting HIV.[56] Lesbians are also at low risk for gonorrhea, chlamydia, and syphilis, and if they have a history of only female partners, they are at low risk for cervical intraepithelial neoplasia (CIN).[56]

***Risk Factors.*** Risk factors for CIN include human papillomavirus, past abnormal Pap smear, heterosexual intercourse before age 20, increased number of sexual partners, partners with increased number of partners, cigarette smoking, and exposure to diethylstilbestrol (DES). Human papillomavirus can be transmitted by genital–genital contact and by sharing sexual toys without first cleaning them. Lesbians may also develop bacterial vaginosis, cytolytic vaginitis, monilia, herpes, and hepatitis A.[56] It is possible to transmit herpes and hepatitis A through oral–genital and genital–genital contact and by sharing sexual toys without first cleaning them.[56,61] Monilia, trichomonas, and bacterial vaginosis can be transmitted through vulva–vulva or finger–vagina contact and by sharing sexual toys without first cleaning them.

***Safer Sex.*** Practices may include use of a dental dam, finger cots, or separate sex toys.

Good hygiene is essential. Dental dams, 6-in. squares of latex used in dental procedures, can also be used during oral sex to prevent spread of sexually transmitted diseases. Plastic wrap can also be used. Dental dams are usually flavored and may be obtained from medical supply stores.

Those using a dental dam must follow a specific procedure: Mark the side of the dental dam that will face the user; cover the entire vulva, as well as anus, holding the edges firmly (the user can stimulate her partner by using mouth and tongue). Dental dams should never be reused or shared. Care should be taken never to move the dam from the anus to the vagina.

## PREGNANCY AND PARENTING

Pregnancy and parenting are real issues for lesbian women. Lesbian women who desire parenthood have several options available.

### Pregnancy by Intercourse

A cooperative or unsuspecting man may participate, although it is not the preferred method.

***Disadvantages and Risks.*** The woman may contract a sexually transmitted disease. Legal complications may arise if the father seeks custody or parental rights at a future date. Nonbiological lesbian parents may have no legal rights in parenting the child if the biological mother dies; the biological father or grandparents become legal guardians.[56]

***Suggestions and Solutions.*** The biological mother can have a legal document drawn up stating her wishes, although this may not stand up in court. The lesbian woman and cooperative partner may make a contract whereby the partner relinquishes all parental rights and the woman agrees never to seek child support from the father.

### Artificial Insemination

Semen may be obtained from a known or unknown donor.

***Disadvantages and Risks.*** The significant costs for screened donor semen and physician fees are generally not covered by insurance. Bills could exceed thousands of dollars if pregnancy does not occur after the first or second insemination. If the donor is known, the same legal complications previously discussed may arise. If the semen donor is unknown, information is limited regarding paternal genetic diseases. There also exists a risk for infection with HIV through infected semen.[62]

***Suggestions and Solutions.*** The properly trained woman may perform her own inseminations, thereby decreasing costs. If the semen donor is known, he can be asked to sign a legal document waiving all parental rights. The client should consult an attorney.

### Adoption

Adoption of a healthy newborn infant is difficult for a married man and woman and almost impossible for a single woman. In most cases, adoption screening procedures limit the chances of adoption because society views lesbians unfavorably. Private adoption or adoption in another country may be possible.

## PLAN

Health care providers have several responsibilities in planning health care for a lesbian woman. The client must trust the provider. To help develop that trust the provider can:

- Explore her or his own feelings regarding homosexuality. A provider who is unable to provide "physically safe and psychologically comfortable health care for the client" should refer that client to a more accepting provider.[55]

- Assure the client that no adverse effect on quality of health care will result from disclosure.
- Recognize that the community in which the client lives can be a positive influence and source of support or a source of dysfunctional behavior.[63]
- Provide resources in the community that will encourage ongoing and positive experiences with health care.

## NURSING DIAGNOSES

The following nursing diagnoses identified by the author are representative of those used in the health care plan of women with psychosocial health problems; however, these diagnoses by no means constitute an inclusive list.

- Alteration in
  - Comfort
  - Family process, function
  - Thought process, potential for violence to self or others
  - Nutrition, less or more than body requirements
  - Bowel elimination
- Anxiety
- Body image disturbance
- Chronic low self-esteem
- Constipation
- Coping compromised, ineffective, personal or family related
- Denial
- Disturbance in self-esteem and self-concept
- Disturbance in sleep pattern
- Dysfunctional family
- Dysfunctional grieving
- Fatigue
- Fear
- Hopelessness
- Hyperthermia
- Impaired adjustment
- Impaired skin integrity, or potential for impaired skin integrity
- Impaired social interaction, potential isolation
- Impaired verbal communication
- Ineffective denial
- Knowledge deficit related to
  - Disease process
  - Available social, legal, and other community resources
- Pain
- Post-trauma response
- Potential for
  - Injury
  - Poisoning
  - Infection
  - Trauma
  - Aspiration
  - Altered body temperature
- Potential to develop
  - Sexual dysfunction
  - Situational low self-esteem
- Powerlessness
- Rape trauma syndrome (silent reaction), potential for compound reaction
- Spiritual distress

## REFERENCES

1. *Policy on sexual harassment.* (1987–1988). Richmond: Department of Personnel Administration, Virginia Commonwealth University.
2. Shrier, D. (1990). Sexual harassment and discrimination. *New Jersey Medicine, 87,* 105–107.

3. U.S. Merit Systems Protection Board. (1981). *Sexual harassment in the federal workplace: Is it a problem?* Washington, DC: U.S. Government Printing Office.
4. Council on Scientific Affairs, American Medical Association (1992). Council reports violence against women. *Journal of the American Medical Association, 267,* 3184–3189.
5. National Clearinghouse on Domestic Violence. (1981). Family violence: A workshop manual for clergy and other service providers. *Domestic Violence,* Monograph Series 6, 53–62.
6. Strauss, M. & Smith, C. (1993). Family patterns and primary prevention of family violence. *Trends Health Care Law Ethics, Spring 8(2),* 17–25.
7. Walker, L.E. (1984). *The battered woman syndrome.* New York: Springer.
8. Blair, K. (1986). The battered woman: Is she a silent victim? *Nurse Practitioner, 11,* 39–47.
9. Berrios, D., & Grady, D. (1991). Domestic violence risk factors and outcomes. *Western Journal of Medicine, 155,* 133–135.
10. Candib, L. (1990). Naming the contradictions: Family medicine's failure to face violence against women. *Family Community Health, 13,* 47–57.
11. Chez, R. (1988). Woman battering. *American Journal of Obstetrics and Gynecology, 158,* 1–4.
12. Campbell, J., & Sheridan, D. (1989). Emergency nursing interventions with battered women. *Journal of Emergency Nursing, 15,* 12–17.
13. Bullock, L., McFarlane, J., Bateman, L., & Miller, V. (1989). The prevalence and characteristics of battered women in a primary care setting. *Nurse Practitioner, 14,* 47–56.
14. Dunn, S.F., & Guilchrist, V.J. (1993). Sexual assault. *Primary Care, 20*(2), 359–372.
15. Adams, A., & Abarbanel, G. (1988). *Sexual assault on campus: What colleges can do.* Santa Monica, CA: Rape Treatment Center, Santa Monica Medical Center.
16. Robinson, J., (1990). Rape—A crime with health consequences. *The Female Patient, 15,* 25–32.
17. Beckman, C., & Groetzinger, L. (1989). Treating sexual assault victims: A protocol for health professionals. *The Female Patient, 14,* 78–83.
18. Beebe, D. (1991). Emergency management of the adult female rape victim. *American Family Physician, 43,* 2041–2046.
19. American Psychiatric Association. (1987). *Diagnostic and statistical manual of mental disorders* (3rd ed., revised). Washington, DC: Author.
20. Naegle, M. (1988). Substance abuse among women: Prevalence, patterns, and treatment issues. *Issues in Mental Health Nursing, 9,* 127–137.
21. Kinney, J. (1991). *Clinical manual of substance abuse.* St. Louis, MO: Mosby–Yearbook.
22. Bell, K. (1992). Identifying the substance abuser in clinical practice. *Orthopaedic Nursing, 11,* 29–36.
23. U.S. Preventive Services Task Force. (1989). Screening for Etoh and other drug abuse. *American Family Physician, 40,* 137–146.
24. Ewing, J. (1984). Detecting alcoholism: The CAGE questionnaire. *Journal of the American Medical Association, 252,* 1905–1907.
25. Tweeds, S. (1989). Identifying the alcoholic client. *Nursing Clinics of North America, 24,* 13–31.
26. Schroeder, S., Krupp, M., Tiernay, L., & McPhee, S. (Eds.) (1991). *Current medical diagnosis and treatment* (30th ed.). Norwalk, CT: Appleton & Lange.
27. Branch, W., Jr. (Ed.) (1987). *Office practice of medicine* (2nd ed.). Philadelphia: W.B. Saunders.
28. U.S. Department of Health and Human Services, Public Health Service, Agency for Health Care Policy and Research. (1993). *Clinical practice guideline No. 5: Depression in primary care: Detection, diagnosis, and treatment* (Publication No. 93-09553). Rockville, MD: *AMCPR.*
29. Perry, M., & Anderson, G. (1992). Assessment and treatment strategies for depressive disorders commonly encountered in primary care settings. *Nurse Practitioner, 17,* 25–36.
30. Cameron, O., & Hill, E. (1989). Women and

anxiety. *Psychiatric Clinics of North America, 12,* 175–185.

31. Billings, C. (1990). Anxiety and physical illness. *Psychiatric Medicine, 8,* 149–161.
32. Diamond, E., & Grauer, K. (1987). The spectrum of anxiety disorders in family practice. *American Family Physician, 36,* 167–173.
33. Manderino, M., & Brown, M. (1992). A practical, step-by-step approach to stress management for women. *Nurse Practitioner, 17,* 18–28.
34. Freedman, R. (1989). *Bodylove: Learning to like our looks and ourselves.* New York: Harper & Row.
35. Garner, D., & Garfinkel, P. (1985). *Handbook of psychotherapy for anorexia nervosa and bulimia* (pp. 19–51, 391–430, 513–572). New York: Guilford Press.
36. Levine, M.P. (1987). *How schools can help combat student eating disorders: Anorexia and bulimia.* Washington, DC: National Education Association.
37. Rodin, G.M., & Daneman, D. (1992). Eating disorders and insulin dependent diabetes mellitus: A problematic association. *Diabetes Care, 15*(10), 1402–1412.
38. Stewart, D.E., Robinson, G.E., Goldbloom, D.S., & Wright, C. (1990). Infertility and eating disorders. *American Journal of Obstetrics and Gynecology, 163*(4), 1196–1199.
39. McSherry, J. (1984). Diagnostic challenge of anorexia nervosa. *American Family Physician, 29*(2), 141–145.
40. Yeager, K.K., Agostini, R., Nattiv, A., & Drinkwater, B. (1993). Female athlete triad: Disordered eating, amenorrhea, osteoporosis. *Medicine and Science in Sports and Exercise, 25*(7), 775–777.
41. Dresser, L.P., Massey, E.W., Johnson, E.E., & Bossen, E. (1993). Ipecac myopathy and cardiomyopathy. *Journal of Neurology, Neurosurgery, and Psychiatry, 56*(5), 560–562.
42. Bo-Linn, G.W., Santa Anna, C.A., Morowski, S.G., & Fordtram, J.S. (1983). Purging and caloric absorption in bulimic patients and normal women. *Annals of International Medicine, 99*(1), 14–77.
43. National Dairy Council. (1990). *Lifesteps: Weight management—A summary of current theory and practice.*
44. Dunn, M.M. (1987). Guidelines for an effective personal fitness prescription. *Nurse Practitioner, 12*(9), 9–23.
45. Boyle, M.A., & Whitney, E.N. (1989). *Personal nutrition.* St. Paul, MN: West.
46. Speroff, L., Glass, R., & Kase, N. (1989). *Clinical gynecology, endocrinology and infertility* (4th ed.). Baltimore: Williams & Wilkins.
47. Giannini, A.J., Newman, M., & Gold, M. (1990). Anorexia and bulimia. *American Family Physician, 41*(4), 1169–1176.
48. Palmer, T. (1990). Anorexia nervosa, bulimia nervosa: Casual theories and treatment. *Nurse Practitioner, 15*(4), 12–19.
49. Willard, M.D. (1991). Obesity: Types and treatments. *American Family Physician, 43*(6), 2099–2108.
50. Saunders, R., & Saunders, D. (1989). Nonpurging bulimics: An ignored population. *British Review of Bulimia and Anorexia Nervosa, 3*(2), 79–85.
51. Siegel, M., Brisman, J., & Weinshel, M. (1988). *Surviving an eating disorder: New perspectives and strategies for family and friends.* New York: Harper & Row.
52. Lichtman, S.W., Pisarska, K., Berman, E.R., Pestone, M., Dowling, H., Offenbacher, E., Weisel, H., Heshka, S., Matthews, D.E., & Heymsfield, S.B. (1992). Discrepancy between self reported and actual caloric intake and exercise in obese subjects. *The New England Journal of Medicine, 327*(27), 1893–1898.
53. Special report: Choosing a weight-loss program. (1990). *Tufts University Diet and Nutrition Letter, 8*(6), 36.
54. Edmunds, M.W. (1991). Strategies for promoting physical fitness. *Nursing Clinics of North America, 26*(4), 855–866.
55. Hitchcock, J.M., & Wilson, H.S. (1992). Personal risking: Lesbian self-disclosure of sexual orientation to professional health care providers. *Nursing Research, 41*(3), 178–183.
56. Zeidenstein, L. (1990). Gynecological and

childbearing needs of lesbians. *Journal of Nurse-Midwifery, 35*(1), 10–18.

57. Smith, M., Heaton, C., & Seiver, D. (1989). Health concerns of lesbian women. *The Female Patient, 14,* 43–74.
58. Troiden, R. (1988). Homosexual identity development. *Journal of Adolescent Health Care, 9,* 105–113.
59. Trippet, S.E., & Bain, J. (1993). Physical health problems and concerns of lesbians. *Women and Health, 20* (2), 59–70.
60. Sanford, N. (1989). Providing sensitive health care to gay and lesbian youth. *The Nurse Practitioner, 14*(5), 30–47.
61. Stewart, F., Guest, F., & Hatcher, R. (1987). *Understanding your body: Every Woman's Guide to Gynecology and Health.* New York: Bantam Books.
62. Holmes, V., & Fernandez, F. (1989). HIV in women, current impact and future implications. *Physician Assistant, May,* 53–58.
63. Eliason, M.J. (1993). Cultural diversity in nursing care: The lesbian, gay, or bisexual client. *Journal of Transcultural Nursing, 5*(1), 14–19.

## BIBLIOGRAPHY

Brone, R.J., & Fisher, C.B. (1988). Determinants of adolescent obesity: A comparison with anorexia nervosa. *Adolescence, 89,* 155–167.

Cranshaw, J.P. (1985, Oct. 30). Anorexia and bulimia: Earliest cues. *Patient Care,* 81–95.

Ehhrenfeld, P. (Ed.) (1991, Spring). Calling on coaches: Athletes need help. *American Anorexia/Bulimia Association, Inc. newsletter.*

Flood, M. (1989). Addictive eating disorders. *Nursing Clinics of North America, 24*(1),45–53.

Geary, M. (1988). A review of treatment models for eating disorders: Toward a holistic nursing model. *Holistic Nursing Practice, 3*(1), 39–45.

Gilchrist, V.J. (1991). Preventive health care for the adolescent. *American Family Physician, 43*(3), 869–878.

Hall, R.C., & Beresford, T.P. (1989). Anorexia nervosa: Diagnostic, prognostic and clinical features. *Psychiatric Medicine, 7*(3), 3–12.

Hall, R.C., & Beresford, T.P. (1989). Bulimia nervosa: Diagnostic criteria, clinical features and discrete clinical subsyndromes. *Psychiatric Medicine, 7*(3), 13–25.

Herron, D.G. (1991). Strategies for promoting a healthy dietary intake. *Nursing Clinics of North America, 26*(4), 875–884.

Herzog, D.B., Keller, M.B., & Lavori, P.W. (1988). Outcome in anorexia nervosa and bulimia nervosa. A review of the literature. *Journal of Nervous and Mental Disease, 176*(3), 131–143.

Johnson, M. (1992). Tailoring the preparticipation exam to female athletes. *The Physician and Sportsmedicine, 20*(7), 61–72.

Jones, J.K. (1989). Bulimia: Determining prevalence and examining intervention. *Journal of American College Health, 37,* 231–233.

Kano, S. (1989). *Making peace with food.* New York: Harper & Row.

Keller, O. (1986). Bulimia: Primary care approach and intervention. *Nurse Practitioner, 11*(8), 42–51.

Kitay, D.Z., & Lincoln, G.H. (1987, Sept.). When is a patient "obese" and why? *Contemporary Obstetrics and Gynecology,* 96–99.

Lipscomb, P. (1987). Bulimia: Diagnosis and management in the primary care setting. *Journal of Family Practice, 24*(2), 187–194.

Moses, A., & Hawkins, R. (1982). *Counseling lesbian women and gay men.* St. Louis: C.V. Mosby.

Palmer, E.P., & Guay, A.T. (1985). Reversible myopathy secondary to abuse of ipecac in patients with major eating disorders. *New England Journal of Medicine, 313,* 1457–1459.

Plehn, K.W. (1990). Anorexia nervosa and bulimia: Incidence and diagnosis. *Nurse Practitioner, 15*(4), 22–29.

Prewitt, T., & Rogers, M. (1987, Oct.). Giving weight loss advice that patients will heed. *Contemporary Obstetrics and Gynecology,* 81–90.

Provost, F.A. (1989). Eating disorders in college students. *Psychiatric Medicine, 7*(3), 47–58.

Rau, J.H., & Green, R.S. (1975). Compulsive eating: A neuropsychologic approach to certain eating disorders. *Comprehensive Psychiatry, 16*(3), 223–231.

Rosenfield, S. (1988). Family influence on eating behavior and attitudes in eating disorders: A review of the literature *Holistic Nursing Practice, 3*(1), 46–55.

Sanford, L.T., & Donovan, M.E. (1984). *Women and self-esteem.* New York: Penguin Books.

Torem, M.S. (1990). Covert multiple personality underlying eating disorders. *American Journal of Psychotherapy, 44,* 3.

Vanin, J.R., & Saylor, K.E. (1989). Laxative abuse: A hazardous habit for weight control. *Journal of American College Health, 37,* 227–230.

White, J.H. (1986). Behavioral intervention for the obese client. *Nurse Practitioner, 11*(1), 27–34.

Wichmann, S., & Martin, D.R. (1993). Eating disorders in athletes: Weighing the risks. *The Physician and Sportsmedicine, 21*(5), 126–135.

## NATIONAL ORGANIZATIONS FOR EATING DISORDERS

National Anorexia Aid Society (NAAS)
445 East Granville Road
Worthington, OH 43085
(614) 436–1112

National Association of Anorexia Nervosa and Associated Disorders, Inc. (ANAD)
Box 7
Highland Park, IL 60035
(708) 831–3438

Anorexia Nervosa and Related Eating Disorders (ANRED)
P.O. Box 5102
Eugene, OR 97405
(503) 344–1144

CHAPTER 19

# ISSUES FOR WOMEN WITH PHYSICAL DISABILITY AND CHRONIC ILLNESS

*Kathleen J. Sawin*

*Being disabled does not contradict responsible, effective parenting, yet judgmental attitudes continue.*

*Highlights*

- Discrimination
- Negative Attitudes Among Health Care Workers
- Architectural Barriers
- Sexuality: Education, Body Image
  - *Spinal Cord Injury*
  - *Joint Inflexibility and Pain*
  - *Multiple Sclerosis*
  - *Diabetes Mellitus*
  - *Epilepsy*
  - *Urinary and Bowel Appliances*
  - *Pelvic Radiotherapy*
  - *Menarche*
  - *Sexual Activity*
  - *Abuse*
- Eliciting a History; Physical Examination
- Management of Contraception
- Pregnancy; Parenting

## INTRODUCTION

The unmet needs of women* with physical disabilities include accessibility to gynecological care, sexuality and birth control counseling, and accessibility to professionals with a knowledge of how disability impacts primary care.

*"Women" will be used here to denote both adults and adolescents with disability or chronic illness unless otherwise specified.

### DISCRIMINATION

The discrimination that women with disabilities and chronic illness face is twofold: first, they are women, and second, they are individuals with disabilities. Narrow negative social attitudes set unnecessary barriers to the optimal growth and development of these women and the health care they obtain. An example is the stereotypic image of American women as having two major functions—caretaker and object of beauty. The ideal woman is physically "perfect."[1]

The Americans with Disabilities Act (ADA) became law in 1990. Discrimination in employment against qualified persons with disabilities is against the law, enforced by the U.S. Equal Employment Opportunity Commission and related agencies. By July 26, 1994, this law will apply to all employers with 15 or more employees.

***Impact of Disability.*** Specific disabilities (spinal cord injury, cerebral palsy, multiple sclerosis, or disabling arthritis) prevent women, it is thought, from meeting society's major functions. Attractive women who use wheelchairs are seen as less than whole. For example, a comment overheard in a family planning clinic concerned a very attractive 19-year-old woman who had recently sustained a spinal cord injury and now used a wheelchair for mobility: "She used to be so pretty." In fact, the accident left no scar but changed only her mode of mobility.

***Economics.*** Women experience greater effects from disability than men in that they earn less, work less, and are studied less.[2–5] High divorce rates are associated with disability; the highest rates are when the woman is the disabled spouse.[6]

## NEGATIVE ATTITUDES AMONG HEALTH CARE WORKERS

Health care providers have negative attitudes toward women with disabilities[7] and expect less of them.[8] Often, health care providers speak without sensitivity. They are frequently unaware of how many adults with disabilities live independently in the community, use adaptive equipment, modify homes, and use attendant care.[9] Moreover, professionals are more aware of predominately male disabilities and underestimate the frequency of disabilities among women.[2]

***Asexual Misperception.*** Women with disabilities, especially those growing up with a disability, are seen by health care providers as asexual.[10–14] To the contrary, these women have numerous needs. Thirty-two women with disabilities reported, unanimously, their need for health care providers to see them as sexual beings.[8] Denying the sexuality of a woman limits the services that are provided for her.

***Lowered Expectations.*** Health care providers are among those who often send the message that a woman's body is unacceptable.[10,11] Expectations are that women with disabilities are less likely to marry or have children; they may be seen as more dependent, weak, and less able to care for themselves or a child.[15]

- School nurses given the same vignette about young adolescents with and without disabilities starting their menstrual period for the first time at school held different expectations for knowledge, self-care, and independence based only on the adolescents' use of a wheelchair for mobility.[16]
- Characteristically, clinic and hospital personnel talk to the person who is accompanying the individual with a disability, not to the individual herself. In addition, they frequently "talk down" or use language patterns appropriate for a child.[8]

***Surmised Retardation.*** Often women are treated as if physical disability means mental retardation, especially if their speech is impaired. Frequently, inebriation is assumed in addition to low IQ.[17] Talking more loudly or more simply is a frequent reaction to speech disability.

***Perceived Parenthood Conflict.*** Conflict is perceived between carrying out the responsibilities of parenthood and complying with a medical regimen. Mothers report that health care providers seem unable to recognize the profound interrelationship between their mothering responsibilities and chronic illness or disability. Many women hold the opinion that it is a contradiction to be both an effective mother and a "good patient."[18]

***Ineffective Terminology.*** Language is a powerful communicator of negative attitudes. Communication needs to be inclusive, and limiting, stereotypic terms avoided.

### ARCHITECTURAL BARRIERS

Health care clinics that have architectural barriers limit the independence of women with mobility limitations. Access to buildings via appropriately constructed ramps and to elevators is critical to quality care, as is easy access to bathrooms and examination rooms.

### SPECIAL PROBLEMS

***Sight and Hearing Impairment.*** Deaf or blind clients are limited in their ability to communicate with providers if interpreters are not available. If a woman provides an interpreter, she loses the option of having private interaction with the provider. If sign language is used in relating issues of sexuality and sexual intercourse, it should be remembered that sign communication is easily interpreted "across the room"; therefore, attention must be given to interview area.[19]

### GENERAL CONSIDERATIONS

Specific educational resources are listed after the References, at the end of this chapter.

Providers may feel that once a woman experiences a disability, she should return to the homemaker role, even when the disability is not severe. Women who report that their sense of self-esteem is tied to work are least likely to report a specific disability.[21]

***Severe Disability.*** Women institutionalized with severe multiple disabilities, including cognitive impairment, may have such clinical problems as vaginal discharge, menstrual cycle dysfunction, and oligomenorrhea. Sensitive on-site management is essential.[20] The severity of physical impairment, however, is not a good predictor of the impact of a disability on a woman.[8,19,21]

Providers need to assess the assumptions they hold. They may be surprised to learn that the severity of physical impairment is not a good predictor of impact of the disability on women.[8,11,23] In fact, fatigue and pain have been found to be predictors of health outcomes even after the impact of functional ability has been taken into consideration.

## SEXUALITY

### COMMUNICATION AND EDUCATION

Communicating and obtaining information about sexuality are among a woman's greatest concerns. The subject of sexuality and disabled women has been studied little, perhaps because of the erroneous assumption that among clients with a disability, sexuality adjustment is less an issue for women than for men.[6] Women report that professionals rarely initiate discussion of sexuality issues.[8,22]

The health care provider needs to take responsibility for initiating discussions of sexuality, but also important is offering "assistance rather than avoiding or overemphasizing the issue."[6] Assumptions should not be made at either extreme: none of these women have sexuality issues, or all of them do. Instead, assess each individual.

Some authors propose that the primary barriers to full expression of sexuality are the negative attitudes of others, especially family members and medical and rehabilitation professionals. The attitude that the disability has somehow "neutered" the woman interferes with her belief in her right to sexual feelings and expression.[13,19,20]

***Questions on How Sexuality Is Affected.*** The specific effects of a disability on sexual activity need to be communicated to a woman. For example, in some conditions spasticity might be experienced with orgasm.[23]

***The PLISSIT Model.*** This model, used to order levels of intervention for clients with sexual issues, is helpful for health care providers (see Chapter 4). PLISSIT is derived from "Permission giving, provision of Limited Information and Specific Suggestions, Intensive Therapy." All providers need to be skilled in permission giving, reinforcing the ability for a woman with a disability to be a sexual person and involved in sexual activities. The professional needs to understand and convey to women with disabilities that any manifestation of sexuality which is acceptable and satisfying to the individual or individuals involved is normal.

## BODY IMAGE

Concerns about body image exist for some women with disabilities.[16] The reactions of others may suggest to a woman that her body is unacceptable.

***Perceived Lack of Control.*** Issues such as physical dependency, bladder incontinence, spasticity, or other involuntary movements, which are not seen as adult conditions may make the woman with a disability seem like an infant. The lack of control can lead to a mind–body split. "It was like my body belonged to the doctors, it wasn't mine any more." "Once I put my feet up in the stirrups, I had no control—my body belonged to them [examiners]."[8]

***Appliances.*** The need to use appliances or equipment may interfere with a woman's sense of self as sexually desirable.

***Source of Trouble.*** The body may have a history of "causing" trouble. If a child grew up with a disability, her body may have caused parents trouble and could have become the "enemy."

## SPASTICITY

Spasticity can be elicited by a variety of tactile stimulations. Each woman needs to determine the ability of a variety of sexual activities to produce this response. Slow building stimulation may produce less spasticity than more intense stimulation. Women with spasticity might experience spasticity with orgasm.[23] The knee–chest position during sexual activities may facilitate decrease in spasticity.

## SPINAL CORD INJURY

Because a women's fertility is not affected in a spinal cord injury, many providers and researchers have assumed no sexuality problems exist. Spinal cord injury precipitates specific physiological changes that reflect the level of cord injury and the completeness of the lesion. Some authors categorize lesions as above thoracic 10, between thoracic 10 and 12, and distal to thoracic 12.[23] Women with complete lesions experience neither traditional orgasm, nor clitoral or vaginal sensation[21,24–26]; however, women with spinal cord injury do report satisfying pleasurable orgasmlike sensations from stimulation of the breasts, ears, or other sensitive areas.[25] Even women with complete lesions report psychological and even physical sensations of orgasm or "intense pleasure" during sex.[26] In addition, menstrual discomfort may remain, even if altered.[26]

***Change in Patterns.*** Adjustment in the first years after injury are most difficult. Some women report issues revolving around physical problems (bladder control, dry vagina), but issues regarding social interaction (attitudes of others) are numerous.[6] Changes in the reproductive system are listed:

- Temporary cessation of menses is normal for several months following injury.
- Patterns of sexual activity for women with a disability may be decreased. Many women report the lack of a partner. It is important, however, to remember that the problem is universal. Participants in a Sexual Attitude Reassessment (SAR) workshop reported they were not as active as they wished (women without disability 56 percent, women disabled 57 percent).[19]
- Alternative areas of sexual stimulation and strategies for sexual expression need to be identified, including alternative positions, such as side lying, knee–chest positions, and chair sitting, for paraplegics and quadriplegics[23] and the stuffing technique (of flaccid penis) for women whose partner is paraplegic. If graphic depiction of positions for sexual intercourse would be helpful, the health care provider needs to communicate the appropriate resources.[23]
- The normal sexual responses that may occur are opening of the labia, contraction of the outer third of the vagina, expansion of the inner two-thirds of the vagina, and uterine contraction.

***Autonomic Dysreflexia.*** A potentially fatal complication for women with spinal cord injury, autonomic dysreflexia, occurs if the lesion is complete and above T-6 and can lead to a stroke.[13]

Autonomic dysreflexia is a physiological reflex response to stimulation. Stimulation may be caused by conditions such as skin breakdown, bladder hyperdistention often due to kinked tubing, bowel distention, severe constipation, pelvic examination, labor, or intercourse positions.

Patterns of response vary among individuals; however, among all who have a complete lesion, the pathway within the cord that transmits sensations to higher levels is blocked. So, too, is the mechanism that relays messages downward from the brain. Consequently, blood pressure is not suppressed, and blood pressure rises with sustained reflex. As long as the sensation continues, the blood pressure continues to rise. Normal blood pressure for women with spinal injury is often lower than normal, for example, 90/60. Blood pressure in early dysreflexia might be 140/80. At this level a woman could have significant symptoms of dysreflexia.

Dysreflexia is often overlooked by health care providers who do not know about the altered blood pressure norm. Headache, sweating, goose flesh above the level of lesion, flushed face, and nasal stuffiness are other signs of this potentially lethal complication.

Sources of stimulation can be additive. For example, if a client is slightly constipated or sitting or lying on an object, or her urine drainage system is slightly kinked, an additional stimulation such as a pelvic exam, sexual intercourse, or labor contraction could trigger dysreflexia. If dysreflexia occurs, the total situation must be assessed for hidden problems.

- If dysreflexia occurs during a procedure, *have the client sit up immediately.* Blood pressure increases when a person is lying down. A semisitting position is helpful to prevent dysreflexia during pelvic exams. Labor in that position might be helpful if it is comfortable.

- Monitor blood pressure during labor contractions.
- Assist the client in establishing effective bowel and bladder routines, which can prevent or reduce accidents and decrease the chance of additive dysreflexia episodes.
- Take extreme care to protect skin when transferring the client to an examining table.
- May need medication for acute episodes or on a long term basis. Unresponsive dysreflexia is a medical emergency.

A woman with a spinal cord injury who is educated about the symptoms of autonomic dysreflexia needs to be listened to. She may have a card with treatment outlined or a hotline for contacting a rehabilitation consultant. Discuss the pattern of autonomic dysreflexia with all women with spinal cord injury before high-risk situations (pelvic examination, labor, catheter change, etc.) occur.[13] Ask the client about the frequency of the symptoms, triggering factors, and usual treatment. Were there any episodes in which she did not respond? Does she take medications routinely?

***Latex Allergy.*** Since 1991 the Centers for Disease Control and Prevention (CDC) has been receiving an increasing number of reports of latex-related allergy. Individuals (especially children) with spina bifida or myelomeningocele (a congenital spinal cord injury) have the highest incidence of latex allergy, varying from 12% to 40%[26a,26b] of the population. This condition also occurs in some women with multiple congenital malformations especially multiple urinary anomalies and in some health care providers with increased latex exposure. Reaction varies from mild wheal and flare episodes to anaphylatic reactions.[26c] The latter are most frequently related to surgery.

Most children/adolescents who have developed this allergy have reacted to balloons and gloves; however, condoms, dental dams, and urinary catheters have also created allergic response. Women with spina bifida are considered high risk and should be tested for latex allergy (RAST—radioallergosorbent testing).[26d] Health care providers need to be alert to the possibility of latex sensitivities in their clients. Avoidance of latex materials (condoms, diaphragms, latex gloves) may be recommended for all individuals with spina bifida. Individuals with a confirmed allergy should wear a medic alert bracelet and carry an epinephrine autoinjector kit.[26e]

## JOINT INFLEXIBILITY AND PAIN

Arthrogryposis congenita, sickle cell anemia with joint involvement, arthritis, severe scoliosis, amputation, and dwarfism may result in joint inflexibility and pain. With respect to sexual activity, careful assessment of physical parameters, such as range of motion, is helpful. Discussion about alternative positioning may follow. The importance of extended foreplay, possible gentle warming up and stretching, and use of vibration, massage, or masturbation to achieve orgasm may also be considered. Sexual activity may augment an overall sense of comfort, as orgasm releases endorphins. The client may profit from some helpful suggestions.

- Choose the time of day for sexual activity relative to pain history.
- Consider a warm shower or compress in foreplay if effective in pain relief.
- Consider medicine for pain relief before intercourse if pain is limiting.
- Consider referral to a physical therapist for comprehensive muscle assessment in complex cases.

Assess social support. Data indicate that after controlling for physical limitations and social integration, social support was found to influence the outcome in women with arthritis.[27]

Encourage a positive, proactive attitude. Self-assessed health status is a powerful predictor of function.[28]

## MULTIPLE SCLEROSIS

The symptoms of multiple sclerosis may vary greatly and may include spasticity, dry vagina, fatigue, muscle weakness, pain, and bladder and bowel incontinence. No change, however, occurs in fertility or menstruation. Balance and fatigue may necessitate energy-sparing sexual activities and positions for intercourse. A water-soluble lubricant may be used if the vagina is dry. Data indicate that about half of women who have multiple sclerosis report changes in their sexual life.[29]

## DIABETES MELLITUS

The effect of diabetes on the sexuality of women is unclear, although sexual changes have been identified among men who have diabetes. Therefore, because genitosexual innervation appears to be analogous in males and females,[30] the potential for dysfunction among women also exists; however, data indicate that diabetic women do not differ in sexual function from their healthy controls.[30]

Spontaneous remission of sexual dysfunction reported on 6-year follow-up was related to improvement in the overall marital and social situations. Acceptance of illness (as judged by interviewer) and psychological distress were strong predictors of sexual function. From these data, it appears that sexual function is related to psychological adjustment to chronic illness.[31]

## EPILEPSY

Sexual function does not appear to be affected by epilepsy. The condition has only minor impact on hormonal status.[32]

## URINARY AND BOWEL APPLIANCES

Apparatus may discourage sexual activity. Steps, however, can be taken to ease discomforts.

- Foley catheters can be taped out of the way or removed, but may need to be reinserted soon after sexual activity; individuals using intermittent catheterizations should catheterize before sexual activity to prevent urine leakage.
- Stomal appliances can be ignored, changed, covered, or removed before sexual activity, based on what has been ordered and individual preference.
- Clients should be told that masturbation and coitus may stimulate bladder or bowel incontinence.
- Discussing how to tell potential partners about bladder and bowel issues may be critical. Role playing may be helpful.

## PELVIC RADIOTHERAPY

Radiation may cause vaginal constriction,[17] resulting in dyspareunia.

## CHANGES IN MENARCHE

It appears that some variations in menarche occur among women with select disabilities. For example, individuals with Down syndrome and spinal bifida experience menarche 11 months earlier than a comparison group of nondisabled subjects; however, others with genetic disabilities may have delayed menarche.[20,33] Individuals with blindness experience menarche earlier than normal. Head injury is also associated with precocious puberty.[34] Most women with spinal cord injury report the same or more discomfort with their menses after injury.[26]

## PERSONAL CARE ATTENDANT

Many women with mobility or sensory limitations employ a personal care attendant. She may address some unique sexuality issues; for example, she may place the cervical cap or diaphragm and carry out the bowel or bladder program before sexual activity. Spouses and significant others often function as personal care attendants, but it can be difficult to be both care provider and lover. Each couple needs to address this issue. If both the woman and her partner are disabled the attendant may assist in positioning the couple.

### PLANNING SEXUAL ACTIVITIES

Women report a need to avoid spontaneity and instead plan for sexual activity. This need, however, can be seen as a benefit: Because many disabled persons must communicate with their partners about sexual possibilities and restrictions, this opens up avenues for communication in other areas of the relationship. Unfortunately, many people who are totally physically independent may never experience such communication.[11]

### ABUSE

Women with physical and cognitive disabilities may be at higher risk for abuse.[35] Educational programs need to be developed to address skill building in coping with potential or real abuse and orientation to sexuality rights and responsibilities.[36] Assess the woman's history of abuse.

In addition, health care providers need to include sexual assertiveness skills in sex education or family life education curricula. The optimal time for this education is in childhood or adolescence. Professionals need to seek out opportunities to act as a consul-tant to schools and community groups that serve this population (YWCA, Independent Living Center, local school districts, and schools).

### PHARMACOLOGICAL AGENTS

A number of drugs may have a negative impact on sexual function. A full assessment of both prescription and over-the-counter drugs is critical when addressing issues of sexuality with women who have a disability.[13]

## HISTORY

### INSPECTION OF SELF

Examiners should look at their own attitudes and expectations before eliciting a history from women with disabilities, to determine potential problems. Do not vary the history protocol to omit potential issues. If you usually ask about first sexual experiences, birth control, episodes of unwanted intercourse, or satisfaction with intimate relationships, also ask women with disabilities. In doing so, it is important to watch your "handicapism" terms and use inclusive and sensitive language (see Table 19–1).

### SEXUAL EDUCATION HISTORY

The woman's knowledge of sexuality is pertinent. What was her family life while in school? Does she understand what implications her disability has for sexuality, contraception, birth control, and routine health needs? Ask if sexual information given either in adolescence or during rehabilitation was sufficient. From discussions with the client, determine knowledge deficits. In addition, identify unmet sexual and health needs. Include review of condition-specific issues such as dysreflexia for women with spinal cord injury, latex allergy for women with spina bifida, or spasticity issues for women with cerebral palsy. Ask all women about any allergy type reactions to latex products (balloons, rubber products, condoms, for example).

### PROBLEMS PRESENTED

Ask the client what problems the disability has presented and how she has overcome these barriers.

**TABLE 19–1. LANGUAGE GUIDELINES FOR USE WHEN INTERACTING WITH WOMEN WHO HAVE A DISABILITY**

1. Where possible, emphasize an individual, not a disability. Say "people or persons with disabilities" or "person who is blind" rather than "disabled persons" or "blind person." (Many individuals prefer to use the words *physically challenged* to describe this population.)
2. Avoid using emotional descriptors such as unfortunate, pitiful, and so on. Emphasize abilities, such as "walks with crutches (braces)" rather than "is crippled," "is partially sighted" rather than "partially blind."
3. Talk directly to the person with a disability. If using an interpreter, speak facing the person with hearing impairment.
4. Avoid labeling persons into groups, as in "the disabled," "the deaf," "retardate," and "the arthritic." Instead, say "people who are deaf," "person with arthritis," and "persons with disabilities."
5. Do not sensationalize a disability by saying "afflicted with," "victim of," and so on. Instead, say "person who has multiple sclerosis" or "person who has polio."
6. Avoid portraying persons with disabilities who succeed as superhuman. This implies that persons who are disabled have no talents or unusual gifts.
7. Position yourself at eye level with the individual.
8. Avoid use of "confined to wheelchair." Instead, consider "wheelchair user." Indeed many individuals are liberated by a wheelchair rather than limited by the chair.
9. Ask permission before leaning on or moving equipment, such as a wheelchair.

***Specific Language Guidelines***

*Disability (disabled, physically disabled).* General term used for a (semi)permanent condition that interferes with a person's ability to do something independently—walk, see, hear, learn, lift. It may refer to a physical, mental, or sensory condition. Preferred usage is as a descriptive noun or adjective, as in persons who are disabled, people with disabilities, or disabled persons. Terms such as the disabled, crippled, deformed, and invalid are inappropriate.

*Handicap.* Often used as a synonym for disability. However, usage has become less acceptable (one origin is from "cap in hand," as in begging). Except when citing laws or regulations, *handicap* should not be used to describe a disability. This word can be used to describe the society or environment that limits accessibility.

*Down Syndrome.* Preferred over *mongoloid* to describe a form of mental retardation caused by improper chromosomal division during gestation.

*Mute, or Person Who Cannot Speak.* Preferred terms to describe persons who cannot speak. Terms such as *deaf-mute* and *deaf and dumb* are inappropriate. They imply that persons without speech are always deaf.

*Nondisabled.* In a media portrayal of persons with and without disabilities, *nondisabled* is the appropriate term for persons without disabilities. Able-bodied should not be used, as it implies that persons with disabilities are less able. *Normal* is appropriate only in reference to statistical norms.

*Seizure.* Describes an involuntary muscular contraction symptomatic of the brain disorder epilepsy. Rather than saying "epileptic," say a "person with epilepsy" or "person with a seizure disorder." The term *convulsion* should be reserved for seizures involving contractions of the entire body. The term *fit* is used by the medical profession in England, but it has strong negative connotations.

*Spastic.* Describes a muscle with sudden, abnormal involuntary spasms. It is not appropriate for describing a person with cerebral palsy. *Muscles, not people, are spastic.*

*Speech Impaired.* Describes persons with limited or difficult speech patterns.

*Cesarean Birth.* Should be used to describe a surgical birth. Avoid "section," it depersonalizes. Grapefruits get sectioned; women give birth.

*Adapted from* Guidelines for reporting and writing about people with disabilities. *Media Project, Research and Training Center on Independent Living (348 Haworth Hall, University of Kansas, Lawrence, KS 66045) and Sawin, K.J. (1986). Physical disability. In* Contemporary women's health. *Menlo Park, CA: Addison–Wesley.*

# PHYSICAL EXAMINATION

## PHYSICAL ACCESSIBILITY OF CLINIC

***Physical Layout.*** In assessing the physical layout of a clinic, determine wheelchair accessibility, for example, ramp dimensions, bathrooms, and doorways. Using a wheelchair may be helpful in assessing the environment. Lack of accessibility promotes the dependence of clients.[37]

The Americans With Disabilities Act, enacted in 1990, mandates that all new buildings meet minimal accessibility standards. Section 504 of the Persons With Disabilities Act of 1978 applies to all facilities receiving any federal funds. The regulations do not require that a facility have special programs or services.

The regulations do, however, require that the same services offered to women without disabilities must be offered to women with disabilities.[38] For example, if women without disabilities are weighed, accurate mechanisms are needed to weigh women with disabilities. Wheelchair-accessible scales can be used to weigh ambulating women as well. If the clinic offers Pap smears and pelvic examinations, it needs to offer women with disabilities the same services and to make necessary accommodations.

***Accessible Supportive Examination Table.*** A table at wheelchair height facilitates transfer of women with motor disabilities. The Mid-Mark 514 table or equivalent adjusts to wheelchair height to facilitate transfer to the table; it provides arm rests to support women with cerebral palsy and spasticity who may fear falling off the table when severe or unexpected spasms occur. The absence of leg support, however, may be a major drawback for women with leg weakness or paralysis. Examination tables that have leg support but are not at wheelchair height may be preferred in some settings. Each setting needs to assess its target population for services and provide the most accessible examination table.

***Client's Equipment.*** The health care provider must realize that the wheelchair, crutches, and/or other equipment are part of the client's personal space. Ask permission from the client before sitting or leaning on the equipment or moving it, particularly when the client is in it or on the examination table, where she may want her equipment close by.

***Special Equipment.*** Equipment such as non-latex gloves, plastic catheters, and nonlatex pads needs to be available.

## PSYCHOLOGICAL ACCESSIBILITY

It has been suggested that the client may find it more difficult to gain psychological accessibility to the health care provider than physical accessibility to the clinic. Providers must limit stereotypes, actively pursue optimal communication procedures, value mutual problem solving and goal setting, and use every opportunity to reaffirm normalcy. In a clinical setting, guidelines are needed to enhance accessibility, beginning with the first telephone contact. Proposed guidelines have been delineated by the Task Force on Concerns of Physically Disabled Women.[37] When the first appointment is made, clients should be asked:

- Do you have a physical disability? If so, ask the client to specify if it is difficulty getting around, hearing, or seeing, and so on.
- What accommodations will be necessary for your visit to the clinic? Arrangements may need to be made that will allow for a longer visit.

## ALTERED PELVIC EXAMINATION

***Mutual Problem Solving.*** A health care provider must be aware that a client with disabilities may need an altered pelvic examination.[19,22] Discussion with the client should attempt to solve problems she might have had during previous pelvic exams. Ask what positions caused problems and what worked best for her. Additional personnel may be needed to assist in supporting the client (e.g., holding legs) during the exam. The client should collaborate in deciding the need. She may prefer to bring a family member or friend with her to the exam.

***Altered Range of Motion.*** A side-lying position or speculum exam with "handle up" may be necessary because of alterations in range of motion.

***Spasticity.*** Women with cerebral palsy report spasms, especially adductor spasms, which may be controlled if the woman takes the knee–chest position, with an assistant "hugging" her,[19] or the side-lying position, with the bottom leg flexed and upper leg on the examiner's shoulder (similar to left lateral delivery position).[39] Keeping the woman's extremities close to the body decreases movement that may stimulate additional spasms.

***Amputation and Decreased Range of Motion.*** The client may be examined in a semisitting position. She may choose to hold the stump herself and place the other leg on the examiner's shoulder or she may choose to have assistance with holding her stump so she can hold a mirror and participate in the examination.

***Specific Examination.*** Examination of the genitalia must include inspection of the vaginal walls for atrophic changes, determination of intravaginal tone, and assessment of hair distribution in the genital region to help rule out possible endocrinopathies.[13] Some authors suggest select use of the Q-Tip Pap smear for the rare woman with disabilities who is unable to tolerate a speculum examination. This technique is much less accurate, however, and every effort should be made to assist the client and her family to understand the implications of its use.[40]

***Reaffirming Normalcy.*** During the pelvic examination, reaffirm the client's identified normalcy and healthy status. This makes a strong positive impact on her perception of self.

### BREAST SELF-EXAMINATION

In some rehabilitation and primary care settings, breast self-examination is not discussed with women with disabilities, even when they present for gynecological examinations. Women with intact manual dexterity and sensation, however, can be taught breast self-examination. Moreover, some women with impaired sensation can perform a modified examination or an attendant or partner can perform it. If neither of these plans is acceptable, more frequent examination by a health care provider should be considered.[19]

## CONTRACEPTION

### LACK OF INFORMATION

Information on contraception is often not offered to women with disabilities.[22] It is important, however, for health care providers to examine the options with clients. The choice may be a balance of risk factors,[41] for example, the risk of pregnancy versus the risk of the contraceptive method. If oral contraception or an intrauterine device (IUD) is considered and the method carries risk, consultation with or referral to a gynecological specialist needs to be initiated.

Discussion of alternatives needs to take place with the women who is allergic or whose partner is allergic to latex. Contraceptive options may be significantly restricted for women with mobility impairment or with a latex allergy. Joint management with a physician colleague is indicated.

## ADOLESCENTS

To prove that they are normal, adolescents with chronic illness or disability often increase their sexual behavior. Consequently, they are at increased risk of pregnancy, sexually transmitted diseases, and abuse.[17] Primary care of all adolescent women with chronic illness and disability must include assessment of the potential for sexual activity or actual sexual activity and the need for contraception.

## TIMING OF DISABILITY

It is not clear what impact the timing of disability onset has on a woman's satisfaction with contraception and sexuality information. Women whose onset of disability is after menarche are identified by some as having special needs for contraception and sexuality.[22] Other data suggest that women who grow up with their disability do not have adequate sexuality and contraception counseling.[8,19] The need for sexuality and contraception counseling must be assessed regardless of the time of onset.

## BARRIER METHODS

Barrier methods are often an optimal choice. If a client has manual limitations and, consequently, difficulty manipulating a barrier device, it is important to determine the availability of a partner or personal care attendant and their roles. A client may need to explore ways to ask her partner to assist with a barrier method. Many women have not considered asking a personal care attendant to assist with placement of a contraceptive device before sexual activity.

- *Condoms.* Condoms, which also provide protection against AIDS and other sexually transmitted diseases, are an option. Water-soluble lubricants can ease vaginal dryness. Caution should be taken to identify women who have or whose partners have latex allergies. A nonlatex condom (Tactylon), effective against STDs and HIV, is being tested and should be available in 1995.[43]
- *Sponge or cap.* A sponge is easier for some women to insert than a diaphragm. For some women, a cervical cap is more attractive, as it can be inserted in the morning by a personal care attendant and removed 24 hours later, eliminating the need for assistance during lovemaking.[19]
- *Diaphragm.* An increase in urinary infections is associated with the arch diaphragm. It may present particular problems and not be appropriate for women with urinary stasis. Caution should be taken to identify women who have or whose partners have latex allergies.

## IMPLANTED AND INJECTED HORMONAL CONTRACEPTIVES

The literature does not yet discuss the use of Norplant implantation for women with disabilities, but the contraindications to oral hormonal contraception need to be considered in the use of Norplant. If memory or manual dexterity is an issue, Norplant may be a new, efficient option.

In addition, Depo-Provera, although only recently approved for contraceptive use by the Food and Drug Administration, is widely used in other countries. This contraceptive has been prescribed for women, including adolescents, with cognitive impairment; 594 woman-months of experience were reported without pregnancy or side effects.

Parents of youth with cognitive impairment reported high satisfaction with this method.[42] The Committee on Drugs of the American Association of Pharmacists (AAP) has found no evidence that Depo-Provera is harmful.[42] For teens with moderate or severe retardation, the benefits probably outweigh the risks.

An additional benefit of or injected hormones is derived by women with severe mobility restrictions. If these women are dependent on others for menstrual hygiene care, the possible lack or decreased frequency of menstrual periods may increase their functional status.[43]

## SPECIFIC CONDITIONS AND CONTRACEPTIVE NEEDS

Although research is limited, the data that are available for the most frequent disabilities and chronic illnesses are reported here and may be presented in discussions with clients. Because women with disabilities are considered high risk medically, joint management with a physician colleague or referral for a form of contraception other than a barrier method is recommended.

***Spinal Cord Injury.*** The fertility of women with spinal cord injury is unaffected. Their decreased mobility and the increased incidence of deep vein thrombosis place them at high risk with respect to hormonal contraceptives, especially those containing estrogen. Birth control pills and Norplant are absolutely contraindicated if the woman is receiving antihypertensive medication or if she is known to have circulatory problems.[10]

Many women have healthy pregnancies and vaginal births. Some complications (urinary tract infections, immobility, skin breakdown) do occur, but in studies that have been conducted, the incidence is low.[6,10]

Intrauterine devices pose a risk because of the woman's decreased sensation and ability to determine warning signs of infection. Some women, however, indicate that dysreflexia is triggered by the "pain" that the patient is unable to perceive. The women may thus be able to "identify" infection with the occurrence of dysreflexia. In addition, they propose that checking the IUD string placement could be carried out by their partners.

Most women with paraplegia can usually manage barrier methods with no or minimal assistance in positioning legs for effective insertion. Women with higher spinal cord lesions require assistance from a partner or an attendant.

***Multiple Sclerosis.*** The menstrual and fertility patterns of women with multiple sclerosis show no change.[10]

The risk of pregnancy is controversial. Data are conflicting. Some studies show no effect on multiple sclerosis; others indicate exacerbation of the condition during pregnancy and postpartum.[43]

At present, there is significant evidence that hormonal therapy alters the course of multiple sclerosis.[44] Such therapy is, however, contraindicated for women with paralysis or restricted mobility.[10] Of concern is one study that reported that 54 percent of subjects used no contraception because of fear of side effects.[44]

***Cystic Fibrosis.*** Women with cystic fibrosis now live until their thirties, and with increasing technology, the age of survival may increase even further in the next few years. Pregnancy can be a significant risk for both mother and infant.

Data on hormonal contraception are conflicting. The method may cause bronchial mucus to become scant, and it may support the development of endocervical polyps.[44] Pulmonary function and respiratory symptoms were not affected in a small study of 10 young women 15 to 24 years old. Nevertheless, hormonal contraception should be used only with extreme caution and very close monitoring of pulmonary status. There is no contraindication to the use of barrier methods among women with cystic fibrosis.[44]

***Rheumatoid Arthritis.*** Rheumatoid arthritis is known to improve during pregnancy. Some evidence is reported that the onset of arthritis may be delayed by hormonal contraceptives.[43,44] Hormonal therapy, however, has not been shown to affect active disease.

Barrier methods may be difficult for some women to use if they experience weakness and decreased manual dexterity.[44] An intrauterine device may worsen existing anemia.[17]

***Cerebral Palsy.*** The effect of cerebral palsy on contraception varies greatly. If the client is paralyzed or has decreased mobility, hormonal contraception is risky. Independent use of barrier methods, especially the diaphragm or cervical cap, may be troublesome for women with spasticity; however, these methods are viable with partner participation.

***Epilepsy.*** Estrogen levels are related to seizure threshold in women with epilepsy. Seizures vary during the menstrual cycle: incidence is highest during the estradiol spike before ovulation and the rapid drop in progesterone immediately before and during menstruation.

The relationship between oral hormonal therapy and seizures is less evident; however, no strong evidence has been found against the use of hormonal contraception.[44] Most reports of interaction between hormonal agents and seizure medication indicate accelerated breakdown of estrogens and recommend the use of 50 μg estrogen.[43,44]

An intrauterine device should be used with extreme caution. Two reports indicate grand mal seizures with insertion.[44]

***Inflammatory Bowel Disease.*** Data are limited on the relationship between inflammatory bowel disease and use of contraception. It is, however, known that the majority of women with inflammatory bowel disease worsen with pregnancy.[42] It is therefore important that the disease be stable for a year before pregnancy is even considered.

Barrier methods are recommended for contraception. A review of the literature indicates that the use of oral hormonal contraceptives is advised only with reservations; that is, low-dose estrogen or progestin-only oral contraceptives may be taken with close monitoring of the disease by the consulting physician. With active disease or in the presence of malabsorption, hormonal therapy may be ineffective or dangerous.[42]

***Down Syndrome.*** Fertility is unaffected. For many women with Down syndrome, the choice of contraception is affected by mobility, chronic illness, and cognitive factors. In the use of contraception, informed consent is a critical aspect.

- Oral hormonal contraception requires that a woman's memory skills be adequate for the regimen.
- Implants may be attractive to some.
- Women who have multiple disabilities (motor and cognitive) may not be able to manage a diaphragm.
- Adolescents and young women need comprehensive ongoing sex education and accessible adults to assist with problem solving and skill development.

## PREGNANCY

### CONFRONTING NEGATIVE ATTITUDES AND BARRIERS

Disability is not a contraindication to responsible, effective parenting, yet judgmental attitudes continue.[8,19,39,45] Moreover, few agencies exist to assist the increasing number of pregnant women and mothers with disabilities. The majority (81 percent) of registered nurses, nurse practitioners, and occupational and physical therapists indicate their experience, education, and training have not prepared them adequately for this high-risk population.[39]

***Education of Health Care Providers.*** Programs must be developed to address health care providers' lack of information about the needs of mothers with disabilities. Information that is modified to answer questions about the unique situation of women with disabilities is needed. What are the emotional and physical changes of pregnancy? What are the special demands of labor and delivery? What are the adaptive parenting skills and equipment necessary for responsible parenting?

***Consumer Guidance.*** Little information is provided to parents by professionals. One study found that women with rheumatoid arthritis depended on lay resources rather than health professionals for guidance in nutrition; use of alcohol, tobacco, and nonprescription drugs; sexuality; consequences of a pregnancy on their disability or disease; and infant care techniques, equipment, and devices.[39] Health care providers who are involved in coordinating care and have no disability-related experience must consult with others. For example, consideration should be given to speaking with a colleague in rehabilitation or an experienced, active consumer with disabilities.

***Case Management.*** During pregnancy, case management may be indicated for a woman with disabilities. The case manager is responsible for assuring that the client's unique health care needs are being met, especially if numerous agencies are involved.

***Partner Preparation.*** It is important for the health care provider to assess whether a woman's partner needs preparation. The partner may require information from the provider about the woman's special needs in order to give realistic support and avoid unnecessary restrictions. A typical concern of any couple experiencing pregnancy—hesitancy to have sexual relations for fear of hurting the baby—may be expanded for couples in which the woman has a disability; they may be afraid of hurting the woman.[39]

Although it is especially important for health care providers to interact with partners, data indicate that women with disabilities feel their partners are unwanted by health care providers during labor and delivery.[6,45] A prenatal care provider or case manager may need to initiate educational sessions to discuss attitudinal barriers. These activities should be organized well before delivery. If the partner also has a disability, special considerations may be needed to facilitate his involvement.

## ACCESSIBILITY TO LABOR AND DELIVERY FACILITIES

Several questions should be asked about the structure of health care facilities and their accessibility to women with mobility and sensory impairment. Are labor and delivery rooms and bathrooms large enough to transfer women from a wheelchair? Are large showers available without a raised lip, which would prevent a woman from rolling her wheelchair into the shower? Are select rooms large enough to accommodate wheelchairs, consumer-owned specially padded commode chairs, leg braces, crutches, and other equipment?

***Specific Adaptive Needs of Client.*** Determine what the client needs with respect to her condition. Is a pressure relief mattress or raised toilet seat needed? Does she want to bring equipment from home? Plan a tour of the hospital during the fifth or sixth month of pregnancy so that the need for special equipment can be identified, and the equipment ordered.

***Accessibility to Equipment.*** Having necessary equipment within reach is critical to the well-being and comfort of the client.[39]

***Education for All Staff.*** Housekeeping personnel may need to know that a wheelchair positioned in a particular way next to a bed allows a woman to be independent. To move the chair essentially makes the woman a prisoner, as it removes her independence. Nursing staff may need to review prevention of skin shearing, management of dysreflexia, and implications of contraction monitoring.

### PRENATAL AND PERINATAL PERIODS

The effects of a disability on the course of pregnancy are summarized in Table 19–2. Generally, in perinatal management, a health care provider needs to determine if a woman with a disability has access to a role model who has the same disability as she or if the client needs case management services.[46]

***Self-Assessment.*** The client should be able to identify the stressors and fears, both general and specific, that are related to her disability.

***Staff Assessment.*** A woman's muscle strength, activities of daily living, and child care skills must be assessed. Determinations may be made by direct observation, reports of activities, and a child care activity assessment tool.[47,48] Or, referral may be made to a physical or occupational therapist, depending on resources and the severity of the woman's limitations. Assessment needs to be made early in pregnancy in order to design adaptive equipment. For example, one woman with minimal distal muscle strength who wished to breastfeed was able to place the child at the breast and initiate nursing, but did not have the strength to hold the child throughout nursing. Believing that she could not breastfeed, she switched to formula. If she had been assessed early in pregnancy, her strength deficiency might have been identified and referral made to a rehabilitation engineer to design or modify a fabric infant carrier that would support the child during nursing. Most women with a disability are able to nurse their newborn. Indeed, the convenience of breastfeeding can be an advantage for women with mobility limitations.[49]

***Dependency Increase.*** If a woman's dependency increases during pregnancy, there is a need to assess her specific level of function. Similarly, assess the body image issues generated by pregnancy.

***Normal Emotional Changes.*** Reassure the client of the normalcy of emotional fluctuations during pregnancy.

***Cesarean Birth.*** If cesarean birth is a possibility, discuss the options available, including father participation.[19,47]

## PARENTING

Health care providers unfamiliar with the adaptive skills of women with disabilities often question the ability of these women to care for their babies. Availability of a role model with a disability similar to the woman's can be very helpful to both the health care provider and the client. The roles of the parents and other caregivers must be assessed. Moreover, for the provider without expertise in infant care issues, consultation with a pediatric nurse practitioner, pediatrician, occupational therapist, rehabilitation consultant, or rehabilitation engineer may be helpful. In addition, an independent living center or a program that focuses on promoting positive parenting for women with disabilities, such as Through the Looking Glass, may be consulted.[47,48]

### ADAPTATION OF THE FAMILY

***Videotaped Evidence.*** A videotape study of parents with disabilities was conducted and several findings were reported.[47]

**TABLE 19–2. EFFECT OF DISABILITY ON COURSE OF PREGNANCY AND LABOR, DELIVERY, AND POSTPARTUM PERIOD**

| Disability/Disease | Pregnancy | Labor/Delivery/Postpartum |
|---|---|---|
| Spinal cord injury (SCI) | May increase risk for skin problems. Women with SCI have the same problems as nondisabled women (urinary tract infections, constipation, incontinence).[48] Data are scarce. Not clear if frequency of these problems is increased in women with SCI. Anemia may occur. | No premature deliveries, no major complications.[48] Vaginal delivery the norm. Cesarean birth reserved for obstetric indications. Lochial flow and sanitary pads put skin at risk. Frequent perinatal care necessary.[11] Silk sutures should be considered for women having episiotomies.[42] Equilibrium restored and pregnancy-exacerbated bladder, bowel, and skin circulatory problems improved in postpartum.[42] If environment not accessible may need extra assistance in dressing and transferring.[42] |
| | Autonomic dysreflexia increased. 85% of clients with SCI at T-6 or above will experience at some time.[51] Medication may be needed to control condition. Nonresponsive dysreflexia needs immediate medical referral. | Labor/birth in semisitting position.[48] Autonomic dysreflexia increased in second-stage labor.[48] Early identification and treatment essential for maternal/fetal health. Can lead to subarachnoid hemorrhage.[50] In labor, aggressive management critical. Epidural anesthesia often effective.[50] If client does not respond to regional anesthesia, potent short-acting hypotensive appropriate (trimethaphan).[50,51] Blood pressure monitoring frequently if not continuously. Take BP during contraction. Critical to avoid known causes.[48] Often misinterpreted as preeclampsia. Treatment is different. Can be triggered by catheterization, enema, insertion of uterine catheter if fetal monitor used, contractions, or insertion of IV lines.[49] May also occur if woman sits on episiotomy[6] or during breastfeeding.[48] |
| | Nausea and vomiting can be especially uncomfortable with limited mobility. Women who use wheelchairs may already experience orthostatic edema, which may be accentuated, not only increasing edema but increasing risk of skin problems. Frequency of weight shifts and position changes may need to increase. Need close monitoring of skin daily.[42] | Assess labor and delivery bed/table for skin risks. |
| | Psychosocial issues common in pregnancy (not specific to some with SCI but comparable frequency not documented).[6,48] | Report being victims of inadequate environmental design that hindered mobility.[48] |

(continued)

**TABLE 19–2. CONTINUED**

| Disability/Disease | Pregnancy | Labor/Delivery/Postparum |
|---|---|---|
| | Report feelings of powerlessness.[6] | Increased if partner blocked from participation in labor and delivery.[6,48] |
| Rheumatoid arthritis | 75% experience remission of disease. Activities of daily living easier to perform due to decreased joint stiffness, swelling, and increase in grip strength.[42] May have overwhelming fatigue. Need to continue supervised exercise routine. For those with hand/shoulder involvement, dressing may become difficult.[48] | Joint contracture may limit positioning. Pain needs to be carefully assessed. 95% will experience flareup of symptoms.[42] |
| Multiple sclerosis | Pregnancy and postpregnancy stress may increase symptoms, but reports are conflicting.[14] | Risk for exacerbation of symptoms may be greater in the postpartum. |
| Impaired vision | Changing body may dramatically affect ability to function (as the center of gravity changes, client may have difficult time with body space and her relation to object). Use tactile models. Assist to palpate abdomen. Lack of material in Braille or audiotape on anatomy/physiology/pregnancy/infant care necessitates increased individual teaching. Birth rehearsal in labor room helps orient self to room, bed, and bathroom. | Needs lots of labeling of people and equipment. Introduce self and identify function. Elicit woman's input on amount of light needed in labor/delivery areas. Important to describe infant and his/her specific reactions, behaviors, and facial expressions; will assist mom to attach.[42] May use tactile calibrated bottle.[42] |
| Impaired hearing | Talk to woman even if interpreter uses eye-to-eye contact; get attention before proceeding. | Visual interaction critical. Assess light needed. Assess if client needs to be in room where nurses' station can be seen.[42] |

- Infants adapt extremely early to their mothers who have physical disabilities.
- Mothers develop the ability to read their infants' states and teach them to assist with necessary movement.
- Children differentiate between care providers. For example, an active toddler lies still during a long diapering by the blind father, but resists and struggles from the outset with the sighted mother.

***Equipment as Part of the Environment.*** It is common for children to consider a parent's equipment, such as wheelchairs and reachers, as ordinary parts of their environment without negative connotations. A toddler was overheard talking with her mom during a basketball tournament in which there was a wheelchair division. While observing a game played by nondisabled college students, she said, "Mom, what are they doing?" "Playing basketball, Honey." "But Mom, where are their wheelchairs?"

***Animals.*** If a woman with a disability uses a guide dog or other animal to assist with impaired mobility, close assessment must be made of its impact on child care.

***Equipment Adaptation for Child Care.*** A woman with impaired mobility can alter equipment or procedures to assist with child care.[39]

- Women with mobility impairment may face special adaptation needs as parents.[39] Women who previously used an manual wheelchair may choose to use an electrical wheelchair to free hands for child care.
- Furniture may need to be altered so that the woman can wheel up to the crib, changing table, or reclined stroller and be able to change the baby without moving it. Furniture may also be altered to create firm raised edges for infant safety and to assist the woman with decreased hand or arm strength.
- Velcro can be sewn on the clothes of both mother and baby for necessary alterations. For example, breastfeeding may be made easier if the mother's bra and blouse have Velcro fasteners. Also, Velcro fasteners on the infant's clothes assist the mother in dressing her baby.[45]
- Bottle holders and bottle devices, such as a tactile calibrated bottle, may be helpful, as may adapting a breastfeeding position in the wheelchair.[39]

***Impaired Vision and Hearing.*** A woman with impaired vision or hearing can also adapt procedures for child care.[39] The provider may need to facilitate the mother's interaction with her infant. The Brazelton tool is used to teach a mother about the states of the infant.[50] For a woman with impaired vision, the focus is on her hearing and touching and how they increase interaction with the infant. On the other hand, for women with hearing impairment, a visual role model, tactile stimulation, and musical toys are used. If both parents have sensory impairment, referral to an infant stimulation program should be considered.

Monitoring devices in a room or on a child can be helpful. Audiovisual resources may be useful.

## REFERENCES

1. Deegan, M.J. (1981). Multiple minority groups: A case study of physically disabled women. *Journal of Sociology and Social Welfare, 8,* 274–297.
2. Westbrook, M.T., & Adamson, B.J. (1989). Gender differences in allied health student's knowledge of disabled women and men. *Women Health, 15*(4), 93–110.
3. Vash, C.L. (1982). Employment issues for women with disabilities. *Rehabilitation Literature, 43,* 198–207.
4. Perlman, L., & Arneson, D. (1982). *Women and rehabilitation of disabled persons.* A report of the sixth Annual Mary E. Switzer Memorial Seminar. Washington, DC: National Rehabilitation Association.
5. Brooks, N.A. (1981). *Independent living and women with disabilities.* Unpublished paper, Wichita State University.
6. Drew, J. (1990). *Implications for nursing practice: A five-year review of recent spinal injury research.* Paper presented at 16th Annual Conference, Association of Rehabilitation Nursing, Phoenix, AZ.
7. Zwerner, J. (1982). Yes we have troubles but nobody's listening: Sexual issues of women with spinal cord injury. *Sexuality and Disability, 5*(3), 158–171.
8. Sawin K.J. (1982). *Disabled women's perception on a health care visit for a physical examination.* Paper presented at 8th Annual Conference, Association of Rehabilitation Nursing, Denver, CO.
9. Kirshbaum, M. (1988). Parents with physical disabilities and their babies. *Zero to Three, 8*(5), 7–11.

10. The Boston Women's Health Book Collective. (1984). *The New Our Bodies, Ourselves.* New York: Simon & Schuster.
11. Bogle, J.E., & Shaul, S.L. (1981). Body image and the woman with a disability. In D.G. Bullard & S.E. Knight (Eds.), *Sexuality and Physical Disability.* St. Louis: C.V. Mosby.
12. DeHaan, C.B., & Wallander, J.L. (1988). Self concept, sexual knowledge and attitudes, and parental support in the sexual adjustment of women with early- and late-onset physical disability. *Archives of Sexual Behavior, 17,* 145–161.
13. Zasler, N.D. (1991). Sexuality in neurologic disability: An overview. *Sexuality and Disability, 9,* 11–27.
14. Drench, M.E. (1992). Impact of altered sexuality and sexual function in spinal cord injury: A review. *Sexuality and Disability, 10,* 3–14.
15. Duffy, Y. (1981). *All things are possible.* Ann Arbor, MI: A. J. Garvin & Associates.
16. Tsy, A.M., & Opie, N.D. (1986). Menarche in the severely disabled adolescent: School nurses' attitudes, perceptions and perceived teaching responsibilities. *Journal of School Health, 56*(10), 443–447.
17. Greydanus, D., Demarest, D.S., & Sears, M.J. (1985). Sexual dysfunction in adolescents. *Seminars in Adolescent Medicine, 1*(3), 177–187.
18. Thorne, S.E. (1990). Mothers with chronic illness: A predicament of social construction. *Health Care Women International, 11*(2), 209–221.
19. Sawin, K.J. (1986). Physical disability. In J. Griffith-Kinney (Ed.), *Contemporary Women's Health.* Reading, MA: Addison–Wesley.
20. Furman, L.M. (1989). Institutionalized disabled adolescents: Gynecologic care. *Clinical Pediatrics, 28,* 163–170.
21. Mudrick, N.R. (1988). Predictors of disability among midlife men and women: Differences by severity of impairment. *Community Health, 13*(2), 70–84.
22. Beckmann, C.R., Gittler, M., Barzansky, B.M., & Beckmann, C.A. (1989). Gynecologic health care of women with disabilities. *Obstetrical Gynecology, 74*(1), 75–79.
23. Berhard, E.J. (1989). The sexuality of spinal cord injured women: Physiology and pathophysiology. A review. *Paraplegia, 27*(2), 99–112.
24. Cole, T.M. (1975). Sexuality and the spinal cord injured. In R. Green (Ed.), *Human sexuality: A health practitioner's text* (2nd ed.), pp. 146–169. Baltimore: Williams & Wilkins.
25. Page, R.C., Cheng, H., Pate, T.C., Mathus, B., Pryor, D., & Ko, J. (1987). The perception of spinal cord injured persons toward sex. *Sexuality and Disability Journal, 8*(2) 112–132.
26. Kettl, P., Zarefoss, S., Jacoby, K., German, C., Hulse, C., Rowley, F., Corey, R., Sredy, M., Bixler, E., & Tyson, K. (1991). Female sexuality after spinal cord injury. *Sexuality and Disability, 9,* 287–295.
26a. Pearson, M.L., Cole, J.S., & Jarvis, W.R. (1994). How common is latex allergy? A survey of children with myelodysplasia. *Developmental Medicine and Child Neurology, 36,* 64–69.
26b. Banta, J.V., Bonanni, C., & Prebluda, J. (1993). Latex anaphylaxis during spinal surgery in children with myelomeningocele. *Developmental Medicine and Child Neurology, 35*(6), 543–548.
26c. Barton, E.C. (1993). Latex allergy: Recognition and management of a modern problem. *Nurse Practitioner, 18*(11), 54–85.
26d. Tosi, L., Slater, J.E., Shaer, C., & Mostello, L.A. (1993). Latex allergy in spina bifida patients: Prevalence and surgical implications. *Journal of Pediatric Orthopedics, 13*(6) 709–712.
27. Goodenow, C., Reisine, S.T., & Grady, K.E. (1990). Quality of social support and associated social and psychological functioning in women with rheumatoid arthritis. *Health Psychology, 9,* 226–284.
28. Reisine, S.T., Grady, K.E., Goodenow, C., & Fifield, J. (1989). Work disability and women with RA: The importance of disability, social, work and family factors. *Arthritis and Rheumatism, 32*(5), 538–543.
29. Stenager, E., Stenager, E.N., Jensen, K., & Boldsen, J. (1990). Multiple sclerosis: Sexual

dysfunctions. *Journal of Sex Education and Therapy, 16,* 262–269.

30. Kolodny, R.C. (1980). *Sexual problems in diabetes and selected endocrine disorders.* Paper presented at 1st Annual Conference on Sexuality and Physical Disabilities: Medical Aspects and Clinical Care, Ann Arbor, MI.
31. Jensen, S.B. (1986). The natural history of sexual dysfunction in diabetic women. A 6-year follow-up study. *Acta Medica Scandinavia, 219*(1), 73–8.
32. Jensen, P., Jensen, S.B., Sorensen, P.S., Bjerre, B.D., Rizzi, D.A., Sorenesen, A.S., Klysner, R., Brinch, K., & Jespersen, B. (1990). Sexual dysfunction in male and female patients with epilepsy: A study of 86 outpatients. *Archives of Sexual Behavior, 19*(1), 1–14.
33. Evans, A.L. (1988). Sexual maturation in girls with severe mental handicap. *Child Care, Health and Development, 14,* 59–69.
34. Sockalosky, J.J., & Kriel, R.L. (1987). Precocious puberty after traumatic brain injury. *Journal of Pediatrics, 110,* 373.
35. Cole, S. (1986). Facing the challenges of sexual abuse in persons with disabilities. *Sexuality and Disability, 7,* 71–87.
36. Elvik, S.L., Berkowitz, C.D., Nichols, E.L., & Inkelis, S.H. (1990). Sexual abuse in the developmentally disabled: Dilemmas of diagnosis. *Child Abuse Neglect, 14*(4), 497–502.
37. Task Force on Concerns of Physically Disabled Women. (1978). *Within reach: Providing family planning services to physically disabled women.* New York: Human Sciences Press.
38. Enforcement of nondiscrimination on the basis of handicap in federally assisted programs. *Federal Register,* December 19, 1990, *55*(244), 52136.
39. Carty, E.M., Tali, C.A., & Hall, L.H. (1990). Comprehensive health promotion for the pregnant women who has disabilities. *Journal of Nurse-Midwifery, 35*(3), 133–190.
40. Ware, L., Muram, D., & Gale, C.L. (1992). Q-Tip Pap smear: Should it be done routinely in patients who have developmental disabilities? *Sexuality and Disability, 10,* 189–192.
41. Pope, A. M., & Tarlov, A. R. (1991). *Disability in America: Summary and recommendations: Toward a national agenda for prevention.* Washington, DC: National Academy Press.
42. Neinstein, L.S., & Katz, B. (1986). Contraceptive use in the chronically ill adolescent female: Part II. *Journal of Adolescent Health Care, 7,* 350–360.
43. Hatcher, R.A., Trussel, J., Stewart, F., Stewart, G.K., Kowal, D., Guest, F., & Cates, W. (1994). *Contraceptive technology* (16th rev. ed.). New York: Irvington.
44. Neinstein, L.S., & Katz, B. (1986). Contraceptive use in the chronically ill adolescent female: Part I. *Journal of Adolescent Health Care, 7,* 123–133.
45. Craig, D.I. (1990). The adaptation to pregnancy of spinal cord injured women. *Rehabilitation Nursing, 15*(1), 6–9.
46. Corbin, J.M. (1987). Women's perceptions and management of pregnancy complicated by chronic illness. *Health Care Women International, 8*(5–6), 317–337.
47. Kirshbaum, M. (1988). Parents with physical disabilities and their babies. *Zero to Three, 8*(5), 7–11.
48. Connie, T.A. (1988). *Aids and adaptations for disabled parents: An illustrated manual for service providers and parents with physical or sensory disabilities* (2nd ed.). Vancouver: School of Rehabilitation Medicine, University of British Columbia.
49. Asreal, W. (1987). The rehabilitation team's role during the childbearing year for disabled women. *Sexuality and Disability, 8,* 47–62.
50. Brazelton, T.B. (1973). *Neonatal behavioral assessment scale.* Philadelphia: J.B. Lippincott.

## RESOURCE LIST

### Physical Accessibility of Health Care Setting

Duffy, Y. (1981). *All things are possible.* Ann Arbor, MI: Garvin & Associates.

Ferreyra, S., & Hughes, K. (1982). *Table manners: Guide to the pelvic examination for dis-*

*abled women and health care providers.* 477 Fifteenth Street, Oakland, CA 94612. Sex Education for Disabled People ($3.50). Written by two differently abled women. Advocates a cooperative approach.

Task Force on Concerns of Physically Disabled Women. (1978). *Within reach: Providing family planning services to physically disabled women.* New York: Human Sciences Press.

Task Force on Concerns of Physically Disabled Sexuality. (1978). *Toward intimacy: Family planning and sexuality concerns of physically disabled women.* New York: Human Sciences Press.

## Parenting and Infant Care

Campion, M.J. (1990). *The baby challenge: A handbook on pregnancy for women with a physical disability.* New York: Tavistock/Routledge.

Cochrane, G.M., & Wilshere, E.R. (Eds.) (1988). *Parents with disabilities.* Oxford, England: Nuffield Orthopaedic Center.

Conine, T.A., Carty, E., & Safarik, P. (1988). *Aids and adaptations for disabled parents: An illustrated manual for service providers and parents with physical or sensory disabilities* (2nd ed.). Vancouver: School of Rehabilitation Medicine, University of British Columbia.

Mathews, J. (1992). *A mother's touch: The Tiffany Callo story.* New York: Henry Holt & Company.

National Newsletter for disabled parents and concerned professionals. Through the Looking Glass, 801 Peralta Avenue, Berkeley, CA 94707.

Ware, N.A., & Schwab, L.O. (1971). The blind mother providing care for an infant. *New Outlook Blind, 65,* 169–173.

## Abuse

Berkowitz, C.D. (1990). Sexual abuse in the physically and developmentally disabled. *Nurse Practitioner Forum, 1*(2), 98–101.

Cole, S. (1986). Facing the challenges of sexual abuse in persons with disabilities. *Sexuality and Disability, 7,* 71–87.

Schor, D.P. (1987). Sex and sexual abuse in developmentally disabled adolescents. *Seminars in Adolescent Medicine, 3*(1), 1–7.

White, R., Benedict, M.I., Wulff, L., & Kelley, M. (1986). Physical disabilities as risk factors for child maltreatment: A selected review. *American Journal of Orthopsychiatry, 57*(1), 93–101.

Woodhead, H.C., & Murph, J.R. (1985). Influence of chronic illness and disability on adolescent sexual development. *Seminars in Adolescent Medicine, 1*(3), 171–176.

## Sex Education

Baugh, R.J. (1984). Sexuality education for the visually and hearing impaired child in the regular classroom. *Journal of School Health, 54*(10), 407–409.

Dickman, I.R. (Ed.). (1975). *Sex education and family life for visually handicapped children and youth: A resource guide.* New York: Siecus.

George Washington University. (1979). *Who cares? A handbook on sex education and counseling services for disabled people.* Washington, DC: Author.

Krajicek, M.J. (1982). Developmental disability and human sexuality. *Nursing Clinics of North America, 17*(3), 377–386.

Kroll, K., & Klein, E.L. (1992). *Enabling romance: A guide to love, sex, and relationships for the disabled (and the people who care about them).* New York: Harmony Books.

McKown, J.M. (1986). Disabled teenagers: Sexual identification and sexual counseling. *Sexual Disability, 7,* 17–27.

McNab, W.L. (1978). The sexual needs of the handicapped. *Journal of School Health, 48,* 301–306.

Rabin, B.J. (1980). *The sensuous wheeler: Sexual adjustment for the spinal cord injured.* San Francisco: Multi Media Resource Center.

Sandowski, C. (1989). *Sexual concerns when illness or disability strikes.* Springfield, IL: Charles C. Thomas.

Spica, M.M. (1992). Educating the client on the effects of COPD on sexuality: The role of the nurse. *Sexuality and Disability, 10,* 91–101.

## Recognizing Accomplishment

Driedger, D., & Gray, S. (1992). *Imprinting our image: An international anthology by women with disabilities.* Charlottetown, Prince Edward Island: Gynergy Books.

National Clearinghouse on Women and Girls With Disabilities. (1990). *Bridging the gap: A national directory of services for women and girls with disabilities.* New York: Education Equity Concepts, Inc.

Shapiro, J.P. (1993). *No pity: People with disabilities forging a new civil rights movement.* New York: Times Books, Random House.

## Organizations

There are national groups for most chronic illness or disability conditions. Contact your local library for current addresses.

APPENDIX A

# EMERGENCY CHILDBIRTH

*Mary Beth Bryant McGurin*

## INTRODUCTION

When a woman presents complaining of labor pains, the health care provider must quickly perform an assessment appropriate to the specific needs of the client; that is, the provider must determine whether delivery of the infant is imminent or if there is time for further assistance to be obtained. The nature of the assessment and interventions depends on the resources available. Blood pressure, pulse, and respirations should be checked and recorded every 15 minutes if possible. Arrangements should be made for car or ambulance transportation to the nearest facility equipped for maternal and newborn care.[1,2]

## ASSESSMENT OF LABOR STATUS

### MOTHER'S HISTORY AND SUBJECTIVE ASSESSMENT OF CURRENT STATUS

Ask the client if she feels the urge to bear down or to have a bowel movement during contractions; this would indicate that the fetal presenting part is in the vaginal vault (putting pressure on the wall of the rectum) and that birth is imminent. Ask her how many infants she has delivered; if this is not the first, anticipate faster labor and delivery. Ask her if she thinks she is near her due date and if she feels like the infant is ready to be born (regardless of the due date). Experienced mothers can often tell you when birth is imminent, but may be confused if labor is occurring too early in pregnancy. Ask if her amniotic sac (bag of water) has broken, and if so, when. Membranes ruptured longer than 24 hours place mother and infant at great risk for infection and sepsis. Ask what color the fluid was. Brownish-green amniotic fluid indicates that the fetus has been stressed and has passed the meconium plug; the infant may need airway clearance and resuscitation immediately after birth. Ask if she has medical problems or if special tests were done for her or the fetus during pregnancy. Some complications that can impact delivery are not viewed as such by women, especially if they do not feel ill (i.e., hypertension, urinary tract infection, twins, fetal abnormalities).

### ANXIETY LEVEL

Determine the client's ability to cooperate during examination and delivery by her response to questions and directions, degree of physical relaxation (resting between contractions) versus tension and fear (thrashing, uncontrolled bearing down), and tone of verbalizations (calm versus frantic).

### PHYSICAL ASSESSMENT

1. *Is the infant's head visible?* Inspect the vulva: bulging of the perineum, anal

sphincter, or both, with separation of labia, revealing protruding membranes or crowning of the fetal head, indicates that birth is imminent.

2. *Is amniotic fluid or blood present?* Leaking amniotic fluid, bloody show (blood-tinged mucus), or both indicate only that labor is in progress, not necessarily that birth is imminent. As discussed earlier, note the color of the amniotic fluid if the sac appears to have ruptured. Test the fluid with nitrozine paper; a blue change in color indicates saline (alkaline) amniotic fluid is present rather than urine. Frank vaginal bleeding (blood flowing like a menstrual period) or dried blood on the legs indicates a possible abnormality of the placenta. *Do not* insert the fingers, a speculum, or any other object into the vagina (see Abnormal Bleeding later in this appendix).
3. *Are uterine contractions effectively dilating the cervix?* Palpate the abdomen. Uterine contractions that begin every 2 minutes, last 60 to 90 seconds, and are hard (indentation is not elicited by fingertips pressing on abdomen during peak of contraction) indicate that active labor is in progress. If the client is bearing down and pushing with contractions, the fetal head is probably already out of the uterus (i.e., the cervix is fully dilated) and into the vaginal vault. Delivery is probably imminent. If sterile gloves are available and there is no frank vaginal bleeding, gently insert the index and middle fingers of one hand into the vagina until the fetal presenting part or cervix is palpable. Instruct the client to breathe slowly during the exam and to relax her buttocks; tell her what you are checking for. A gravid cervix is very soft, often indiscernible from the vaginal wall, but easily distinguishable from the fetal presenting part, which is firmer. If the cervix can be felt between your fingers and the fetal presenting part, then you may have time to attempt transport to the closest facility offering maternity services. If only the fetal head is palpable deep in the vagina close to the perineum, the cervix is completely dilated, and delivery is imminent.
4. *Is the fetus tolerating the intrauterine environment?* Fetal well-being is assessed to ascertain measures that need to be taken before birth, to decrease stress to the fetus, and after delivery, to facilitate the transition to extrauterine life. If not already known, ask when the infant is due to be born and if there are any known or suspected problems with the infant. The gestational age of the fetus and any physical challenges will determine how much stress the infant can tolerate. (*Note:* Estimation of the gestational age of the fetus by measurement of fundal height is not accurate during the late stages of labor.) Between contractions, perform Leopold's maneuvers to determine which side of the abdomen to listen to for fetal heart sounds; that is, the side where you can feel a smooth, firm fetal back. Listen with the bell side of the stethoscope in the lower abdomen on that side. Count heartbeats for 15 to 30 seconds and multiply to obtain the beats per minute. If the fetal heartrate is less than 100 bpm or if amniotic fluid is meconium stained (green or brown), the fetus is or has been stressed; be prepared to resuscitate the infant immediately after birth. If birth does not seem imminent, turn the client onto her side (preferably left) to allow better blood flow to her uterus and the fetus. Auscultate the fetal heartbeat every 5 to 10 minutes. Also ask the client if the fetus has been moving in the last few hours, another measure of fetal well-being. A stressed, compromised fetus will not be as active as usual.

## PROVISION OF EMOTIONAL SUPPORT AND RELAXATION COACHING

Enhance the client's ability to cooperate during the examination and delivery by teaching her how to gain some measure of control with her breathing. Encourage her to open her mouth and pant or blow slowly during contractions. She is probably frightened and uncomfortable. Acknowledge that everything possible will be done to help her. Ask her to keep her eyes open and to watch for directions. Maintain eye contact, speak calmly, and give simple directions. Have any available support person stay by her upper body to hold her hands and assist with instructions. Give frequent feedback and reassurance that they are both doing a good job. If in the process of transport, when expulsion of the fetus begins stop the vehicle; this facilitates balance and concentration for you and mother.

## PREPARATION FOR DELIVERY

### ASSEMBLY OF AVAILABLE SUPPLIES

Where delivery is taking place will determine the type and amount of assistance and equipment available. If a readymade delivery kit is available, open it and place it to one side within easy reach. If no kit is readily available, have someone get the following items for you if possible: eight or more towels, sheets, or blankets (warm two of them); bulb syringe; sterile scissors; three cord clamps, kelly clamps, or shoestrings; two pair of sterile gloves; bowl or sealable plastic bag; sanitary pads; 3-cc syringe with needle; alcohol wipes; 1000 mL 5% dextrose in half-normal saline or in lactated Ringer's; intravenous catheters; intravenous tubing; other intravenous start supplies; two vials oxytocin (Pitocin, 10 units each) or 0.2 mg (1 cc) of methylergonovine maleate (Methergine); hot water bottle (filled) or heat pack. *Note:* If no supplies are available, use whatever cloth is available to protect your hands from contact with body fluids.

### POSITIONING OF MOTHER AND DRAPING

Wash hands. Position the client lying on her back on a firm surface, with her knees bent and spread apart and her upper body elevated if possible. (This position provides maximum control in an emergency situation.) Observe the perineum while maintaining intermittent eye contact with the client and her support person.

### INTRAVENOUS INFUSION

Start an intravenous infusion at a keep-vein-open rate; draw up both vials of oxytocin to be added to the intravenous fluid immediately following delivery of placenta.

## DELIVERY OF THE INFANT

### DELIVERY OF PRESENTING PART AND CLEARANCE OF AIRWAY

To avoid explosive delivery of the head (causing perineal tears), have the client pant or blow during contractions and give gentle, short pushes only between contractions. Place your right hand on the infant's presenting part, usually the crown of the head, as it protrudes from the vagina during each contraction. Maintain gentle, even pressure on the head, with the length of the fingers allowing the head to slide out of the vagina slowly. (It may take several contractions to complete delivery of the head.) If the amniotic sac is intact over the infant's face, remove it with your fingers. As the head is born, turn it gently to one side, dry it, and suction the nose and mouth gently with a bulb syringe. If one is not available, use a clean towel to wipe away fluids. Check around the neck for a loop(s) of cord; if found, pull it gently over the head. If the loop is too tight, have the mother pant or blow while you clamp the cord in two places; cut between the two clamps.

### DELIVERY OF BODY

Shift slightly toward the back of the infant's head. Place your hands on each side of the head so that your fingers point toward the face, with the little fingers closest to the perineum. With contraction, or gentle pushes from the mother, exert downward and outward pressure on the side of the head with your top hand until the infant's anterior shoulder has slipped out from under the mother's symphysis pubis bone and can be seen. Then apply upward and outward pressure on the sides of the head with your bottom hand, and with both hands lift the infant's head toward the ceiling. As the infant is being born, slide your bottom hand down close to the perineum so that the shoulder, arm, elbow, and hand are held close to the infant's body, controlled, and born into the palm of your hand. The thumb on your bottom hand will be on the infant's back, your fingers will be across the infant's chest, and the infant's head will be resting on your wrist. Slide your top hand down the infant's back, slip your index finger between the infant's legs as the buttocks clear the perineum, and grasp the infant by the ankles. *Note the time of delivery.*

### IMMEDIATE INFANT CARE

Move the infant in a smooth arc into a football hold by allowing the head and shoulders to pivot in your hand while swinging the legs and torso around; the infant's back is supported by your lower arm, and the lower half of the infant's body is tucked between your upper arm and side. Keep the infant's head in a downward position and turned to the side. Stay close enough to the mother so that there is no tension on the umbilical cord.

Suction the infant's nose and mouth gently with a bulb syringe (or wipe out with a cloth) and dry the infant. If you did not do so earlier, clamp the umbilical cord in two places about 6 in. from the infant's body and cut between the clamps. If clamps are not available, tie with shoestrings. (Not with thread!) If the infant does not breathe spontaneously and start to cry, dry the skin vigorously, rub the back, and flick the foot with your finger. Initiate infant CPR (rescue breathing and chest compressions) if necessary. When the infant does cry, place her or him on the mother's chest, skin to skin, and cover with warm blankets so that the infant's scalp is covered but the face can be seen. Use a hot water bottle or heat pack covered with a towel, if necessary and available, to keep the infant warm. Observe the infant for cyanosis or lethargy; stimulate as above if needed. Assign APGAR scores at 1 and 5 minutes. (Refer to Appendix B.)

## DELIVERY OF PLACENTA

Observe the vaginal opening for lengthening of the cord or increased bleeding, which indicate placental separation. Do *not* pull on the cord; instead, wait for uterine contractions to push out the placenta with attached membranes, and place it in a bowl or plastic bag. Transport to the hospital with the infant. Note any tears in the perineum.

## IMMEDIATE POSTDELIVERY CARE OF MOTHER

### CONTROL OF BLEEDING

Locate the grapefruit-sized uterine fundus under the umbilicus and massage it with one hand to keep it firm while supporting the uterus with the other hand just above the symphysis pubis. If oxytocin is available and an IV is running, introduce 20 units of oxytocin into the bag, and allow the IV to run open for about 5 minutes or until the uterus remains firm. If no IV is running, give 10 units (1 cc) oxytocin or 0.2 mg (1 cc) methylergonovine maleate IM into the buttocks or thigh. Even if medications are not available, vaginal bleeding should be minimal if the infant is put to breast, and the uterus is kept well contracted with massage every 10 to 15 minutes. Place a sanitary pad or folded cloth firmly against the perineum. Record blood pressure, pulse, and respirations every 15 minutes; the urinary bladder should be checked for distention and emptied if needed. If the uterus is soft or is above the umbilicus, it has lost its muscle tone and is full of clots. The fundus needs to be massaged (with support from the opposite hand right above the pubic bone to prevent eversion of the uterus into the vagina) until clots are expelled and the fundus is firm. If the uterus is displaced to one side of the midline, the urinary bladder is distended and needs to be emptied.

### PHYSICAL AND EMOTIONAL RECOVERY

If the mother experiences severe shaking chills, reassure her that this reaction is normal after the hard work and anxiety of delivery. Cover her with available blankets. Reinforce what a wonderful job she did during her labor and delivery. Encourage her to breathe slowly to try to relax, while interacting with the infant and support person. Assist the mother to breastfeed if she is planning to nurse. Notify the receiving health care facility of the impending arrival and condition of the mother and infant.

## ABNORMAL CONDITIONS

### BREECH PRESENTATION

When initially assessing the client's vaginal opening, instead of the top of the infant's head, the buttocks may present first (breech presentation), often accompanied by meconium. Prepare the client and supplies as usual; allow the infant's legs, buttocks, and trunk to deliver spontaneously. Support the body in the palm of your gloved hand and on your lower arm, and try to bring the infant's arms out with the other gloved hand. Allow the head to deliver slowly with support. If the head is not delivered in 3 minutes, take action to prevent suffocation, as the umbilical cord is being compressed by the head in the birth canal. Place a gloved hand in the vagina with your palm toward the infant's face. Form a V with fingers on either side of the infant's nose, and push the vaginal wall away from the face until the head is delivered. Transport to the nearest hospital's obstetric unit with the mother's buttocks elevated; be prepared to resuscitate the infant if the head does deliver en route. Alert the receiving facility of impending arrival.

### OTHER ABNORMAL PRESENTATION SITUATIONS

If the infant's arm protrudes from the vagina, transport the mother immediately to the nearest hospital's obstetric unit. This woman will not deliver spontaneously.

If a loop of umbilical cord protrudes from the vagina, cover it with moistened cloth (preferably with normal saline). Have the client assume the knee–chest position on the stretcher or car seat. (This is difficult to do, and the client and her support person will need much reassurance!) Insert your gloved hand into the vagina, and attempt to hold the infant's head up off of the prolapsed cord until you reach the delivery room, where staff are prepared to perform a Cesarean delivery.

If the mother is carrying more than one fetus, deliver subsequent infants just as the first. Remember that twin babies are likely to be smaller and in need of warmth and possible resuscitation.

## ABNORMAL BLEEDING

If before or during delivery you observe blood flow rather than blood-tinged mucus, suspect a placental abnormality. Transport the client to the nearest hospital's obstetric unit while maintaining her in shock position (head down, hips elevated, covered with blankets). Record blood pressure, pulse, respirations, and fetal heart rate every 10 minutes. Monitor contractions and deliver the infant as indicated, being prepared to resuscitate the infant as needed and to treat the mother for shock if pulse rises and blood pressure drops. If the mother bleeds after delivery despite breastfeeding or nipple stimulation and your best efforts to keep her fundus firm, look for perineal lacerations, and apply a peripad or folded cloth snugly to the vulva. Bring all blood-soaked pads or material to the hospital. Always call the receiving facility to alert them of the arrival time and condition of the client and infant.

## REFERENCES

1. Bidwell, D. (1990). Congratulations—It's a baby! *Emergency Medical Services, 19*(10), 21–24.
2. Varney, H. (1987). *Nursery midwifery* (2nd ed.). Boston: Blackwell Scientific.

APPENDIX B

# IMMEDIATE ASSESSMENT OF THE NEWBORN

*Martha Edwards Hart*

## INTRODUCTION

Newborn assessment is an ongoing process incorporating the basic principles of health care and promotion.

- *Purposes*
  a. To provide baseline information.
  b. To identify problems with transition from intra- to extrauterine life.
  c. To document individual variation and reactivity.
- *Principles*
  a. Follow a systematic approach, progressing from noninvasive to invasive, clean to dirty, and head to toe.
  b. Anticipate, on the basis of history.
  c. Do no harm.
  d. Attend to instinctive feelings that something may be wrong.
- *General Guidelines*
  a. Maintain universal precautions and neutral thermal environment.
  b. Focus on ABCs of cardiopulmonary resuscitation.
  c. Assess symmetry.
  d. If an external abnormality is visible, closely assess internal organs.
  e. Measure lesions, graph vital statistics, and document and interpret findings.

## REVIEW OF HISTORY FOR RISK FACTORS (SEE CHAPTER 12)

- *Maternal.* Age; past medical history; social, developmental, and occupational history.
- *Obstetric.* Parity; last menstrual period (LMP); previous menstrual period (PMP); history of prematurity; medical complications and outcome of previous or current pregnancy.
- *Perinatal.* Intrapartum events; gestational age; condition at birth.

## APGAR SCORES

### EVALUATION OF INITIAL NEONATAL TRANSITION PERIOD

The acronym *APGAR*[1,2] facilitates assessment of five components of neonates' responses: appearance, pulse, grimace, activity, and respiration.

### INTERPRETATION

- The APGAR is scored at 1 and 5 minutes of life.

**APGAR SIGNS**

| Signs | 0 | 1 | 2 |
|---|---|---|---|
| Appearance (color) | Blue/pale | Body pink<br>Extremities blue | Completely pink |
| Pulse (heart rate) | Absent | <100 | >100 |
| Grimace (reflex irritability) | No response | Grimace | Cough, sneeze, cry |
| Activity (muscle tone) | Limp | Some flexion | Flexed, active motion |
| Respiration (breathing efforts) | Absent | Weak, irregular gasping | Strong cry |

- Five signs are evaluated and scored 0, 1, or 2.
- *10–10, Best Possible Condition.* As most healthy newborns are acrocyanotic, expect a score of 8 or 9.
- When the 5-minute score is 6 or less, some states require a 10-minute score. It is useful to obtain additional scores every 5 minutes until 20 minutes has passed or until two successive scores of 7 or higher are obtained.
- *0–2, Severe Asphyxia.* Infant is at high risk; requires resuscitation and further evaluation.
- *3–4, Moderate Asphyxia.* Infant is at moderate risk; probable resuscitation and further evaluation.
- *5–7, Mild Asphyxia.* Infant is at risk; possible intermittent resuscitation, and with or without further evaluation.
- *8–10, No Asphyxia.* Infant is at minimal risk; routine elective procedures.

# PHYSICAL EXAMINATION

Abnormal findings are noted in parentheses.

## GENERAL SURVEY

- *State.*[3] Deep or light sleep; drowsy; quiet or active alert; crying.
- *Reactivity.* State changes, interactive capacity, self-consolability.
- *Color.* Pink, acrocyanosis; mottling (plethora, pallor, jaundice, cyanosis).
- *Posture.* Flexed (asymmetry, restricted movement).
- *Skin.* Smooth, elastic, warm, moist; vernix; lanugo; desquamation; Mongolian spots; milia; nevi; edema or petechiae over presenting part (pustules, lacerations, ecchymosis, rashes, café-au-lait spots, hemangiomas, meconium staining, pitting edema, poor turgor, scaling, sweating).
- *Respirations at Rest.* Rate = 30–60; symmetric; diaphragmatic or abdominal (flaring; grunting; intercostal, supraclavicular, or substernal retractions).

## HEENT, MOUTH, AND NECK

- *Head.* Occipitofrontal circumference: 32.5–37 cm. Round; symmetric; molding; overriding or slightly open sutures; caput succedaneum = scalp edema, may cross suture line; cephal hematoma = subperiosteal hemorrhage, does not cross suture line (irregularities; craniotabes; depressions; asymmetry; fracture; fixed, widely spaced/closed sutures). Fontanelles soft, flat, may bulge with crying; anterior = diamond; posterior = triangle (sunken; bulging at rest; enlarged; absent anterior; third fontanelle).
- *Face.* Symmetric; intact (asymmetry with movement, micrognathia; clefts).
- *Eyes.* Symmetric; lids easily open; posi-

tive blink; pupils round, equal, and reactive to light; positive red reflex; blue-gray or brown iris; no discharge; cornea and lens clear and intact; sclera bluish white; minor hemorrhages; pale pink conjunctiva; subconjunctival hemorrhage; chemical conjunctivitis; nystagmus; strabismus (asymmetry; short palpebral fissures; hypertelorism; fused, edematous, drooping, or inflamed lids; setting sun sign; unequal, constricted, or poorly reactive pupils; pinkish or clefted iris; blue or jaundiced sclera; corneal opacities or ulcerations; purulent discharge; persistent uncoordinated movements).

- *Ears.* Well formed; symmetric; upper pinna at or above outer canthus of eye; curved pinna, firm cartilage; patent canals; positive response to noise (asymmetric; low-set; rotated; very large or small; malformed; preauricular, auricular skin tags, sinuses).
- *Nose.* Midline; intact; no discharge; bilateral nasal patency; obligatory nose breather (flattened nasal bridge; flaring; clefts; chloanal atresia).
- *Mouth and Throat.* Pink, moist mucosa; sucking blisters; positive suck, root, and gag reflexes; transient circumoral cyanosis; midline mobile tongue; well-formed palate and gums; Epstein's pearls; inclusion cysts; teeth; scant saliva (clefts; thrush; tongue protrusion; long frenulum; macroglossia; high arched palate; excessive mucus).
- *Neck.* Short, straight, full range of motion; intact clavicles (webbing; masses; edema, venous distention; limited range of motion; torticollis; crepitation; fractures; opisthotonus).

## CHEST

- *Thorax.* Symmetric; cylindrical; circumference at nipple line = 30–33 cm (bulging, depressed sternum; retractions; tachypnea; apnea).
- *Nipples.* Present; symmetric placement; supernumerary; enlarged; milky secretion (asymmetry; purulent drainage).
- *Breath Sounds.* Auscultate for vesicular or clear bilaterally (expiratory grunting; rales/crackles; rhonchi/wheezes; decreased, unequal).
- *Heart Sounds.* Rate = 120–160; auscultate for two clear, distinct sounds: $S_2$ slightly sharper, higher pitched than $S_1$; regular rhythm; point of maximal impulse (PMI) = lower left sternal border (displaced, distant, muffled, extra sounds; bradycardia/tachycardia; irregular rhythm; hyperactive precordium).

## ABDOMEN

- *Contour.* Protuberant; symmetric; cylindrical shape; diastasis recti; prominent superficial veins (asymmetry; distention; flat; scaphoid; masses; visible peristalsis).
- *Bowel Sounds Present in All Four Quadrants.* Intermittent tinkling (hyperactive or absent).
- *Liver.* Palpate 1–2 cm below right costal margin; sharp edge (enlarged; round edge).
- *Kidneys.* Palpate oval structure in posterior flanks 1–2 cm above umbilicus; often difficult to palpate (enlarged; absent).
- *Umbilical Cord and Umbilicus.* Two arteries; one vein; gelatinous, bluish-white; skin clear and dry; umbilical hernia (two vessels; thin cord; foul odor; discharge; meconium stained).
- *Femoral Pulses and Lymph Nodes.* Palpate strong, regular pulses bilaterally (absent, irregular, weak, bounding, absent pulses; enlarged nodes).
- *Rectum and Anus.* Patent; positive anal wink (imperforate anus; fistulas; decreased tone); document passage and character of stools: meconium = dark green, tarry, thick

viscous; mucus plug (foul odor; diarrhea; mucus; blood).

## GENITOURINARY TRACT

- *Urination.* Confirm; clear; yellow; full stream (bladder distention; abnormal stream; blood-tinged).
- *External Genitalia.* Confirm appropriate for given gender (ambiguous; fecal urethral discharge).
  - *Male:* Observe urinary stream; meatus at tip of penis, glans covered by prepuce (epispadias = dorsal; hypospadias = ventral surface; phimosis); scrotum—pink to brown; symmetric; pendulous; rugation; testes descended or descending bilaterally; edema or bruising if breech (hydrocele = positive transillumination; hernia = negative transillumination; undescended or absent testes).
  - *Female:* Observe presence and position of urethra; introitus posterior to clitoris; labia majora meet midline; labia minora prominent; edema; hymenal tags; pseudomenstruation; mucoid, milky discharge (absent vagina or meatus).

## BACK

- *Back and Spine.* Midline; straight; intact; easily flexed; symmetric; lanugo; pilonidal dimple (asymmetry; abnormal curvature; masses; pilonidal cyst, sinus, dimple, hair tufts; spina bifida).
- *Buttocks.* Symmetry; Mongolian spots (asymmetric gluteal folds).

## EXTREMITIES

- *General.* Appearance, symmetry, size, length, and range of motion.
- *Fingers and Toes.* All present.
- *Hands and Feet.* Palmar and plantar creases; fisted hands (Simian crease; dysplastic nails; tightly fisted hands, obligatory palmar thumb; metatarsus varus; club feet; rocker-bottom feet; absent digits, abnormal spacing).
- *Arms.* Occasional tremors; easily adduct from trunk; full range of motion at elbow (fracture; palsy; paralysis).
- *Legs.* Mild medial rotation; transient in utero positioning = breech, "frogs legs"; symmetry of medial thigh skinfolds (asymmetric size/appearance; limited range of motion).
- *Hips.* Tests[2] to evaluate:
  - *Ortolani's Maneuver—Abduct, Up and Out.* Flex knees and hips, placing fingers bilaterally on greater trochanters, thumbs gripping medial aspect of femurs; adduct and abduct (positive jerking motion as femur passes over acetabulum).
  - *Barlow's Test—Up and Back, "Piston."* Flex hip and knee 90 degrees; gently attempt to slip femur head onto posterior tip of acetabulum by lateral pressure of thumb and by rocking knee medially with knuckle of index finger (palpable or audible hip click; movement is not normally felt).
- *Peripheral Pulses.* Present; symmetric; strong (absent; varied strength).

## NERVOUS SYSTEM

- *Character of Cry.* Strong, lusty (weak, high-pitched, constant or none).
- *Reflexes.* Assess symmetry and strength of responses.
  - *Asymmetric Tonic Neck ("Fencing").* With the infant supine, turn head to one side. The infant may extend arm and leg on side head is turned toward with flexion of opposite arm and leg.
  - *Moro or Startle.* Abrupt position change or noise elicits extension and abduction of arms and extension of fingers with

subsequent flexion or drawing in; infant may habituate or diminish response with repeated attempts.

- *Rooting.* Stroke side of cheek, lips, or mouth with finger or nipple and head turns toward the stimulus, mouth opens, and sucking begins.
- *Sucking.* Finger or nipple in mouth elicits sucking movements.
- *Swallow.* Assess coordination of suck or swallow with first oral feeding.
- *Extrusion.* Solid object placed on tongue causes tongue to push outward to remove it.
- *Palmar and Plantar Grasp.* Finger placed in palm and base of toes elicits grasp of finger and brief downward curling of toes.
- *Babinski.* Stroke up lateral aspect of feet and toes fan up and out.
- *Pull to Sit or Traction.* With the infant supine, grasp the arms and pull to sitting position; the head lags, then is brought up and held briefly; note position and tone.
- *Glabellar or Blink.* Tap forehead at bridge of nose with finger to elicit bilateral blink.
- *Galant or Trunk Incurvation.* With infant in ventral suspension over examiner's hand, gently stroke, with finger of other hand, paravertebral portion of spine to elicit curvature toward stimulus.
- *Placing or Stepping.* Holding infant upright on flat surface elicits "stepping" movements with alternating flexion and extension of feet (may also elicit this response by stroking dor-sum of foot while holding infant upright).

## ESTIMATION OF GESTATIONAL AGE

Use Dubowitz or Ballard clinical assessments of physical characteristics and neuromuscular maturity[4,5] to classify neonates by gestational age and to determine potential mortality and morbidity risks.

### REFERENCES


1. Apgar, V. (1966). The newborn (Apgar) scoring system: Reflections and advice. *Pediatric Clinics of North America, 13,* 645.
2. NAACOG. (1991). *OGN Nursing Practice Resource: Physical assessment of the neonate.* Washington, DC: Author.
3. Brazelton, T.B. (1973). *Neonatal behavioral assessment scale.* Philadelphia: J.B. Lippincott/Spastics International Medical Publishers.
4. Dubowitz, L.M.S., Dubowitz, V., & Goldberg, C. (1970). Clinical assessment of gestational age in the newborn infant. *Journal of Pediatrics, 77,* 1.
5. Ballard, J.L., Khoury, J.C., Wedig, K., Wang, L., Eilers-Walsman, B.L., Lipp, R. (1991). New Ballard score, expanded to include extremely premature infants. *Journal of Pediatrics, 3,* 417.


### BIBLIOGRAPHY


Chow, M.P., Durand, B.A., Feldman, M.N., & Mills, M.N. (1984). *Handbook of pediatric primary care* (2nd ed.). New York: John Wiley & Sons.

Golden, S.M., & Peters, D.Y. (1989). Delivery room care. In *Handbook of neonatal intensive care* (2nd ed.). St. Louis: C.V. Mosby.

Lepley, C.J., Gardner, S.L., and Lubchenco, L.O. (1989). Initial nursery care. In *Handbook of neonatal intensive care* (2nd ed.). St. Louis: C.V. Mosby.

APPENDIX C

# SELECTED LABORATORY VALUES

*Ellis Quinn Youngkin*

**Chem 6 (1)a**

| | |
|---|---|
| Sodium | 135–145 mEq/L (mmol/L) |
| Potassium | 3.6–5.1 mEq/L (mmol/L) |
| Chloride | 101–111 mEq/L (mmol/L) |
| Carbon dioxide | 21–31 mEq/L (mmol/L) |
| Glucose (fasting) | 65–110 mg/dL |
| Blood urea nitrogen | 6–22 mg/dL |

**Chem 12 (1)**

| | |
|---|---|
| Creatinine (2) | 0.6–0.9 mg/dL (in females) |
| Urate | 2.3–6.9 mg/dL |
| Calcium | 8.9–10.5 mg/dL |
| Phosphate | 2.5–4.6 mg/dL |
| Anion gap (2) | 8–14 mEq/L (mmol/L) |
| Osmolality | 280–295 mmol/kg |
| Iron (2) | 80–150 μg/dL |
| Cholesterol | ≤200 mg/dL |
| Alkaline Phosphatase (2) | 30–120 U/L |
| AST (SGOT) (2)[b] | 8–40 U/L |
| ALT (SGPT) (2) | 9–24 U/L (in females) |
| Protein (total) | 6–8 g/dL |

**Lipid Profile (3)**

| | |
|---|---|
| Cholesterol | 150–200 mg/dL |
| Triglycerides | 40–150 mg/dL |
| Phospholipids | 150–380 mg/dL |
| LDL-CHO (1) | <130 mg/dL |
| HDL-CHO (1) | >35 mg/dL |
| Cholesterol/HDL ratio (1) | ≤4.4 |

**Thyroid Profile (1)**

| | |
|---|---|
| TSH | 0.32–5.00 μIU/mL |
| $T_3$ uptake | 30–42% |
| $T_4$ total | 4.5–12 μg/dL |
| FTI (calc) | 5–12 μg/dL |
| Free $T_4$ | 1–3 ng/dL |
| Free $T_3$ | 0.2–0.6 ng/dL |

**Other Values (2)**

| | |
|---|---|
| Prolactin | 0–20 ng/dL |
| FSH | 5–30 mIU/mL |
| LH | 5–15 mIU/mL (follicular and luteal/stages)<br>30–60 mIU/mL (midcycle/ovulation) |
| Progesterone | <150 ng/dL (follicular)<br>approx. 300 ng/dL (luteal)<br>2000 mg/dL (midluteal) |
| Estrogen | 24–68 pg/mL (days 1–10 of menstrual cycle)<br>50–186 pg/mL (days 11–20 of menstrual cycle)<br>73–149 pg/mL (days 21–30 of menstrual cycle) |
| Testosterone | 30–95 ng/dL (females) |
| Free testosterone (4) | 1–2% of total testosterone |
| DHEA-S (4) | <250 ng/dL (ranges vary with age) |
| Androstenedione (4) | 65–270 ng/mL |
| 17-Hydroxyprogesterone (4) | 80 ng/dL (follicular)<br>30–290 ng/dL (luteal) |
| Cortisol (random) (4) | 5–25 μg/dL[c] |
| Dexamethasone suppression test | 5+ μg/dL cortisone = test failure |
| Albumin (3) | 3.2–4.5 g/dL |

| ***Anemia Workup (3)*** | | | |
|---|---|---|---|
| Complete blood count | | Reticulocyte count | 0.5–2% |
| Red blood cells | 4.2–5.4 × $10^6$/$mm^3$ | Iron | 60–190 μg/dL |
| Hemoglobin | 12–16 g/dL | Total iron binding capacity | 250–420 μg/dL |
| Hematocrit | 37–43% | Transferrin saturation | 30–40% |
| MCV | 80–95 μ$g^3$ | Ferritin (2) | 20–120 ng/mL (in females) |
| MCH | 27–31 pg | | |
| MCHC | 32–36% or g/dL | Hemoglobin electrophoresis | |
| White blood cells | 5000–10,000/$mm^3$ | Hgb $A_1$ | 95–98% |
| Differential | | Hgb $A_2$ | 2–3% |
| Neutrophils | 55–70% | Hgb F | 0.8–2% |
| Lymphocytes | 20–40% | Hgb S | 0 |
| Monocytes | 2–8% | Hgb C | 0 |
| Eosinophils | 1–4% | | |
| Basophils | 0.5–1% | | |

[a](1) Medical College of Virginia, Virginia Commonwealth University Hospitals Laboratory, September 1992. (2) *Clinical laboratory tests*, Springhouse: Springhouse Corp., 1991. (3) Pagana, K., & Pagana, T. (1986). *Diagnostic testing and nursing implications* (2nd ed.). St. Louis: C.V. Mosby. (4) Sue Wood, MS, RNC, OGNP. Author of Chapter 7.

[b]AST(SGOT), aspartate aminotransferase (serum glutamic–oxaloacetic transaminase; ALT(SGPT), alanine aminotransferase (serum glutamic–pyruvic transaminase; LDL-CHO, low-density lipoprotein cholesterol; HDL-CHO, high-density lipoprotein cholesterol; TSH, thyroid-stimulating hormone; $T_3$, triiodothyronine; $T_4$, thyroxine; FTI (calc), free thyroxine index (calculated); FSH, follicle-stimulating hormone; LH, luteinizing hormone; DHEA-$SO_4$, dehydroepiandrosterone sulfate; MCV, mean corpuscular volume; MCH, mean corpuscular hemoglobin; MCHC, mean corpuscular hemoglobin concentration; Hgb, hemoglobin.

[c]After adrenocorticotropin (ACTH) stimulation: AM, 5–25 μg/dL; PM, 2–12 μg/dL.

# INDEX

Page numbers followed by *t* and *f* indicate tables and figures respectively